Pearson MyLab

MyLab Math for *Calculus and Its Applications, Brief Version, 12e*

(access code required)

MyLab™ Math is the teaching and learning platform that empowers instructors to reach every student. By combining trusted author content with digital tools and a flexible platform, MyLab Math for *Calculus and Its Applications, Brief Version*, 12e, personalizes the learning experience and improves results for each student.

Integrated Review

The MyLab Math course contains premade, assignable quizzes to assess the prerequisite skills needed for each chapter, plus personalized remediation for any gaps in skills that are identified. Each student, therefore, receives just the help that he or she needs—no more, no less.

Get Ready for Chapter 5

This page is designed to help you with prerequisite skills that are needed to be successful with this chapter's content.

Skills Check

Check that you have the skills needed for this chapter by taking the Chapter 5 Skills Check Quiz.

Skills Review

Brush up skills you need to review by watching the videos below.

Convert between radicals and rational exponents.	Video
Simplify complex rational expressions.	Video
Find the composition of functions.	Video
Decompose functions.	Video
Solve exponential equations.	Video
Solve logarithmic equations.	Video
Graph basic polynomial functions.	Video

Skills Practice

After taking the quiz, practice the skills you need to master on the Chapter 5 Skills Check Homework.

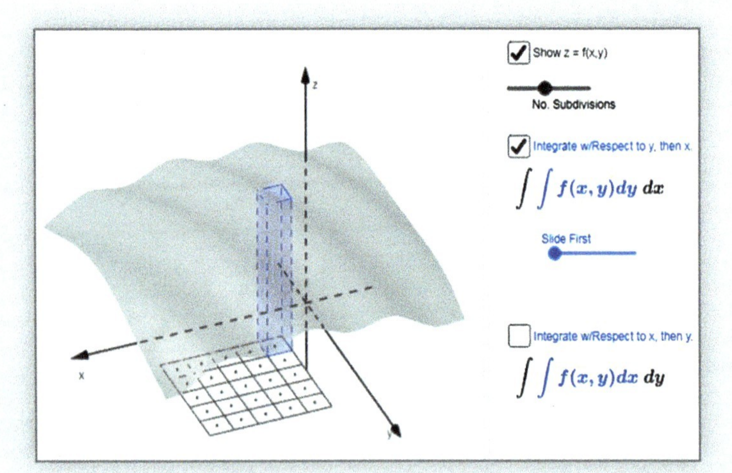

Interactive Figures

An expanded full suite of Interactive Figures illustrates key concepts and allow manipulation. They are designed to be used in lecture as well as by students independently.

Questions That Deepen Understanding

MyLab Math includes a variety of question types designed to help students succeed in the course. In **Setup & Solve** questions, students show how they set up a problem as well as the solution, better mirroring what is required on tests. **Additional Conceptual Questions** provide support for assessing concepts and vocabulary. Many of these questions are application oriented.

Find the area of the region enclosed by the curves $y^2 - 5x = 1$ and $x - y = 1$.

Set up the integral that gives the area of the shaded region.

$$\int_{-1}^{6}\left[y + 1 - \frac{y^2 - 1}{5}\right]dy$$

Find the area by evaluating the integral

$\frac{343}{30}$ (Type an integer or a simplified fraction.)

pearson.com/mylab/math

Algebra Review

Properties of Exponents

$$a^n = \underbrace{a \cdot a \cdot a \cdot \cdots \cdot a}_{n \text{ factors}}$$

$a^0 = 1$, for $a \neq 0$

$a^1 = a$

$a^{-n} = \frac{1}{a^n}$, for $a \neq 0$

$a^m a^n = a^{m+n}$

$\frac{a^n}{a^m} = a^{n-m}$, for $a \neq 0$

$(a^n)^m = a^{nm}$

$(ab)^n = a^n b^n$

$a^{1/n} = \sqrt[n]{a}$, where $a \geq 0$ when n is even

Common Multiplication and Factoring Forms

Distributive Law: $a(b \pm c) = ab \pm ac$

Difference of Squares: $a^2 - b^2 = (a + b)(a - b)$

Squared Binomials:

$(a + b)^2 = a^2 + 2ab + b^2$

$(a - b)^2 = a^2 - 2ab + b^2$

Linear Equations

Slope of a Line: $m = \frac{y_2 - y_1}{x_2 - x_1}$, where (x_1, y_1) and (x_2, y_2) are two points on the line such that $x_1 \neq x_2$

Point–Slope Equation of a Line with Slope *m* Passing through (x_1, y_1):

$y - y_1 = m(x - x_1)$

Slope–Intercept Equation of a Line with Slope *m* and *y*-Intercept $(0, b)$:

$y = mx + b$

The Quadratic Formula

The solutions of a quadratic equation of the form $y = ax^2 + bx + c$ are given by

$$x = \frac{-b \pm \sqrt{b^2 - 4ac}}{2a}.$$

Geometric Formulas

Rectangles

Area: $A = lw$

Perimeter: $P = 2(l + w)$

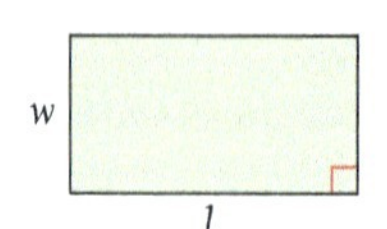

Parallelograms

Area: $A = bh$

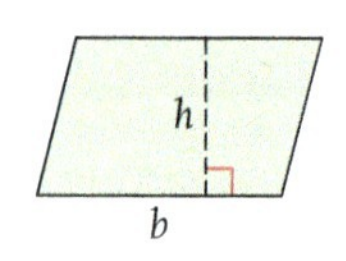

Trapezoids

Area: $A = \frac{1}{2}h(b_1 + b_2)$

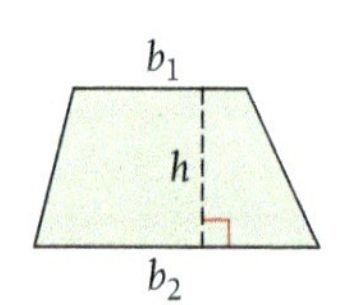

Circles

Area: $A = \pi d = 2\pi r$

Circumference: $C = 2\pi r$

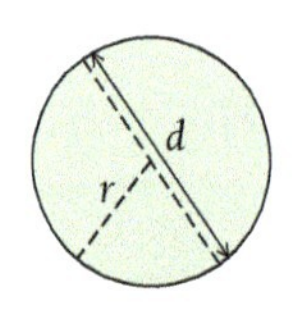

Triangles

Area: $A = \frac{1}{2}bh$

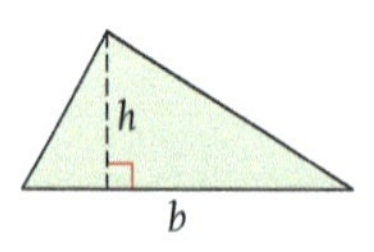

Pythagorean Theorem:

$$c^2 = a^2 + b^2,$$

where a and b are the legs and c is the hypotenuse of a right triangle

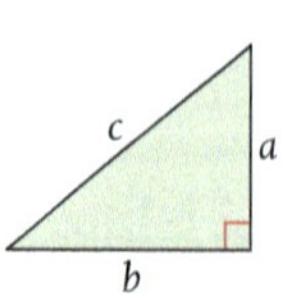

Rectangular Solids

Volume: $V = lwh$

Surface Area:

$$A = 2(lw + lh + wh)$$

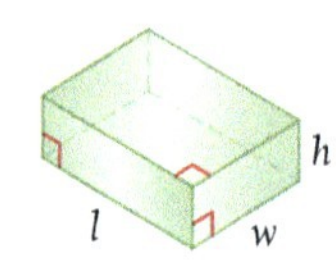

Spheres

Volume: $V = \frac{4}{3}\pi r^3$

Surface Area: $A = 4\pi r^2$

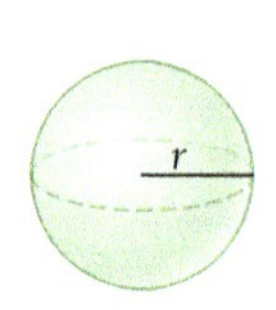

Circular Cylinders

Volume: $V = \pi r^2 h$

Surface Area: $A = 2\pi r^2 + 2\pi rh$

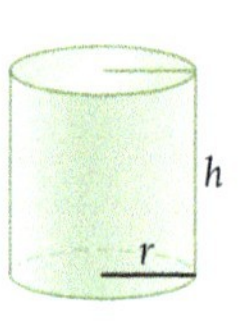

Cones

Volume: $V = \frac{1}{3}\pi r^2 h$

Surface Area (Including the Base):

$$A = \pi r^2 + \pi r\sqrt{r^2 + h^2}$$

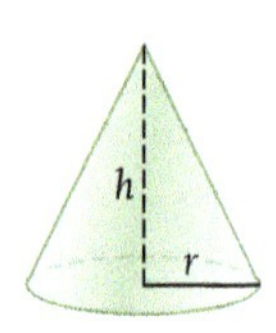

Calculus

AND ITS APPLICATIONS

BRIEF VERSION

TWELFTH EDITION

Marvin L. Bittinger
Indiana University Purdue University Indianapolis

David J. Ellenbogen
Community College of Vermont

Scott A. Surgent
Arizona State University

with the assistance of
Gene F. Kramer
University of Cincinnati Blue Ash

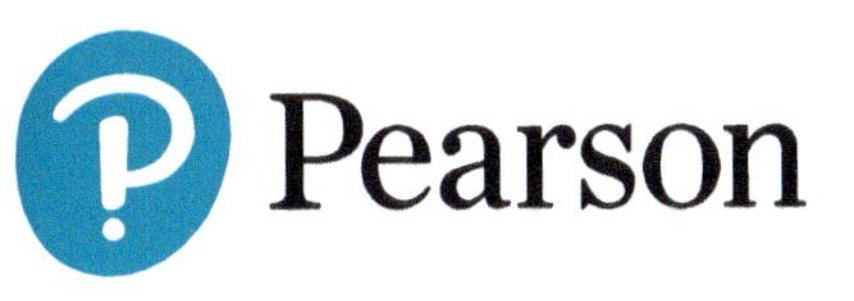

Director, Portfolio Management	Deirdre Lynch	*Marketing Assistant*	Shannon McCormack
Executive Editor	Jeff Weidenaar	*Senior Author Support/ Technology Specialist*	Joe Vetere
Editorial Assistant	Jon Krebs	*Manager, Rights and Permissions*	Gina Cheselka
Content Producer	Ron Hampton	*Manufacturing Buyer*	Carol Melville, LSC Communications
Managing Producer	Karen Wernholm	*Text Design*	The Davis Group, Inc.
Senior Producer	Stephanie Green	*Cover Design*	Pearson CSC
Associate Producer	Shannon Bushee	*Production Coordination*	Jane Hoover/Lifland et al., Bookmakers
Manager, Courseware QA	Mary Durnwald	*Composition*	Pearson CSC
Manager, Content Development	Kristina Evans	*Cover Image*	Leungchopan/Shutterstock
Product Marketing Manager	Emily Ockay		
Field Marketing Manager	Evan St. Cyr		

Acknowledgments of third-party content appear on page 646, which constitutes an extension of this copyright page.

Library of Congress Cataloging-in-Publication Data is on file with the publisher.

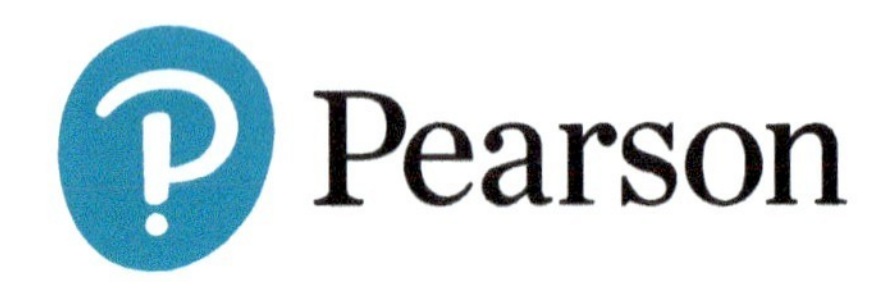

Student Edition ISBNs: 0135164885; 9780135164884
Instructor's Edition ISBNs: 0135165903; 9780135165904

16 2020

To Elaine, Kit, Beth, and Julie

Contents

The following chapters are included in the longer version of this text (entitled *Calculus and Its Applications*):

Preface

Calculus and Its Applications, Brief Version, is designed for a one-semester course in calculus for students majoring in business, economics, social sciences, or health/life sciences. We have strived to produce the most student-oriented applied calculus text on the market. We believe that appealing to students' intuition and writing in a direct, down-to-earth manner make this text accessible to any student possessing the prerequisite math skills. By presenting more topics in a conceptual and often visual manner and adding student self-assessment and teaching aids to this edition of the text, we address students' needs better than ever before. Tapping into areas of student interest, we provide motivation through an abundant supply of examples and exercises rich in real-world data from business, economics, environmental studies, health care, and the life sciences.

New examples cover a variety of applications designed to appeal to students taking the course. Found in every chapter, realistic applications draw students into the discipline and help them to generalize the material and apply it to new situations. To further spark student interest, hundreds of meticulously rendered graphs and illustrations appear throughout the text, making it a favorite among students who are visual learners.

A course in intermediate algebra is a prerequisite to this applied calculus text, although "Appendix A: Review of Basic Algebra" and "Chapter R: Functions, Graphs, and Models" provide a sufficient foundation to unify the diverse backgrounds of most students. Note the availability of two different versions of this text by the same authors:

- The **brief version** contains Chapters R–6 and is generally used for a one-semester course.
- The **complete** *Calculus and Its Applications* contains Chapters R–12 and is generally used for a two-semester course.

New to This Edition

We welcome to this edition co-author Gene Kramer of University of Cincinnati Blue Ash. Gene's primary focus was updating the contents of the MyLab Math course for the text.

This is a substantial revision of the text and its associated technology. The revisions were informed by feedback from users of the text and the accompanying MyLab Math course as well as our own classroom experiences.

New to MyLab Math

Many improvements have been made to the overall functionality of MyLab Math since the previous edition. However, beyond that, we have also increased and improved the content specific to this text.

- All MyLab Math **exercises have been reviewed and edited** where necessary by author Gene Kramer for improved quality and fidelity to the text.
- Instructors now have **more exercises** than ever to choose from when assigning homework. Most new questions are application-oriented. There are approximately 3270 assignable exercises in MyLab Math for this text. New exercise types include:
  - Setup and Solve exercises require students to show how they set up a problem as well as giving the solution, better mirroring what is required of students on tests.
  - Additional Conceptual Questions (labeled ACQ) provide support for assessing concepts and vocabulary. Many of these questions are application-oriented.

- About **90% of the instructional videos are brand-new**. The new videos were made using the latest technology and feature authors Gene Kramer and Scott Surgent along with instructors Mary Ann Barber (University of North Texas) and Thomas Hartfield (University of North Georgia).
    - The Guide to Video-Based Assignments shows which MyLab Math exercises can be assigned for each video. This resource is especially useful for online or flipped classes.
- The **suite of interactive figures has been expanded** to support teaching and learning. These figures (created in GeoGebra) illustrate key concepts and can be manipulated by users. They have been designed to be used in lectures as well as by students independently.
- **Enhanced Sample Assignments** are section-level assignments that (1) address gaps in precalculus skills with personalized prerequisite review, (2) help keep skills fresh with spaced practice of key calculus concepts, and (3) provide opportunities to work exercises without learning aids so that students can check their understanding. They are assignable and editable.
- **Study skills modules** help students with the life skills that can make the difference between passing and failing.
- The **Graphing Calculator Manual** and **Excel Spreadsheet Manual**, both specific to this course, have been updated to support the TI-84 Plus CE (color display) and Excel 2016, respectively. Both manuals also contain additional topics to support the course.
- We heard from users that the Annotated Instructor's Edition for the previous edition required too much flipping of pages to find answers, so MyLab Math now contains a **downloadable Instructor's Answers** document—*with all the answers in one place*. (This augments the downloadable Instructor Solutions Manual, which contains all *solutions*.)

Content Updates

Our overall goals in revising the text were as follows:

- Tighten language and consolidate examples and exercises whenever possible.
- Help students master exponential and logarithmic functions and realize their utility by introducing them earlier and using them more often.
- Bolster themes that endure throughout the book—for example, by adding material in Section R.3 on disjoint intervals, which is something students apply later when considering appropriate intervals of domain.
- Incorporate spreadsheets as a means of explaining concepts, when appropriate.
- Remove unnecessary or out-of-date Technology Connection features.
- Add new examples or subsections to pre-existing examples or sections and reference earlier examples or themes wherever appropriate.

Detailed changes to each chapter are as follows:

Chapter R

- In Section R.3, material on disjoint intervals, which are used elsewhere in the book, has been added.
- In Section R.4, the presentation of lines has been reordered, building from the most basic to the most general form.
- In Section R.5, all supply-demand curves have been revised so that price now sits on the vertical axis. This matches what students see in business and economics courses.
- New Section R.6 provides a deeper treatment of logarithms and exponentials. Some material from the previous edition's Section R.5 is used here but a significant portion is brand-new.

Chapter 1

- In Section 1.1, the introduction to limits along the number line has been rewritten to explain the idea of left- and right-hand approaches, thus setting up the general limit approach more intuitively.
- Section 1.2 contains added material on limits at infinity, to better set the stage for the introduction of asymptotic behavior in Chapter 3.

- In Section 1.7, composition of functions is discussed earlier, and the Extended Power Rule is treated as a special case of the general case. (Previously, we treated it as its own theorem.)

Chapters 2 and 3

Based on the feedback we received on the importance of exponential and logarithmic functions to the students in this class (particularly business students), we now introduce exponential and logarithmic functions (and their derivatives) in Chapter 2, then cover applications of the derivative in Chapter 3 (including applications involving exponential and logarithmic functions). This change helps students better learn exponential and logarithmic functions by introducing them earlier and providing increased opportunities to practice and apply them in both chapters.

- New Section 2.1 has increased coverage of how the natural base *e* is derived, including new examples and significant expansion of the exercise set.
- Former Section 3.2 is split into two new sections (2.2 and 2.3), which discuss the derivatives of the natural base and natural logarithmic functions, respectively. This allowed us to add more examples and give greater depth to the discussion of these topics.
- In Section 2.6 (formerly 3.5), discussion of models where base 10 or base *e* are not used has been expanded. We use general bases and show how one can go back and forth, the advantages of each, and so on.
- In new Sections 3.1–3.4, exponential and logarithmic functions have been added to the curve-sketching discussions. This is significant because we now have a richer set of examples and can go deeper into these topics.
- Optimization questions involving exponentials and logarithms have been added to Section 3.5. We include some discussion of the use of spreadsheets to show how a student could "solve" a maximum–minimum problem in this manner.
- New material on linearization has been included in Section 3.6.
- Exponential models are now covered in the discussion of elasticity of demand in Section 3.7, which includes three examples (rather than just one, as in the previous edition).
- Former Section 2.8 has been split into two sections (3.8 and 3.9) to lighten the content load. Section 3.8 covers implicit differentiation (including a subsection on logarithmic differentiation), and Section 3.9 covers related rates and includes more examples than in the previous edition.

Chapters 4 and 5

- Section 4.1 has increased focus on antidifferentiation as accumulation, using easy intuitive examples to appeal to students' familiarity with real life.
- Section 4.4 has a new subsection on moving averages.
- In Section 4.6, a new example involving exponential decay provides a life sciences application.
- New Section 4.7 covers numerical methods of integration.
- The previous edition's little-used section on integral tables is now Appendix E.
- Section 5.1 has been expanded to include material on price ceilings, price floors, and deadweight loss. This material is a natural extension of the topic of consumer and producer surplus, and the level of mathematics is a perfect fit.
- Problems in Section 5.2 have been updated with more realistic interest rates and current real-world data.

Chapter 6

- New material on differentials and tolerances is included in Section 6.2. This expands on ideas developed in Section 3.6.
- Section 6.3 includes new content on constrained optimization in three variables, showing how a constraint reduces a problem to a two-variable maximum–minimum problem. This sets the stage for Section 6.5.
- In Section 6.5, a new example (and exercises) shows how Lagrange multipliers can be used to solve constrained maximum–minimum problems in three variables.
- Examples in Section 6.6 have been revised to eliminate unnecessary fractions.

Our Approach

Intuitive Presentation

Although the word *intuitive* has many meanings and interpretations, we use it to mean "experience based, without proof." Throughout the text, when a concept is discussed, its presentation is designed so that the students' learning process is based on their earlier mathematical experience. This is illustrated by the following situations.

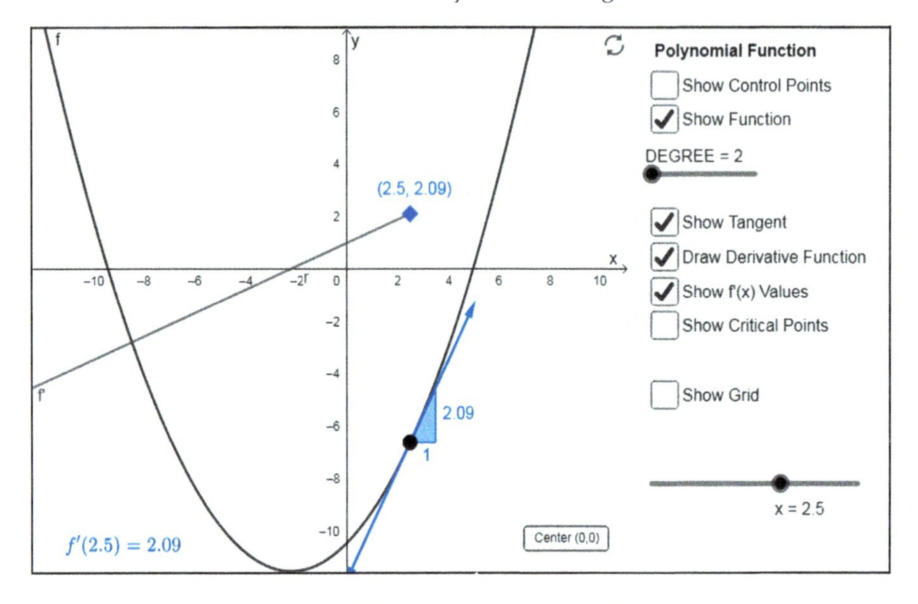

- Within MyLab Math, students and instructors have access to interactive figures that illustrate concepts and allow manipulation so that students can better predict and understand the underlying concepts.
- Before the formal definition of *continuity* is presented, an informal explanation is given, complete with graphs that take advantage of student intuition about ways in which a function could be discontinuous (see pp. 120–121).
- The definition of *derivative*, in Chapter 1, is presented in the context of a discussion of average rates of change (see p. 139). This presentation is more accessible and realistic than the strictly geometric idea of slope.
- When maximization problems involving volume are introduced (see pp. 318–319), a function that is to be maximized is derived. Instead of forging ahead with the standard calculus solution, the text first asks students to make a table of function values, graph the function, and then estimate the maximum value. This experience provides students with more insight into the problem. They recognize not only that different dimensions yield different volumes, but also that the dimensions yielding the maximum volume may be conjectured or estimated as a result of the calculations.

Timely Help for Gaps in Algebra Skills

One of the most critical factors underlying success in this course is a strong foundation in algebra skills. We recognize that students start this course with varying degrees of skills, so we have included multiple opportunities in both the text and MyLab Math to help students target their weak areas and remediate or refresh the needed skills.

In the Text

- **Prerequisite Skills Diagnostic Test (Part A).** This portion of the diagnostic test assesses skills refreshed in "Appendix A: Review of Basic Algebra." Answers to the questions (provided at the back of the book) reference specific examples within the appendix.
- **Appendix A: Review of Basic Algebra.** This 13-page appendix provides examples on topics such as exponents, equations, and inequalities and applied problems. It ends with an exercise set, for which answers are provided at the back of the book so students can check their understanding.
- **Prerequisite Skills Diagnostic Test (Part B).** This portion of the diagnostic test assesses skills that are reviewed in "Chapter R: Functions, Graphs, and Models," and the answers (provided at the back of the book) reference specific examples in that chapter. Some instructors may choose to cover these topics thoroughly in class, making this assessment less critical. Other instructors may use some or all of the questions in this test to determine whether there is a need to spend time remediating before moving on with Chapter 1.

- **Chapter R: Functions, Graphs, and Models.** This chapter covers basic concepts related to functions, graphing, and modeling. It can be an optional chapter, depending on students' prerequisite skills.

In MyLab Math

You can diagnose weak prerequisite skills through built-in diagnostic quizzes. By coupling these quizzes with personalized homework, MyLab Math provides remediation for just those skills a student lacks. Even if you choose not to assign the diagnostic quizzes with personalized homework, students can self-remediate through videos and practice exercises provided at the objective level. MyLab Math provides the just-in-time help that students need, so you can focus on the course content.

Exercises and Applications

There are 4114 assignable homework exercises in this edition. A large percentage of these exercises are rendered algorithmically in MyLab Math. All exercise sets are enhanced by the inclusion of real-world applications, detailed figures, and illustrative graphs. There are a variety of types of exercises, too, so different levels of understanding and varying approaches to problems can be assessed. In addition to applications, the exercise sets include Thinking and Writing, Synthesis, Technology Connection, and Concept Reinforcement exercises. The exercises in MyLab Math reflect the depth and variety of those in the printed text.

The authors also provide Quick Check exercises following selected examples to give students the opportunity to check their understanding of new concepts or skills as soon as they learn them and one skill at a time. Instructors may include these as part of a lecture as a means of gauging skills and gaining immediate student feedback. Answers to the Quick Check exercises are provided following the exercise set at the end of each section.

Relevant and factual applications drawn from a broad spectrum of fields are integrated throughout the text as applied examples and exercises, and are also featured in separate application subsections. Applications have been updated and expanded in this edition to include even more real-world data. In addition, each chapter opener features an application that serves as a preview of what students will learn in the chapter. The Index of Applications at the back of the book provides students and instructors with a comprehensive list of the many different fields featured in examples and exercises throughout the text.

The applications in the exercise sets in the text and within MyLab Math are grouped under headings that identify them as reflecting real-world situations: Business and Economics, Life and Physical Sciences, Social Sciences, and General Interest (abbreviated as BE, LS, PS, SS, and GI within MyLab Math). This organization allows the instructor to gear the assigned exercises to specific students and also allows each student to know whether a particular exercise applies to his or her major.

Opportunities to Incorporate Technology

This edition continues to emphasize mathematical modeling, utilizing the advantages of technology as appropriate. The use of Excel as a tool for solving problems has been expanded in this edition. Though the use of technology is optional with this text, its use meshes well with the text's more intuitive approach to applied calculus.

Technology Connections

Technology Connections are included throughout the text to illustrate the use of technology, including graphing calculators and Excel spreadsheets. Whenever appropriate, figures that simulate graphs or tables generated by a graphing calculator are included. The goal is to take advantage of technology to which many students have access, wherever it makes sense, given the mathematical situation.

Four types of Technology Connections allow students and instructors to explore key ideas:

1. **Lesson/Teaching**—provide students with an example, followed by exercises to work within the lesson.
2. **Checking**—tell the students how to verify a solution within an example by using a graphing calculator.

3. **Exploratory/Investigation**—provide questions to guide students through an investigation.
4. **Technology Connection Exercises**—found in most section exercise sets, Chapter Review Exercises, and Chapter Tests.

Extended Technology Applications at the ends of all chapters use real applications and real data. They require a step-by-step analysis that encourages group work. More challenging in nature, the exercises in these features often involve the use of regression to create models on a graphing calculator.

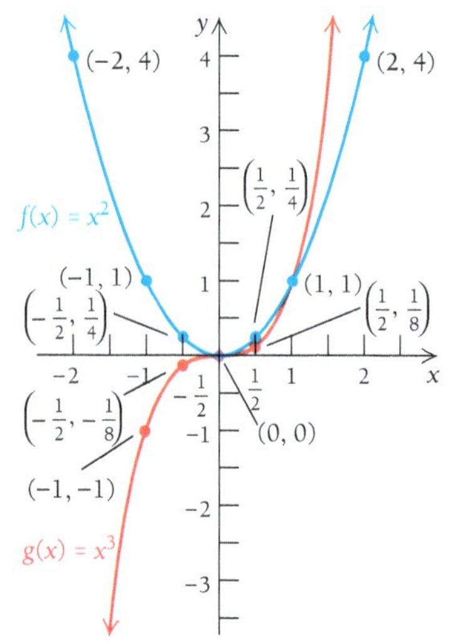

Use of Art and Color

One of the hallmarks of this text is the pervasive use of color as a pedagogical tool. Color is used in a methodical and precise manner that enhances the readability of the text for students and instructors.

- When two curves are graphed using the same set of axes, one is usually red and the other blue, with the red graph being the curve of major importance. As in the graph to the left, equation labels are the same color as the curve for clarity.
- When the instructions say "Graph," the dots match the color of the curve. When dots are used for emphasis other than just for plotting, they are black.
- Throughout the text, blue is used for secant lines and red for tangent lines (see p. 138).
- Red denotes substitution in equations while blue highlights the corresponding outputs, and the specific use of color is carried out in related figures (see pp. 282–284).
- Beginning with the discussion of integration, an amber color is used to highlight areas in graphs (see p. 408).

Opportunity for Review and Synthesis

Recognizing that it is often while preparing for exams that concepts gel for students, this text offers abundant opportunities for students to review, analyze, and synthesize recently learned concepts and skills.

- A **Section Summary** precedes every exercise set to assist students in identifying the key topics for each section and to serve as a mini-review.
- A **Chapter Summary** at the end of every chapter includes a section-by-section list of key definitions, concepts, and theorems, with examples for further clarification.
- **Chapter Review Exercises**, which include bracketed references to the section in which the related concept is first introduced, provide comprehensive coverage and appropriate referencing of each chapter's material.
- A **Chapter Test** at the end of every chapter and a **Cumulative Review** at the end of the text give students an authentic exam-like environment for testing their mastery. Answers to the chapter tests and the Cumulative Review are at the back of the text and include section references so students can diagnose their mistakes while preparing for exams.

Acknowledgments

As authors, we have taken many steps to ensure the accuracy of this text. Many devoted individuals comprised the team that was responsible for monitoring the revision and production process in a manner that makes this a work of which we can all be proud. We are thankful for our publishing team at Pearson, as well as all of the Pearson representatives who share our book with educators across the country. We would like to thank Jane Hoover for her many helpful suggestions, proofreading, and checking of art. Geri Davis deserves credit for both the attractive design of the text and the coordination of the many illustrations, photos, and graphs. Many thanks also to John Samons and Laurie Hurley for their careful checking of the manuscript and typeset pages and to Sal Sciandra for his work on the Solutions Manuals. Special thanks go to Cara McDaniel of Arizona State University for her thoughtful insights on the new material in the text. We are grateful to all those who have contributed to the improvement of this text over the years, including those who were instrumental in helping us to shape this 12th edition.

The following individuals provided terrific insights and meaningful suggestions for improving this text. We thank them:

Olusola Akinyele, *Bowie State University*
Karen Appel, *Mesa Community College*
Kristen A. Ceballos, *Southern Illinois University–Carbondale*
Manny Decena, *American Heritage School*
Tim Doyle, *University of Illinois at Chicago*
Justin Dunham, *Johnson County Community College*
Sharon L. Giles, *Grossmont Community College*
H. Ray Hendrickson, *Bucks County Community College*
Dwight Jackson, *Brunswick School*
Dynechia M. Jones, *Baton Rouge Community College*
Cheryl Kane, *University of Nebraska–Lincoln*
Tatyana Kravchuk, *Northern Virginia Community College*
Mariana Lowe, *Arizona State University*
James Martin, *Christopher Newport University*
Tamara Miller, *Ivy Tech Community College of Indiana*
Michael R. Payne, *Pueblo Community College*
Brendan Patrick Purdy, *Moorpark College*
Thomas C. Redd, *North Carolina A&T State University*
Shumaila Saeed, *Indiana University Purdue University Indianapolis*
Scott R. Sykes, *University of West Georgia*
Maria Jane Thoundayil, *Prince George's Community College*
Jacob Tschume, *Mississippi State University*
Robert Vilardi, *Troy University*
Kimberly W. Walters, *Mississippi State University*

The following individuals provided insights and meaningful suggestions for improving the MyLab Math course for this text. We thank them:

Majid Bani-Yaghoub, *University of Missouri–Kansas City*
Gerry Baygents, *University of Missouri–Kansas City*
Mary Beth Headlee, *MiraCosta College*
Joy St. John Johnson, *Calhoun Community College*
Cheryl Kane, *University of Nebraska–Lincoln*
Joseph Londino, *University of Memphis*
Raquel Lopez, *Arizona State University*
Emma Lozowski, *Lewis and Clark Community College*
Rick Pugsley, *Ivy Tech Community College*
Cassandra Scott, *Bowie State University*
Ilham Tayahi, *University of Memphis*
Ben Tschida, *North Idaho College*
Cheryl Van Rhein, *University of Missouri–Kansas City*
Mehrdad Mahmoudi Zarandi, *Ivy Tech Community College of Indiana*

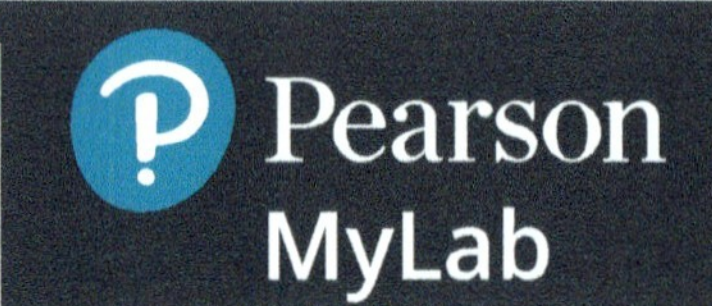

MyLab Math Online Course for *Calculus and Its Applications, Brief Version,* 12th edition

(access code required)

MyLab™ Math is available to accompany Pearson's market-leading text offerings. To give students a consistent tone, voice, and teaching method, each text's flavor and approach are tightly integrated throughout the accompanying MyLab Math course, making learning the material as seamless as possible.

PREPAREDNESS

One of the biggest challenges in applied calculus courses is making sure students are adequately prepared with the prerequisite skills needed to successfully complete their course work. MyLab Math supports students with just-in-time remediation and key-concept review.

Integrated Review

The MyLab Math course contains pre-made, assignable quizzes to assess the prerequisite skills needed for each chapter, plus personalized remediation for any gaps in skills that are identified. Each student, therefore, receives just the help that he or she needs—no more, no less.

NEW! Study Skills Modules

Study skills modules help students with the life skills that can make the difference between passing and failing.

DEVELOPING DEEPER UNDERSTANDING

MyLab Math provides content and tools that help students build a deeper understanding of course content than would otherwise be possible.

Exercises with Immediate Feedback

The approximately 3270 homework and practice exercises for this text regenerate algorithmically to give students unlimited opportunity for practice and mastery. MyLab Math provides helpful feedback when students enter incorrect answers and includes several optional learning aids: Help Me Solve This, View an Example, Video, and Textbook (links to the eText). All exercises have been reviewed and edited for this edition by author Gene Kramer.

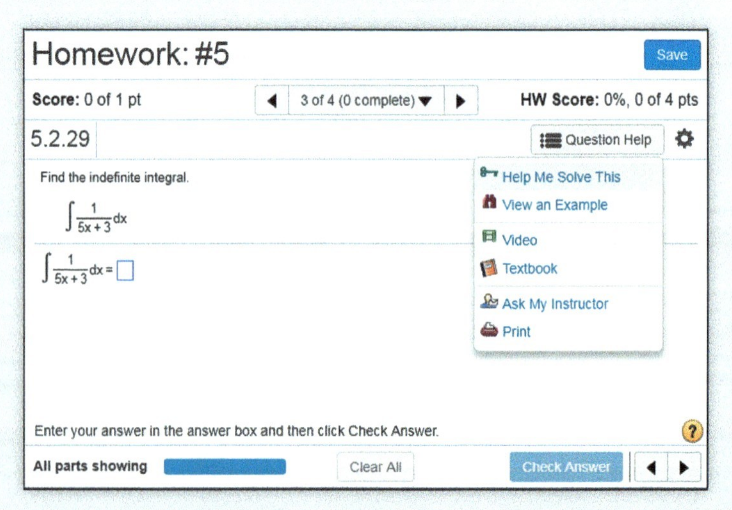

Pearson MyLab

NEW! Setup and Solve Exercises

These exercises require students to show how they set up a problem as well as giving the solution, better mirroring what is required on tests.

Find the area of the region enclosed by the curves $y^2 - 5x = 1$ and $x - y = 1$.

Set up the integral that gives the area of the shaded region.

$$\int_{-1}^{6} \left[y + 1 - \frac{y^2 - 1}{5} \right] dy$$

Find the area by evaluating the integral

$\frac{343}{30}$ (Type an integer or a simplified fraction.)

NEW! Additional Conceptual Questions

Additional Conceptual Questions provide support for assessing concepts and vocabulary. Many of these questions are application-oriented. They are clearly labeled ACQ in the Assignment Manager.

EXPANDED! Instructional Videos

About 90% of the instructional videos are brand-new. The new videos were made using the latest technology and feature authors Gene Kramer and Scott Surgent along with instructors Mary Ann Barber (University of North Texas) and Thomas Hartfield (University of North Georgia). In addition, there are MathTalk videos that highlight applications of the content of the course to business and are supported by assignable exercises.

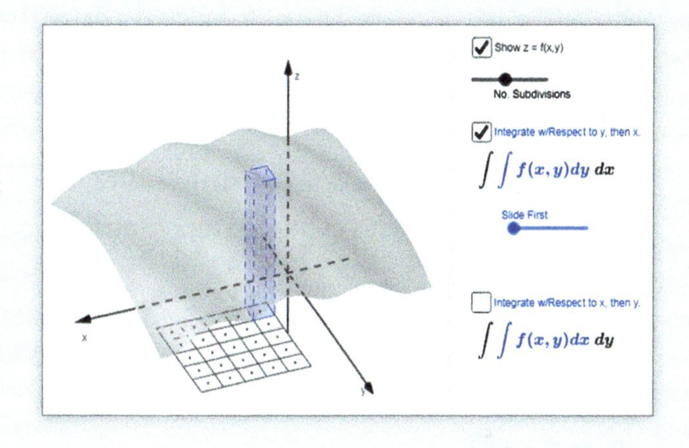

EXPANDED! Interactive Figures

An expanded full suite of interactive figures illustrate key concepts and allow manipulation. They are designed to be used in lecture as well as by students independently.

NEW! Enhanced Sample Assignments

These assignments include just-in-time prerequisite review, help keep skills fresh with spaced practice of key concepts, and provide opportunities to work exercises without learning aids so that students can check their understanding. They are assignable and editable within MyLab Math.

UPDATED! Graphing Calculator and Excel Spreadsheet Manuals (downloadable)

Graphing Calculator Manual by Chris True, University of Nebraska
Excel Spreadsheet Manual by Stela Pudar-Hozo, Indiana University–Northwest
These manuals, both specific to this course, have been updated to support the TI-84 Plus CE (color display) and Excel 2016, respectively. Instructions are ordered by mathematical topic.

Student's Solutions Manual (softcover or downloadable)

ISBN: 0-13-516568-7 | 978-0-13-516568-3
The Student's Solutions Manual contains worked-out solutions to all the odd-numbered exercises and all Chapter Test exercises. This manual is available in print and can be downloaded from within MyLab Math.

A Complete eText

Students get unlimited access to the eText within any MyLab Math course using that edition of the textbook. The Pearson eText app allows existing subscribers to access their titles on an iPad or Android tablet for either online or offline viewing.

pearson.com/mylab/math

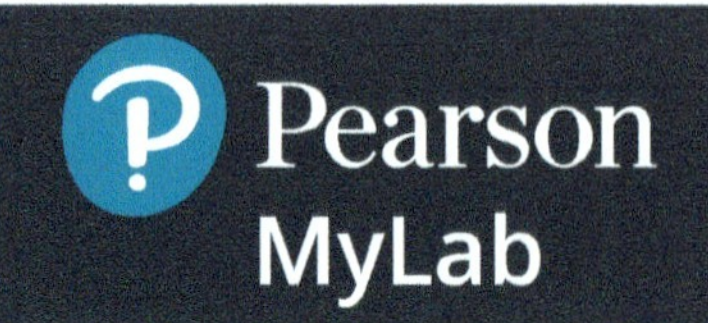

SUPPORTING INSTRUCTION

MyLab Math comes from an experienced partner with educational expertise and an eye on the future. It provides resources to help you assess and improve students' results at every turn and unparalleled flexibility to create a course tailored to you and your students.

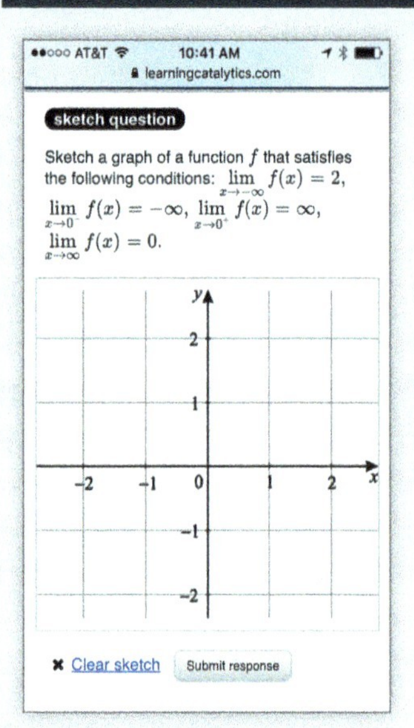

NEW! Learning Catalytics™

Now included in all MyLab Math courses, this student response tool uses students' smartphones, tablets, or laptops to engage them in more interactive tasks and thinking during lecture. Learning Catalytics fosters student engagement and peer-to-peer learning with real-time analytics. Access pre-built exercises created specifically for this course.

PowerPoint® Lectures (downloadable)

Slides contain presentation resources such as key concepts, examples, definitions, figures, and tables from this text. They can be downloaded from within MyLab Math or from Pearson's online catalog at **www.pearson.com**.

Comprehensive Gradebook

The gradebook includes enhanced reporting functionality such as item analysis and a reporting dashboard to allow you to efficiently manage your course. Student performance data is presented at the class, section, and program levels in an accessible, visual manner, providing the information you need to keep your students on track.

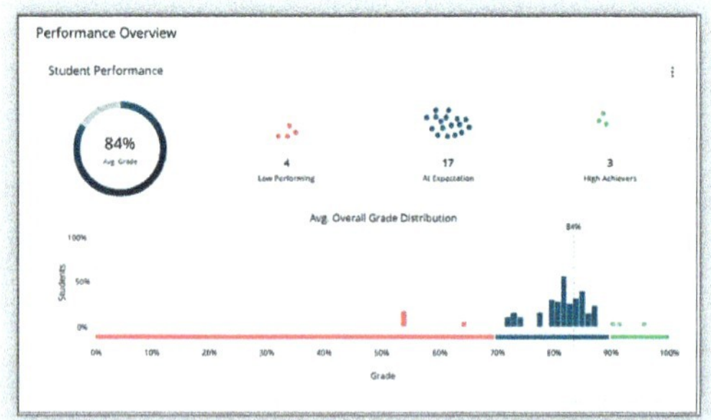

TestGen®

TestGen (**www.pearson.com/testgen**) enables instructors to build, edit, print, and administer tests using a computerized bank of questions developed to cover all the objectives of the text. TestGen is algorithmically based, allowing instructors to create multiple but equivalent versions of the same question or test with the click of a button. Instructors can also modify test bank questions or add new questions. The software and test bank are available for download from Pearson's online catalog at **www.pearson.com**. The questions are also assignable in MyLab Math.

Instructor's Solutions Manual and NEW! Instructor's Answers (downloadable)

Solutions Manual ISBN: 0-13-518244-1 | 978-0-13-518244-4
Answers ISBN: 0-13-522497-7 | 978-0-13-522497-7
The Instructor's Solutions Manual contains worked-out solutions to all text exercises. The Instructor's Answers contain just the answers to exercises. Both of these can be downloaded *by instructors only* from within MyLab Math or from Pearson's online catalog at **www.pearson.com**.

Accessibility

Pearson works continuously to ensure our products are as accessible as possible to all students. We are working toward achieving WCAG 2.0 Level AA and Section 508 standards, as expressed in the Pearson Guidelines for Accessible Educational Web Media, **www.pearson.com/mylab/math/accessibility**. Please see the "Accessibility" tab within the MyLab Math course for accessible student resources for this text.

pearson.com/mylab/math

Prerequisite Skills Diagnostic Test

To the Student and the Instructor

This diagnostic test can be used to assess student needs for this course. Part A covers algebra concepts discussed in Appendix A. Part B covers topics discussed in Chapter R, most of which come from a course in intermediate or college algebra. (This diagnostic test does not cover regression, though it is considered in Section R.7 and used throughout the text.) Students who have difficulty with the questions in part A should study Appendix A before moving to Chapter R. Those who have difficulty with the questions in part B should study Chapter R. Students who miss just a few questions might study the related topics in either Appendix A or Chapter R before continuing with the calculus chapters.

Part A: *Answers and locations of step-by-step solutions appear on p. A-1.*

Write an equivalent expression for each of the following without an exponent.

1. 4^3 **2.** $(-2)^5$ **3.** $(\frac{1}{2})^3$ **4.** $(-2x)^1$ **5.** e^0

Write an equivalent expression for each of the following without a negative exponent.

6. x^{-5} **7.** $(\frac{1}{4})^{-2}$ **8.** t^{-1}

Multiply.

9. $x^5 \cdot x^6$ **10.** $x^{-2} \cdot x^9$ **11.** $2x^{-3} \cdot 5x^{-4} \cdot 4x^{10}$

Divide.

12. $\dfrac{a^3}{a^2}$ **13.** $\dfrac{b^3}{b^{-5}}$

Simplify. Express each answer without a negative exponent.

14. $(x^{-2})^3$ **15.** $(2x^4y^{-5}z^3)^{-3}$

Multiply.

16. $3(x - 5)$ **17.** $(x - 5)(x + 3)$

18. $(a + b)(a + b)$ **19.** $(2x - t)^2$

20. $(3c + d)(3c - d)$

Factor.

21. $2xh + h^2$ **22.** $x^2 - 6xy + 9y^2$

23. $x^2 - 5x - 14$ **24.** $6x^2 + 7x - 5$

25. $x^3 - 7x^2 - 4x + 28$

Solve.

26. $-\frac{5}{6}x + 10 = \frac{1}{2}x + 2$ **27.** $3x(x - 2)(5x + 4) = 0$

28. $4x^3 = x$ **29.** $\dfrac{2x}{x-3} - \dfrac{6}{x} = \dfrac{18}{x^2 - 3x}$

30. $17 - 8x \geq 5x - 4$

31. After a 5% gain in weight, a grizzly bear weighs 693 lb. What was the bear's original weight?

32. Raggs, Ltd., a clothing firm, determines that its total revenue, R, in dollars, from the sale of x suits is given by $R = 350x + 500$. Find the number of suits that must be sold so that total revenue is more than $70,050.

Part B: *Answers and locations of step-by-step solutions appear on p. A-1.*

Graph.

1. $y = 2x + 1$ **2.** $3x + 5y = 10$

3. $y = x^2 - 1$ **4.** $x = y^2$

5. A function g is given by $g(x) = 3x^2 - 2x + 8$. Find each of the following: $g(0)$, $g(-5)$, and $g(7a)$.

6. A function f is given by $f(x) = 3x - 12$. Find all x such that $f(x) = 0$.

7. Graph the function f:

$$f(x) = \begin{cases} 4, & \text{for } x \leq 0, \\ 3 - x^2, & \text{for } 0 < x \leq 2, \\ 2x - 6, & \text{for } x > 2. \end{cases}$$

8. Write interval notation for $\{x \mid -4 < x \leq 5\}$.

9. Find the domain of f: $f(x) = \dfrac{3}{2x - 5}$.

10. Find the slope and y-intercept of the graph of $2x - 4y - 7 = 0$.

11. Find an equation of the line with slope 3 containing the point $(-1, -5)$.

12. Find the slope of the line containing the points $(-2, 6)$ and $(-4, 9)$.

13. Solve for x: $\log_2 x = 32$. **14.** Solve for x: $7^x = \dfrac{1}{49}$.

Graph.

15. $f(x) = x^2 - 2x - 3$ **16.** $g(x) = x^3$

17. $f(x) = \dfrac{1}{x}$ **18.** $f(x) = |x|$

19. $f(x) = -\sqrt{x}$

20. Suppose that $1000 is earning 5% interest, compounded annually. How much is the investment worth at the end of 2 yr?

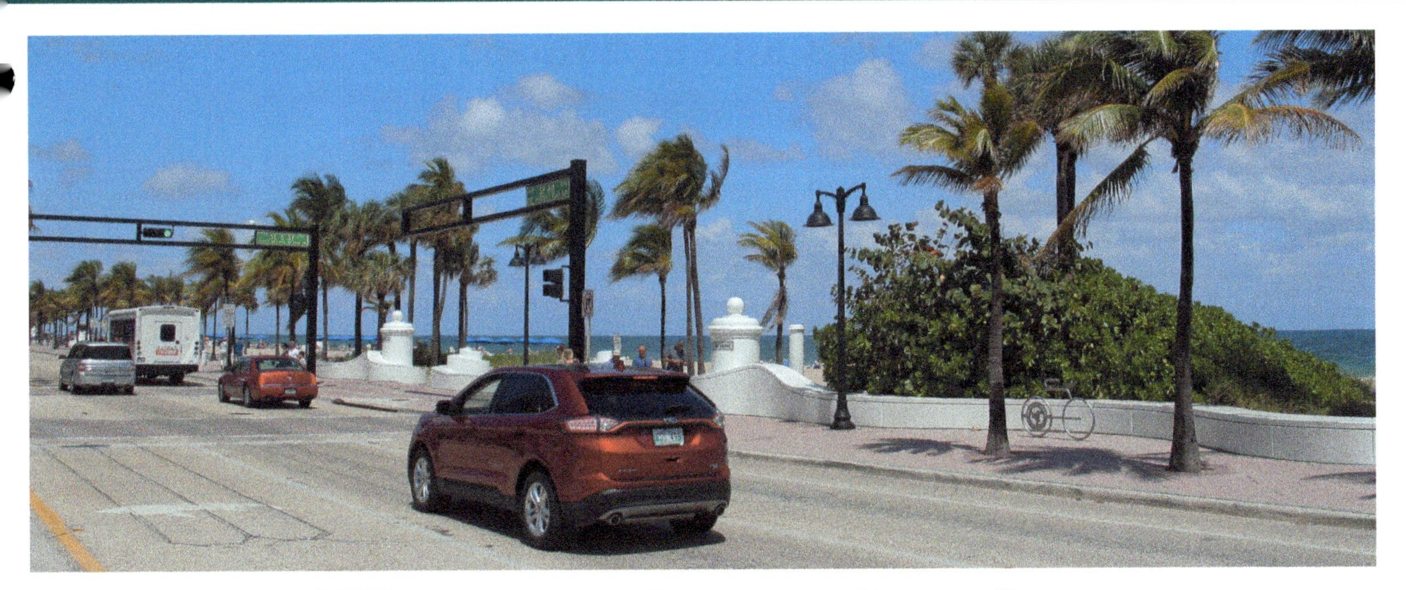

R Functions, Graphs, and Models

What You'll Learn

Why It's Important

This chapter introduces functions and their notation, graphs, and applications. Also presented are many topics considered often throughout the text: supply and demand; total cost, revenue, and profit; the concept of a mathematical model; and curve fitting.

Skills in using a graphing calculator and other forms of technology are introduced and discussed in the Technology Connections. Details on keystrokes are given in the *Graphing Calculator Manual* (GCM).

Part A of the diagnostic test (p. xvii), on basic algebra concepts, allows students to determine whether they need to review Appendix A (p. 615) before studying this chapter. Part B, on college algebra topics, assesses the need to study this chapter before the calculus chapters.

Where It's Used

Rental Car Rates: What would be the total cost of renting a minivan in Florida for 36 hr?

(This problem appears as Example 8 in Section R.3.)

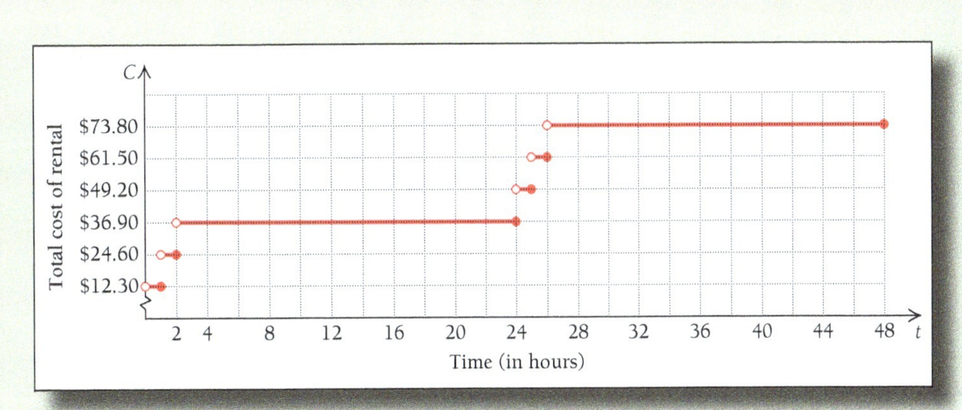

R.1

- Graph equations.
- Use graphs as mathematical models to make predictions.
- Carry out calculations involving compound interest.

Graphs and Equations

What Is Calculus?

What is calculus? How does calculus differ from algebra? These are common questions at the start of a course like this. Consider the following problems that one might encounter in an algebra course:

- A hotel manager charges \$120 per room per night. In one night, she had total revenue of \$5160. How many rooms did she rent that night?
- Juanita's car is moving at 40 mi/hr (58.67 ft/sec) when she applies the brakes. The car's velocity, t seconds after Juanita applies the brakes, is given by $v = -1.197t^2 + 58.67$, where v is in feet per second and $0 \leq t \leq 7$. How fast is the car traveling at $t = 3$ sec?
- A cylindrical soup can has a volume of 250 cm^3. If its height is twice the length of its radius, find the dimensions of the can.

Now, consider similar problems one might encounter in a calculus course:

- At \$120 per room per night, a hotel manager typically rents 50 rooms each night. For every \$10 decrease in the price per room per night, she will rent 5 more rooms per night. Find the price per room that will maximize total nightly revenue.
- Juanita's car is moving at 40 mi/hr (58.67 ft/sec) when she applies the brakes. The car's velocity, t seconds after Juanita applies the brakes, is given by $v = -1.197t^2 + 58.67$, where v is in feet per second and $0 \leq t \leq 7$. How far does the car travel during the 7 sec it takes to come to a stop?
- A cylindrical soup can has a volume of 250 cm^3. If the cost of material for the top and bottom of the can is \$0.0008 per square centimeter, and the cost of material for the side is \$0.0015 per square centimeter, what dimensions minimize the cost of material for the can?

Problems about minimizing, maximizing, or finding a total accumulation of a quantity can be solved using calculus. A hotel manager might want to find the price that *maximizes* nightly revenue. A traffic engineer might want to determine a *total* distance traveled based on information about a vehicle's velocity. A manufacturer might want to find the dimensions that *minimize* the cost of producing a can.

Let's model this last problem using algebra. The combined area of the top and bottom of the soup can is $2\pi r^2$, and the area of the side is $2\pi rh$. Using the earlier information on material cost, the cost, C, of material for one can is

$$C = 0.0008(2\pi r^2) + 0.0015(2\pi rh),$$
$$= 0.0016\pi r^2 + 0.003\pi rh. \quad \text{Simplifying}$$

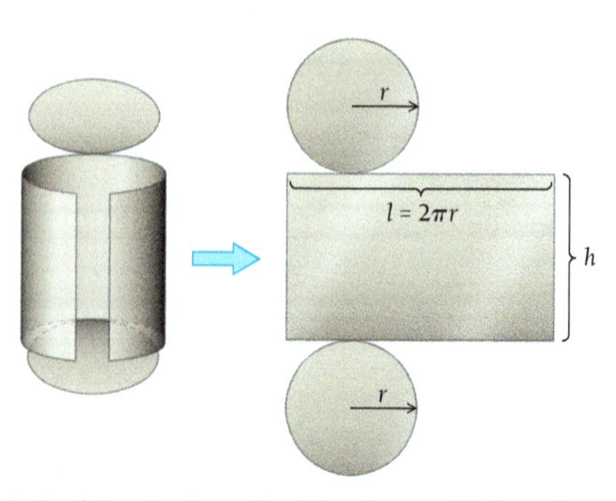

Each of the circular ends of the disassembled can has an area of πr^2, and the side has an area of $2\pi rh$.

The volume V of a circular cylinder with radius r and height h is given by $V = \pi r^2 h$. Using $V = 250 \text{ cm}^3$, we have $h = \frac{250}{\pi r^2}$. Thus,

$$C = 0.0016\pi r^2 + 0.003\pi r\left(\frac{250}{\pi r^2}\right) \quad \text{Replacing } h \text{ with } \frac{250}{\pi r^2}$$

$$= 0.0016\pi r^2 + \frac{0.75}{r}. \quad \text{Simplifying}$$

Using the above formula in a spreadsheet, we see how values of C, the cost of material for one can, vary with values of r, the radius, and from this, infer the value of r that results in the possible lowest cost C:

	A	B
1	radius	cost
2	r	C
33	3.5	0.275868914
34	3.6	0.273485845
35	3.7	0.271525071
36	3.8	0.269961189
37	3.9	0.268771404
38	4	0.267924772
39	4.1	0.267423105
40	4.2	0.26723974 ← Possible lowest cost
41	4.3	0.267359482
42	4.4	0.267768519
43	4.5	0.268454269
44	4.6	0.26941903
45	4.7	0.270625316
46	4.8	0.272076688
47	4.9	0.273764296
48	5	0.27568

When the radius of the can is 4.2 cm, the cost of material for the can is about \$0.26724. This appears to be the radius that results in the lowest cost. *But how can we be certain that no other dimensions will give a lower cost?* This is a question that algebra alone cannot answer. We need the tools of calculus to answer this. In Chapter 3, we study such maximum-minimum problems, including a complete solution to this one about the material cost for a can, which appears as Example 3 in Section 3.5.

Other topics we consider in calculus are the slope of a line touching a curve at a point, rates of change, areas under curves, accumulations of quantities, and statistical applications such as finding lines that best "fit" data (regression) and finding probabilities using certain distribution models.

Ordered Pairs and Graphs

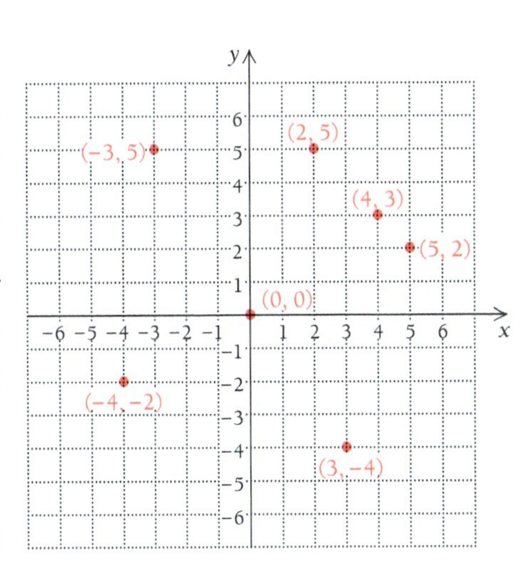

Each point in a plane corresponds to an ordered pair of numbers. Note in the figure at the right that the point corresponding to the pair (2, 5) is different from the point corresponding to the pair (5, 2). This is why we call a pair like (2, 5) an *ordered pair*. The first number is called the *first coordinate* of the point, and the second number is called the *second coordinate*. Together these are the *coordinates of the point*. The horizontal line is often labeled as the *x-axis*, and the vertical line is often labeled as the *y-axis*. The two axes intersect at the *origin*, (0, 0). The use of axes to display all points in the plane is often called the *xy-coordinate system*, the *xy-coordinate plane*, or simply the Cartesian plane.

Graphs

The study of graphs is an essential aspect of calculus. A graph allows us to visualize relationships between two variables. For instance, the graph below shows how the annual inflation rate in the United States changed from 2000 to 2016. A graph can be a powerful aid in understanding how change in one variable affects change in another.

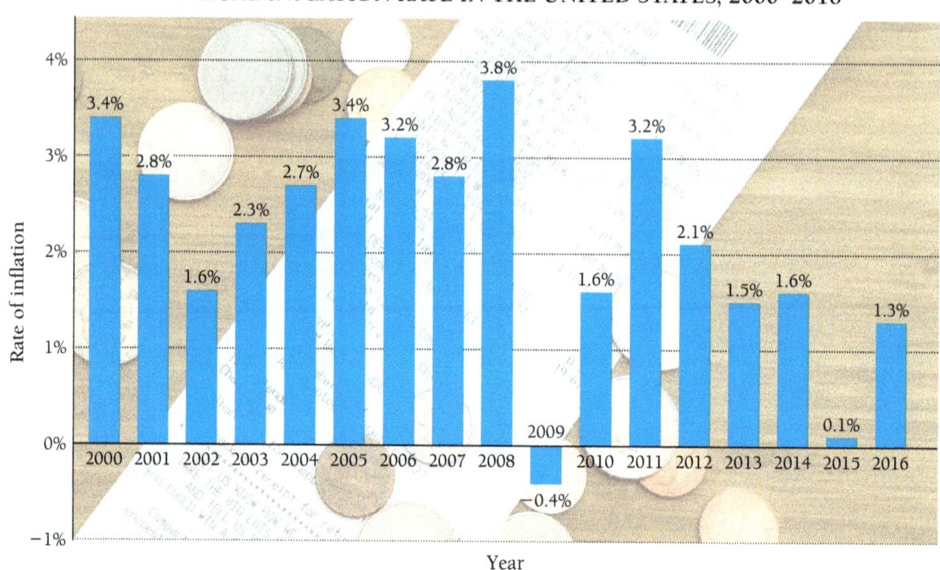

(*Source*: Bureau of Labor Statistics.)

Graphs of Equations

Equations such as $y = 2x - 1$ and $v = 125t^2 + 25$ are called *equations in two variables*. A *solution* of an equation in two variables is an ordered pair of numbers that, when substituted for the variables, forms a true statement. If not directed otherwise, we usually take the variables in *alphabetical* order. For example, $(-1, 2)$ is a solution of the equation $3x^2 + y = 5$, because when we substitute -1 for x and 2 for y, we get a true statement:

$$\begin{array}{r|l} 3x^2 + y & = 5 \\ \hline 3(-1)^2 + 2 & ?\ 5 \\ 3 + 2 & \ 5 \\ 5 & \ 5 \quad \text{TRUE} \end{array}$$

> **DEFINITION**
>
> The **graph** of an equation is a drawing that represents all ordered pairs that are solutions of the equation.

We obtain the graph of an equation by plotting enough ordered pairs (that are solutions) to see a pattern.

EXAMPLE 1 Graph: $y = 2x + 1$.

Solution We first find ordered pairs that are solutions and arrange them in a table. To find an ordered pair, we choose a number for x and then determine y.

For example, if we choose -2 for x and substitute that value in $y = 2x + 1$, we find that $y = 2(-2) + 1 = -4 + 1 = -3$. Thus, $(-2, -3)$ is a solution. We can select both negative numbers and positive numbers, as well as 0, for x.

x	y	(x, y)
-2	-3	$(-2, -3)$
-1	-1	$(-1, -1)$
0	1	$(0, 1)$
1	3	$(1, 3)$
2	5	$(2, 5)$

(1) Choose any x.
(2) Compute y.
(3) Form the pair (x, y).
(4) Plot the points.

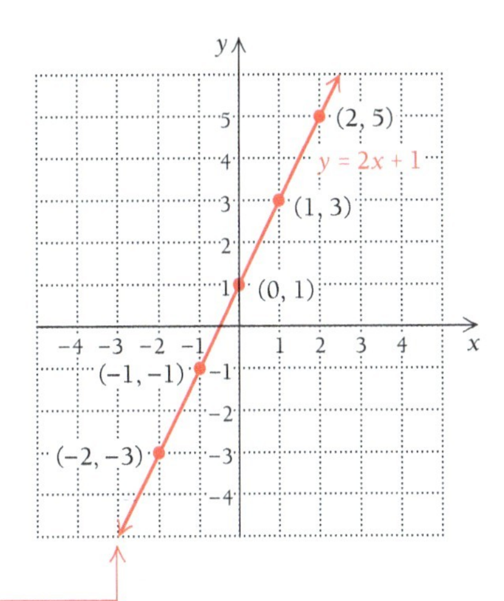

Quick Check 1 ✓
Graph: $y = 3 - x$.

After we plot the points, we look for a pattern in the graph. In this case, the points suggest a line. We draw the line with a straightedge and label it $y = 2x + 1$. **1 ✓**

EXAMPLE 2 Graph: $3x + 5y = 10$.

Solution We could choose x-values, substitute, and determine corresponding y-values, but it is easier to first solve for y.*

$$
\begin{aligned}
3x + 5y &= 10 \\
3x + 5y - 3x &= 10 - 3x && \text{Subtracting } 3x \text{ from both sides} \\
5y &= 10 - 3x && \text{Simplifying} \\
\tfrac{1}{5} \cdot 5y &= \tfrac{1}{5} \cdot (10 - 3x) && \text{Multiplying both sides by } \tfrac{1}{5} \\
y &= \tfrac{1}{5} \cdot (10) - \tfrac{1}{5} \cdot (3x) && \text{Using the distributive law} \\
y &= 2 - \tfrac{3}{5}x && \text{Simplifying} \\
y &= -\tfrac{3}{5}x + 2
\end{aligned}
$$

Next we use $y = -\frac{3}{5}x + 2$ to find solutions that are ordered pairs. Choosing multiples of 5 for x avoids obtaining fractions as values of y.

x	y	(x, y)
0	2	$(0, 2)$
5	-1	$(5, -1)$
-5	5	$(-5, 5)$

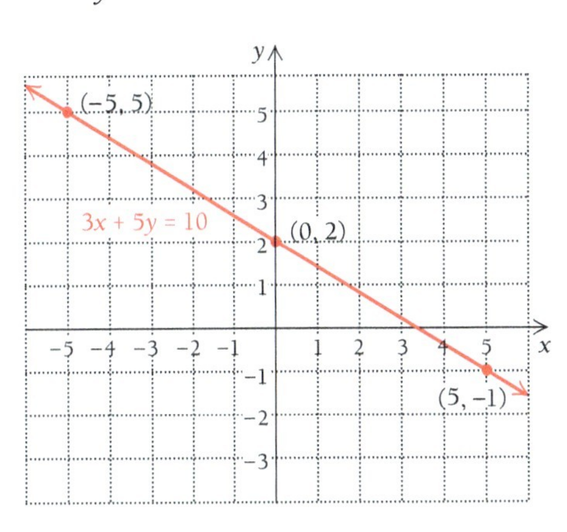

Quick Check 2 ✓
Graph: $3x - 5y = 10$.

We plot the points, draw the line, and label the graph as shown. **2 ✓**

*Be sure to consult Appendix A, as needed, for a review of algebra.

Examples 1 and 2 show graphs of linear equations. Such graphs are considered in greater detail in Section R.4.

EXAMPLE 3 Graph: $y = x^2 - 1$.

Solution

x	y	(x, y)
-2	3	$(-2, 3)$
-1	0	$(-1, 0)$
0	-1	$(0, -1)$
1	0	$(1, 0)$
2	3	$(2, 3)$

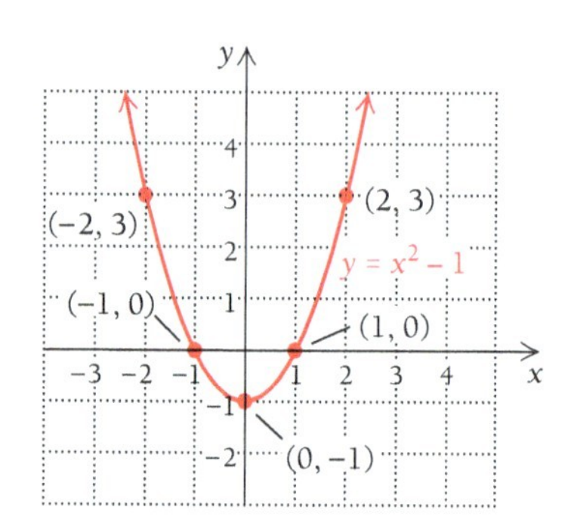

Quick Check 3 ✓
Graph: $y = 2 - x^2$.

This time the pattern of the points is a curve called a *parabola*. We plot enough points to see a pattern and draw the graph. **3 ✓**

EXAMPLE 4 Graph: $x = y^2$.

Solution In this case, x is expressed in terms of the variable y, making it simpler to first choose numbers for y and then compute x.

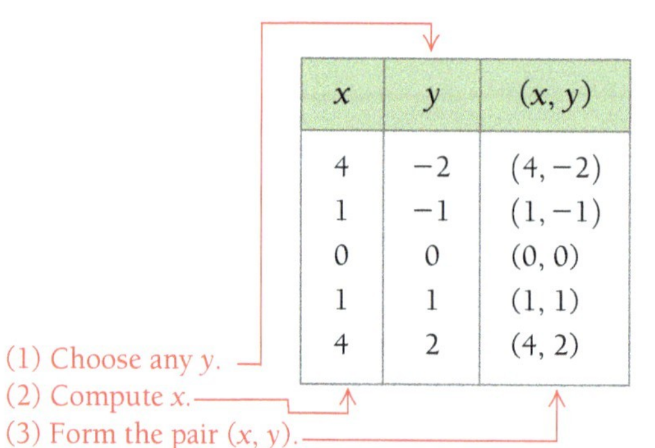

x	y	(x, y)
4	-2	$(4, -2)$
1	-1	$(1, -1)$
0	0	$(0, 0)$
1	1	$(1, 1)$
4	2	$(4, 2)$

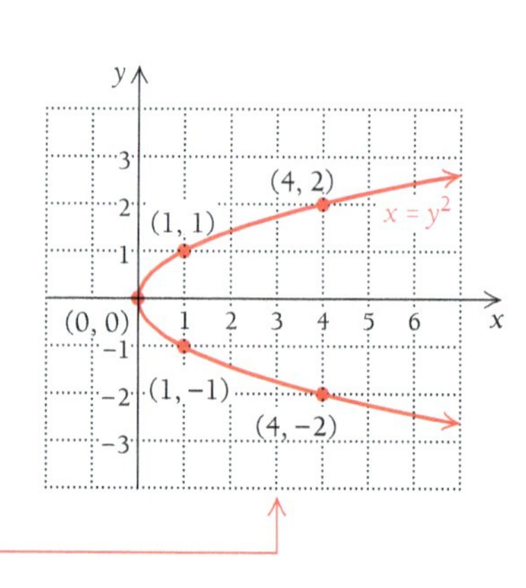

Quick Check 4 ✓
Graph: $x = 1 + y^2$.

We plot these points, keeping in mind that x is still the first coordinate and y the second. We look for a pattern and complete the graph by connecting the points. **4 ✓**

In calculus, we often study how the change in one variable affects the change in the other variable in the equation.

Mathematical Models

A real-world situation described using mathematics is called a **mathematical model**. For example, the speed at which a body falls due to gravity can be described using a mathematical model.

Mathematical models often allow us to predict what will happen in the real world. If the predictions are too inaccurate or if actual results do not conform to the model, the model must be changed or discarded.

Technology Connection 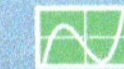

Introduction to the Graphing Calculator: Windows and Graphs

Viewing Windows

In this first of the optional Technology Connections, we begin to create graphs using a graphing calculator. Although some keystrokes are listed, exact keystrokes can be found in the owner's manual for your calculator or in the *Graphing Calculator Manual* (GCM) that accompanies this text.

The **viewing window** is the rectangular screen in which a graph appears. Windows are described by four numbers in the format [L, R, B, T], representing the **L**eft and **R**ight endpoints of the x-axis and the **B**ottom and **T**op endpoints of the y-axis. The WINDOW feature is used to set these dimensions. Below is a window setting of $[-20, 20, -5, 5]$ with axis scaling denoted as Xscl = 5 and Yscl = 1, which produces 5 units between tick marks from -20 to 20 on the x-axis and 1 unit between tick marks from -5 to 5 on the y-axis.

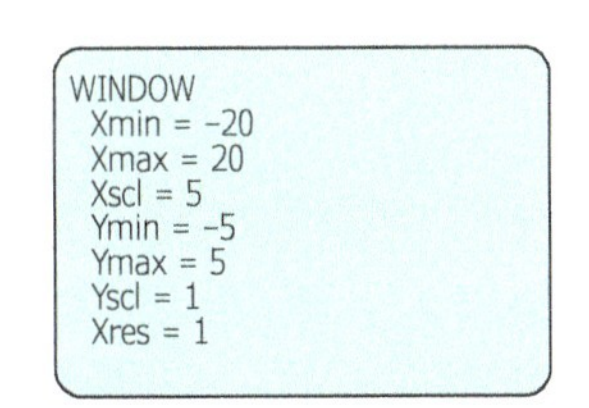

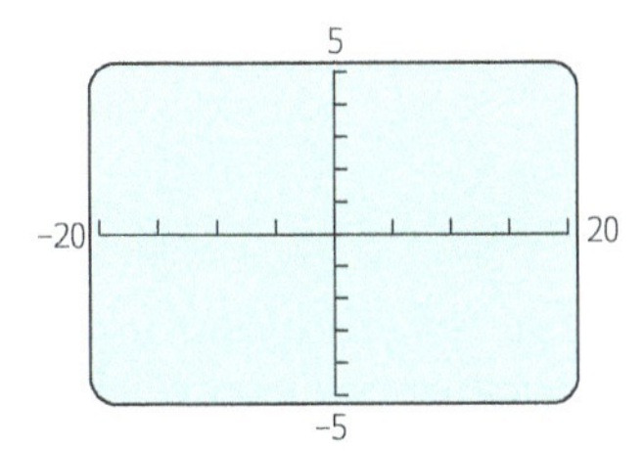

Scales should be chosen with care, since tick marks become indistinguishable when too many appear. On most graphing calculators, a window setting of $[-10, 10, -10, 10]$, Xscl = 1, Yscl = 1, Xres = 1 is considered **standard**.

Graphs

To graph the equation $y = x^3 - 5x + 1$, we press Y= and enter x^3–5x+1. We obtain the following graph in the standard viewing window.

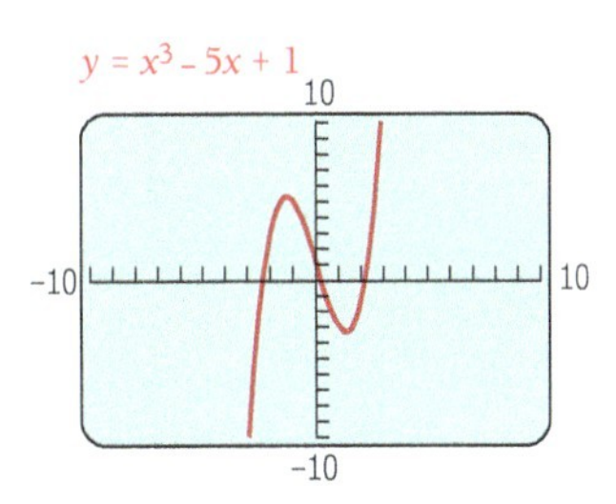

It is often necessary to change viewing windows in order to get the best display of a graph. For example, each of the following is a graph of $y = 3x^5 - 20x^3$, but with a different viewing window. Which best displays the curvature of the graph?

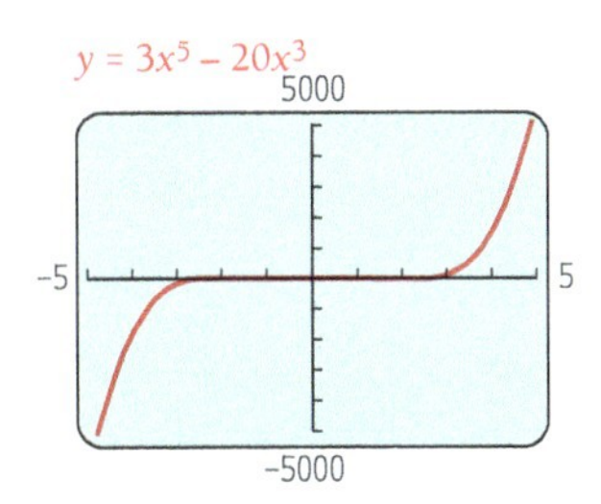

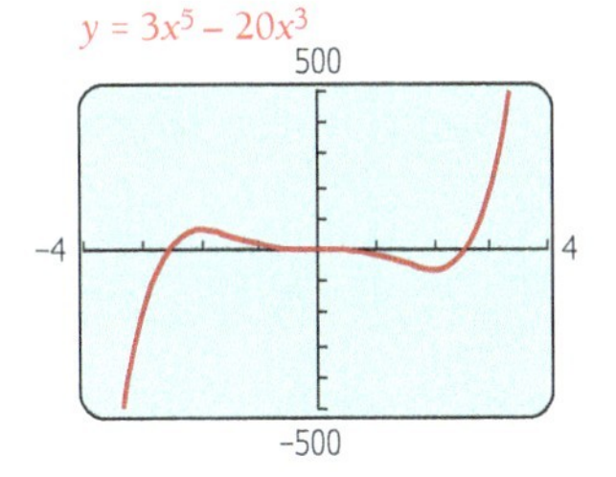

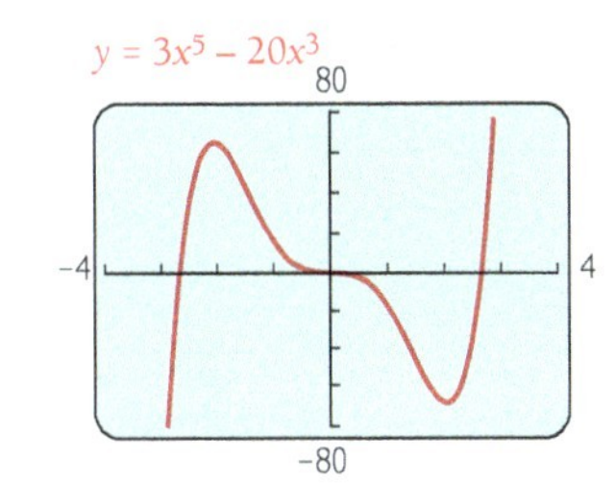

Often, choosing a window that best reveals a graph's characteristics involves some trial and error and, in some cases, knowledge about the shape of the graph.

EXERCISE

Using your graphing calculator, reproduce the graphs shown in Examples 1, 2, and 3 of this section and those on this page. Adjust the viewing window in each case until you obtain a satisfactory graph.

Creating a mathematical model is a process involving several steps.

CREATING A MATHEMATICAL MODEL

1. Recognize a real-world problem. → 2. Collect data. → 3. Analyze the data. → 4. Construct a model. → 5. Test and refine the model. → 6. Explain and predict.

Mathematical modeling is often an ongoing process. For example, finding a mathematical model that will accurately predict earnings is not simple. Most models will need to be reshaped as further information is acquired.

EXAMPLE 5 The following graph shows the mean (average) yearly earnings of individuals in the United States who have a bachelor's degree but no higher degree.

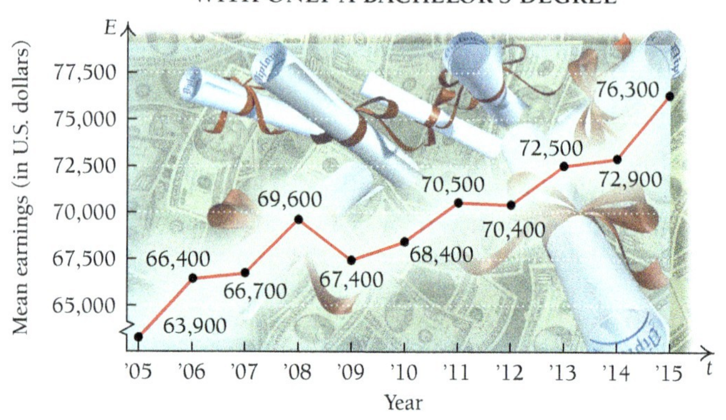

(*Source*: U.S. Census Bureau.)

Use the model $E = 1000t + 64{,}540$, where t is the number of years after 2005 and E is the yearly earnings, in dollars, to predict the yearly earnings in 2020 of an individual who holds a bachelor's degree but no higher degree.

Solution Since 2020 is 15 years after 2005, we substitute 15 for t:

$$\begin{aligned} E &= 1000(15) + 64{,}540 \\ &= 15{,}000 + 64{,}540 \\ &= 79{,}540. \end{aligned}$$

According to this model, the expected yearly earnings in 2020 of an individual with a bachelor's degree but no higher degree will be \$79,540. **5 ✓**

Quick Check 5 ✓

Using the model in Example 5, determine the year in which earnings of the individual will first exceed \$82,000.

As is the case with most models, the model in Example 5 is not perfect. For example, for $t = 10$, we get $E = \$74{,}540$, a number slightly different from the \$76,300 in the original data. But, for purposes of estimating, the model is adequate.

Compound Interest

One important model that is extremely precise involves **compound interest**. Suppose we invest P dollars at interest rate r, expressed as a decimal, and compounded annually. The amount A_1 in the account at the end of the first year is given by

$$A_1 = P + Pr = P(1 + r).$$

The original amount invested, P, is called the *principal*.

Going into the second year, we have $P(1 + r)$ dollars, so by the end of the second year, we will have the amount A_2 given by

$$A_2 = A_1 \cdot (1 + r) = [P(1 + r)](1 + r) = P(1 + r)^2.$$

Going into the third year, we have $P(1 + r)^2$ dollars, so by the end of the third year, we will have the amount A_3 given by

$$A_3 = A_2 \cdot (1 + r) = [P(1 + r)^2](1 + r) = P(1 + r)^3.$$

In general, we have the following theorem.

THEOREM 1

If an amount P is invested at interest rate r, expressed as a decimal, and compounded annually, then in t years it will grow to an amount A, where

$$A = P(1 + r)^t.$$

EXAMPLE 6 **Business: Compound Interest.** Suppose \$1000 is invested in Fibonacci Investment Fund at 5%, compounded annually. How much is in the account at the end of the second year?

Solution We substitute 1000 for P, 0.05 for r, and 2 for t in $A = P(1 + r)^t$ and get

$$\begin{aligned} A &= 1000(1 + 0.05)^2 && \text{Substituting} \\ &= 1000(1.05)^2 && \text{Adding terms in parentheses} \\ &= 1000(1.1025) && \text{Squaring} \\ &= \$1102.50. && \text{Multiplying} \end{aligned}$$

There is \$1102.50 in the account after 2 yr. 6 ✓

Quick Check 6 ✓

Business. Repeat Example 6 for an interest rate of 6%.

For interest compounded quarterly (four times per year), we can find a formula like the one above, as illustrated in the following diagram.

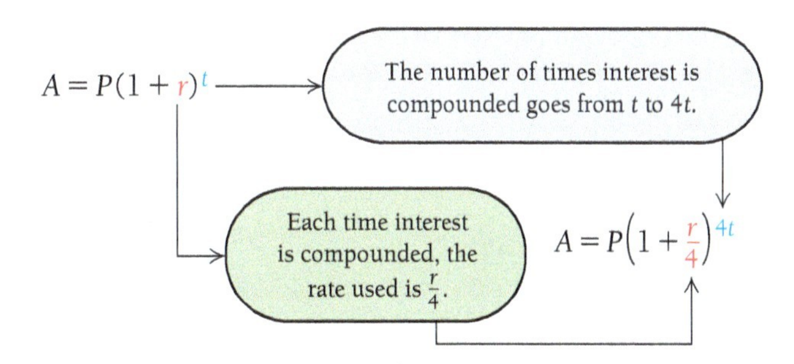

Compounding Frequency	n
Annually	1
Semiannually	2
Quarterly	4
Monthly	12
Daily	365
Hourly	8760

"Compounded quarterly" means that the given interest rate is divided by 4 and compounded four times per year. In general, the following theorem applies.

THEOREM 2

If a principal P is invested at interest rate r, expressed as a decimal, and compounded n times a year, in t years it grows to an amount A given by

$$A = P\left(1 + \frac{r}{n}\right)^{nt}.$$

EXAMPLE 7 **Business: Compound Interest.** Jan invests \$1000 in the Green View Fund at 2.75%, compounded quarterly. How much is in the account at the end of 3 yr?

Solution We use $A = P(1 + r/n)^{nt}$, substituting 1000 for P, 0.0275 for r, 4 for n (compounding quarterly), and 3 for t:

$$\begin{aligned} A &= 1000\left(1 + \frac{0.0275}{4}\right)^{4\cdot 3} && \text{Substituting} \\ &= 1000(1 + 0.006875)^{12} \\ &= 1000(1.006875)^{12} \\ &= 1000(1.085692139) && \text{Using a calculator to approximate } (1.006875)^{12} \\ &= 1085.692139 \\ &\approx \$1085.69. && \text{The symbol} \approx \text{means "approximately equal to."} \end{aligned}$$

There is \$1085.69 in the account after 3 yr. 7 ✓

Quick Check 7 ✓

Business. Repeat Example 7 with a principal of \$25,000 and an interest rate of 3.25%, compounded monthly ($n = 12$), for 5 yr.

A calculator with a y^x or ^ key and a ten-digit display was used to find $(1.006875)^{12}$ in Example 7. The number of places on a calculator may affect the accuracy of the answer. Thus, you may occasionally find that your answers do not agree with those at the back of the text, which were found on a calculator with a ten-digit display. In general, when using a calculator, do all computations and round only at the end, as in Example 7. Usually, your answer will agree to at least four digits. It is a good idea to consult with your instructor about the accuracy required.

Section Summary

- Most graphs can be created by plotting points and looking for patterns. A graphing calculator creates graphs rapidly.
- Mathematical equations can serve as models in a wide variety of applications.
- An example of a mathematical model is the formula for compound interest. If P dollars are invested at interest rate r, compounded n times a year for t years, then the amount A in the account at the end of the t years is given by

$$A = P\left(1 + \frac{r}{n}\right)^{nt}.$$

R.1 Exercise Set

Exercises designated by the symbol ✎ are thinking and writing exercises. They should be answered using one or two English sentences. Because answers to many such exercises will vary, solutions are not given at the back of the book.

In Exercises 1–22, graph each equation. Use a graphing calculator only as a check.

1. $y = x - 1$
2. $y = x + 4$
3. $y = -\frac{1}{4}x$
4. $y = -3x$
5. $y = -\frac{5}{3}x + 3$
6. $y = \frac{2}{3}x - 4$
7. $x + y = 5$
8. $x - y = 4$
9. $6x + 3y = -9$
10. $8y - 2x = 4$
11. $2x + 5y = 10$
12. $5x - 6y = 12$
13. $y = x^2 - 5$
14. $y = x^2 - 3$
15. $x = y^2 + 2$
16. $x = 2 - y^2$
17. $y = 5$
18. $y = -2$
19. $y = 7 - x^2$
20. $y = 5 - x^2$
21. $y - 7 = x^3$
22. $y + 1 = x^3$

APPLICATIONS

23. Medicine. Ibuprofen is a medication used to relieve pain. The model given by

$$A = 0.5t^4 + 3.45t^3 - 96.65t^2 + 347.7t, 0 \leq t \leq 6,$$

can be used to estimate the number of milligrams, A, of ibuprofen in the bloodstream t hours after 400 mg of the medication has been swallowed. (*Source*: Based on data from Dr. P. Carey, Burlington, VT.) How many milligrams of ibuprofen are in the bloodstream 2 hr after 400 mg has been swallowed?

24. Running records. According to at least one study, the world record in any running race can be modeled by a linear equation. In particular, the world record R, in minutes, for the mile run in year x can be modeled by

$$R = -0.006x + 15.714.$$

Use this model to estimate the world records for the mile run in 1954, 2000, and 2025. Round your answers to the nearest hundredth of a minute.

25. Optimum solar panel angle. The optimum angle A, in degrees, to tilt a solar panel to capture the most sunlight is approximated by $A = -0.002x^2 + 0.924x - 0.152$, where x is the location of the panel in degrees latitude north of the equator. (*Source*: Based on data from solarpaneltilt.com.)

a) At what angle should a solar panel tilt in Honolulu (21.3° N)?
b) At what angle should a solar panel tilt in Kansas City (39.1° N)?
c) At what angle should a solar panel tilt in Edmonton (53.5° N)?

26. Rise in sea level. The rise in sea level t years after 1993 can be modeled by $S = -0.00173t^2 + 3.477t + 0.924$, where S is in millimeters. (*Source*: Based on data from climate.nasa.gov.)

a) How much had the sea level risen by 2003?
b) Estimate the rise in sea level in 2020.
c) When will sea level have risen 100 mm over the 1993 level?

27. The graph below shows participation by females in high school athletics from 2007 to 2016.

PARTICIPATION OF FEMALES IN HIGH SCHOOL ATHLETICS

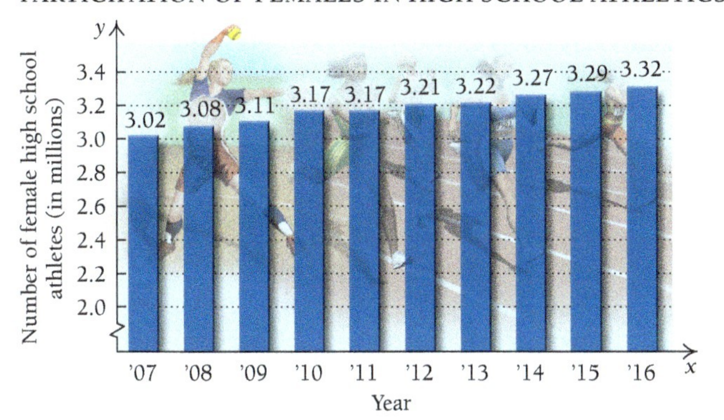

(*Source*: National Federation of State High School Associations.)

a) Use the model $N = 0.0319t + 3.081$, where t is the number of years since 2007 and N is the number of participants, in millions, to predict the number of female high school athletes in 2020.

b) Use the model from part (a) to predict the year in which the number of female high school athletes exceeds 3.6 million.

28. Use the model $N = -0.0011t^2 + 0.0412t + 3.032$, where t is the number of years since 2007 and N is the number, in millions, of female high school athletes (see the graph in Exercise 27).

a) Use this model to predict the number of female high school athletes in 2020. Compare your answer to the number found in part (a) of Exercise 27.

b) Use this model to predict the number of female high school athletes in 2037.

c) Which of the two models better predicts the number of female high school athletes in the future? Why?

29. Snowboarding in the half-pipe. Shaun White, "The Flying Tomato," won a gold medal in the 2010 Winter Olympics for snowboarding in the half-pipe. He soared an unprecedented 25 ft above the edge of the half-pipe (which was still the world record in 2017). His speed $v(t)$, in miles per hour, upon reentering the pipe can be approximated by $v(t) = 10.9t$, where t is the number of seconds for which he was airborne. White was airborne for 2.5 sec. (*Source*: "White Rides to Repeat in Halfpipe, Lago Takes Bronze," Associated Press, 2/18/2010.) How fast was he going when he reentered the half-pipe?

30. Skateboard bomb drop. The distance $s(t)$, in feet, traveled by a body falling freely from rest in t seconds is approximated by

$$s(t) = 16t^2.$$

On April 6, 2006, pro skateboarder Danny Way smashed the world record for the "bomb drop" by free-falling 28 ft from the Fender Stratocaster guitar atop the Hard Rock Hotel & Casino in Las Vegas onto a ramp below (as of 2017 this was still the world record). (*Source*: www.skateboardingmagazine.com.) How long did it take until he hit the ramp?

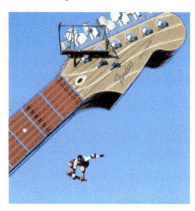

31. Compound interest. Southside Investments purchases a \$100,000 certificate of deposit from Newton Bank, at 2.8%. How much is the investment worth (rounded to the nearest cent) at the end of 1 yr, if interest is compounded:

a) annually? **b)** semiannually?
c) quarterly? **d)** daily?
e) hourly?

32. Compound interest. Greenleaf Investments purchases a \$300,000 certificate of deposit from Descartes Bank, at 2.2%. How much is the investment worth (rounded to the nearest cent) at the end of 1 yr, if interest is compounded:

a) annually? **b)** semiannually?
c) quarterly? **d)** daily?
e) hourly?

33. Compound interest. Stateside Brokers deposit \$30,000 in Godel Municipal Bond Funds, at 4%. How much is the investment worth (rounded to the nearest cent) at the end of 3 yr, if interest is compounded:

a) annually? **b)** semiannually?
c) quarterly? **d)** daily?
e) hourly?

34. Compound interest. The Kims deposit \$1000 in Wiles Municipal Bond Funds, at 5%. How much is the investment worth (rounded to the nearest cent) at the end of 4 yr, if interest is compounded:

a) annually? **b)** semiannually?
c) quarterly? **d)** daily?
e) hourly?

Determining monthly loan payments. *If P dollars are borrowed at an annual interest rate r, expressed as a decimal, the payment M made each month for a total of n months is*

$$M = P\frac{\frac{r}{12}\left(1 + \frac{r}{12}\right)^n}{\left(1 + \frac{r}{12}\right)^n - 1}.$$

35. Fermat's Last Bank makes a car loan of \$18,000, at 4.6% interest and with a loan period of 3 yr. What is the monthly payment?

36. At Haken Bank, Ken Appel takes out a \$100,000 mortgage at an interest rate of 2.4% for a loan period of 30 yr. What is the monthly payment?

Annuities. *If P dollars are invested annually in an annuity (investment fund), after n years, the annuity is worth*

$$W = P\left[\frac{(1 + r)^n - 1}{r}\right],$$

where r is the interest rate, expressed as a decimal and compounded annually.

37. Kate invests \$3000 annually in an annuity from Mersenne Fund that earns 3.05% interest. How much is the investment worth after 18 yr? Round to the nearest cent.

38. Paulo establishes an annuity that earns $4\frac{1}{4}\%$ interest and wants it to be worth \$50,000 in 20 yr. How much will he need to invest annually to achieve this goal?

39. Unemployment rate. The unemployment rate in the United States from 2006 to 2016 is shown in the graph below.

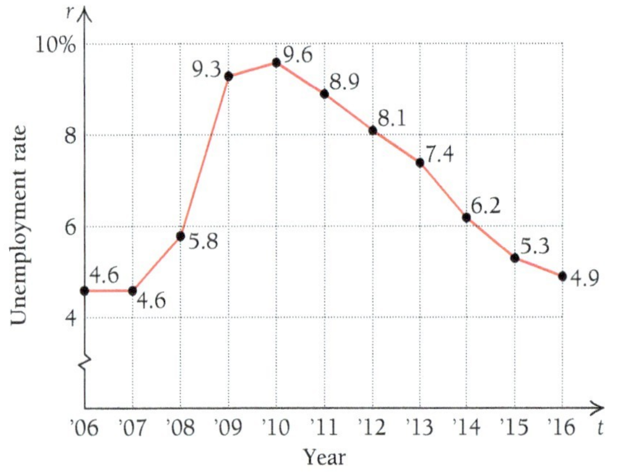

(*Source*: Bureau of Labor Statistics.)

a) In what years was the unemployment rate at or above 5.8%?

b) In what years was the unemployment rate below 7%?

c) When was unemployment highest? What was the rate?

d) When was unemployment lowest? What was the rate?

40. Assuming that U.S. unemployment follows the trend shown between 2010 and 2016 (see Exercise 39), estimate the unemployment rate in 2019. Would you use this same trend to estimate the unemployment rate in 2025? Why or why not?

SYNTHESIS

Retirement account. *Sally makes deposits into a retirement account every year from age 30 until she retires at age 65.*

41. a) If Sally deposits \$1200 per year and the account earns interest at a rate of 4% per year, compounded annually, how much will she have in the account when she retires? (*Hint*: Use the annuity formula given for Exercises 37 and 38.)

b) How much of that total amount is from Sally's deposits? How much is interest?

42. a) Sally plans to take regular monthly distributions from her retirement account from the time she retires until she is 80 years old, when the account will have a value of \$0. How much should she take each month? Assume an interest rate of 4% per year, compounded monthly. (*Hint*: Use the formula given for Exercises 35 and 36 that calculates the monthly payments on a loan.)

b) What is the total of the payments Sally will receive? How much of the total will be her own money (see part b of Exercise 41), and how much will be interest?

Annual yield. *The annual interest rate r, when compounded more than once a year, results in a slightly higher yearly interest rate; this is called the* annual (or effective) yield *and denoted as Y. For example, \$1000 deposited at 5%, compounded monthly for 1 yr (12 months), will have a value given by* $A = 1000(1 + \frac{0.05}{12})^{12} = \$1051.16$. *The interest earned is \$51.16/\$1000, or 0.05116, which is 5.116% of the original deposit. Thus, we say that this account has a yield of* $Y = 0.05116$, *or 5.116%. The formula for annual yield depends on the annual interest rate r and the compounding frequency n:*

$$Y = \left(1 + \frac{r}{n}\right)^n - 1.$$

For Exercises 43–46, find the annual yield as a percentage, to two decimal places, given the annual interest rate and the compounding frequency.

43. Annual interest rate of 5.3%, compounded monthly

44. Annual interest rate of 4.1%, compounded quarterly

45. Annual interest rate of 3.75%, compounded weekly

46. Annual interest rate of 4%, compounded daily

47. Lena is considering two savings accounts: Western Bank offers 2.5%, compounded annually, on savings accounts, while Commonwealth Savings offers 2.43%, compounded monthly.

a) Find the annual yield for both accounts.

b) Which account has the higher annual yield?

48. Chris is considering two savings accounts: Sierra Savings offers 3%, compounded annually, on savings accounts, while Foothill Bank offers 2.97%, compounded weekly.

a) Find the annual yield for both accounts.

b) Which account has the higher annual yield?

49. Stockman's Bank will pay 2.2%, compounded annually, on a savings account. A competitor, Mesalands Savings, offers monthly compounding on savings accounts. What is the minimum annual interest rate that Mesalands needs to pay to make its annual yield exceed that of Stockman's?

50. Belltown Bank offers a certificate of deposit at 3.75%, compounded annually. Shea Savings offers savings accounts with interest compounded quarterly. What is the minimum annual interest rate that Shea needs to pay to make its annual yield exceed that of Belltown?

Technology Connection 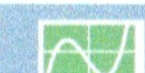

The Technology Connection heading indicates exercises that provide practice using a graphing calculator.

51. Graph $y = x^3 - x^2$ in the standard window, then in the window $[-2, 2, -2, 2]$. Which window shows better detail? Why?

52. Graph $y = 2^x$ in the standard window. Does the graph actually touch the x-axis? Why or why not?

Answers to Quick Checks

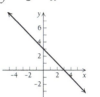

1. $y = 3 - x$

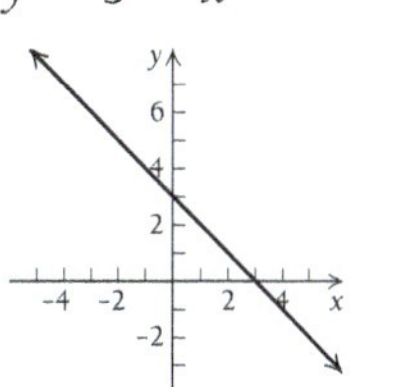

2. $3x - 5y = 10$

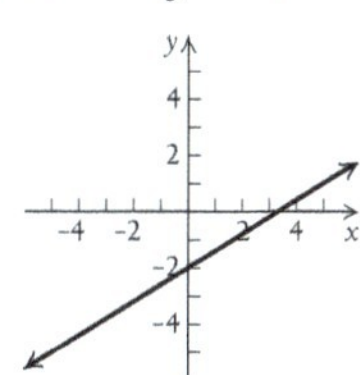

3. $y = 2 - x^2$

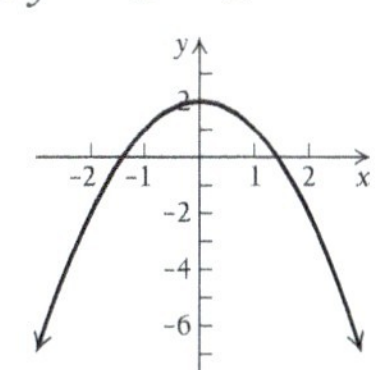

4. $x = 1 + y^2$

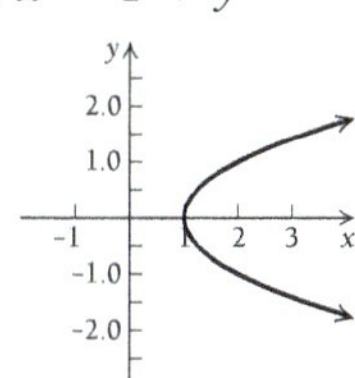

5. In 2022 **6.** There is $1123.60 in the account after 2 yr. **7.** There is $29,404.75 in the account after 5 yr.

R.2

- Determine whether a correspondence is a function.
- Find function values.
- Graph functions and determine whether a graph represents a function.
- Graph functions that are piecewise-defined.

Functions and Models

Identifying Functions

A function is a special kind of correspondence between two sets that is a fundamental concept in mathematics. Consider the following situations:

- For each weekday, there corresponds the closing value of the Dow Jones Industrial Average.
- For each student at a university, there corresponds the student's identification number.
- For each letter on a phone's keypad, there corresponds a number.
- For each real number x, there corresponds that number's square, x^2.

In each of these examples, the first set is called the *domain* and the second set is called the *range*. For any member of the domain, there is *exactly one* member of the range to which it corresponds (is matched). This type of correspondence is called a *function*.

Correspondence

Domain Range

DEFINITION

A **function** is a correspondence between a first set, called the **domain**, and a second set, called the **range**, such that each member of the domain corresponds to *exactly one* member of the range.

Each correspondence in the list on the preceding page is a function. On a phone's keypad, each of the 26 letters corresponds to exactly one number. For example, the letter H corresponds to the number 4. However, the reverse situation is not a function. The number 4 does not correspond to exactly one letter, since it corresponds to *three* letters: G, H, and I.

EXAMPLE 1 Determine whether or not each correspondence is a function.

a) *Number of iPhones sold yearly (in millions)*

Domain		Range
2014	→	169.2
2015	→	231.7
2016	→	211.9
2017	→	216.8

(*Source:* Apple Inc.)

b) *Squaring*

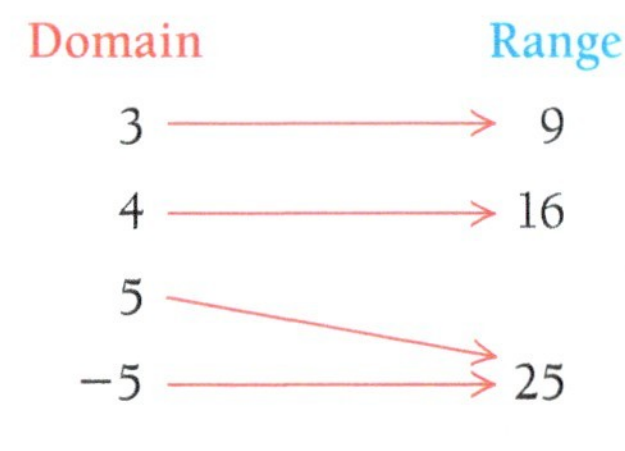

c) *Basketball teams*

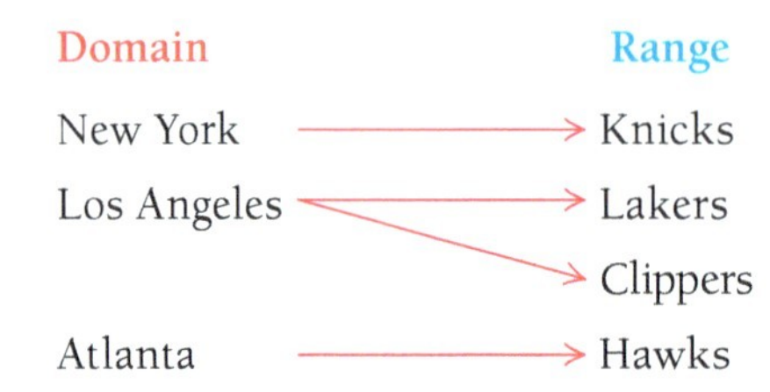

Solution

a) The correspondence *is* a function because each member of the domain corresponds to only one member of the range.

b) The correspondence *is* a function because each member of the domain corresponds to only one member of the range, even though two members of the domain correspond to 25.

c) The correspondence is *not* a function because one member of the domain, Los Angeles, corresponds to two members of the range, Lakers and Clippers.

EXAMPLE 2 Determine whether or not each correspondence is a function.

	Domain	Correspondence	Range
a)	A group of people in an elevator	Each person's weight	A set of positive numbers
b)	The integers $\{\ldots, -3, -2, -1, 0, 1, 2, 3, \ldots\}$	Each number's square	A set of nonnegative integers: $\{0, 1, 4, 9, 16, 25, \ldots\}$
c)	The set of all states	Each state's U.S. Senators	The set of all 100 U.S. Senators

Solution

a) The correspondence is a function because each person has *only one* weight.

b) The correspondence is a function because each integer has *only one* square.

c) The correspondence is *not* a function because each state has *two* U.S. Senators.

1 ✓

Quick Check 1 ✓

Determine whether or not each correspondence is a function.

a) The domain is the books in a library, the range is the set of positive integers, and the correspondence is the page count of each book.

b) The domain is the letters of the alphabet, the range is the set of all Americans, and the correspondence is the first letter of a person's last name.

Consistent with the definition on p. 13, we can regard a function as a set of ordered pairs, such that no two pairs have the same first coordinate paired with different second coordinates. When a function is written as a set of ordered pairs, the domain is the set of all first coordinates, and the range is the set of all second coordinates. Function names are usually represented by lowercase letters. Thus, if f represents the function in Example 2(b), we have

$$f = \{\ldots, (-3, 9), (-2, 4), (-1, 1), (0, 0), (1, 1), (2, 4), (3, 9), \ldots\},$$

and

$$\text{domain of } f = \{\ldots, -3, -2, -1, 0, 1, 2, 3, \ldots\}; \quad \text{range of } f = \{0, 1, 4, 9, \ldots\}.$$

Finding Function Values

Functions can be described by equations such as $y = 2x + 3$ and $y = 4 - x^2$. To graph the function given by $y = 2x + 3$, we find ordered pairs by performing calculations for selected x values:

for $x = 4$, $y = 2 \cdot 4 + 3 = 11$; The graph includes (4, 11).

for $x = -5$, $y = 2 \cdot (-5) + 3 = -7$; The graph includes $(-5, -7)$.

for $x = 0$, $y = 2 \cdot 0 + 3 = 3$; and so on. The graph includes (0, 3).

The **inputs** (members of the domain) are the values of x substituted into the equation. The **outputs** (members of the range) are the resulting values of y. If we call the function f, we can use x to represent an arbitrary input and $f(x)$, read "f of x" or "f at x" or "the value of f at x," to represent the corresponding output. In this notation, the function given by $y = 2x + 3$ is written as $f(x) = 2x + 3$, and the calculations above can be written more concisely as

$$f(4) = 2 \cdot 4 + 3 = 11;$$

$$f(-5) = 2 \cdot (-5) + 3 = -7;$$

$$f(0) = 2 \cdot 0 + 3 = 3; \text{ and so on.}$$

Thus, instead of writing "when $x = 4$, the value of y is 11," we can simply write "$f(4) = 11$," which is most commonly read as "f of 4 is 11." Note that $f(4)$ *does not mean* "f times 4."

It helps to think of a function as a machine. Think of $f(4) = 11$ as the result of putting a member of the domain (an input), 4, into the machine. The machine knows the correspondence $f(x) = 2x + 3$, computes $2 \cdot 4 + 3$, and produces a member of the range (the output), 11.

Function: $f(x) = 2x + 3$

Input	Output
4	11
-5	-7
0	3
t	$2t + 3$
$a + h$	$2(a + h) + 3$

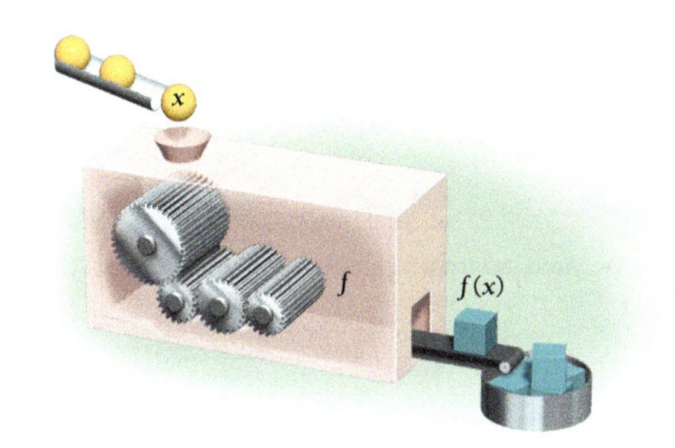

EXAMPLE 3 The squaring function f is given by $f(x) = x^2$. Find $f(-3), f(1), f(k)$, $f(\sqrt{k})$, and $f(x + h)$.

Solution We have

$$f(-3) = (-3)^2 = 9;$$
$$f(1) = 1^2 = 1;$$
$$f(k) = k^2 = k^2;$$
$$f(\sqrt{k}) = (\sqrt{k})^2 = k;$$
$$f(x + h) = (x + h)^2 = x^2 + 2xh + h^2.$$

For a review of algebra, see Appendix A .

To find $f(x + h)$, remember what the function does: It squares the input. Thus, $f(x + h) = (x + h)^2 = x^2 + 2xh + h^2$. This amounts to replacing x on both sides of $f(x) = x^2$ with $x + h$. **2 ✓**

Quick Check 2 ✓

A function f is given by $f(x) = 3x + 5$. Find $f(4), f(-5), f(0)$, and $f(x + h)$.

EXAMPLE 4 A function g is given by $g(x) = 3x^2 - 2x + 8$. Find $g(0), g(-5)$, and $g(7a)$.

Solution One way to find function values when a formula is given is to think of the formula with blanks, or placeholders, as follows:

$$g(\quad) = 3 \cdot \quad^2 - 2 \cdot \quad + 8.$$

To find an output for a given input, we think: "Whatever goes in the blank on the left goes in the blank(s) on the right."

$$g(0) = 3 \cdot 0^2 - 2 \cdot 0 + 8 = 8$$
$$g(-5) = 3(-5)^2 - 2 \cdot (-5) + 8 = 3 \cdot 25 + 10 + 8 = 75 + 10 + 8 = 93$$
$$g(7a) = 3(7a)^2 - 2(7a) + 8 = 3 \cdot 49a^2 - 14a + 8 = 147a^2 - 14a + 8$$

3 ✓

Quick Check 3 ✓

A function h is given by $h(x) = 3x^2 + 2x - 7$. Find $h(4), h(-5), h(0), h(a)$, and $h(5a)$.

Technology Connection

The TABLE Feature

The TABLE feature is one way to find ordered pairs of inputs and outputs of functions. Consider the function given by $f(x) = x^3 - 5x + 1$, entered as $y_1 = x^3 - 5x + 1$. To use the TABLE feature, we access the TABLE SETUP screen and enter the x-value at which the table will start and an increment for the x-value. For this equation, we let TblStart = 0.3 and ΔTbl = 1. This means that the table's x-values will start at 0.3 and increase by 1.

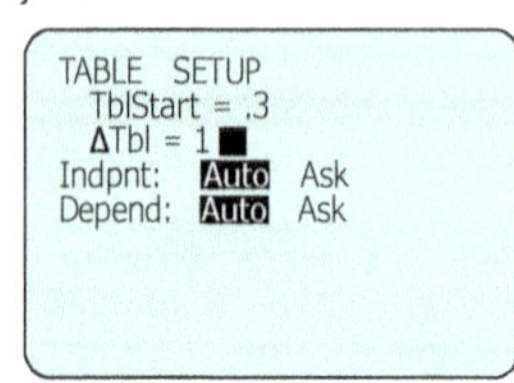

We next set Indpnt and Depend to Auto and then press TABLE. The result is shown below.

X	Y1
.3	−.473
1.3	−3.303
2.3	1.667
3.3	20.437
4.3	59.007
5.3	123.38
6.3	219.55

X = .3

The arrow keys, ⌃ and ⌄, allow us to scroll up and down to view other values.

X	Y1
12.3	1800.4
13.3	2287.1
14.3	2853.7
15.3	3506.1
16.3	4250.2
17.3	5092.2
18.3	6038

X = 18.3

If we set Indpnt to Ask, leave Depend set to Auto, and press TABLE, we can enter any value for x.

EXERCISES

Use the function given by $f(x) = x^3 - 5x + 1$ for Exercises 1 and 2.

1. Use the TABLE feature to construct a table starting with $x = 10$ and ΔTbl = 5. Find the value of y when x is 10. Then find the value of y when x is 35.
2. Adjust the table settings to Indpnt: Ask. How does the table change? Enter a number of your choice and see what happens. Use this setting to find the value of y when x is 28.

EXAMPLE 5 A function f subtracts the square of an input from the input:

$$f(x) = x - x^2.$$

Find $f(4), f(x+h)$, and $\frac{f(x+h) - f(x)}{h}$. Simplify your results.

Solution We have

$$f(4) = 4 - 4^2 = 4 - 16 = -12;$$

and
$$\begin{aligned} f(x+h) &= (x+h) - (x+h)^2 \\ &= x + h - (x^2 + 2xh + h^2) \quad \text{Squaring the binomial} \\ &= x + h - x^2 - 2xh - h^2. \end{aligned}$$

For the expression $\frac{f(x+h) - f(x)}{h}$, we have

$$\begin{aligned} \frac{f(x+h) - f(x)}{h} &= \frac{\overbrace{x + h - x^2 - 2xh - h^2}^{f(x+h),\text{ found above}} - \overbrace{(x - x^2)}^{f(x)}}{h} \\ &= \frac{h - 2xh - h^2}{h} \quad \text{Simplifying} \\ &= \frac{h(1 - 2x - h)}{h} \quad \text{Factoring} \\ &= 1 - 2x - h, \quad \text{for } h \neq 0. \end{aligned}$$

4 ✓

Quick Check 4 ✓

A function f is given by $f(x) = 2x - x^2$. Find $f(4), f(x+h)$, and $\frac{f(x+h) - f(x)}{h}$. Simplify your results.

Graphs of Functions

Consider again the function given by $f(x) = x^2$. The input 3 is associated with the output 9. The input–output pair (3, 9) is one point on the *graph* of this function.

DEFINITION

The **graph** of a function f is a drawing that represents all the input–output pairs, $(x, f(x))$. When the function is given by an equation, the graph of the function is the graph of the equation, $y = f(x)$.

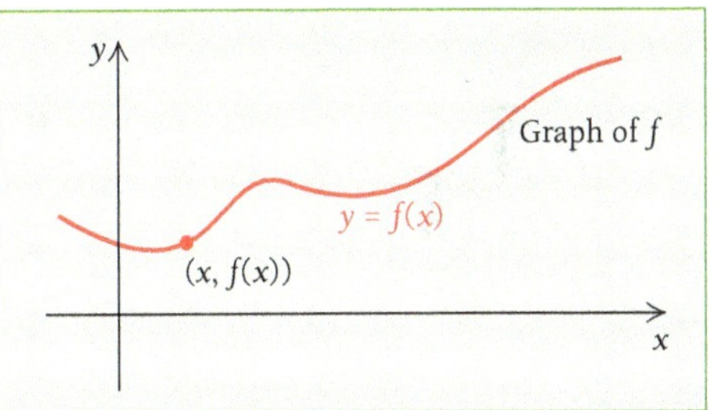

It is customary to locate input values (the domain) on the horizontal axis and output values (the range) on the vertical axis.

EXAMPLE 6 Graph: $f(x) = x^2 + 1$.

Solution

x	$f(x)$	$(x, f(x))$
-2	5	$(-2, 5)$
-1	2	$(-1, 2)$
0	1	$(0, 1)$
1	2	$(1, 2)$
2	5	$(2, 5)$

(1) Choose any x.
(2) Compute y.
(3) Form the pair (x, y).
(4) Plot the points.

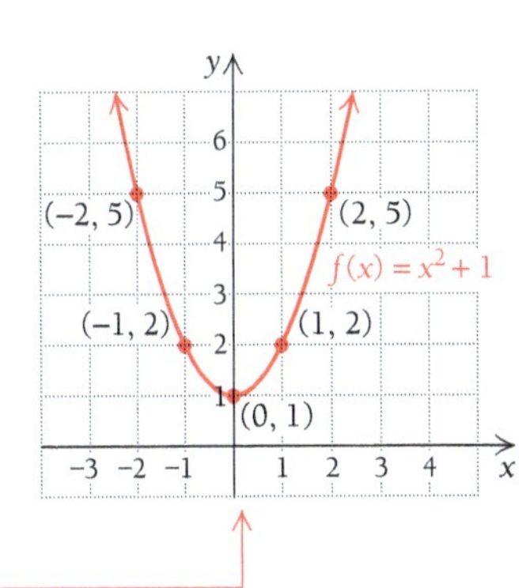

Quick Check 5 ✓

Graph: $f(x) = 2 - x^2$.

We plot the input–output pairs from the table and, in this case, draw a curve to complete the graph.

5 ✓

The Vertical-Line Test

Let's now determine how to look at a graph and decide whether it represents a function. In the graph at the right, note that x_1 has *two* outputs. Since a function must have exactly *one* output for every input, this graph cannot represent a function. The fact that a vertical line can intersect the graph in more than one place demonstrates that the graph does not represent a function.

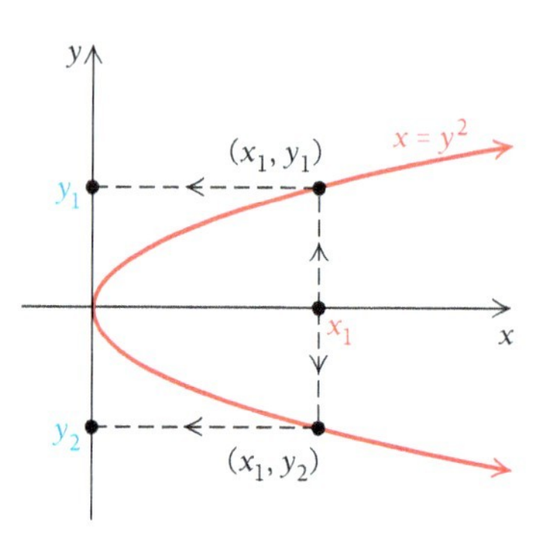

> **The Vertical-Line Test**
>
> A graph represents a function if it is impossible to draw a vertical line that intersects the graph more than once.

Equivalently, if a vertical line intersects a graph more than once, then the graph does not represent a function.

EXAMPLE 7 Determine whether each of the following is the graph of a function.

a)

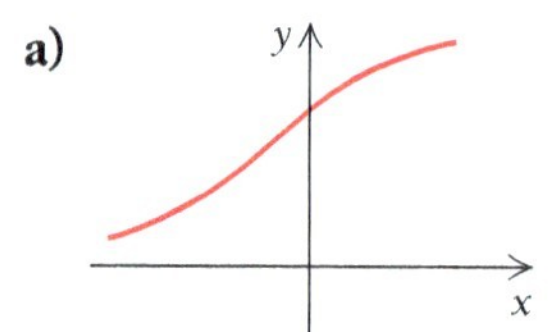

b)

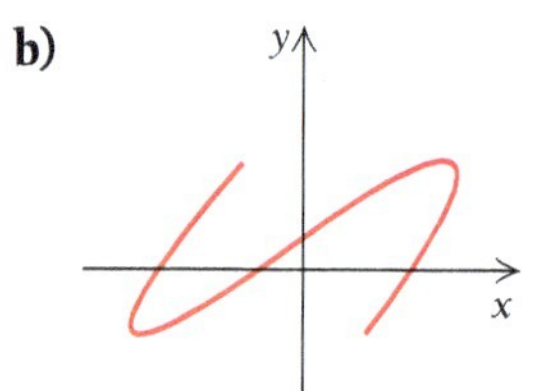

c)

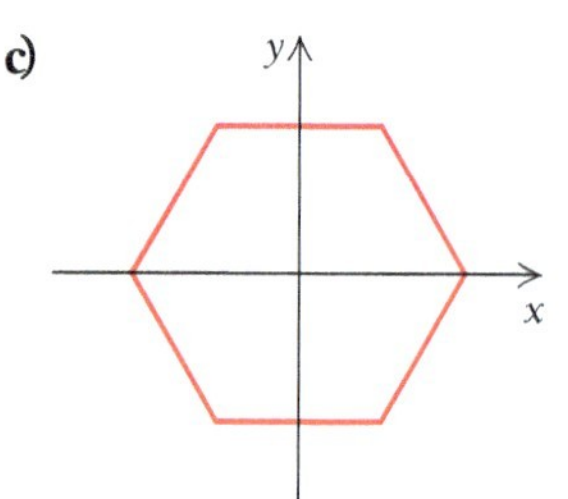

d)

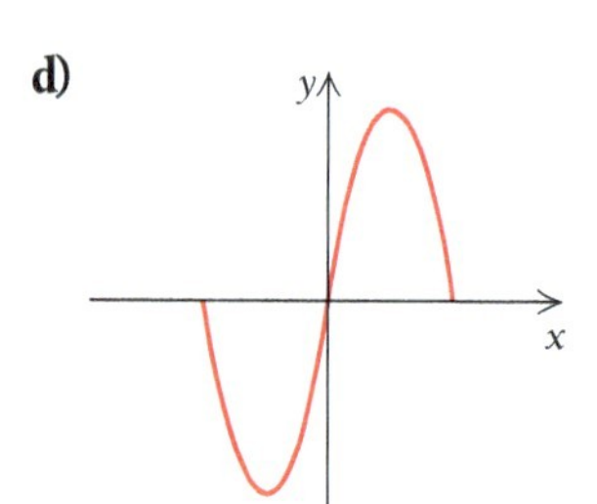

e)

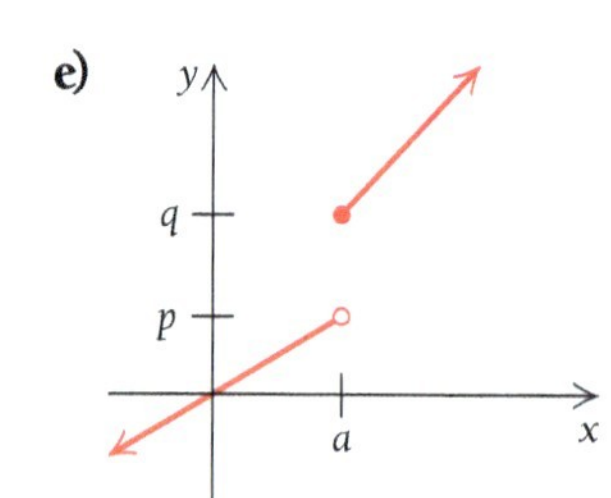

f)

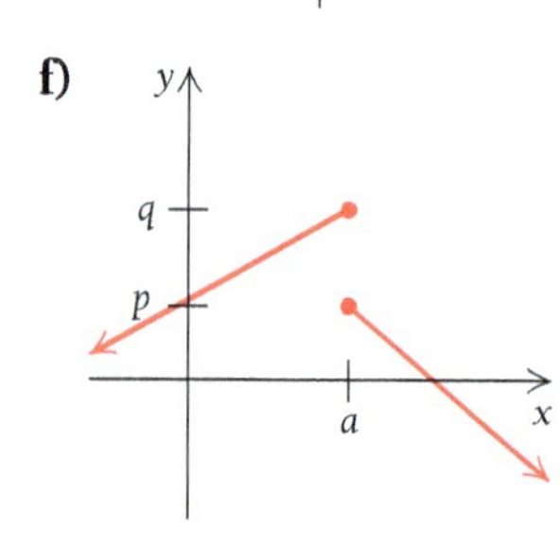

Quick Check 6 ✓

Determine whether each of the following is the graph of a function.

a)

b)

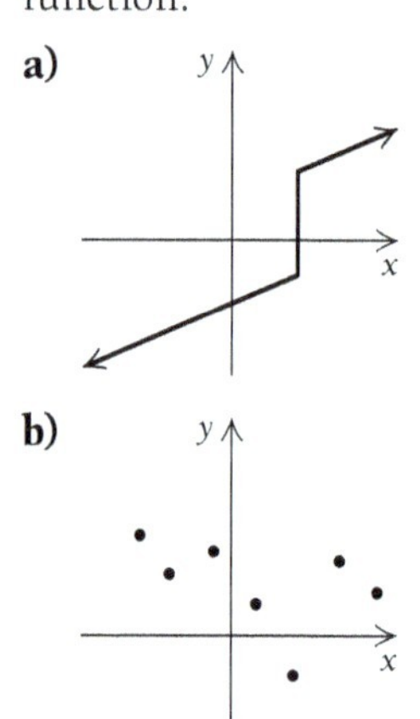

Solution

a) The graph is that of a function. Any vertical line that is drawn will intersect the graph no more than once.

b) The graph is not that of a function. Some vertical lines will intersect the graph more than once.

c) The graph is not that of a function.

d) The graph is that of a function.

e) The graph is that of a function. Note that a vertical line at $x = a$ will intersect the graph once.

f) The graph is not that of a function. Note that a vertical line at $x = a$ will intersect the graph more than once.

In parts (e) and (f), an open dot represents an ordered pair that is not part of the graph, and a solid dot represents an ordered pair that is part of the graph. Thus, in part (e), the ordered pair (a, p) is not part of the graph, but the ordered pair (a, q) is. 6 ✓

Functions Defined Piecewise

Some functions are defined *piecewise*, using different output formulas for different parts of the domain, as in parts (e) and (f) of Example 7. To graph a piecewise-defined function, we use the correspondence specified for each part of the domain.

EXAMPLE 8 Graph the function defined as follows:

$$f(x) = \begin{cases} 4, & \text{for } x \le 0, \\ 3 - x^2, & \text{for } 0 < x \le 2, \\ 2x - 6, & \text{for } x > 2. \end{cases}$$

This means that for any input x less than or equal to 0, the output is 4.

This means that for any input x greater than 0 and less than or equal to 2, the output is $3 - x^2$.

This means that for any input x greater than 2, the output is $2x - 6$.

Solution Working from left to right, note that for all x-values less than or equal to 0, the graph is the horizontal line $y = 4$. For example,

$$f(-2) = 4;$$
$$f(-1) = 4;$$
and $$f(0) = 4.$$

The solid dot at (0, 4) indicates that (0, 4) is part of the graph.

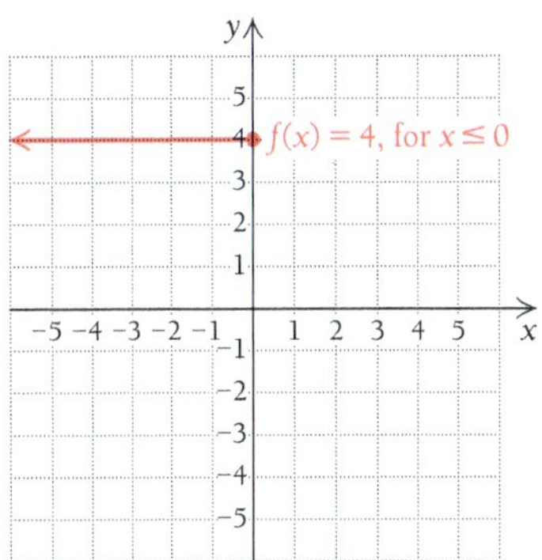

Next, observe that for x-values greater than 0 but not greater than 2, the graph is a portion of the parabola given by $y = 3 - x^2$. Note that for $f(x) = 3 - x^2$,

$$f(0.5) = 3 - 0.5^2 = 2.75;$$
$$f(1) = 2;$$
and $$f(2) = -1.$$

The open dot at (0, 3) indicates that this point is *not* part of the graph.

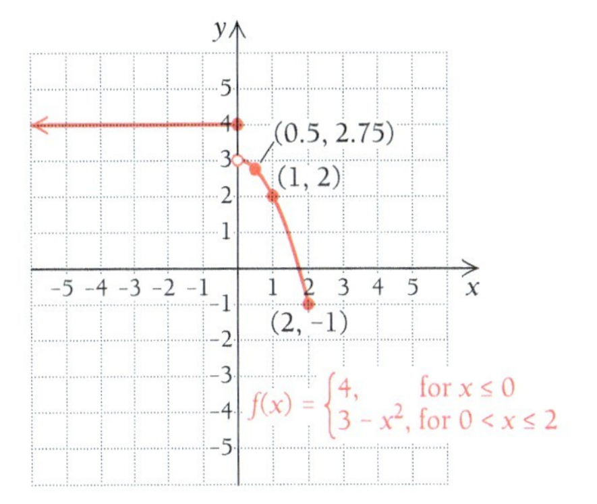

Finally, note that for x-values greater than 2, the graph is the line $y = 2x - 6$.

$$f(2.5) = 2 \cdot 2.5 - 6 = -1;$$
$$f(4) = 2;$$
and $$f(5) = 4.$$

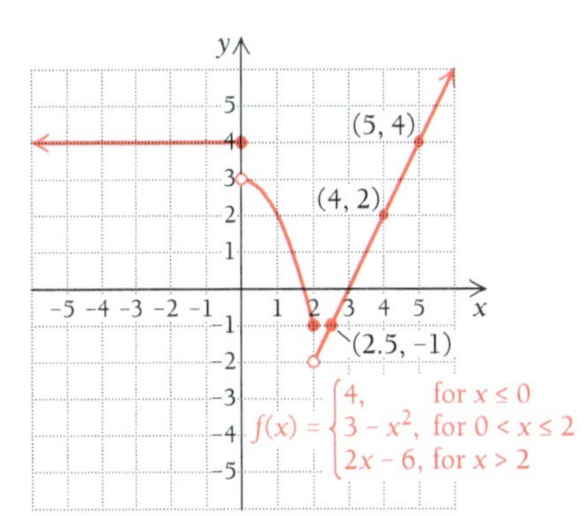

7 ✓

Quick Check 7 ✓

Graph the function defined as follows:

$$f(x) = \begin{cases} 4, & \text{for } x \le 0, \\ 4 - x^2, & \text{for } 0 < x \le 2, \\ 2x - 6, & \text{for } x > 2. \end{cases}$$

EXAMPLE 9 Graph the function defined as follows:

$$g(x) = \begin{cases} 3, & \text{for } x = 1, \\ -x + 2, & \text{for } x \neq 1. \end{cases}$$

Solution The function is defined such that $g(1) = 3$ and for all other x-values (that is, for $x \neq 1$), we have $g(x) = -x + 2$. Thus, to graph this function, we graph the line given by $y = -x + 2$, but with an open dot at the point corresponding to $x = 1$. To complete the graph, we plot the point $(1, 3)$ since $g(1) = 3$.

x	$g(x)$	$(x, g(x))$
-3	$-(-3) + 2$	$(-3, 5)$
0	$-0 + 2$	$(0, 2)$
1	3	$(1, 3)$
2	$-2 + 2$	$(2, 0)$
3	$-3 + 2$	$(3, -1)$

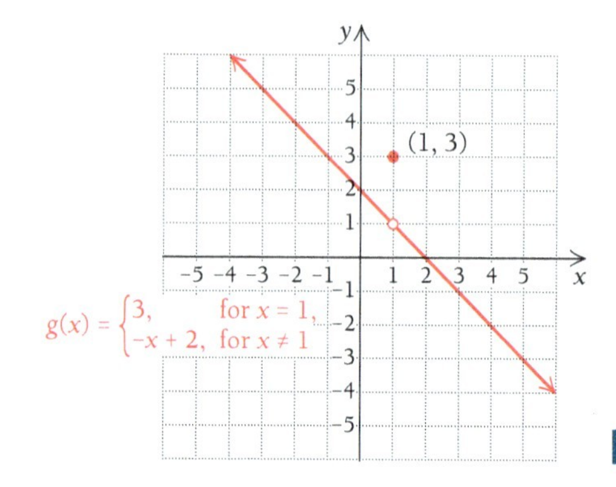

8 ✓

Quick Check 8 ✓

Graph the function defined as follows:

$$f(x) = \begin{cases} 1, & \text{for } x = -2, \\ 2 - x, & \text{for } x \neq -2. \end{cases}$$

Some Final Remarks

We sometimes use the terminology *y is a function of x*. This means that x is an input and y is an output. It also means that x is the **independent variable** because it represents inputs and y is the **dependent variable** because it represents outputs. We may refer to "a function $y = x^2$" without naming it using a letter f.

Section Summary

- A *function* is a correspondence between two sets such that for each member of the first set (the *domain*), there corresponds exactly one member of the second set (the *range*).
- A function's domain represents *inputs*, and its range represents *outputs*.
- A function given as an equation can be written using function notation: $y = f(x)$, where f is the name of the function. Ordered pairs are of the form $(x, f(x))$.

R.2 Exercise Set

Note: A review of algebra can be found in Appendix A.

Determine whether each correspondence is a function.

1.

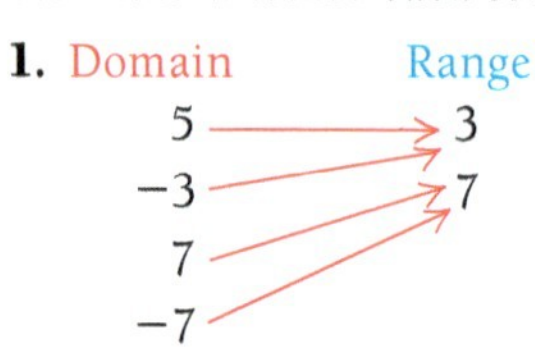

2.

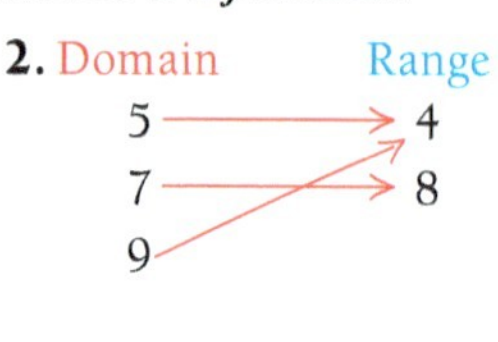

3.

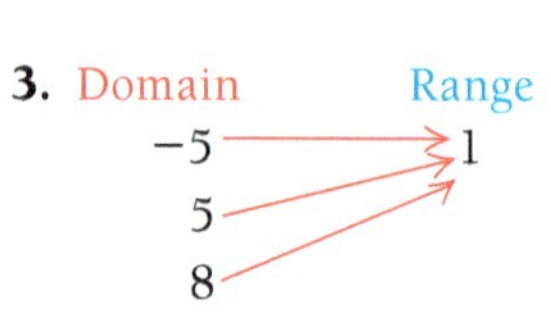

4.

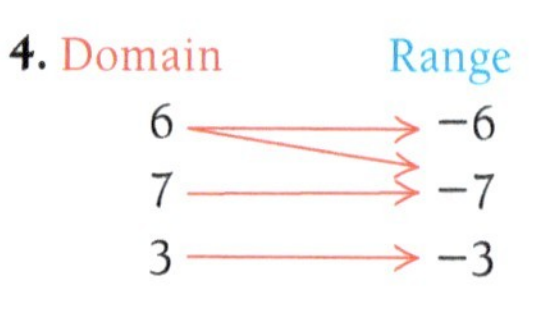

5. Sandwich prices.

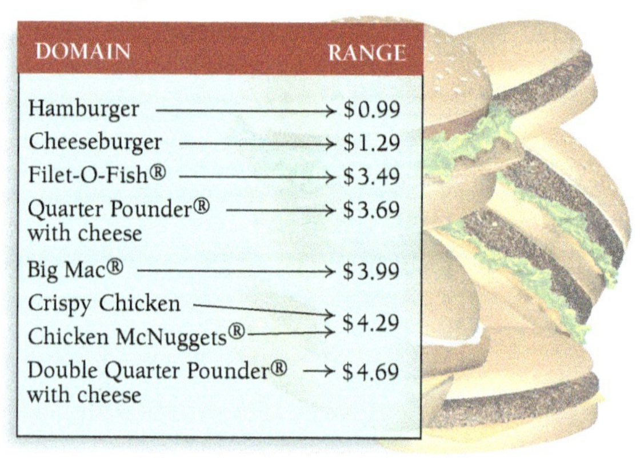

DOMAIN	RANGE
Hamburger	$0.99
Cheeseburger	$1.29
Filet-O-Fish®	$3.49
Quarter Pounder® with cheese	$3.69
Big Mac®	$3.99
Crispy Chicken	$4.29
Chicken McNuggets®	$4.29
Double Quarter Pounder® with cheese	$4.69

(*Source*: www.mcdonalds.com.)

6. **Sandwich calorie content.**

DOMAIN	RANGE
Hamburger	→ 250
Cheeseburger	→ 300
Quarter Pounder®	→ 410
Double Cheeseburger®	→ 440
Filet-O-Fish®	→ 380
Big Mac®	→ 540
Double Quarter Pounder® with cheese	→ 740

(*Source*: www.mcdonalds.com.)

Determine whether each of the following is a function.

	Domain	Correspondence	Range
7.	A set of numbers	A number doubled	A set of numbers
8.	A set of numbers	Two less than the number	A set of numbers
9.	A set of positive numbers	The square root of a number	A set of positive numbers
10.	A set of numbers	The cube root of a number	A set of numbers
11.	A set of positive numbers	Positive integers that are less than or equal to a number	A set of numbers
12.	A set of numbers	Odd integers that are less than or equal to a number	A set of numbers
13.	A set of books in a bookstore	A book's Library of Congress Catalog Number	A set of numeric codes
14.	A set of books in a bookstore	A book's ISBN	A set of numeric codes
15.	A set of people	A person's birthdate	A set of numerical codes of the form mm/dd/yyyy
16.	A set of people	A person's weight	A set of numbers
17.	A set of numerical codes of the form mm/dd/yyyy	A person's birthdate	A set of people
18.	A set of numbers	A person's weight	A set of people
19.	A set of rectangles	A rectangle's area	A set of numbers
20.	A set of rectangles	A rectangle's perimeter	A set of numbers
21.	A set of numbers	A rectangle with that area	A set of rectangles
22.	A set of numbers	A rectangle with that perimeter	A set of rectangles

23. A function f is given by

$$f(x) = 4x - 3.$$

This function takes a number x, multiplies it by 4, and subtracts 3.

a) Complete this table.

x	5.1	5.01	5.001	5
$f(x)$				

b) Find $f(4), f(3), f(-2), f(k)$, and $f(x + h)$.

24. A function f is given by

$$f(x) = 3x + 2.$$

This function takes a number x, multiplies it by 3, and adds 2.

a) Complete this table.

x	4.1	4.01	4.001	4
$f(x)$				

b) Find $f(5), f(-1), f(k)$, and $f(x + h)$.

25. A function g is given by

$$g(x) = x^2 - 3.$$

Find $g(-1), g(0), g(1), g(5), g(a + h)$, and

$$\frac{g(x + h) - g(x)}{h}.$$

26. A function g is given by

$$g(x) = x^2 + 4.$$

Find $g(-3), g(0), g(-1), g(7), g(a + h)$, and

$$\frac{g(x + h) - g(x)}{h}.$$

27. A function f is given by

$$f(x) = \frac{1}{(x + 3)^2}.$$

Find $f(4), f(0), f(a), f(x + h)$, and

$$\frac{f(x + h) - f(x)}{h}.$$

28. A function f is given by

$$f(x) = \frac{1}{(x - 5)^2}.$$

This function takes a number x, subtracts 5 from it, squares the result, and takes the reciprocal of the square. Find $f(3), f(-1), f(k)$, and $f(x + h)$.

29. A function f takes a number x, multiplies it by 4, and adds 2.

a) Write f as an equation. **b)** Graph f.

30. A function g takes a number x, multiplies it by -3, and subtracts 4.

a) Write g as an equation. **b)** Graph g.

31. A function h takes a number x, squares it, and adds x.

a) Write h as an equation.
b) Graph h.

32. A function k takes a number x, squares it, and subtracts 3 times x.

a) Write k as an equation.
b) Graph k.

Graph each function.

33. $f(x) = 2x - 5$
34. $f(x) = 3x - 1$
35. $g(x) = -4x$
36. $g(x) = -2x$
37. $f(x) = x^2 - 2$
38. $f(x) = x^2 + 4$
39. $f(x) = 6 - x^2$
40. $g(x) = -x^2 + 1$
41. $g(x) = x^3$
42. $g(x) = \frac{1}{2}x^3$

Use the vertical-line test to determine whether each graph is that of a function. (In Exercises 51–55, the dashed lines are not part of the graphs.)

43.

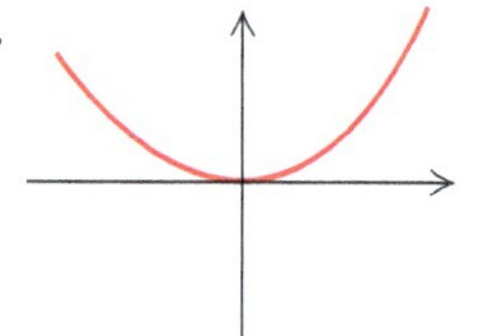

44.

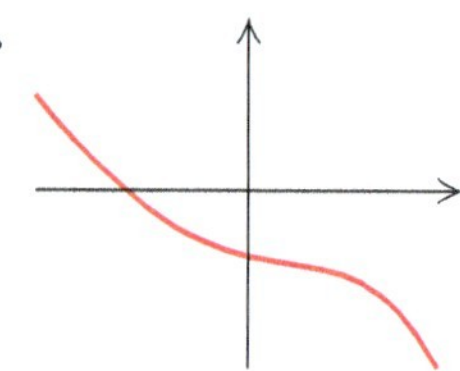

45.

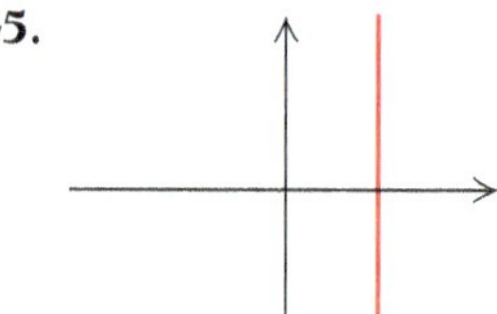

46.

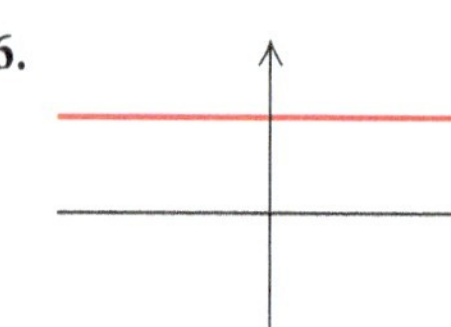

47.

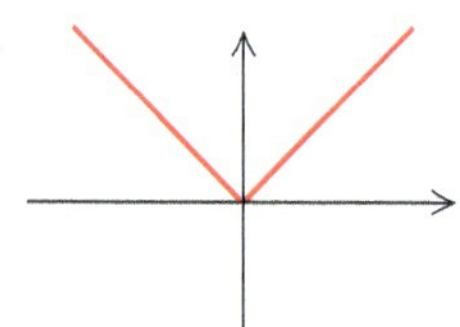

48.

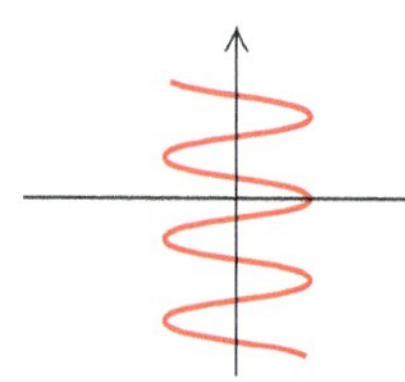

49.

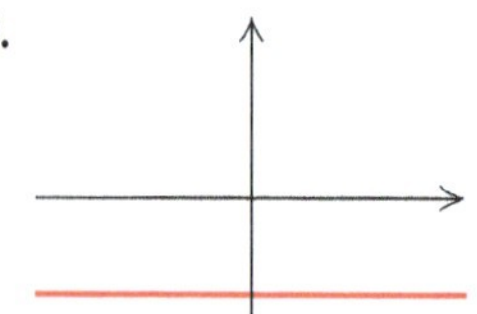

50.

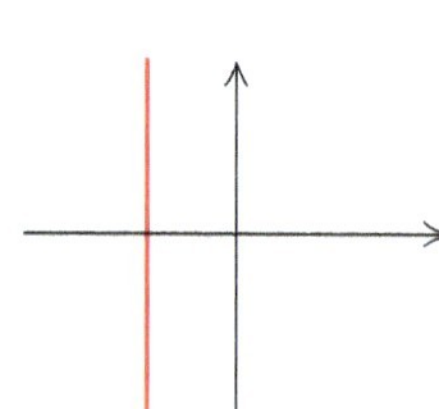

51.

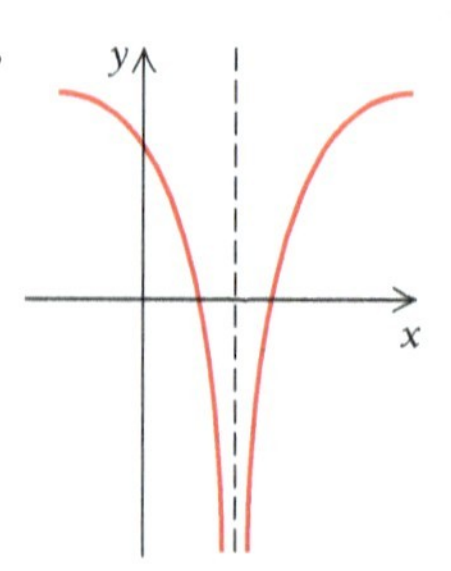

52.

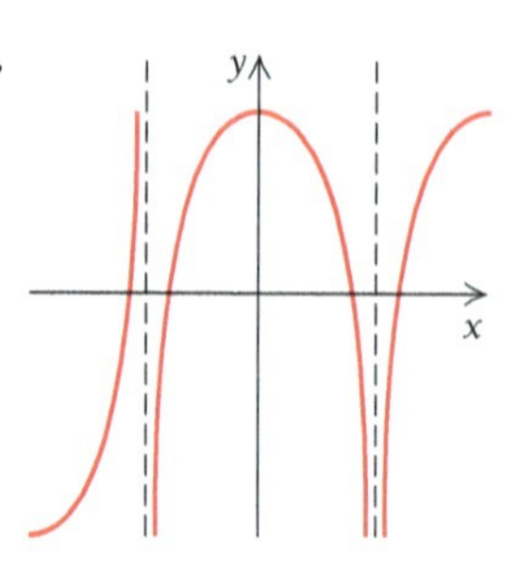

53.

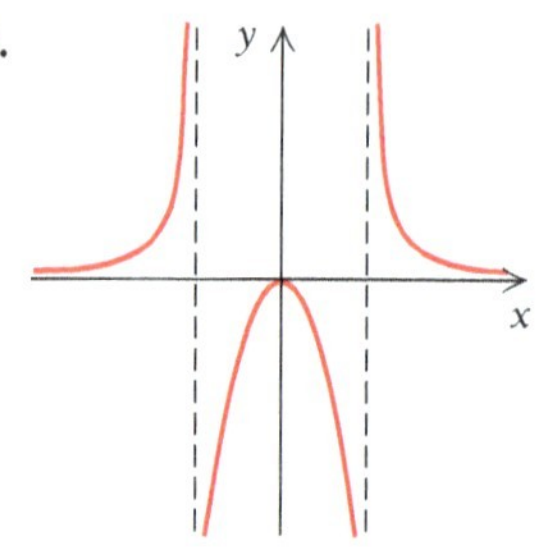

54.

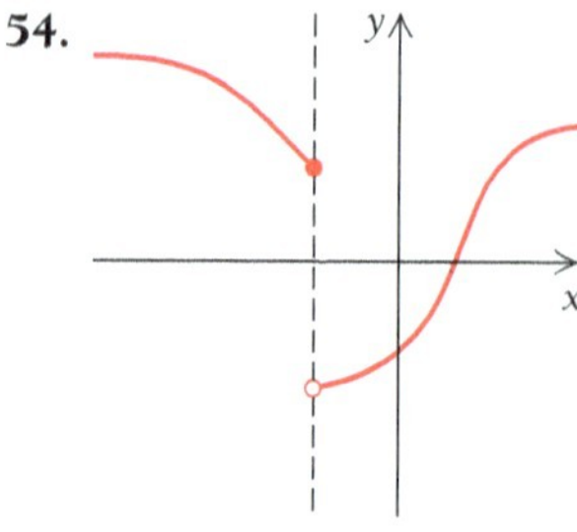

55.

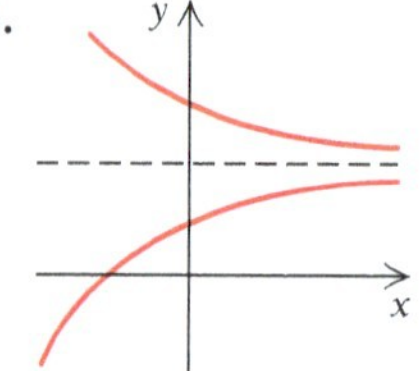

56.

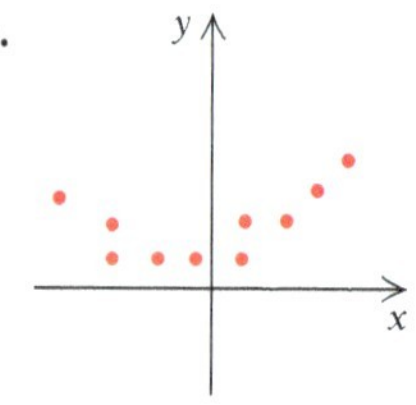

In Exercises 57 and 58, assume that x is the input and y is the output.

57. a) Graph $x = y^2 - 2$.
b) Is this a function? Why or why not?

58. a) Graph $x = y^2 - 3$.
b) Is this a function? Why or why not?

59. For $f(x) = x^2 - 3x$, find $\dfrac{f(x + h) - f(x)}{h}$.

60. For $f(x) = x^2 + 4x$, find $\dfrac{f(x + h) - f(x)}{h}$.

For Exercises 61–64, consider the function f given by

$$f(x) = \begin{cases} -2x + 1, & \text{for } x < 0, \\ 17, & \text{for } x = 0, \\ x^2 - 3, & \text{for } 0 < x < 4, \\ \frac{1}{2}x + 1, & \text{for } x \geq 4. \end{cases}$$

61. Find $f(-1)$ and $f(1)$.
62. Find $f(-3)$ and $f(3)$.
63. Find $f(0)$ and $f(10)$.
64. Find $f(-5)$ and $f(5)$.

Graph.

65. $f(x) = \begin{cases} 1, & \text{for } x < 0, \\ -1, & \text{for } x \geq 0 \end{cases}$

66. $f(x) = \begin{cases} 2, & \text{for } x \leq 3, \\ -2, & \text{for } x > 3 \end{cases}$

67. $f(x) = \begin{cases} 6, & \text{for } x = -2, \\ x^2, & \text{for } x \neq -2 \end{cases}$

68. $f(x) = \begin{cases} 5, & \text{for } x = 1, \\ x^3, & \text{for } x \neq 1 \end{cases}$

69. $f(x) = \begin{cases} -x, & \text{for } x < 0, \\ 4, & \text{for } x = 0, \\ x + 2, & \text{for } x > 0 \end{cases}$

70. $g(x) = \begin{cases} 2x - 3, & \text{for } x < 1, \\ 5, & \text{for } x = 1, \\ x - 2, & \text{for } x > 1 \end{cases}$

71. $g(x) = \begin{cases} \frac{1}{2}x - 1, & \text{for } x < 2, \\ -4, & \text{for } x = 2, \\ x - 3, & \text{for } x > 2 \end{cases}$

72. $g(x) = \begin{cases} x^2, & \text{for } x < 0, \\ -3, & \text{for } x = 0, \\ -2x + 3, & \text{for } x > 0 \end{cases}$

73. $f(x) = \begin{cases} -7, & \text{for } x = 2, \\ x^2 - 3, & \text{for } x \neq 2 \end{cases}$

74. $f(x) = \begin{cases} -6, & \text{for } x = -3, \\ -x^2 + 5, & \text{for } x \neq -3 \end{cases}$

Compound interest. *The amount of money, $A(t)$, in a savings account that pays 3% interest, compounded quarterly for t years, with an initial investment of P dollars, is given by*

$$A(t) = P\left(1 + \frac{0.03}{4}\right)^{4t}.$$

75. If \$500 is invested at 3%, compounded quarterly, how much will the investment be worth after 2 yr?

76. If \$800 is invested at 3%, compounded quarterly, how much will the investment be worth after 3 yr?

Chemotherapy. *In computing the dosage for some chemotherapy patients, the measure of a patient's body surface area is needed. A good approximation of this area s, in square meters (m^2), is given by*

$$s = \sqrt{\frac{hw}{3600}},$$

where w is the patient's weight in kilograms (kg) and h is the patient's height in centimeters (cm). (Source: U.S. Oncology.) Use this information for Exercises 77 and 78. Round your answers to the nearest thousandth.

77. If a patient's height is 170 cm, approximate the patient's surface area assuming that:
   a) The patient's weight is 70 kg.
   b) The patient's weight is 100 kg.
   c) The patient's weight is 50 kg.

78. If a patient's weight is 70 kg, approximate the patient's surface area assuming that:
   a) The patient's height is 150 cm.
   b) The patient's height is 180 cm.

79. **Business: monthly payments.** The table below shows the monthly payment for a \$20,000 auto loan at a rate of 2.5% for a term of 5, 6, or 7 yr.

Term (in years)	Interest Rate	Monthly Payment (in dollars)
5	0.025	354.95
6	0.025	299.42
7	0.025	259.78

   a) If the inputs are the term and the outputs are the monthly payment, is this correspondence a function?
   b) If the inputs are the monthly payment and the outputs are the term, is this correspondence a function?
   c) If the input is the interest rate and the outputs are the monthly payments, is this correspondence a function?
   d) If the inputs are the monthly payments and the output is the rate, is this correspondence a function?

80. **Scaling stress factors.** In psychology, a process called *scaling* is used to attach numerical ratings to a group of life experiences. In the following table, various events have been rated on a scale from 1 to 100 according to their stress levels.

Event	Scale of Impact
Death of spouse	100
Divorce	73
Jail term	63
Marriage	50
Lost job	47
Pregnancy	40
Death of close friend	37
Loan over \$10,000	31
Child leaving home	29
Change in schools	20
Loan less than \$10,000	17
Christmas	12

(*Source:* Thomas H. Holmes, University of Washington School of Medicine.)

   a) Does the table represent a function? Why or why not?
   b) What are the inputs? What are the outputs?

SYNTHESIS

Solve for y in terms of x, and determine if the resulting equation represents a function.

81. $2x + y - 16 = 4 - 3y + 2x$

82. $2y^2 + 3x = 4x + 5$

83. $(4y^{2/3})^3 = 64x$

84. $(3y^{3/2})^2 = 72x$

85. Explain why the vertical-line test works.

86. A function f is given by

$$f(x) = |x - 2| + |x + 1| - 5.$$

Find $f(-3)$, $f(-2)$, $f(0)$, and $f(4)$.

Technology Connection

In Exercises 87 and 88, use the TABLE *feature to construct a table for the function under the given conditions.*

87. $f(x) = x^3 + 2x^2 - 4x - 13$; TblStart $= -3$; ΔTbl $= 2$

88. $f(x) = \dfrac{3}{x^2 - 4}$; TblStart $= -3$; ΔTbl $= 1$

89. Graph the function in each of Exercises 87 and 88.

90. Use the TRACE feature to find several ordered-pair solutions of the function $f(x) = \sqrt{10 - x^2}$.

91. A function f takes a number x, adds 2, and then multiplies the result by 5, while a function g takes a number x, multiplies it by 5, and then adds 2.

a) Express f and g as equations.
b) Graph f and g on the same axes.
c) Are f and g the same function?

92. A function f takes a number x, subtracts 4, and then squares the result, while a function g takes a number x, squares it, and then subtracts 4.

a) Express f and g as equations.
b) Graph f and g on the same axes.
c) Are f and g the same function?

93. A function f takes a number x, multiplies it by 3, and then adds 6, while a function g takes a number x, adds h to it, and then multiplies the result by 3. Find h if f and g are the same function.

94. A function f takes a number x, adds 3, and then squares the result, while a function g takes a number x, squares it, adds 6 times x, and then adds h to the result. Find h if f and g are the same function.

Answers to Quick Checks

1. (a) The correspondence is a function since each book has one page count associated with it.
(b) The correspondence is not a function since more than one person will have a last name that starts with any particular letter. That is, each letter has more than one last name associated with it.
2. $17, -10, 5, 3x + 3h + 5$
3. $49, 58, -7, 3a^2 + 2a - 7, 75a^2 + 10a - 7$
4. $-8, 2x + 2h - x^2 - 2xh - h^2, 2 - 2x - h$
5. $f(x) = 2 - x^2$

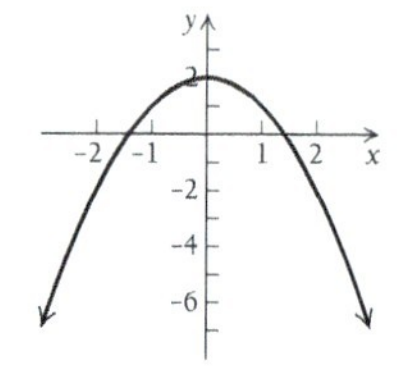

6. (a) The graph is not that of a function. **(b)** The graph is that of a function.

7.

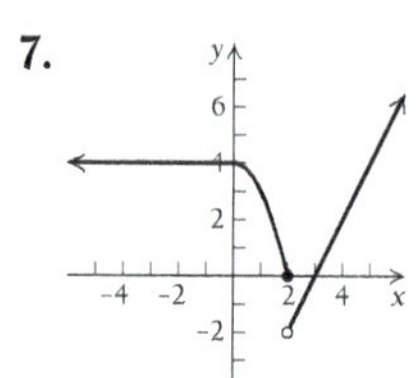

8.

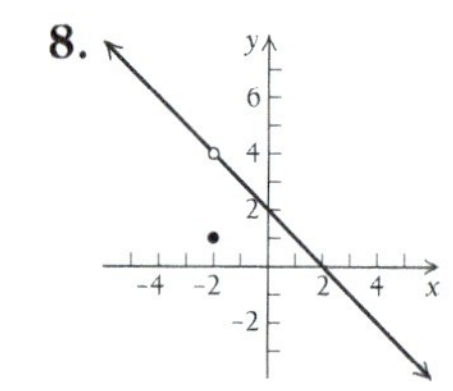

R.3 Finding Domain and Range

- Write interval notation for a set of points.
- Find the domain and the range of a function.

Set Notation

A **set** is any collection of objects, such as numbers. The set of numbers we consider most often in calculus is the set of **real numbers**, denoted ℝ. The real numbers can be represented by a line, called the **real number line**. Every point on the line represents a real number.

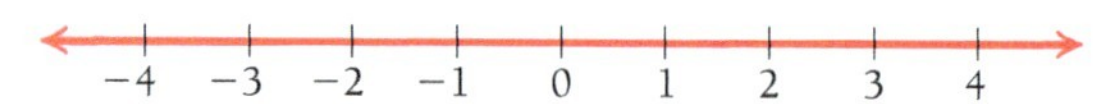

For example, the set consisting of 2, $-\frac{1}{2}$, and π can be written $\{2, -\frac{1}{2}, \pi\}$. On the real number line, a dot is placed at each number's location:

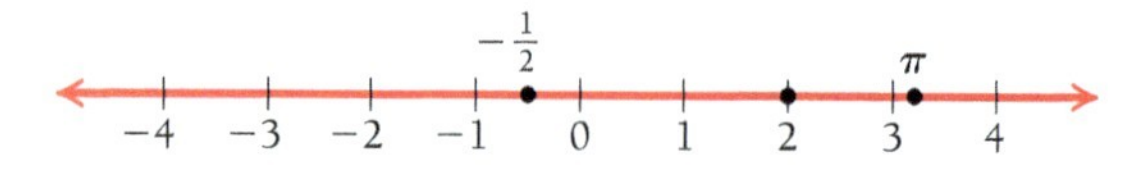

The method of describing a set by listing its members within braces { } is known as the **roster method**. Larger sets can be described using **set-builder notation**, which specifies conditions for which an object is a member of the set. For example, the set of all real numbers less than 4 can be described in set-builder notation as follows:

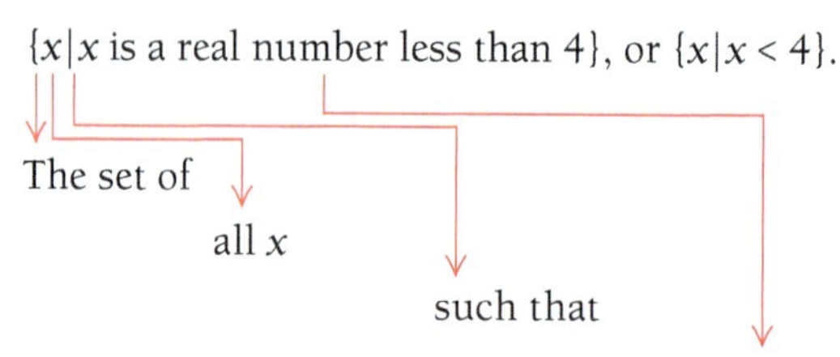

Interval Notation

We can also describe certain sets using **interval notation**. If a and b are real numbers, with $a < b$, we define the interval (a, b) as the set of all numbers between but not including a and b, that is, the set of all x for which $a < x < b$. Thus,

the set $(a, b) = \{x | a < x < b\}$
is displayed on the number line as

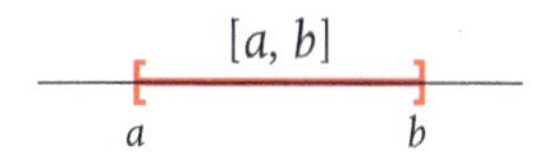

The points a and b are the **endpoints** of the interval. The parentheses indicate that the endpoints are *not* included in the interval.

The interval $[a, b]$ is defined as the set of all x for which $a \le x \le b$. Thus,

the set $[a, b] = \{x | a \le x \le b\}$
is displayed on the number line as

The brackets indicate that the endpoints *are* included in the interval.*

Do not confuse the *interval* (a, b) with the *ordered pair* (a, b) used to represent a point in the plane, as in Section R.1. The context in which the notation appears makes the meaning clear.

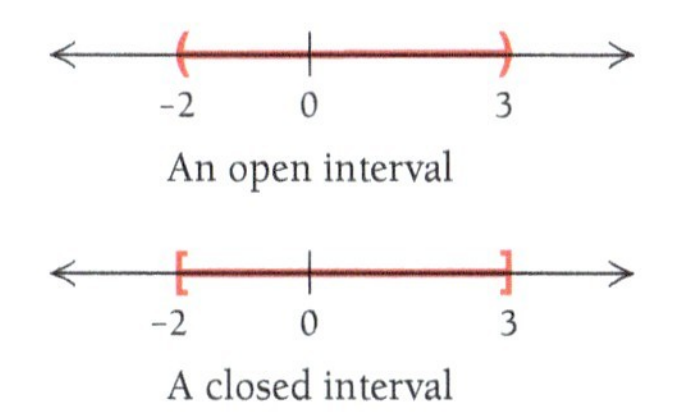

An open interval

A closed interval

Intervals like $(-2, 3)$, in which neither endpoint is included, are called **open intervals**; intervals like $[-2, 3]$, which include both endpoints, are called **closed intervals**. Thus, (a, b) is read "the open interval a, b," and $[a, b]$ is read "the closed interval a, b."

Intervals that are **half-open** include one endpoint but not the other:

$(a, b] = \{x | a < x \le b\}$. The graph excludes a and includes b.

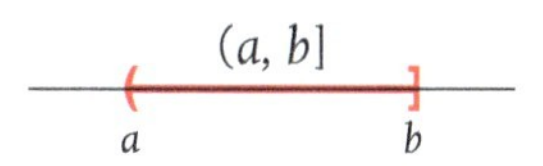

$[a, b) = \{x | a \le x < b\}$. The graph includes a and excludes b.

Intervals may extend without bound in one or both directions. We use the symbols ∞, read "infinity," and $-\infty$, read "negative infinity," to describe these intervals. The notation $(5, \infty)$ represents the set of all real numbers greater than 5. That is,

$$(5, \infty) = \{x | x > 5\}.$$

Similarly, the notation $(-\infty, 5)$ represents the set of all real numbers less than 5. That is,

$$(-\infty, 5) = \{x | x < 5\}.$$

The notations $[5, \infty)$ and $(-\infty, 5]$ are used when we want to include an endpoint. The interval $(-\infty, \infty)$ describes the set of all real numbers.

$(-\infty, \infty) = \{x | x \text{ is a real number}\}$

*The representations (open dots at a, b) and (closed dots at a, b) are sometimes used instead of, respectively, (parentheses at a, b) and (brackets at a, b).

Union and Intersection of Intervals

The *union* of two (or more) intervals consists of all real numbers x that are contained in one interval *or* the other *or* both. We use the symbol $\cup$ to represent the union of intervals. For example, $[-2, 1) \cup [4, 7]$ represents all real numbers x such that $-2 \leq x < 1$ *or* $4 \leq x \leq 7$. That is,

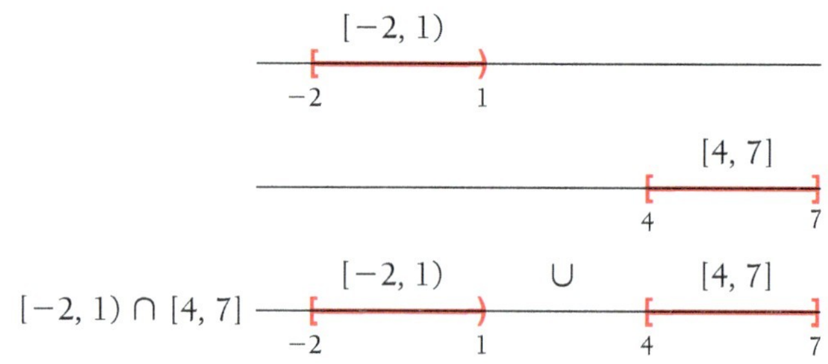

The *intersection* of two (or more) intervals consists of all real numbers x that are contained in both (or all) intervals simultaneously. We use the symbol $\cap$ to represent the intersection of intervals. For example, $(0, 5) \cap [2, 7)$ represents all real numbers x such that $0 < x < 5$ *and* $2 \leq x < 7$, and simplifies as the interval $[2, 5)$.

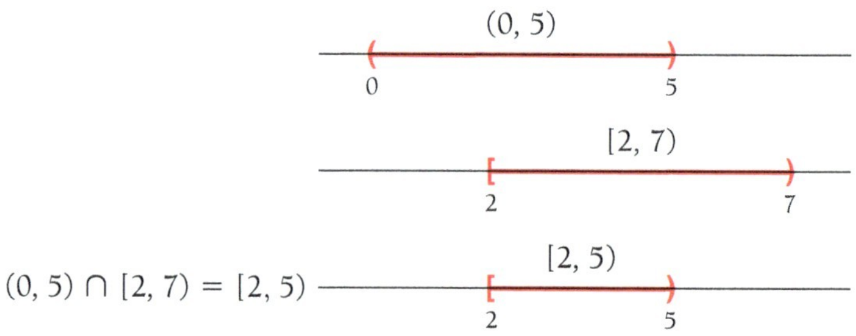

When two intervals do not contain any common elements, then their intersection is empty, denoted by $\varnothing$. For example, the intervals $[-2, 1)$ and $[4, 7]$ shown above do not have any real numbers in common (numbers that are in both intervals simultaneously), so $[-2, 1) \cap [4, 7] = \varnothing$. Such intervals are called *disjoint*.

Interval notation is summarized in the table on the next page.

EXAMPLE 1 Write interval notation for each set or graph:

a) $\{x \mid -4 < x < 5\}$

b) $\{x \mid x \geq -2\}$

c) 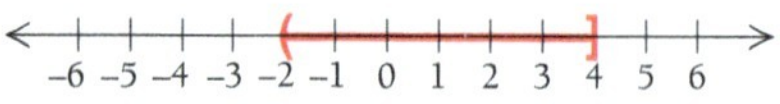

d) 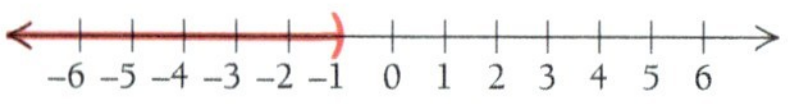

e) $\{x \mid -3 < x < 1 \text{ or } x \geq 2\}$

f) $\{x \mid x \leq 2 \text{ and } x > 0\}$

Solution

a) $\{x \mid -4 < x < 5\} = (-4, 5)$

b) $\{x \mid x \geq -2\} = [-2, \infty)$

c) $(-2, 4]$

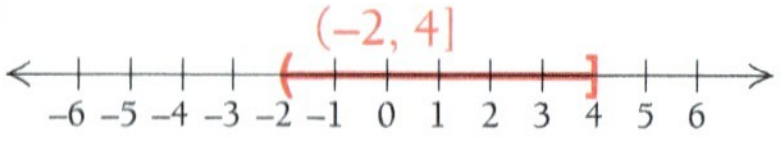

d) $(-\infty, -1)$

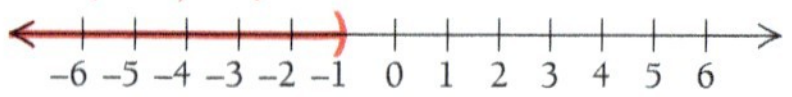

e) $(-3, 1) \cup [2, \infty)$

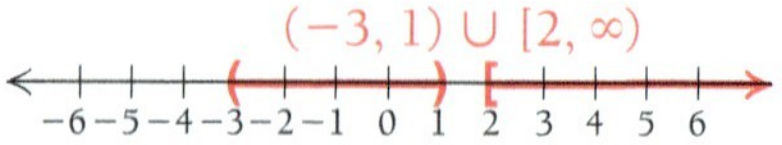

f) $(-\infty, 2] \cap (0, \infty) = (0, 2]$

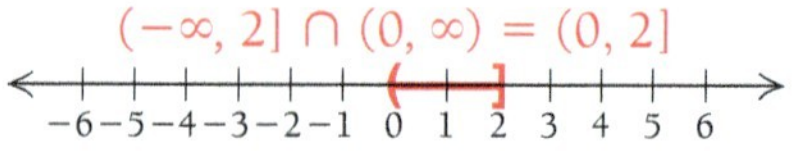

1 ✓

Quick Check 1 ✓

Write interval notation for each set, and show it on a graph.

a) $\{x \mid -2 \leq x \leq 5\}$

b) $\{x \mid -2 \leq x < 5\}$

c) $\{x \mid -2 < x \leq 5\}$

d) $\{x \mid -2 < x < 5\}$

e) $\{x \mid x < 0 \text{ or } 2 \leq x < 5\}$

f) $\{x \mid 2 < x < 5 \text{ and } 4 \leq x\}$

Finding Domain and Range

Recall that a set of ordered pairs in which no two different pairs share a common first coordinate is a function. The **domain** is the set of all first coordinates, and the **range** is the set of all second coordinates.

Intervals: Notation and Graphs

Interval Notation	Set Notation	Graph
(a, b)	$\{x \mid a < x < b\}$	
$[a, b]$	$\{x \mid a \le x \le b\}$	
$[a, b)$	$\{x \mid a \le x < b\}$	
$(a, b]$	$\{x \mid a < x \le b\}$	
(a, ∞)	$\{x \mid x > a\}$	
$[a, \infty)$	$\{x \mid x \ge a\}$	
$(-\infty, b)$	$\{x \mid x < b\}$	
$(-\infty, b]$	$\{x \mid x \le b\}$	
$(-\infty, \infty)$	$\{x \mid x \text{ is a real number}\}$	
$(a, b) \cup (c, d)$	$\{x \mid a < x < b \text{ or } c < x < d\}$	If (a, b) and (c, d), then $(a, b) \cup (c, d)$:
$(a, b) \cap (c, d)$	$\{x \mid a < x < b \text{ and } c < x < d\}$ If (a, b) and (c, d) have no common elements, then $(a, b) \cap (c, d) = \varnothing$.	If (a, b) and (c, d), then $(a, b) \cap (c, d) = (c, b)$:

EXAMPLE 2 For the function f shown in the graph to the right, determine the domain and the range.

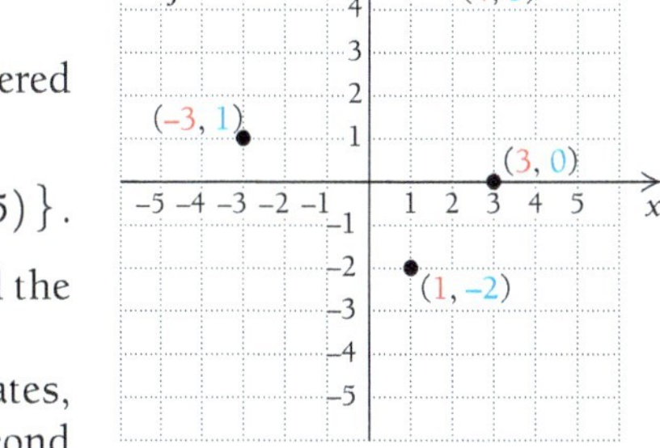

Solution This function consists of just five ordered pairs and can be written as

$$f = \{(-3, 1), (-2, 5), (1, -2), (3, 0), (4, 5)\}.$$

To determine the domain and the range, we read the x- and the y-values directly from the graph.

The domain is the set of all first coordinates, $\{-3, -2, 1, 3, 4\}$. The range is the set of all second coordinates, $\{-2, 0, 1, 5\}$. The ordering of the numbers within the set is not important, and repeated numbers are not listed. Although 5 appears twice as a second coordinate, we list it only once. **2 ✓**

Quick Check 2 ✓

For the function shown in the graph below, determine the domain and the range.

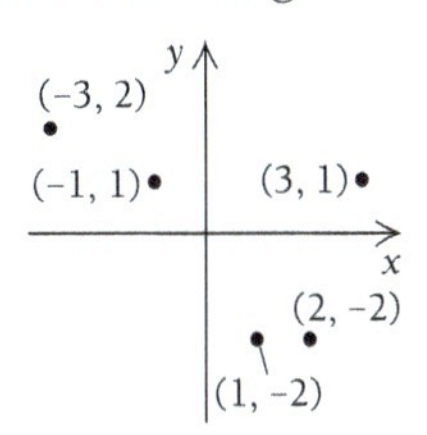

EXAMPLE 3 For the function f shown in the graph to the right, determine each of the following.

a) The number in the range that is paired with the input 1. That is, find $f(1)$.

b) The domain of f

c) The number(s) in the domain that is (are) paired with the output 1. That is, find all x-values for which $f(x) = 1$.

d) The range of f

Solution

a) To determine which number is paired with the input 1, we locate 1 on the horizontal axis. Next, we identify the point on the graph of f for which 1 is the first coordinate. From that point, we look to the vertical axis to find the corresponding y-coordinate, 2. The input 1 has the output 2; that is, $f(1) = 2$.

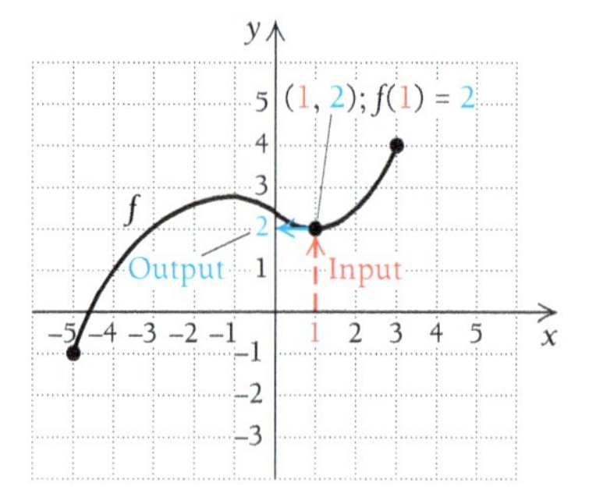

b) The domain of the function is the set of all x-values, or inputs, of the points on the graph. These extend from -5 to 3 and can be viewed as the curve's shadow on the x-axis. Thus, the domain is the set $\{x|-5 \leq x \leq 3\}$, or, in interval notation, $[-5, 3]$.

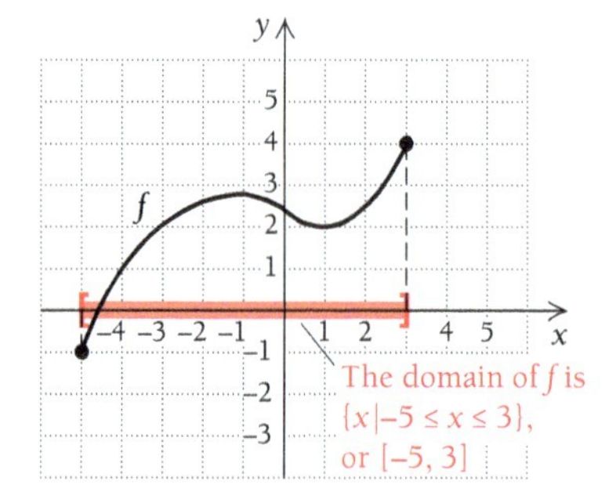

c) To determine which number(s) in the domain is (are) paired with the output 1, we locate 1 on the vertical axis. From there, we look left and right to the graph of f to identify any points for which 1 is the second coordinate. One such point exists: $(-4, 1)$. For this function, we note that $x = -4$ is the only member of the domain paired with the range value 1. There may be more than one member of the domain paired with a member of the range. For example, the output 2 appears to be paired with more than one input.

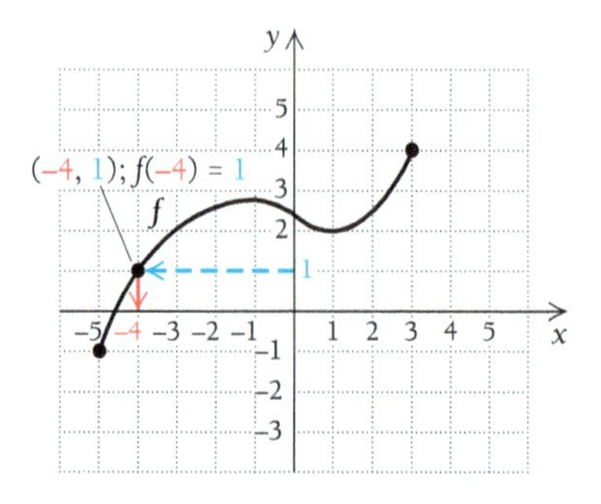

d) The range of the function is the set of all y-values, or outputs, of the points on the graph. These extend from -1 to 4 and can be viewed as the curve's shadow on the y-axis. Thus, the range is the set $\{y|-1 \leq y \leq 4\}$, or, in interval notation, $[-1, 4]$.

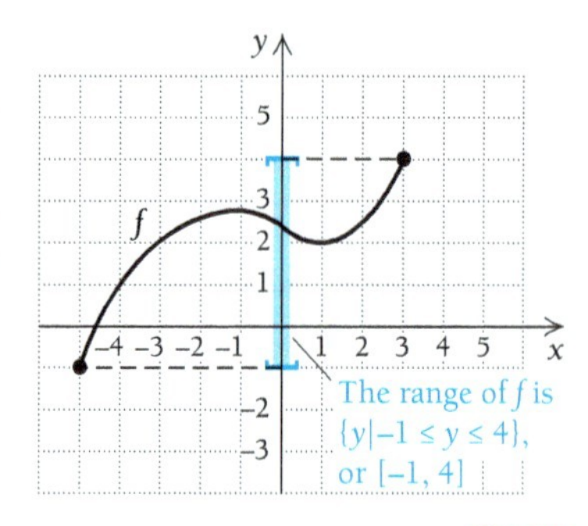

Quick Check 3 ✓

For the function f, shown in the graph below, determine each of the following:

a) $f(-1)$

b) $f(1)$

c) the domain

d) the range

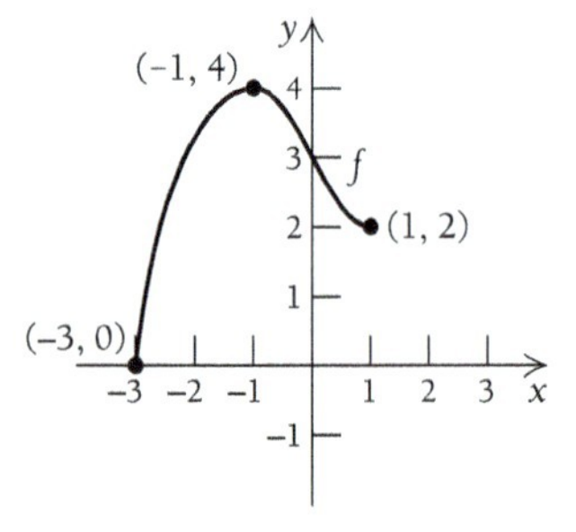

3 ✓

When a function is given by an equation or formula, the domain is understood to be the largest set of real numbers (inputs) for which function values (outputs) can be calculated. That is, the domain is the set of all allowable inputs into the formula. To find the domain, we think, "For what input values does the function have an output?"

EXAMPLE 4 Find and graph the domain: $f(x) = 3x + 2$.

Solution Is there any number x for which we cannot calculate $3x + 2$? The answer is no. Thus, the domain of f is the set of all real numbers: $(-\infty, \infty)$. The graph of the domain of f is shown below.

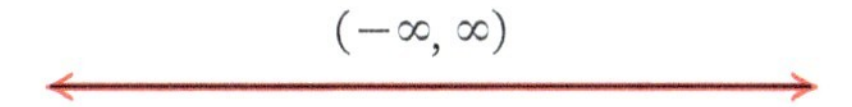

EXAMPLE 5 Find and graph the domain: $f(x) = \dfrac{3}{2x - 5}$.

Solution We recall that a denominator cannot equal zero. Since $3/(2x - 5)$ cannot be calculated when the denominator, $2x - 5$, is 0, we solve $2x - 5 = 0$ to find those real numbers that must be excluded from the domain of f:

$$2x - 5 = 0 \quad \text{Setting the denominator equal to 0}$$
$$2x = 5 \quad \text{Adding 5 to both sides}$$
$$x = \tfrac{5}{2}. \quad \text{Dividing both sides by 2}$$

Thus, $\frac{5}{2}$ is not in the domain, whereas all other real numbers are. We say that *f is not defined at $\frac{5}{2}$*, or *$f(\frac{5}{2})$ does not exist.*

The domain of f is $\{x | x \text{ is a real number } \textit{and } x \neq \frac{5}{2}\}$, or, in interval notation, $(-\infty, \frac{5}{2}) \cup (\frac{5}{2}, \infty)$. The graph of the domain is shown below; only $\frac{5}{2}$ is not part of the domain.

$(-\infty, \frac{5}{2}) \cup (\frac{5}{2}, \infty)$

$\frac{5}{2}$

EXAMPLE 6 Find and graph the domain: $g(x) = \sqrt{4 + 3x}$.

Solution Since radicands in even roots cannot be negative, $\sqrt{4 + 3x}$ is not a real number when $4 + 3x$ is negative. The domain is all real numbers for which $4 + 3x \geq 0$. We find the domain by solving the inequality. (See Appendix A for a review of solving inequalities.)

$$4 + 3x \geq 0$$
$$3x \geq -4 \quad \text{Adding } -4 \text{ to both sides}$$
$$x \geq -\tfrac{4}{3} \quad \text{Dividing both sides by 3}$$

The domain is $\{x | -\frac{4}{3} \leq x < \infty\}$, or, in interval notation, $[-\frac{4}{3}, \infty)$. Its graph is shown below.

$[-\frac{4}{3}, \infty)$

$-\frac{4}{3}$

4 ✓

Quick Check 4 ✓

Find and graph the domain of each function.

a) $f(x) = \dfrac{5}{x - 8}$

b) $f(x) = \sqrt{2x - 8}$

EXAMPLE 7 Find and graph the domain: $h(x) = \sqrt{x} + \sqrt{3 - x}$.

Solution The radicands of both square root terms must be nonnegative. From the term $\sqrt{x}$, we see that x must be in the interval $[0, \infty)$, and from the term $\sqrt{3 - x}$, we see that x must be in the interval $(-\infty, 3]$. The domain of h is the set of real numbers x that are included in both intervals; that is, the domain is the intersection of the intervals $[0, \infty)$ and $(-\infty, 3]$. Thus, the domain of h is

$$(-\infty, 3] \cap [0, \infty) = [0, 3].$$

The graph of the domain is shown below.

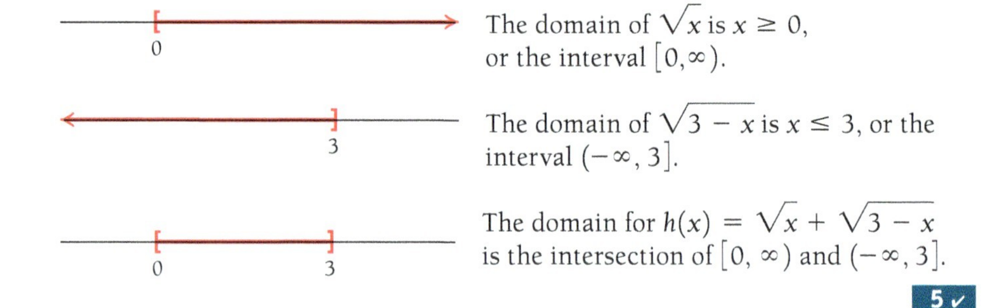

0
The domain of $\sqrt{x}$ is $x \geq 0$, or the interval $[0, \infty)$.
3
The domain of $\sqrt{3 - x}$ is $x \leq 3$, or the interval $(-\infty, 3]$.
0
3
The domain for $h(x) = \sqrt{x} + \sqrt{3 - x}$ is the intersection of $[0, \infty)$ and $(-\infty, 3]$.

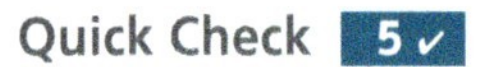

Quick Check 5 ✓

Find and graph the domain: $m(x) = \sqrt{x + 2} + \sqrt{4 - x}$.

5 ✓

Domains and Ranges in Applications

The domain and the range of a function given by a formula are sometimes affected by the context of an application. In such cases, we consider the function's practical domain and range. For example, for the function $y = 15x$, the domain is $\{x | x \text{ is any real number}\}$ and the range is $\{y | y \text{ is any real number}\}$. However, if this function represents the pay, y, for someone who works x hours at \$15 per hour, then negative values of x and y do not make sense. In this case, the function's practical domain is $\{x | x \geq 0\}$ and its practical range is $\{y | y \geq 0\}$.

EXAMPLE 8 **Rental Car Rates.** The hourly rate to rent a minivan in Florida is \$12.30 per hour or any part of an hour. For any rental period of more than 2 hr, the daily rate of \$36.90 applies, up to and including a maximum of 24 hr. This pricing also applies to subsequent 24-hr periods. Let $C(t)$ be the cost to rent a minivan for t hours. Disregard any extra taxes or surcharges. (*Sources*: avis.com; dms.myflorida.com.)

a) Find $C(18)$, and explain what this number represents.

b) Find $C(25.5)$, and explain what this number represents.

c) Find $C(30)$, and explain what this number represents.

d) Sketch the graph of C for $0 < t \leq 48$, and state the practical range of C.

Solution

a) Since 18 hr exceeds 2 hr and is less than 24 hr, we have $C(18) = \$36.90$, meaning that the charge to rent a minivan for 18 hr is the daily rate of \$36.90.

b) A rental period of 25.5 hr consists of a 24-hr period for which the daily rate is charged plus two 1-hr periods, since the extra 0.5 hr is considered part of a full second hour. Thus,

$$C(25.5) = \$36.90 + \$12.30 + \$12.30 = \$61.50.$$

c) A rental period of 30 hr consists of a 24-hr period for which the daily rate is charged plus an extra 6 hr for which the daily rate is charged again. Thus,

$$C(30) = \$36.90 + \$36.90 = \$73.80.$$

d) The graph of C, for $0 < t \leq 48$, is shown below.

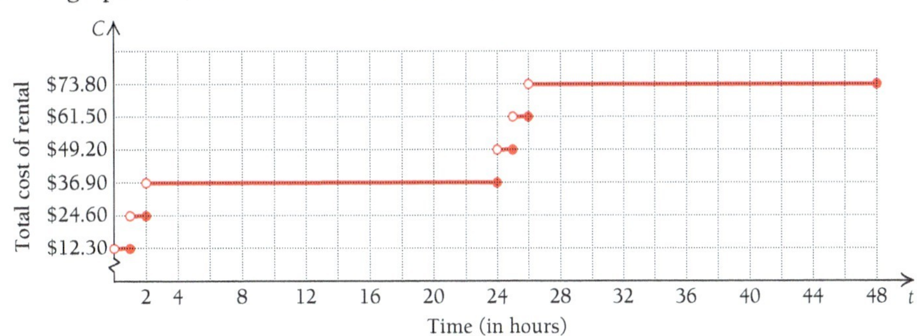

Since the cost is in increments of \$12.30, we use the roster method to write the practical range of C, for $0 < t \leq 48$: $\{12.3, 24.6, 36.9, 49.2, 61.5, 73.8\}$.

Section Summary

The following is a review of function terminology from Sections R.1–R.3.

Function Concepts

- Formula for f: $f(x) = x^2 - 7$
- For every input of f, there is exactly one output.
- For the input 1, the output is -6.
- For the output -3, the inputs are -2 and 2; $f(-2) = -3$ and $f(2) = -3$.
- The domain is the set of all inputs, or in this case, the set of all real numbers, $\mathbb{R}$.
- The range is the set of all outputs, or in this case, the interval $[-7, \infty)$.

Graph

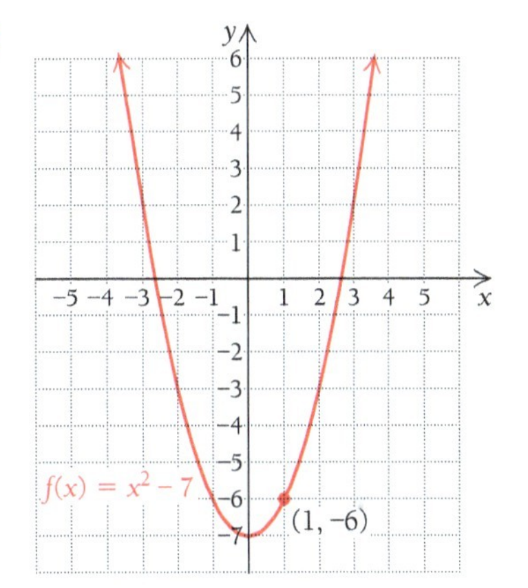

R.3 Exercise Set

In Exercises 1–10, write interval notation for each graph.

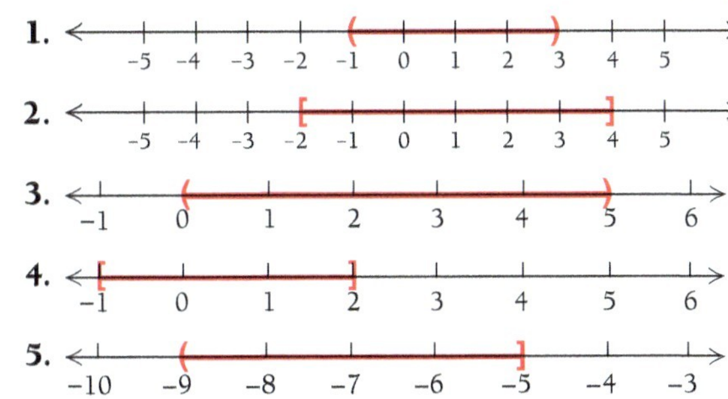

1.

2.

3.

4.

5.

6.

7.

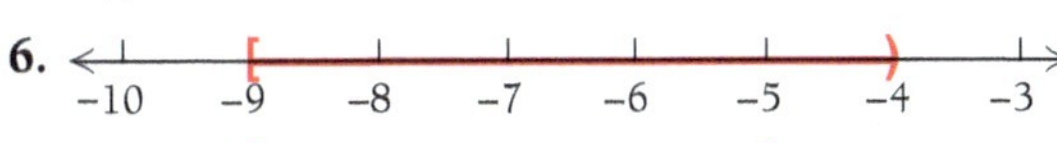

8.

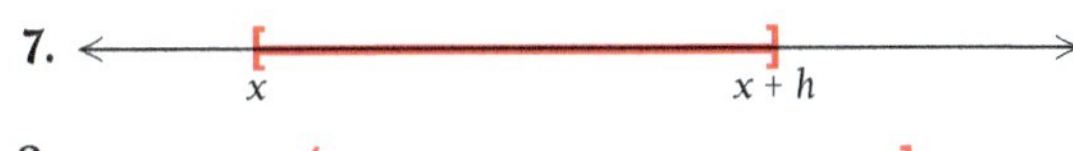

9.

10.

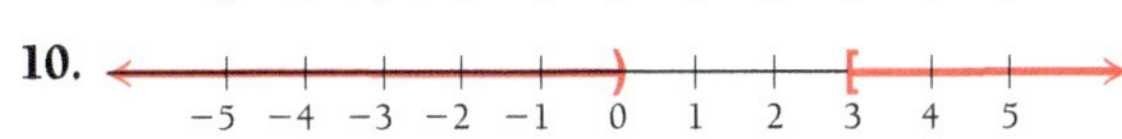

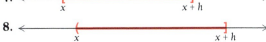

Write interval notation for each of the following. Then graph the interval on a number line.

11. The set of all numbers x such that $-2 \leq x \leq 2$

12. The set of all numbers x such that $-5 < x < 5$

13. $\{x|6 < x \leq 20\}$

14. $\{x|-4 \leq x < -1\}$

15. $\{x|x > -3\}$

16. $\{x|x \leq -2\}$

17. $\{x|-2 < x \leq 3\}$

18. $\{x|-10 \leq x < 4\}$

19. $\{x|-4 \leq x < -3 \text{ or } 0 < x \leq 5\}$

20. $\{x|x < -2 \text{ or } 1 \leq x < 4\}$

In Exercises 21–32, each graph is that of a function, f. Determine (a) $f(1)$; (b) *the domain;* (c) *all x-values such that* $f(x) = 2$; *and* (d) *the range.*

21.

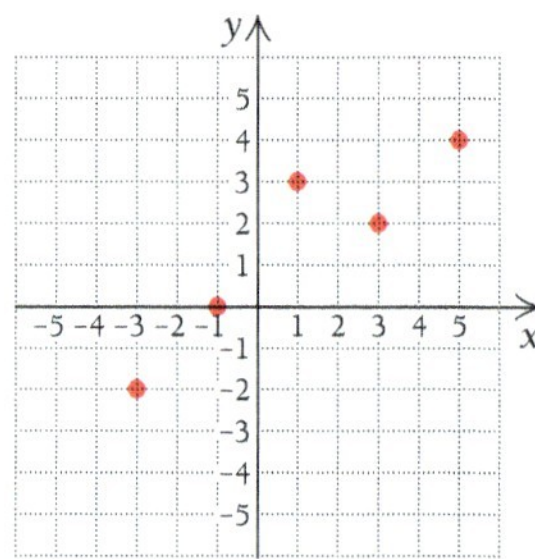

22.

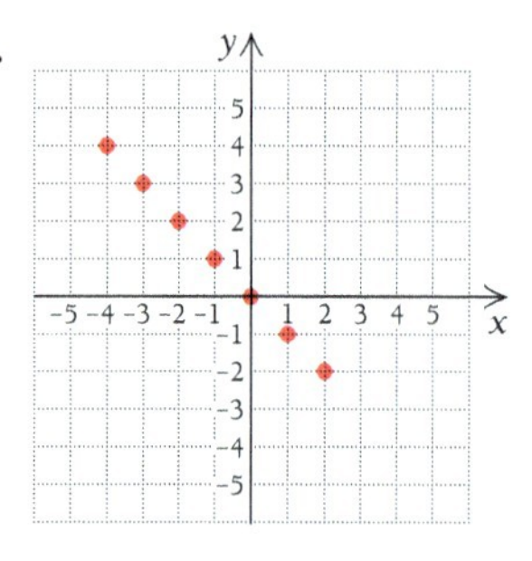

23.

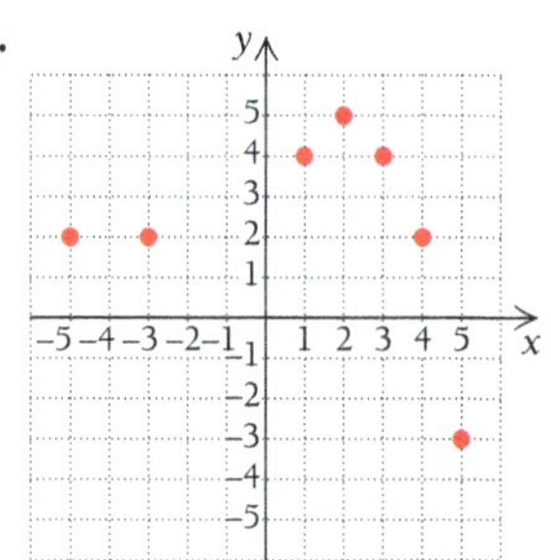

24.

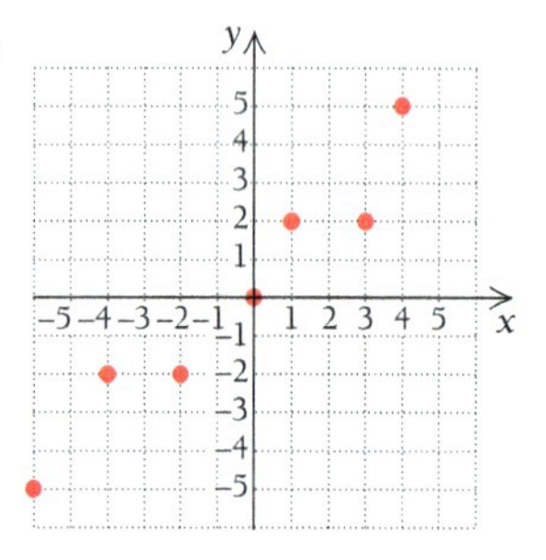

25.

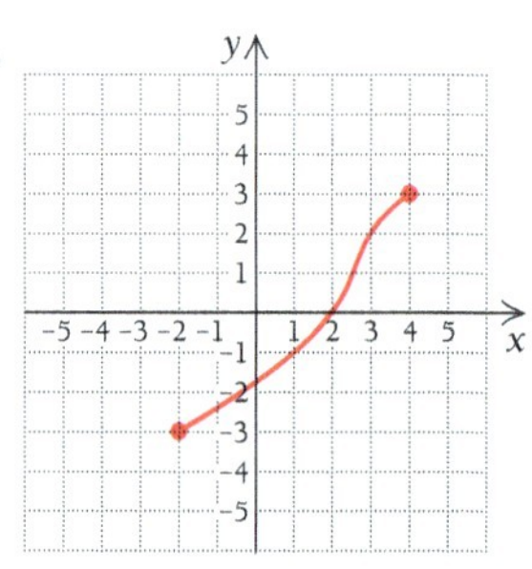

26.

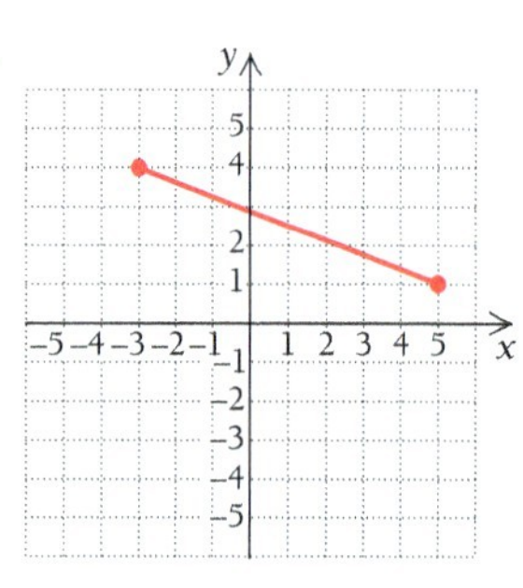

27.

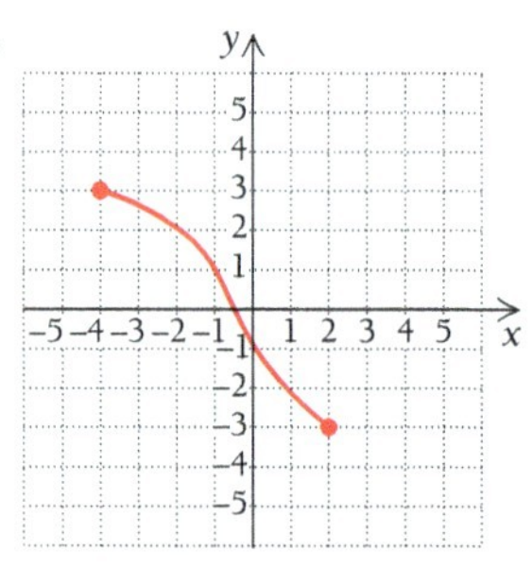

28.

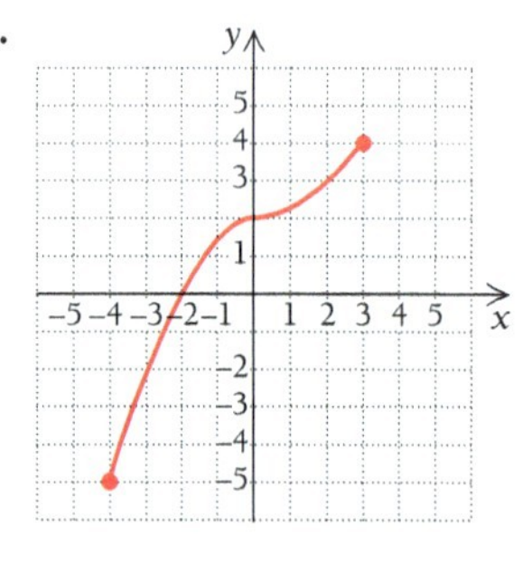

29.

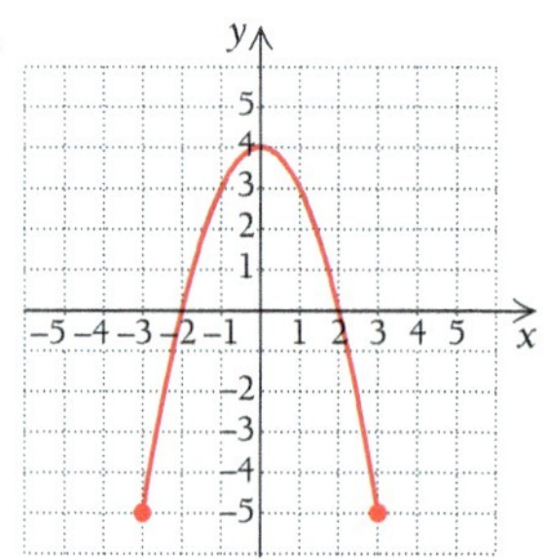

30.

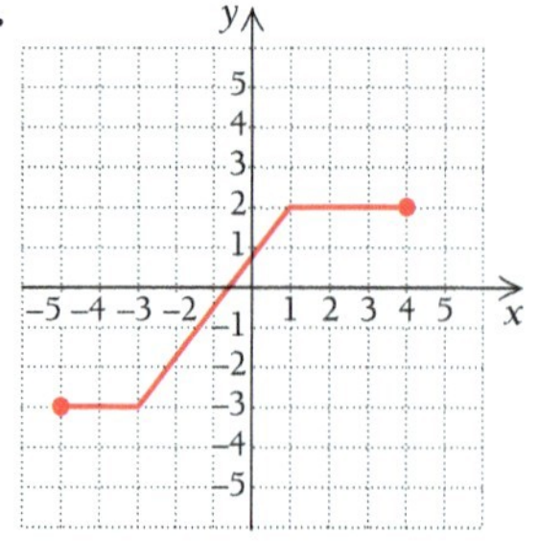

31.

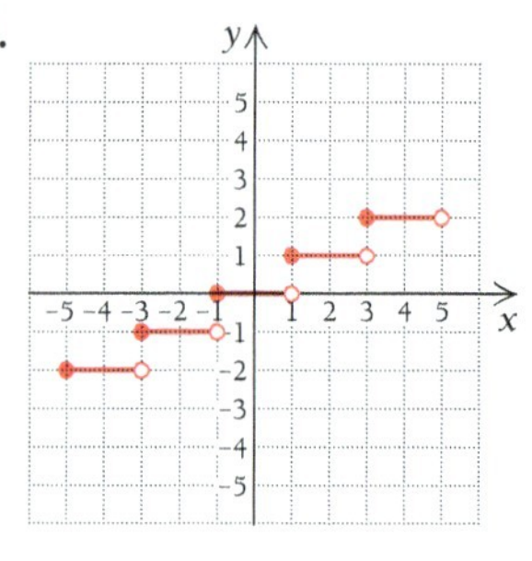

32.

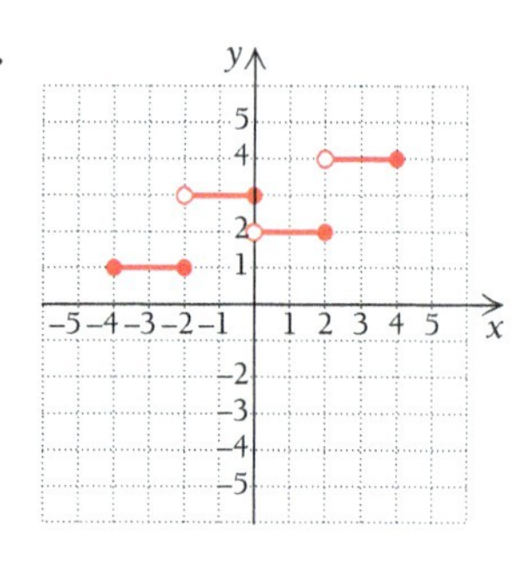

Write the domain of each function given below in interval notation; then graph the domain on a number line.

33. $f(x) = \dfrac{6}{2 - x}$

34. $f(x) = \dfrac{2}{x + 3}$

35. $f(x) = \sqrt{2x}$

36. $f(x) = \sqrt{x - 2}$

37. $f(x) = x^2 - 2x + 3$

38. $f(x) = x^2 + 3$

39. $f(x) = \dfrac{x - 2}{6x - 12}$

40. $f(x) = \dfrac{8}{3x - 6}$

41. $f(x) = x - 4$

42. $f(x) = 3x + 7$

43. $f(x) = \dfrac{3x - 1}{7 - 2x}$

44. $f(x) = \dfrac{2x - 1}{9 - 2x}$

45. $g(x) = \sqrt{4 + 5x}$

46. $g(x) = \sqrt{2 - 3x}$

47. $g(x) = x^2 - 2x + 1$

48. $g(x) = 4x^3 + 5x^2 - 2x$

49. $g(x) = \dfrac{2x}{x^2 - 25}$ (*Hint*: Factor the denominator.)

50. $g(x) = \dfrac{x - 1}{x^2 - 36}$ (*Hint*: Factor the denominator.)

51. $g(x) = \dfrac{1}{x^2 + 9}$

52. $g(x) = \dfrac{x}{x^2 + 1}$

53. $f(x) = \sqrt{x + 1} + \sqrt{6 - 2x}$

54. $k(x) = \sqrt{2x + 3} - \sqrt{12 - 5x}$

55. For the function f shown in the graph, find all x-values for which $f(x) \leq 0$.

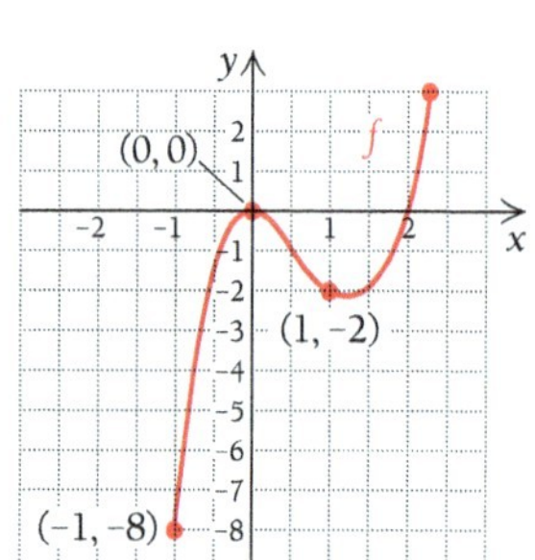

56. For the function g shown in the graph, find all x-values for which $g(x) = 1$.

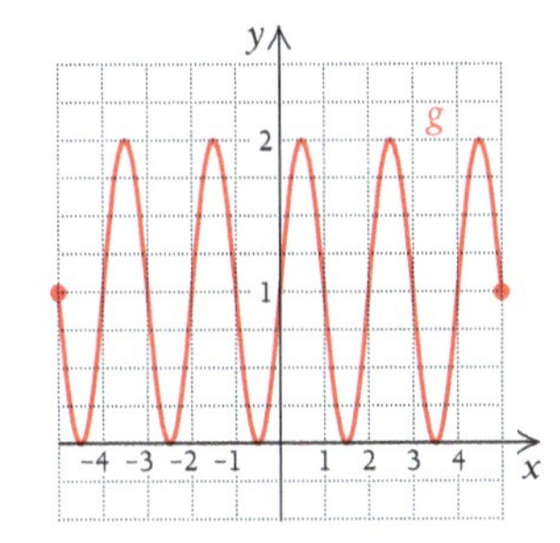

57. For the function h shown in the graph, find all x-values for which $h(x) = 2$.

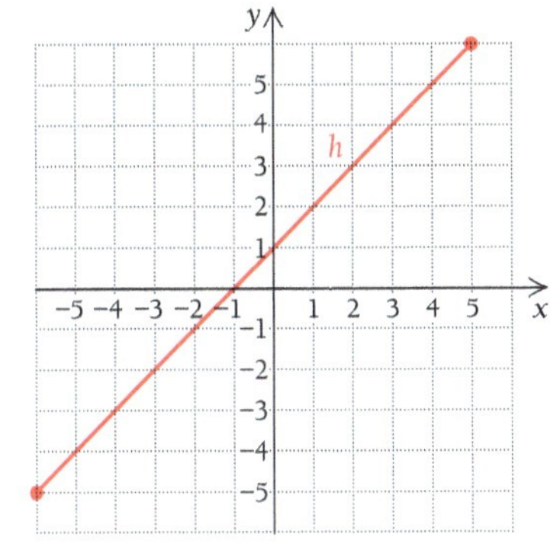

58. For the function G shown in the graph, find all x-values for which $G(x) > -4$.

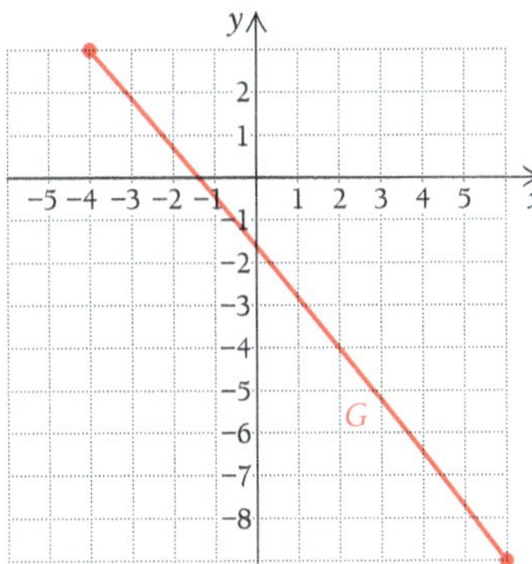

59. For the function W shown in the graph, find all x-values for which $W(x) = 0$.

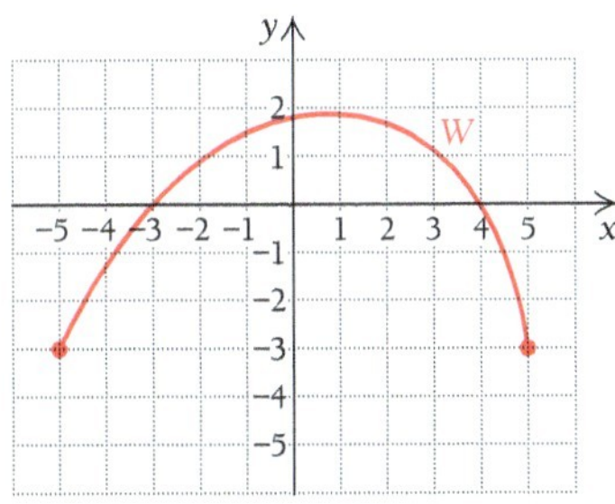

60. For the function k shown in the graph, find all x-values for which $k(x) \geq 0$.

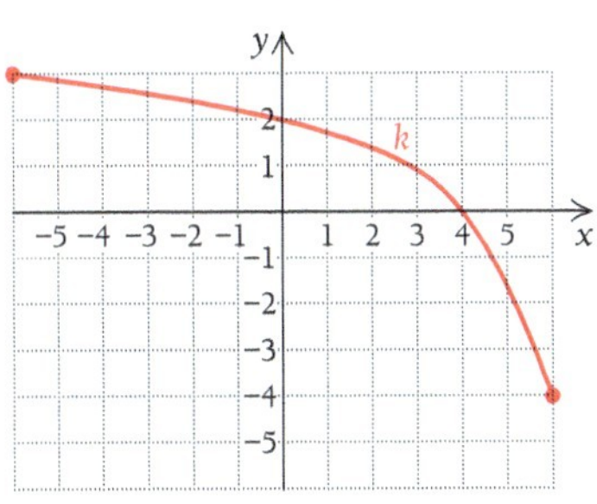

APPLICATIONS

Business and Economics

61. Hourly earnings. Karen works as a contractor, earning \$40 per hour. She will work at most 10 days, for at most 8 hours per day. Her total earnings P after working t hours are given by $P(t) = 40t$. Find the practical domain and range of this function.

62. Sales tax. Marcus plans to spend at most \$200 at the electronics store. The sales tax rate is 5% per dollar spent. The total tax T on x dollars spent is given by $T(x) = 0.05x$. Find the practical domain and range of this function.

Life and Physical Sciences

63. Incidence of breast cancer. The following graph approximates the incidence of breast cancer I, per 100,000 women, as a function of age x, in years. The equation for this graph is

$$I(x) = -0.0000554x^4 + 0.0067x^3 - 0.0997x^2 - 0.84x - 0.25.$$

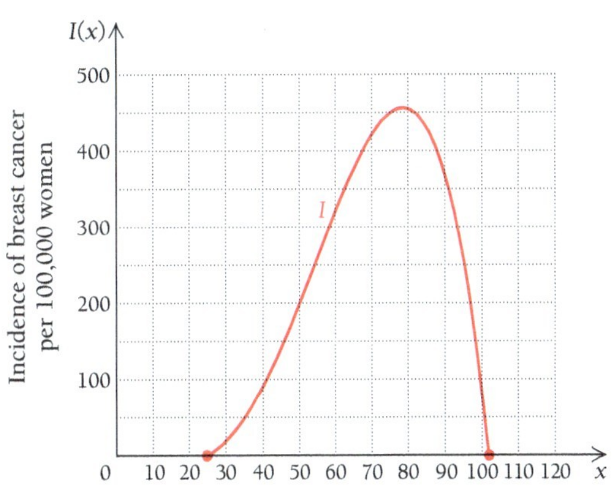

(*Source*: Based on data from the National Cancer Institute.)

a) Use the graph to estimate the domain of I.
b) Use the graph to estimate the range of I.
c) What 10-yr age interval sees the greatest increase in the incidence of breast cancer? Explain how you determined this.

64. Hearing-impaired Americans. The following graph approximates the number N, in millions, of hearing-impaired Americans who are x years old. The equation for this graph is

$$N(x) = -0.000065x^3 + 0.0072x^2 - 0.133x + 2.062.$$

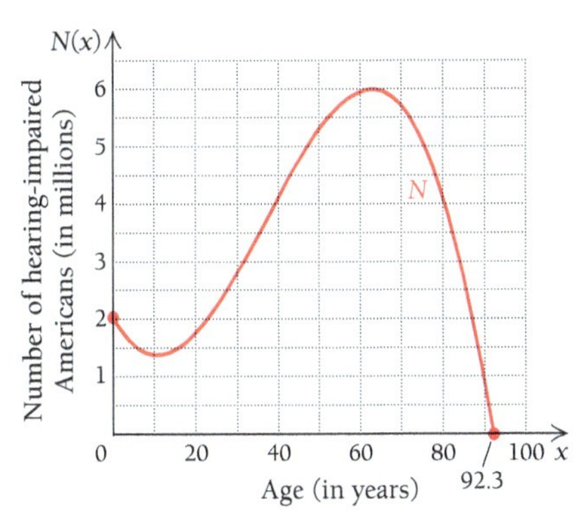

(*Source*: Better Hearing Institute.)

a) Use the graph to determine the domain of N.
b) Use the graph to approximate the range of N.
c) If you were marketing a new type of hearing aid, at what age group (expressed as a 10-yr interval) would you target advertisements? Why?

65. Taxi fares. Goldenrod TaxiCab charges \$5 for the first mile and \$3.50 for each additional mile or part of a mile. Let $f(x)$ represent the fare, in dollars, for a trip of x miles.

a) Find $f(4)$, and explain what that value represents.
b) Find $f(4.25)$, and explain what that value represents.
c) Find the range of f for $0 < x \leq 10$.

66. Shipping charges. Online Couture charges \$20 to ship orders for which the total amount spent is any amount up to and including \$100. For every extra \$20 spent, the shipping rate is reduced by \$5, with the possibility of free shipping if the total amount of the order is large enough. Let $S(x)$ be the shipping charge, in dollars, for an order totaling x dollars.

a) Find $S(95)$, and explain what that value represents.
b) Find $S(102)$, and explain what that value represents.
c) What is the minimum order total to receive free shipping?
d) Find the range of S when $0 < x \leq 200$.

SYNTHESIS

67. Determine the domain of $f(x) = \dfrac{\sqrt{x}}{\sqrt{5 - x}}$.

68. Determine the domain of $g(x) = \dfrac{\sqrt{3 - x}}{x}$.

69. Determine the domain of $f(x) = \dfrac{1}{x(x^2 - 9)}$.

70. Determine the domain of $g(x) = \dfrac{4}{x(x^2 - x - 12)}$.

71. Write an equation for a function whose domain is all of the real numbers except $x = -2, 0, 2$. (*Hint*: See Exercise 69.)

72. Write an equation for a function whose domain is all of the real numbers except $x = -1, 0, 7$. (*Hint*: See Exercise 70.)

73. Explain why the domain of $f(x) = \sqrt{1 - x} + \sqrt{x - 3}$ is $\varnothing$.

Technology Connection

In Exercises 74 and 75, use a graphing calculator to find the domain of the function.

74. $f(x) = \sqrt{x^2 - 25}$

75. $g(x) = \sqrt{x^2 - 3x - 4}$

76. The function $P(t) = 2500(1.02)^t$ gives the population $P(t)$ of a city, t years after 2010 (where $t = 0$ represents 2010). Could the domain include negative values for t? If so, describe a situation in which a negative value of t makes sense within the context of the problem. How would the range be affected if negative values of t are included?

Answers to Quick Checks

1. (a) $[-2, 5]$, 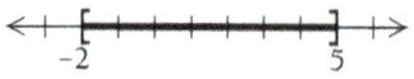

(b) $[-2, 5)$, 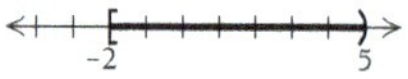

(c) $(-2, 5]$, 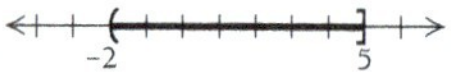

(d) $(-2, 5)$, 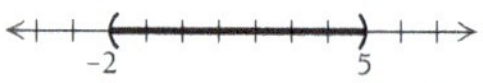

(e) $(-\infty, 0) \cup [2, 5)$, 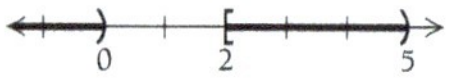

(f) $[4, 5)$, 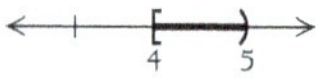

2. Domain is $\{-3, -1, 1, 2, 3\}$, and range is $\{-2, 1, 2\}$.
3. (a) $f(-1) = 4$ **(b)** $f(1) = 2$ **(c)** domain is $[-3, 1]$ **(d)** range is $[0, 4]$
4. (a) $(-\infty, 8) \cup (8, \infty)$, 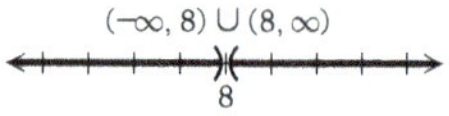

(b) $[4, \infty)$, 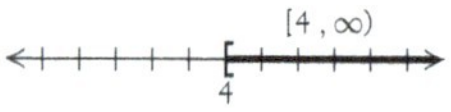

5. $[-2, 4]$, 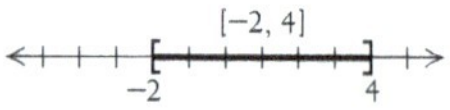

R.4

- Find and interpret the slope of a line.
- Graph equations of the form $y = c$ and $x = a$.
- Graph linear functions.
- Find an equation of a line when given the slope and one point on the line and when given two points on the line.
- Solve applied problems involving slope and linear functions.

Slope and Linear Functions

Given any two points $P_1 = (x_1, y_1)$ and $P_2 = (x_2, y_2)$, we can draw a line containing these points. A measure of the line's steepness is called the **slope**, denoted by the letter m.

DEFINITION

The **slope** of a line containing points $P_1 = (x_1, y_1)$ and $P_2 = (x_2, y_2)$ is

$$m = \frac{y_2 - y_1}{x_2 - x_1} = \frac{\text{change in } y}{\text{change in } x}.$$

EXAMPLE 1 Find the slope of the line containing the points $(-2, 6)$ and $(-4, 9)$.

Solution We have

$$m = \frac{y_2 - y_1}{x_2 - x_1} = \frac{6 - 9}{-2 - (-4)} \qquad \text{Regarding } (-2, 6) \text{ as } P_2 \text{ and } (-4, 9) \text{ as } P_1$$

$$= \frac{-3}{2} = -\frac{3}{2}.$$

It does not matter which point is regarded as P_1 or P_2, as long as we subtract the coordinates in the same order. Thus, we can also find m as follows:

$$m = \frac{9 - 6}{-4 - (-2)} = \frac{3}{-2} = -\frac{3}{2}. \qquad \text{Here, } (-4, 9) \text{ serves as } P_2, \text{ and } (-2, 6) \text{ serves as } P_1.$$

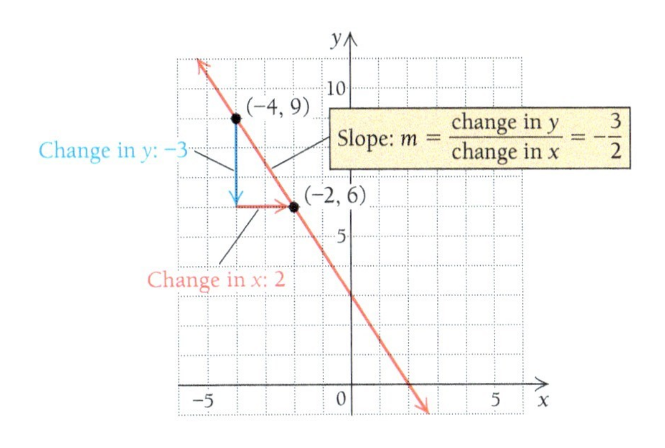

In the graph above, the points $(-2, 6)$ and $(-4, 9)$ are plotted, and a line is drawn through them. The slope $m = -\frac{3}{2}$ indicates that for each horizontal change of 2 units, the corresponding vertical change is -3 units. This line slopes down from left to right.

Quick Check 1 ✓

Find the slope of the line containing the points $(2, 3)$ and $(1, -4)$.

1 ✓

If a line is horizontal, the vertical change between any two points is 0. Thus, a horizontal line has slope 0. If a line is vertical, the horizontal change between any two points is 0. In this case, the slope is *not defined* because we cannot divide by 0. A vertical line has undefined slope. Thus, "0 slope" and "undefined slope" are two very different concepts.

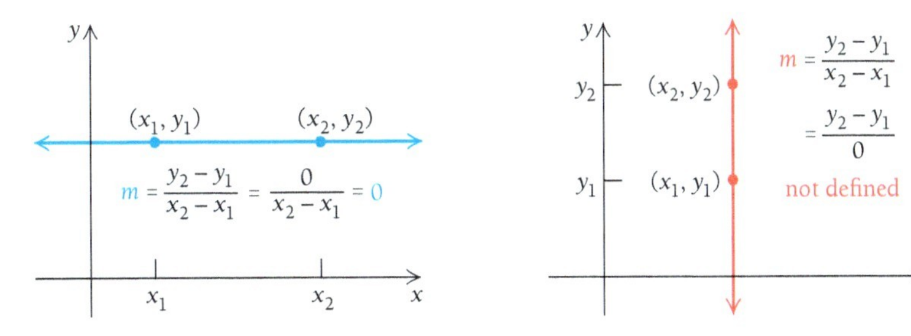

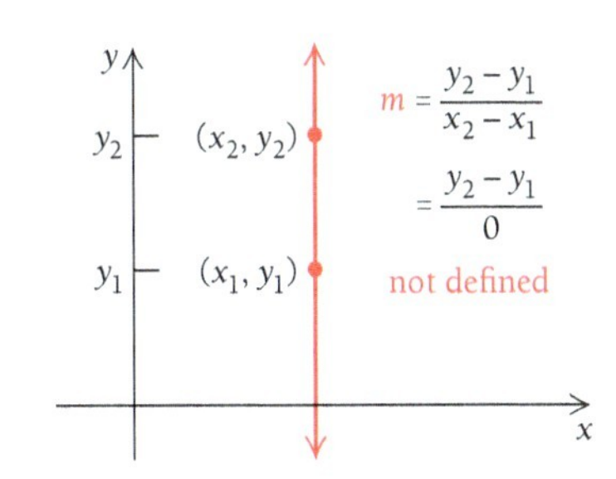

Applications of Slope

Slope has many real-world applications. For example, numbers like 2%, 3%, and 6% are often used to represent the *grade*, or steepness, of a road. A 3% grade $(3\% = \frac{3}{100})$ means that for every horizontal distance of 100 ft, the road rises 3 ft. In solar arrays, photovoltaic panels are tilted to optimize solar gain, based on geography and weather patterns. Wheelchair-ramp design also involves slope: Building codes rarely allow the steepness of a wheelchair ramp to exceed $\frac{1}{12}$.

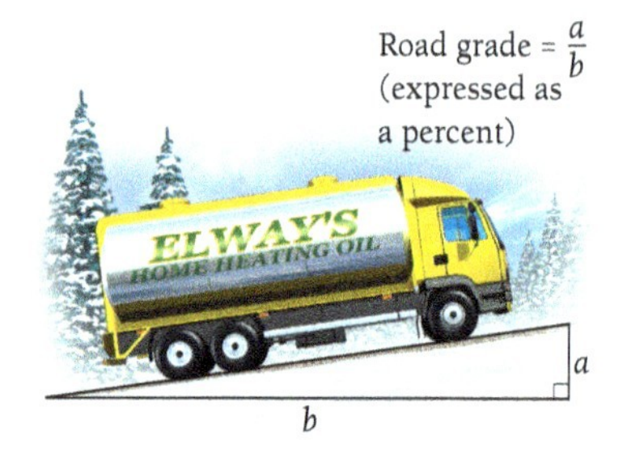

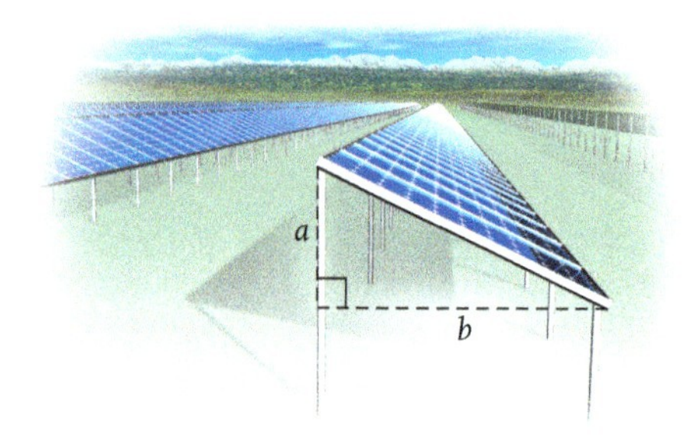

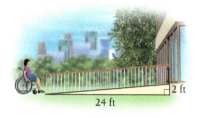

Ski trail difficulty ratings, or *gradients*, are yet another application of slope. The following table presents examples.

Ski Trail Difficulty Ratings in North America

Trail Rating	Symbol	Level of Difficulty	Description
Green Dot	●	Easiest	A Green Dot trail is the easiest. These trails typically have slope gradients ranging from 6% to 25% (a 100% slope is a 45° angle).
Blue Square	■	Intermediate	A Blue Square trail is of intermediate difficulty. These trails have gradients ranging from 25% to 40%.
Black Diamond	◆	Difficult	Black Diamond trails tend to be steep—typically 40% and up.

Slope can also be considered as an **average rate of change**.

EXAMPLE 2 **Life Science: Amount Spent on Cancer Research.** The amount spent on cancer research has increased steadily over the years and is approximated in the following graph. Find the average rate of change of the amount spent on the research.

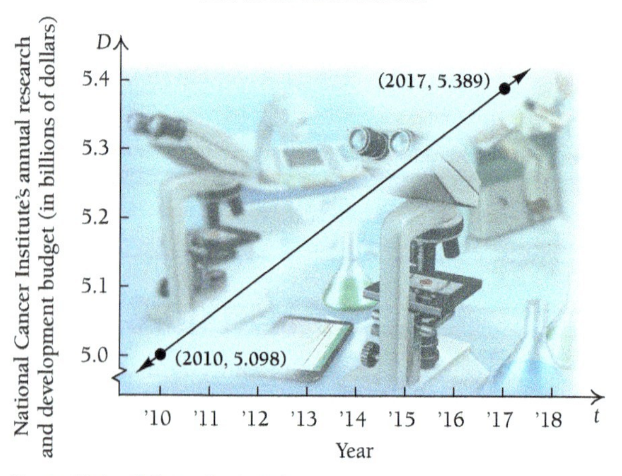

(*Source*: National Cancer Institute.)

Solution First, we determine the coordinates of two points on the graph, which are given as (2010, \$5.098) and (2017, \$5.389). Then we compute the slope, or rate of change, as follows:

$$\text{Slope} = \text{average rate of change} = \frac{\text{change in } D}{\text{change in } t}$$

$$= \frac{\$5.389 - \$5.098}{2017 - 2010} = \frac{\$0.291}{7} \approx \$0.0416 \text{ billion/yr.}$$

Horizontal and Vertical Lines

Let's consider the graphs of $y = c$ and $x = a$, where c and a are real numbers.

EXAMPLE 3

a) Graph $y = 4$.

b) Does the graph represent a function? Why or why not?

c) What is the line's slope?

Solution

a) The graph consists of all ordered pairs whose second coordinate is 4. For example, $(-2, 4)$ and $(1, 4)$ are two points on the graph, since their second coordinate is 4. The resulting graph is a horizontal line.

b) No vertical line will cross the graph more than once. The graph represents a function, since it passes the vertical-line test.

c) Since there is no change in y, the line's slope is 0.

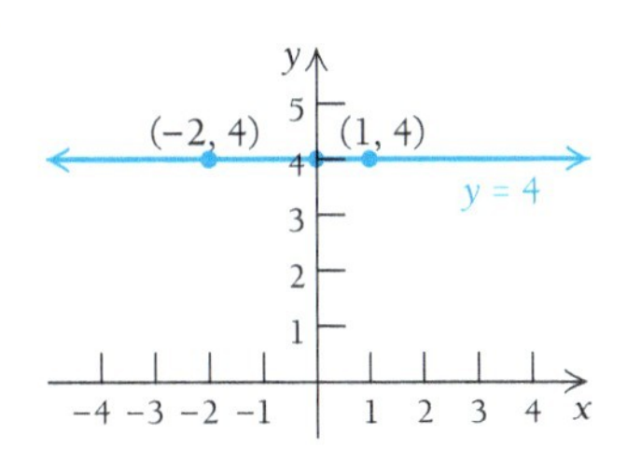

EXAMPLE 4

a) Graph $x = -3$.

b) Does the graph represent a function? Why or why not?

c) What is the line's slope?

Solution

a) The graph consists of all ordered pairs whose first coordinate is -3. For example, $(-3, 1)$ and $(-3, 4)$ are two points on the graph, since their first coordinate is -3. The resulting graph is a vertical line.

b) This graph does not represent a function because it fails the vertical-line test. A vertical line at $x = -3$ crosses the graph more than once—in fact, infinitely many times.

c) Since there is no change in x, this line's slope is undefined.

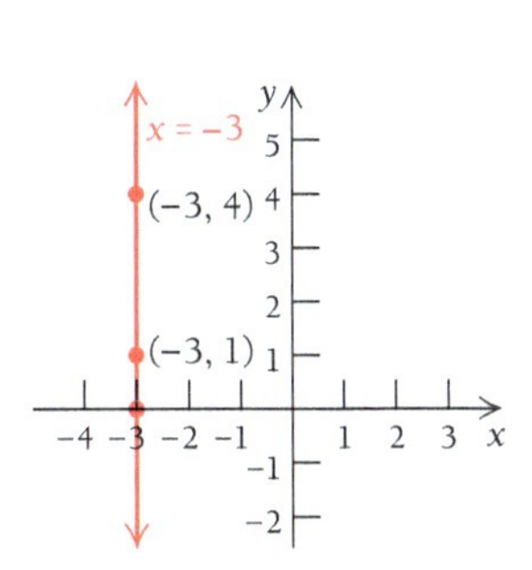

Quick Check 2

Graph each equation:

a) $x = 4$; **b)** $y = -3$.

In general, we have the following.

DEFINITION

The graph of $y = c$, or $f(x) = c$, a horizontal line, is the graph of a function. Such a function is referred to as a **constant function**.

The graph of $x = a$ is a vertical line and does not represent a function.

Equations of the Form $y = mx$ or $y = mx + b$

Consider the following table of numbers and look for a pattern.

x	0	1	-1	$-\frac{1}{2}$	2	-2	3	-7	5
y	0	3	-3	$-\frac{3}{2}$	6	-6	9	-21	15

Note that the ratio of the y-value to the x-value is 3 to 1. That is,

$$y = 3x.$$

Ordered pairs from the table can be used to graph $y = 3x$ (see the figure at the left). Note that this is a function and that 3 is the slope between any two pairs of points in the table.

DEFINITION

The graph of the function given by

$$y = mx \quad \text{or} \quad f(x) = mx$$

is the straight line through the origin $(0, 0)$ and the point $(1, m)$.

Various graphs of $y = mx$ for $m > 0$ are shown on the left below. Such graphs slant up from left to right and rise faster when m is larger.

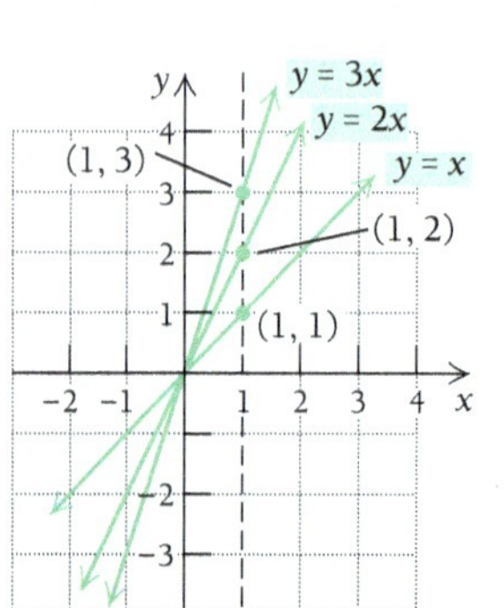

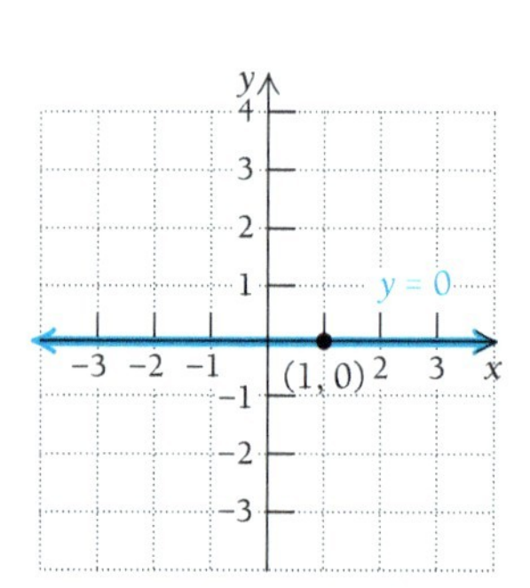

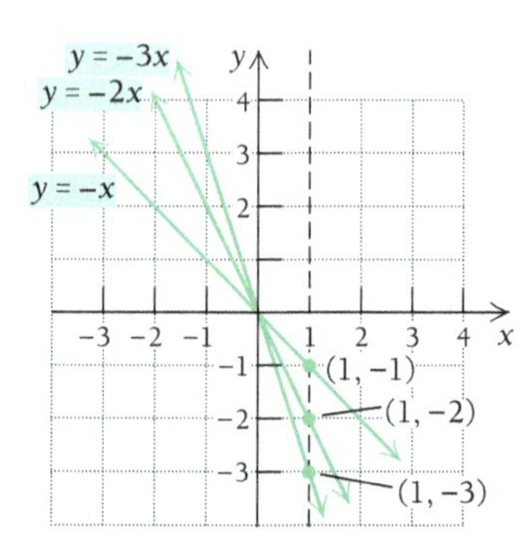

When $m = 0$, we have $y = 0x$, or $y = 0$. In the middle above is a graph of $y = 0$. Note that this is both the x-axis and a horizontal line. Graphs of $y = mx$ for $m < 0$ are shown on the right above. Note that such graphs slant down from left to right.

Quick Check 3 ✓

Graph each equation:

a) $y = \frac{1}{2}x$;

b) $y = -\frac{1}{2}x$.

3 ✓

For equations of the form $y = mx$, where $m > 0$, $x \geq 0$, and $y \geq 0$, we say that y is **proportional** to x (or that y *varies directly* with x) and that m is the **constant of proportionality** (or the *constant of variation*).

EXAMPLE 5 **Physical Science: Weight on Earth and the Moon.** The weight M, in pounds, of an object on the moon is proportional to the weight E of that object on Earth. An astronaut who weighs 180 lb on Earth will weigh 28.8 lb on the moon.

a) Find an equation that relates weight on the moon, M, to weight on the Earth, E.

b) An astronaut weighs 120 lb on Earth. How much will the astronaut weigh on the moon?

Solution

a) The equation has the form $M = mE$. To find m, we substitute:

$$28.8 = m \cdot 180$$
$$\frac{28.8}{180} = m$$
$$0.16 = m.$$

Thus, $M = 0.16E$, where $E \geq 0$ and $M \geq 0$.

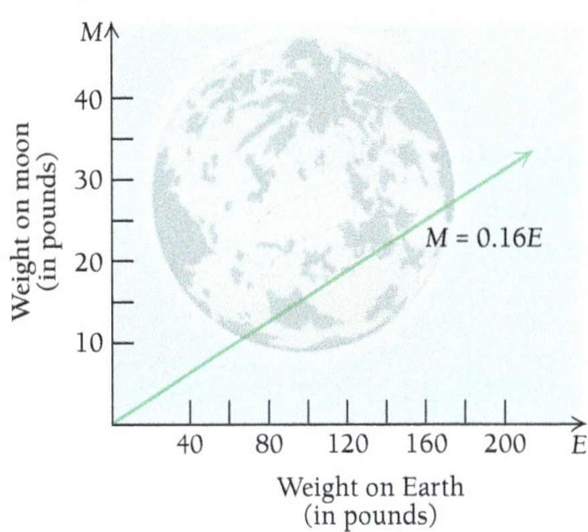

b) To find the weight on the moon of an astronaut who weighs 120 lb on Earth, we substitute 120 for E in the equation of variation,

$$M = 0.16 \cdot 120 \quad \text{Substituting 120 for } E$$
$$M = 19.2.$$

Thus, an astronaut who weighs 120 lb on Earth weighs 19.2 lb on the moon. 4 ✓

Quick Check 4 ✓

Measurements in inches and centimeters are proportional. For example, a length of 12 in. is the same as a length of 30.48 cm.

a) Find an equation that relates a length in centimeters to a length in inches.

b) The height of a table is 90 cm. Find this measurement in inches.

Compare the graphs of the equations

$$y = 3x \quad \text{and} \quad y = 3x - 2,$$

shown at the right. Note that the graph of $y = 3x - 2$ is shifted 2 units down from the graph of $y = 3x$, and that $y = 3x - 2$ has the y-*intercept* $(0, -2)$. Both graphs represent functions.

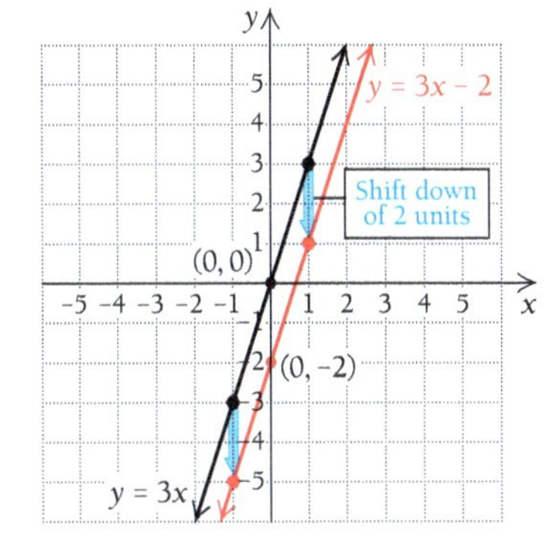

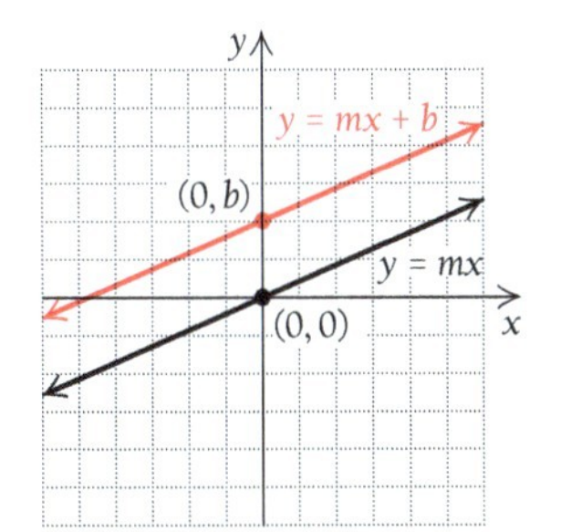

DEFINITION

A **linear function** is any function that can be written in the form

$$y = mx + b \quad \text{or} \quad f(x) = mx + b.$$

Its graph has the same slope, m, as the graph of $y = mx$ and crosses the y-axis at $(0, b)$. The point $(0, b)$ is called the **y-intercept**. (See the figure at the left.)

Two lines that have the same slope but different y-intercepts are **parallel**. The graphs of $y = mx$ and $y = mx + b$ (for $b \neq 0$) are parallel lines for any value of m.

The Slope–Intercept Equation

Every nonvertical line is uniquely determined by its slope m and its y-intercept $(0, b)$. In other words, the slope describes the "slant" of the line, and the y-intercept locates the point at which the line crosses the y-axis. Thus, we have the following.

DEFINITION

$y = mx + b$ is called the **slope–intercept equation** of a line.

EXAMPLE 6 Find the slope and the y-intercept of the graph of $2x - 4y - 7 = 0$.

Solution We solve for y:

$$2x - 4y - 7 = 0$$

$$4y = 2x - 7 \quad \text{Adding } 4y \text{ to both sides and reversing the equation}$$

$$y = \frac{2}{4}x - \frac{7}{4} \quad \text{Dividing both sides by 4}$$

Slope: $\frac{1}{2}$ y-intercept: $(0, -\frac{7}{4})$ **5 ✓**

Quick Check 5 ✓

Find the slope and the y-intercept of the graph of $3x - 6y - 7 = 0$.

Technology Connection

Exploring *b*

To explore the effect of b when graphing $y = mx + b$, let $y_1 = x$, $y_2 = x + 3$, and $y_3 = x - 4$.

EXERCISES

1. Graph y_1, y_2, and y_3. Then, without drawing them, describe how the graphs of $y = x$ and $y = x - 5$ compare.
2. Use the TABLE feature to compare the values of y_1, y_2, and y_3 when $x = 0$. Then scroll through other values and describe a pattern.

The Point–Slope Equation

Suppose we know the slope of a line and any point on the line. We can use these to find an equation of the line.

EXAMPLE 7 Find an equation of the line with slope 3 containing the point $(-1, -5)$.

Solution The slope is given as $m = 3$. From the slope–intercept equation, we have

$$y = 3x + b. \quad (1)$$

To determine b, we substitute -5 for y and -1 for x:

$$-5 = 3(-1) + b$$

$$-5 = -3 + b,$$

so $$-2 = b$$

Then, replacing b in equation (1) with -2, we get $y = 3x - 2$.

There is a faster way to find an equation for a line when we know the slope and any point on the line. Suppose (x_1, y_1) is on the line given by

$$y = mx + b. \quad (2)$$

Then it follows that

$$y_1 = mx_1 + b. \quad (3)$$

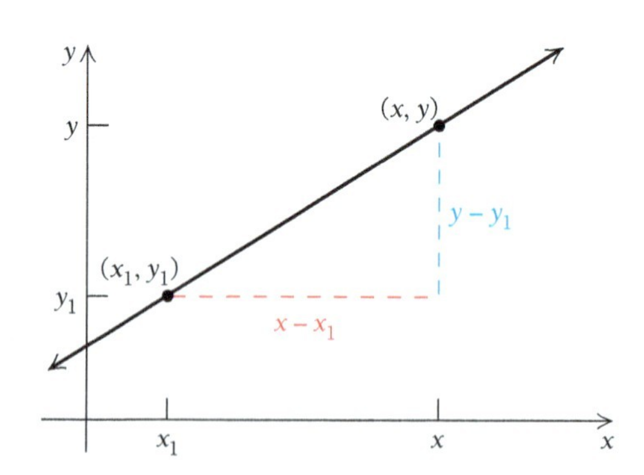

Subtracting the left and right sides of equation (3) from the left and right sides of equation (2), we have

$$y - y_1 = (mx + b) - (mx_1 + b)$$

$$= mx + b - mx_1 - b \quad \text{Simplifying}$$

$$= mx - mx_1 \quad \text{Combining like terms}$$

$$= m(x - x_1). \quad \text{Factoring}$$

DEFINITION

$y - y_1 = m(x - x_1)$ is called the **point–slope equation** of a line. The graph includes the point (x_1, y_1), and the slope is m.

EXAMPLE 8 Find the equation of the line containing the points $(-1, 4)$ and $(3, -6)$. Then, determine the line's y-intercept and express it as an ordered pair.

Solution We first find the slope:

$$m = \frac{-6 - 4}{3 - (-1)} \quad \text{Substituting}$$

$$= -\frac{10}{4}, \text{ or } -\frac{5}{2}.$$

Now, we use the point–slope equation of the line with $m = -\frac{5}{2}$ and either of the two given points as (x_1, y_1). Let's use $(-1, 4)$:

$$y - 4 = -\frac{5}{2}[x - (-1)] \quad \text{Substituting}$$

$$y - 4 = -\frac{5}{2}(x + 1)$$

$$y - 4 = -\frac{5}{2}x - \frac{5}{2} \quad \text{Distributing}$$

$$y - 4 + 4 = -\frac{5}{2}x - \frac{5}{2} + 4 \quad \text{Adding 4 to both sides}$$

$$y = -\frac{5}{2}x + \frac{3}{2} \quad \text{Simplifying to the slope–intercept form}$$

If we used the other point, $(3, -6)$, we would get the same result. We leave this for the student to confirm. The line's y-intercept is $(0, \frac{3}{2})$. 6 ✓

Quick Check 6 ✓

Find the equation of the line containing the points $(2, 7)$ and $(4, -9)$, and determine its y-intercept expressed as an ordered pair.

Applications of Linear Functions

Many applications are modeled by linear functions.

EXAMPLE 9 **Business: Total Cost.** Raggs, Ltd., a clothing firm, has **fixed costs** of \$10,000 per month. These costs, such as rent, maintenance, and so on, must be paid no matter how much the company produces. To produce x units of a certain kind of suit, it costs \$20 per suit (unit) in addition to the fixed costs. That is, the **variable costs** for producing x of these suits are $20x$ dollars. These costs are due to the amount produced and cover material, wages, fuel, and so on. The **total cost** $C(x)$ of producing x suits in a month is given by

$$C(x) = (\text{Variable costs}) + (\text{Fixed costs}) = 20x + 10{,}000.$$

a) Graph the variable-cost, fixed-cost, and total-cost functions.

b) What is the total cost of producing 100 suits? 400 suits?

Solution

a) The variable-cost and fixed-cost functions are graphed on the left below.

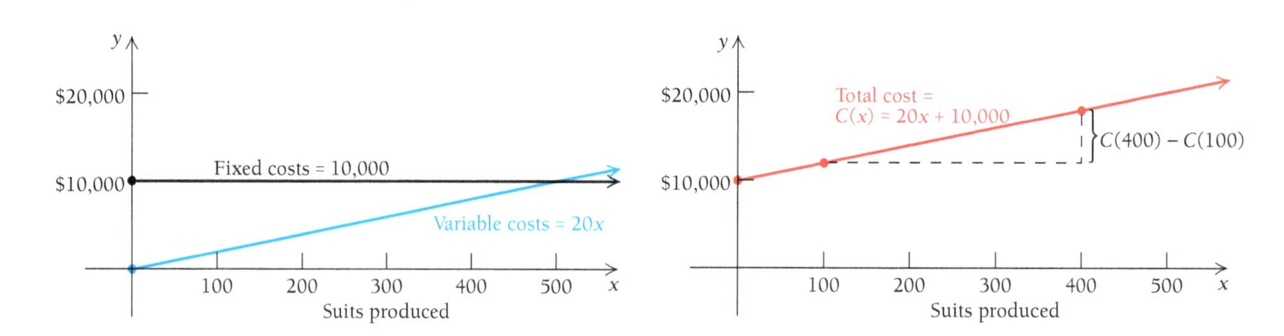

The total-cost function is shown in the graph on the right. From a practical standpoint, the domains of these functions are nonnegative integers 0, 1, 2, 3, and so on, since it does not make sense to make either a negative number or a fractional number of suits. It is common practice to draw such graphs as though the domains were the entire set of nonnegative real numbers.

b) The total cost of producing 100 suits is

$$C(100) = 20 \cdot 100 + 10{,}000 = \$12{,}000.$$

The total cost of producing 400 suits is

$$C(400) = 20 \cdot 400 + 10{,}000 = \$18{,}000.$$

EXAMPLE 10 **Business: Profit-and-Loss Analysis.** When a business sells an item, it receives the *price* paid by the consumer (this is normally greater than the *cost* to the business of producing the item).

a) The **total revenue** that a business receives is the product of the number of items sold and the price paid per item. Thus, if Raggs, Ltd., sells x suits at \$80 per suit, the total revenue $R(x)$, in dollars, is given by

$$R(x) = \text{Unit price} \cdot \text{Quantity sold} = 80x.$$

If $C(x) = 20x + 10{,}000$ (see Example 9), graph R and C using the same set of axes.

b) The **total profit** that a business makes is the amount left after all costs have been subtracted from the total revenue. Thus, if $P(x)$ represents the total profit when x items are produced and sold, we have

$$P(x) = (\text{Total revenue}) - (\text{Total costs}) = R(x) - C(x).$$

Determine $P(x)$, and draw its graph using the same set of axes used for the graph in part (a).

c) The company will *break even* at that value of x for which $P(x) = 0$ (that is, no profit and no loss). This is the point at which $R(x) = C(x)$. Find the **break-even value** of x.

Solution

a) The graphs of $R(x) = 80x$ and $C(x) = 20x + 10{,}000$ are shown on the next page. When $C(x)$ is above $R(x)$, a loss occurs. This is shown by the region shaded red. When $R(x)$ is above $C(x)$, a gain occurs. This is shown by the region shaded gray.

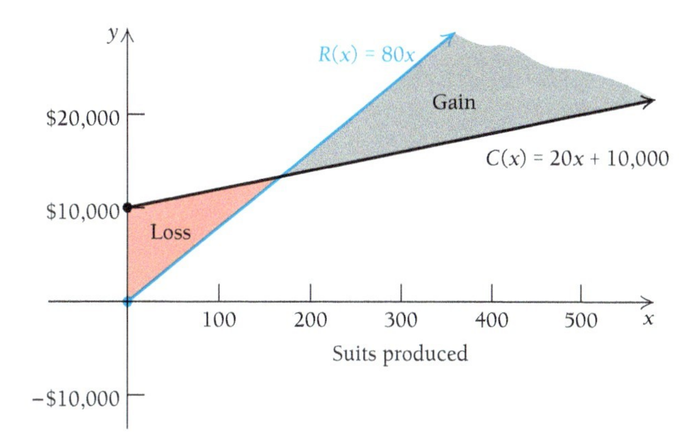

b) To find P, the profit function, we have

$$P(x) = R(x) - C(x) = 80x - (20x + 10{,}000)$$
$$= 60x - 10{,}000.$$

The graph of $P(x) = 60x - 10{,}000$ is shown by the heavy line. The red portion of the line shows a "negative" profit, or a loss. The black portion of the heavy line shows a "positive" profit, or a gain.

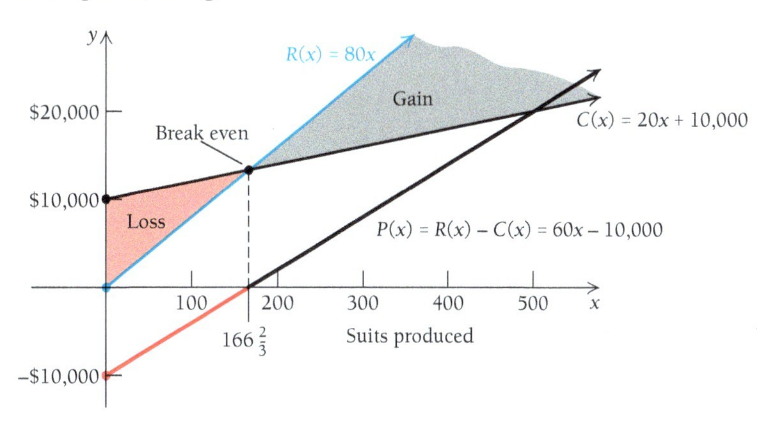

c) To find the break-even value, we solve $R(x) = C(x)$:

$$R(x) = C(x)$$
$$80x = 20x + 10{,}000$$
$$60x = 10{,}000$$
$$x = 166\tfrac{2}{3}.$$

How do we interpret the fractional answer, since it does not make sense to produce $\frac{2}{3}$ of a suit? We can round to 167, assuming that an estimated break-even value is sufficient. **7 ✓**

Quick Check 7 ✓

Business. Suppose that in Examples 9 and 10 fixed costs are increased to $20,000. Find:

a) the total-cost, total-revenue, and total-profit functions;

b) the break-even value.

Section Summary

- The slope m of a line containing the points (x_1, y_1) and (x_2, y_2) is given by $m = \dfrac{y_2 - y_1}{x_2 - x_1}$.
- The slope of a line can be interpreted as $\dfrac{\text{change in } y}{\text{change in } x}$.
- A horizontal line has slope $m = 0$, and a vertical line has an undefined slope.
- Graphs of functions that are straight lines (*linear functions*) are characterized by an equation of the type $f(x) = mx + b$, where m is the slope and $(0, b)$ is the *y-intercept*, the point at which the graph crosses the y-axis.
- The form $y = mx + b$ is called the *slope–intercept equation* of a line.
- The *point–slope equation* of a line is $y - y_1 = m(x - x_1)$, where (x_1, y_1) is a point on the line and m is the slope.

R.4 Exercise Set

Graph. List the slope and y-intercept.

1. $y = -2x$
2. $y = -3x$
3. $f(x) = -0.5x$
4. $f(x) = 0.5x$
5. $y = 3x - 4$
6. $y = 2x - 5$
7. $g(x) = x - 2.5$
8. $g(x) = -x + 3$
9. $y = 7$
10. $y = -5$

Find the slope and y-intercept.

11. $y - 4x = 1$
12. $y - 3x = 6$
13. $2x + y - 3 = 0$
14. $2x - y + 3 = 0$
15. $3x - 3y + 6 = 0$
16. $2x + 2y + 8 = 0$
17. $x = 3y + 7$
18. $x = -4y + 3$

For Exercises 19–28, use the given point and slope to write (a) an equation of the line in point–slope form and (b) an equivalent equation of the line in slope–intercept form.

19. With $m = 7$, containing $(1, 7)$
20. With $m = -5$, containing $(-2, -3)$
21. With $m = -2$, containing $(2, 3)$
22. With $m = -3$, containing $(5, -2)$
23. With slope -5, containing $(5, 0)$
24. With slope 2, containing $(3, 0)$
25. With y-intercept $(0, -6)$ and slope $\frac{1}{2}$
26. With y-intercept $(0, 7)$ and slope $\frac{4}{3}$
27. With slope 0, containing $(4, 8)$
28. With slope 0, containing $(2, 3)$

For Exercises 29–50, find (a) the slope (if it is defined) of a line containing the two given points, (b) the equation of the line containing the two points in the slope–intercept form, and (c) the ordered pair identifying the line's y-intercept, assuming that it exists. If appropriate, state whether the line is vertical or horizontal.

29. $(1, 5)$ and $(3, 9)$
30. $(2, -11)$ and $(5, 1)$
31. $(0, 4)$ and $(-3, 1)$
32. $(5, 1)$ and $(0, 21)$
33. $(2, -3)$ and $(-3, -5)$
34. $(-11, 2)$ and $(1, 4)$
35. $(-8, -3)$ and $(-3, -12)$
36. $(-5, 13)$ and $(-2, -6)$
37. $(4, 6)$ and $(7, 6)$
38. $(3, -1)$ and $(8, -1)$
39. $(6, 0)$ and $(10, 0)$
40. $(1, 0)$ and $(100, 0)$
41. $(4, 4)$ and $(4, 9)$
42. $(-6, 3)$ and $(-6, 7)$
43. $(0, 1)$ and $(0, -9)$
44. $(0, 0)$ and $(0, 50)$
45. $\left(\frac{3}{2}, -\frac{1}{2}\right)$ and $\left(2, -\frac{1}{3}\right)$
46. $\left(\frac{1}{4}, 5\right)$ and $\left(-\frac{3}{4}, \frac{5}{4}\right)$
47. $\left(\frac{1}{2}, \frac{1}{3}\right)$ and $\left(\frac{1}{4}, \frac{1}{5}\right)$
48. $\left(-\frac{3}{4}, \frac{4}{3}\right)$ and $\left(\frac{2}{5}, -\frac{5}{2}\right)$
49. (h, k) and $(h + 2, k + 3)$
50. $(u, v + 3)$ and $(u - 3, v)$
51. Find the slope (or grade) of the treadmill.

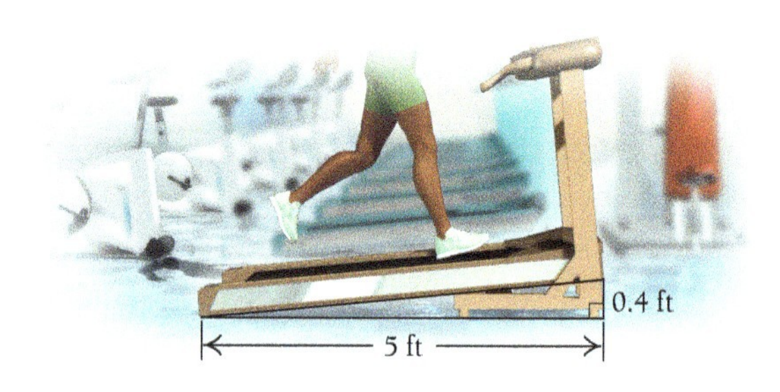

52. Find the slope of the skateboard ramp.

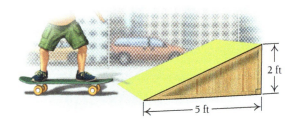

53. Find the slope (or head) of the river. Express the answer as a percentage.

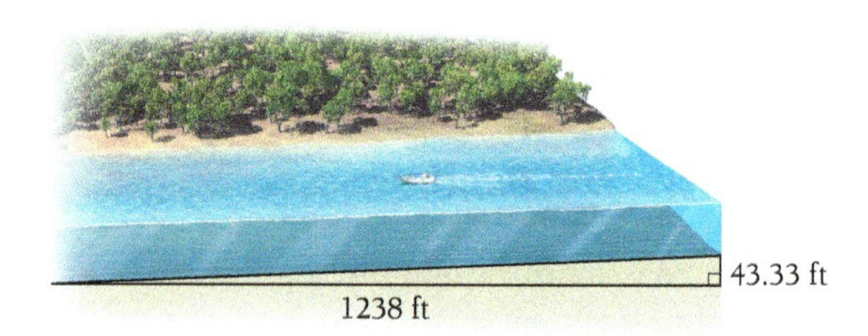

54. Find the slope (or rake) of the stairway.

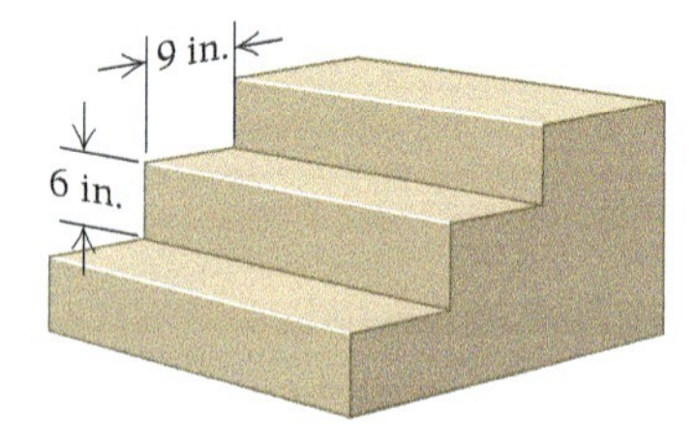

55. **Solar panel tilt.** Find the slope for the optimum tilt of a solar panel at latitude 35° N. (*Source:* solarpaneltilt.com.)

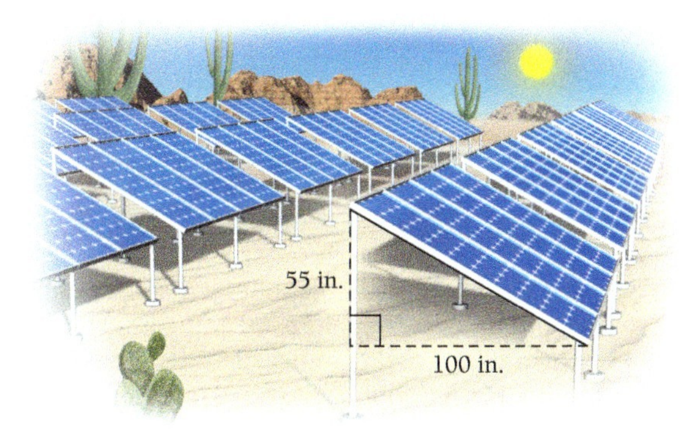

56. **Solar panel tilt.** Find the slope for the optimum tilt of a solar panel at latitude 50° N. (*Source:* solarpaneltilt.com.)

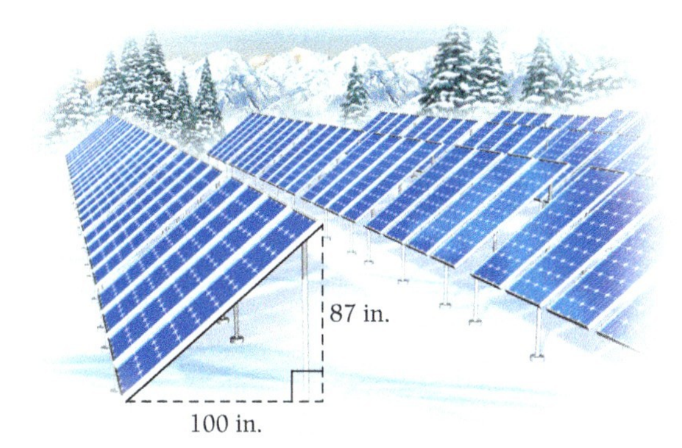

APPLICATIONS

Business and Economics

57. **Highway tolls.** It has been suggested that since heavier vehicles are responsible for more wear and tear on highways, drivers should pay tolls in direct proportion to the weight of their vehicles. Suppose a Toyota Camry weighing 3350 lb is charged $2.70 for traveling an 80-mi stretch of highway.
   a) Find an equation in slope–intercept form that expresses the amount of the toll T as a function of the vehicle's weight w.
   b) What is the toll if a 3700-lb Jeep Cherokee travels the same 80-mi stretch of highway?

58. **Inkjet cartridges.** A registrar's office finds that the number of inkjet cartridges, I, required each year for its copiers and printers varies directly with the number of students enrolled, s.
   a) Find an equation in slope–intercept form that expresses I as a function of s, if the office requires 16 cartridges when 2800 students enroll.
   b) How many cartridges would be required if 3100 students enrolled?

59. **Profit-and-loss analysis.** Boxowitz, Inc., is planning to produce a new graphing calculator. For the first year, the fixed costs for setting up the new production line are $1,000,000. The variable costs for each calculator are $3. The sales department projects that 150,000 calculators will be sold during the first year at a price of $75 each.
   a) Find and graph $C(x)$, the total cost of producing x calculators.
   b) Using the same axes as in part (a), find and graph $R(x)$, the total revenue from the sale of x calculators.
   c) Using the same axes as in part (a), find and graph $P(x)$, the total profit from the production and sale of x calculators.
   d) What profit or loss will the firm realize if the expected sale of 150,000 calculators occurs?
   e) How many calculators must the firm sell in order to break even?

60. **Profit-and-loss analysis.** Red Tide is planning a new line of skis. For the first year, the fixed costs for setting up production are $45,000. The variable costs for producing each pair of skis are estimated at $80, and the selling price will be $450 per pair. It is projected that 3000 pairs will sell the first year.
   a) Find and graph $C(x)$, the total cost of producing x pairs of skis.
   b) Find and graph $R(x)$, the total revenue from the sale of x pairs of skis. Use the same axes as in part (a).
   c) Using the same axes as in part (a), find and graph $P(x)$, the total profit from the production and sale of x pairs of skis.
   d) What profit or loss will the company realize if the expected sale of 3000 pairs occurs?
   e) How many pairs must the company sell in order to break even?

61. **Profit-and-loss analysis.** Jamal decides to mow lawns to earn money. The initial cost of his electric lawnmower is $250. Electricity and maintenance costs are $4 per lawn.
   a) Formulate a function $C(x)$ for the total cost of mowing x lawns.
   b) Jamal determines that the total-profit function for the lawn-mowing business is given by $P(x) = 16x - 250$. Find a function for the total revenue from mowing x lawns. How much does Jamal charge per lawn?
   c) How many lawns must Jamal mow before he begins making a profit?

62. **Profit-and-loss analysis.** Raven Entertainment rents an auditorium that seats 3000 people for a performance by a musical act. The rent is $25,000, and Raven Entertainment calculates that the variable cost is $5 per patron.
   a) Formulate a function $C(x)$ for the total cost of renting the auditorium.
   b) Raven Entertainment determines that the total-profit function is given by $P(x) = 20x - 25{,}000$. Find a function for the total revenue from selling x tickets. How much does each ticket cost?
   c) How many tickets must be sold for Raven Entertainment to break even?

63. **Straight-line depreciation.** Quick Copy buys an office machine for $5200 on January 1 of a given year.

The machine is expected to last for 8 yr, at the end of which time its *salvage value* will be \$1100. If the company figures the decline in value to be the same each year, then the *straight-line depreciation value*, $V(t)$, after t years, $0 \leq t \leq 8$, is given by

$$V(t) = C - t\left(\frac{C - S}{N}\right),$$

where C is the original cost of the item, N is the number of years of expected life, and S is the salvage value. $V(t)$ is also called the *book value*.

a) Find the linear function for the straight-line depreciation of the machine.
b) Find the book value of the machine after 0 yr, 1 yr, 2 yr, 3 yr, 4 yr, 7 yr, and 8 yr.

64. Straight-line depreciation. (See Exercise 63.) Hanna's Photography spends \$40 per square foot on improvements to a 25,000-ft^2 office space. Suppose that according to tax guidelines for straight-line depreciation, these improvements will depreciate completely—that is, have zero salvage value—after 39 yr. Find the depreciated value of the improvements after 10 yr.

65. Straight-line depreciation. The Video Game Wizard buys a new computer system for \$60,000 and projects that its book value will be \$2000 after 5 yr. Using straight-line depreciation (see Exercise 63), find the book value after 3 yr.

66. Straight-line depreciation. Tyline Electric uses the function $B(t) = -700t + 3500$ to find the book value, $B(t)$, in dollars, of a photocopier t years after its purchase.

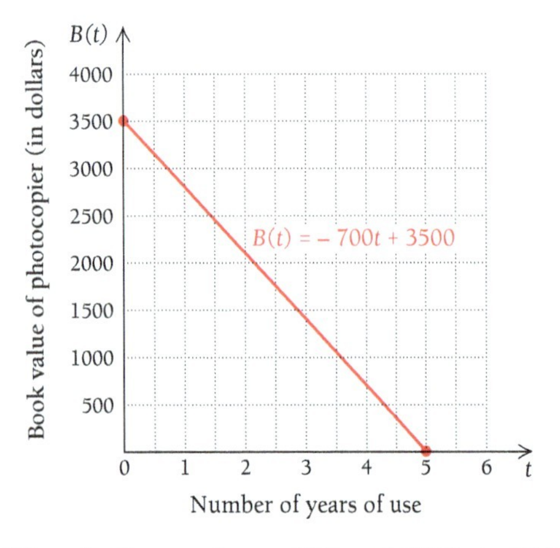

a) What do the numbers -700 and 3500 signify?
b) How long will it take the copier to depreciate completely?
c) What is the practical domain of B? Explain.

General Interest

67. Stair requirements. A North Carolina state law requires that stairs have minimum treads of 9 in. and maximum risers of 8.25 in. (*Source*: North Carolina Office of the State Fire Marshal.) According to this law, what is the maximum grade of stairs in North Carolina?

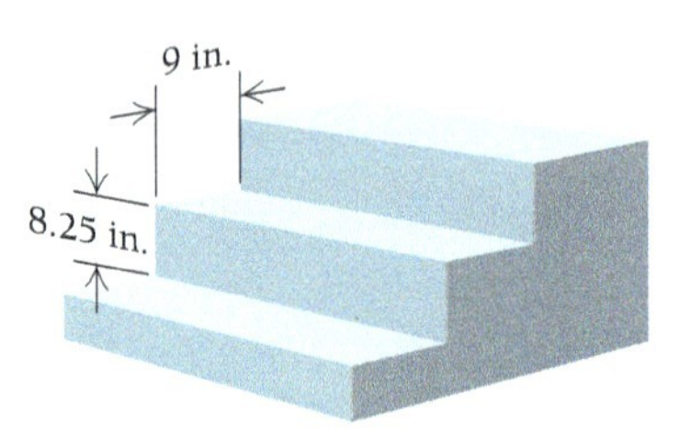

68. Low-pitch roof. Shingles cannot be installed on roofs with a pitch lower than 4:12, meaning a vertical rise of 4 ft over a horizontal distance of 12 ft. What is the minimum pitch a roof has to have in order for shingles to be installed?

ROOF PITCH

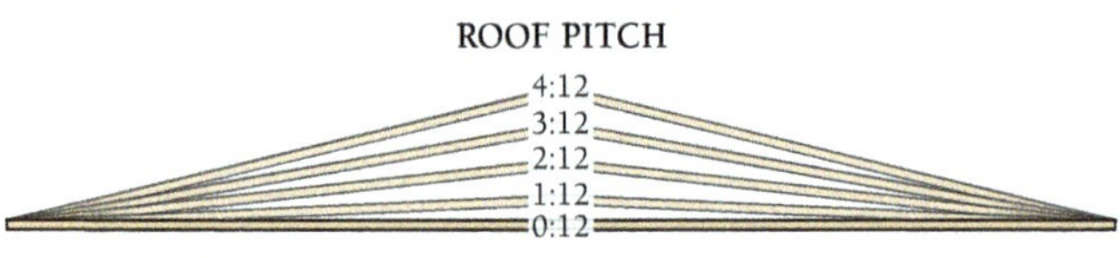

(*Source*: www.inspectapedia.com.)

69. Health insurance premiums. Find the average rate of change in the annual premium for a family's health insurance.

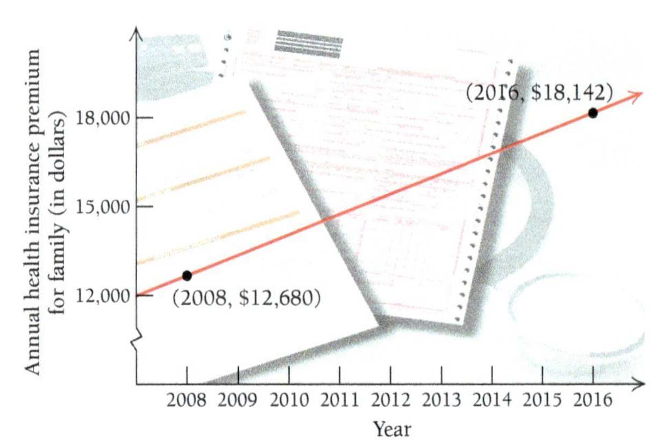

(*Source*: The Kaiser Family Foundation; time.com/money.)

70. Health insurance premiums. Find the average rate of change in the annual premium for a single person.

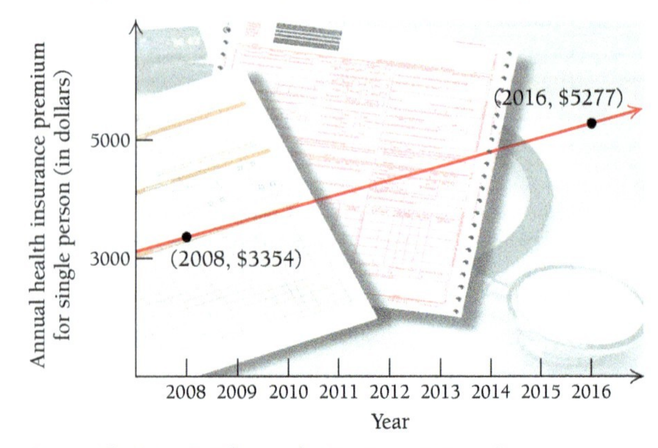

(*Source*: The Kaiser Family Foundation; time.com/money.)

71. Two-year college tuition. Find the average rate of change of the tuition and fees at public two-year colleges.

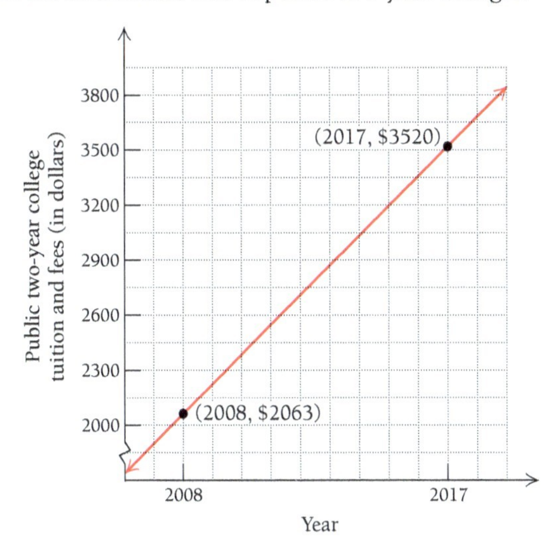

(*Source*: U.S. National Center for Education Statistics, *Digest of Education Statistics*, annual.)

72. Organic food sales. Find the average rate of change of organic food sales in the United States.

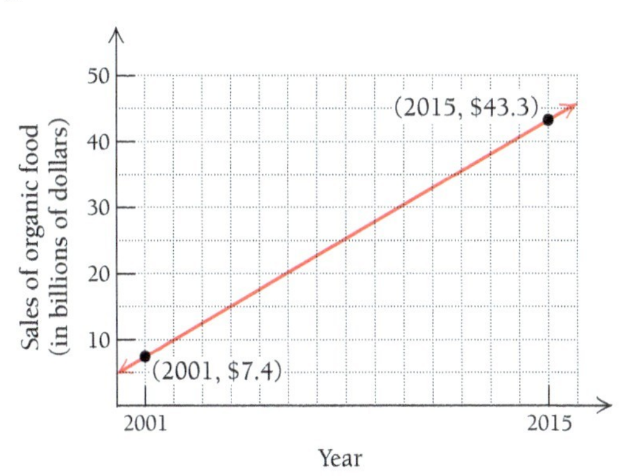

(*Source*: www.ota.com.)

73. Energy conservation. The R-factor of home insulation is proportional to its thickness T.

a) Find an equation of the form $R = mT$ if $R = 12.51$ when $T = 3$ in.

b) What is the R-factor for insulation that is 6 in. thick?

74. Nerve impulse speed. Impulses in nerve fibers travel at a speed of 293 ft/sec. The distance D, in feet, traveled in t sec is given by $D = 293t$. How long would it take an impulse to travel from the brain to the toes of a person who is 6 ft tall?

75. Muscle weight. The weight M of a person's muscles is proportional to the person's body weight W.

a) It is known that a person weighing 200 lb has 80 lb of muscles. Find an equation expressing M as a function of W.

b) Express the slope as a percentage, and interpret the resulting equation.

c) What is the muscle weight of a person weighing 120 lb?

76. Brain weight. The weight B of a person's brain is proportional to the person's body weight W.

a) It is known that a person weighing 120 lb has a brain that weighs 3 lb. Find an equation expressing B as a function of W.

b) Express the slope as a percentage, and interpret its meaning.

c) What is the weight of the brain of a person weighing 160 lb?

77. Stopping distance on glare ice. The stopping distance (at some fixed speed) of regular tires on glare ice is a linear function of the air temperature F,

$$D(F) = 2F + 115,$$

where $D(F)$ is the stopping distance, in feet, when the air temperature is F, in degrees Fahrenheit.

a) Find $D(0°)$, $D(-20°)$, $D(10°)$, and $D(32°)$.

b) Interpret the meaning of the slope in the context of this problem.

c) Explain why the domain should be restricted to the interval $[-57.5°, 32°]$.

78. Reaction time. While driving a car, you see a child suddenly crossing the street. Your brain registers the emergency and sends a signal to your foot to hit the brake. The car travels a reaction distance D, in feet, during the time it takes you to react, where D is a function of the car's speed r, in miles per hour. That reaction distance is a linear function given by

$$D(r) = \frac{11r + 5}{10}.$$

a) Find $D(5)$, $D(10)$, $D(20)$, $D(50)$, and $D(65)$.

b) Graph $D(r)$.

c) Interpret the meaning of the slope in the context of this problem.

d) What is the domain of the function? Explain.

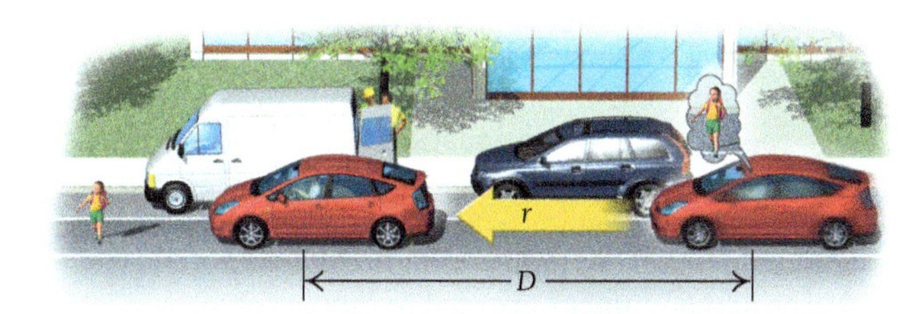

79. Estimating heights. An anthropologist can use certain linear functions to estimate the height of a male or female, given the length of certain bones. The *humerus* is the bone from the elbow to the shoulder. Let x = the length of the humerus, in centimeters. Then the height, in centimeters, of a male with a humerus of length x is given by

$$M(x) = 2.89x + 70.64.$$

The height, in centimeters, of a female with a humerus of length x is given by

$$F(x) = 2.75x + 71.48.$$

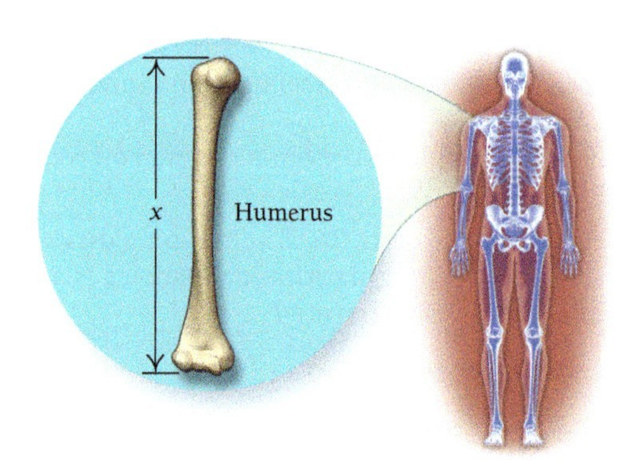

A 26-cm humerus was uncovered in some ruins.

a) If we assume it was from a male, how tall was he?
b) If we assume it was from a female, how tall was she?

80. Mobile-only Facebook users. At the end of 2013, 296 million people accessed Facebook using a mobile device only. By the end of 2015, that figure had risen to 823 million people. (*Source*: facebook.com.)

a) Letting the year be the x-coordinate and the number of mobile-only users, in millions, be the y-coordinate, find the equation of the line that contains the data points.
b) Use the equation in part (a) to estimate the number of people who will access Facebook using only a mobile device in 2020.
c) Explain why a linear equation is not a good model for estimating the number of mobile-only Facebook users in 2030, 2040, and so on.

81. Manatee population. In January 2005, 3143 manatees were counted in an aerial survey of Florida. In January 2017, 6620 manatees were counted. (*Source*: Florida Fish and Wildlife Conservation Commission.)

a) Letting the number of years since 2005 be the x-coordinate and the number of manatees be the y-coordinate, find an equation of the line that contains the two data points.
b) Use the equation in part (a) to estimate the number of manatees counted in January 2011.
c) The actual number counted in January 2011 was 4834. Does the equation found in part (a) give an accurate representation of the number of manatees counted each year? Why or why not?

82. Urban population. The population of Woodland is P. After growing 2%, the new population is N.

a) Assuming that N is proportional to P, find an equation that expresses N as a function of P.
b) Find N when $P = 200{,}000$.
c) Find P when $N = 367{,}200$.

83. Median age of women at first marriage. In general, people in our society are marrying at a later age. The median age, $A(t)$, of women at first marriage can be approximated by

$$A(t) = 0.08t + 19.7,$$

where t is the number of years after 1950. Thus, $A(0)$ is the median age of women at first marriage in 1950, $A(50)$ is the median age in 2000, and so on.

a) Find $A(0)$, $A(1)$, $A(10)$, $A(50)$, and $A(60)$.
b) What is the median age of women at first marriage in 2020?
c) Graph $A(t)$.

SYNTHESIS

84. Suppose (2, 5), (4, 13), and (7, y) all lie on the same line. Find y.

85. Describe one situation in which you would use the slope–intercept equation rather than the point–slope equation.

86. Business: daily sales. Match each sentence below with the most appropriate of the following graphs (I, II, III, or IV).

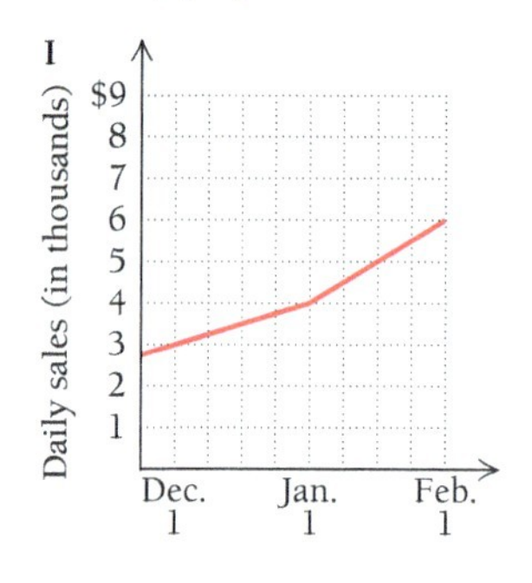

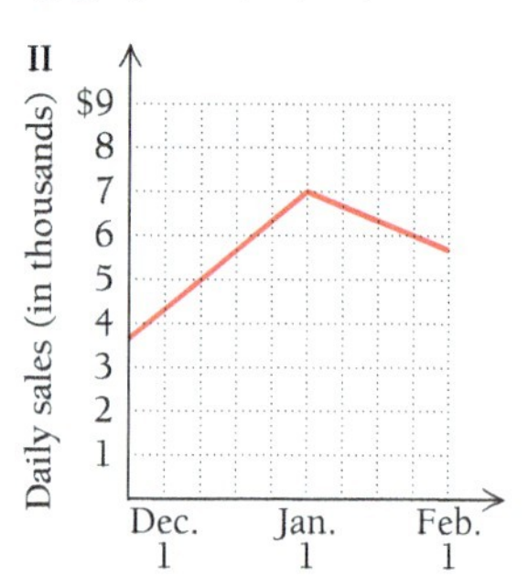

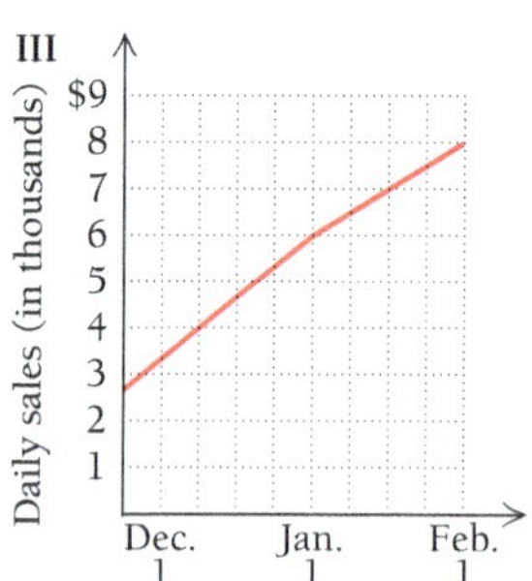

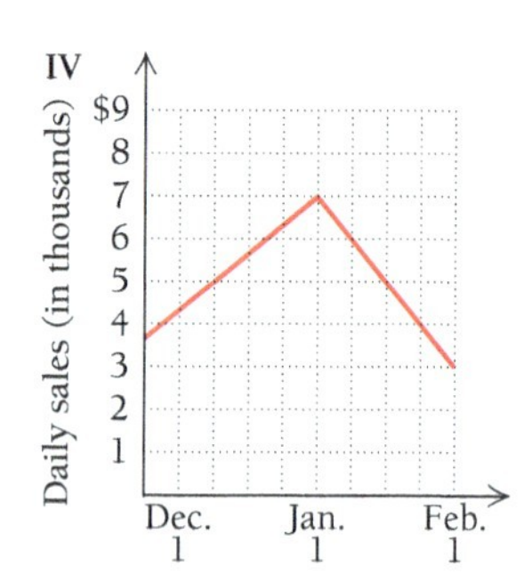

a) After January 1, daily sales continued to rise, but at a slower rate.
b) After January 1, sales decreased faster than they ever grew.
c) The rate of growth in daily sales doubled after January 1.
d) After January 1, daily sales decreased at half the rate that they grew in December.

87. Business: depreciation. A large crane is being depreciated according to the model $V(t) = 900 - 60t$, where $V(t)$ is in thousands of dollars and t is the number of years since 2005. If the crane is to be depreciated until its value is \$0, what is the practical domain of this model?

Technology Connection 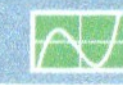

88. Graph some of the total-revenue, total-cost, and total-profit functions in this exercise set using the same set of axes. Identify regions of profit and loss.

Answers to Quick Checks

1. $m = 7$

2. (a) **(b)**

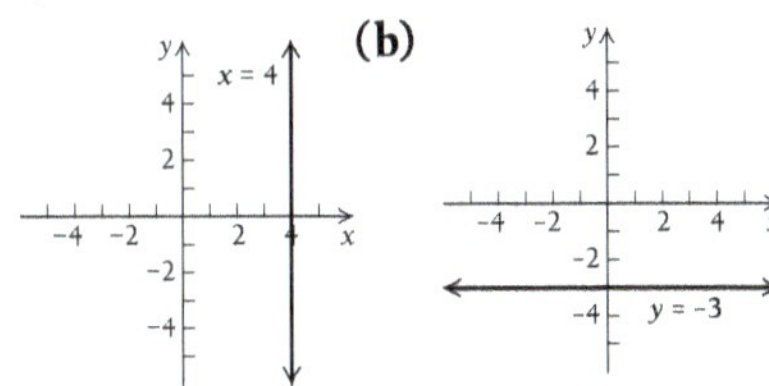

3. (a)

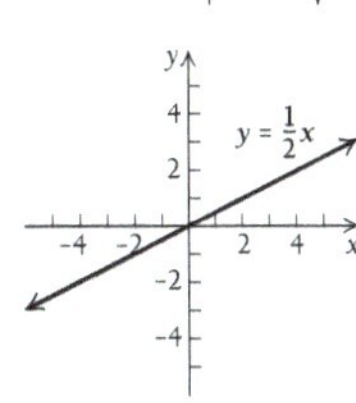

(b)

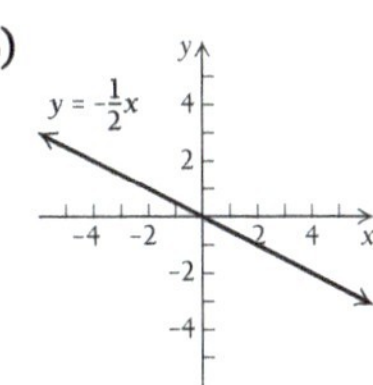

4. (a) Let x be a measurement in inches and y be a measurement in centimeters. Then $y = 2.54x$. **(b)** 35.4 in. **5.** $m = \frac{1}{2}$, y-intercept: $\left(0, -\frac{7}{6}\right)$ **6.** $y = -8x + 23$; $(0, 23)$ **7. (a)** $C(x) = 20x + 20{,}000$; $R(x) = 80x$; $P(x) = R(x) - C(x) = 60x - 20{,}000$; **(b)** 333 suits

R.5 Nonlinear Functions and Models

- Graph nonlinear functions and solve applied problems.
- Manipulate radical expressions and rational exponents.
- Determine the domain of a rational function and graph certain rational functions.
- Find the equilibrium point given a supply function and a demand function.

Many functions have graphs that are not lines. In this section, we study some of these **nonlinear functions** that we will use throughout this text.

Quadratic Functions

DEFINITION

A **quadratic function** f is given by

$$f(x) = ax^2 + bx + c, \quad \text{where } a \neq 0.$$

We have already encountered some quadratic functions—for example, $f(x) = x^2$ and $g(x) = x^2 - 1$. We can create hand-drawn graphs of quadratic functions using the following information.

The graph of a quadratic function given by $f(x) = ax^2 + bx + c$, where $a \neq 0$, is called a **parabola**.

a) It is always a cup-shaped curve, like those in Examples 1 and 2 that follow.

b) It opens upward if $a > 0$ and opens downward if $a < 0$.

c) Its turning point, or **vertex**, has a first coordinate given by $x = -\dfrac{b}{2a}$.

d) The vertical line $x = -b/(2a)$ is the **line of symmetry**, although it is not part of the graph.

EXAMPLE 1 Graph $f(x) = x^2 - 2x - 3$, and determine and label the vertex and the line of symmetry.

Solution Note that for $f(x) = 1x^2 - 2x - 3$, we have $a = 1$, $b = -2$, and $c = -3$. Since $a > 0$, the graph opens upward. The x-coordinate of the vertex is

$$\begin{aligned} x &= -\frac{b}{2a} \\ &= -\frac{-2}{2(1)} = 1. \end{aligned}$$

Substituting 1 for x, we find the second coordinate of the vertex, $f(1)$:

$$\begin{aligned} f(1) &= 1^2 - 2(1) - 3 \\ &= 1 - 2 - 3 \\ &= -4. \end{aligned}$$

The vertex is $(1, -4)$, and the line $x = 1$ is the line of symmetry of the graph. We choose x-values on each side of the vertex, compute y-values, plot the points, and graph the parabola.

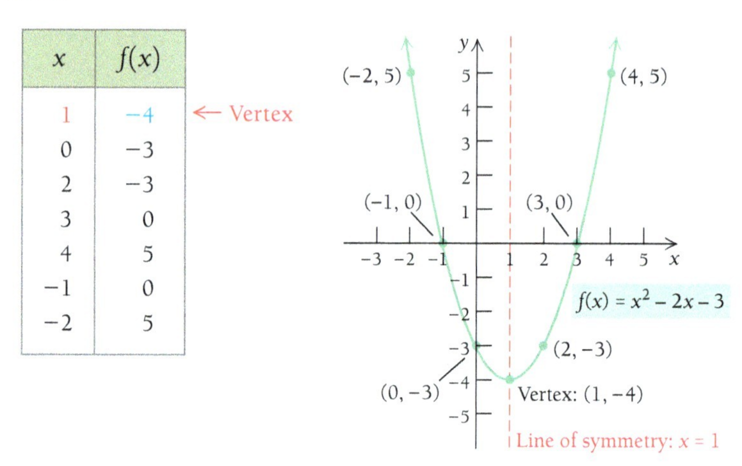

x	$f(x)$
1	−4
0	−3
2	−3
3	0
4	5
−1	0
−2	5

EXAMPLE 2 Graph $f(x) = -2x^2 + 10x - 7$, and determine and label the vertex and the line of symmetry.

Solution Note that $a = -2$, and since $a < 0$, the graph opens downward. The x-coordinate of the vertex is

$$\begin{aligned} x &= -\frac{b}{2a} \\ &= -\frac{10}{2(-2)} = \frac{5}{2}. \end{aligned}$$

Substituting $\frac{5}{2}$ for x in the equation, we calculate $f(\frac{5}{2})$, the second coordinate of the vertex:

$$\begin{aligned} y = f(\tfrac{5}{2}) &= -2(\tfrac{5}{2})^2 + 10(\tfrac{5}{2}) - 7 \\ &= -2(\tfrac{25}{4}) + 25 - 7 \\ &= \tfrac{11}{2}. \end{aligned}$$

The vertex is $(\frac{5}{2}, \frac{11}{2})$, and the line of symmetry is $x = \frac{5}{2}$. We choose x-values on each side of the vertex, compute y-values, plot the points, and graph the parabola:

x	$f(x)$
$\frac{5}{2}$	$\frac{11}{2}$
0	−7
1	1
2	5
3	5
4	1
5	−7

← Vertex

Vertex: $\left(\frac{5}{2}, \frac{11}{2}\right)$

$f(x) = -2x^2 + 10x - 7$

Line of symmetry: $x = \frac{5}{2}$

1 ✓

Quick Check 1 ✓

Graph each function:

a) $f(x) = x^2 + 2x - 3$;

b) $f(x) = -2x^2 - 10x - 5$.

The **x-intercepts** of any graph are those points, if they exist, where the graph intersects the x-axis. To find the x-intercepts of a quadratic function, we solve the quadratic equation:

$$ax^2 + bx + c = 0.$$

To solve such an equation, we first try to factor and use the Principle of Zero Products (see Appendix A at the end of the text). When factoring seems difficult or impossible, we use the quadratic formula. (See Appendix A for additional review of this important result.)

THEOREM 3 The Quadratic Formula

The solutions of any quadratic equation $ax^2 + bx + c = 0, a \neq 0$, are given by

$$x = \frac{-b \pm \sqrt{b^2 - 4ac}}{2a}.$$

Note that for $b^2 - 4ac < 0$, there are no real-number solutions and thus no x-intercepts.

Technology Connection

EXERCISES

1. a) Below is the graph of

$f(x) = x^2 - 6x + 8.$

Using *only* the graph, find the solutions of $x^2 - 6x + 8 = 0$.

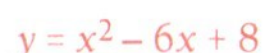

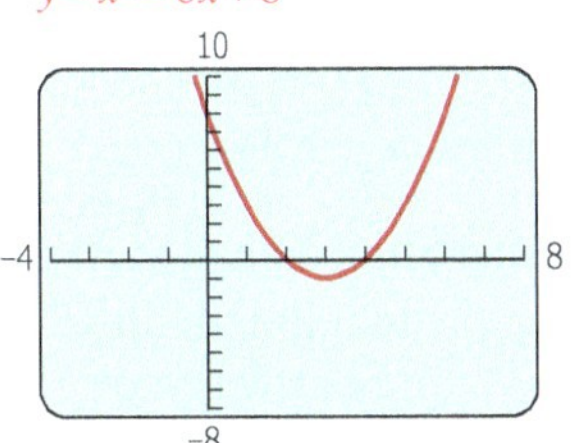

b) Use the TABLE feature to check your answer to part (a).

Algebraic–Graphical Connection

To make an algebraic–graphical connection between the solutions of a quadratic equation and the x-intercepts of a quadratic function, consider the graph of $f(x) = x^2 + 6x + 8$ and its x-intercepts, shown to the right.

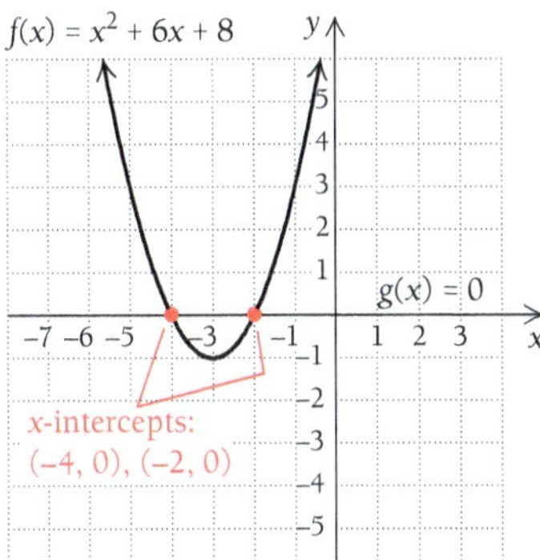

The x-intercepts, $(-4, 0)$ and $(-2, 0)$, are the points of intersection of the graphs of $f(x) = x^2 + 6x + 8$ and $g(x) = 0$ (the x-axis). The x-values, -4 and -2, can be found by solving $f(x) = g(x)$:

$$x^2 + 6x + 8 = 0$$

$$(x + 4)(x + 2) = 0 \quad \text{Factoring; there is no need for the quadratic formula here.}$$

$$x + 4 = 0 \quad or \quad x + 2 = 0 \quad \text{Principle of Zero Products}$$

$$x = -4 \quad or \quad x = -2.$$

The solutions of $x^2 + 6x + 8 = 0$ are -4 and -2, the first coordinates of the x-intercepts, $(-4, 0)$ and $(-2, 0)$. (A brief review of factoring is presented in Appendix A at the end of the text.)

EXAMPLE 3 Solve: $3x^2 - 4x - 2 = 0$.

Solution We first determine a, b, and c:

$$a = 3, \quad b = -4, \quad c = -2.$$

Next we use the quadratic formula:

$$x = \frac{-b \pm \sqrt{b^2 - 4ac}}{2a}$$

$$= \frac{-(-4) \pm \sqrt{(-4)^2 - 4(3)(-2)}}{2 \cdot 3} \quad \text{Substituting}$$

$$= \frac{4 \pm \sqrt{16 + 24}}{6} = \frac{4 \pm \sqrt{40}}{6} \quad \text{Simplifying}$$

$$= \frac{4 \pm \sqrt{4 \cdot 10}}{6} = \frac{4 \pm 2\sqrt{10}}{6}$$

$$= \frac{2(2 \pm \sqrt{10})}{2 \cdot 3} \qquad \text{Factoring}$$

$$= \frac{2 \pm \sqrt{10}}{3}.$$

The solutions are $(2 + \sqrt{10})/3$ and $(2 - \sqrt{10})/3$, or approximately 1.721 and -0.387, respectively. The x-intercepts are shown on the graph of the parabola.

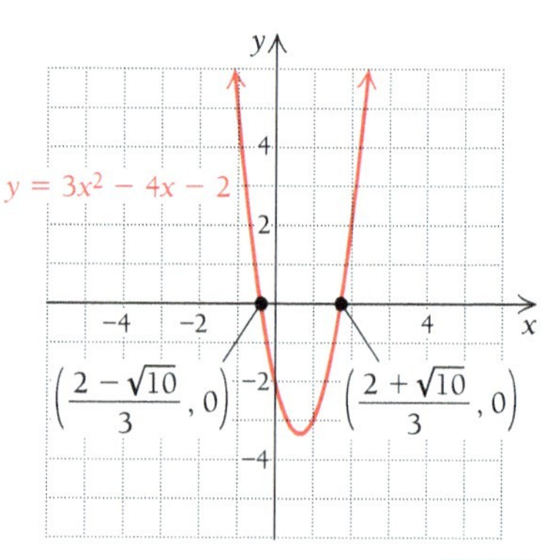

Quick Check 2 ✓

Solve: $3x^2 + 2x = 7$.

Polynomial Functions

Linear and quadratic functions are part of a general class of *polynomial functions.*

DEFINITION

A **polynomial function** f is given by

$$f(x) = a_n x^n + a_{n-1}x^{n-1} + \cdots + a_2 x^2 + a_1 x^1 + a_0,$$

where n is a nonnegative integer and $a_n, a_{n-1}, \ldots, a_1, a_0$ are real numbers, called **coefficients**.

The following are examples of polynomial functions:

$f(x) = -5,$ (A constant function)

$f(x) = 4x + 3,$ (A linear function)

$f(x) = -x^2 + 2x + 3,$ (A quadratic function)

$f(x) = 2x^3 - 4x^2 + x + 1.$ (A cubic, or third-degree, function)

In general, drawing graphs of polynomial functions other than linear and quadratic functions by hand is difficult. Calculus will help us sketch such graphs in Chapter 3. However, some **power functions**, of the form $f(x) = ax^n$, are relatively easy to graph.

EXAMPLE 4 Using the same set of axes, graph $f(x) = x^2$ and $g(x) = x^3$.

Solution We set up a table of values, plot the points, and then draw the graphs.

x	x^2	x^3
-2	4	-8
-1	1	-1
$-\frac{1}{2}$	$\frac{1}{4}$	$-\frac{1}{8}$
0	0	0
$\frac{1}{2}$	$\frac{1}{4}$	$\frac{1}{8}$
1	1	1
2	4	8

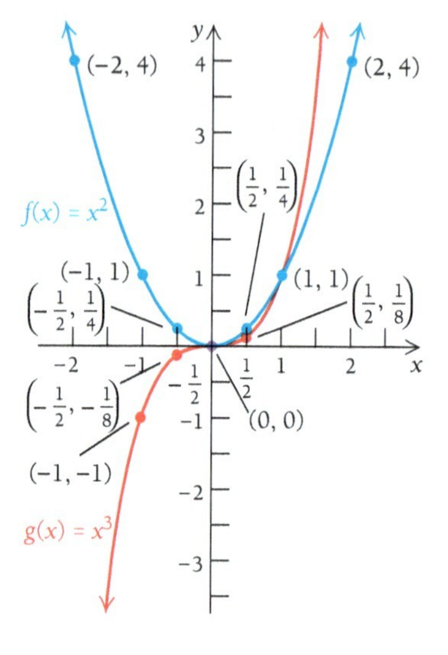

Quick Check 3 ✓

Graph each function using the same set of axes:

$f(x) = -x^2$ and

$g(x) = \frac{1}{3}x^3.$

Technology Connection 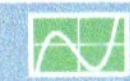

Solving Polynomial Equations

The INTERSECT *Feature*

Solving $x^3 = 3x + 1$ amounts to finding the x-coordinates of the point(s) of intersection of the graphs of

$$f(x) = x^3 \quad \text{and} \quad g(x) = 3x + 1.$$

We enter the functions as

$$y_1 = x^3 \quad \text{and} \quad y_2 = 3x + 1$$

and then graph. We use a $[-3, 3, -5, 8]$ window to see the curvature and possible points of intersection.

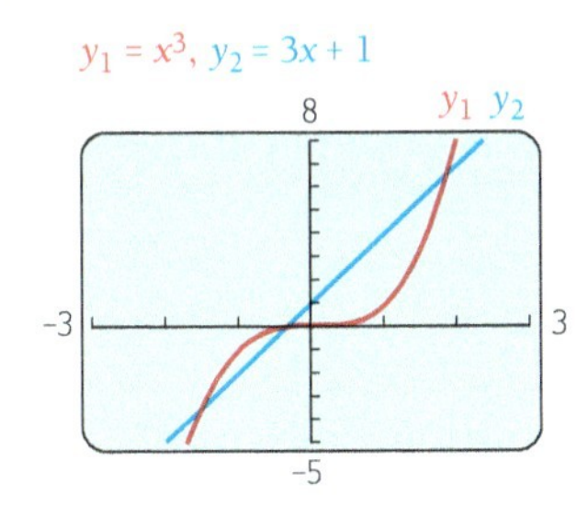

There appear to be at least three points of intersection. Using the INTERSECT feature in the CALC menu, we see that the point of intersection on the left is at about $(-1.53, -3.60)$.

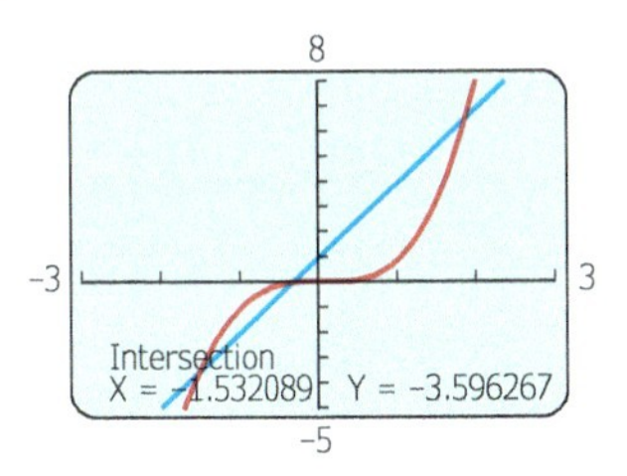

In a similar manner, we approximate the other points of intersection as $(-0.35, -0.04)$ and $(1.88, 6.64)$. The solutions of $x^3 = 3x + 1$ are the x-coordinates of these points, approximately

$$-1.53, -0.35, \text{ and } 1.88.$$

The ZERO *Feature*

The ZERO, or ROOT, feature can be used to solve an equation. The word "zero" in this context refers to an input, or x-value, for which the output of a function is 0. That is, c is a **zero** of the function f if $f(c) = 0$.

To use such a feature requires a 0 on one side of the equation. Thus, to solve $x^3 = 3x + 1$, we obtain $x^3 - 3x - 1 = 0$ by subtracting $3x + 1$ from both sides. Graphing $y = x^3 - 3x - 1$ and using the ZERO feature to find the zeros, we view a screen like the following.

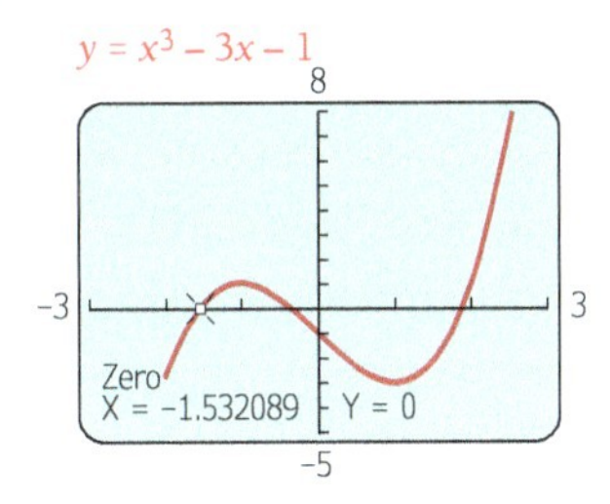

We see that $x^3 - 3x - 1 = 0$ when $x \approx -1.53$, so -1.53 is an approximate solution of $x^3 = 3x + 1$. In a similar manner, we can approximate the other solutions as -0.35 and 1.88. Note that the points of intersection of the graphs of f and g, shown to the left, have the same x-values as the zeros of $x^3 - 3x - 1$.

EXERCISES

Using the INTERSECT feature, solve each equation.

1. $x^3 = 3x - 2$

2. $x^4 - 2x^2 = 0$

Using the ZERO feature, solve each equation.

3. $0.4x^2 = 280x$

(*Hint*: Use the window $[-200, 800, -100{,}000, 200{,}000]$.)

4. $\frac{1}{3}x^3 - \frac{1}{2}x^2 = 2x - 1$

Find the zeros of each function.

5. $f(x) = 3x^2 - 4x - 2$

6. $g(x) = x^4 + x^3 - 4x^2 - 2x + 4$

Rational Functions

DEFINITION

Functions that can be expressed as the quotient, or ratio, of two polynomials are called **rational functions**.

The following are examples of rational functions:

$$f(x) = \frac{x^2 - 9}{x - 3}, \qquad h(x) = \frac{x - 3}{x^2 - x - 2},$$

$$g(x) = \frac{3x^2 - 4x}{2x + 10}, \qquad k(x) = \frac{x^3 - 2x + 7}{1} = x^3 - 2x + 7.$$

As the function k illustrates, every polynomial function is also a rational function.

The domain of a rational function cannot include any input value that results in division by zero. Thus, for $f(x) = \dfrac{x^2 - 9}{x - 3}$, the domain consists of all of the real numbers except 3, that is, $\{x \mid (-\infty, 3) \cup (3, \infty)\}$. To determine the domain of h, we set the denominator equal to 0 and solve:

$$x^2 - x - 2 = 0$$
$$(x + 1)(x - 2) = 0$$
$$x = -1 \quad or \quad x = 2.$$

Neither -1 nor 2 is in the domain of h. The domain of h is therefore $\{x \mid (-\infty, -1) \cup (-1, 2) \cup (2, \infty)\}$. Similarly, the domain of g is $\{x \mid (-\infty, -5) \cup (-5, \infty)\}$, and the domain of k is $\mathbb{R}$, the set of all real numbers, since the denominator is never 0.

Graphing rational functions can be complicated and is best done using tools of calculus covered in Chapters 1 and 2. For now, we focus on graphs that are fairly basic.

One important class of rational functions is given by $f(x) = k/x$, where k is a constant.

EXAMPLE 5 Graph: $f(x) = 1/x$.

Solution We make a table of values, plot the corresponding points, and then draw the graph. Note that $x = 0$ is not in the domain of f.

x	$f(x)$
-3	$-\frac{1}{3}$
-2	$-\frac{1}{2}$
-1	-1
$-\frac{1}{2}$	-2
$-\frac{1}{4}$	-4
$\frac{1}{4}$	4
$\frac{1}{2}$	2
1	1
2	$\frac{1}{2}$
3	$\frac{1}{3}$

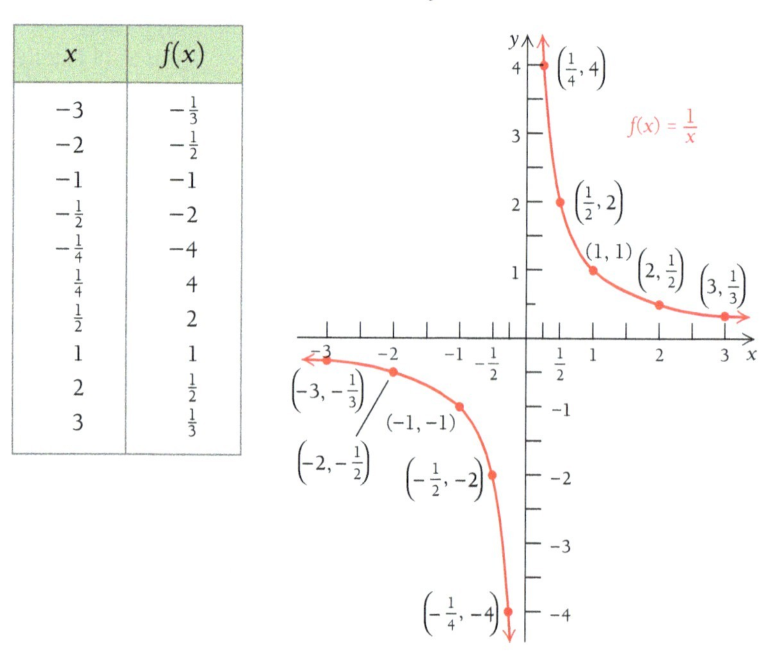

In Example 5, note that 0 is not in the domain of f because it would yield a denominator of zero. The function given by $f(x) = 1/x$ is an example of **inverse proportion**. Note that as the value of x increases, the value of $f(x)$ decreases.

DEFINITION

y is **inversely proportional** to x if there is some positive number k for which $y = k/x$.

EXAMPLE 6 **Ticket Sales.** A minor league baseball team notices that as the average ticket price increases, the number of tickets sold decreases, and as the average ticket price decreases, the number of tickets sold increases. Suppose 10,000 tickets are sold when the average ticket price is \$12. Assuming that the relationship between average ticket price x, in dollars, and the number of tickets sold y is an inverse proportion, find the number of tickets sold when the average price is \$20.

Solution Assuming that $y = \frac{k}{x}$, we substitute 10,000 for y and 12 for x to find k:

$$10{,}000 = \frac{k}{12} \qquad \text{Substituting}$$
$$k = 120{,}000. \qquad \text{Multiplying both sides by 12}$$

Thus, the inversely proportional relationship is given by $y = \frac{120{,}000}{x}$.

Substituting 20 for x, we have

$$y = \frac{120{,}000}{20} = 6000$$

When the average ticket price is \$20, about 6000 tickets will be sold. **4 ✓**

Quick Check 4 ✓

Joanna orders 30 reams of copier paper at a cost of \$5 per ream. Assuming an inversely proportional relationship between the number of reams of copier paper and the cost per ream, how much can Joanna expect to pay per ream when she orders 50 reams?

Absolute-Value Functions

The *absolute value* of a number is its distance from 0 on the number line. We denote the absolute value of a number x as $|x|$. The absolute-value function, given by $f(x) = |x|$, is important in calculus, and its graph has a distinctive V shape.

Technology Connection 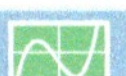

Absolute value is entered as ABS and is often accessed from the NUM option of the MATH menu.

EXERCISES

Graph.

1. $f(x) = |\frac{1}{2}x|$
2. $g(x) = |x + 2| - 3$

EXAMPLE 7 Graph: $f(x) = |x|$.

Solution We make a table of values, plot the points, and then draw the graph. The domain of f is the set of all real numbers, or $(-\infty, \infty)$.

x	$f(x)$
-3	3
-2	2
-1	1
0	0
1	1
2	2
3	3

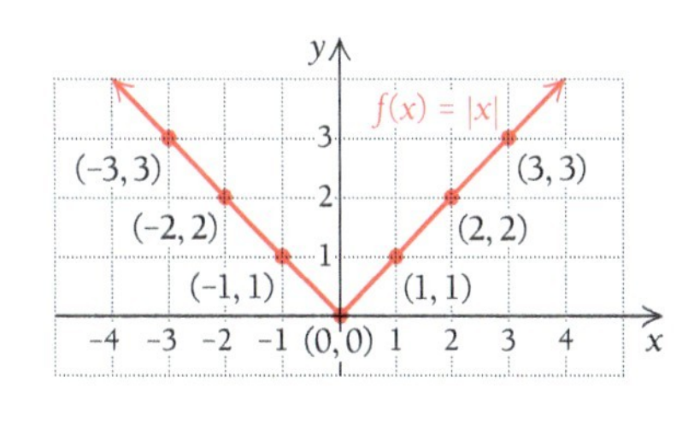

We regard this function as being defined piecewise as follows:

$$f(x) = |x| = \begin{cases} x, & \text{if } x \geq 0, \\ -x, & \text{if } x < 0. \end{cases}$$

Square-Root Functions

The following is an example of a square-root function and its graph.

EXAMPLE 8 Graph: $f(x) = \sqrt{x}$.

Solution The domain of this function is the set of all nonnegative numbers, or the interval $[0, \infty)$. Values of x are chosen to allow convenient calculations.

We make a table of values, plot the points, and then draw the graph.

x	0	1	4	9	16	25
$f(x) = \sqrt{x}$	0	1	2	3	4	5

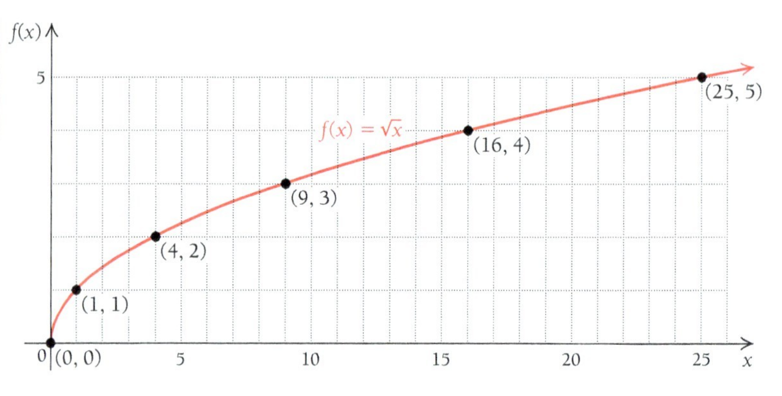

Quick Check 5 ✓

Graph each function and state the domain:

a) $f(x) = |x + 2|$;

b) $f(x) = \sqrt{x + 4}$.

5 ✓

Power Functions with Rational Exponents

We are motivated to define rational exponents so that the following laws of exponents still hold (also see Appendix A):

> For any nonzero real number a and any integers n and m,
>
> $$a^n \cdot a^m = a^{n+m}; \quad \frac{a^n}{a^m} = a^{n-m}; \quad (a^n)^m = a^{n \cdot m}; \quad a^{-m} = \frac{1}{a^m}.$$

This suggests that $a^{1/2}$ be defined so that $(a^{1/2})^2 = a^{(1/2)\cdot 2} = a^1$. Thus, we define $a^{1/2}$ as $\sqrt{a}$. Similarly, in order to have $(a^{1/3})^3 = a^{(1/3)\cdot 3} = a^1$, we define $a^{1/3}$ as $\sqrt[3]{a}$. In general,

$$a^{1/n} = \sqrt[n]{a}, \quad \text{provided } \sqrt[n]{a} \text{ is defined.}$$

Again, for the laws of exponents to hold, and assuming that $\sqrt[n]{a}$ exists, we have

$$a^{m/n} = (a^m)^{1/n} = \sqrt[n]{a^m} = (\sqrt[n]{a})^m.$$

Similarly, $a^{-m/n}$ is defined by

$$a^{-m/n} = \frac{1}{a^{m/n}} = \frac{1}{\sqrt[n]{a^m}}.$$

EXAMPLE 9 Rewrite each of the following as an equivalent expression using radical notation: **a)** $x^{1/3}$; **b)** $t^{6/7}$; **c)** $x^{-2/3}$; **d)** $r^{-1/4}$.

Solution

a) $x^{1/3} = \sqrt[3]{x}$

b) $t^{6/7} = \sqrt[7]{t^6}$

c) $x^{-2/3} = \dfrac{1}{x^{2/3}} = \dfrac{1}{\sqrt[3]{x^2}}, \quad x \neq 0$

d) $r^{-1/4} = \dfrac{1}{r^{1/4}} = \dfrac{1}{\sqrt[4]{r}}, \quad r > 0$

EXAMPLE 10 Rewrite each of the following as an equivalent expression with a rational exponent:

a) $\sqrt[4]{x}$, for $x \geq 0$

b) $\sqrt[3]{r^2}$

c) $\sqrt{x^{10}}$, for $x \geq 0$

d) $\dfrac{1}{\sqrt[3]{b^5}}$, for $b \neq 0$

Solution

a) $\sqrt[4]{x} = x^{1/4}, \quad x \geq 0$

b) $\sqrt[3]{r^2} = r^{2/3}$

c) $\sqrt{x^{10}} = x^{10/2} = x^5, \quad x \geq 0$

d) $\dfrac{1}{\sqrt[3]{b^5}} = \dfrac{1}{b^{5/3}} = b^{-5/3}, \quad b \neq 0$

Because even roots (square roots, fourth roots, sixth roots, and so on) of negative numbers are not real numbers, the domain of a radical function often has restrictions.

EXAMPLE 11 Find the domain of the function given by

$$f(x) = \sqrt[4]{2x - 10}.$$

Solution For $f(x)$ to be a real number, the radicand, $2x - 10$, cannot be negative. Thus, to find the domain of f, we solve $2x - 10 \geq 0$:

$$2x - 10 \geq 0$$

$$2x \geq 10 \quad \text{Adding 10 to both sides}$$

$$x \geq 5. \quad \text{Dividing both sides by 2}$$

The domain of f is $\{x | x \geq 5\}$, or, in interval notation, $[5, \infty)$. 6 ✓

Quick Check 6 ✓

Find the domain of each function:

a) $f(x) = \sqrt[4]{x + 3}$;

b) $g(x) = \sqrt[3]{x + 7}$.

EXAMPLE 12 **Life Science: Home Range.** The *home range* of an animal is defined as the region to which the animal confines its movements. It has been shown that for carnivorous mammals the area of that region can be approximated by

$$H(w) = 0.11w^{1.36},$$

where w is the mass of the animal, in grams, and $H(w)$ is the area of the home range, in hectares. Graph the function. (*Source:* Based on information in Emlen, J. M., *Ecology: An Evolutionary Approach*, p. 200 (Reading, MA: Addison-Wesley, 1973), and Harestad, A. S., and Bunnel, F. L., "Home Range and Body Weight—A Reevaluation," *Ecology*, Vol. 60, No. 2 (April, 1979), pp. 389–402.)

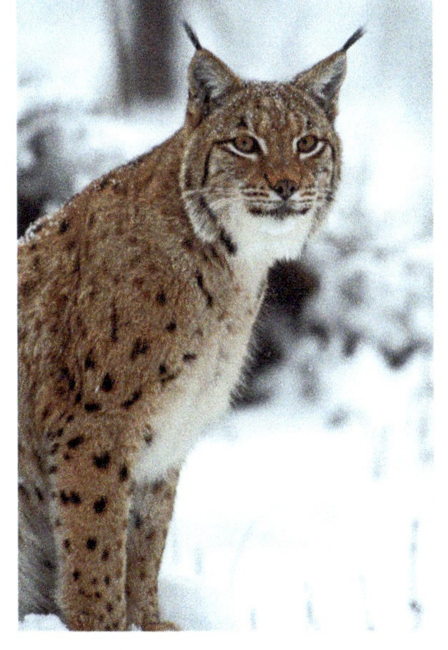

A lynx in its territorial area.

Solution We can approximate function values using a power key, usually labeled ^ or y^x. Note that $w^{1.36} = w^{136/100} = \sqrt[100]{w^{136}}$.

w	0	700	1400	2100	2800	3500
$H(w)$	0	814.2	2089.9	3627.5	5364.5	7266.5

The graph is shown below. Note that function values increase from left to right. As body weight increases, the area of an animal's home range increases.

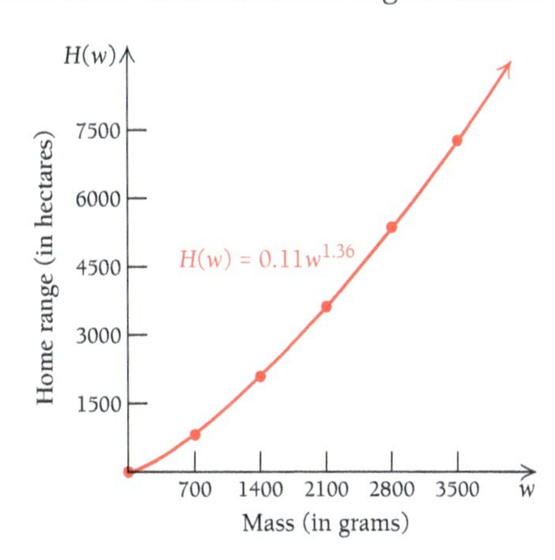

Supply and Demand Functions

In economics, *demand* is modeled by a decreasing function; as the quantity q demanded by consumers gets larger, the price p gets smaller. However, supply is modeled by an increasing function; as the quantity q supplied by sellers increases, so does the price p.

Graphs of supply and demand functions are usually labeled with q on the horizontal axis and p on the vertical axis. However, in some situations, we use p to label the horizontal axis (see Section 3.7).

Demand Functions

Suppose the relationship between the price p of a 1-lb box of sugar and the quantity q of boxes that consumers will demand at that price is given in the table and graph below.

Demand Schedule

Quantity, q, of 1-lb Boxes (in millions)	Price, p, per 1-lb Box
4	$5
5	4
7	3
10	2
15	1

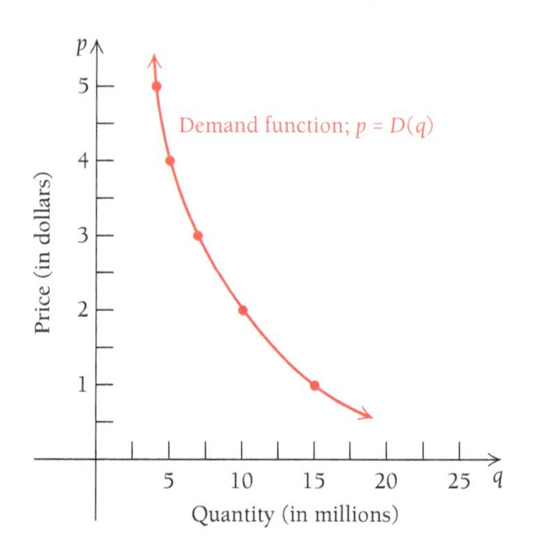

Supply Functions

Furthermore, suppose the relationship between the price p of a 1-lb box of sugar and the quantity q of boxes that sellers are willing to supply, or sell, at that price is given in the table and graph below.

Supply Schedule

Quantity, q, of 1-lb Boxes (in millions)	Price, p, per 1-lb Box
1	$1
10	2
16	3
20	4
22	5

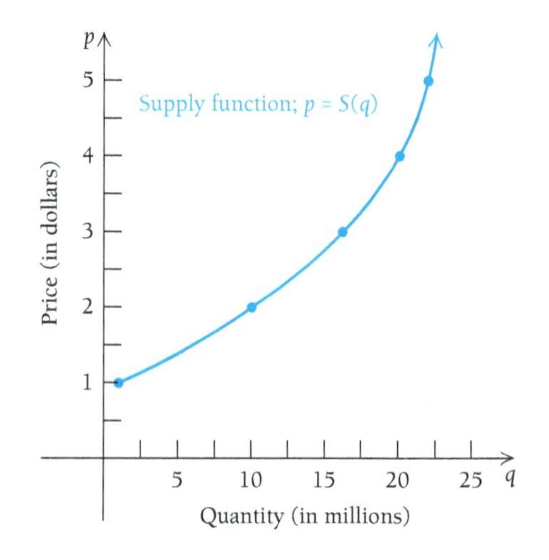

Note that sellers want to supply greater quantities at higher unit prices, and consumers demand greater quantities at lower prices.

Let's now look at these curves together. As price increases, supply increases and demand decreases; and as price decreases, demand increases but supply decreases. The point of intersection (q_E, p_E) is called the **equilibrium point**. The equilibrium price p_E (in this case, \$2 per box) corresponds to an equilibrium quantity q_E (in this case, 10, or 10 million boxes). Sellers are willing to sell 10 million boxes at \$2 per box, and consumers are willing to buy 10 million boxes at that price. The situation is a bit like a buyer and a seller haggling over the price of an item. The equilibrium point, or selling price, is what they finally agree on.

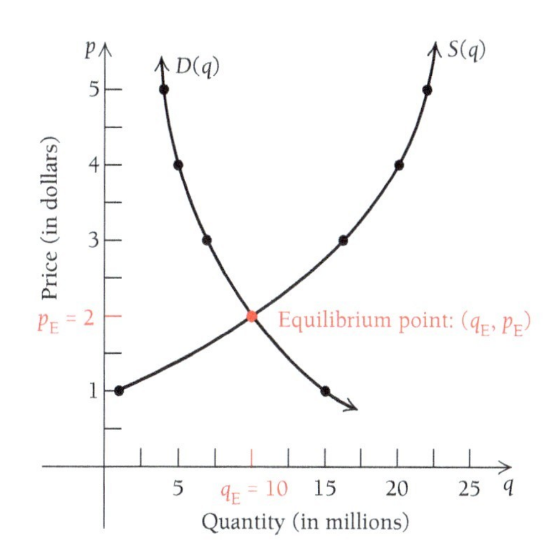

EXAMPLE 13 **Economics: Equilibrium Point.** Find the equilibrium point for the demand and supply functions for the Ultra-Fine coffee maker. Here q represents the number of coffee makers produced, in millions, and p is the price of a coffee maker, in dollars.

Demand: $p = 200 - 4q$

Supply: $p = q + 25$

Solution To find the equilibrium point, the quantity demanded must match the quantity produced:

$$200 - 4q = q + 25 \quad \text{Setting demand equal to supply}$$
$$200 = 5q + 25 \quad \text{Adding } 4q \text{ to both sides}$$
$$175 = 5q \quad \text{Subtracting 25 from both sides}$$
$$175 \cdot \frac{1}{5} = q \quad \text{Multiplying both sides by } \frac{1}{5}$$
$$35 = q.$$

Thus, $q_E = 35$, or 35 million units. To find p_E, we substitute q_E into either function. We select the supply function:

$$p_E = q_E + 25 = 35 + 25 = 60.$$

Thus, the equilibrium price is \$60, and the equilibrium point is (35, \$60), where q_E is in millions. **7 ✓**

Quick Check 7 ✓

Economics: Equilibrium Point. Repeat Example 13 for the following functions.

Demand: $p = 350 - 5q$

Supply: $p = q + 20$

Section Summary

- Many types of functions have graphs that are not straight lines; among these are *quadratic functions, polynomial functions, power functions, rational functions, the absolute-value function*, and *square-root functions*.
- Demand is modeled by a decreasing function; that is, as the demand q gets larger, the price p gets smaller.
- Supply is modeled by an increasing function; that is, as the quantity supplied gets larger, so does the price p. The point of intersection of the graphs of demand and supply functions for the same product is called the *equilibrium point*.

R.5 Exercise Set

Graph each pair of equations on one set of axes, and state the domain of each equation.

1. $y = \frac{1}{4}x^2$ and $y = -\frac{1}{4}x^2$

2. $y = \frac{1}{2}x^2$ and $y = -\frac{1}{2}x^2$

3. $y = x^2$ and $y = x^2 - 1$

4. $y = x^2$ and $y = x^2 - 3$

5. $y = -3x^2$ and $y = -3x^2 + 2$

6. $y = -2x^2$ and $y = -2x^2 + 1$

7. $y = |x|$ and $y = |x - 3|$

8. $y = |x|$ and $y = |x - 1|$

9. $y = |x|$ and $y = |x + 2| + 1$

10. $y = |x|$ and $y = |x - 3| - 4$

11. $y = x^3$ and $y = x^3 + 1$

12. $y = x^3$ and $y = x^3 + 2$

13. $y = \sqrt{x}$ and $y = \sqrt{x - 1}$

14. $y = \sqrt{x}$ and $y = \sqrt{x - 2}$

15. $y = \sqrt{x}$ and $y = \sqrt{x + 2} - 1$

16. $y = \sqrt{x}$ and $y = \sqrt{x - 3} + 4$

For each of the following quadratic functions, (a) find the vertex and the line of symmetry, (b) state whether the parabola opens upward or downward, and (c) find its x-intercept(s), if they exist.

17. $f(x) = x^2 + 4x + 3$

18. $g(x) = x^2 - 6x + 5$

19. $k(t) = t^2 + 8t$

20. $u(t) = -t^2 - 12t$

21. $m(s) = -2s^2 + s + 4$

22. $v(r) = -3r^2 + 2r + 2$

23. $a(x) = 0.5x^2 + 1.2x - 1.7$

24. $b(x) = \frac{1}{3}x^2 + \frac{2}{5}x - \frac{11}{15}$

Graph, and state the domain using interval notation.

25. $y = \dfrac{3}{x}$

26. $y = \dfrac{2}{x}$

27. $y = -\dfrac{2}{x}$

28. $y = -\dfrac{3}{x}$

29. $y = \dfrac{1}{x - 1}$

30. $y = \dfrac{1}{x^2}$

31. $y = \sqrt[3]{x}$

32. $y = \dfrac{1}{|x|}$

33. $g(x) = \dfrac{x^2 + 7x + 10}{x + 2}$

34. $f(x) = \dfrac{x^2 + 5x + 6}{x + 3}$

Solve.

35. $x^2 - 2x = 2$

36. $x^2 - 2x + 1 = 5$

37. $x^2 + 6x = 1$

38. $x^2 + 4x = 3$

39. $4x^2 = 4x + 1$

40. $-4x^2 = 4x - 1$

41. $3y^2 + 8y + 2 = 0$

42. $2p^2 - 5p = 1$

43. $x + 7 + \dfrac{9}{x} = 0$ (*Hint*: Multiply both sides by x.)

44. $1 - \dfrac{1}{w} = \dfrac{1}{w^2}$

Rewrite each of the following as an equivalent expression using radical notation.

45. $x^{1/5}$

46. $t^{1/7}$

47. $y^{2/3}$

48. $t^{2/5}$

49. $t^{-2/5}$

50. $y^{-2/3}$

51. $b^{-1/3}$

52. $b^{-1/5}$

53. $(x^2 + 3)^{-1/2}$

54. $(y^2 + 7)^{-1/4}$

Rewrite each of the following as an equivalent expression with rational exponents.

55. $\sqrt{x^3}$, $x \geq 0$

56. $\sqrt{x^5}$, $x \geq 0$

57. $\sqrt[5]{a^3}$

58. $\sqrt[4]{b^2}$, $b \geq 0$

59. $\sqrt[4]{x^{12}}$, $x \geq 0$

60. $\sqrt[3]{t^6}$

61. $\dfrac{1}{\sqrt[3]{t^5}}$, $t \neq 0$

62. $\dfrac{1}{\sqrt{m^4}}$, $m \neq 0$

63. $\dfrac{1}{\sqrt{x^2 + 7}}$

64. $\sqrt{x^3 + 4}$

Simplify.

65. $9^{3/2}$

66. $16^{5/2}$

67. $64^{2/3}$

68. $8^{2/3}$

Determine the domain of each function.

69. $f(x) = \dfrac{x^2 - 25}{x - 5}$

70. $f(x) = \dfrac{x^2 - 4}{x + 2}$

71. $f(x) = \dfrac{x^3}{x^2 - 5x + 6}$

72. $f(x) = \dfrac{x^4 + 7}{x^2 + 6x + 5}$

73. $f(x) = \sqrt{5x + 4}$

74. $f(x) = \sqrt{2x - 6}$

75. $f(x) = \sqrt[4]{7 - x}$

76. $f(x) = \sqrt[6]{5 - x}$

APPLICATIONS

Business and Economics

Find the equilibrium point for each pair of demand and supply functions.

77. Demand: $p = 1000 - 10q$; Supply: $p = 250 + 5q$

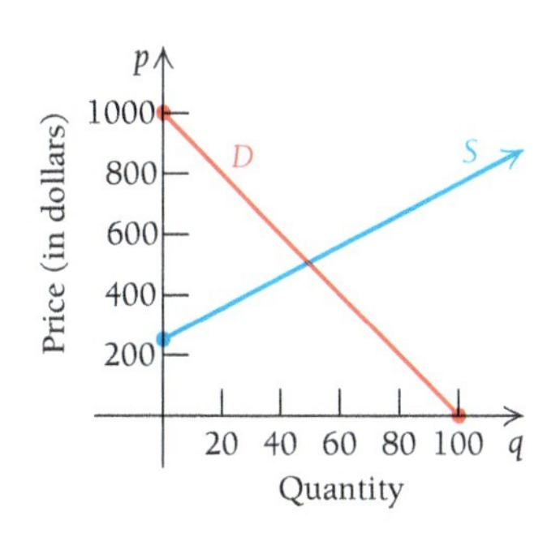

78. Demand: $p = 8800 - 30q$; Supply: $p = 7000 + 15q$

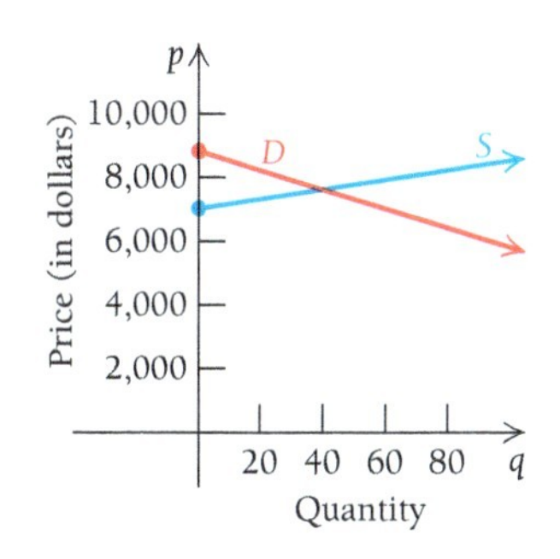

79. Demand: $p = \dfrac{5}{q}$; Supply: $p = \dfrac{q}{5}$

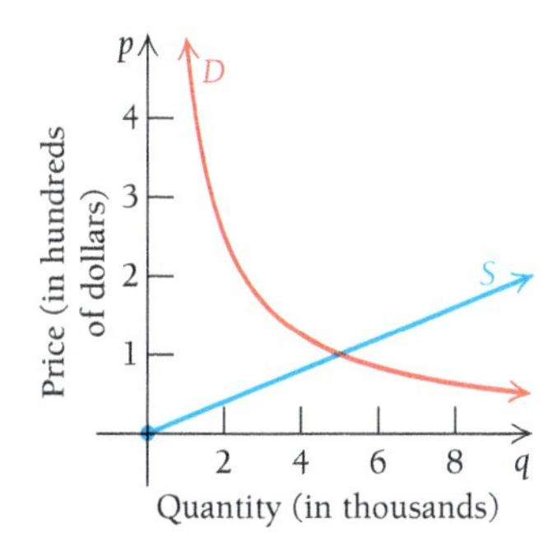

80. Demand: $p = \dfrac{4}{q}$; Supply: $p = \dfrac{q}{4}$

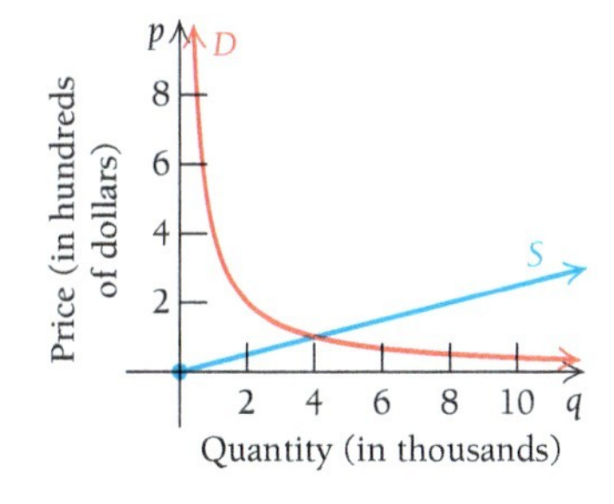

81. Demand: $p = (q - 3)^2$; Supply: $p = q^2 + 2q + 1$ (assume $q \le 3$)

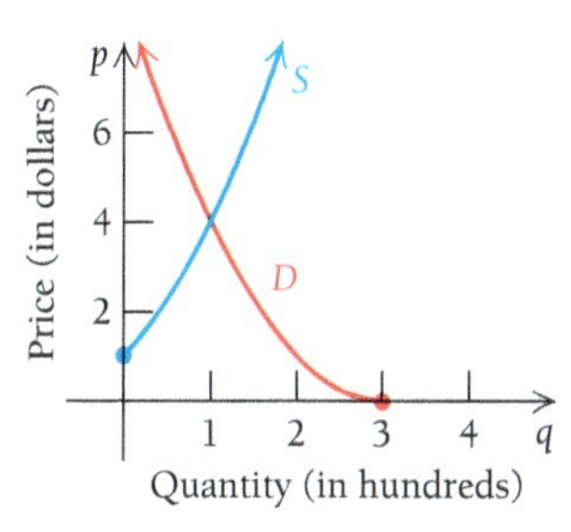

82. Demand: $p = (q - 4)^2$; Supply: $p = q^2 + 2q + 6$ (assume $q \le 4$)

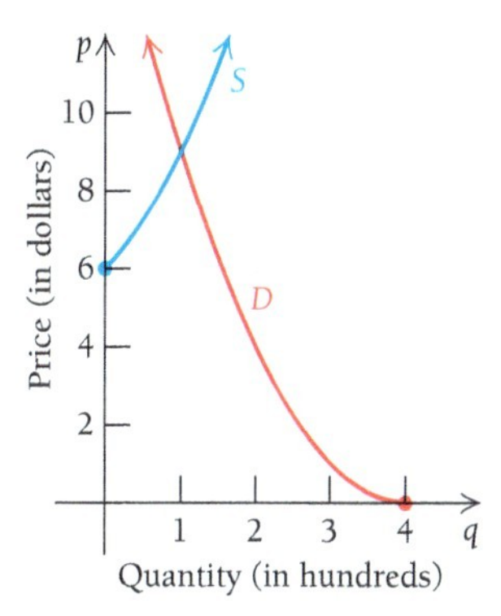

83. Demand: $p = 5 - q$; Supply: $p = \sqrt{q + 7}$

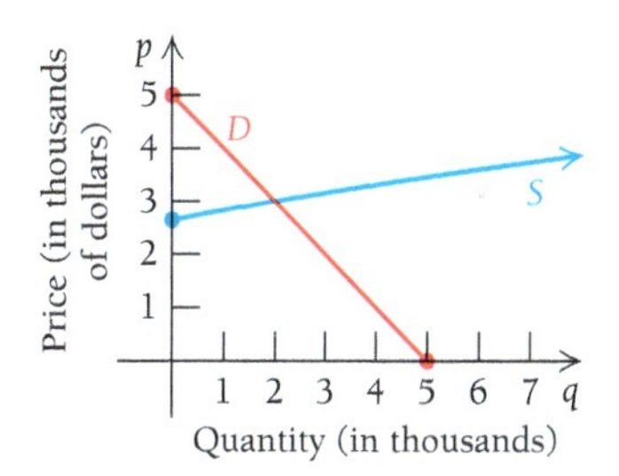

84. Demand: $p = 7 - q$; Supply: $p = 2\sqrt{q + 1}$

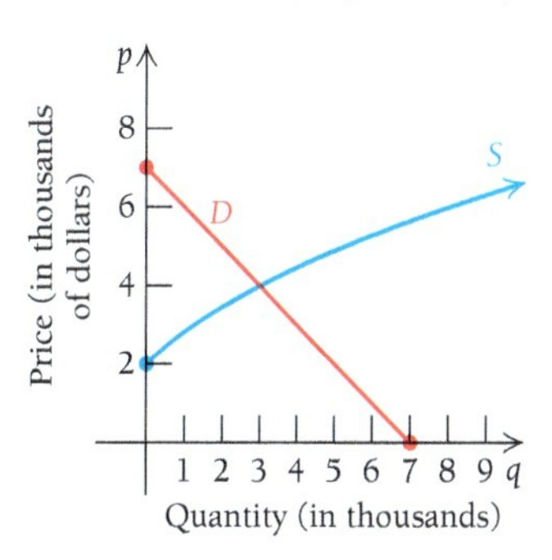

85. Price of admission. The number of tickets sold for a humane society fund-raiser is inversely proportional to the price of a ticket, p. If 175 tickets can be sold for \$20 each, how many tickets will be sold if the price is \$25 each?

86. Demand. The quantity sold q of a high-definition TV is inversely proportional to the price p. If 85,000 high-definition TVs sold for \$1200 each, how many will be sold if the price is \$850 each?

Life and Physical Sciences

87. Radar range. The function given by

$$R(x) = 11.74x^{0.25}$$

can be used to approximate the maximum range, $R(x)$, in miles, of ARSR-3 surveillance radar with a peak power of x watts.

a) Determine the maximum radar range when the peak power is 40,000 watts, 50,000 watts, and 60,000 watts.
b) Graph the function.

88. Home range. Refer to Example 12. The home range, in hectares, of an omnivorous mammal of mass w grams is given by

$$H(w) = 0.059w^{0.92}.$$

(*Source:* Harestad, A. S., and Bunnel, F. L., "Home Range and Body Weight—A Reevaluation," *Ecology*, Vol. 60, No. 2 (April, 1979), pp. 389–402.) Complete the table of approximate function values and graph the function.

w	0	1000	2000	3000	4000	5000	6000	7000
$H(w)$	0	34.0						

89. Life science: pollution control. Pollution control is an important concern worldwide. The function

$$p(t) = 12.85t^{-0.077}$$

describes the average pollution, in micrograms per cubic meter of air, t years after 2000. (*Source*: epa.gov/airtrends/pm.html)

a) Predict the pollution in 2015, 2020, and 2025.
b) Graph the function over the interval $[0, 50]$.

90. Surface area and mass. The surface area of a person whose mass is 75 kg can be approximated by

$$f(h) = 0.144h^{1/2},$$

where $f(h)$ is measured in square meters and h is the person's height in centimeters. (*Source*: *U.S. Oncology*.)

a) Find the approximate surface area of a person whose mass is 75 kg and whose height is 180 cm.
b) Find the approximate surface area of a person whose mass is 75 kg and whose height is 170 cm.
c) Graph the function f for $0 \leq h \leq 200$.

SYNTHESIS

91. Zipf's Law. According to Zipf's Law, the number of cities N with a population greater than S is inversely proportional to S. In 2015, there were 304 U.S. cities with a population greater than 100,000. Estimate the number of U.S. cities with a population between 350,000 and 500,000; between 300,000 and 600,000.

92. At most, how many y-intercepts can a function have? Why?

93. What is the difference between a rational function and a polynomial function?

Technology Connection 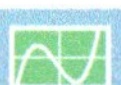

Use the ZERO *feature or the* INTERSECT *feature to approximate the zeros of each function to three decimal places. To graph an absolute-value function, press* MATH *and then select* NUM *followed by* abs(. *For example,* $y = |x + 1|$ *is entered as* abs(x+1).

94. $f(x) = x^3 - x$
(Also use algebra to find the zeros of this function.)

95. $f(x) = 2x^3 - x^2 - 14x - 10$

96. $f(x) = \frac{1}{2}(|x - 4| + |x - 7|) - 4$

97. $f(x) = x^4 + 4x^3 - 36x^2 - 160x + 300$

98. $f(x) = \sqrt{7 - x^2} - 1$

99. $f(x) = |x + 1| + |x - 2| - 5$

100. $f(x) = |x + 1| + |x - 2|$

101. $f(x) = |x + 1| + |x - 2| - 3$

102. $f(x) = x^8 + 8x^7 - 28x^6 - 56x^5 + 70x^4 + 56x^3 - 28x^2 - 8x + 1$

103. Find a positive number x such that adding 1 gives its square.

104. Find a positive number x such that adding 1, then taking the square root of the result, gives x.

105. Find a positive number x such that its reciprocal added to 1 gives x.

106. Explain why Exercises 103, 104, and 105 are equivalent.

Answers to Quick Checks

1. (a) **(b)**

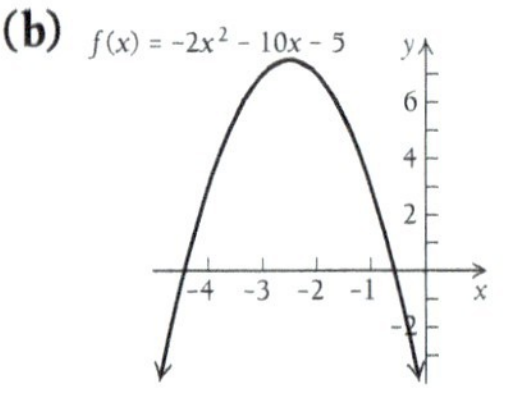

2. 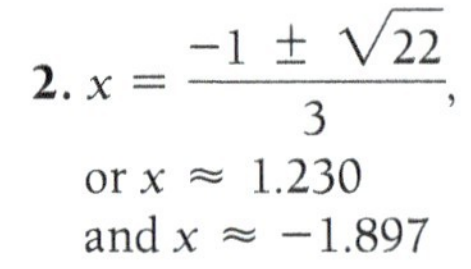
$x = \dfrac{-1 \pm \sqrt{22}}{3}$, or $x \approx 1.230$ and $x \approx -1.897$

3.

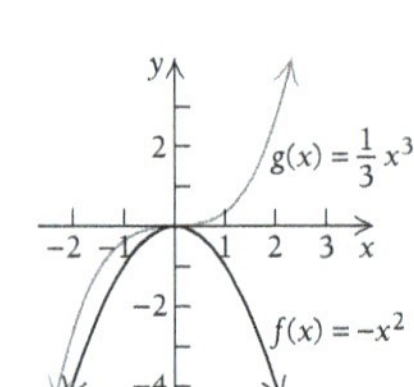

4. \$3 per ream

5. (a) Domain: $(-\infty, \infty)$

(b)

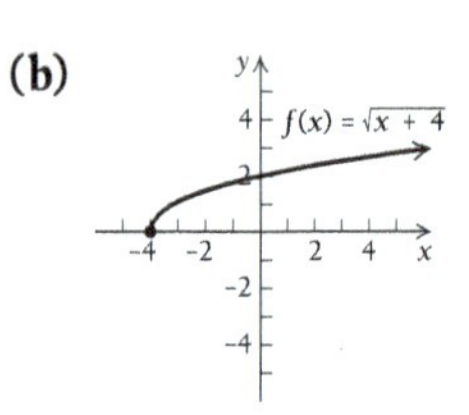

Domain: $[-4, \infty)$

6. (a) $[-3, \infty)$ **(b)** $(-\infty, \infty)$ **7.** Equilibrium point is $(55, 75)$; price is \$75, and quantity is 55,000,000.

R.6 Exponential and Logarithmic Functions

- Graph exponential functions.
- Graph logarithmic functions.
- Convert an exponential equation into an equivalent logarithmic equation.
- Convert a logarithmic equation into an equivalent exponential equation.
- Find the domain of a logarithmic function.
- Use exponential and logarithmic functions to solve certain applied problems.

Exponential Functions

Every term in a polynomial function can be written in the form of a variable raised to a power. Here we consider exponential functions, in which the exponent is a variable (or an expression containing a variable). Exponential functions are used to model real-world problems that include heating/cooling rates, population growth and decay, compound interest, and much more. Every exponential function has the property that its outputs change at a rate that is a constant percentage.

DEFINITION

An **exponential function** f is given by

$$f(x) = a_0 \cdot a^x,$$

where x is any real number and $a > 0$ and $a \neq 1$. The number a is the **base**, and the y-intercept is $(0, a_0)$.

The following are examples of exponential functions:

$$f(x) = 2^x, \quad f(x) = \left(\frac{1}{2}\right)^x, \quad f(x) = 3(0.4)^x.$$

Note that in contrast to a power function like $y = x^2$, an exponential function has the variable in the exponent, not the base.

In Section R.1, an exponential model was expressed as

$$A = P(1 + r)^t.$$

This equation is of the form $f(x) = a_0 \cdot a^x$, where

$$a = 1 + r.$$

Here, r represents the percent increase (if $r > 0$) or percent decrease (if $-1 < r < 0$) of the quantity over a fixed period of time.

EXAMPLE 1 Graph $y = f(x) = \left(\frac{5}{4}\right)^x = 1.25^x$, and state the percent change in y per unit increase in x.

Solution First, we find some function values. Note that 1.25^x is always positive:

$$x = -3, y = 1.25^{-3} = \frac{64}{125};$$

$$x = -2, y = 1.25^{-2} = \frac{16}{25};$$

$$x = -1, y = 1.25^{-1} = \frac{4}{5};$$

$$x = 0, y = 1.25^{0} = 1;$$

$$x = 1, y = 1.25^{1} = \frac{5}{4};$$

$$x = 2, y = 1.25^{2} = \frac{25}{16};$$

$$x = 3, y = 1.25^{3} = \frac{125}{64}.$$

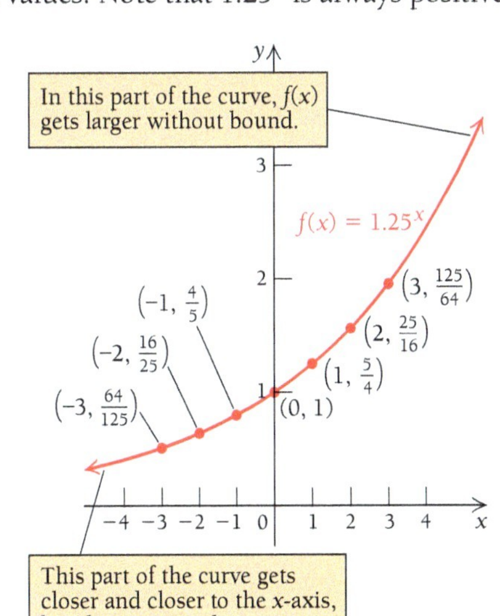

Quick Check 1 ✓

For $f(x) = 3^x$, complete this table of function values.

x	$f(x) = 3^x$
-3	
-2	
-1	
0	
1	
2	
3	

Graph $f(x) = 3^x$, and state the percent change in y per unit increase in x.

x	-3	-2	-1	0	1	2	3
$y = f(x) = \left(\frac{5}{4}\right)^x = 1.25^x$	$\frac{64}{125}$	$\frac{16}{25}$	$\frac{4}{5}$	1	$\frac{5}{4}$	$\frac{25}{16}$	$\frac{125}{64}$

Here, we have $a = 1 + r = 1.25$, so $r = 0.25$, or 25%. The value of y is increasing by 25% for every unit increase in x. **1 ✓**

EXAMPLE 2 Graph: $y = g(x) = 3 \cdot \left(\frac{1}{4}\right)^x$, and state the percent change in y per unit increase in x.

Solution We find some function values:

$$x = -3, \quad y = 3 \cdot \left(\frac{1}{4}\right)^{-3} = 192;$$

$$x = -2, \quad y = 3 \cdot \left(\frac{1}{4}\right)^{-2} = 48;$$

$$x = -1, \quad y = 3 \cdot \left(\frac{1}{4}\right)^{-1} = 12;$$

$$x = 0, \quad y = 3 \cdot \left(\frac{1}{4}\right)^{0} = 3;$$

$$x = 1, \quad y = 3 \cdot \left(\frac{1}{4}\right)^{1} = \frac{3}{4};$$

$$x = 2, \quad y = 3 \cdot \left(\frac{1}{4}\right)^{2} = \frac{3}{16};$$

$$x = 3, \quad y = 3 \cdot \left(\frac{1}{4}\right)^{3} = \frac{3}{64}.$$

x	-3	-2	-1	0	1	2	3
$y = g(x) = 3 \cdot \left(\frac{1}{4}\right)^x$	192	48	12	3	$\frac{3}{4}$	$\frac{3}{16}$	$\frac{3}{64}$

Quick Check 2 ✓

For $g(x) = 2 \cdot \left(\frac{1}{3}\right)^x$, complete this table of function values.

x	$g(x) = 2 \cdot \left(\frac{1}{3}\right)^x$
-3	
-2	
-1	
0	
1	
2	
3	

Graph $g(x) = 2 \cdot \left(\frac{1}{3}\right)^x$, and state the percent change in y per unit increase in x.

In this example, we have $a = 1 + r = \frac{1}{4}$, so $r = -\frac{3}{4} = -75\%$. The value of y is decreasing by 75% for every unit increase in x. **2 ✓**

In general, when $0 < a < 1$, as x gets larger, $f(x)$ gets smaller. When $a > 1$, as x gets larger, $f(x)$ also gets larger. The domain of an exponential function is all of the real numbers. The range is the set of all nonnegative real numbers.

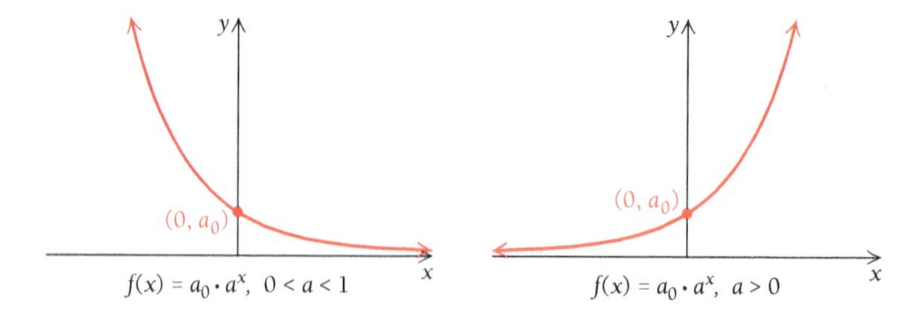

When $x = 0$, we have $f(0) = a_0$. In many applications, this is considered the *initial quantity*. Exponential functions have many applications, such as growth of the value of a savings account, growth of a population, and decay of radioactive elements.

EXAMPLE 3 **Business: Compound Interest.** Bert invests \$10,000 in an account that earns 3.25% interest per year.

a) Find the function that gives the value A of Bert's investment after t years.

b) Find $A(10)$, and interpret this result.

c) Graph $A(t)$ for $0 \leq t \leq 10$.

Solution

a) We know that an amount P invested at interest rate r, compounded annually for t years, grows to an amount A, given by

$$A = P(1 + r)^t.$$

For $P = \$10{,}000$ and $r = 3.25\% = 0.0325$, we have

$$A = 10{,}000(1 + 0.0325)^t \quad \text{Substituting}$$

$$A(t) = 10{,}000(1.0325)^t.$$

Note that when $t = 0$, we have $A(0) = 10{,}000(1.0325)^0 = 10{,}000 \cdot 1 = \$10{,}000$, the initial value of Bert's investment.

b) We have

$$A(10) = 10{,}000(1.0325)^{10} = 13{,}768.94. \quad \text{Using a calculator and rounding to two decimal places}$$

After 10 years, Bert's investment of \$10,000 will be worth \$13,768.94.

c) The graph is shown below.

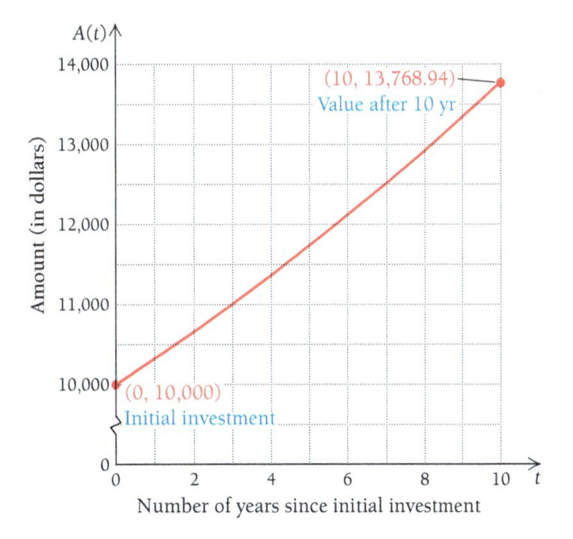

3 ✓

Quick Check 3 ✓

Michele invests \$75,000 at an annual interest rate of 4.5%.

a) Find the function that gives the value A of Michele's investment after t years.

b) Find $A(15)$, and interpret this result.

EXAMPLE 4 **Population Decay.** The city of Cuprite had a population of 15,000 people in 2012, when the closing of a mine initiated a decrease in population that persists to the present. Assume that the population decreases by the same percentage each year and that in 2017 the population was 11,250.

a) Find $P(t)$, the population of Cuprite t years after 2012.

b) Estimate Cuprite's population in 2022.

c) Graph $P(t)$ for $0 \leq t \leq 10$.

d) Find the annual percent change in Cuprite's population.

Solution

a) Here, $P(t) = P_0a^t$, where $P_0 = 15{,}000$, the population at $t = 0$, representing the year 2012. To find the base a, we use the fact that when $t = 5$, the population is 11,250:

$$11{,}250 = 15{,}000a^5 \quad \text{Substituting}$$

$$\frac{11{,}250}{15{,}000} = a^5$$

$$\left(\frac{11{,}250}{15{,}000}\right)^{1/5} = a \quad \text{Raising both sides to the } \tfrac{1}{5}\text{th power to isolate } a$$

$$0.944 \approx a. \quad \text{Using a calculator, and rounding to three decimal places}$$

Thus, the function that models Cuprite's population t years after 2012 is given by

$$P(t) = 15{,}000(0.944)^t.$$

b) In 2022, Cuprite's estimated population will be

$$P(10) = 15{,}000(0.944)^{10} \approx 8430.$$

c) The graph is shown below. Note the downward trend in population as t increases.

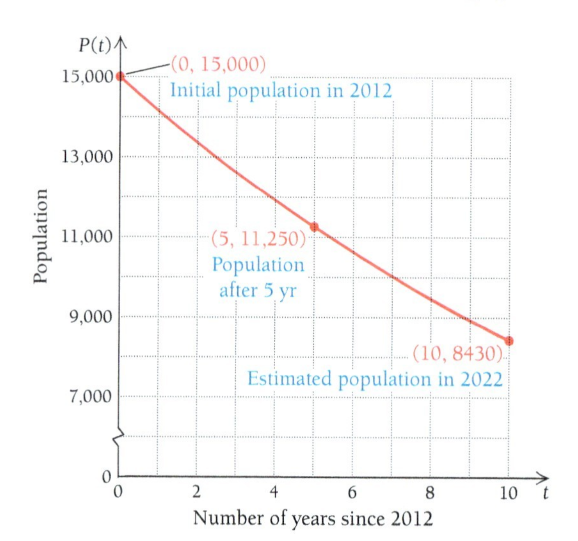

Quick Check 4 ✓

A sample of 15 g of an element is decaying exponentially. After 10 days, the mass of this sample is 14.2 g.

a) Find $M(t)$, the mass of this sample after t days.

b) Find $M(50)$, and interpret this result.

c) State the percent change in the amount of this element per day.

d) Since $a = 1 + r$, we have $1 + r = 0.944$, so $r = -0.056$. Cuprite's population is *decreasing* at a rate of 5.6% per year. **4 ✓**

Logarithms

A *logarithm* is an exponent. For example, because $3^2 = 9$, we say "the logarithm, base 3, of 9 is 2." Using logarithm notation, we write

$$\log_3 9 = 2.$$

In general, if $a^x = y$, then $\log_a y = x$.

DEFINITION

The **logarithm**, base a, of y is the number x for which $a^x = y$.

Equivalently, $a^x = y$, if and only if $\log_a y = x$.

The base a must be positive and not equal to 1, that is, $a > 0$ and $a \neq 1$.

We can rewrite exponential equations as equivalent logarithmic equations, and logarithmic equations as equivalent exponential equations.

EXAMPLE 5 Rewrite each exponential equation as an equivalent logarithmic equation:

a) $2^5 = 32$; **b)** $4^2 = 16$; **c)** $6^1 = 6$; **d)** $3^{-2} = \frac{1}{9}$; **e)** $7^0 = 1$.

Solution We use the definition of logarithm: The logarithm, base a, of y is the number x for which $a^x = y$.

a) Since $2^5 = 32$, we have $\log_2 32 = 5$.

b) Since $4^2 = 16$, we have $\log_4 16 = 2$.

c) Since $6^1 = 6$, we have $\log_6 6 = 1$.

d) Since $3^{-2} = \frac{1}{9}$, we have $\log_3\left(\frac{1}{9}\right) = -2$.

e) Since $7^0 = 1$, we have $\log_7 1 = 0$.

5 ✓

Quick Check 5 ✓

Rewrite each exponential equation as an equivalent logarithmic equation:

a) $8^2 = 64$;

b) $3^{-4} = \frac{1}{81}$;

c) $12^0 = 1$.

EXAMPLE 6 Rewrite each logarithmic equation as an equivalent exponential equation:

a) $\log_5 25 = 2$; **b)** $\log_3 243 = 5$; **c)** $\log_{10} 100 = 2$; **d)** $\log_4 0.25 = -1$.

Solution We use the definition of logarithm: the logarithm, base a, of y is the number x for which $a^x = y$.

a) Since $\log_5 25 = 2$, we identify the base as 5 and the exponent as 2. Thus, we have $5^2 = 25$.

b) Since $\log_3 243 = 5$, we have $3^5 = 243$.

c) Since $\log_{10} 100 = 2$, we have $10^2 = 100$.

d) Since $\log_4 0.25 = -1$, we have $4^{-1} = \frac{1}{4} = 0.25$.

6 ✓

Quick Check 6 ✓

Rewrite each logarithmic equation as an equivalent exponential equation:

a) $\log_2\left(\frac{1}{8}\right) = -3$;

b) $\log_9 81 = 2$;

c) $\log_{11} 11 = 1$.

EXAMPLE 7 Solve for x in each logarithmic equation.

a) $\log_2 x = 6$ **b)** $\log_3\left(\frac{1}{3}\right) = x$ **c)** $\log_x 49 = 2$ **d)** $\log_{16} x = -\frac{1}{2}$

Solution

a) Since $\log_2 x = 6$, we identify the base as 2 and the exponent as 6. Thus, we have $2^6 = x$, so $x = 64$. The solution is 64.

b) Since $\log_3\left(\frac{1}{3}\right) = x$, we have $3^x = \frac{1}{3}$, so $x = -1$. The solution is –1.

c) Since $\log_x 49 = 2$, we have $x^2 = 49$, so $x = 7$ or $x = -7$. Because the base must be positive, we conclude that $x = 7$. The solution is 7.

d) Since $\log_{16} x = -\frac{1}{2}$, we have $x = 16^{-1/2} = \frac{1}{16^{1/2}} = \frac{1}{\sqrt{16}} = \frac{1}{4}$. The solution is $\frac{1}{4}$.

7 ✓

Quick Check 7 ✓

Solve for x in each logarithmic equation:

a) $\log_{10} 1000 = x$;

b) $\log_2 x = -4$;

c) $\log_x 9 = 2$.

Basic Properties of Logarithms

The following are some basic properties of logarithms. Properties P4, P5, P7, and P8 follow directly from the definition of a logarithm, and the proof of P6 is left as Exercise 89.

THEOREM 4 Properties of Logarithms

P1. $\log_a (MN) = \log_a M + \log_a N$

P2. $\log_a \left(\frac{M}{N}\right) = \log_a M - \log_a N$

P3. $\log_a (M^b) = b \log_a M$

P4. $\log_a a = 1$

P5. $\log_a 1 = 0$

P6. $\log_a M = \frac{\log_b M}{\log_b a}$ (the change-of-base formula)

P7. $\log_a a^k = k$

P8. For any $x > 0$, $a^{\log_a x} = x$.

The proof of Property P1, $\log_a (MN) = \log_a M + \log_a N$, is shown below.

Proof: Let $x = \log_a M$ and $y = \log_a N$. Writing these as exponential equations, we have $a^x = M$ and $a^y = N$, respectively. It follows that $a^x a^y = MN$. By Theorem 1 in Appendix A, we have

$$MN = a^x a^y = a^{x+y}.$$

Since $a^{x+y} = MN$, it follows that

$$x + y = \log_a (MN).$$

Since $x = \log_a M$ and $y = \log_a N$, we have

$$\log_a M + \log_a N = \log_a (MN). \quad \text{Substituting}$$

The proofs of Properties P2 and P3 are similar and are left as Exercises 87 and 88. ■

Let's illustrate these properties.

EXAMPLE 8 Given

$$\log_a 2 = 0.301 \quad \text{and} \quad \log_a 3 = 0.477,$$

find each of the following:

a) $\log_a 6$; **b)** $\log_a \frac{2}{3}$; **c)** $\log_a 81$; **d)** $\log_a \frac{1}{3}$;

e) $\log_a \sqrt{a}$; **f)** $\log_a (2a)$; **g)** $\frac{\log_a 3}{\log_a 2}$; **h)** $\log_a 5$.

Solution

a)
$$\begin{aligned} \log_a 6 &= \log_a (2 \cdot 3) \\ &= \log_a 2 + \log_a 3 && \text{Using Property P1} \\ &= 0.301 + 0.477 \\ &= 0.778 \end{aligned}$$

b)
$$\begin{aligned} \log_a \tfrac{2}{3} &= \log_a 2 - \log_a 3 && \text{Using Property P2} \\ &= 0.301 - 0.477 \\ &= -0.176 \end{aligned}$$

c)
$$\begin{aligned} \log_a 81 &= \log_a 3^4 && \text{Recognizing 81 as a power of 3} \\ &= 4 \log_a 3 && \text{Using Property P3} \\ &= 4(0.477) \\ &= 1.908 \end{aligned}$$

d) $\log_a \frac{1}{3} = \log_a 1 - \log_a 3$ Using Property P2

$= 0 - 0.477$ Using Property P5

$= -0.477$

e) $\log_a \sqrt{a} = \log_a (a^{1/2}) = \frac{1}{2}$ Using Property P7

f) $\log_a (2a) = \log_a 2 + \log_a a$

$= 0.301 + 1$ Using Properties P1 and P4

$= 1.301$

g) $\dfrac{\log_a 3}{\log_a 2} = \dfrac{0.477}{0.301} \approx 1.58$

Here we simply divided and used none of the properties.

h) It is not possible to find $\log_a 5$ using the properties of logarithms (note that $\log_a 5 \neq \log_a 2 + \log_a 3$).

8 ✓

Quick Check 8 ✓

Assume that $\log_b 2 = 0.356$ and $\log_b 5 = 0.827$. If possible, find each of the following:

a) $\log_b 10$; **b)** $\log_b \frac{2}{5}$;

c) $\log_b \frac{5}{2}$; **d)** $\log_b 16$;

e) $\log_b 5b$; **f)** $\log_b \sqrt{b}$.

Common Logarithms

The number $\log_{10} x$ is the **common logarithm** of x and is abbreviated $\log x$.

DEFINITION

For any positive number x, $\log x = \log_{10} x$.

Thus, when we write "$\log x$" with no base indicated, base 10 is assumed. Note the following comparison of common logarithms and powers of 10.

$1000 = 10^3$	The common logarithms at the right follow from the powers at the left.	$\log 1000 = 3$
$100 = 10^2$		$\log 100 = 2$
$10 = 10^1$		$\log 10 = 1$
$1 = 10^0$		$\log 1 = 0$
$0.1 = 10^{-1}$		$\log 0.1 = -1$
$0.01 = 10^{-2}$		$\log 0.01 = -2$
$0.001 = 10^{-3}$		$\log 0.001 = -3$

Since $\log 100 = 2$ and $\log 1000 = 3$, it seems reasonable that $\log 500$ is somewhere between 2 and 3. Using a calculator with a LOG key, we find that $\log 500 \approx 2.6990$.

Before calculators became readily available, common logarithms were listed in tables and used extensively to do certain computations. In fact, computation is the reason logarithms were developed. Since standard notation for numbers is based on 10, it was logical to use base-10, or common, logarithms for computations.

For a logarithm with a base other than 10, we can use the change-of-base formula (Property P6) to rewrite the logarithm as a quotient of two common logarithms:

$$\log_a x = \frac{\log x}{\log a}.$$

EXAMPLE 9 Use common logarithms and the change-of-base formula to find the following:

a) $\log 45$; **b)** $\log_5 12$; **c)** $\log_6 27$.

Solution We use the change-of-base formula, and let the base $b = 10$ so that we can use a calculator's common logarithm feature to solve.

a) $\log 45 = 1.65321\ldots$. As a check, we note that $10^{1.65321} = 44.99973953 \approx 45$. Since we rounded the exponent, the result of our check has a small amount of error.

b) Using the change-of-base formula, we have $\log_5 12 = \dfrac{\log 12}{\log 5} \approx 1.54396$.

Check: $5^{1.54396} = 12.00001331 \approx 12$.

c) $\log_6 27 = \dfrac{\log 27}{\log 6} \approx 1.83944$

Check: $6^{1.83944} = 26.99992 \approx 27$. **9 ✓**

Quick Check 9 ✓

Find: $\log_9 18$ and $\log_{20} 10$.

Graphs of Logarithmic Functions

The graph of a logarithmic function of the form $g(x) = \log_a x$ can be drawn by considering the graph of $f(x) = a^x$ and reversing the coordinates in each ordered pair. For example, the graph of $f(x) = 2^x$ is shown below, along with an input-output table:

x	-3	-2	-1	0	1	2	3
$y = f(x) = 2^x$	$\frac{1}{8}$	$\frac{1}{4}$	$\frac{1}{2}$	1	2	4	8

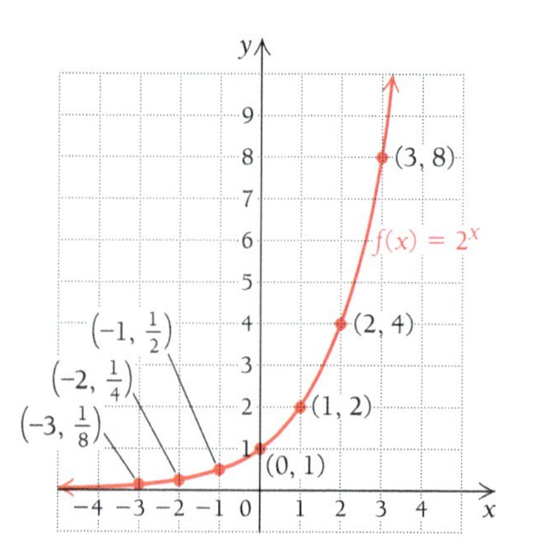

To graph $g(x) = \log_2 x$, we reverse the coordinates of each ordered pair:

x	$\frac{1}{8}$	$\frac{1}{4}$	$\frac{1}{2}$	1	2	4	8
$y = g(x) = \log_2 x$	-3	-2	-1	0	1	2	3

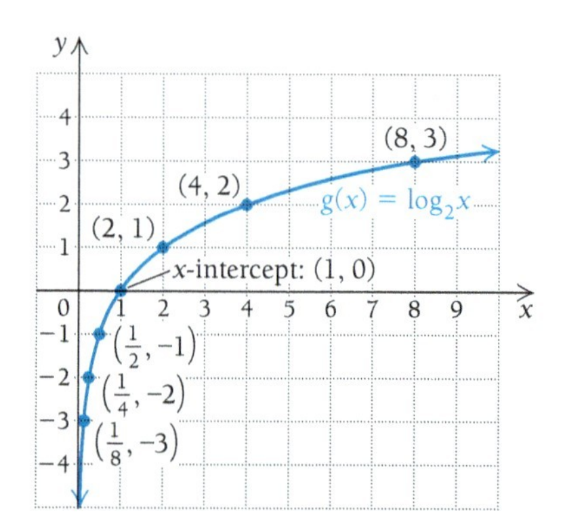

All functions of the form $g(x) = \log_a x$, where $a > 1$, have the following characteristics:

- The domain is $\{x|x > 0\}$.
- The range is $\{y|-\infty < y < \infty\}$.
- The x-intercept is $(1, 0)$.
- There is no y-intercept.
- As x approaches infinity, so does y, but more slowly.
- As x approaches 0, y decreases toward negative infinity.

EXAMPLE 10 Graph $y = \log_5 (x + 2)$, and state its domain.

Solution We rewrite the given equation, $y = \log_5 (x + 2)$, as an equivalent exponential equation:

$$5^y = x + 2, \qquad \text{or} \qquad x = 5^y - 2.$$

We now choose convenient values for y and find x:

y	-2	-1	0	1	2
$x = 5^y - 2$	$5^{-2} - 2 = -1.96$	$5^{-1} - 2 = -1.8$	$5^0 - 2 = -1$	$5^1 - 2 = 3$	$5^2 - 2 = 23$

Next, we write these ordered pairs as (x, y) to create an input-output table for $y = \log_5 (x + 2)$:

x	-1.96	-1.8	-1	3	23
$y = \log_5 (x + 2)$	-2	-1	0	1	2

We plot these ordered pairs and draw a smooth curve joining them.

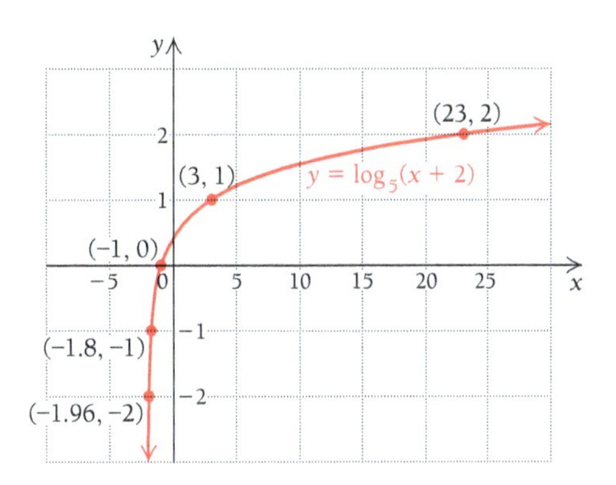

Note that the domain of $y = \log_5 (x + 2)$ is $\{x | x > -2\}$. **10 ✓**

Quick Check 10 ✓

Graph $y = 4 \log_2 (x - 1)$, and state its domain.

Applications of Logarithms

EXAMPLE 11 **Business: Compound Interest.** Bert deposits \$10,000 in a savings account that earns 3.25% interest per year. When will his account have a value of \$20,000?

Solution In Example 3, we found that the value, A, of Bert's account t years after his initial deposit is given by

$$A(t) = 10{,}000(1.0325)^t.$$

To find when his account will have a value of \$20,000, we substitute 20,000 for A and solve for t:

$$20{,}000 = 10{,}000(1.0325)^t \quad \text{Substituting 20,000 for } A$$

$$2 = (1.0325)^t \quad \text{Dividing both sides by 10,000}$$

$$t = \log_{1.0325} 2 \quad \text{Rewriting as an equivalent logarithmic equation}$$

$$t = \frac{\log 2}{\log (1.0325)} \approx 21.67 \quad \text{Using the change-of-base formula}$$

Bert's savings account will reach a value of \$20,000 after about 21.67 yr. **11 ✓**

Quick Check 11 ✓

Michele invests \$75,000 at an annual interest rate of 4.5%. When will her investment be worth \$125,000? (*Hint*: Use the result from Quick Check 3.)

Section Summary

- An *exponential function* is of the form $f(x) = a_0 \cdot a^x$, where $a > 0$ and $a \neq 1$. The y-intercept is $(0, a_0)$; there are no x-intercepts; the domain is all of the real numbers, $\{x \mid -\infty < x < \infty\}$; and the range is $\{y \mid y > 0\}$.
- Consider $A = P(1 + r)^t$. If we write $a = 1 + r$, then r represents the fixed percent increase (if $r > 0$) or decrease (if $-1 < r < 0$) of the quantity over a fixed period of time. Note that when $-1 < r < 0$, then $0 < a < 1$, and when $r > 0$, then $a > 1$.
- The *logarithm*, base a, of y is the number x for which $a^x = y$. Equivalently, $a^x = y$, if and only if $\log_a y = x$. The base a must be positive and not equal to 1, that is, $a > 0$ and $a \neq 1$.
- The properties of logarithms include the following:
  - **P1.** $\log_a (MN) = \log_a M + \log_a N$;
  - **P2.** $\log_a \left(\frac{M}{N}\right) = \log_a M - \log_a N$;
  - **P3.** $\log_a (M^b) = b \log_a M$;
  - **P4.** $\log_a a = 1$;
  - **P5.** $\log_a 1 = 0$;
  - **P6.** $\log_a M = \frac{\log_b M}{\log_b a}$;
  - **P7.** $\log_a a^k = k$;
  - **P8.** For any $x > 0$, $a^{\log_a x} = x$.
- The *common logarithm* has the base 10. The expression $\log x$ is understood to be the same as $\log_{10} x$.
- A logarithmic function is of the form $f(x) = \log_a x$, where $a > 0$ and $a \neq 1$. Its domain is $\{x \mid x > 0\}$. Its x-intercept is $(1, 0)$, and there is no y-intercept.

R.6 Exercise Set

For Exercises 1–10, (a) complete an input-output table for $x = -3, -2, -1, 0, 1, 2, 3$; (b) state the percent increase or decrease per unit x, (c) identify the y-intercept, and (d) sketch the graph.

1. $f(x) = 4^x$
2. $g(x) = 5^x$
3. $h(x) = 2 \cdot 1.5^x$
4. $k(x) = 6 \cdot 1.2^x$
5. $m(x) = -3 \cdot 2.15^x$
6. $n(x) = -2 \cdot 3.04^x$
7. $p(x) = 12{,}000(0.95)^x$
8. $q(x) = 75{,}000{,}000(0.875)^x$
9. $r(x) = r_0(0.233)^x$
10. $s(x) = s_0(0.752)^x$

Write an equivalent logarithmic equation.

11. $4^3 = 64$
12. $5^4 = 625$
13. $10^{-2} = 0.01$
14. $7^{-2} = \frac{1}{49}$
15. $\sqrt{25} = 5$
16. $\sqrt{36} = 6$
17. $\sqrt[3]{216} = 6$
18. $\sqrt[5]{32} = 2$
19. $P^n = Q$
20. $r^v = z$

Write an equivalent exponential equation.

21. $\log_2 128 = 7$
22. $\log_4 1024 = 5$
23. $\log 10{,}000{,}000 = 7$
24. $\log 100{,}000 = 5$
25. $\log_{16} 4 = \frac{1}{2}$
26. $\log_{100} 10 = \frac{1}{2}$
27. $\log_7 \sqrt[3]{7} = \frac{1}{3}$
28. $\log_{15} \sqrt[4]{15} = \frac{1}{4}$
29. $\log_9 1 = 0$
30. $\log_\pi 1 = 0$

Solve for x without using a calculator.

31. $\log_2 x = 8$
32. $\log_2 x = 10$
33. $\log_x 125 = 3$
34. $\log_x 64 = 2$
35. $\log_{13} 13 = x$
36. $\log_{25} 25 = x$
37. $\log_5 \frac{1}{25} = x$
38. $\log_6 \frac{1}{36} = x$
39. $\log_6 6^\pi = x$
40. $\log_7 7^{\sqrt{2}} = x$

Use the change-of-base formula to find each logarithm. Give the answers to five decimal places.

41. $\log_2 7$
42. $\log_5 8$
43. $\log_3 16$
44. $\log_7 14$
45. $\log_4 25$
46. $\log_8 30$
47. $\log_9 45$
48. $\log_2 9$
49. $\log_6 3$
50. $\log_9 2$

Solve each equation for x. Give the answers to five decimal places.

51. $7^x = 28$
52. $11^x = 33$
53. $5^x = 50$
54. $9^x = 63$
55. $(1.055)^x = 1.78$
56. $(1.0325)^x = 3.5$
57. $(0.45)^x = 0.22$
58. $(0.87)^x = 0.59$
59. $3 \cdot 6^x = 19$
60. $5 \cdot 7^x = 42$

Given $\log_a 2 = 0.483$ and $\log_a 3 = 0.766$, use the properties of logarithms to find each of the following.

61. $\log_a 8$
62. $\log_a 9$
63. $\log_a 12$
64. $\log_a 18$
65. $\log_a 1.5$
66. $\log_a 4.5$

67. $\log_a 4a$

68. $\log_a 6a$

69. $\log_a \frac{1}{2}$

70. $\log_a \frac{1}{3}$

Sketch the graph of each logarithmic function, and state its domain.

71. $f(x) = \log_3 x$

72. $m(x) = \log_5 x$

73. $t(x) = \log_4 (x - 3)$

74. $v(x) = \log_3 (x + 5)$

75. $k(x) = \log (2x - 1)$

76. $r(x) = \log_2 (2 - 3x)$

APPLICATIONS

General Interest

77. Casa Grande Technical School had a total enrollment of 900 students in 2015, and the student population is increasing by 4.5% yearly.
   a) Find the exponential function A that gives the population t years after 2015.
   b) Find $A(5)$, and interpret this result.
   c) When will the student population first reach 1200?

78. Parker Valley had a population of 12,500 in 2015, and the population is increasing by 2.75% yearly.
   a) Find the exponential function P that gives the population t years after 2015.
   b) Find $P(8)$, and interpret this result.
   c) When will the population of Parker Valley first reach 20,000?

79. An element undergoes natural radioactive decay. The original sample had a mass of 50 mg, and it is losing 1.25% of its mass daily.
   a) Find an exponential function M that gives the mass of the sample t days after the original sample was set aside for observation.
   b) Find $M(15)$, and interpret this result.
   c) When will the sample have a mass of 20 mg?

80. Tonopah Acres had a population of 2500 in 2011 but has been losing 2.4% of its population yearly.
   a) Find the exponential function q that gives the population t years after 2011.
   b) Find $q(11)$, and interpret this result.
   c) When will the population be 1250?

81. The online program at Accent University had an enrollment of 550 students at its inception and an enrollment of 1750 students 3 yr later. Assume that the enrollment increases by the same percentage per year.
   a) Find the exponential function E that gives the enrollment t years after the online program's inception.
   b) Find $E(10)$, and interpret this result.
   c) When will the program's enrollment reach 5000 students?

82. The startup GorePoint Inc. had 15 employees initially and 50 employees 6 months later. Assume that the number of employees increases by the same percentage per month.
   a) Find the exponential function G that gives the number of employees t months after the company started operations.
   b) Find $G(12)$, and interpret this result.
   c) When will the number of employees at GorePoint Inc. reach 250?

Business and Economics

83. Hank deposits \$100,000 into a retirement fund that earns 2.5% annual interest. When will his initial investment have doubled in value?

84. Jenny deposits \$5000 into a savings account that earns 3% annual interest. When will her savings account have tripled in value?

85. A stock originally worth \$50 per share is losing 1% of its value per week. When will a share of the stock be worth \$45?

86. A property originally worth \$12,000 is losing 3% of its value every month. When will the property be worth \$10,000?

SYNTHESIS

87. Prove that $\log_a \left(\frac{M}{N}\right) = \log_a M - \log_a N$.
$\left(\textit{Hint}: \text{Use the fact that } \frac{a^x}{a^y} = a^{x-y}.\right)$

88. Prove that $\log_a (M^b) = b \log_a M$. [*Hint*: Use Property P1, where $M^b = M \cdot M \cdot M \cdot \cdots \cdot M$ (there are b factors).]

89. Prove that $\log_a M = \frac{\log_b M}{\log_b a}$. (*Hint*: Use Property P3 and the fact that if $x = y$, then $\log_b x = \log_b y$.)

90. Prove that $\log_a \left(\frac{N}{M}\right) = -\log_a \left(\frac{M}{N}\right)$.

In Exercises 91 and 92, use the fact that if $M < N$, then $\log_a M < \log_a N$ when $a > 1$.

91. Which is larger, 80^{90} or 90^{80}?

92. Which is larger, 125^{200} or 200^{125}?

93. Find the domain of $f(x) = \log_4 (x^2 - 1)$.

Answers to Quick Checks

1.

x	$f(x) = 3^x$
-3	$\frac{1}{27}$
-2	$\frac{1}{9}$
-1	$\frac{1}{3}$
0	1
1	3
2	9
3	27

200%

(continued)

Answers to Quick Checks (*cont.*)

2.

x	$g(x) = 2\cdot\left(\frac{1}{3}\right)^x$
-3	54
-2	18
-1	6
0	2
1	$\frac{2}{3}$
2	$\frac{2}{9}$
3	$\frac{2}{27}$

(0, 2)

66.7%

3. (a) $A(t) = 75{,}000(1.045)^t$; **(b)** $A(15) = 145{,}146.18$, which means that in 15 years, Michele's account will be worth \$145,146.18. **4. (a)** $M(t) = 15(0.9945)^t$; **(b)** $M(50) = 11.38$, which means that after 50 days, 11.38 g remain; **(c)** -0.55% per day **5. (a)** $\log_8 64 = 2$; **(b)** $\log_3\left(\frac{1}{81}\right) = -4$; **(c)** $\log_{12} 1 = 0$

6. (a) $2^{-3} = \frac{1}{8}$; **(b)** $9^2 = 81$; **(c)** $11^1 = 11$

7. (a) $x = 3$; **(b)** $x = \frac{1}{16}$; **(c)** $x = 3$

8. (a) 1.183; **(b)** -0.471; **(c)** 0.471; **(d)** 1.424; **(e)** 1.827; **(f)** $\frac{1}{2}$ **9.** 1.31546 . . . ; 0.76862 . . .

10. $y = 4\log_2(x-1)$ $\{x|x > 1\}$ **11.** In 11.6 yr

R.7

- Use curve fitting to find a mathematical model for a set of data, and use the model to make predictions.

Mathematical Modeling and Curve Fitting

Fitting Functions to Data

We now have a library of functions that can serve as models for applications, and they are shown below. Cubic and quartic functions are covered in detail in Chapter 2, but we show them here for reference. In this section, we will not consider rational functions.

Linear function: $f(x) = mx + b$

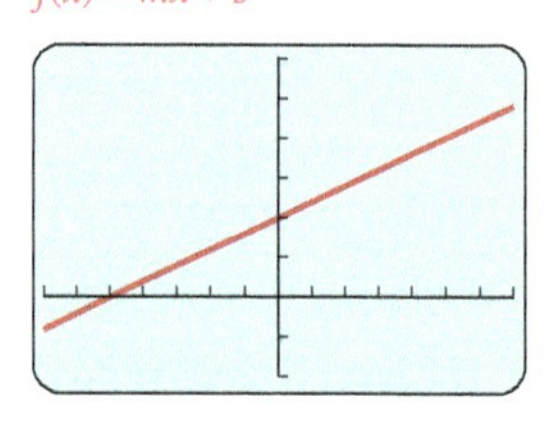

Quadratic function: $f(x) = ax^2 + bx + c,\ a > 0$

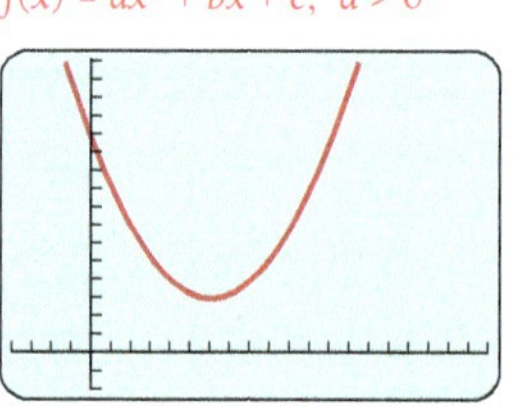

Quadratic function: $f(x) = ax^2 + bx + c,\ a < 0$

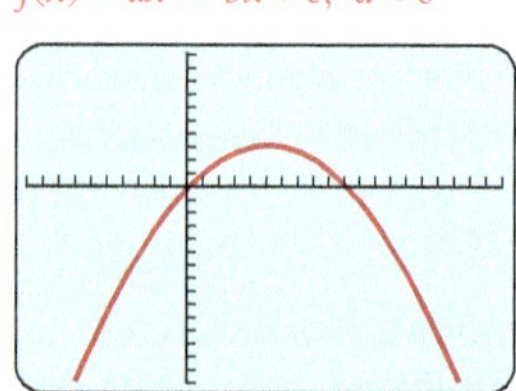

Absolute-value function: $f(x) = |x|$

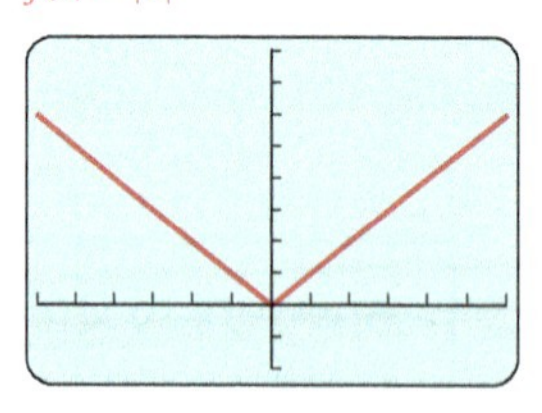

Cubic function: $f(x) = ax^3 + bx^2 + cx + d,\ a > 0$

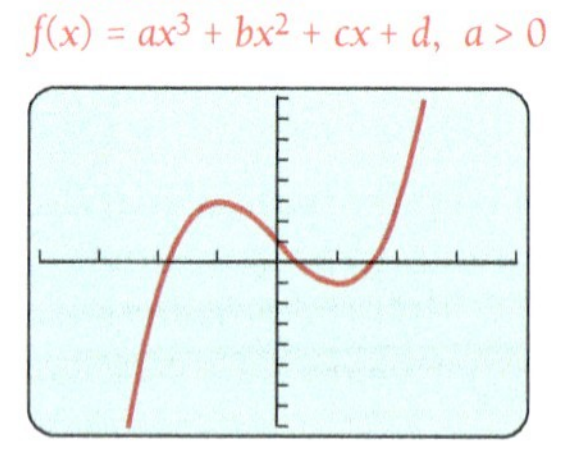

Quartic function: $f(x) = ax^4 + bx^3 + cx^2 + dx + e,\ a > 0$

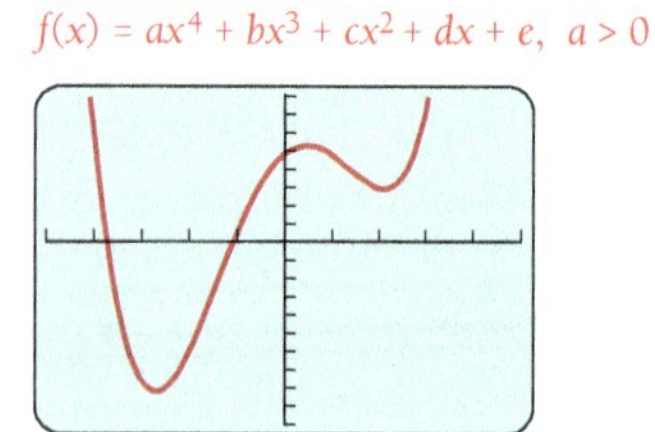

Exponential growth: $f(x) = a_0\cdot a^x,\ a > 1$

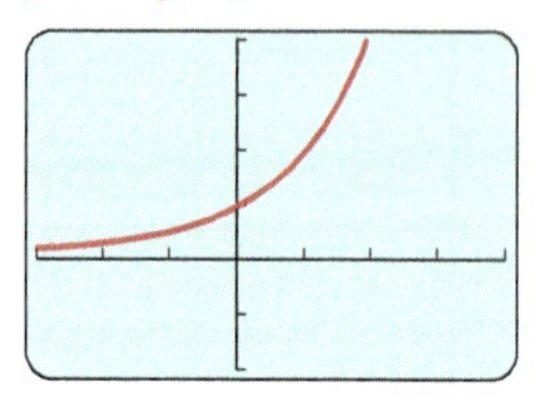

Exponential decay: $f(x) = a_0\cdot a^x,\ 0 < a < 1$

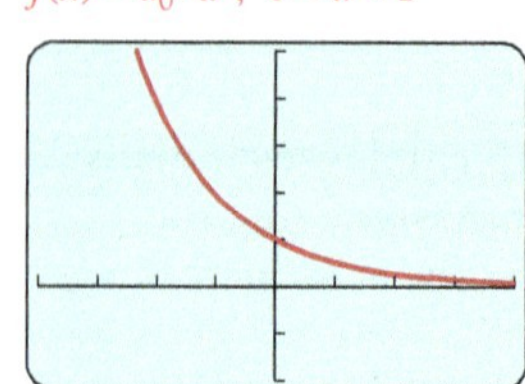

Logarithmic growth: $f(x) = a + b\log x$

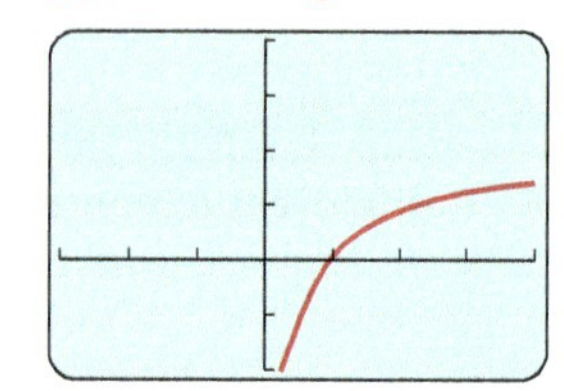

Now let's consider real-world data. How can we decide which, if any, type of function might fit the given data? One way is to examine a graph of the data called a **scatterplot**. Then we look for a pattern resembling one of the preceding graphs. For example, if the graph resembles a straight line, the best model might be a linear function. Other functions may be appropriate if the graph has the form of a curve. More than one type of function might be used to model a set of data.

EXAMPLE 1 **Choosing Models.** For the following scatterplots and graphs, determine which, if any, of the following functions might be used as a model for the data.

Linear: $f(x) = mx + b$

Quadratic: $f(x) = ax^2 + bx + c, \quad a > 0$

Quadratic: $f(x) = ax^2 + bx + c, \quad a < 0$

Polynomial: neither quadratic nor linear

Exponential: $f(x) = a_0 \cdot a^x, \quad 0 < a < 1$ or $a > 1$

Logarithmic: $f(x) = a + b \log x$

a)

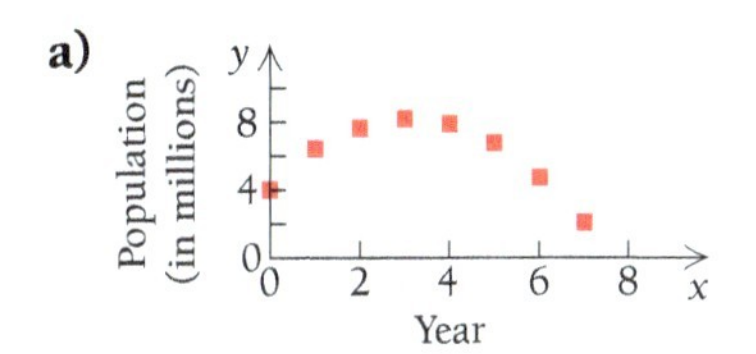

b)

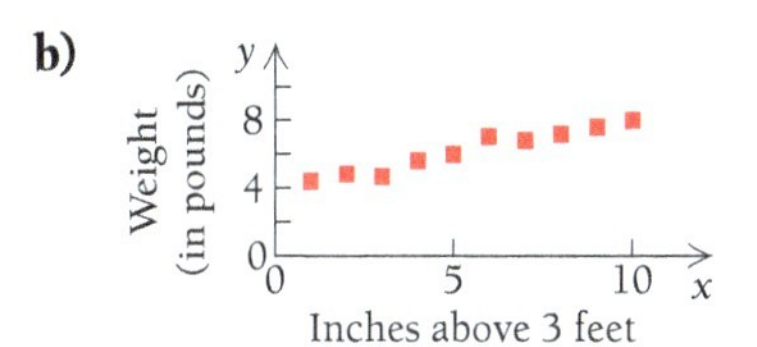

c)

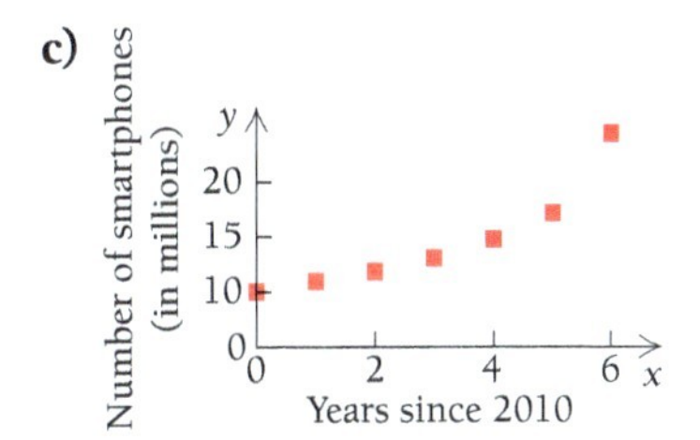

d)

YEARLY AUTO INSURANCE PREMIUMS BY AGE

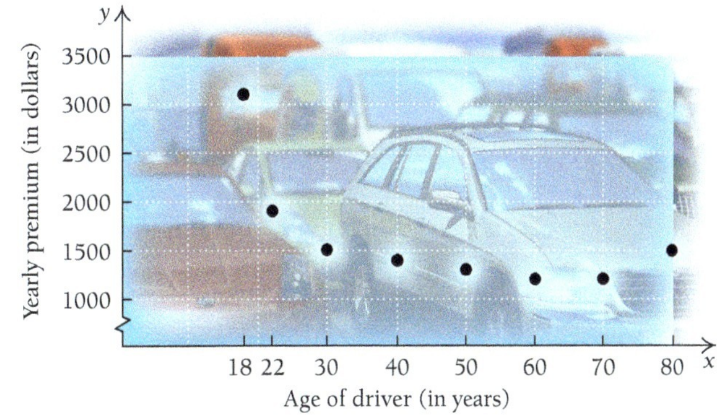

(*Source*: Based on data from insurance.com/auto-insurance, 2016.)

e)

ANNUAL SUIT SALES FOR RAGGS LTD.

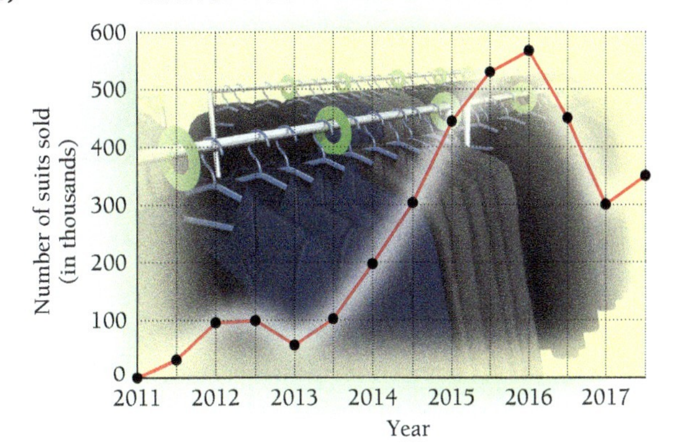

Solution

a) The data rise and then fall in a curved manner suggesting a quadratic function,

$$f(x) = ax^2 + bx + c, \quad a < 0.$$

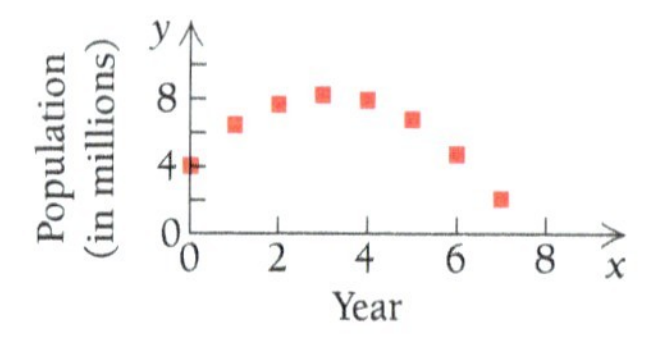

b) The data seem to fit a linear function,

$$f(x) = mx + b.$$

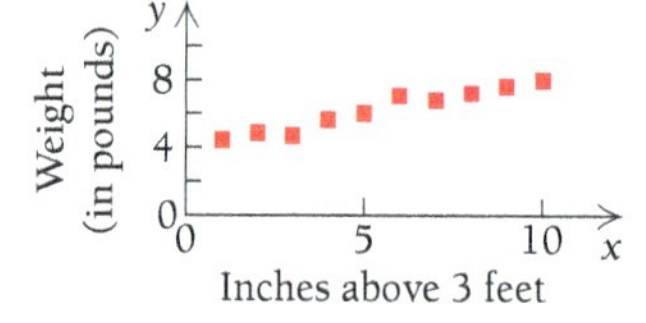

c) The data rise in a manner fitting the right-hand side of a quadratic function,

$$f(x) = ax^2 + bx + c, \quad a > 0.$$

The data may also fit an exponential growth function,

$$f(x) = a_0 \cdot a^x, \quad a > 1.$$

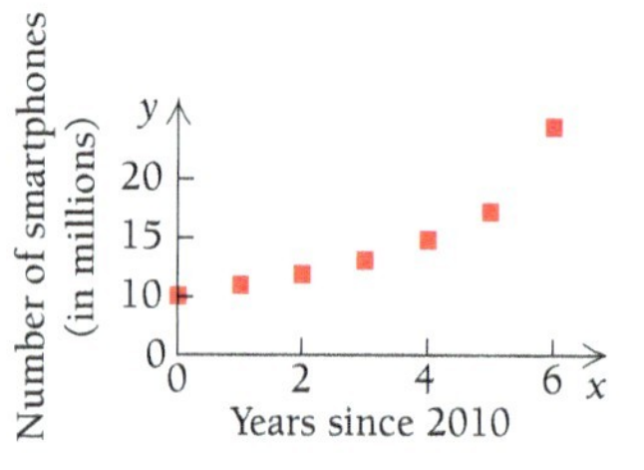

d) The data fall and then rise in a curved manner suggesting a quadratic function,

$$f(x) = ax^2 + bx + c, \quad a > 0.$$

YEARLY AUTO INSURANCE PREMIUMS BY AGE

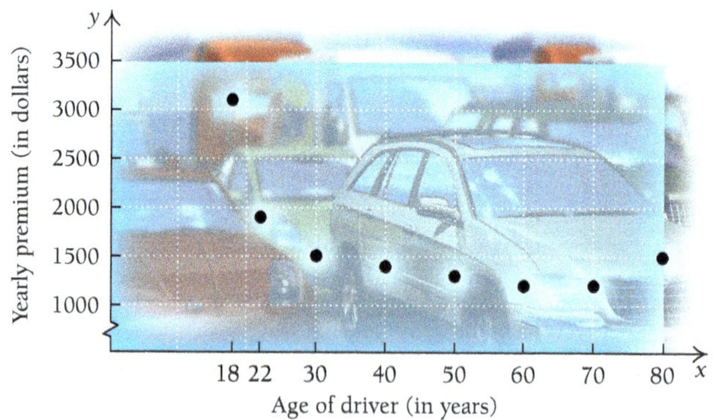

(*Source*: Based on data from insurance.com/auto-insurance, 2016.)

e) The data rise and fall more than once, so they do not fit a linear or quadratic function but might fit a polynomial function that is neither quadratic nor linear.

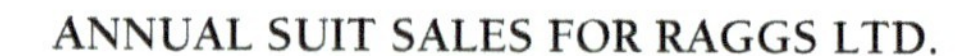

ANNUAL SUIT SALES FOR RAGGS LTD.

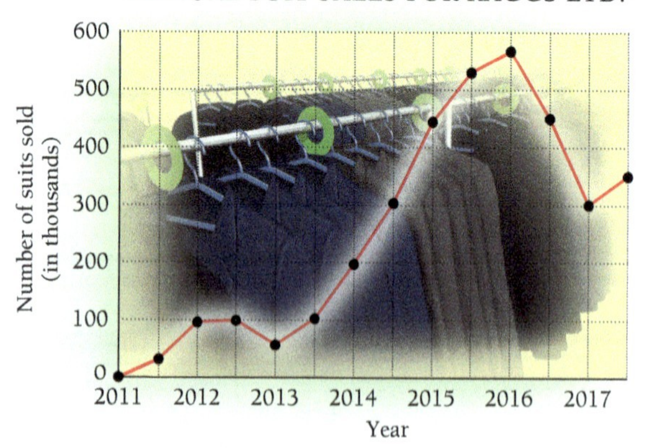

It is sometimes possible to find a mathematical model by graphing a set of data as a scatterplot, inspecting the graph to see if a known type of function seems to fit, and then using the data points to derive the equation of a specific function.

EXAMPLE 2 **Business: Broadband Cable Customers.** The following table and scatterplot show the numbers of broadband cable customers in the United States for several years.

Years since 2011, x	Number of Broadband Cable Customers (in millions), y	Scatterplot
2011, 0	47	Broadband Cable Customers in the United States
2012, 1	49	
2013, 2	51	
2014, 3	55	
2015, 4	58	
2016, 5	60	
2017, 6	66	

(*Source:* Based on data from www.ncta.com.)

a) It appears that the data can be modeled by a linear function. Find a linear function that fits the data.

b) Use the model to predict the number of broadband cable customers in the United States in 2020.

Solution

a) We can choose any two data points to determine an equation. Let's use (1, 49) and (6, 66). (Different pairs of points will yield different results, as we will discuss shortly.)

We first determine the slope of the line:

$$m = \frac{66 - 49}{6 - 1} = \frac{17}{5} = 3.4.$$

We substitute 3.4 for m and either of the points (1, 49) or (6, 66) for (x_1, y_1) in the point–slope equation. Using (1, 49), we get

$$y - 49 = 3.4(x - 1),$$

which is equivalent to

$$y = 3.4x + 45.6,$$

where x is the number of years after 2011 and y is the number of broadband cable customers, in millions. We can then graph $y = 3.4x + 45.6$ on the scatterplot to see how well it fits the data.

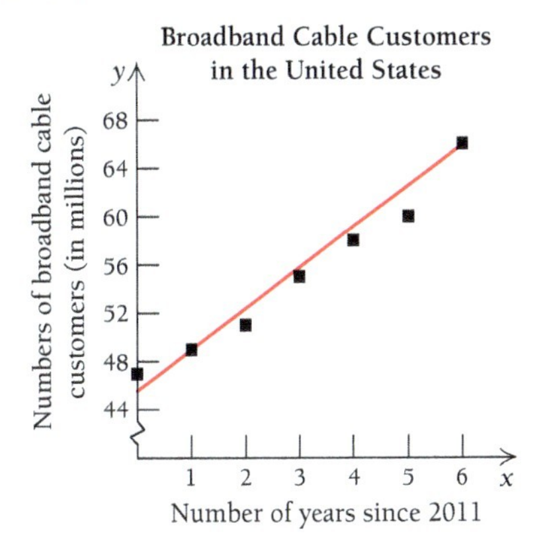

b) We can predict the number of broadband cable customers in 2020 by substituting 9 for x (since $2020 - 2011 = 9$) in the model:

$$\begin{aligned} y &= 3.4x + 45.6 && \text{Model} \\ &= 3.4(9) + 45.6 && \text{Substituting} \\ &= 76.2. \end{aligned}$$

We can predict that there will be about 76.2 million broadband cable customers in the United States in 2020. **1 ✓**

Quick Check 1 ✓

Business. Repeat Example 2 using the data points (0, 47) and (3, 55). Are the model and the result different from those we obtained in Example 2?

Because different pairs of points yield different linear models, a method known as *regression* is used to find a line of *best* fit.

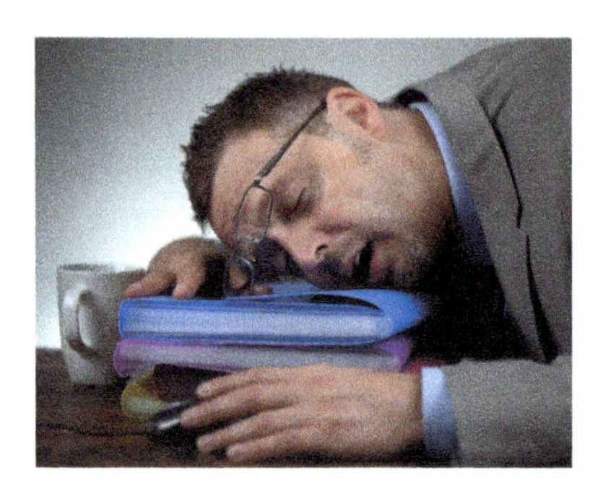

EXAMPLE 3 **Life Science: Hours of Sleep and Death Rate.** From a study by Dr. Harold J. Morowitz of Yale University, the following data show the relationship between the death rate of men and the average number of hours per day that the men slept.

Average Number of Hours of Sleep, x	Death Rate per 100,000 Males, y
5	1121
6	805
7	626
8	813
9	967

(*Source:* Morowitz, Harold J., "Hiding in the Hammond Report," *Hospital Practice.*)

a) Make a scatterplot of the data.

b) Find a function that fits the data.

c) Use the model to estimate the death rate for men who sleep 2 hr, 8 hr, and 10 hr.

Possible quadratic function that "fits" data

Death rate per 100,000 males

Average number of hours of sleep

Solution

a) The scatterplot is shown to the left. Note that the rate drops and then rises, which suggests that a quadratic function might fit the data.

b) We consider the quadratic model,

$$y = ax^2 + bx + c. \tag{1}$$

To determine the constants a, b, and c, we choose three of the data points: (5, 1121), (7, 626), and (9, 967). Since these points are to be solutions of equation (1), it follows that

$$\begin{aligned} 1121 &= a \cdot 5^2 + b \cdot 5 + c, && \text{or} && 1121 = 25a + 5b + c, \\ 626 &= a \cdot 7^2 + b \cdot 7 + c, && \text{or} && 626 = 49a + 7b + c, \\ 967 &= a \cdot 9^2 + b \cdot 9 + c, && \text{or} && 967 = 81a + 9b + c. \end{aligned}$$

This system of three equations can be solved algebraically by using two different pairs of the equations to create a system of two equations in two unknowns and solving that system. The steps used to do this are given in Exercise 27. The solutions are

$$a = 104.5, \quad b = -1501.5, \quad \text{and} \quad c = 6016.$$

Substituting these values into equation (1), we have

$$y = 104.5x^2 - 1501.5x + 6016.$$

Technology Connection 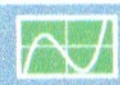

Linear Regression: Fitting a Linear Function to Data

We now consider **linear regression**, the preferred method for fitting a linear function to a set of data. Although the complete basis for this method is discussed in Section 6.4, we introduce it here because we can perform the procedure easily using technology. One advantage of linear regression is that it uses *all* data points rather than just two.

EXAMPLE Business: Broadband Cable Customers. Consider the data in Example 2.

a) Find the equation of the regression line for the given data. Then graph both the regression line and the data.

b) Use the model to predict the number of broadband cable customers in 2020. Compare your answer to that found in Example 2.

Solution

a) To fit a linear function using regression, select the EDIT option of the STAT menu. Then enter each first coordinate for L1 and the corresponding second coordinate for L2.

(0, 47), (1, 49), (2, 51), (3, 55), (4, 58), (5, 60), (6, 66)

L1	L2	L3
0	47	------
1	49	
2	51	
3	55	
4	58	
5	60	
6	66	

L2(6) = 66

To view the data points, press 2ND Y=, then select PLOT 1, highlight ON, and press ENTER and then QUIT. Next, select [0, 15, 0, 100] as the window size, because this will allow the given data to be displayed along with the forecasted point for 2020.

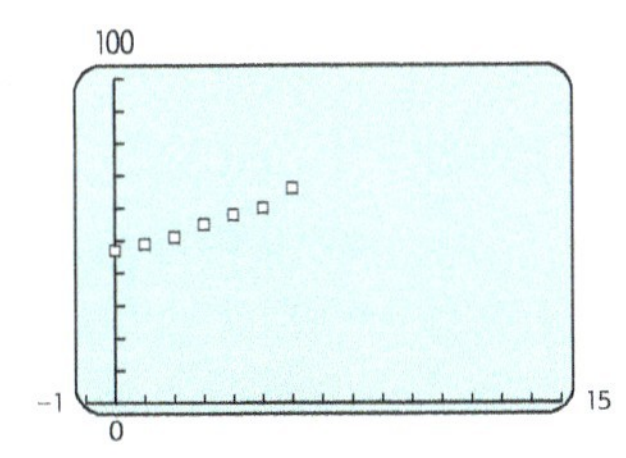

To find the line that best fits the data, press STAT, select CALC, then LinReg(ax+b), and then press ENTER.

LinReg
y = ax + b
a = 3.071428571
b = 45.92857143

To copy a regression function onto the Y= screen, press Y=, move the cursor to Y2 (or wherever the function is to appear), press VARS, and select STATISTICS and then EQ and RegEq.

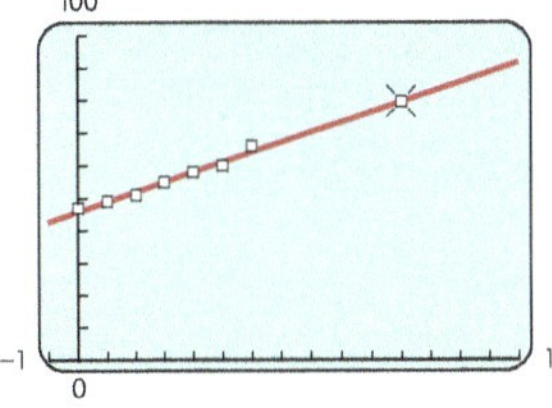

b) To find, or predict, the number of broadband cable customers in 2020, press 2ND, CALC, 1, and enter 11.

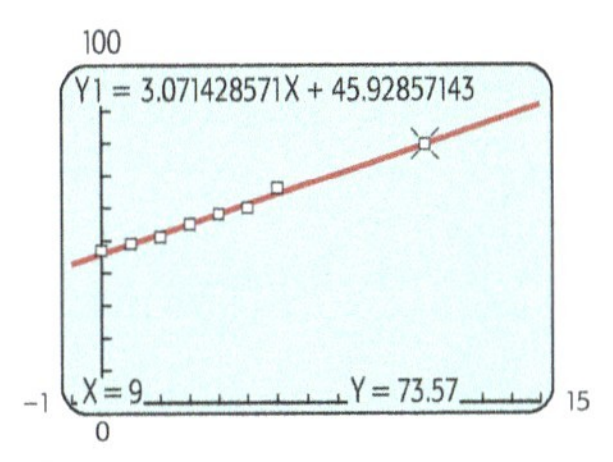

Note that the result, 73.57 million, is slightly less than the 76.2 million found in Example 2. Researchers generally give more credence to the regression value because more data points are used to construct the equation.

EXERCISE

1. Study time and test scores. The data in the following table relate study time and test scores.

Study Time (in hours)	Test Score (in percent)
7	83
8	85
9	88
10	91

a) Make a scatterplot of the data, fit a regression line to the data, and graph the line with the scatterplot.

b) Use the linear model to predict the test score received when study time is 11 hr.

c) What are some of the limitations of a linear model for this application?

Quick Check 2 ✓

Life Science. See the data on live births in the following Technology Connection. Use the data points (16, 9.9), (27, 104.3), and (37, 51.8) to find a quadratic function that fits the data. Then predict the average number of live births to women age 20.

c) The estimated death rate for men who sleep 2 hr is

$$y = 104.5(2)^2 - 1501.5(2) + 6016 = 3431 \text{ deaths per 100,000 men.}$$

The estimated death rate for men who sleep 8 hr is

$$y = 104.5(8)^2 - 1501.5(8) + 6016 = 692 \text{ deaths per 100,000 men.}$$

The estimated death rate for men who sleep 10 hr is

$$y = 104.5(10)^2 - 1501.5(10) + 6016 = 1451 \text{ deaths per 100,000 men.}$$

2 ✓

Note that choosing a different set of three points in Example 3 would yield a different quadratic function. Using regression, as discussed in the preceding Technology Connection, allows us to use *all* of the data points to find a function that is generally more reliable.

Exponential Models

Data that increase quickly as x increases may fit an exponential model of the form $f(x) = a_0 \cdot a^x$, where $a > 1$. When data decrease in such a way that they "level off" to zero as x increases, then the exponential model $f(x) = a_0 \cdot a^x$, where $0 < a < 1$, may fit the data well.

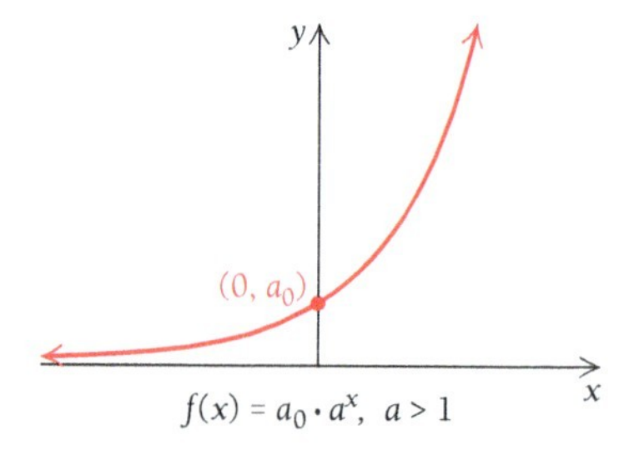

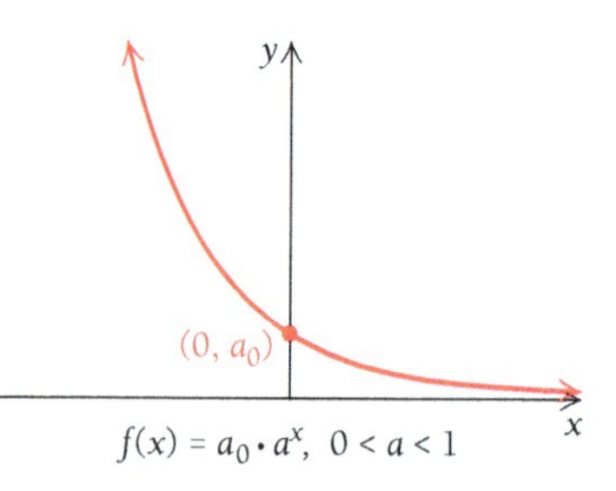

EXAMPLE 4 **Business: Annual Sales of Compact Discs.** The graph below illustrates the annual sales (in millions of dollars) of compact discs in the United States between 2011 and 2015.

ANNUAL SALES OF COMPACT DISCS

Year	2011	2012	2013	2014	2015
Annual sales (in millions of dollars)	224	193	165	141	126

(*Source*: Based on data from Glorious Noise and Neilsen.)

a) Using regression, find a quadratic model, $f(x) = ax^2 + bx + c$, that fits the data, and use it to estimate annual sales in 2020. Let x be the number of years since 2011.

b) Using regression, find an exponential model, $f(x) = a_0 \cdot a^x$, that fits the data, and use it to estimate annual sales in 2020.

c) Which model better predicts future annual sales of compact discs?

Technology Connection 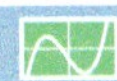

Mathematical Modeling Using Regression: Fitting Quadratic and Other Polynomial Functions to Data

Regression extends to quadratic, cubic, and quartic polynomial functions.

EXAMPLE **Life Science: Live Births to Women of Age x.** The chart below relates the average number of live births to women of a particular age.

Age, x (in years)	Average Number of Live Births per 1000 Women
16	9.9
18.5	40.7
22	76.8
27	104.3
32	101.5
37	51.8
42	11.0

(*Source:* CDC, *National Vital Statistics*, Vol. 66, No. 1, January 5, 2017.)

a) Fit a quadratic function to the data using REGRESSION. Then make a scatterplot of the data and graph the quadratic function with the scatterplot.

b) Fit a cubic function to the data using REGRESSION. Then make a scatterplot of the data and graph the cubic function with the scatterplot.

c) Which function seems to fit the data better?

d) Use the function from part (c) to estimate the average number of live births to women of ages 20 and 30.

Solution We proceed as follows.

a) To fit a quadratic function using REGRESSION, the procedure is similar to what is outlined in the Extended Technology Application at the end of this chapter. We enter the data and select QuadReg. In this case, we use ZoomStat to set the window. Here y_1 uses approximations of a, b, and c from the QuadReg screen.

$y_1 = -0.560178106x^2 + 32.29165009x - 363.0632803$

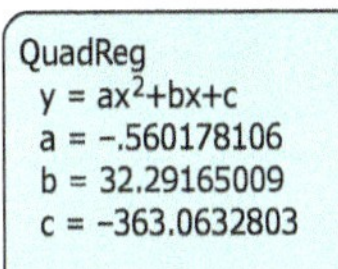

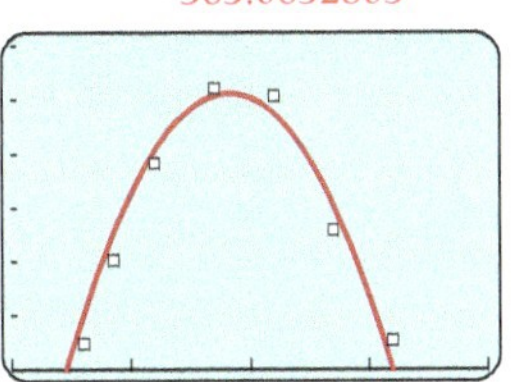

b) To fit a cubic function, we select the CALC option on the STAT menu and then select CubicReg. We obtain the following, which we enter as y_2.

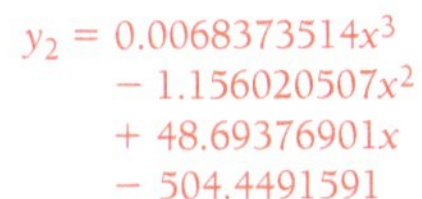

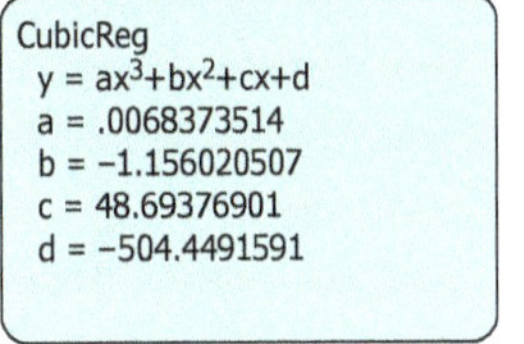

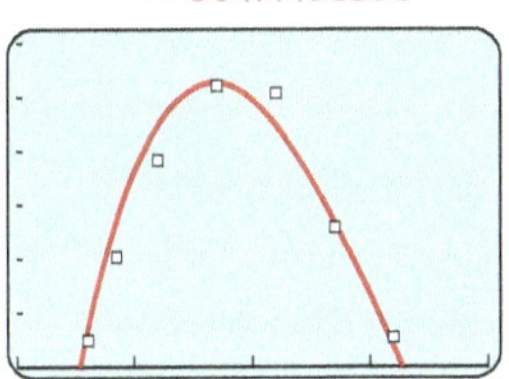

c) Both regression curves fit the data well. We'll use the cubic function for part (d).

d) We press 2ND QUIT to leave the graph screen. Pressing VARS and selecting Y-VARS and then FUNCTION and Y2, we have $y_2(20) = 61.7$ and $y_2(30) = 100.6$, as shown.

Y2(20) 61.71682992
Y2(30) 100.5539439

Thus, the average number of live births is about 62 per 1000 women age 20 and about 101 per 1000 women age 30.

EXERCISES

1. **Life science: live births.** Use REGRESSION to fit a quartic equation to the live-birth data. Graph both the scatterplot of the data and the quartic function. Does the quartic function appear to give a better fit than either the quadratic or the cubic function?

2. **Business: median household income by age.**

Age, x	Median Income in 2015*
19.5	\$36,000
29.5	57,500
39.5	71,000
49.5	73,000
59.5	62,500
69.5	38,000

*Rounded to the nearest \$500.

(*Source:* Based on data from the U.S. Census Bureau.)

a) Make a scatterplot of the data and fit a quadratic function to the data using QuadReg. Then graph the quadratic function with the scatterplot.

b) Fit a cubic function to the data using CubicReg. Then graph the cubic function with the scatterplot.

c) Fit a quartic function to the data using QuartReg. Then graph the quartic function with the scatterplot.

d) Which of the quadratic, cubic, or quartic functions seems to best fit the data?

e) Using the function from part (d), estimate the median household income of people age 25; of people age 45.

Solution

a) We find that $f(x) = 2.5714x^2 - 35.0857x + 224.5429$ fits the data. Since 2020 is 9 years after 2011, we use $x = 9$. The estimate of annual sales of compact discs for 2020 is $f(9) = 117.06$, or approximately $117 million.

b) We find that $f(x) = 222.7381(0.8638)^x$ also fits the data. Using this model, the estimated annual sales of compact discs for 2020 is $f(9) = 59.6$, or approximately $59.6 million.

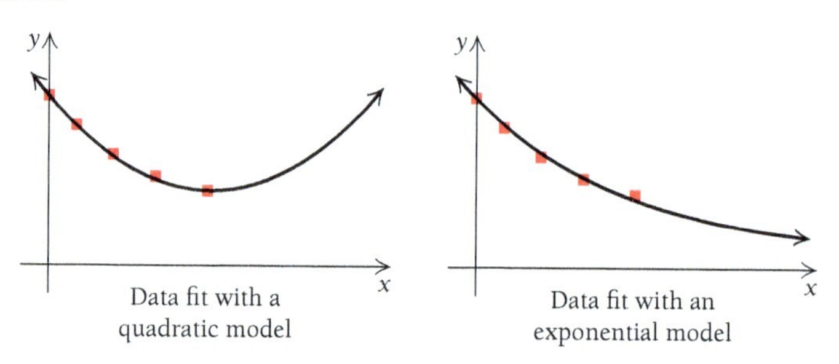

c) With the quadratic model, annual sales eventually increase over time, so it is probably not a very accurate model for predicting future sales of compact discs. The exponential model yields decreasing sales as x increases. Thus, it is probably a more accurate predictor of future sales of compact discs.

R.7 Exercise Set

Choosing models. *For the scatterplots and graphs in Exercises 1–9, determine which, if any, of the following functions might be the best model for the data:*

Linear, $f(x) = mx + b$

Quadratic, $f(x) = ax^2 + bx + c, a > 0$

Quadratic, $f(x) = ax^2 + bx + c, a < 0$

Polynomial, neither quadratic nor linear

Exponential, $f(x) = a_0 \cdot a^x, 0 < a < 1$ or $a > 1$

1.

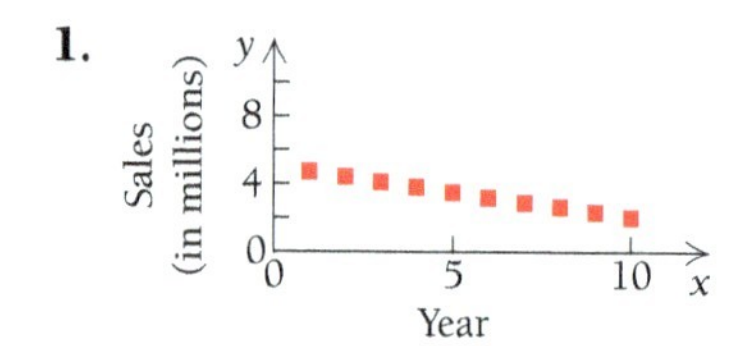

2.

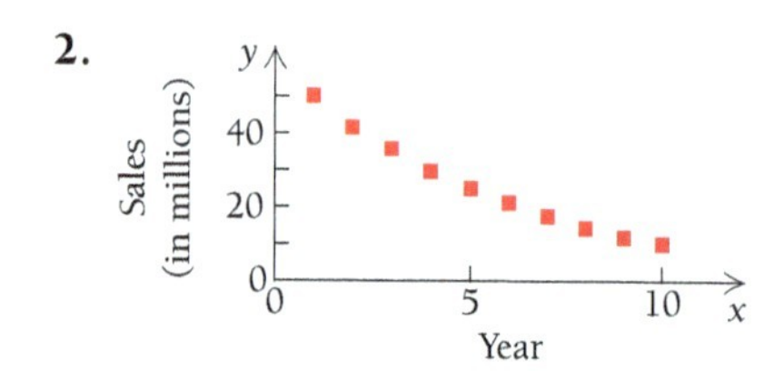

3.

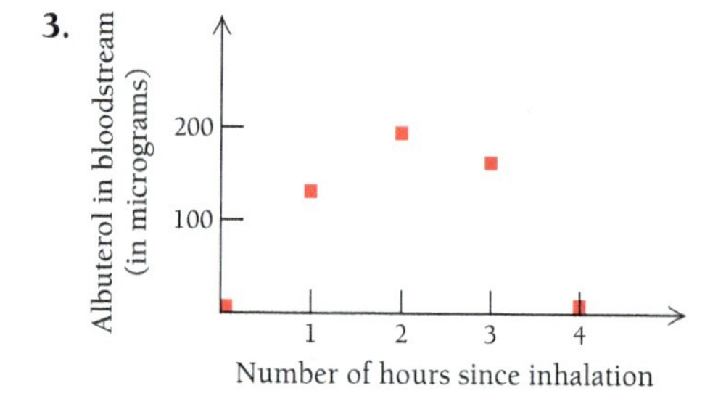

4.

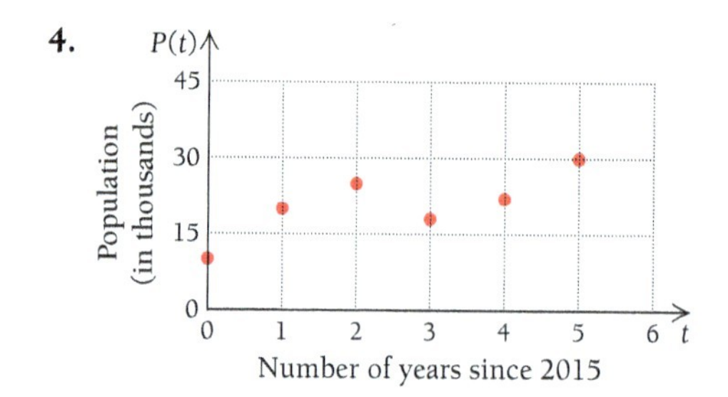

Business and Economics

5. MEDIAN HOUSEHOLD INCOME IN THE UNITED STATES

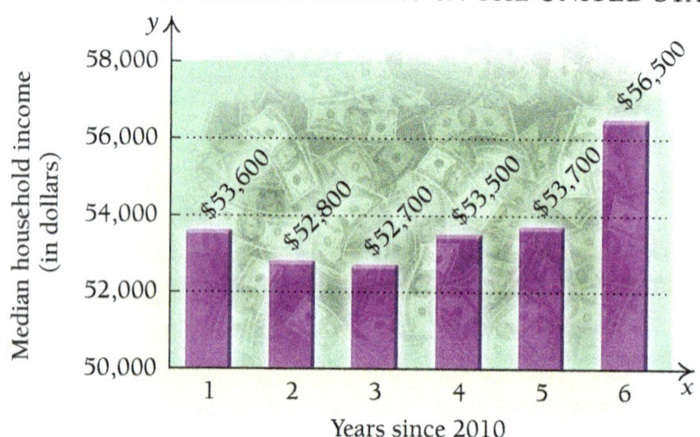

(*Source*: census.gov.)

6.

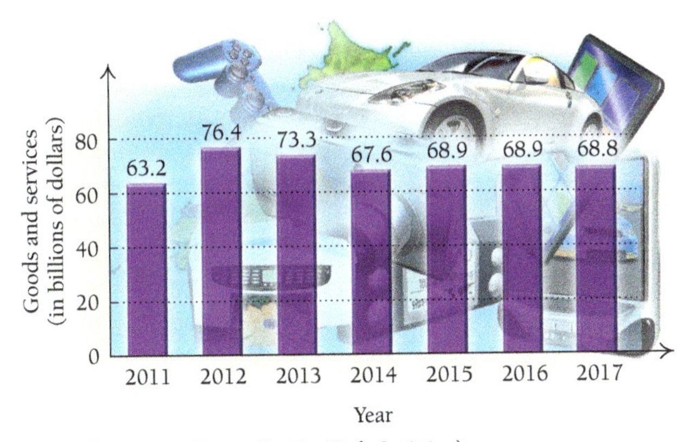

(*Source*: U.S. Census Bureau, Foreign Trade Statistics.)

7.

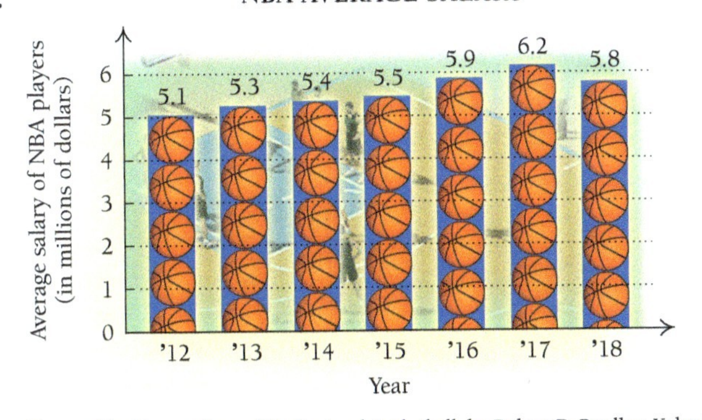

(*Source*: *The Compendium of Professional Basketball*, by Robert D. Bradley, Xaler Press, 2010; personal communication with author, 2017; basketball-reference.com, 2018.)

8.

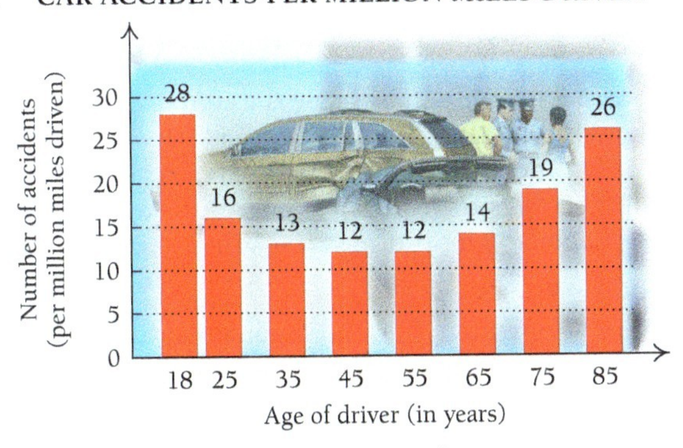

(*Source*: Based on data at qualityplanning.com.)

9.

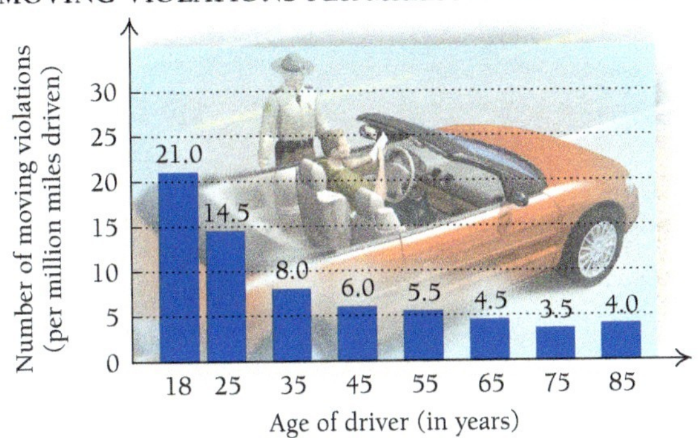

(*Source*: Based on data at qualityplanning.com.)

APPLICATIONS

Business and Economics

10. Average salary in NBA. Use the data from the bar graph in Exercise 7.

a) Find a linear function that fits the data using the average salaries given for the years 2012 and 2018. Use 0 for 2012 and 6 for 2018.

b) Use the linear function to predict average salaries in 2020 and 2025.

c) In what year will the average salary in the NBA reach \$7.0 million?

11. U.S. trade deficit with Japan.

a) For the data shown in Exercise 6, find a linear function that fits the data using the values for 2011 and 2017. Let x represent the number of years since 2011.

b) Use the linear function from part (a) to estimate the trade deficit with Japan in 2020.

Life and Physical Sciences

12. Absorption of an asthma medication. Use the data from Exercise 3.

a) Find a quadratic function that fits the data using the data points (0, 0), (2, 200), and (3, 167).

b) Use the function to estimate the amount of albuterol in the bloodstream 4 hr after inhalation.

c) Does it make sense to use this function for $t = 6$? Why or why not?

13. Median household income. Use the data given in Exercise 5.

a) Find a quadratic function that fits the data using the data points (1, 53,600), (3, 52,700), and (5, 53,700).

b) Use the function to estimate the median household income, rounded to the nearest hundred, in 2020.

14. Braking distance.

a) Find a quadratic function that fits the following data.

Travel Speed (mph)	Braking Distance (ft)
20	25
40	105
60	300

(*Source*: New Jersey Department of Law and Public Safety.)

b) Use the function to estimate the braking distance of a car traveling at 50 mph.

c) Does it make sense to use this function when speeds are less than 15 mph? Why or why not?

15. High blood pressure in women.

a) Use the first and last data points in the following table to find a linear function in which y represents the percentage of women with high blood pressure and x is the women's age, in years.

Age of Women, x	Percentage of Women with High Blood Pressure, y
27	6.7
40	17.6
50	34.3
60	52.0
70	70.8

(*Source:* Based on data from www.heart.org.)

b) Use the function from part (a) to estimate the percentage of 50-year-old women with high blood pressure.

c) How accurate is the estimate from part (b) compared to the actual value given in the table?

16. High blood pressure in men.

a) Use the first and last data points in the following table to find a linear function in which y represents the percentage of men with high blood pressure and x is the men's age, in years.

Age of Men, x	Percentage of Men with High Blood Pressure, y
27	9.1
40	24.4
50	37.7
60	52.0
70	63.9

(*Source:* Based on data from www.heart.org.)

b) Use the function from part (a) to estimate the percentage of 40-year-old men with high blood pressure.

c) How accurate is the estimate from part (b) compared to the actual value given in the table?

In Exercises 17–20, round the numbers in each exponential function to three decimal places.

17. Population.

a) Using regression, find the exponential function that best fits the following data.

Years since 1970	Population of Texas (in millions)
0	11.2
10	14.2
20	17.0
30	20.9
40	25.3
45	27.5

(*Source:* www.census.gov.)

b) Use the function to estimate the population of Texas in 2025.

18. Population.

a) Using regression, find the exponential function that best fits the following data.

Years since 1970	Population of Detroit (in millions)
0	1.5
10	1.2
20	1.0
30	0.95
40	0.71
45	0.68

(*Source:* www.census.gov.)

b) Use the function to estimate the population of Detroit in 2025.

19. Buying power.

a) Using regression, find the exponential function that best fits the following data.

Years since 1980	Equivalent Buying Power of $100 (in 1980 dollars)
0	$100.00
10	$158.62
20	$208.98
30	$264.63
37	$312.13

(*Source:* http://data.bls.gov/cgi-bin/cpicalc.pl.)

b) Use the function to estimate the equivalent buying power of $100 (in 1980 dollars) in 2020.

c) What other models also fit the data? Which model best predicts the equivalent buying power of $100 (in 1980 dollars) for future years? Why?

20. Stock prices.

a) Using regression, find the exponential function that best fits the following data.

Years since 2012	Price of One Share of Microsoft Stock at Beginning of January
0	$29.53
1	$27.45
2	$37.84
3	$40.40
4	$55.09
5	$64.65

(*Source:* yahoo.finance; Nasdaq.)

b) Use the function to estimate the price of one share of Microsoft stock in 2022.

c) What other models also fit the data? Which model best predicts the price of one share of Microsoft stock in future years? Why?

SYNTHESIS

21. Under what conditions might it make better sense to use a linear function rather than a quadratic or cubic function that fits a few data points more closely?

22. For modeling the number of moving violations per million miles driven as a function of drivers' age (see Exercise 9), which type of function would be the better choice: quadratic or exponential? Why?

23. Consider this set of three data points: (0, 1), (1, 3), and (2, 4).

    a) Find the slope between the first and second points, between the first and third points, and between the second and third points; then find the average of these slopes.

    b) Use regression to find a linear function that best fits these three points.

    c) What can you conclude about the slope found using regression and the slope found by the method in part (a)?

24. Explain why more than one type of function may be used to model the data in Exercise 8. For example, why might the first data point be ignored when using regression? Would this result in different forecasts?

Technology Connection

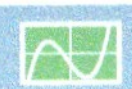

25. **Moving violations.**

    a) Use regression to fit a quadratic function to the data shown in Exercise 9.

    b) Use the function to estimate the number of moving violations per million miles driven for drivers aged 50.

    c) Fit an exponential function to the data and use it to estimate the number of moving violations per million miles driven for drivers aged 50.

    d) Is a quadratic or an exponential model more appropriate for this set of data? Why?

26. **Business: trade deficit with Japan.**

    a) Use regression to fit a quartic function to the data in Exercise 6. Let x be the number of years after 2011.

    b) Use the function to estimate the trade deficit with Japan in 2020.

    c) Why might a linear function be a more logical choice than a quartic function for modeling this set of data?

27. **Solving a three-variable, three-equation system.** The system of equations obtained in Example 3 can be solved using a process called *row reduction*. The first step is to write the system, giving each equation a number:

$$25a + 5b + c = 1121 \quad (1)$$
$$49a + 7b + c = 626 \quad (2)$$
$$81a + 9b + c = 967 \quad (3)$$

    a) Next, multiply both sides of equation (2) by -1, and then add its terms to those on each side of equation (1). This is new equation (4). What is equation (4)?

    b) Multiply both sides of equation (2) by -1, and then add its terms to those on each side of equation (3). This is new equation (5). What is equation (5)?

    c) Add the terms on each side of equation (4) to the terms on each side of equation (5). This gives the value of a. What is a?

    d) Evaluate equation (4) or (5) using the value of a found in part (c). This gives the value of b. What is b?

    e) Evaluate equation (1), (2), or (3) using the values of a and b. This gives the value of c. What is c?

Answers to Quick Checks

1. $y = \frac{8}{3}x + 47$; 71 million broadband cable customers. The model and the result are close to those found in Example 2.

2. $y = -0.659x^2 + 36.904x - 411.949$; 62.7 live births per 1000 women age 20.

Chapter R Summary

KEY TERMS AND CONCEPTS	EXAMPLES

SECTION R.1

In an **ordered pair** (x, y), the first number is called the **first coordinate** and the second number is called the **second coordinate**. Together, they are the **coordinates** of the point.

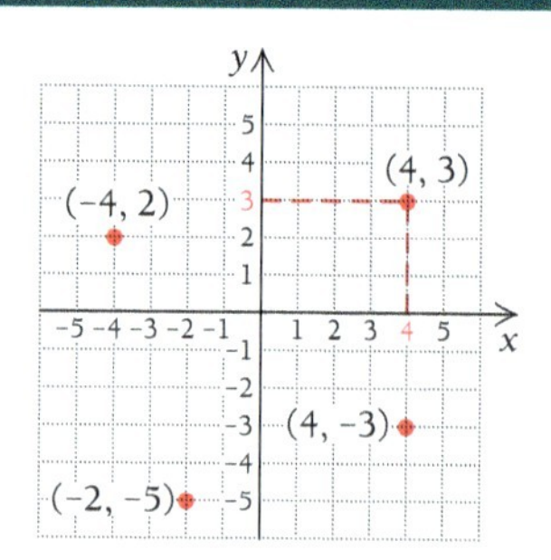

A **solution** of an equation in two variables is an ordered pair of numbers that, when substituted for the variables, forms a true statement.

The ordered pair $(1, -1)$ is a solution of $y = x^4 - 2x^2$ because substituting 1 for x and -1 for y results in a true statement:

$$\begin{array}{c|l} y & = x^4 - 2x^2 \\ \hline -1 & ?\ (1)^4 - 2(1)^2 \\ -1 & 1 - 2 \\ -1 & -1 \end{array} \quad \text{TRUE}$$

The **graph** of an equation is a drawing that represents all ordered pairs that are solutions of the equation.

This is the graph of the equation $y = x^4 - 2x^2$.

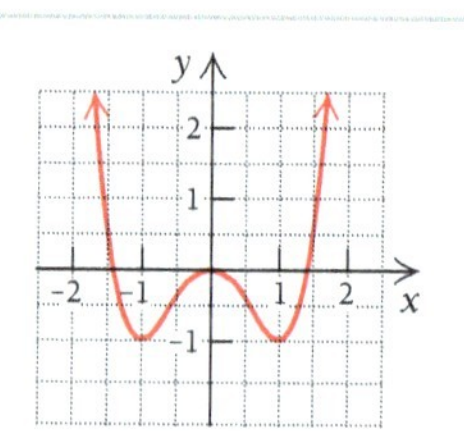

The mathematics used to represent the essential features of a real-world problem comprise a **mathematical model**.

Business. A hotel owner normally rents 200 rooms per night at \$100 per room. The equation

$$R(x) = (100 - x)(200 + 2x)$$

estimates the total nightly revenue, $R(x)$, in dollars, when for every x dollars the price of a room is reduced, $2x$ more rooms are rented per night.

SECTION R.2

A **function** is a correspondence between a first set, called the **domain**, and a second set, called the **range**, for which each member of the domain corresponds to *exactly one* member of the range.

- The domain is the set of 15 players on a softball team, the range is the set of integers from 1 to 15, and the function is the correspondence between a player and her uniform number.
- The domain is the set of real numbers, the range is the set of real numbers, and the function is the correspondence between a number x and half of that number's value, $x/2$.
- The set $\{(0, 5), (1, 4), (2, 3), (3, 4)\}$ is a function. The domain is $\{0, 1, 2, 3\}$ and the range is $\{3, 4, 5\}$. Note that the number 4 in the range corresponds to both 1 and 3 in the domain.

KEY TERMS AND CONCEPTS	EXAMPLES
SECTION R.2 (*continued*)	
A graph represents a function if it is impossible to draw a vertical line that crosses the graph more than once.	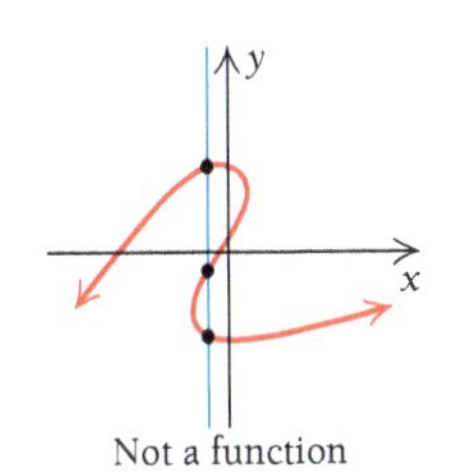 Not a function 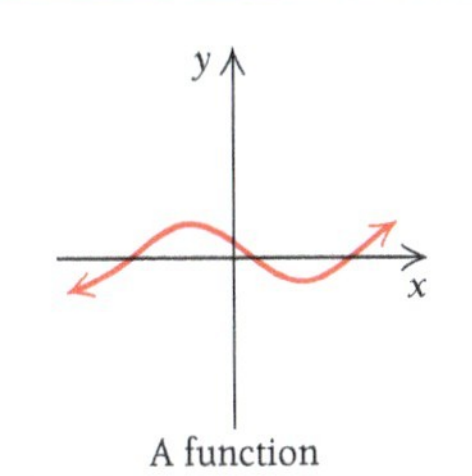 A function 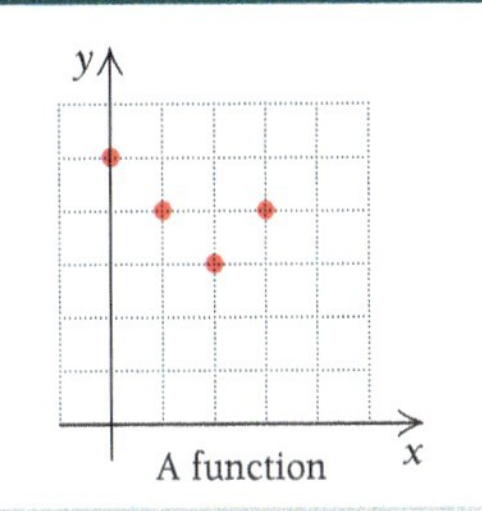 A function
Function notation permits us to easily indicate the **output**, or member of the range, that is paired with a given **input**, or member of the domain.	For $f(x) = x^2 - 5x - 8$, the notation $f(2)$ indicates the member of the range that is paired with the number 2 of the domain: $f(x) = x^2 - 5x - 8$; $f(2) = 2^2 - 5(2) - 8 = 4 - 10 - 8 = -14$.
In calculus, it is important to be able to simplify an expression like $\frac{f(x+h) - f(x)}{h}$ for a given function f.	For $f(x) = x^2 - 5x - 8$, $\frac{f(x+h) - f(x)}{h} = \frac{[(x+h)^2 - 5(x+h) - 8] - f(x)}{h} = \frac{x^2 + 2xh + h^2 - 5x - 5h - 8 - [x^2 - 5x - 8]}{h} = \frac{x^2 + 2xh + h^2 - 5x - 5h - 8 - x^2 + 5x + 8}{h} = \frac{2xh + h^2 - 5h}{h} = \frac{h(2x + h - 5)}{h} = 2x + h - 5,\ h \neq 0.$
A function that is defined **piecewise** states specific rules for different parts of the domain.	To graph $g(x) = \begin{cases} \frac{1}{3}x + 3, & \text{for } x < 3, \\ -x, & \text{for } x \geq 3, \end{cases}$ we graph $y = \frac{1}{3}x + 3$ for all inputs x less than 3 and graph $y = -x$ for all inputs x greater than or equal to 3. 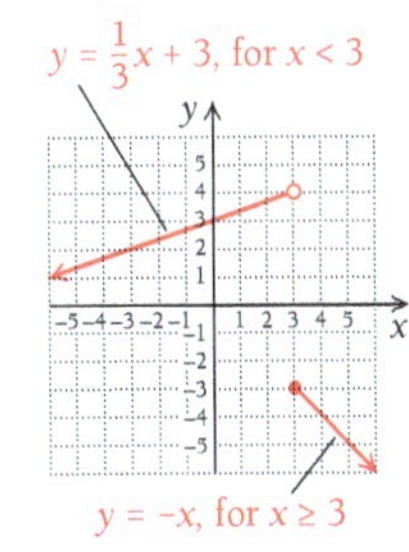

KEY TERMS AND CONCEPTS / EXAMPLES

SECTION R.3

A set of numbers can be represented using **roster notation**, in which the members of the set are listed.

Roster Notation: $\{-2, 5, 9, \pi\}$

In **set-builder notation**, the members of a set are described.

Set-Builder Notation: $\{x \mid x \text{ is a real number and } x \geq 3\}$

If the numbers in a set form an interval on the real number line, then **interval notation** can be used.

Intervals of real numbers can be represented using interval notation.

Closed interval: includes the endpoints

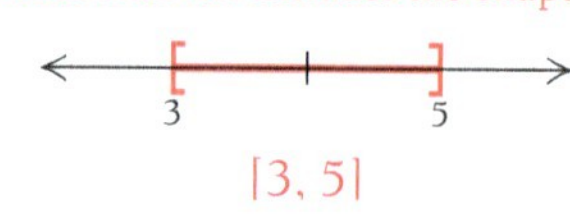

Open interval: excludes the endpoints

3 5

(3, 5)

Half-open interval: includes one endpoint but excludes the other

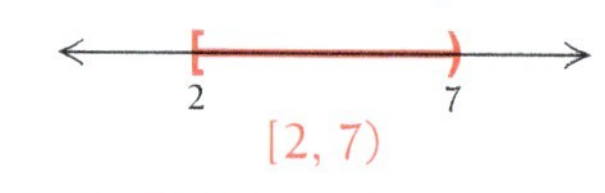

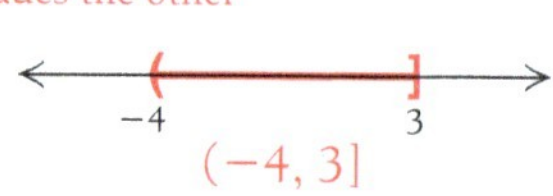

Unless otherwise specified, for a function given by an equation, the domain is the largest set of real numbers (inputs) for which function values (outputs) can be calculated.

Function	Domain
$f(x) = \dfrac{8x}{x^2 - 9} = \dfrac{8x}{(x-3)(x+3)}$	The set of all real numbers except -3 and 3, or $(-\infty, -3) \cup (-3, 3) \cup (3, \infty)$.
$g(x) = \sqrt{10 - 5x}$	The set of all real numbers x for which $10 - 5x \geq 0$ or $2 \geq x$. The domain is $(-\infty, 2]$.
$h(x) = 3x^2 + 5x - 1$	The set of all real numbers, $\mathbb{R}$.

SECTION R.4

The **slope** m of the line containing the points (x_1, y_1) and (x_2, y_2) is given by $m = \dfrac{y_2 - y_1}{x_2 - x_1}$ and can be regarded as the **average rate of change** between (x_1, y_1) and (x_2, y_2). An equation of the form $f(x) = mx + b$ is in **slope–intercept form**. Its graph has **slope** m and **y-intercept** $(0, b)$.

An equation of the form $y - y_1 = m(x - x_1)$ is in **point–slope form**. Its graph is a line with slope m passing through the point (x_1, y_1).

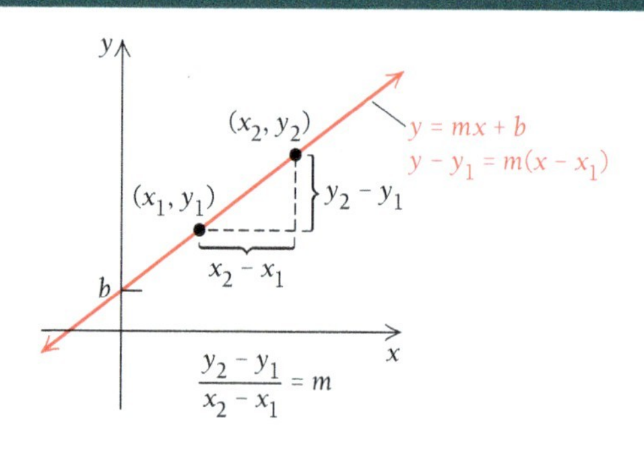

The graph of a **constant function**, given by $f(x) = c$, is a horizontal line. Its slope is 0.

y

c $f(x) = c$

x

The graph of an equation of the form $x = a$ is a vertical line and is not a function. Its slope is undefined.

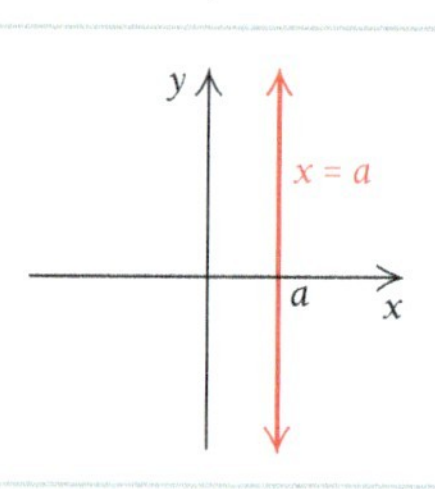

KEY TERMS AND CONCEPTS	EXAMPLES
SECTION R.4 (*continued*)	
The variable y is **proportional** to x (or *varies directly* with x) if there exists some positive constant m for which $y = mx$. We say that m is the **constant of proportionality** (or the *constant of variation*).	$y = 3.14x, \quad A = 1.08t, \quad I = kR, \quad y = \frac{1}{3}x$
Total profit, $P(x)$, is the difference between **total revenue**, $R(x)$, and total cost, $C(x)$, where x is the number of units produced. The value x for which $P(x) = 0$ is the **break-even value**.	If $R(x) = 84x$ and $C(x) = 28x + 56{,}000$, then the break-even value is found by setting $P(x)$ equal to 0: $P(x) = 0$; $R(x) - C(x) = 0$; $R(x) = C(x)$; $84x = 28x + 56{,}000$ (Substituting); $56x = 56{,}000$; $x = 1000.$
SECTION R.5	
The graph of a **quadratic function** $f(x) = ax^2 + bx + c$ is a **parabola** with a **vertex** at $\left(-\frac{b}{2a}, f\left(-\frac{b}{2a}\right)\right)$. The graph opens **upward** for $a > 0$ and **downward** for $a < 0$. It is an example of a **nonlinear** function. The vertical line $x = -\frac{b}{2a}$ is the **line of symmetry**.	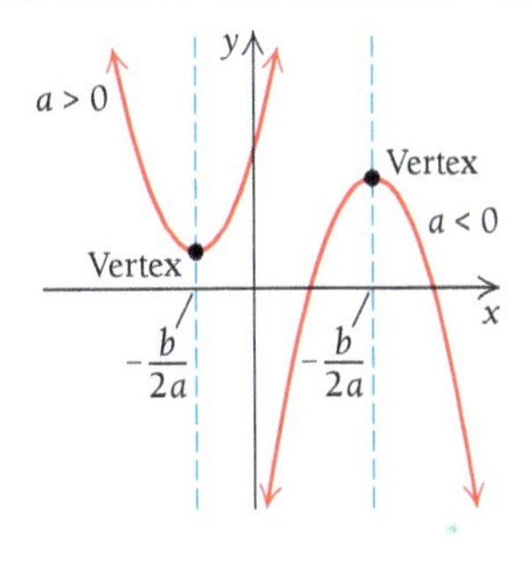
Any **x-intercepts** of the graph of a quadratic function, $f(x) = ax^2 + bx + c$, are the solutions of $ax^2 + bx + c = 0$ and are given by the quadratic formula $x = \frac{-b \pm \sqrt{b^2 - 4ac}}{2a}.$	The x-intercepts of $f(x) = x^2 - 6x - 10$ are found by solving $x^2 - 6x - 10 = 0$: $\frac{-b + \sqrt{b^2 - 4ac}}{2a} = \frac{-(-6) + \sqrt{(-6)^2 - 4(1)(-10)}}{2(1)} = 3 + \sqrt{19},$ and $\frac{-b - \sqrt{b^2 - 4ac}}{2a} = \frac{-(-6) - \sqrt{(-6)^2 - 4(1)(-10)}}{2(1)} = 3 - \sqrt{19}.$ 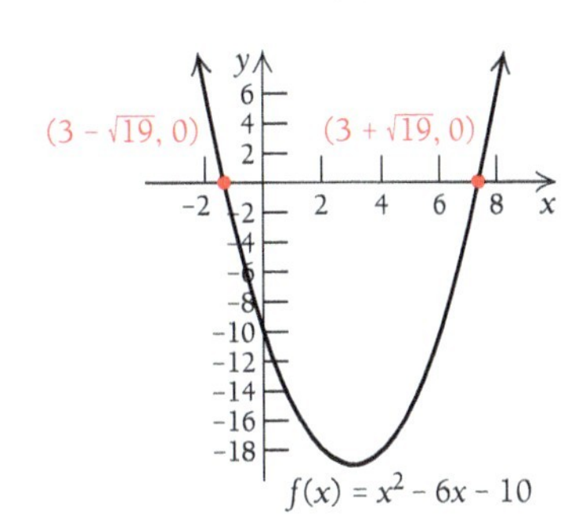

KEY TERMS AND CONCEPTS	EXAMPLES
SECTION R.5 (*continued*)	

A **polynomial function** f is given by

$$f(x) = a_n x^n + a_{n-1} x^{n-1} + \cdots + a_2 x^2 + a_1 x^1 + a_0,$$

where n is a nonnegative integer and $a_n, a_{n-1}, \ldots, a_2, a_1, a_0$ are real numbers, called **coefficients**.

- $f(x) = -8$, constant
- $g(x) = 3x - 7$, linear
- $h(x) = x^2 - 6x - 10$, quadratic
- $p(x) = 2x^3 - 7x^2 + 0.23x - 10$, cubic

Power functions are polynomial functions of the form $f(x) = ax^n$, where n is a positive integer.

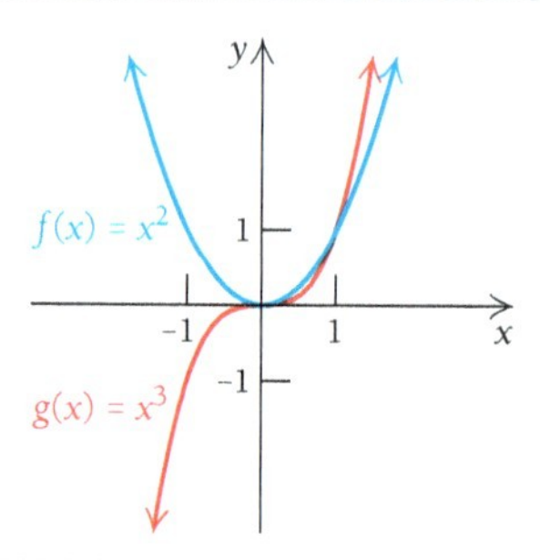

A **rational function** is a function that can be expressed as the quotient of two polynomials.

$$g(x) = \frac{x^2 - 9}{x + 3}, \quad h(x) = \frac{x^3 - 4x^2 + x - 5}{x^2 - 6x - 10},$$

$$f(x) = \frac{x^3 - 4x^2 + x - 5}{1} = x^3 - 4x^2 + x - 5$$

The domain of a rational function is the set of all input values that do not result in division by zero.

For $f(x) = \dfrac{1}{x - 3}$, the domain is the set of all real numbers except 3: $(-\infty, 3) \cup (3, \infty)$.

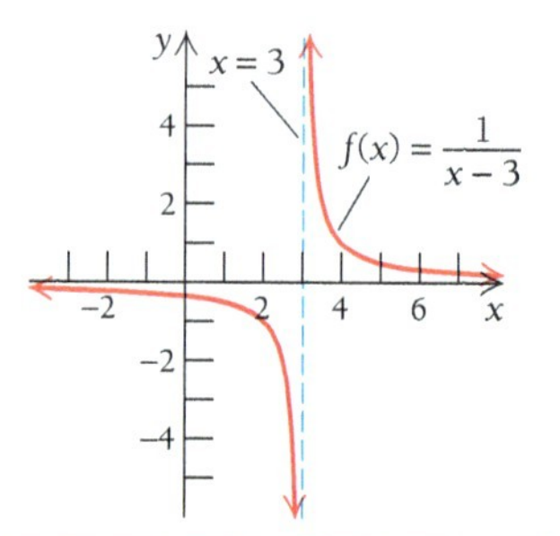

An **absolute-value** function is described using absolute value symbols.

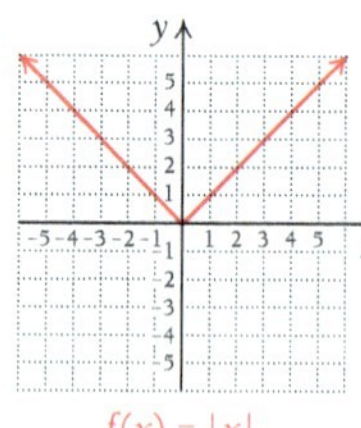
$f(x) = |x|$

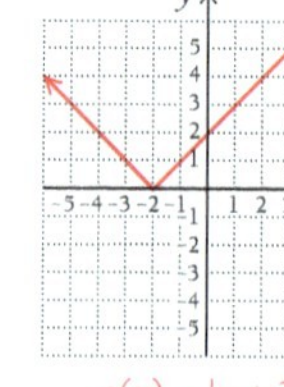
$g(x) = |x + 2|$

A **square-root function** is a function described using a square root symbol.

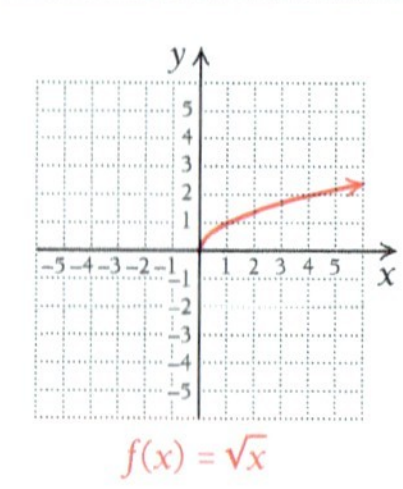
$f(x) = \sqrt{x}$

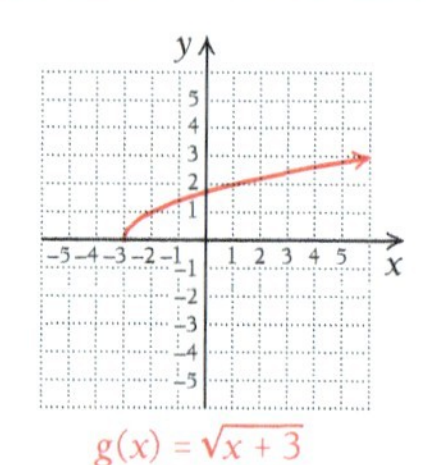
$g(x) = \sqrt{x + 3}$

KEY TERMS AND CONCEPTS	EXAMPLES
SECTION R.5 (*continued*)	
The point at which demand and supply are the same is called an **equilibrium point**.	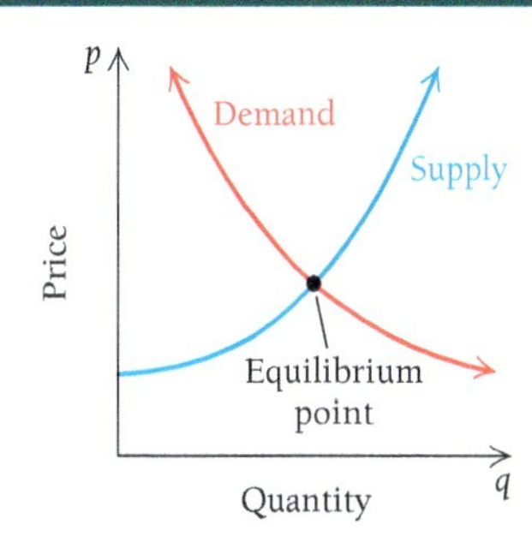
SECTION R.6	
An **exponential function** can be written in the form $f(x) = a_0 \cdot a^x$, where $a > 0$, $a \neq 1$. The domain of an exponential function is the set of all real numbers. The range is the set of all positive numbers, $(0, \infty)$, and the y-intercept is $(0, a_0)$. There is no x-intercept.	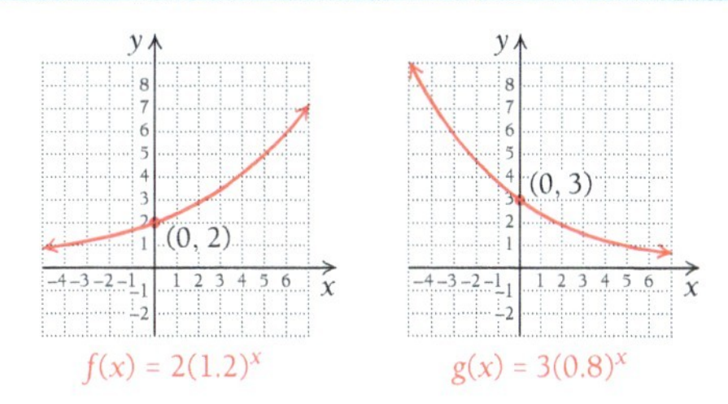
The **logarithm**, base a, of y is the number x such that $a^x = y$. Equivalently, $a^x = y$, if and only if $\log_a y = x$. The base a must be positive and not equal to 1; that is, $a > 0$ and $a \neq 1$.	• Since $2^5 = 32$, we have $\log_2 32 = 5$. • Since $5^{-1} = \frac{1}{5}$, we have $\log_5\left(\frac{1}{5}\right) = -1$. • Since $\log_3 9 = 2$, we have $3^2 = 9$. • Since $\log_5 125 = 3$, we have $5^3 = 125$.
The common logarithm has base 10 and is written log (without a subscript).	• $\log 1000 = 3$ **Check:** $10^3 = 1000$ • $\log 0.01 = -2$ **Check:** $10^{-2} = \frac{1}{100} = 0.01$ • $\log 16 \approx 1.204$ **Check:** $10^{1.204} = 15.9955\ldots \approx 16$
Properties of Logarithms: **P1.** $\log_a (MN) = \log_a M + \log_a N$ **P2.** $\log_a \left(\frac{M}{N}\right) = \log_a M - \log_a N$ **P3.** $\log_a (M^b) = b \log_a M$ **P4.** $\log_a a = 1$ **P5.** $\log_a 1 = 0$ **P6.** $\log_a M = \frac{\log_b M}{\log_b a}$ (change-of-base formula) **P7.** $\log_a a^k = k$ **P8.** For any $x > 0$, $a^{\log_a x} = x$	• $\log_4 64 = \log_4 (4 \cdot 16) = \log_4 4 + \log_4 16 = 1 + 2 = 3$ • $\log_2 32 = \log_2 2^5 = 5$ • $\log_5 5 = 1$ • $\log_8 1 = 0$ • $\log_3 5 = \frac{\log_b 5}{\log_b 3}$. For $b = 10$, we have $\log_3 5 = \frac{\log 5}{\log 3} \approx 1.465$. **Check:** $3^{1.465} = 5.000145\ldots \approx 5$ • $7^{\log_7 3} = 3$

KEY TERMS AND CONCEPTS	EXAMPLES

SECTION R.6 (*continued*)

A logarithmic function is given by $f(x) = \log_a x$, where $a > 0$ and $a \neq 1$. Its domain is $\{x | x > 0\}$, its x-intercept is $(1, 0)$, and there is no y-intercept.

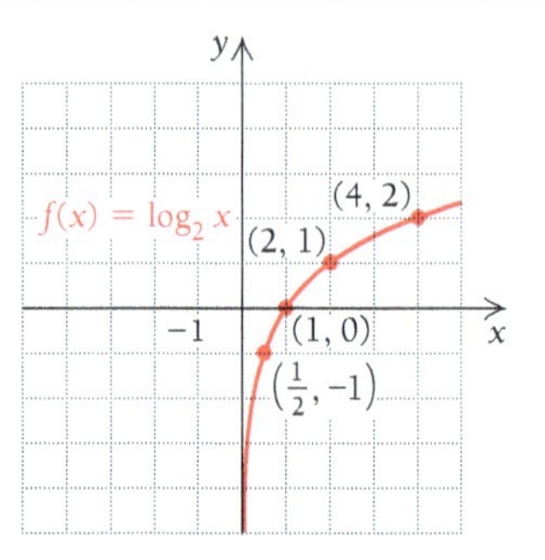

SECTION R.7

When real-world data are available, we can make a **scatterplot** and decide which, if any, of the graphs in this chapter best models the situation. Then we can use an appropriate model to make predictions.

Business.

Average Gasoline Prices, 2012–2017

Years since 2012	Price per Gallon (in dollars)
0	3.62
1	3.51
2	3.36
3	2.43
4	2.14
5	2.42

(*Source:* eia.gov.)

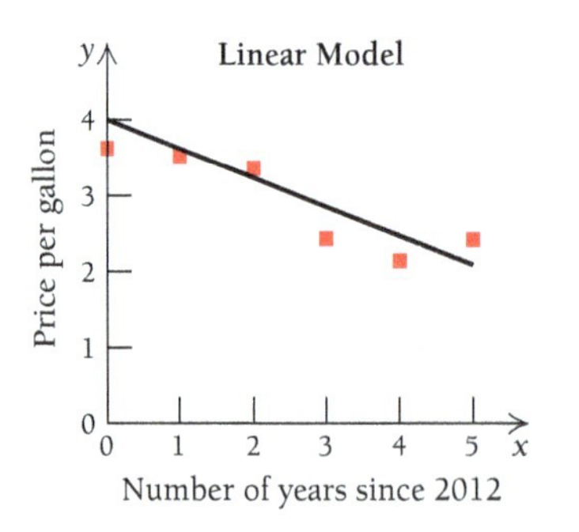

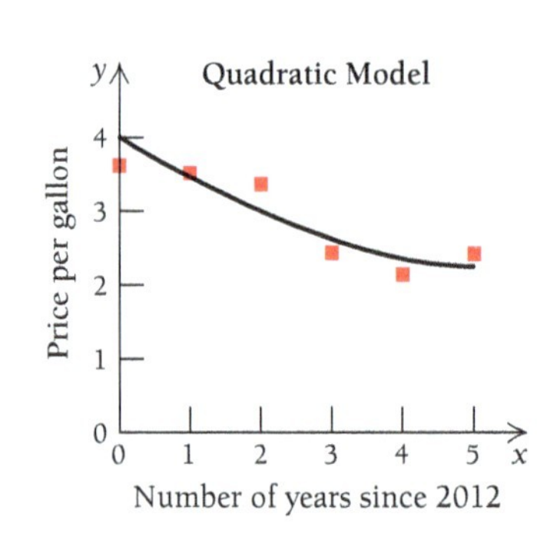

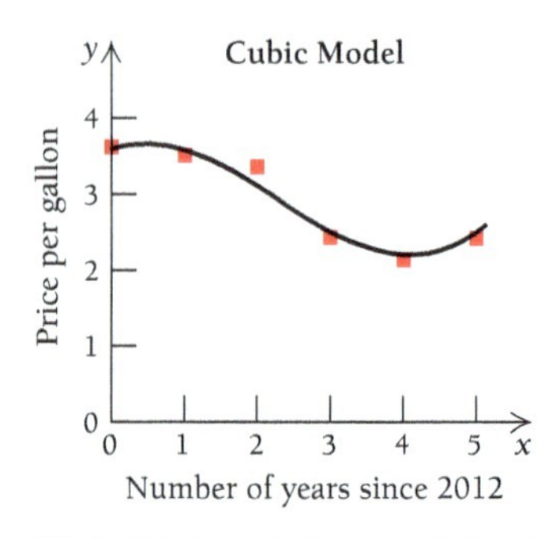

Chapter R Review Exercises

These review exercises are for test preparation. They can also serve as a practice test. Answers are at the back of the book. Red bracketed section references indicate the part(s) of the chapter to restudy if your answer is incorrect.

For each equation in column A, select the most appropriate graph in column B. [R.1, R.4, R.5, R.6]

Column A

Column B

1. $y = |x + 1|$

a)

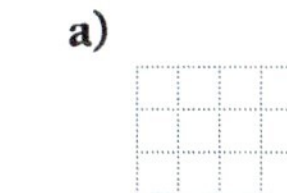

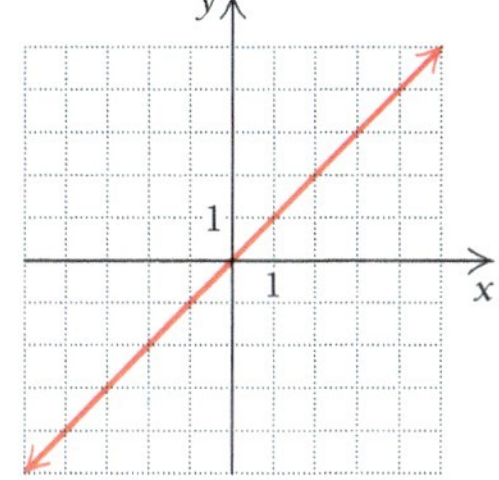

2. $f(x) = x^2 - 1$

b)

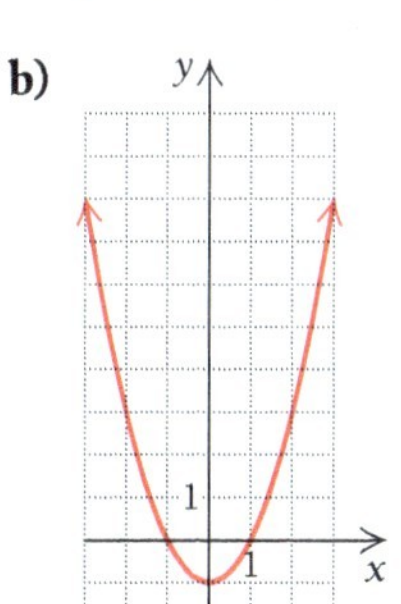

3. $y = -2x - 1$

c)

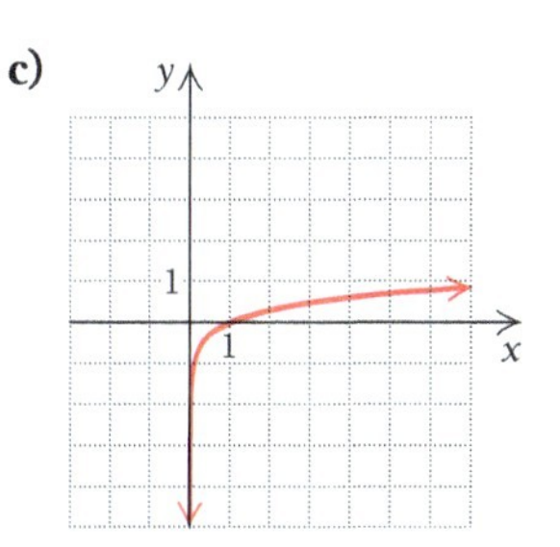

4. $y = x$

d)

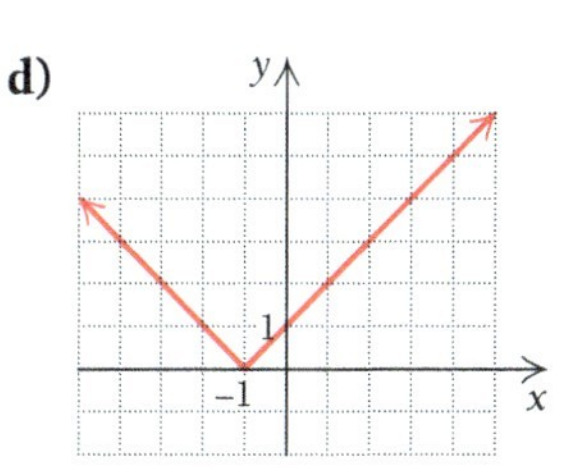

5. $g(x) = \sqrt{x + 2} - 1$

e)

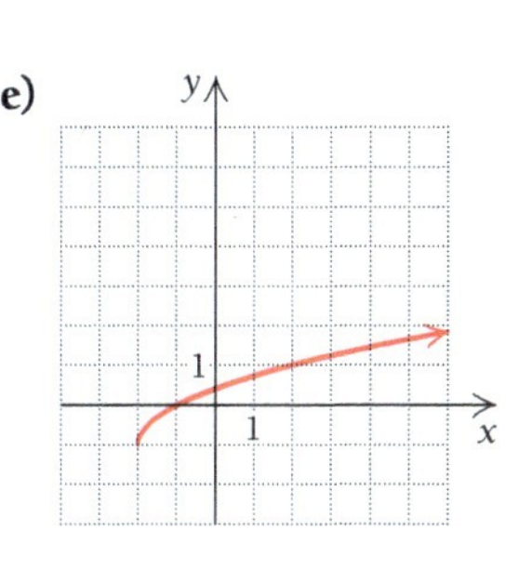

6. $f(x) = 0.5(1.2)^x$

f)

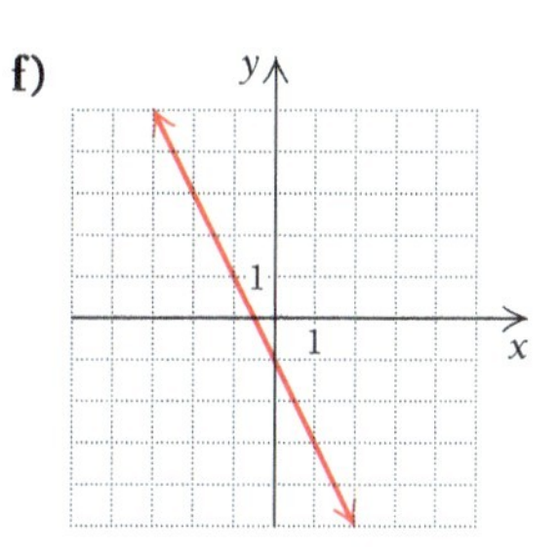

7. $f(x) = \dfrac{1}{x}$

g)

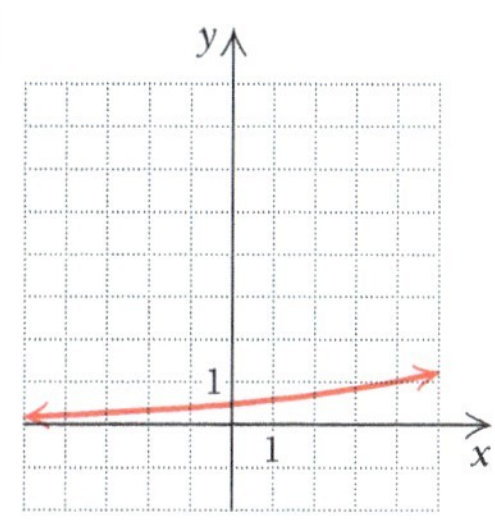

8. $f(x) = \log x$

h)

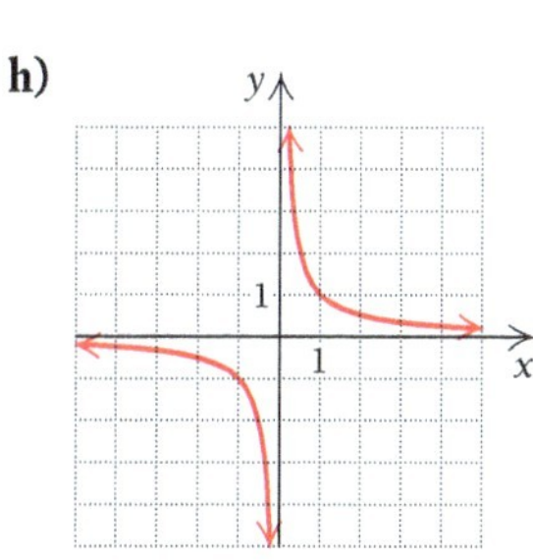

In Exercises 9–15, classify each statement as either true or false.

9. The graph of an equation represents all ordered pairs that are solutions of the equation. [R.1]

10. If $f(-3) = 5$ and $f(3) = 5$, then f cannot be a function. [R.2]

11. The notation (3, 7) can represent a point or an interval. [R.1, R.3]

12. An equation of the form $y - y_1 = m(x - x_1)$ has a graph that is a line of slope m passing through the point (x_1, y_1). [R.4]

13. The graph of an equation of the form $f(x) = ax^2 + bx + c$ has its vertex at $x = b/(2a)$. [R.5]

14. The graph of the exponential function $y = 10(1.05)^x$ has a slope of 0.05. [R.6]

15. Unless stated otherwise, the domain of a polynomial function is the set of all real numbers. [R.5]

16. Hearing-impaired Americans. The following graph shows the number of hearing-impaired Americans who are x years old. (*Source:* Better Hearing Institute.) [R.1, R.5]

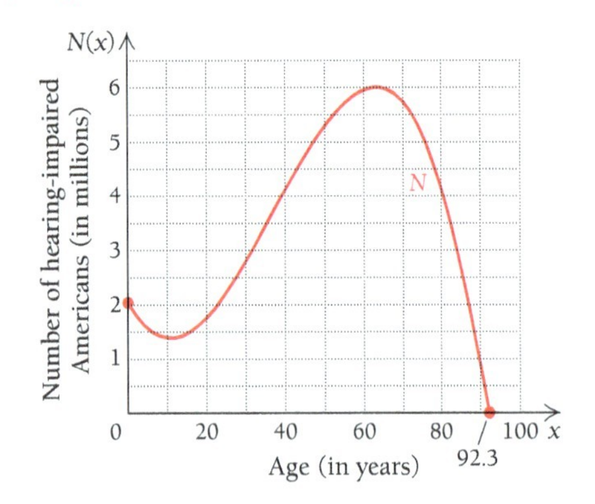

a) What is the number of hearing-impaired Americans aged 40?

b) For what age(s) are about 3,000,000 Americans hearing-impaired?

c) What is a reasonable estimate of the domain of this function? Why?

17. Finance: compound interest. Sam borrows \$4000 at 2.2%, compounded annually. How much does she owe at the end of 2 yr? [R.1]

18. Business: compound interest. Lucinda invests \$11,000 at 5%, compounded semiannually. How much is her investment worth at the end of 4 yr? [R.1]

19. Is the following correspondence a function? Why or why not? [R.2]

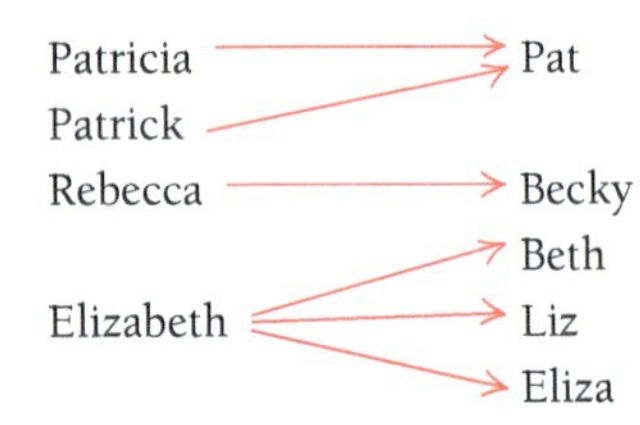

20. A function is given by $f(x) = -x^2 + x$. Find each of the following. [R.2]

a) $f(3)$

b) $f(-5)$

c) $f(a)$

d) $f(x + h)$

Graph. [R.5]

21. $f(x) = (x - 2)^2$

22. $y = |x - 1|$

23. $f(x) = \dfrac{3 - x}{x + 4}$

24. $g(x) = \sqrt{x} + 1$

Use the vertical-line test to determine whether each of the following is the graph of a function. [R.2]

25.

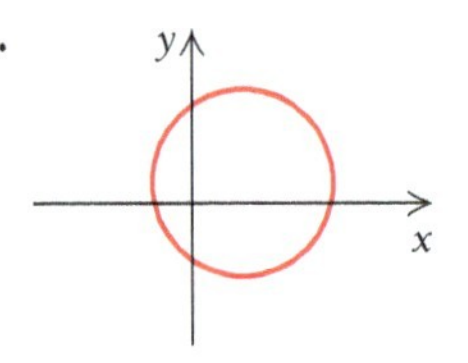

26.

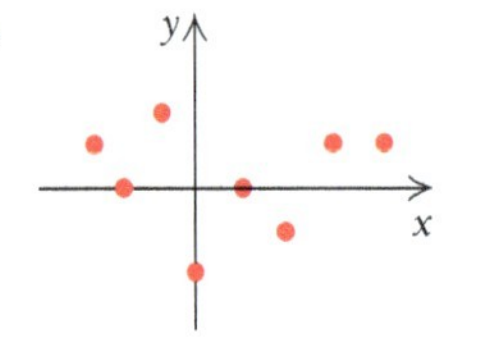

27.

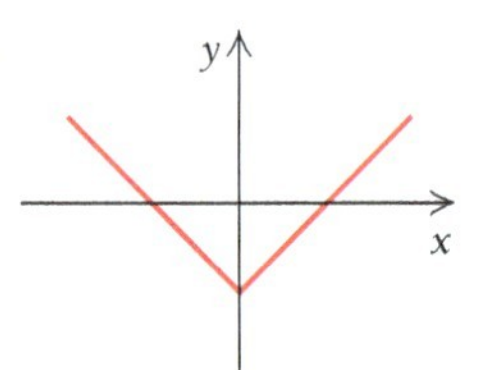

28.

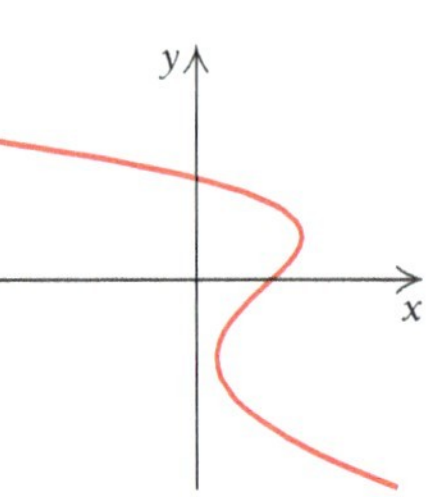

29. For the graph of function f shown to the right, determine (a) $f(2)$; (b) the domain; (c) all x-values for which $f(x) = 2$; and (d) the range. [R.3]

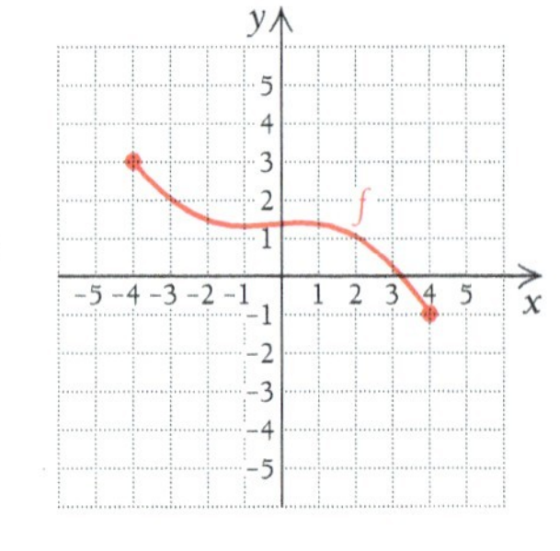

30. Consider the function given by

$$f(x) = \begin{cases} -x^2 + 2, & \text{for } x < 1, \\ 4, & \text{for } 1 \le x < 2, \\ \frac{1}{2}x, & \text{for } x \ge 2. \end{cases}$$

a) Find $f(-1)$, $f(1.5)$, and $f(6)$. [R.2]

b) Graph the function. [R.2]

31. Write interval notation for each graph. [R.3]

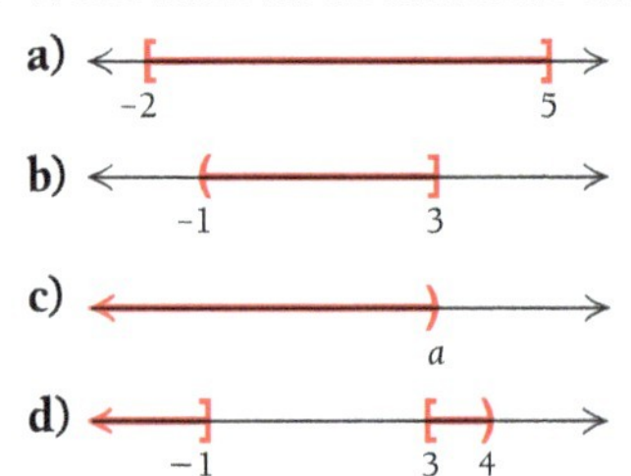

32. Write interval notation for each of the following. Then graph each interval on a number line. [R.3]

a) $\{x \mid -4 \le x < 5\}$

b) $\{x \mid x > 2\}$

33. For the function graphed below, determine (a) $f(-3)$; (b) the domain; (c) all x-values for which $f(x) = 4$; (d) the range. [R.3]

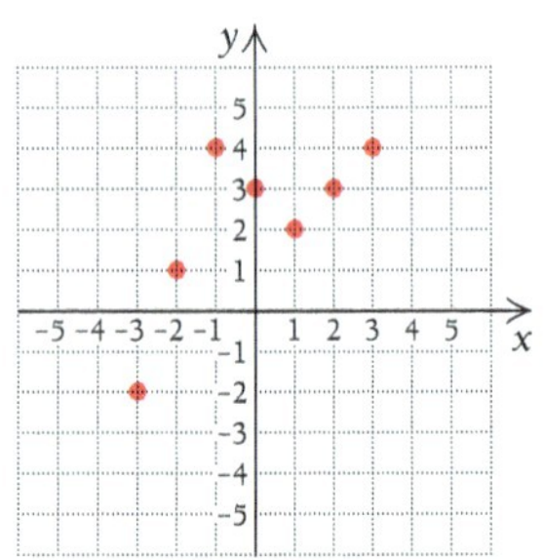

34. Find the domain of f. [R.3, R.5, R.6]

a) $f(x) = \dfrac{7}{2x - 10}$

b) $f(x) = \sqrt{x + 6}$

c) $f(x) = \log_3 (x - 2)$

d) $f(x) = \sqrt{x} + \sqrt{5 - x}$

35. What are the slope and the y-intercept of $y = -3x + 2$? [R.4]

36. Find an equation in slope–intercept form of the line with slope $\frac{1}{4}$, containing the point $(8, -5)$. [R.4]

37. Find the slope of the line containing the points $(2, -5)$ and $(-3, 10)$. [R.4]

Find the average rate of change. [R.4]

38.

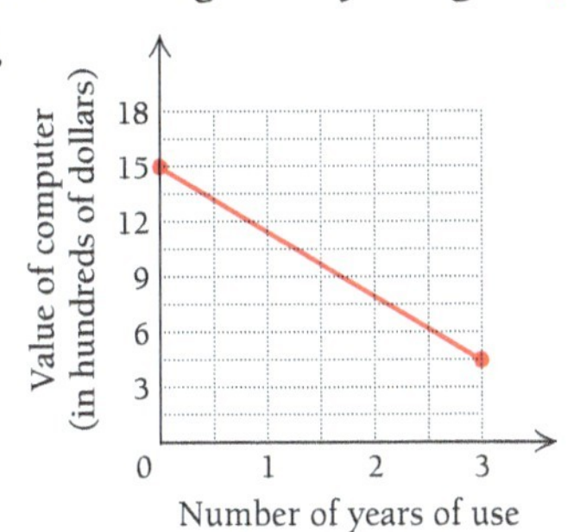

39.

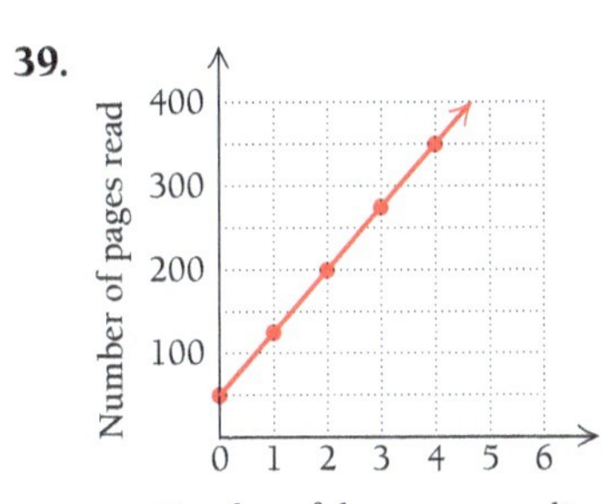

40. **Business: shipping charges.** The amount A that Pet-Treats-to-U charges for shipping is proportional to the value V of the item(s) being shipped. If the business charges \$6.00 to ship a \$60 gift basket, find an equation expressing A as a function of V. [R.4]

41. **Business: profit-and-loss analysis.** The band Soul Purpose has fixed costs of \$4000 for producing a new CD. Thereafter, the variable costs are \$0.50 per CD, and the CD will sell for \$10. [R.4]

a) Find and graph $C(x)$, the total cost of producing x CDs.

b) Find and graph $R(x)$, the total revenue from the sale of x CDs. Use the same axes as in part (a).

c) Find and graph $P(x)$, the total profit from the production and sale of x CDs. Use the same axes as in part (b).

d) How many CDs must the band sell in order to break even?

42. Graph each pair of equations on one set of axes. [R.5]

a) $y = \sqrt{x}$ and $y = \sqrt{x} - 3$

b) $y = x^3$ and $y = (x - 1)^3$

43. Graph each of the following. If the graph is a parabola, identify the vertex. [R.5]

a) $f(x) = x^2 - 6x + 8$ b) $g(x) = \sqrt[3]{x} + 2$

c) $y = -\dfrac{1}{x}$ d) $y = \dfrac{x^2 + x - 6}{x - 2}$

44. Solve each of the following. [R.5]

a) $5 + x^2 = 4x + 2$

b) $2x^2 = 4x + 3$

45. Rewrite each of the following as an equivalent expression with a rational exponent. [R.5]

a) $\sqrt[5]{x^4}$ b) $\sqrt{t^8}$

c) $\dfrac{1}{\sqrt[3]{m^2}}$ d) $\dfrac{1}{\sqrt{x^2 - 9}}$

46. Rewrite each of the following as an equivalent expression using radical notation. [R.5]

a) $x^{2/5}$ b) $m^{-3/5}$

c) $(x^2 - 5)^{1/2}$ d) $\dfrac{1}{t^{-1/3}}$

47. Determine the domain of the function given by $f(x) = \sqrt[8]{2x - 9}$. [R.5]

48. Graph each of the following, and identify the y-intercept. [R.6]

a) $y = \dfrac{1}{2}\cdot(4)^x$ b) $y = 3\cdot\left(\dfrac{1}{4}\right)^x$

49. The population of Arvon Hill is given by $A(t) = 22{,}500(1.023)^t$, where t is the number of years after 2018. [R.6]

a) State the annual percent change in the population.

b) Find $A(5)$, and explain what that value represents.

c) When will the population of Arvon Hill be 35,000?

50. A chemist has a 125-g sample of a radioactive substance that undergoes exponential decay. After 8 weeks, 112 g of the substance remains. [R.6]

a) Find a function $M(t)$ that gives the mass of the substance remaining after t weeks.

b) State the weekly percent change in the mass of the substance.

c) When will 50 g of the substance remain?

51. Given $\log_b 2 = 0.314$ and $\log_b 3 = 0.497$: [R.6]

a) Find $\log_b 16$.

b) Find $\log_b 1.5$.

c) Find $\log_b 3b$.

52. Find $\log_3 81$, and interpret the result. [R.6]

53. **Economics: equilibrium point.** Find the equilibrium point for the given demand and supply functions. [R.5]

Demand: $p = (q - 7)^2$

Supply: $p = q^2 + q + 4$ (assume $q \leq 7$)

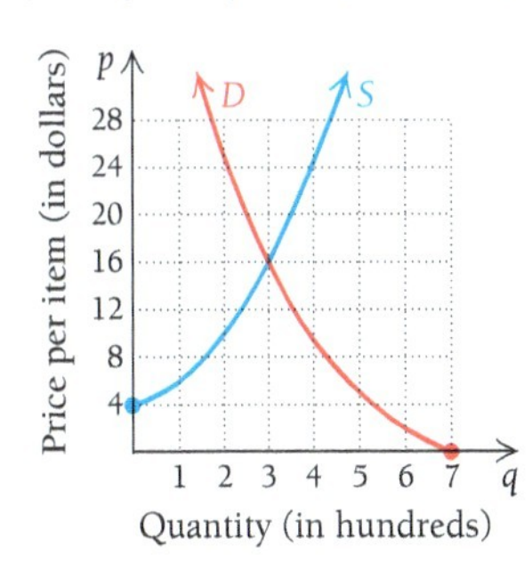

54. **Trail maintenance.** The amount of time required to maintain a section of the Pacific Crest Trail varies

inversely with the number of volunteers working. If a particular section of trail can be cleared in 4 hr by 9 volunteers, how long would it take 11 volunteers to clear the same section? [R.5]

55. Life science: maximum heart rate. A person exercising should not exceed a maximum heart rate, which depends on his or her gender, age, and resting heart rate. The following table shows data relating resting heart rate and maximum heart rate for a 20-yr-old woman. [R.7]

Resting Heart Rate, r (in beats per minute)	Maximum Heart Rate, M (in beats per minute)
50	170
60	172
70	174
80	176

(*Source:* American Heart Association.)

a) Using the data points (50, 170) and (80, 176), find a linear function.

b) Graph the scatterplot and the function from part (a) on the same set of axes.

c) Use the function from part (a) to predict the maximum heart rate of a woman whose resting heart rate is 67.

56. Business: ticket profits. The Spring Valley Drama Troupe is performing a new play. Data relating daily profit P to the number of days after opening night appear below. [R.7]

Days, x	0	9	18	27	36	45
Profit, P (in dollars)	870	548	−100	−100	510	872

a) Make a scatterplot of the data.

b) Do the data appear to fit a quadratic function?

c) Fit a quadratic function to the data points (0, 870), (18, −100), and (45, 872).

d) Use the function from part (c) to estimate the profit made on the 30th day.

e) Estimate the domain of this function. Why must it have restrictions?

SYNTHESIS

57. Economics: demand. The demand function for Clifton American Cheese is given by

$$\text{Demand: } p = \sqrt[3]{800 - q},\ 0 \le q \le 800,$$

where p is the price per pound and q is in thousands of pounds. [R.5]

a) Find the number of pounds sold when the price per pound is \$6.50.

b) Find the price per pound when 720,000 lb are sold.

58. Find the domain of $f(x) = \sqrt{25 - x^2}$. [R.3, R.5]

59. Find the domain of $g(x) = \sqrt{x - 1} + \sqrt{2 - x}$. [R.3, R.5]

60. The points (3, 5), (5, 8), and $(a, a/2)$ lie on the same line. Find a. [R.4]

Technology Connection

Graph each function and find the zeros, the domain, and the range. [R.5]

61. $f(x) = x^3 - 9x^2 + 27x + 50$

62. $f(x) = \sqrt[3]{|4 - x^2|} + 1$

63. Approximate the point(s) of intersection of the graphs of the two functions in Exercises 61 and 62. [R.5]

64. Business: ticket profits. Use the data in Exercise 56. [R.7]

a) Use regression to fit a quadratic function to the data.

b) Use the function from part (a) to estimate the profit made on the 30th day.

c) What factors might cause the Spring Valley Drama Troupe's profit to drop and then rise?

65. Social sciences: friends on Facebook. The data in the table below relate A, the average number of friends on Facebook, to x, a person's age. [R.7]

a) Use regression to fit linear, quadratic, cubic, and quartic functions to the data.

b) Make a scatterplot of the data, and graph each function on the scatterplot.

c) Which function provides the best model for the data? Why?

Age, x (in years)	Average Number of Facebook Friends, A (rounded to nearest 10)
14	520
21	650
30	360
40	280
50	220
60	130
70	100

(*Source:* Marketingcharts.com; Edison Research.)

Chapter R Test

1. **Business: compound interest.** Cecilia invests funds at 6.5% compounded annually. The investment grows to \$798.75 in 1 yr. How much was originally invested?

2. A function is given by $f(x) = -x^2 + 5$. Find:
   a) $f(-3)$;
   b) $f(x + h)$.

3. Find the slope and the y-intercept of the graph of $y = \frac{4}{5}x - \frac{2}{3}$.

4. Find an equation in slope–intercept form of the line with slope $\frac{1}{4}$, containing the point $(-3, 7)$.

5. Find the slope of the line containing the points $(-9, 2)$ and $(3, -4)$.

Find the average rate of change.

6.

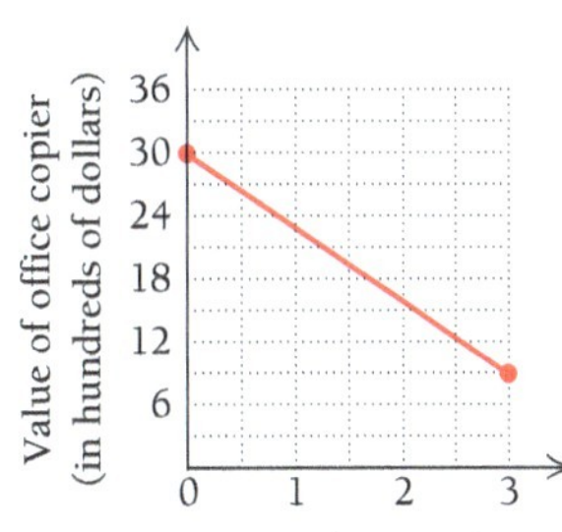

7.

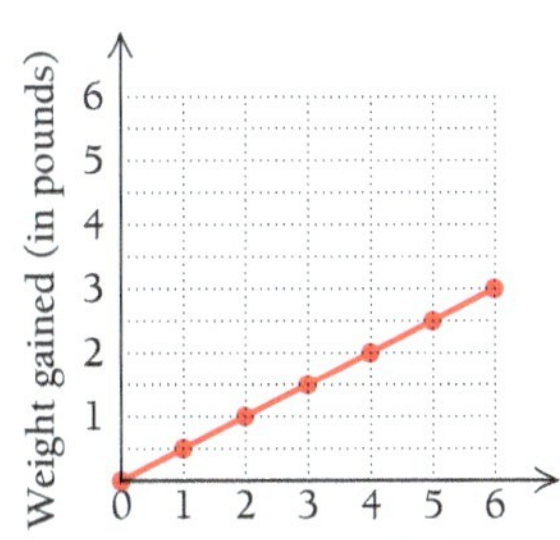

8. **Life science: body fluids.** The weight F of fluids in a human is directly proportional to body weight W. It is known that a 180-lb person has 120 lb of fluids. Find an equation of variation expressing F as a function of W.

9. **Business: profit-and-loss analysis.** Prentice Printing has fixed costs of \$8000 for producing a newly designed note card. The variable costs are \$0.08 per card. The revenue from each card will be \$0.50.
   a) Find $C(x)$, the total cost of producing x cards.
   b) Find $R(x)$, the total revenue from the sale of x cards.
   c) Find $P(x)$, the total profit from the production and sale of x cards.
   d) How many cards must Prentice Printing sell in order to break even?

10. **Economics: equilibrium point.** Find the equilibrium point for these demand and supply functions:

$$\text{Demand: } p = (q - 8)^2, 0 \le q \le 8,$$

$$\text{Supply: } p = q^2 + q + 13,$$

given that q is the quantity demanded or supplied, in thousands, and p is the unit price, in dollars.

Use the vertical-line test to determine whether each of the following is the graph of a function.

11.

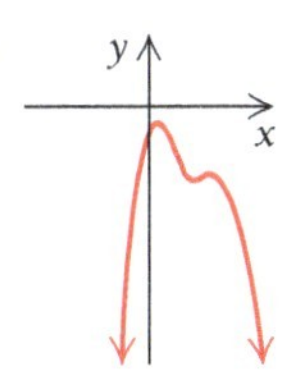

12.

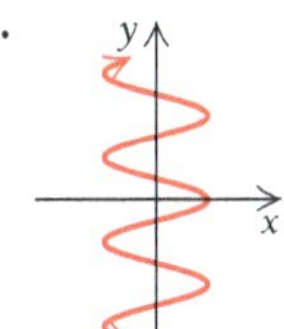

13. For the following graph of a quadratic function f, determine (a) $f(1)$; (b) the domain; (c) all x-values for which $f(x) = 4$; and (d) the range.

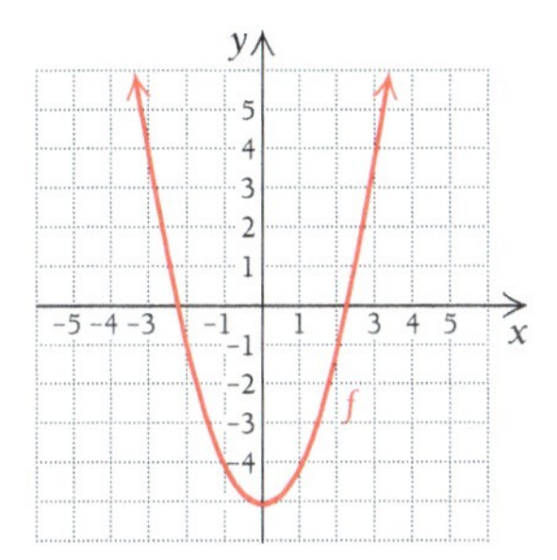

14. Graph: $f(x) = 8/x$.

15. Write $\dfrac{1}{\sqrt{t}}$ as an equivalent expression using a rational exponent.

16. Write $t^{-3/5}$ as an equivalent expression using radical notation.

17. Solve for x: $\log_9 \dfrac{1}{3} = x$.

18. Graph: $f(x) = \sqrt{x - 4} + 1$.

19. Write interval notation for the following graph.

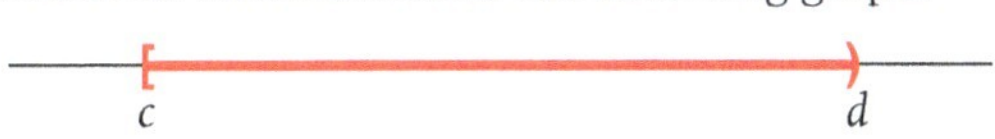

Write the domain of each function using interval notation.

20. $f(x) = \dfrac{x}{\sqrt{3x + 6}}$

21. $f(x) = \dfrac{x^2 + 20}{x^2 + 5x - 14}$

22. Graph:

$$f(x) = \begin{cases} x^2 + 2, & \text{for } x \ge 0, \\ x^2 - 2, & \text{for } x < 0. \end{cases}$$

23. Graph, and identify the y-intercept:

$$f(x) = \frac{1}{2} \cdot (3)^x.$$

24. The value of Joe's investment is given by

$$A(t) = 50{,}000\,(1.041)^t,$$

where t is the number of years since his initial deposit.

a) State the annual percent increase in the value of the investment.

b) When will the investment be worth \$75,000?

25. Nutrition. As people age, their daily caloric needs change. The following table shows data for physically active females, relating age, in years, to number of calories needed daily.

Age	Number of Calories Needed Daily
6	1800
11	2200
16	2400
24	2400
41	2200

(*Source:* Based on data from U.S. Department of Agriculture.)

a) Make a scatterplot of the data.

b) Do the data appear to fit a quadratic function?

c) Using the data points (6, 1800), (16, 2400), and (41, 2200), find a quadratic function that fits the data.

d) Use the function from part (c) to predict the number of calories needed daily by a physically active 30-yr-old woman.

e) What restrictions are reasonable for the domain of the function from part (c)? Why?

SYNTHESIS

26. Simplify: $(64^{4/3})^{-1/2}$.

27. Find the domain and the zeros of the function given by

$$f(x) = (5 - 3x)^{1/4} - 7.$$

28. Write an equation that has exactly three solutions: -3, 1, and 4. Answers may vary.

29. A function's average rate of change over the interval $[1, 5]$ is $-\frac{3}{7}$. If $f(1) = 9$, find $f(5)$.

Technology Connection 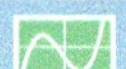

30. Graph f and find its zeros, domain, and range:

$$f(x) = \sqrt[3]{|9 - x^2|} - 1.$$

31. Nutrition. Use the data in Exercise 25.

a) Use REGRESSION to fit a quadratic function to the data.

b) Use the function from part (a) to predict the number of calories needed daily by a physically active 30-yr-old woman.

c) Compare your answer from part (b) with that from part (d) of Exercise 25. Which answer do you feel is more accurate? Why?

EXTENDED TECHNOLOGY APPLICATION

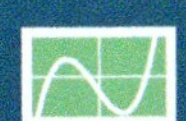

Average Price of a Movie Ticket

Extended Technology Applications occur at the end of every chapter. They consider certain applications in greater depth, make use of calculator skills, and allow for possible group or collaborative learning.

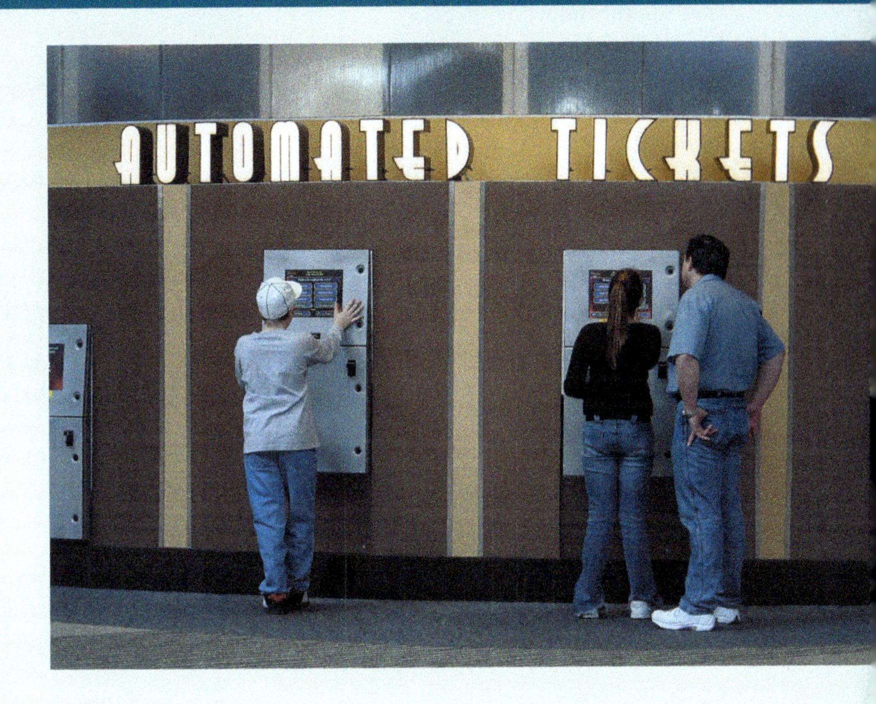

Have you noticed that the price of a movie ticket seems to increase over time? The table and graph that follow show the average price of a movie ticket for the years 1950 to 2015.

How much did you pay the last time you went to an evening movie? The average prices in the table may seem low, but they reflect discounts for matinees, children, and senior citizens. Let's use REGRESSION to analyze the data.

Year, t	Average Ticket Price, $P(t)$
1950, 0	\$0.46
1955, 5	0.58
1960, 10	0.76
1965, 15	1.01
1970, 20	1.55
1975, 25	2.05
1980, 30	2.69
1985, 35	3.55
1990, 40	4.23
1995, 45	4.35
2000, 50	5.39
2005, 55	6.41
2010, 60	8.01
2015, 65	8.43

(*Source:* Motion Picture Association of America.)

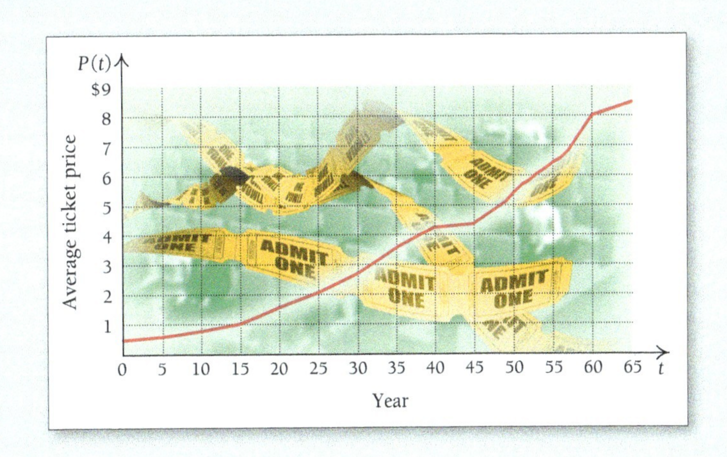

Exercises

1. a) Using REGRESSION, find a linear function that fits the data.
   b) Graph the linear function.
   c) Use the linear function to predict the average price of a movie ticket in 2020 and in 2025. Do these estimates appear reasonable?
   d) Use the function to predict the year in which the average price of a ticket will reach \$20. Does this estimate seem reasonable?

2. a) Using REGRESSION, find a quadratic function,
   $$y = ax^2 + bx + c,$$
   that fits the data.
   b) Graph the quadratic function.
   c) Use the quadratic function to predict the average price of a movie ticket in 2020 and in 2025. Do these estimates appear reasonable?
   d) Use the function to predict the year in which the average price of a ticket will reach \$20. Does this estimate seem reasonable?

3. a) Using REGRESSION, find a cubic function,

$$y = ax^3 + bx^2 + cx + d,$$

that fits the data.

b) Graph the cubic function.

c) Use the cubic function to predict the average price of a movie ticket in 2020 and in 2025. Do these estimates appear reasonable?

d) Use the function to predict the year in which the average price of a ticket will reach $20. Does this estimate seem reasonable?

4. a) Using REGRESSION, find a quartic function,

$$y = ax^4 + bx^3 + cx^2 + dx + e,$$

that fits the data.

b) Graph the quartic function.

c) Use the quartic function to predict the average price of a movie ticket in 2020 and in 2025. Do these estimates appear reasonable?

d) Use the function to predict the year in which the average price of a ticket will reach $20. Does this estimate seem reasonable?

5. a) Using REGRESSION, find an exponential function,

$$y = a_0 \cdot a^x,$$

that fits the data.

b) Graph the exponential function.

c) Use the exponential function to predict the average price of a movie ticket in 2020 and 2025. Do these estimates appear reasonable?

d) Use the function to predict the year when the average price of a ticket will reach $20. Does this estimate seem reasonable?

6. You are a research statistician assigned the task of making an accurate prediction of movie ticket prices.

a) Why might you not use the linear function?

b) Why might you use the quadratic function rather than the linear function?

c) Why might you use the exponential function rather than the quadratic function?

There are other procedures statisticians use to create predictive functions but they are beyond the scope of this text.

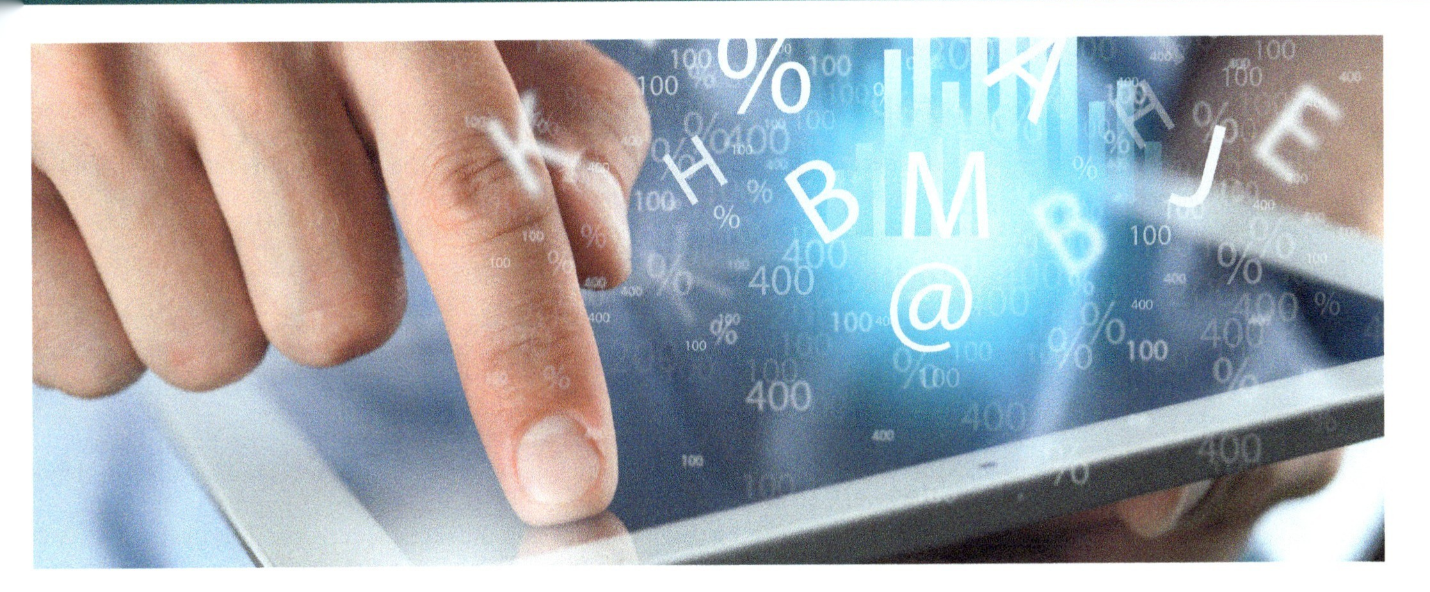

1 Differentiation

What You'll Learn

Why It's Important

In this chapter, we begin our study of calculus. The first concepts we consider are *limits* and *continuity*. We apply those concepts to establishing the first of the two main building blocks of calculus: differentiation.

Differentiation is a process that takes a formula for a function and derives another function, called a *derivative*. A derivative represents an instantaneous rate of change. Throughout this chapter, we develop techniques for finding derivatives and explore their many applications.

Where It's Used

Sales of iPads: The number of Apple iPads sold per year, in millions of units, t years after 2010, can be approximated by

$N(t) = 0.106t^4 - 1.452t^3 + 5.659t^2 + 1.946t + 20.714.$

Find the number of iPads sold, and the rate at which sales were increasing, in 2017.

(*This problem appears in Example 5 of Section 1.8.*)

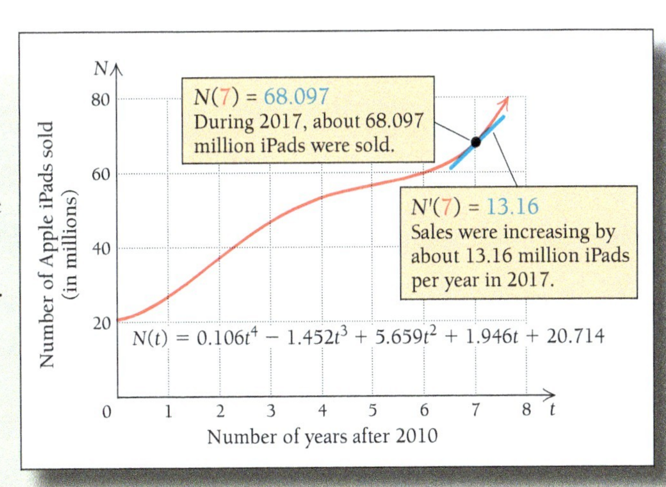

1.1 Limits: A Numerical and Graphical Approach

- Find limits of functions, if they exist, using numerical or graphical methods.

In this section, we discuss the concept of a *limit*. The discussion is intuitive—that is, it relies on prior experience and lacks formal proof.

Limits on the Number Line

Consider the pattern formed by the following sequence of numbers:

0.9, 0.99, 0.999, 0.9999, 0.99999, and so on.

The numbers appear to be getting close to the number 1, yet never equal 1 exactly. Assuming that the sequence continues in the same manner, we could say that the *limit* of this sequence of numbers is 1. Note that this sequence of numbers approaches 1 "from the left," meaning that all numbers in the sequence are less than the limit, 1. We write $x \to a^-$, read "x approaches a from the left," to represent a sequence of numbers that approaches a from the left. Thus, the sequence 0.9, 0.99, 0.999, 0.9999, 0.99999, and so on, is written $x \to 1^-$.

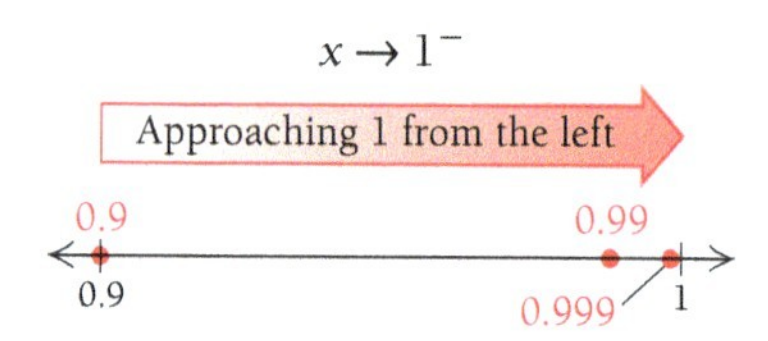

The following sequence approaches 1 "from the right":

1.1, 1.01, 1.001, 1.0001, 1.00001, and so on.

Numbers in this sequence are all greater than 1.

We write $x \to a^+$, read "x approaches a from the right," to represent a sequence of numbers that approaches a from the right. Thus, the sequence 1.1, 1.01, 1.001, 1.0001, 1.00001, and so on, is written $x \to 1^+$.

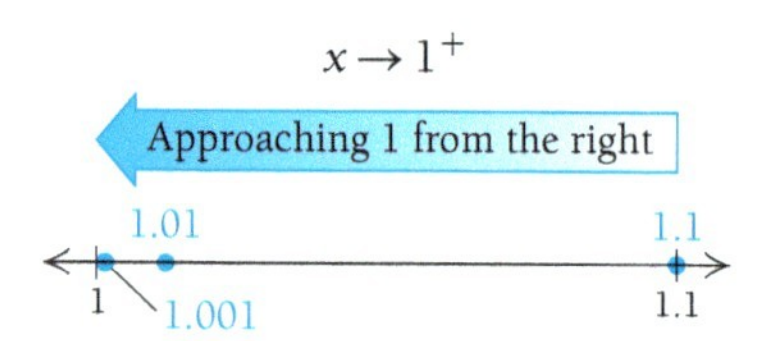

EXAMPLE 1 For each sequence, determine its limit, and rewrite the sequence in the form $x \to a^-$ or $x \to a^+$.

a) 2.24, 2.249, 2.2499, 2.24999, . . .

b) 5.51, 5.501, 5.5001, 5.50001, . . .

c) $\frac{1}{2}, \frac{3}{4}, \frac{7}{8}, \frac{15}{16}, \frac{31}{32}, \frac{63}{64}, \ldots$

Solution

a) These numbers are approaching the limit 2.25. Since each number in the sequence is less than 2.25, we write $x \to 2.25^-$, read "x approaches 2.25 from the left."

b) These numbers are approaching the limit 5.5. Since each number in the sequence is greater than 5.5, we write $x \to 5.5^+$, read "x approaches 5.5 from the right."

c) These numbers are approaching the limit 1. Since each number in the sequence is less than 1, we write $x \to 1^-$, read "x approaches 1 from the left." **1 ✓**

Quick Check 1 ✓

Determine the limit of 0.3, 0.33, 0.333, 0.3333, 0.33333, . . . , and rewrite the sequence in the form $x \to a^-$ or $x \to a^+$.

Numerical Limits of Functions

Suppose $f(x) = 2x + 1$, and let x assume the values in the sequence 0.9, 0.99, 0.999, 0.9999, 0.99999, and so on. Evaluating $f(x)$ for each of these values, we have

$$f(0.9) = 2(0.9) + 1 = 2.8,$$
$$f(0.99) = 2(0.99) + 1 = 2.98,$$
$$f(0.999) = 2(0.999) + 1 = 2.998,$$
$$f(0.9999) = 2(0.9999) + 1 = 2.9998,$$
$$f(0.99999) = 2(0.99999) + 1 = 2.99998, \quad \text{and so on.}$$

As x approaches the number 1 from the left, the sequence of outputs, $f(x)$, approaches the number 3. This is an example of a *left-hand limit* and is written

$$\lim_{x \to 1^-} f(x) = 3.$$ This is read "the limit of $f(x)$, as x approaches 1 from the left, is 3."

Now, let x assume the values in the sequence 1.1, 1.01, 1.001, 1.0001, 1.00001, and so on. Evaluating $f(x)$ for each of these values, we have

$$f(1.1) = 2(1.1) + 1 = 3.2,$$
$$f(1.01) = 2(1.01) + 1 = 3.02,$$
$$f(1.001) = 2(1.001) + 1 = 3.002,$$
$$f(1.0001) = 2(1.0001) + 1 = 3.0002,$$
$$f(1.00001) = 2(1.00001) + 1 = 3.00002, \quad \text{and so on.}$$

As x approaches the number 1 from the right, the sequence of outputs, $f(x)$, also approaches 3. This is an example of a *right-hand limit* and is written

$$\lim_{x \to 1^+} f(x) = 3.$$ This is read "the limit of $f(x)$, as x approaches 1 from the right, is 3."

Writing $x \to 1$ with no superscript, $^+$ or $^-$, on 1 indicates that "x approaches 1 from both sides." If both the left-hand limit and the right-hand limit exist and are equal to the same real number L, then the *general limit* (or simply, *the limit*) is L. In the above discussion, since $\lim_{x \to 1^-} f(x) = 3$ and $\lim_{x \to 1^+} f(x) = 3$, the general limit as x approaches 1 from both sides exists and is written $\lim_{x \to 1} f(x) = 3$.

This leads to the following theorem.

THEOREM 1

As x approaches a, the limit of $f(x)$ is L, where L is a real number, if the left-hand limit exists and the right-hand limit exists and if both limits are L. That is,

$$\text{if } \lim_{x \to a^+} f(x) = \lim_{x \to a^-} f(x) = L, \text{ then } \lim_{x \to a} f(x) = L.$$

The converse of this theorem is also true: If $\lim_{x \to a} f(x) = L$, then it follows that $\lim_{x \to a^-} f(x) = L$ and $\lim_{x \to a^+} f(x) = L$

If the left-hand or right-hand limit does not exist, or if the right-hand and left-hand limits exist but are different, then the limit itself does not exist.

Graphical Limits

To view limits graphically, we let $f(x) = 2x + 3$ and select x-values that get close to 4. In the table and graph below, we see that as input values approach 4 from the left (that is, are less than 4), output values approach 11, and as input values approach 4 from the right (that is, are greater than 4), output values also approach 11. Thus, we say:

As x approaches 4 from either side, the function $f(x) = 2x + 3$ approaches 11.

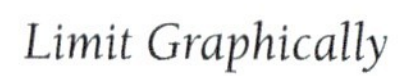
Limit Graphically

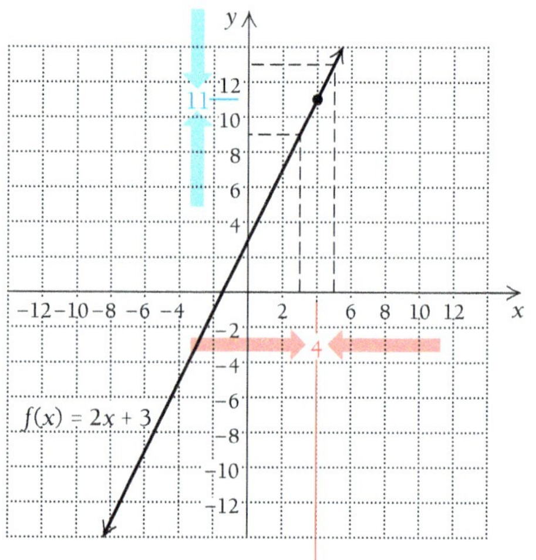
f(x) = 2x + 3
These input values approach 4 from the left.
These input values approach 4 from the right.

Limit Numerically

x	3.9	3.99	3.999	4	4.001	4.01	4.1
$f(x)$	10.8	10.98	10.998	11	11.002	11.02	11.2

These output values approach 11. These output values approach 11.

Since $\lim_{x \to 4^-} f(x) = 11$ and $\lim_{x \to 4^+} f(x) = 11$, it follows that the limit of $f(x)$, as x approaches 4, is 11. That is, $\lim_{x \to 4} f(x) = 11$.

EXAMPLE 2 Let $f(x) = -3x + 4$. Find the following limits:

a) $\lim_{x \to 2^-} f(x)$; **b)** $\lim_{x \to 2^+} f(x)$; **c)** $\lim_{x \to 2} f(x)$.

Solution

a) We choose values of x that approach 2 from the left, and evaluate $f(x)$:

$$f(1.9) = -3(1.9) + 4 = -1.7,$$
$$f(1.99) = -3(1.99) + 4 = -1.97,$$
$$f(1.999) = -3(1.999) + 4 = -1.997, \quad \text{and so on.}$$

We see that as x approaches 2 from the left, the function values approach -2. Thus, we have a left-hand limit, $\lim_{x \to 2^-} f(x) = -2$

b) We choose values of x that approach 2 from the right, and evaluate $f(x)$:

$$f(2.1) = -3(2.1) + 4 = -2.3,$$
$$f(2.01) = -3(2.01) + 4 = -2.03,$$
$$f(2.001) = -3(2.001) + 4 = -2.003, \quad \text{and so on.}$$

We see that as x approaches 2 from the right, the function values approach -2. Thus, we have a right-hand limit, $\lim_{x \to 2^+} f(x) = -2$.

c) Since the left-hand limit and the right-hand limit exist and are both equal to -2, we conclude that the limit as x approaches 2 exists and is -2: $\lim_{x \to 2} f(x) = -2$.

2 ✓

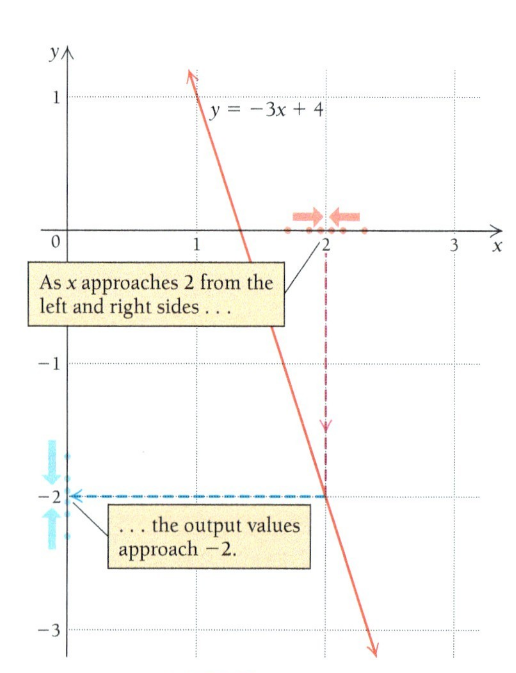
y = −3x + 4
As x approaches 2 from the left and right sides . . .
. . . the output values approach −2.

Quick Check 2 ✓

Let $f(x) = \frac{1}{2}x$. Find the following limits, if they exist:

a) $\lim_{x \to 3^-} f(x)$; **b)** $\lim_{x \to 3^+} f(x)$;

c) $\lim_{x \to 3} f(x)$.

In Example 2, note that $f(2) = -3(2) + 4 = -2$. Is it true that in some cases, finding the limit of $f(x)$ as x approaches a can be as simple as evaluating f at a directly? This "shortcut" is permissible under certain conditions, which we discuss in Section 1.2. For now, we explore limits using numerical and graphical methods that examine the behavior of a function *near* an x-value a.

EXAMPLE 3 Let $f(x) = \frac{x^2 - 1}{x - 1}$. Find $\lim_{x\to 1} f(x)$.

Solution Note that $f(x)$ does not exist at $x = 1$. Thus, we cannot find this limit by evaluating f at $x = 1$ directly. Instead, we use numerical and graphical methods to find this limit.

Using numerical methods, we choose values of x that approach 1 from the left, and values of x that approach 1 from the right. The tables below show selected values of x and the resulting limits, which are 2 in both cases:

Limit Numerically

Left-hand limit

$x \to 1^-$ $(x < 1)$	$f(x)$
0.9	1.9
0.99	1.99
0.999	1.999

$\lim_{x\to 1^-} f(x) = 2$

Right-hand limit

$x \to 1^+$ $(x > 1)$	$f(x)$
1.1	2.1
1.01	2.01
1.001	2.001

$\lim_{x\to 1^+} f(x) = 2$

Since the left-hand and right-hand limits exist and are equal, we conclude that the limit of $f(x)$ as x approaches 1 is

$$\lim_{x\to 1} f(x) = 2.$$

To graph f, we have

$$f(x) = \frac{x^2 - 1}{x - 1}$$

$$= \frac{(x + 1)(x - 1)}{x - 1} \qquad \text{Factoring the numerator}$$

$$= x + 1, \quad x \neq 1. \qquad \text{Note that } \frac{x - 1}{x - 1} = 1 \text{ for } x \neq 1.$$

Thus, the graph of $f(x) = \frac{x^2 - 1}{x - 1}$ is the line given by $f(x) = x + 1$ where the point corresponding to $x = 1$ has been removed.

The graph has a "hole" at the point $(1, 2)$. Thus, even though the function is not defined at $x = 1$, the limit *does* exist as $x \to 1$, and its value is 2.

Limit Graphically

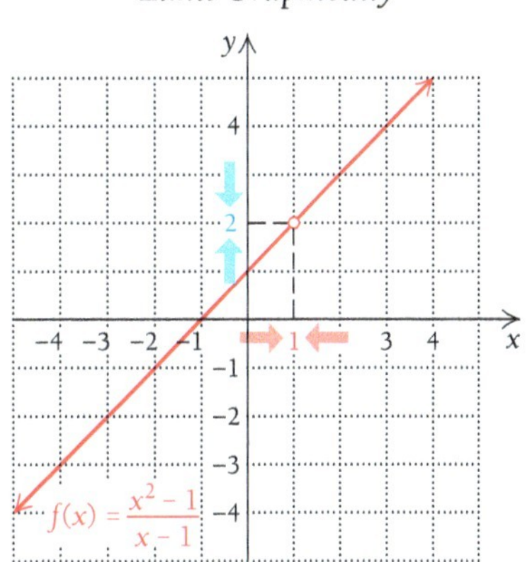

3 ✓

Technology Connection

Exploratory: Finding Limits Using the TABLE Feature

Consider the function given by $f(x) = 3x - 1$. To use the TABLE feature to explore the limit of this function as x approaches 6, we use TblSet and select Indpnt and Ask mode. Then we enter the inputs shown and the corresponding outputs automatically complete the table.

$$f(x) = 3x - 1$$

x	$f(x)$
5.9	16.7
5.99	16.97
5.999	16.997
6	?
6.001	17.003
6.01	17.03
6.1	17.3

Quick Check 3 ✓

Let

$$f(x) = \frac{x^2 - 9}{x - 3}.$$

a) Does $f(3)$ exist? Why or why not?

b) What is the limit of $f(x)$ as x approaches 3?

To summarize:

- When $x = 1$ exactly, $f(x)$ is undefined. The value $x = 1$ is not in the domain of f.
- When x approaches 1 from both sides, the output values approach 2.

Limits are also useful when considering piecewise-defined functions.

EXAMPLE 4 Consider the function H given by

$$H(x) = \begin{cases} 2x + 2, & \text{for } x < 1, \\ 2x - 4, & \text{for } x \geq 1. \end{cases}$$

Find $\lim_{x \to 1} H(x)$.

Solution We check the limits from the left and from the right both numerically, with an input–output table, and graphically.

Limit Numerically

$x \to 1^-$ $(x < 1)$	$H(x)$
0.9	3.8
0.99	3.98
0.999	3.998

These choices can vary.

$x \to 1^+$ $(x > 1)$	$H(x)$
1.01	−1.98
1.001	−1.998
1.0001	−1.9998

Limit Graphically

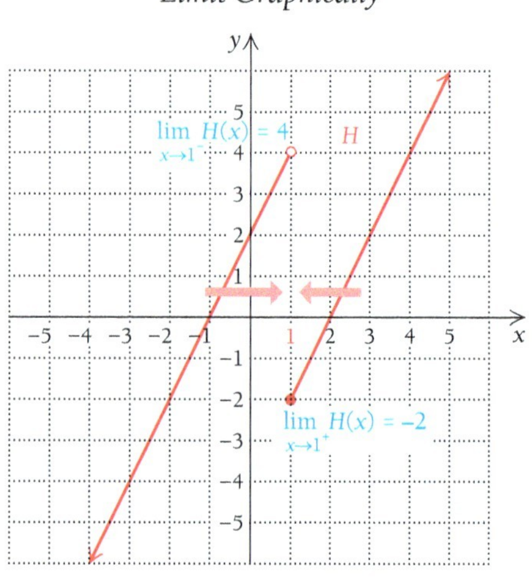

As inputs x approach 1 from the left (see the upper table), outputs $H(x)$ approach 4. Thus, the left-hand limit is 4. That is,

$$\lim_{x \to 1^-} H(x) = 4.$$

As inputs x approach 1 from the right (see the lower table), outputs $H(x)$ approach −2. Thus, the right-hand limit is −2. That is,

$$\lim_{x \to 1^+} H(x) = -2.$$

Since the left-hand limit, 4, is not the same as the right-hand limit, −2, we say that

$$\lim_{x \to 1} H(x) \textit{ does not exist.}$$

Note that $H(1) = -2$. In this example, the function value exists for $x = 1$, but the limit as $x \to 1$ does not exist. **4 ✓**

Quick Check 4 ✓

Let

$$k(x) = \begin{cases} -x + 4, & \text{for } x \leq 3, \\ 2x + 1, & \text{for } x > 3. \end{cases}$$

Graph k and then find $\lim_{x \to 3^-} k(x)$, $\lim_{x \to 3^+} k(x)$, and, if it exists, $\lim_{x \to 3} k(x)$.

> The existence of $\lim_{x \to a} f(x)$ does not require that $f(a)$ exists. If $f(a)$ does exist, it does not automatically follow that $\lim_{x \to a} f(x) = f(a)$. (See Example 5.)

The "Wall" Method

An alternative approach for Example 4 is to draw a "wall" at $x = 1$, as shown in blue on the graph to the left below. We then trace the graph from left to right with a pencil until we hit the wall and mark the location with an ×, assuming it can be determined. Then we trace the graph from right to left until we hit the wall and mark that location with an ×. If the locations are not the same, as shown in the graph to the left, a limit does not exist. Thus, for Example 4,

$$\lim_{x \to 1} H(x) \textit{ does not exist.}$$

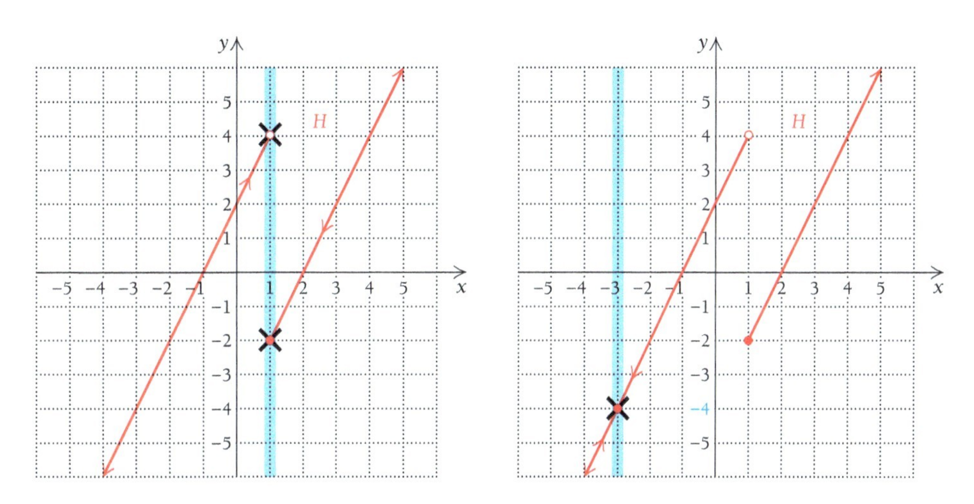

However, for any other value a, $\lim_{x \to a} H(x)$ does exist. For example, as x approaches -3, we see in the graph to the right that the wall method gives -4 whether -3 is approached from the left or from the right. Thus,

$$\lim_{x \to -3} H(x) = -4.$$

EXAMPLE 5 Consider the piecewise function defined as follows:

$$G(x) = \begin{cases} 5, & \text{for } x = 1, \\ x + 1, & \text{for } x \neq 1. \end{cases}$$

Graph the function, and find each of the following:

a) $G(1)$ **b)** $\lim_{x \to 1} G(x)$

Solution The graph of G follows.

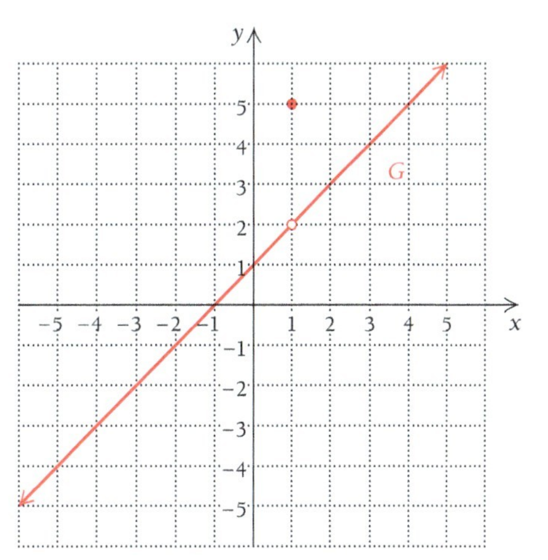

a) From the definition of G, we see that

$$G(1) = 5.$$

b) As inputs x approach 1 from the left, outputs $G(x)$ approach 2, so the limit from the left is 2. As inputs x approach 1 from the right, outputs $G(x)$ also approach 2, so the limit from the right is 2. Both limits are the same, so

$$\lim_{x \to 1} G(x) = 2.$$

Note that the limit, 2, is not the same as the function value at 1.

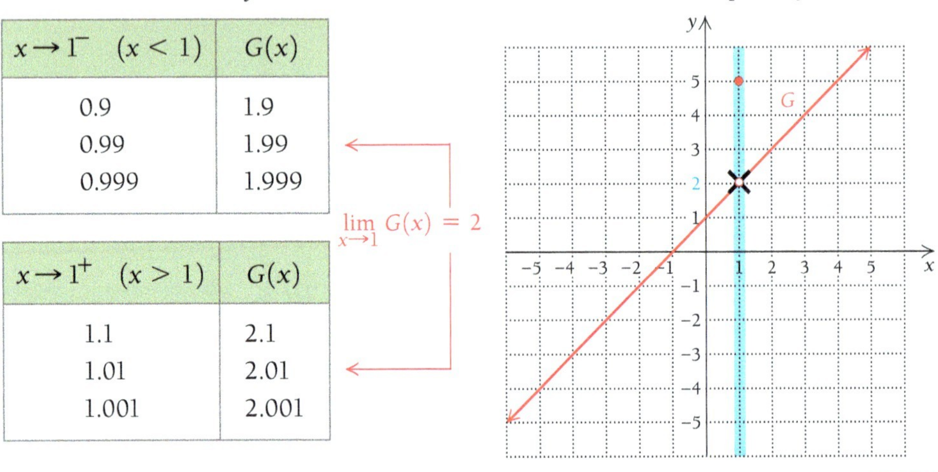

Limit Numerically

$x \to 1^-$ $(x < 1)$	$G(x)$
0.9	1.9
0.99	1.99
0.999	1.999

$x \to 1^+$ $(x > 1)$	$G(x)$
1.1	2.1
1.01	2.01
1.001	2.001

5 ✓

Quick Check 5 ✓

Find the following based on the graph of f.

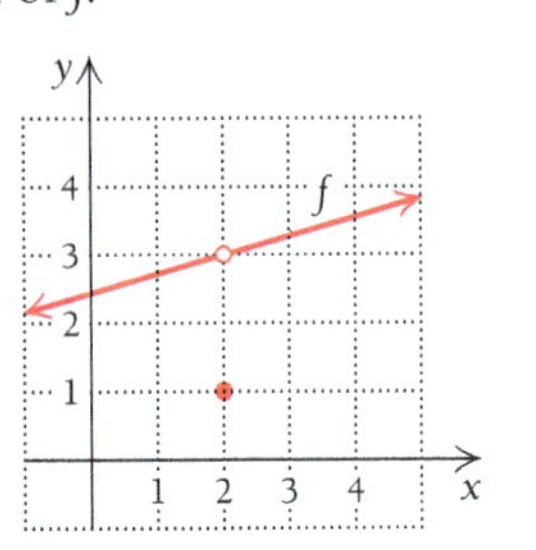

a) $f(2)$ **b)** $\lim_{x \to 2} f(x)$

Limits Involving Infinity

Limits also help us understand the role of infinity with respect to some functions.

EXAMPLE 6 Let $f(x) = \dfrac{1}{x - 2}$.

a) Find $\lim_{x \to 2^-} f(x)$. **b)** Find $\lim_{x \to 2^+} f(x)$.

c) Does $\lim_{x \to 2} f(x)$ exist? Why or why not?

Solution Although the limits may exist, note first that $f(2)$ does not exist, since 2 is not in the domain of f.

Limit Numerically

$x \to 2^-$ $(x < 2)$	$f(x)$
1.9	−10
1.99	−100
1.999	−1000
1.9999	−10,000

$x \to 2^+$ $(x > 2)$	$f(x)$
2.1	10
2.01	100
2.001	1000
2.0001	10,000

Limit Graphically

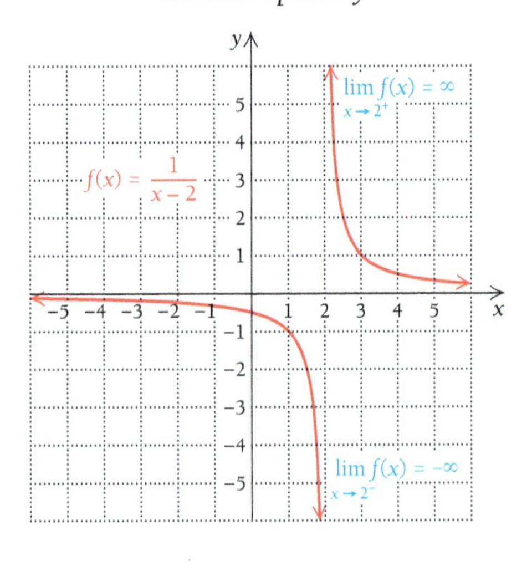

a) The table and graph show that as x approaches 2 from the left, $f(x)$ decreases without bound. We conclude that the left-hand limit is negative infinity; that is, $\lim_{x \to 2^-} f(x) = -\infty$. We symbolize the notion of "infinity" with ∞. The symbol ∞ *does not represent* a real number.

b) The table and graph show that as x approaches 2 from the right, $f(x)$ increases without bound toward positive infinity. Thus, $\lim_{x \to 2^+} f(x) = \infty$.

c) Since the left-hand and right-hand limits are not equal, $\lim_{x \to 2} f(x)$ does not exist.

Sometimes we need to determine limits as inputs approach positive or negative infinity. In such cases, we say that we are finding *limits at infinity*. Such a limit is expressed as

$$\lim_{x \to \infty} f(x) \quad \text{or} \quad \lim_{x \to -\infty} f(x).$$

These limits are approached from one side only: from the left if approaching positive infinity or from the right if approaching negative infinity.

EXAMPLE 7 Let $f(x) = \frac{1}{x}$. Find $\lim_{x \to \infty} f(x)$ and $\lim_{x \to -\infty} f(x)$.

Solution The table shows that as x increases toward positive infinity, $f(x)$ approaches 0. Thus, $\lim_{x \to \infty} f(x) = 0$. As x decreases toward negative infinity, $f(x)$ again approaches 0. Thus, $\lim_{x \to -\infty} f(x) = 0$.

Limit Numerically

$x \to \infty$	$f(x)$
100	0.01
1,000	0.001
10,000	0.0001

$\lim_{x \to \infty} f(x) = 0$

$x \to -\infty$	$f(x)$
−100	−0.01
−1,000	−0.001
−10,000	−0.0001

$\lim_{x \to -\infty} f(x) = 0$

Limit Graphically

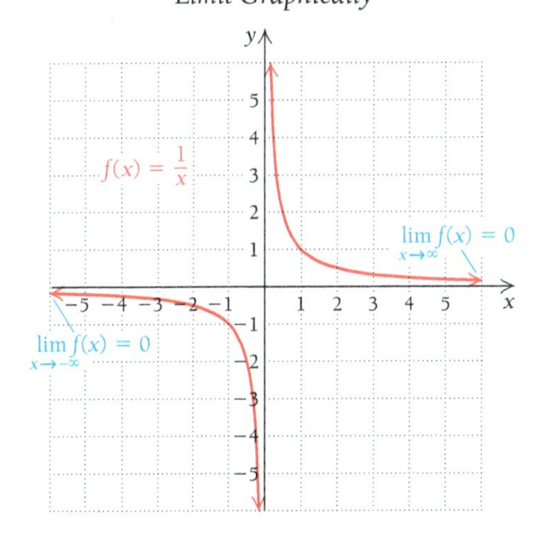

We will use the fact that $\lim_{x \to -\infty} \left(\frac{1}{x}\right) = 0$ and $\lim_{x \to \infty} \left(\frac{1}{x}\right) = 0$, or, more succinctly, that $\lim_{x \to \pm\infty} \left(\frac{1}{x}\right) = 0$, to evaluate other limits. In general, $\lim_{x \to \pm\infty} \left(\frac{k}{x}\right) = 0$, for any real number k.

EXAMPLE 8 Consider the function f given by

$$f(x) = \frac{3x - 5}{x - 2}.$$

Graph the function, and find each limit, if it exists.

a) $\lim_{x \to 3} f(x)$ **b)** $\lim_{x \to 2} f(x)$ **c)** $\lim_{x \to \infty} f(x)$ **d)** $\lim_{x \to -\infty} f(x)$

Solution The graph of f is shown to the right.

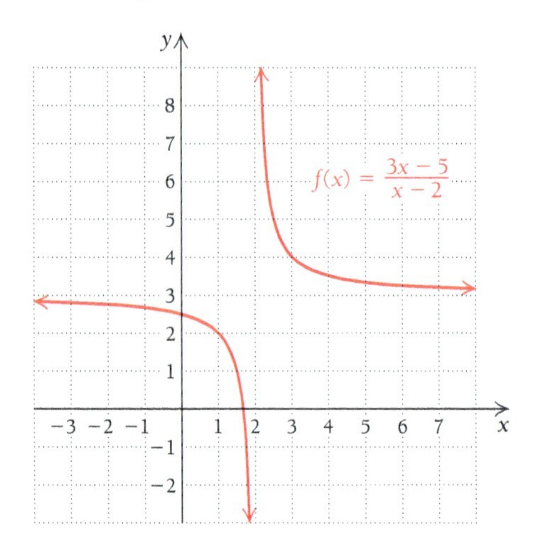

a) As x approaches 3 from the left, $f(x)$ approaches 4, so the left-hand limit is 4. As x approaches 3 from the right, $f(x)$ also approaches 4, so the right-hand limit is also 4. Since the left-hand limit is the same as the right-hand limit, we have

$$\lim_{x \to 3} f(x) = 4.$$

Limit Numerically

$x \to 3^-$ $(x < 3)$	$f(x)$
2.9	4.1111. . .
2.99	4.0101. . .
2.999	4.001. . .

$\lim_{x \to 3} f(x) = 4$

$x \to 3^+$ $(x > 3)$	$f(x)$
3.1	3.9090. . .
3.01	3.99009900. . .
3.001	3.9990. . .

Limit Graphically

b) As inputs x approach 2 from the left, outputs $f(x)$ approach negative infinity. That is,

$$\lim_{x \to 2^-} f(x) = -\infty.$$

As inputs x approach 2 from the right, outputs $f(x)$ approach positive infinity. That is,

$$\lim_{x \to 2^+} f(x) = \infty.$$

Because the left-hand limit differs from the right-hand limit,

$$\lim_{x \to 2} f(x) \text{ does not exist.}$$

Limit Numerically

$x \to 2^-$ $(x < 2)$	$f(x)$
1.9	−7
1.99	−97
1.999	−997

$\lim\limits_{x \to 2} f(x)$ does not exist.

$x \to 2^+$ $(x > 2)$	$f(x)$
2.1	13
2.01	103
2.001	1003

Limit Graphically

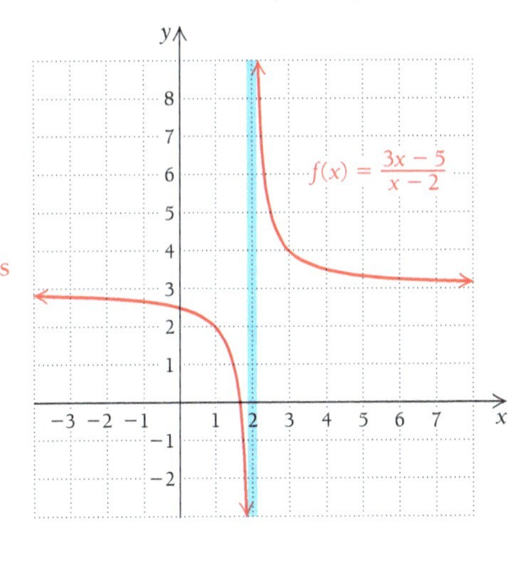

c) As shown in the table and graph below, as inputs x approach positive infinity, the outputs approach 3. Thus,

$$\lim_{x \to \infty} f(x) = 3.$$

d) As inputs x approach negative infinity, much as in part (c), the outputs again approach 3. Thus,

$$\lim_{x \to -\infty} f(x) = 3.$$

Limit Numerically *Limit Graphically*

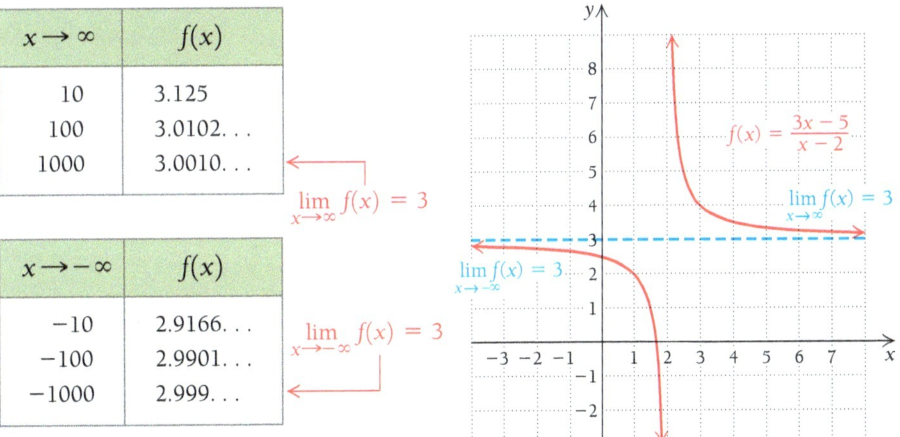

$x \to \infty$	$f(x)$
10	3.125
100	3.0102. . .
1000	3.0010. . .

$\lim\limits_{x \to \infty} f(x) = 3$

$x \to -\infty$	$f(x)$
−10	2.9166. . .
−100	2.9901. . .
−1000	2.999. . .

$\lim\limits_{x \to -\infty} f(x) = 3$

Quick Check 6 ✓

Let $h(x) = \dfrac{7 - 6x}{1 - x}$. Find each limit, if it exists.

a) $\lim\limits_{x \to 1} h(x)$; **b)** $\lim\limits_{x \to 2} h(x)$;

c) $\lim\limits_{x \to \infty} h(x)$; **d)** $\lim\limits_{x \to -\infty} h(x)$.

6 ✓

Section Summary

- The notation $x \to a^-$ represents a sequence of numbers that approach a limit value a from the left. The notation $x \to a^+$ represents a sequence of numbers that approach a limit value a from the right.
- The *limit* of $f(x)$, as x approaches a, is written $\lim\limits_{x \to a} f(x) = L$. This means that as the values of x approach a, the corresponding values of $f(x)$ approach L. The value L must be a unique real number.
- A *left-hand limit* is written $\lim\limits_{x \to a^-} f(x)$. Values of x approach a from the left, that is, $x < a$.
- A *right-hand limit* is written $\lim\limits_{x \to a^+} f(x)$. Values of x approach a from the right, that is, $x > a$.

- If the left-hand and right-hand limits (as x approaches a) are *not* equal, the limit does *not* exist at a. If the left-hand and right-hand limits are equal and not infinite, the limit does exist.
- A limit $\lim_{x \to a} f(x)$ can exist even though the function value $f(a)$ might not exist. (See Example 3.)
- A limit $\lim_{x \to a} f(x)$ can exist and be different from the function value $f(a)$. (See Example 5.)
- Graphs and tables are useful tools in determining limits.

1.1 Exercise Set

For each sequence of numbers, determine the limit and then rewrite the sequence using the notation $x \to a^-$ or $x \to a^+$.

1. 0.29, 0.299, 0.2999, 0.29999, . . .

2. 1.71, 1.701, 1.7001, 1.70001, . . .

3. −3.5, −3.05, −3.005, −3.0005, . . .

4. −4.89, −4.899, −4.8999, −4.89999, . . .

5. 0.6, 0.66, 0.666, 0.6666, . . .

6. 1.3, 1.33, 1.333, 1.3333, . . .

7. 0.29, 0.299, 0.2999, 0.29999, . . .

8. 1.19, 1.199, 1.1999, 1.19999, . . .

9. $\frac{3}{2}, \frac{5}{4}, \frac{9}{8}, \frac{17}{16}, \frac{33}{32}, \ldots$

10. $-\frac{3}{10}, -\frac{3}{100}, -\frac{3}{1000}, -\frac{3}{10{,}000}, \ldots$

Complete each of the following statements.

11. As x approaches ________, the value of $-3x$ approaches 6.

12. As x approaches ________, the value of $x - 2$ approaches 5.

13. The notation ________ is read "the limit, as x approaches 2 from the right."

14. The notation ________ is read "the limit, as x approaches 3 from the left."

15. The notation ________ is read "the limit as x approaches 5."

16. The notation ________ is read "the limit as x approaches $\frac{1}{2}$."

17. The notation $\lim_{x \to 4} f(x)$ is read ________.

18. The notation $\lim_{x \to 1} g(x)$ is read ________.

19. The notation $\lim_{x \to 5^-} F(x)$ is read ________.

20. The notation $\lim_{x \to 4^+} G(x)$ is read ________.

For Exercises 21 and 22, consider the function f given by

$$f(x) = \begin{cases} x - 2, & \text{for } x \leq 3, \\ x - 1, & \text{for } x > 3. \end{cases}$$

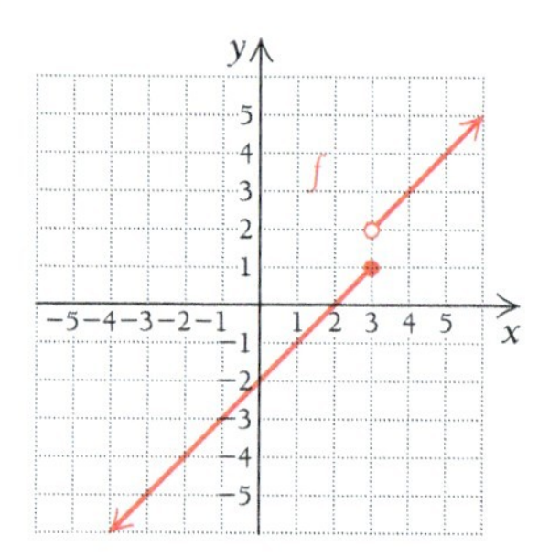

If a limit does not exist, state that fact.

21. Find **(a)** $\lim_{x \to -1^-} f(x)$; **(b)** $\lim_{x \to -1^+} f(x)$; **(c)** $\lim_{x \to -1} f(x)$.

22. Find **(a)** $\lim_{x \to 3^-} f(x)$; **(b)** $\lim_{x \to 3^+} f(x)$; **(c)** $\lim_{x \to 3} f(x)$.

For Exercises 23 and 24, consider the function g given by

$$g(x) = \begin{cases} x + 6, & \text{for } x < -2, \\ -\frac{1}{2}x + 1, & \text{for } x \geq -2. \end{cases}$$

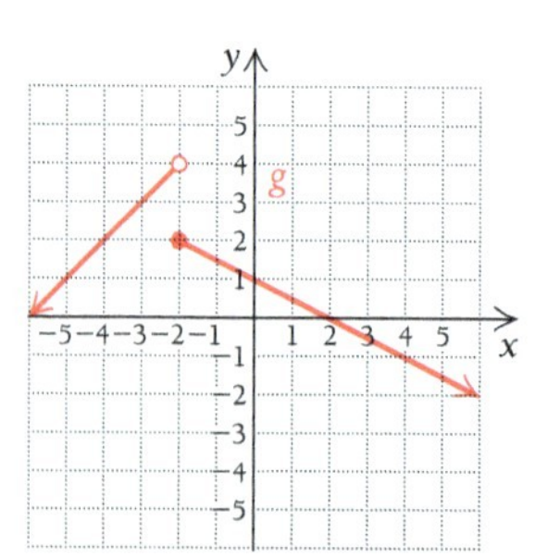

If a limit does not exist, state that fact.

23. Find **(a)** $\lim_{x \to 4^-} g(x)$; **(b)** $\lim_{x \to 4^+} g(x)$; **(c)** $\lim_{x \to 4} g(x)$.

24. Find **(a)** $\lim_{x \to -2^-} g(x)$; **(b)** $\lim_{x \to -2^+} g(x)$; **(c)** $\lim_{x \to -2} g(x)$.

For Exercises 25–32, use the following graph of F to find each limit. When necessary, state that the limit does not exist.

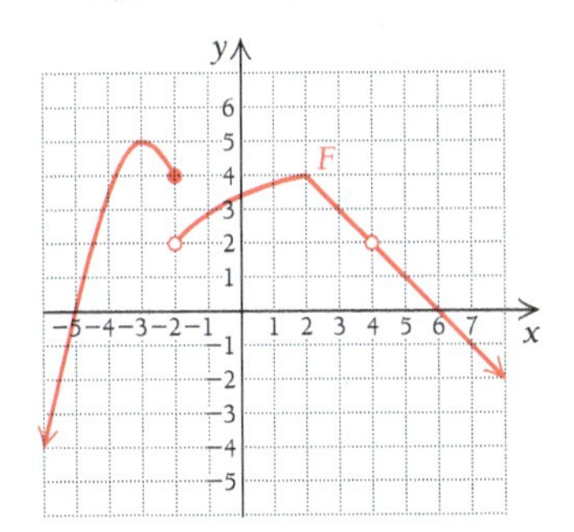

25. $\lim_{x \to -3} F(x)$
26. $\lim_{x \to 2} F(x)$
27. $\lim_{x \to -2} F(x)$
28. $\lim_{x \to -5} F(x)$
29. $\lim_{x \to 4} F(x)$
30. $\lim_{x \to 6} F(x)$
31. $\lim_{x \to -2^+} F(x)$
32. $\lim_{x \to -2^-} F(x)$

For Exercises 33–40, use the following graph of G to find each limit. When necessary, state that the limit does not exist.

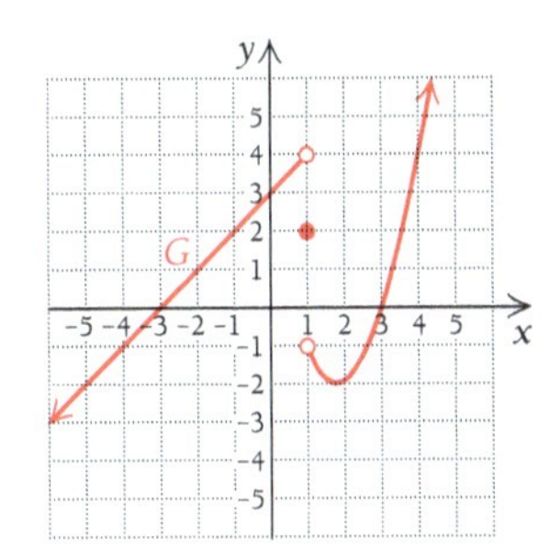

33. $\lim_{x \to -2} G(x)$
34. $\lim_{x \to 0} G(x)$
35. $\lim_{x \to 1^-} G(x)$
36. $\lim_{x \to 1^+} G(x)$
37. $\lim_{x \to 3^-} G(x)$
38. $\lim_{x \to 1} G(x)$
39. $\lim_{x \to 3^+} G(x)$
40. $\lim_{x \to 3} G(x)$

For Exercises 41–50, use the following graph of H to find each limit. When necessary, state that the limit does not exist.

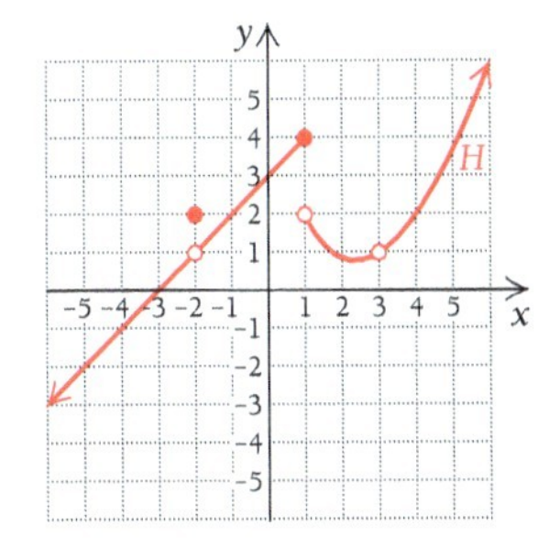

41. $\lim_{x \to -3} H(x)$
42. $\lim_{x \to -2^-} H(x)$
43. $\lim_{x \to -2^+} H(x)$
44. $\lim_{x \to -2} H(x)$
45. $\lim_{x \to 1^-} H(x)$
46. $\lim_{x \to 1^+} H(x)$
47. $\lim_{x \to 3^-} H(x)$
48. $\lim_{x \to 1} H(x)$
49. $\lim_{x \to 3^+} H(x)$
50. $\lim_{x \to 3} H(x)$

For Exercises 51–60, use the following graph of f to find each limit. When necessary, state that the limit does not exist.

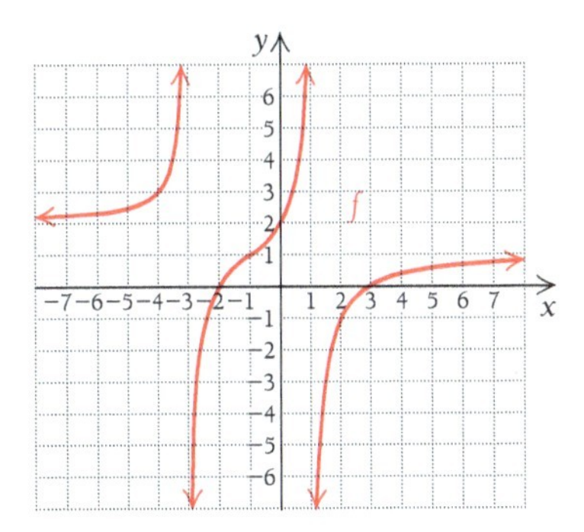

51. $\lim_{x \to 2} f(x)$
52. $\lim_{x \to -1} f(x)$
53. $\lim_{x \to 0} f(x)$
54. $\lim_{x \to -3} f(x)$
55. $\lim_{x \to 1} f(x)$
56. $\lim_{x \to 3} f(x)$
57. $\lim_{x \to -2} f(x)$
58. $\lim_{x \to -4} f(x)$
59. $\lim_{x \to -\infty} f(x)$
60. $\lim_{x \to \infty} f(x)$

For Exercises 61–78, graph each function and then find the specified limits. When necessary, state that the limit does not exist.

61. $f(x) = |x|$; find $\lim_{x \to 0} f(x)$ and $\lim_{x \to -2} f(x)$.

62. $f(x) = x^2$; find $\lim_{x \to -1} f(x)$ and $\lim_{x \to 0} f(x)$.

63. $g(x) = x^2 - 5$; find $\lim_{x \to 0} g(x)$ and $\lim_{x \to -1} g(x)$.

64. $g(x) = |x| + 1$; find $\lim_{x \to -3} g(x)$ and $\lim_{x \to 0} g(x)$.

65. $G(x) = \dfrac{4}{x + 2}$; find $\lim_{x \to -1} G(x)$ and $\lim_{x \to -2} G(x)$.

66. $F(x) = \dfrac{2}{x - 3}$; find $\lim_{x \to 3} F(x)$ and $\lim_{x \to 4} F(x)$.

67. $f(x) = \dfrac{1 - 2x}{x}$; find $\lim_{x \to \infty} f(x)$ and $\lim_{x \to 0} f(x)$.

68. $f(x) = \dfrac{1 + 3x}{x}$; find $\lim_{x \to \infty} f(x)$ and $\lim_{x \to 0} f(x)$.

69. $g(x) = \dfrac{2x - 5}{x - 3}$; find $\lim_{x \to \infty} g(x)$ and $\lim_{x \to 3} g(x)$.

70. $g(x) = \dfrac{4x + 9}{x + 2}$; find $\lim_{x \to \infty} g(x)$ and $\lim_{x \to -2} g(x)$.

71. $F(x) = \begin{cases} 2x + 1, & \text{for } x < 1, \\ x, & \text{for } x \geq 1. \end{cases}$

Find $\lim_{x \to 1^-} F(x)$, $\lim_{x \to 1^+} F(x)$, and $\lim_{x \to 1} F(x)$.

72. $G(x) = \begin{cases} -x + 3, & \text{for } x < 2, \\ x + 1, & \text{for } x \geq 2. \end{cases}$

Find $\lim_{x \to 2^-} G(x)$, $\lim_{x \to 2^+} G(x)$, and $\lim_{x \to 2} G(x)$.

73. $g(x) = \begin{cases} -x + 4, & \text{for } x < 3, \\ x - 3, & \text{for } x > 3. \end{cases}$

Find $\lim_{x \to 3^-} g(x)$, $\lim_{x \to 3^+} g(x)$, and $\lim_{x \to 3} g(x)$.

74. $f(x) = \begin{cases} 3x - 4, & \text{for } x < 1, \\ x - 2, & \text{for } x > 1. \end{cases}$

Find $\lim_{x \to 1^-} f(x)$, $\lim_{x \to 1^+} f(x)$, and $\lim_{x \to 1} f(x)$.

75. $F(x) = \begin{cases} -2x - 3, & \text{for } x < -1, \\ x^3, & \text{for } x > -1. \end{cases}$ Find $\lim_{x \to -1} F(x)$.

76. $G(x) = \begin{cases} x^2, & \text{for } x < -1, \\ x + 2, & \text{for } x > -1. \end{cases}$ Find $\lim_{x \to -1} G(x)$.

77. $H(x) = \begin{cases} x + 1, & \text{for } x < 0, \\ 2, & \text{for } 0 \leq x < 1, \\ 3 - x, & \text{for } x \geq 1. \end{cases}$

Find $\lim_{x \to 0} H(x)$ and $\lim_{x \to 1} H(x)$.

78. $G(x) = \begin{cases} 2 + x, & \text{for } x \leq -1, \\ x^2, & \text{for } -1 < x < 3, \\ 9, & \text{for } x \geq 3. \end{cases}$

Find $\lim_{x \to -1} G(x)$ and $\lim_{x \to 3} G(x)$.

APPLICATIONS

Business and Economics

Taxicab fares. *In New York City, taxicabs charge passengers \$2.50 for entering a cab and then \$0.50 for each one-fifth of a mile (or fraction thereof) traveled. (There are additional charges for slow traffic and idle times, but these are not considered in this problem.) If x represents the distance traveled in miles, then C(x) is the cost of the taxi fare, where*

$$C(x) = \$2.50, \quad \text{if} \quad x = 0,$$
$$C(x) = \$3.00, \quad \text{if} \quad 0 < x \leq 0.2,$$
$$C(x) = \$3.50, \quad \text{if} \quad 0.2 < x \leq 0.4,$$
$$C(x) = \$4.00, \quad \text{if} \quad 0.4 < x \leq 0.6,$$

and so on. The graph of C is shown below. (Source: New York City Taxi and Limousine Commission.)

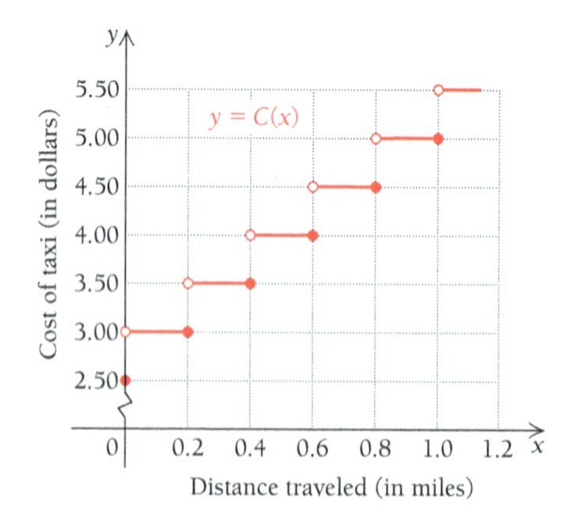

Using the graph of the taxicab fare function, find each of the following limits, if it exists.

79. $\lim_{x \to 0.25^-} C(x)$, $\lim_{x \to 0.25^+} C(x)$, $\lim_{x \to 0.25} C(x)$

80. $\lim_{x \to 0.2^-} C(x)$, $\lim_{x \to 0.2^+} C(x)$, $\lim_{x \to 0.2} C(x)$

81. $\lim_{x \to 0.6^-} C(x)$, $\lim_{x \to 0.6^+} C(x)$, $\lim_{x \to 0.6} C(x)$

The postage function. *The cost of sending a large envelope via U.S. first-class mail in 2018 was \$1.00 for the first ounce and \$0.21 for each additional ounce (or fraction thereof). (Source: www.usps.com.) If x represents the weight of a large envelope, in ounces, then p(x) is the cost of mailing it, where*

$$p(x) = \$1.00, \quad \text{if} \quad 0 < x \leq 1,$$
$$p(x) = \$1.21, \quad \text{if} \quad 1 < x \leq 2,$$
$$p(x) = \$1.42, \quad \text{if} \quad 2 < x \leq 3,$$

and so on, up through 13 ounces. The graph of p is shown below.

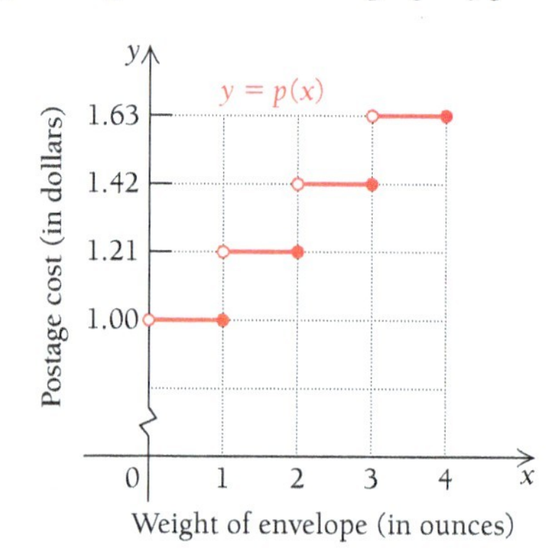

Using the graph of the postage function, find each of the following limits, if it exists.

82. $\lim_{x \to 1^-} p(x)$, $\lim_{x \to 1^+} p(x)$, $\lim_{x \to 1} p(x)$

83. $\lim_{x \to 2^-} p(x)$, $\lim_{x \to 2^+} p(x)$, $\lim_{x \to 2} p(x)$

84. $\lim_{x \to 2.6^-} p(x)$, $\lim_{x \to 2.6^+} p(x)$, $\lim_{x \to 2.6} p(x)$

85. $\lim_{x \to 3} p(x)$

86. $\lim_{x \to 3.4} p(x)$

Tax rate schedule. *The federal tax rate for single filers is given as a percentage of taxable income in the graph below. (Source: troweprice.com, 2018.) Use the graph for Exercises 87–89.*

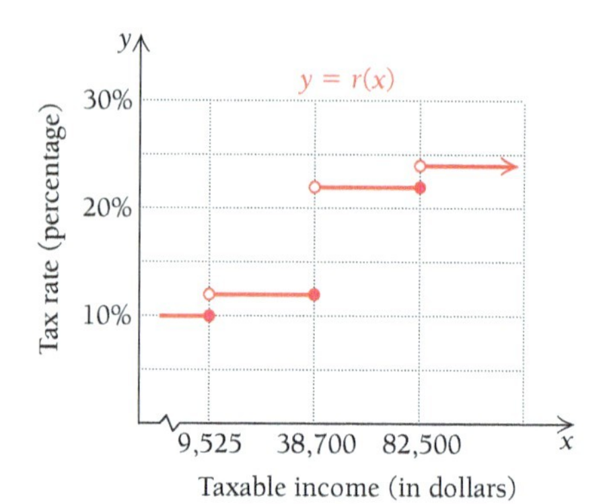

87. Find $\lim_{x \to 9525^-} r(x)$, $\lim_{x \to 9525^+} r(x)$, and $\lim_{x \to 9525} r(x)$.

88. Find $\lim_{x \to 10,000^-} r(x)$, $\lim_{x \to 10,000^+} r(x)$, and $\lim_{x \to 10,000} r(x)$.

89. Find $\lim_{x \to 50,000} r(x)$ and $\lim_{x \to 82,500} r(x)$.

Tax rate schedule. *The federal tax rate for heads of household is given in the graph below. (Source: troweprice.com, 2018.) Use the graph for Exercises 90–92.*

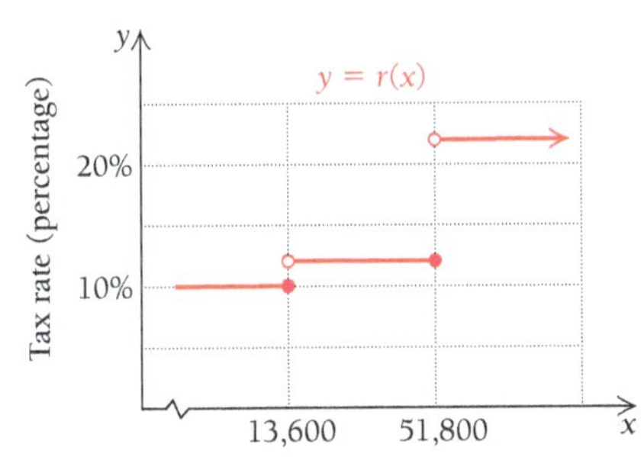

90. Find $\lim_{x \to 9000^-} r(x)$, $\lim_{x \to 9000^+} r(x)$, and $\lim_{x \to 9000} r(x)$.

91. Find $\lim_{x \to 51,800^-} r(x)$, $\lim_{x \to 51,800^+} r(x)$, and $\lim_{x \to 51,800} r(x)$.

92. Find $\lim_{x \to 60,000} r(x)$ and $\lim_{x \to 13,600} r(x)$.

SYNTHESIS

In Exercises 93–95, fill in each blank so that $\lim_{x \to 2} f(x)$ exists.

93. $f(x) = \begin{cases} \frac{1}{2}x + \_\_, & \text{for } x < 2, \\ -x + 6, & \text{for } x > 2 \end{cases}$

94. $f(x) = \begin{cases} -\frac{1}{2}x + 1, & \text{for } x < 2, \\ \frac{3}{2}x + \_\_, & \text{for } x > 2 \end{cases}$

95. $f(x) = \begin{cases} x^2 - 9, & \text{for } x < 2, \\ -x^2 + \_\_, & \text{for } x > 2 \end{cases}$

96. **Supremums.** At the start of this section, we determined that the sequence of numbers 0.9, 0.99, 0.999, 0.9999, . . . approaches 1 as a limit, since it can be argued that each number in the sequence is "closer" to 1 than the previous number in the sequence. A *supremum* is any number that is greater than all numbers of a sequence. Thus, 1 is a supremum of this sequence. In fact, any number $S > 1$ is a supremum of this sequence.

   a) Consider the sequence $1 - 0.9, 1 - 0.99, 1 - 0.999, \ldots$. What is the limit of this sequence?

   b) Now consider the sequence $3 - 0.9, 3 - 0.99, 3 - 0.999, \ldots$. What is the limit of this sequence?

   c) Based on parts (a) and (b), what extra requirement should be placed on a supremum S in order for it to be the limit of a sequence?

Technology Connection

97. Graph the function f given by

$$f(x) = \begin{cases} -3, & \text{for } x = -2, \\ x^2, & \text{for } x \neq -2. \end{cases}$$

Use GRAPH and TRACE to find each of the following limits. When necessary, state that the limit does not exist.

a) $\lim_{x \to -2^+} f(x)$
b) $\lim_{x \to -2^-} f(x)$
c) $\lim_{x \to -2} f(x)$
d) $\lim_{x \to 2^+} f(x)$
e) $\lim_{x \to 2^-} f(x)$
f) Does $\lim_{x \to -2} f(x) = f(-2)$?
g) Does $\lim_{x \to 2} f(x) = f(2)$?

In Exercises 98–100, use GRAPH and TRACE to find each limit. When necessary, state that the limit does not exist.

98. For $f(x) = \begin{cases} x^2 - 2, & \text{for } x < 0, \\ 2 - x^2, & \text{for } x \geq 0, \end{cases}$ find $\lim_{x \to 0} f(x)$ and $\lim_{x \to -2} f(x)$.

99. For $g(x) = \dfrac{20x^2}{x^3 + 2x^2 + 5x}$, find $\lim_{x \to \infty} g(x)$ and $\lim_{x \to -\infty} g(x)$.

100. For $f(x) = \dfrac{x - 5}{x^2 - 4x - 5}$, find $\lim_{x \to -1} f(x)$ and $\lim_{x \to 5} f(x)$.

Answers to Quick Checks

1. $\frac{1}{3}$; $x \to \left(\frac{1}{3}\right)^-$ **2. (a)** $\frac{3}{2}$; **(b)** $\frac{3}{2}$; **(c)** $\frac{3}{2}$
3. (a) $f(3)$ does not exist because 3 is not in the domain of f; **(b)** 6
4. 1, 7, does not exist

$k(x) = \begin{cases} -x + 4, & \text{for } x \leq 3, \\ 2x + 1, & \text{for } x > 3 \end{cases}$

5. (a) 1; **(b)** 3
6. (a) Limit does not exist; **(b)** 5; **(c)** 6; **(d)** 6

1.2

- Develop and use the Limit Properties to calculate limits.
- Determine whether a function is continuous at a point.

Algebraic Limits and Continuity

In this section, we develop methods to quickly evaluate limits of certain functions. We then use algebraic limits to study *continuity*, a concept of great importance in calculus.

Algebraic Limits

Consider the functions given by $f(x) = x$, $g(x) = 3$, and $F(x) = x + 3$, displayed in the following graphs. Note that function F is the sum of functions f and g.

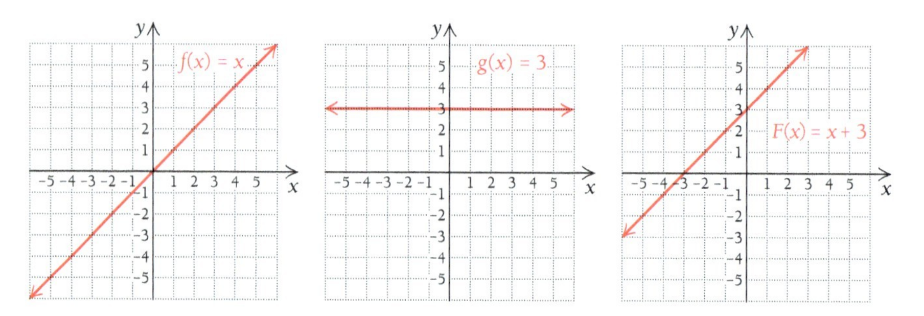

Suppose we are interested in the limits of $f(x)$, $g(x)$, and $F(x)$ as x approaches 2. In Section 1.1, we learned numerical and graphical techniques that can be used to show that

$$\lim_{x\to 2} f(x) = 2, \quad \lim_{x\to 2} g(x) = 3, \quad \text{and} \quad \lim_{x\to 2} F(x) = 5.$$

These techniques work for any value of a in $\lim_{x\to a} f(x)$. For example, if we choose $a = -1$, we can compute the following limits:

$$\lim_{x\to -1} f(x) = -1, \quad \lim_{x\to -1} g(x) = 3, \quad \text{and} \quad \lim_{x\to -1} F(x) = 2.$$

From these results, the following observations can be made:

1. For any real number a, $\lim_{x\to a} x = a$.
2. For any real number a, $\lim_{x\to a} 3 = 3$.

Recalling that $F(x) = f(x) + g(x)$, we make this reasonable conclusion:

3. For any real number a, $\lim_{x\to a} (x + 3) = a + 3$.

We determined the limits of these functions by observing patterns and making a reasonable generalization. For what other functions can limits (as x approaches a) be found by evaluating the function at $x = a$, rather than using numerical or graphical methods? The following list summarizes important limit properties that allow us to calculate limits of certain functions more efficiently.

Limit Properties

If $\lim_{x\to a} f(x) = L$ and $\lim_{x\to a} g(x) = M$, and c is any constant, then we have the following limit properties.

L1. The limit of a constant function is the constant itself:

$$\lim_{x\to a} c = c.$$

L2. The limit of a power function is the limit of the base, raised to that power.

$$\lim_{x\to a} [f(x)]^n = [\lim_{x\to a} f(x)]^n = L^n, \quad \text{and} \quad \lim_{x\to a} \sqrt[n]{f(x)} = \sqrt[n]{\lim_{x\to a} f(x)} = \sqrt[n]{L}$$

In the case of the power, we must have $L \neq 0$ if n is negative, and in the case of the root, we must have $L \geq 0$ if n is an even integer.

L3. The limit of a sum or difference is the sum or difference of the limits:

$$\lim_{x \to a} [f(x) \pm g(x)] = \lim_{x \to a} f(x) \pm \lim_{x \to a} g(x) = L \pm M.$$

L4. The limit of a product is the product of the limits:

$$\lim_{x \to a} [f(x) \cdot g(x)] = [\lim_{x \to a} f(x)] \cdot [\lim_{x \to a} g(x)] = L \cdot M.$$

L5. The limit of a quotient is the quotient of the limits:

$$\lim_{x \to a} \frac{f(x)}{g(x)} = \frac{\lim_{x \to a} f(x)}{\lim_{x \to a} g(x)} = \frac{L}{M}, \quad \text{assuming } M \neq 0.$$

L6. The limit of a constant times a function is the constant times the limit of the function:

$$\lim_{x \to a} c \cdot f(x) = c \cdot \lim_{x \to a} f(x) = c \cdot L.$$

Property L6 combines L1 and L4 but is stated separately because it is used so frequently.

EXAMPLE 1 Use the Limit Properties to find $\lim_{x \to 4} (x^2 - 3x + 7)$.

Solution We know that $\lim_{x \to 4} x$ is 4.

By Limit Property L2,

$$\lim_{x \to 4} x^2 = [\lim_{x \to 4} x]^2 = 4^2 = 16;$$

by Limit Property L6,

$$\lim_{x \to 4} (-3x) = -3 \cdot \lim_{x \to 4} x = -3 \cdot 4 = -12;$$

and by Limit Property L1,

$$\lim_{x \to 4} 7 = 7.$$

Using Limit Property L3 to combine these results, we have

$$\lim_{x \to 4} (x^2 - 3x + 7) = 16 - 12 + 7 = 11.$$

The result of Example 1 is extended in the following theorem.

THEOREM 2 Limits of Rational Functions

For any rational function F, with a in the domain of F,

$$\lim_{x \to a} F(x) = F(a).$$

Rational functions include all polynomial functions (which include constant functions and linear functions) and ratios composed of such functions (see Section R.5). Thus, the Limit Properties allow us to evaluate limits of rational functions, for values in a function's domain, quickly without tables or graphs, as illustrated in the following examples.

EXAMPLE 2 Find $\lim_{x \to 2} (x^4 - 5x^3 + x^2 - 7)$.

Solution It follows from the Theorem on Limits of Rational Functions that we can find the limit by substitution:

$$\begin{aligned}\lim_{x \to 2} (x^4 - 5x^3 + x^2 - 7) &= 2^4 - 5 \cdot 2^3 + 2^2 - 7 \\ &= 16 - 40 + 4 - 7 \\ &= -27.\end{aligned}$$

EXAMPLE 3 Find $\lim_{x \to -3} \dfrac{x^2 + 3x - 1}{2x + 4}$.

Solution Since -3 is in the domain of $f(x) = \dfrac{x^2 + 3x - 1}{2x + 4}$, we can use the Theorem on Limits of Rational Functions to find the limit by substitution:

$$\lim_{x \to -3} \frac{x^2 + 3x - 1}{2x + 4} = \frac{(-3)^2 + 3(-3) - 1}{2(-3) + 4} = \frac{1}{2}.$$

Quick Check 1 ✓

Find these limits and note the Limit Property you use at each step.

a) $\lim_{x \to 1} (2x^3 + 3x^2 - 6)$

b) $\lim_{x \to 4} \dfrac{2x^2 + 5x - 1}{3x - 2}$

c) $\lim_{x \to -2} \sqrt{1 + 3x^2}$

EXAMPLE 4 Find $\lim_{x \to 0} \sqrt{x^2 - 3x + 2}$.

Solution The Theorem on Limits of Rational Functions can be used to evaluate the expression under the radical:

$$\lim_{x \to 0} (x^2 - 3x + 2) = 0^2 - 3 \cdot 0 + 2 = 2.$$

By Limit Property L2, we have

$$\lim_{x \to 0} \sqrt{x^2 - 3x + 2} = \sqrt{\lim_{x \to 0} (x^2 - 3x + 2)} = \sqrt{2}.$$

1 ✓

In the following example, the function is rational, but a is not in the domain of the function, since it would result in a zero in the denominator. Nevertheless, we can still find the limit.

EXAMPLE 5 Let $r(x) = \dfrac{x^2 - x - 12}{x + 3}$. Find $\lim_{x \to -3} r(x)$.

Solution Note that $r(-3)$ does not exist, because -3 is not in the domain of r. Since it is impossible to determine this limit by direct evaluation (the assumption for Limit Property L5 is not met), we use a table and a graph.

Limit Numerically

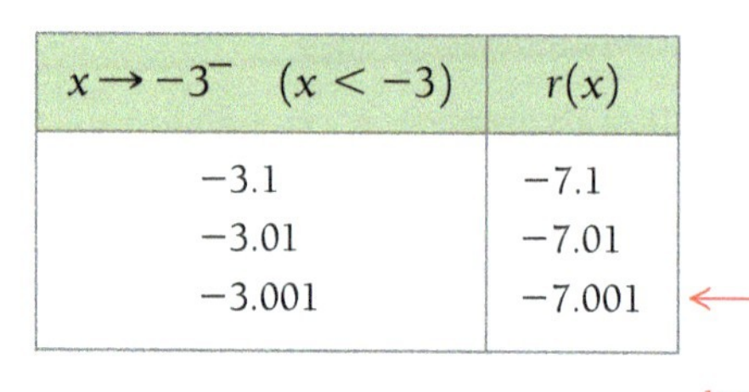

$x \to -3^-$ $(x < -3)$	$r(x)$
-3.1	-7.1
-3.01	-7.01
-3.001	-7.001

$\lim_{x \to -3} r(x) = -7$

$x \to -3^+$ $(x > -3)$	$r(x)$
-2.9	-6.9
-2.99	-6.99
-2.999	-6.999

Limit Graphically

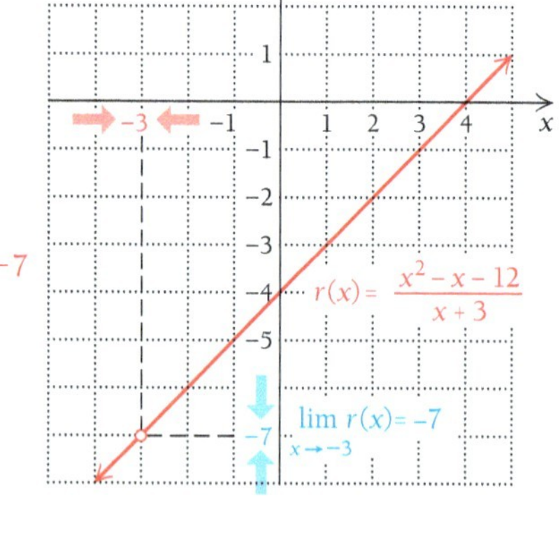

Both the table and the graph suggest that the limit is

$$\lim_{x \to -3} \left(\frac{x^2 - x - 12}{x + 3} \right) = -7.$$

Limit Algebraically. The function is simplified by factoring and noting that the factor $(x + 3)$ is present in both numerator and denominator. As long as $x \neq -3$, the expression can be simplified:

$$\frac{x^2 - x - 12}{x + 3} = \frac{(x + 3)(x - 4)}{(x + 3)} = x - 4, \quad \text{for } x \neq -3.$$

We then evaluate the limit using the simplified form:

$$\lim_{x \to -3} (x - 4) = (-3) - 4 = -7.$$

The graph of r is a line with a "hole" at $(-3, -7)$. Even though $r(-3)$ does not exist, the limit *does* exist since we are concerned about the behavior of $r(x)$ as x approaches -3. The decision to simplify was made by noting that $[(-3)^2 - (-3) - 12]/[(-3) + 3] = 0/0$. This *indeterminate form* indicates that the polynomials in the numerator and the denominator share a common factor, in this case, $(x + 3)$. The $0/0$ form is a hint that a limit may exist. Look for ways to simplify algebraically, or use a table or a graph to determine a limit in cases like this. **2 ✓**

Quick Check 2 ✓

Using a table, a graph, and algebra, find:

$$\lim_{x \to 2} \frac{x^2 + 4x - 12}{x^2 - 4}.$$

A common error in determining limits is to assume that all limits can be found by direct evaluation. Students may attempt to find the limit of a function like the one in Example 5, get a zero in the denominator, and then mistakenly conclude that the limit does not exist. Remember, finding a limit as x approaches a focuses on x *close* to a, not *at* a. As Example 5 shows, a function may not be defined at a certain a-value, but its limit as $x \to a$ may still exist.

The Limit Properties can also be used to evaluate limits of rational functions as x approaches infinity.

EXAMPLE 6 Find $\lim_{x \to \infty} \left(\frac{x^2 + 4x - 5}{2x^2 + x + 1} \right)$.

Solution We multiply the numerator and denominator by the expression $\frac{1}{x^2}$:

$$\frac{(x^2 + 4x - 5) \cdot \frac{1}{x^2}}{(2x^2 + x + 1) \cdot \frac{1}{x^2}} = \frac{1 + \frac{4}{x} - \frac{5}{x^2}}{2 + \frac{1}{x} + \frac{1}{x^2}}.$$

In Section 1.1, we saw that $\lim_{x \to \pm\infty} \left(\frac{k}{x} \right) = 0$, for any nonzero real number k. Thus, using Limit Property L2, we can conclude that

$$\lim_{x \to \pm\infty} \left(\frac{k}{x} \right)^2 = \left(\lim_{x \to \pm\infty} \frac{k}{x} \right)^2 = 0^2 = 0.$$

Using a combination of the Limit Properties, we have

$$\begin{aligned}
\lim_{x \to \infty} \left(\frac{x^2 + 4x - 5}{2x^2 + x + 1} \right) &= \lim_{x \to \infty} \left(\frac{1 + \frac{4}{x} - \frac{5}{x^2}}{2 + \frac{1}{x} + \frac{1}{x^2}} \right) \\
&= \frac{\lim_{x \to \infty} 1 + \lim_{x \to \infty} \frac{4}{x} - \lim_{x \to \infty} \frac{5}{x^2}}{\lim_{x \to \infty} 2 + \lim_{x \to \infty} \frac{1}{x} + \lim_{x \to \infty} \frac{1}{x^2}} \\
&= \frac{1 + 0 - 0}{2 + 0 + 0} \\
&= \frac{1}{2}.
\end{aligned}$$

3 ✓

Quick Check 3 ✓

Find

$$\lim_{x \to \infty} \left(\frac{2x^3 + 5x^2 + 4x - 1}{3x^3 + 6x^2 - 7} \right).$$

The limit properties can be used to show that if $f(x) = \dfrac{ax^m + \cdots}{bx^n + \cdots}$, then

$$\lim_{x \to \pm\infty} f(x) = \frac{a}{b} \text{ if } m = n$$

$$\lim_{x \to \pm\infty} f(x) = 0 \text{ if } m < n$$

and $$\lim_{x \to \pm\infty} f(x) \text{ does not exist if } m > n.$$

In calculus, we often consider expressions containing more than one variable.

EXAMPLE 7 Find $\lim_{h \to 0} (3x^2 + 3xh + h^2)$.

Solution We treat x as a constant since we are interested only in how the expression changes as h approaches 0. We use the Limit Properties to find that

$$\lim_{h \to 0} (3x^2 + 3xh + h^2) = 3x^2 + 3x(0) + 0^2$$
$$= 3x^2.$$

4 ✓

Quick Check 4 ✓

Find $\lim_{h \to 0} \dfrac{1}{2x(x + h)}$.

Continuity

The following are graphs of *continuous* functions. For now, we use an intuitive definition of continuity, which we will soon refine.

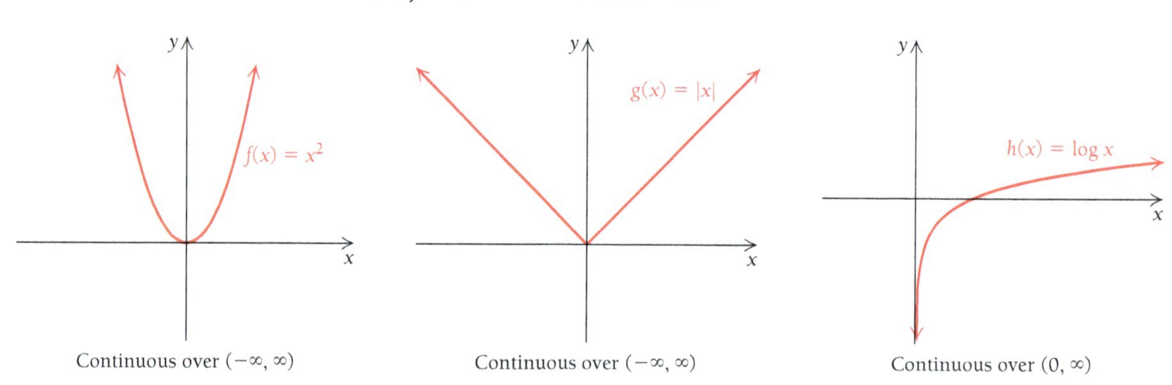

Continuous over $(-\infty, \infty)$ Continuous over $(-\infty, \infty)$ Continuous over $(0, \infty)$

Note that there are no "jumps" or "holes" in the graphs. We say that a function is **continuous over**, or **on**, **some interval** of the real number line if its graph can be traced without lifting a pencil off the graph. If there is any point in an interval where a "jump" or a "hole" occurs, then we say that the function is *not continuous*, or is *discontinuous*, over that interval. The functions F, G, and H in the following graphs are examples of functions that are *not* continuous over $(-\infty, \infty)$.

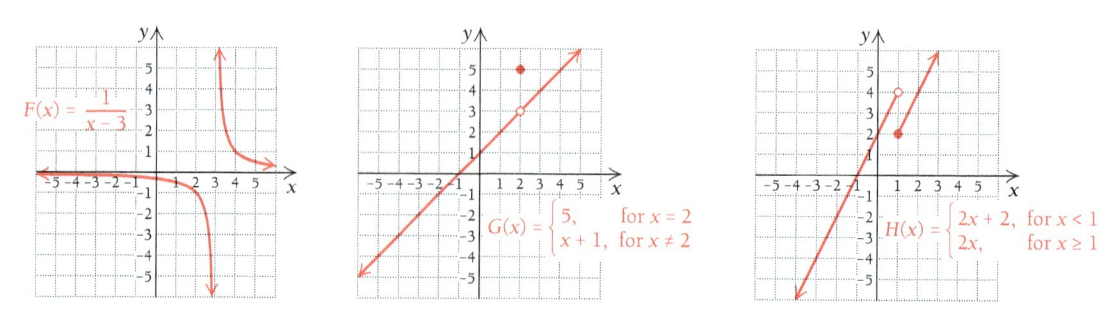

In each case, the graph *cannot* be traced without lifting the pencil off the graph. However, each case represents a different situation:

- F is not continuous over $(-\infty, \infty)$ because 3 is not in the domain of F. Thus, there is no point to trace at $x = 3$. Note that F is continuous for all x in its domain, $(-\infty, 3) \cup (3, \infty)$.

- G is not continuous over $(-\infty, \infty)$ because it is not continuous at $x = 2$. To see this, note that, as x approaches 2 from either side, $G(x)$ approaches 3. However, *at* $x = 2$, $G(x)$ *jumps* up to 5. Note that G is continuous for all other x in $(-\infty, 2) \cup (2, \infty)$.
- H is not continuous over $(-\infty, \infty)$ because it is not continuous at $x = 1$. To see this, trace the graph and note that, as x approaches 1 from the left, $H(x)$ approaches 4. However, as x approaches 1 from the right, $H(x)$ approaches 2. Note that H is continuous for all other x in $(-\infty, 1) \cup (1, \infty)$.

Each of the above graphs has a *point of discontinuity*. The graph of F is discontinuous at 3, because $x = 3$ is not in the domain of F; G is discontinuous at 2, because $\lim_{x \to 2} G(x) \neq G(2)$; and H is discontinuous at 1, because $\lim_{x \to 1} H(x)$ does not exist.

DEFINITION

A function f is **continuous** at $x = a$ if:

a) $f(a)$ exists, (The input a is in the domain of f.)

b) $\lim_{x \to a} f(x)$ exists, (The limit as x approaches a exists.)

and

c) $\lim_{x \to a} f(x) = f(a)$. (The limit is the same as the output.)

A function is **continuous over an open interval** I if it is continuous at each point a in I. If f is not continuous at $x = a$, we say that f is **discontinuous**, or has a **discontinuity**, at $x = a$.

We can define continuity at the endpoint of a closed interval by allowing for a one-sided limit, instead of the general limit, in part (b) of the definition of continuity. For example, the function $f(x) = \sqrt{x}$ is continuous over $[0, \infty)$ since $f(0) = \sqrt{0} = 0$, the right-hand limit is $\lim_{x \to 0^+} f(x) = 0$, and we have $\lim_{x \to 0^+} f(x) = f(0)$.

A visualization of the function in Example 8

EXAMPLE 8 Determine whether the function given by

$$f(x) = 2x + 3$$

is continuous at $x = 4$.

Solution This function is continuous at $x = 4$ because:

a) $f(4)$ exists, The input 4 is in the domain of f.

b) $\lim_{x \to 4} f(x)$ exists, We found $\lim_{x \to 4} f(x) = 11$ in Section 1.1.

and

c) $\lim_{x \to 4} f(x) = 11 = f(4)$.

In fact, $f(x) = 2x + 3$ is continuous over its domain, $\mathbb{R}$.

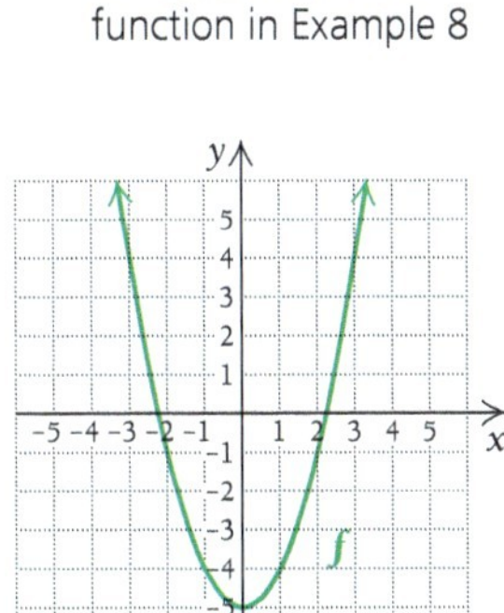

A visualization of the function in Example 9

EXAMPLE 9 Is the function f given by

$$f(x) = x^2 - 5$$

continuous at $x = 3$? Why or why not?

Solution By the Theorem on Limits of Rational Functions, we have

$$\lim_{x \to 3} f(x) = 3^2 - 5 = 9 - 5 = 4. \quad \text{The limit exists.}$$

Since $f(3) = 3^2 - 5 = 4$, $f(3)$ exists.

we have

$$\lim_{x\to 3} f(x) = f(3).$$

Thus, f is continuous at $x = 3$. This function is also continuous over its domain, $\mathbb{R}$.

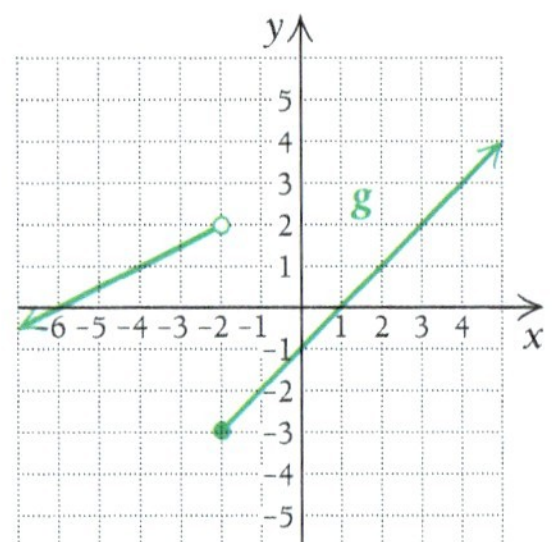

A visualization of the function in Example 10

EXAMPLE 10 Is the function g, given by

$$g(x) = \begin{cases} \frac{1}{2}x + 3, & \text{for } x < -2, \\ x - 1, & \text{for } x \geq -2, \end{cases}$$

continuous at $x = -2$? Why or why not?

Solution To find out if g is continuous at -2, we must determine whether $\lim_{x\to -2} g(x) = g(-2)$. Thus, we first note that $g(-2) = -2 - 1 = -3$. To find $\lim_{x\to -2} g(x)$, we look at left-hand and right-hand limits:

$$\lim_{x\to -2^-} g(x) = \frac{1}{2}(-2) + 3 = -1 + 3 = 2; \quad \lim_{x\to -2^+} g(x) = -2 - 1 = -3.$$

Since $\lim_{x\to -2^-} g(x) \neq \lim_{x\to -2^+} g(x)$, we see that $\lim_{x\to -2} g(x)$ does not exist. Thus, g is not continuous at -2. It is continuous at all other x-values. **5 ✓**

Quick Check 5 ✓

Let

$$g(x) = \begin{cases} 3x - 5, & \text{for } x < 2, \\ 2x + 1, & \text{for } x \geq 2. \end{cases}$$

Is g continuous at $x = 2$? Why or why not?

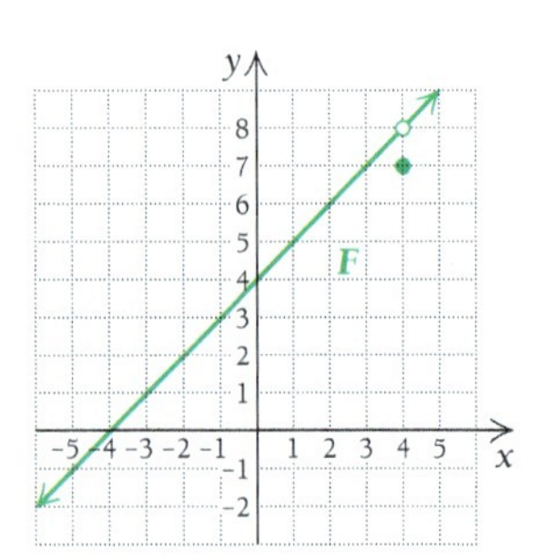

A visualization of the function in Example 11

EXAMPLE 11 Is the function F, given by

$$F(x) = \begin{cases} \dfrac{x^2 - 16}{x - 4}, & \text{for } x \neq 4, \\ 7, & \text{for } x = 4, \end{cases}$$

continuous at $x = 4$? Why or why not?

Solution For F to be continuous at 4, we must have $\lim_{x\to 4} F(x) = F(4)$. We are given $F(4) = 7$. To find $\lim_{x\to 4} F(x)$, note that, for $x \neq 4$,

$$\frac{x^2 - 16}{x - 4} = \frac{(x - 4)(x + 4)}{x - 4} = x + 4.$$

Thus,

$$\lim_{x\to 4} F(x) = 4 + 4 = 8.$$

We see that F is *not* continuous at $x = 4$ since

$$\lim_{x\to 4} F(x) \neq F(4).$$

The Limit Properties and the Theorem on Limits of Rational Functions can be used to show that if $f(x)$ and $g(x)$ are two arbitrary polynomial functions, then f and g are both continuous. Furthermore, $f + g$, $f - g$, $f \cdot g$, and, assuming $g(x) \neq 0$, f/g are also continuous. We can also use the Limit Properties to show that for n, an integer greater than 1, $\sqrt[n]{f(x)}$ is continuous, provided that $f(x) \geq 0$ when n is even.

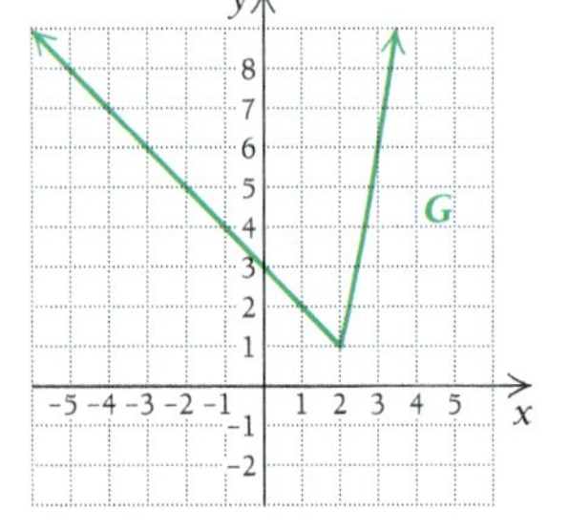

A visualization of the function in Example 12

EXAMPLE 12 Is the function G, given by

$$G(x) = \begin{cases} -x + 3, & \text{for } x \leq 2, \\ x^2 - 3, & \text{for } x > 2, \end{cases}$$

continuous for all x? Why or why not?

Solution For G to be continuous, it must be continuous for all real numbers. Since $y = -x + 3$ is continuous on $(-\infty, 2]$ and $y = x^2 - 3$ is continuous on $(2, \infty)$, we only need to determine whether $\lim_{x \to 2} G(x) = G(2)$, that is, whether G is continuous at $x = 2$:

$$G(2) = -2 + 3 = 1;$$

$$\lim_{x \to 2^-} G(x) = -2 + 3 = 1 \quad \text{and} \quad \lim_{x \to 2^+} G(x) = (2)^2 - 3 = 4 - 3 = 1,$$

so $\lim_{x \to 2} G(x) = 1.$

Since $\lim_{x \to 2} G(x) = G(2)$, we have shown that G is continuous at $x = 2$, and we can conclude that G is continuous for all x in its domain. **6 ✓**

Quick Check 6 ✓

Let

$$h(x) = \begin{cases} \dfrac{x^2 - 9}{x - 3}, & \text{for } x \neq 3, \\ 6, & \text{for } x = 3. \end{cases}$$

Is h continuous at $x = 3$? Why or why not?

EXAMPLE 13 **Business: Price Breaks.** Righteous Rocks sells decorative landscape rocks in bulk quantities. For quantities up to and including 500 lb, the company charges \$2.50 per pound. For quantities over 500 lb, it charges \$2 per pound. The price function can be stated as a piecewise function:

$$p(x) = \begin{cases} 2.50x, & \text{for } 0 \leq x \leq 500, \\ 2x, & \text{for } x > 500, \end{cases}$$

where p is the price in dollars and x is the quantity in pounds. Is p continuous at $x = 500$? Why or why not?

Solution The graph of $p(x)$ follows.

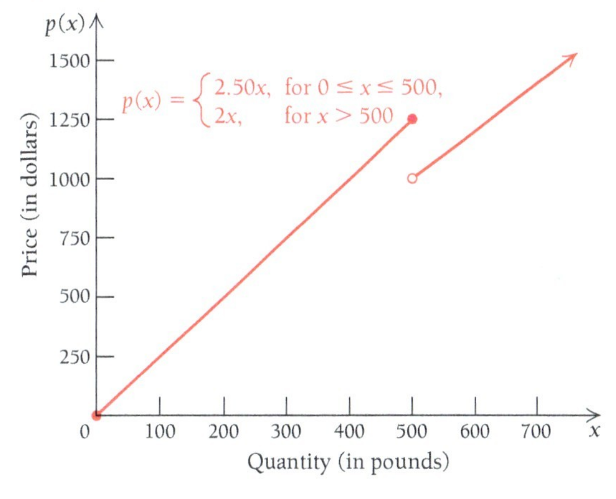

As x approaches 500, we have $\lim_{x \to 500^-} p(x) = 1250$ and $\lim_{x \to 500^+} p(x) = 1000$. Since the left-hand and right-hand limits are not equal, $\lim_{x \to 500} p(x)$ does not exist. Thus, p is *not* continuous at $x = 500$. The graph literally shows a price "break." **7 ✓**

Quick Check 7 ✓

A water tank is empty at time $t = 0$ minutes. It then fills at a rate of 3 gallons of water per minute for 30 min. At 30 min, the tank is no longer being filled and a valve is opened, allowing water to escape at a rate of 4 gallons per minute. The volume of water in the tank v, in gallons, after t minutes is given by

$$v(t) = \begin{cases} 3t, & \text{for } 0 \leq t \leq 30, \\ 210 - 4t, & \text{for } t > 30. \end{cases}$$

Find $\lim_{t \to 30^-} v(t)$, $\lim_{t \to 30^+} v(t)$, and $\lim_{t \to 30} v(t)$.

Section Summary

- For a rational function with a in its domain, the limit as x approaches a can be found by evaluating the function at a.
- When evaluating a limit leads to the *indeterminate form* $0/0$, the limit may still exist: algebraic simplification and/or a table and graph are used to find the limit.
- Informally, a function is *continuous* if its graph can be traced without lifting pencil from paper.
- Formally, a function f is continuous at $x = a$ if
  (1) the function value $f(a)$ exists (a is in the domain of f),
  (2) the limit as x approaches a exists, and
  (3) the function value and the limit are equal.
  This is summarized as $\lim_{x \to a} f(x) = f(a)$.
- If any part of the continuity definition fails, then the function is *discontinuous* at $x = a$.
- If f is a rational function in which the degrees of the numerator and the denominator are the same, then the limit of f, as x approaches positive or negative infinity, is the ratio of the leading coefficients. That is, if $f(x) = \dfrac{ax^n + \cdots}{bx^n + \cdots}$, then $\lim_{x \to \pm\infty} f(x) = \dfrac{a}{b}$.

1.2 Exercise Set

Classify each statement as either true or false.

1. If $\lim_{x\to 2} f(x) = 9$, then $\lim_{x\to 2} \sqrt{f(x)} = 3$.
2. $\lim_{x\to 3} 7 = 3$
3. If $\lim_{x\to 1} g(x) = 5$, then $\lim_{x\to 1} [g(x)]^2 = 25$.
4. If $\lim_{x\to 4} F(x) = 7$, then $\lim_{x\to 4} [c \cdot F(x)] = 7c$.
5. If f is continuous at $x = 2$, then $f(2)$ must exist.
6. If g is discontinuous at $x = 3$, then $g(3)$ must not exist.
7. If $\lim_{x\to 4} F(x)$ exists, then F must be continuous at $x = 4$.
8. If $\lim_{x\to 7} G(x)$ equals $G(7)$, then G must be continuous at $x = 7$.

Use the Theorem on Limits of Rational Functions to find each limit. When necessary, state that the limit does not exist.

9. $\lim_{x\to 1} (3x + 2)$
10. $\lim_{x\to 2} (4x - 5)$
11. $\lim_{x\to -1} (x^2 - 4)$
12. $\lim_{x\to -2} (x^2 + 3)$
13. $\lim_{x\to 3} (x^2 - 4x + 7)$
14. $\lim_{x\to 5} (x^2 - 6x + 9)$
15. $\lim_{x\to 2} (2x^4 - 3x^3 + 4x - 1)$
16. $\lim_{x\to -1} (3x^5 + 4x^4 - 3x + 6)$
17. $\lim_{x\to 3} \dfrac{x^2 - 8}{x - 2}$
18. $\lim_{x\to 3} \dfrac{x^2 - 25}{x^2 - 5}$

For Exercises 19–30, the initial substitution of $x = a$ yields the form $0/0$. Simplify the function algebraically, or use a table or graph to determine the limit. When necessary, state that the limit does not exist.

19. $\lim_{x\to 5} \dfrac{x^2 - 25}{x - 5}$
20. $\lim_{x\to 3} \dfrac{x^2 - 9}{x - 3}$
21. $\lim_{x\to 1} \dfrac{x^2 + 5x - 6}{x^2 - 1}$
22. $\lim_{x\to -2} \dfrac{x^2 - 2x - 8}{x^2 - 4}$
23. $\lim_{x\to -3} \dfrac{2x^2 - x - 21}{9 - x^2}$
24. $\lim_{x\to 2} \dfrac{3x^2 + x - 14}{x^2 - 4}$
25. $\lim_{x\to 1} \dfrac{x^3 - 1}{x - 1}$
26. $\lim_{x\to 2} \dfrac{x^3 - 8}{2 - x}$
27. $\lim_{x\to 9} \dfrac{9 - x}{\sqrt{x} - 3}$
28. $\lim_{x\to 25} \dfrac{\sqrt{x} - 5}{x - 25}$
29. $\lim_{x\to -1} \dfrac{x^2 + 5x + 4}{x^2 + 2x + 1}$
30. $\lim_{x\to 2} \dfrac{x^2 + 3x - 10}{x^2 - 4x + 4}$

Use the Limit Properties to find the following limits, if they exist.

31. $\lim_{x\to \infty} \left(\dfrac{5x - 2}{4x + 1}\right)$
32. $\lim_{x\to \infty} \left(\dfrac{7x + 5}{3x}\right)$
33. $\lim_{x\to -\infty} \left(\dfrac{x + 2}{6x - 10}\right)$
34. $\lim_{x\to -\infty} \left(\dfrac{12x}{4x - 7}\right)$
35. $\lim_{x\to \infty} \left(\dfrac{x^2 + 2x + 3}{3x^2 + 5}\right)$
36. $\lim_{x\to \infty} \left(\dfrac{5x^2 + 5x + 2}{10x^2 + x + 1}\right)$
37. $\lim_{x\to \infty} \left(\dfrac{8x + 1}{x^2}\right)$
38. $\lim_{x\to \infty} \left(\dfrac{2x^2 + 6x - 1}{x^3 + x + 7}\right)$
39. $\lim_{x\to -\infty} \left(\dfrac{x^3 + x^2 + x + 1}{x^2 + x + 1}\right)$
40. $\lim_{x\to \infty} \left(\dfrac{x^5}{x^3 + 4x + 10}\right)$

Use the Limit Properties to find the following limits. If a limit does not exist, state that fact.

41. $\lim_{x\to 5} \sqrt{x^2 - 16}$
42. $\lim_{x\to 4} \sqrt{x^2 - 9}$
43. $\lim_{x\to 2} \sqrt{x^2 - 9}$
44. $\lim_{x\to 3} \sqrt{x^2 - 16}$
45. $\lim_{x\to -4^-} \sqrt{x^2 - 16}$
46. $\lim_{x\to 3^+} \sqrt{x^2 - 9}$

Determine whether each of the functions shown in Exercises 47–51 is continuous over the interval $(-6, 6)$.

47.

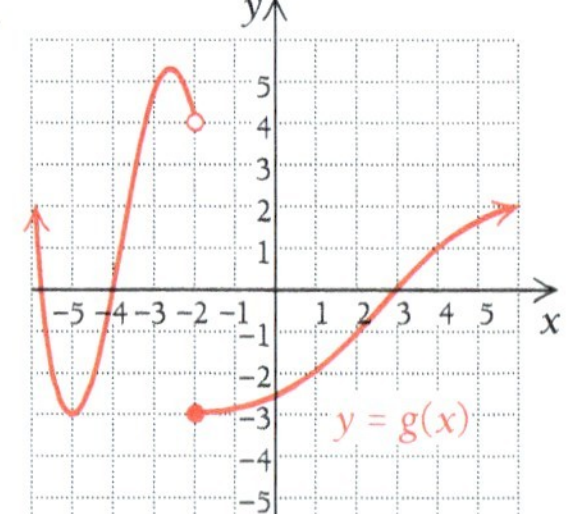

48.

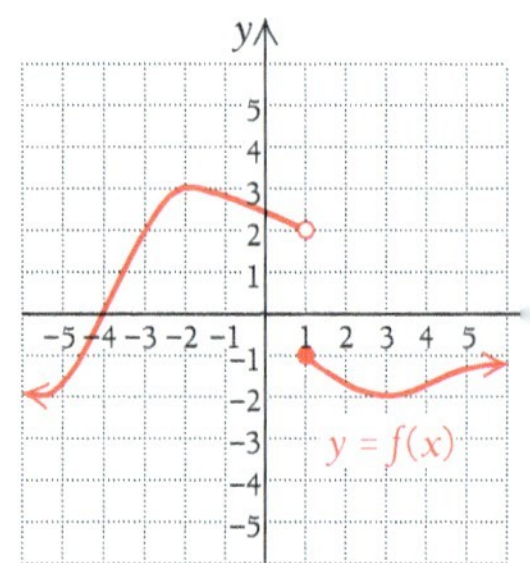

49.

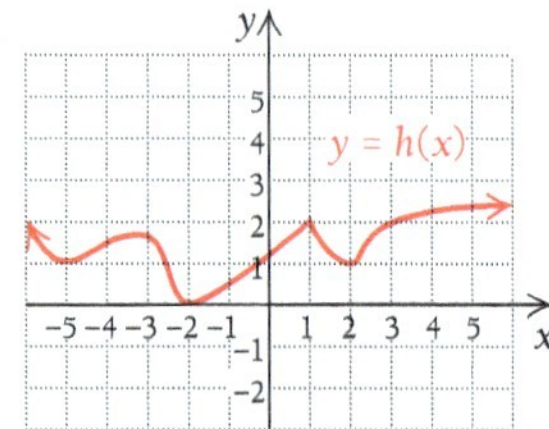

50.

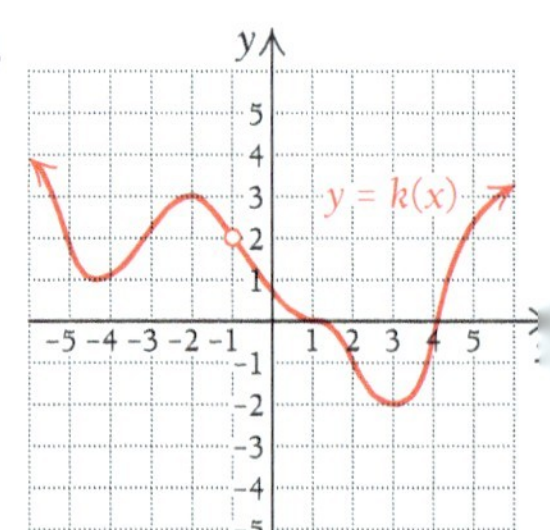

51.

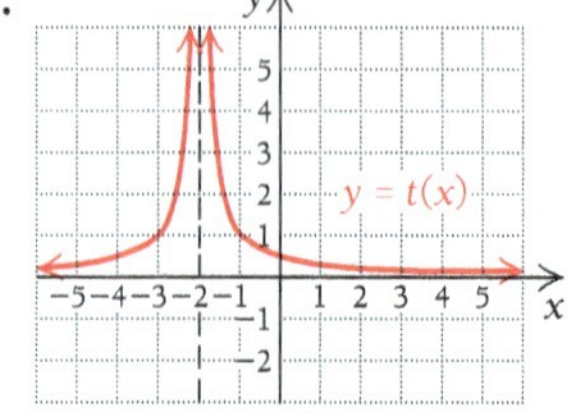

Use the graphs and functions in Exercises 47–51 to answer each of the following. If a function value or limit does not exist, state that.

52. a) Find $\lim_{x\to 1^+} g(x)$, $\lim_{x\to 1^-} g(x)$, and $\lim_{x\to 1} g(x)$.
    b) Find $g(1)$.
    c) Is g continuous at $x = 1$? Why or why not?

d) Find $\lim_{x \to -2} g(x)$.

e) Find $g(-2)$.

f) Is g continuous at $x = -2$? Why or why not?

53. a) Find $\lim_{x \to 1^+} f(x)$, $\lim_{x \to 1^-} f(x)$, and $\lim_{x \to 1} f(x)$.

b) Find $f(1)$.

c) Is f continuous at $x = 1$? Why or why not?

d) Find $\lim_{x \to -2} f(x)$.

e) Find $f(-2)$.

f) Is f continuous at $x = -2$? Why or why not?

54. a) Find $\lim_{x \to 1} h(x)$.

b) Find $h(1)$.

c) Is h continuous at $x = 1$? Why or why not?

d) Find $\lim_{x \to -2} h(x)$.

e) Find $h(-2)$.

f) Is h continuous at $x = -2$? Why or why not?

55. a) Find $\lim_{x \to -1} k(x)$.

b) Find $k(-1)$.

c) Is k continuous at $x = -1$? Why or why not?

d) Find $\lim_{x \to 3} k(x)$.

e) Find $k(3)$.

f) Is k continuous at $x = 3$? Why or why not?

56. a) Find $\lim_{x \to 1} t(x)$.

b) Find $t(1)$.

c) Is t continuous at $x = 1$? Why or why not?

d) Find $\lim_{x \to -2} t(x)$.

e) Find $t(-2)$.

f) Is t continuous at $x = -2$? Why or why not?

Answer Exercises 57 and 58 using the graphs provided.

57.

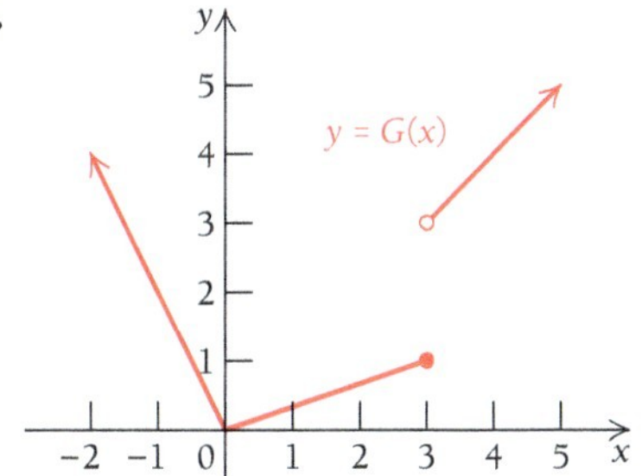

a) Find $\lim_{x \to 3^+} G(x)$.

b) Find $\lim_{x \to 3^-} G(x)$.

c) Find $\lim_{x \to 3} G(x)$.

d) Find $G(3)$.

e) Is G continuous at $x = 3$? Why or why not?

f) Is G continuous at $x = 0$? Why or why not?

g) Is G continuous at $x = 2.9$? Why or why not?

58. Consider the function C given by

$$C(x) = \begin{cases} -1, & \text{for } x < 2, \\ 1, & \text{for } x \geq 2. \end{cases}$$

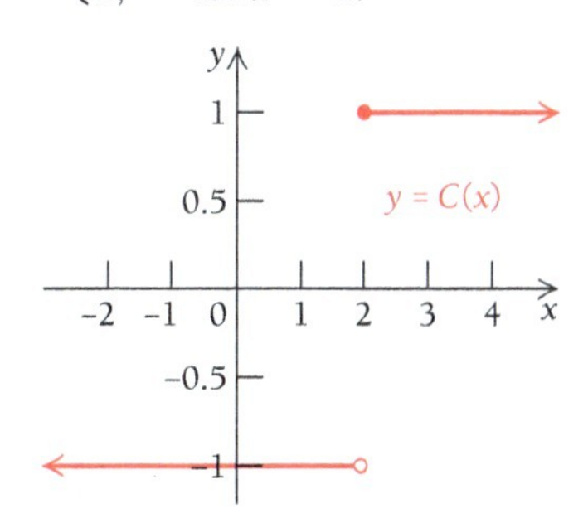

a) Find $\lim_{x \to 2^+} C(x)$.

b) Find $\lim_{x \to 2^-} C(x)$.

c) Find $\lim_{x \to 2} C(x)$.

d) Find $C(2)$.

e) Is C continuous at $x = 2$? Why or why not?

f) Is C continuous at $x = 1.95$? Why or why not?

59. Is the function given by $g(x) = x^2 - 3x$ continuous at $x = 4$? Why or why not?

60. Is the function given by $f(x) = 3x - 2$ continuous at $x = 5$? Why or why not?

61. Is the function given by $G(x) = \frac{1}{x}$ continuous at $x = 0$? Why or why not?

62. Is the function given by $F(x) = \sqrt{x}$ continuous at $x = -1$? Why or why not?

63. Is the function given by

$$f(x) = \begin{cases} \frac{1}{2}x + 1, & \text{for } x < 4, \\ -x + 7, & \text{for } x \geq 4, \end{cases}$$

continuous at $x = 4$? Why or why not?

64. Is the function given by

$$g(x) = \begin{cases} \frac{1}{3}x + 4, & \text{for } x \leq 3, \\ 2x - 1, & \text{for } x > 3, \end{cases}$$

continuous at $x = 3$? Why or why not?

65. Is the function given by

$$F(x) = \begin{cases} x + 2, & \text{for } x \leq 3, \\ 2x - 5, & \text{for } x > 3, \end{cases}$$

continuous at $x = 3$? Why or why not?

66. Is the function given by

$$G(x) = \begin{cases} \frac{1}{2}x + 1, & \text{for } x < 4, \\ -x + 5, & \text{for } x > 4, \end{cases}$$

continuous at $x = 4$? Why or why not?

67. Is the function given by

$$g(x) = \begin{cases} \frac{1}{2}x + 1, & \text{for } x < 4, \\ -x + 7, & \text{for } x > 4, \end{cases}$$

continuous at $x = 4$? Why or why not?

68. Is the function given by

$$f(x) = \begin{cases} x^2 + x, & \text{for } x < 3, \\ 4x, & \text{for } x \geq 3, \end{cases}$$

continuous at $x = 3$? Why or why not?

69. Is the function given by

$$G(x) = \begin{cases} \dfrac{x^2 - 4}{x - 2}, & \text{for } x \neq 2, \\ 5, & \text{for } x = 2, \end{cases}$$

continuous at $x = 2$? Why or why not?

70. Is the function given by

$$F(x) = \begin{cases} \dfrac{x^2 - 1}{x - 1}, & \text{for } x \neq 1, \\ 4, & \text{for } x = 1, \end{cases}$$

continuous at $x = 1$? Why or why not?

71. Is the function given by

$$G(x) = \begin{cases} \dfrac{x^2 - 3x - 4}{x - 4}, & \text{for } x < 4, \\ 2x - 3, & \text{for } x \geq 4, \end{cases}$$

continuous at $x = 4$? Why or why not?

72. Is the function given by

$$f(x) = \begin{cases} \dfrac{x^2 - 4x - 5}{x - 5}, & \text{for } x < 5, \\ x + 1, & \text{for } x \geq 5, \end{cases}$$

continuous at $x = 5$? Why or why not?

73. Is the function given by $g(x) = \dfrac{1}{x^2 - 7x + 10}$ continuous at $x = 5$? Why or why not?

74. Is the function given by $f(x) = \dfrac{1}{x^2 - 6x + 8}$ continuous at $x = 3$? Why or why not?

75. Is the function given by $G(x) = \dfrac{1}{x^2 - 6x + 8}$ continuous at $x = 2$? Why or why not?

76. Is the function given by $F(x) = \dfrac{1}{x^2 - 7x + 10}$ continuous at $x = 4$? Why or why not?

77. Is the function given by $g(x) = \dfrac{1}{x + 5}$ continuous over the interval $(-4, 4)$? Why or why not?

78. Is the function given by $F(x) = -\dfrac{2}{x - 7}$ continuous over the interval $(-5, 5)$? Why or why not?

79. Is the function given by $g(x) = \sqrt{x - 1}$ continuous over the interval $[1, \infty)$? Why or why not?

80. Is the function given by $h(x) = \sqrt{x + 3}$ continuous over the interval $[-3, \infty)$? Why or why not?

81. Is the function given by $F(x) = \sqrt{25 - x^2}$ continuous over the interval $[-5, 5]$? Why or why not?

82. Is the function given by $G(x) = \sqrt{9 - x^2}$ continuous over the interval $[-3, 3]$? Why or why not?

APPLICATIONS

Business and Economics

83. The Candy Factory sells candy by the pound, charging \$1.50 per pound for quantities up to and including 20 pounds. Above 20 pounds, the Candy Factory charges \$1.25 per pound for the entire quantity. If x represents the number of pounds, the price function is

$$p(x) = \begin{cases} 1.50x, & \text{for } x \leq 20, \\ 1.25x, & \text{for } x > 20. \end{cases}$$

Find $\lim_{x \to 20^-} p(x)$, $\lim_{x \to 20^+} p(x)$, and $\lim_{x \to 20} p(x)$.

84. The Copy Shoppe charges \$0.08 per copy for quantities up to and including 100 copies. For quantities above 100, the charge is \$0.06 per copy. If x represents the number of copies, the price function is

$$p(x) = \begin{cases} 0.08x, & \text{for } x \leq 100, \\ 0.06x, & \text{for } x > 100. \end{cases}$$

Find $\lim_{x \to 100^-} p(x)$, $\lim_{x \to 100^+} p(x)$, and $\lim_{x \to 100} p(x)$.

Life and Physical Sciences

85. A lab technician controls the temperature T inside a kiln. From an initial temperature of 0 degrees Celsius (°C), he allows the temperature to increase by 2°C per minute for the next 60 minutes. After the 60th minute, he allows the temperature to cool by 3°C per minute. If t is the number of minutes, the temperature T is given by

$$T(t) = \begin{cases} 2t, & \text{for } t \leq 60, \\ 300 - 3t, & \text{for } t > 60. \end{cases}$$

Find $\lim_{t \to 60^-} T(t)$, $\lim_{t \to 60^+} T(t)$, and $\lim_{t \to 60} T(t)$.

SYNTHESIS

A function for which the definition of continuity is true for all x in its domain is said to be continuous over its domain. For example, $f(x) = \dfrac{1}{x}$ ***is not continuous at*** $x = 0$***, but 0 is not in the domain of f. Thus, f is continuous over its domain,*** $(-\infty, 0) \cup (0, \infty)$.

86. Is the function given by $f(x) = \dfrac{x^2 + 3x}{2x - 1}$ continuous over its domain?

87. Is the function given by $g(x) = \dfrac{3x}{x - 2}$ continuous over its domain?

88. Is the function given by $r(x) = \sqrt{x^2 + 1}$ continuous over its domain?

89. Is the function given by $s(x) = \sqrt{x^2 - 1}$ continuous over its domain?

90. Is the function given by $p(x) = \begin{cases} 2x, & x \leq 0 \\ x - 1, & x > 0 \end{cases}$ continuous over its domain?

91. Is the function given by $q(x) = \begin{cases} 1 - 3x, & x \leq 1 \\ 2x^2, & x > 1 \end{cases}$ continuous over its domain?

92. Is the function given by $u(x) = \begin{cases} 4x - 2, & x < -2 \\ x - 8, & x \geq -2 \end{cases}$ continuous over its domain?

93. Is the function given by $u(x) = \begin{cases} x + 1, & x < 4 \\ x^2 - 11, & x \geq 4 \end{cases}$ continuous over its domain?

94. In Exercise 83, let

$$p(x) = \begin{cases} 1.50x, & \text{for } x \leq 20, \\ 1.25x + k, & \text{for } x > 20. \end{cases}$$

Find k such that the price function p is continuous at $x = 20$.

95. In Exercise 84, let

$$p(x) = \begin{cases} 0.08x, & \text{for } x \leq 100, \\ 0.06x + k, & \text{for } x > 100. \end{cases}$$

Find k such that the price function p is continuous at $x = 100$.

96. Find each limit, if it exists. If a limit does not exist, state that fact.

a) $\lim_{x \to 0} \frac{|x|}{x}$

b) $\lim_{x \to -2} \frac{x^3 + 8}{x^2 - 4}$

97. Find a and b so that p is continuous over all of the real numbers: $p(x) = \begin{cases} -3, & x \leq 0 \\ ax + b, & 0 < x \leq 4. \\ x^2, & x > 4 \end{cases}$

98. Find c so that q is continuous over all of the real numbers: $q(t) = \begin{cases} 3^t, & t \leq 2 \\ c, & t > 2 \end{cases}$.

Technology Connection

In Exercises 99–106, find each limit. Use TABLE *and start with* ΔTbl = 0.1. *Then use* 0.01, 0.001, *and* 0.0001. *When you think you know the limit, graph and use* TRACE *to verify your assertion. Then try to verify each limit algebraically.*

99. $\lim_{x \to 1} \frac{\sqrt{x} - 1}{x - 1}$

100. $\lim_{a \to -2} \frac{a^2 - 4}{\sqrt{a^2 + 5} - 3}$

101. $\lim_{x \to 0} \frac{\sqrt{4 + x} - \sqrt{4 - x}}{x}$

102. $\lim_{x \to 0} \frac{\sqrt{3 - x} - \sqrt{3}}{x}$

103. $\lim_{x \to 0} \frac{\sqrt{7 + 2x} - \sqrt{7}}{x}$

104. $\lim_{x \to 1} \frac{x - \sqrt[4]{x}}{x - 1}$

105. $\lim_{x \to 0} \frac{7 - \sqrt{49 - x^2}}{x}$

106. $\lim_{x \to 4} \frac{2 - \sqrt{x}}{4 - x}$

Answers to Quick Checks

1. (a) -1; L1, L2, L3, L6; (b) $\frac{51}{10}$, or 5.1; L1, L2, L3, L5, L6; (c) $\sqrt{13}$; L1, L2, L3, L6 2. 2 3. $\frac{2}{3}$ 4. $\frac{1}{2x^2}$
5. No, the limit as $x \to 2$ does not exist.
6. Yes, $\lim_{x \to 3} h(x) = 6$ and $h(3) = 6$, so $\lim_{x \to 3} h(x) = h(3)$.
7. 90, 90, 90

1.3 Average Rates of Change

- Compute an average rate of change.
- Find a simplified difference quotient.

A *rate*, or *rate of change*, is a ratio of two quantities. For example, if you drive 110 mi over a 2-hr period, then your *average rate of change* in distance (miles) per unit of time (hours) over the 2-hr period is $\frac{110 \text{ mi}}{2 \text{ hr}}$, or 55 mi/hr. Suppose that at one instant during your drive, you glance at the speedometer and see that at that moment you are traveling at 65 mi/hr. This is an *instantaneous rate of change*. These are two different, yet related, concepts. To understand instantaneous rate of change, we first need to develop a solid understanding of average rate of change.

Quick Check 1 ✓

State the average rate of change for each situation. Be sure to include units.

a) It rained 4 in. over a period of 8 hr. State your answer in inches per hour.

b) Your car travels 250 mi on 10 gallons of gas. State your answer in miles per gallon.

c) At 2 p.m., the temperature was 82 degrees. At 5 p.m., the temperature was 76 degrees. State your answer in degrees per hour.

EXAMPLE 1 State the average rate of change for each situation. Be sure to include units.

a) Jan rode a bicycle 30 mi in 3 hr.

b) It snowed 12 in. between midnight and 8 a.m.

c) Sue earned $250 from selling 8 pieces of jewelry.

Solution

a) Jan averaged $\frac{30 \text{ mi}}{3 \text{ hr}} = 10\frac{\text{mi}}{\text{hr}}$ during the bicycle ride.

b) It snowed an average of $\frac{12 \text{ in.}}{8 \text{ hr}} = 1.5\frac{\text{in.}}{\text{hr}}$ between midnight and 8 a.m.

c) Sue earned an average of $\frac{250 \text{ dollars}}{8 \text{ pieces}} = 31.25\frac{\text{dollars}}{\text{piece}}$ from selling the jewelry.

1 ✓

EXAMPLE 2 **Business: Revenue and Rate of Change.** The graph below shows fourth-quarter revenue for Groupon from 2012 to 2017, rounded to the nearest million dollars. (*Source*: Groupon.)

a) How much did revenue increase between the fourth quarter of 2014 and the fourth quarter of 2015?

b) What was the average change in fourth-quarter revenue between 2013 and 2016?

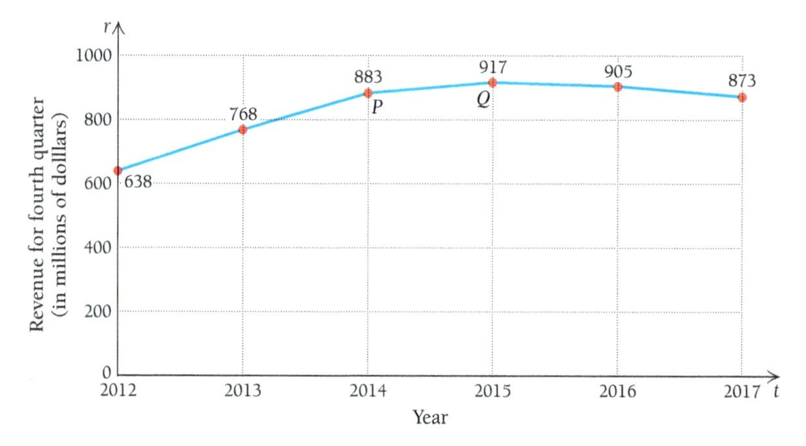

Solution

a) From the graph, we see that Groupon had revenue of $883 million during the fourth quarter of 2014 and $917 million during the fourth quarter of 2015. Thus, over that year, revenue increased by

$$917 - 883 = 34, \quad \text{or} \quad \$34 \text{ million.}$$

Note that 34 (representing $34 million) is the slope of the line segment *PQ*, which is equal to the rate of change in Groupon's revenue between the fourth quarter of 2014 and the fourth quarter of 2015.

b) We have

$$\frac{\$905 \text{ million} - \$768 \text{ million}}{2016 - 2013} = \frac{\$137 \text{ million}}{3 \text{ yr}} = \$45.67\frac{\text{million}}{\text{yr}}.$$

Note in the graph on the next page that 45.67 (representing $45.67 million) is the slope of the line segment *RS*, which indicates that Groupon had an average rate of change of $45.67 million per year in fourth-quarter revenue between 2013 and 2016.

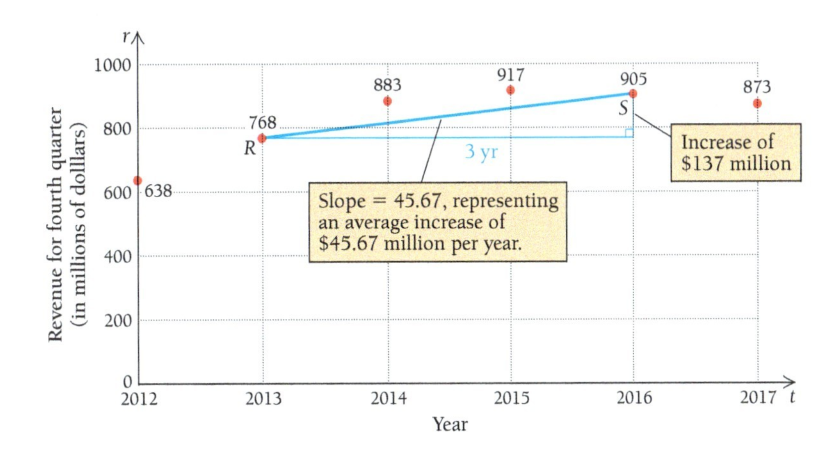

Quick Check 2✓

Using the graph in Example 2, find the average rate of change in fourth-quarter revenue between 2012 and 2014.

2✓

DEFINITION

The **average rate of change of** y, **or** $f(x)$, **with respect to** x, as x changes from x_1 to x_2, is the ratio of the change in output to the change in input:

$$\frac{y_2 - y_1}{x_2 - x_1} \quad \text{or} \quad \frac{f(x_2) - f(x_1)}{x_2 - x_1}, \quad \text{where } x_2 \neq x_1.$$

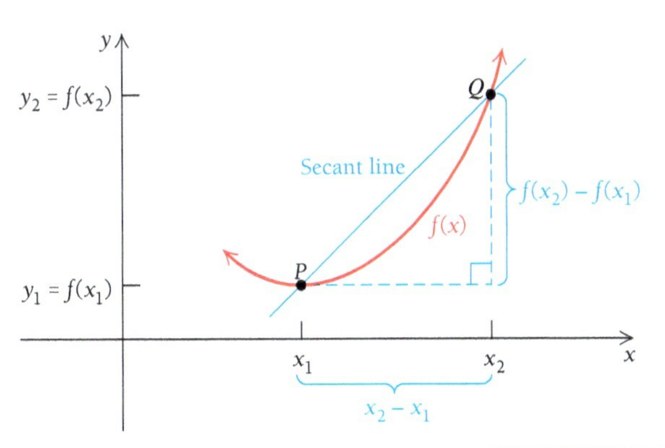

Graphically, this ratio is both the average rate of change and the slope of the line from $P(x_1, y_1)$ to $Q(x_2, y_2)$. The line passing through P and Q, denoted $\overleftrightarrow{PQ}$, is called a **secant line**. The slope of the secant line is interpreted as the average rate of change of $f(x)$ over the interval $[x_1, x_2]$.

EXAMPLE 3 For $y = f(x) = x^2 + 1$, find the average rate of change as:

a) x changes from 1 to 3; **b)** x changes from 1 to 2.

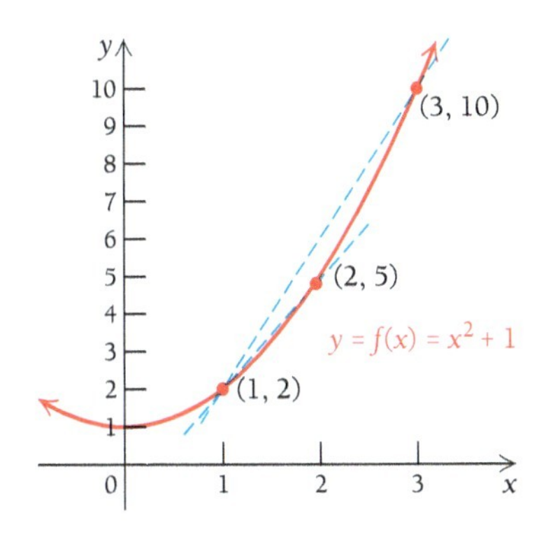

Solution The graph at the left shows the two secant lines for which slopes are being computed.

a) When $x_1 = 1$,

$$y_1 = f(x_1) = f(1) = 1^2 + 1 = 2;$$

and when $x_2 = 3$,

$$y_2 = f(x_2) = f(3) = 3^2 + 1 = 10.$$

The average rate of change is

$$\frac{y_2 - y_1}{x_2 - x_1} = \frac{f(x_2) - f(x_1)}{x_2 - x_1}$$

$$= \frac{10 - 2}{3 - 1}$$

$$= \frac{8}{2} = 4.$$

b) When $x_1 = 1$,

$$y_1 = f(x_1) = f(1) = 1^2 + 1 = 2;$$

and when $x_2 = 2$,

$$y_2 = f(x_2) = f(2) = 2^2 + 1 = 5.$$

The average rate of change is

$$\frac{5-2}{2-1} = \frac{3}{1} = 3.$$

3 ✓

Quick Check 3 ✓

For $f(x) = x^3 + 5$, find the average rate of change between:

a) $x = 1$ and $x = 4$;

b) $x = 1$ and $x = 2$.

For a linear function, the average rate of change (the slope) between any two choices of x_1 and x_2 is constant. As we saw in Example 3, a nonlinear function has average rates of change that generally vary with choices of x_1 and x_2.

Difference Quotient as Average Rate of Change

We now develop a notation for average rate of change that does not require subscripts. Instead of x_1, we write x; in place of x_2, we write $x + h$.

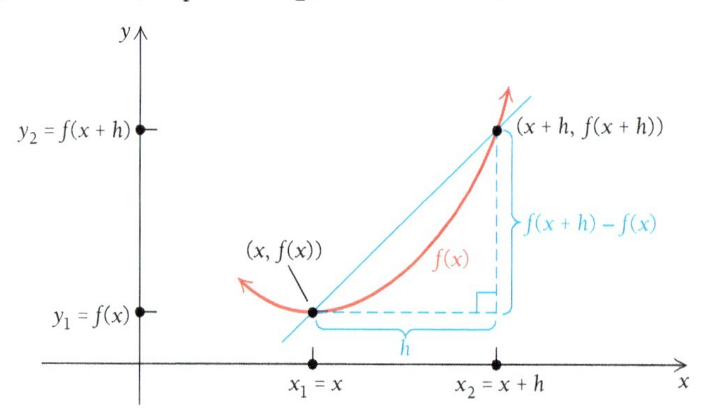

Think of h as a (usually small) horizontal distance between inputs x_1 and x_2. That is, to get from x_1, or x, to x_2, we move a distance h. Thus, $x_2 = x + h$. Then the average rate of change, also called the *difference quotient*, is given by

$$\frac{y_2 - y_1}{x_2 - x_1} = \frac{f(x_2) - f(x_1)}{x_2 - x_1} = \frac{f(x+h) - f(x)}{(x+h) - x} = \frac{f(x+h) - f(x)}{h}.$$

DEFINITION

The average rate of change of $f(x)$ with respect to x is also called the **difference quotient**. It is given by

$$\frac{f(x+h) - f(x)}{h}, \quad \text{where } h \neq 0.$$

The difference quotient is equal to the slope of the secant line passing through $(x, f(x))$ and $(x + h, f(x + h))$.

Although the value of h is never 0, it can be close to 0 or negative, as the following example shows.

EXAMPLE 4 For $f(x) = x^2$, find the difference quotient when:

a) $x = 5$ and $h = 0.1$;

b) $x = 5$ and $h = 0.01$;

c) $x = 5$ and $h = -0.01$.

Solution

a) We substitute $x = 5$ and $h = 0.1$ into the formula:

$$\frac{f(x+h) - f(x)}{h} = \frac{f(5+0.1) - f(5)}{0.1} = \frac{f(5.1) - f(5)}{0.1}.$$

Since $f(5.1) = (5.1)^2 = 26.01$ and $f(5) = 25$, we have

$$\frac{f(5.1) - f(5)}{0.1} = \frac{26.01 - 25}{0.1} = \frac{1.01}{0.1} = 10.1.$$

b) We substitute $x = 5$ and $h = 0.01$ into the formula:

$$\frac{f(x+h) - f(x)}{h} = \frac{f(5+0.01) - f(5)}{0.01} = \frac{f(5.01) - f(5)}{0.01}.$$

Since $f(5.01) = (5.01)^2 = 25.1001$ and $f(5) = 25$, we have

$$\frac{f(5.01) - f(5)}{0.01} = \frac{25.1001 - 25}{0.01} = \frac{0.1001}{0.01} = 10.01.$$

c) We substitute $x = 5$ and $h = -0.01$ into the formula:

$$\frac{f(x+h) - f(x)}{h} = \frac{f(5-0.01) - f(5)}{-0.01} = \frac{f(4.99) - f(5)}{-0.01}.$$

Since $f(4.99) = (4.99)^2 = 24.9001$ and $f(5) = 25$, we have

$$\frac{f(4.99) - f(5)}{-0.01} = \frac{24.9001 - 25}{-0.01} = \frac{-0.0999}{-0.01} = 9.99.$$

For the function in Example 4, let's find a form of the difference quotient that will allow for more efficient computations.

EXAMPLE 5 For $f(x) = x^2$, find a simplified form of the difference quotient. Then evaluate the difference quotient for $x = 5$ and $h = 0.1$ and for $x = 5$ and $h = -0.01$.

Solution

We have

$$f(x) = x^2.$$

Substituting $x + h$ into the function gives us

$$f(x+h) = (x+h)^2 = x^2 + 2xh + h^2.$$ Multiplying $(x+h)(x+h)$

Subtracting $f(x)$, we have

$$f(x+h) - f(x) = (x^2 + 2xh + h^2) - x^2 = 2xh + h^2.$$ The x^2 terms add to 0.

Thus,

$$\begin{aligned}\frac{f(x+h) - f(x)}{h} &= \frac{2xh + h^2}{h} \\ &= \frac{h(2x+h)}{h} && \text{Factoring } h \text{ in the numerator} \\ &= 2x + h, \quad h \neq 0. && h/h = 1\end{aligned}$$

This is the simplified form of this difference quotient. It is important to note that for any difference quotient, we must have $h \neq 0$.

For $x = 5$ and $h = 0.1$, we have

$$\frac{f(x+h) - f(x)}{h} = 2x + h = 2 \cdot 5 + 0.1 = 10 + 0.1 = 10.1.$$

For $x = 5$ and $h = -0.01$, we have

$$\frac{f(x+h) - f(x)}{h} = 2x + h = 2 \cdot 5 - 0.01 = 9.99.$$

Although the expression $2x + h$ is valid only when $h \neq 0$, we may allow h to approach 0 as a limit. Perhaps you can infer the limit of the expression $2x + h$ with $x = 5$ and h approaching 0.

Compare the results of Example 4(a) and 4(c) and Example 5. In general, computations are easier when a simplified form of a difference quotient is found before calculations are performed.

EXAMPLE 6 For $f(x) = x^3$, find the simplified form of the difference quotient.

Solution For $f(x) = x^3$, we have

$$f(x+h) = (x+h)^3 = x^3 + 3x^2h + 3xh^2 + h^3,$$ See Appendix A.

$$f(x+h) - f(x) = (x^3 + 3x^2h + 3xh^2 + h^3) - x^3 = 3x^2h + 3xh^2 + h^3.$$

Substituting this expression into the difference quotient gives us

$$\frac{f(x+h) - f(x)}{h} = \frac{3x^2h + 3xh^2 + h^3}{h}$$ It is understood that $h \neq 0$.

$$= \frac{h(3x^2 + 3xh + h^2)}{h}$$ Factoring h; removing a factor equal to 1

$$= 3x^2 + 3xh + h^2, \quad h \neq 0.$$

Again, this is true *only* for $h \neq 0$. 4✓

Quick Check 4✓

Use the result of Example 6 to calculate the slope of the secant line (average rate of change) at $x = 2$, for $h = 0.1$ and $h = 0.01$.

The next examples illustrate difference quotients that are common in calculus.

EXAMPLE 7 For $f(x) = 1/x$, find the simplified form of the difference quotient.

Solution For $f(x) = 1/x$, we have

$$f(x+h) = \frac{1}{x+h}.$$

Then

$$f(x+h) - f(x) = \frac{1}{x+h} - \frac{1}{x}$$

$$= \frac{1}{x+h} \cdot \frac{x}{x} - \frac{1}{x} \cdot \frac{x+h}{x+h}$$ Multiplying by 1 to get a common denominator

$$= \frac{x - (x+h)}{x(x+h)}$$ Parentheses are important here.

$$= \frac{x - x - h}{x(x+h)}$$

$$= \frac{-h}{x(x+h)}.$$

Thus,

$$\frac{f(x+h)-f(x)}{h} = \frac{\frac{-h}{x(x+h)}}{h} \quad \text{Substituting the expression just obtained}$$

$$= \frac{-h}{x(x+h)} \cdot \frac{1}{h} = \frac{-1}{x(x+h)}, \quad h \neq 0.$$

This is true *only* for $h \neq 0$. This simplified difference quotient appears again in Section 1.4.

EXAMPLE 8 For $f(x) = \sqrt{x}$, find the simplified form of the difference quotient.

Solution For $f(x) = \sqrt{x}$, we have $f(x+h) = \sqrt{x+h}$, so the difference quotient is

$$\frac{f(x+h)-f(x)}{h} = \frac{\sqrt{x+h}-\sqrt{x}}{h}.$$

Algebraic simplification (outlined in Exercise 72) leads to

$$\frac{f(x+h)-f(x)}{h} = \frac{1}{\sqrt{x+h}+\sqrt{x}}, \quad h \neq 0.$$

In all of the above cases, the simplified difference quotient includes two variables: x and h, where h cannot be 0. Although h cannot be 0, we may let h be as small as we desire. In the next section, we take a further step: allowing h to approach 0 as a limit.

Section Summary

- An *average rate of change* is the slope of a line passing through two points. If the points are (x_1, y_1) and (x_2, y_2), then the average rate of change is $\frac{y_2 - y_1}{x_2 - x_1}$.
- If the two points are on the graph of f, an equivalent form of the slope formula is $\frac{f(x+h)-f(x)}{h}$, where h is the horizontal difference between the two x-values. This is called the *difference quotient*.
- The difference quotient gives the *average rate of change* between two points on a graph.
- It is often preferable to simplify a difference quotient algebraically before evaluating it for particular values of x and h.

1.3 Exercise Set

In Exercises 1–10, state the average rate of change for each situation. Be sure to include units.

1. The temperature rose from 72 degrees at 3 p.m. to 78 degrees at 5 p.m.
2. Jennifer hiked 6 mi in 2 hr.
3. Marcus delivered 28 packages in 4 hr.
4. The population of Felton was 2500 in 2012 and 3000 in 2017.
5. Tanya scored 125 points in 5 basketball games.
6. Chris grew from 150 cm tall at age 13 to 180 cm tall at age 17.
7. Burnham Industries had $20,000,000 in revenue over a 4-month period.
8. Juan spent $33.75 to buy 15 gallons of gasoline.
9. Unemployment changed from 6% to 4% over a 6-month period.
10. Shannon's electric bill for April (30 days) was $93.

In Exercises 11–20, find the average rate of change for the indicated values of x.

11. $f(x) = 3x + 2, x_1 = 4, x_2 = 6$
12. $g(x) = 5x - 4, x_1 = 8, x_2 = 11$
13. $F(x) = 2x^2, x_1 = -1, x_2 = 2$
14. $G(x) = -3x^2, x_1 = -2, x_2 = 0$
15. $h(x) = \frac{1}{x}, x_1 = 4, x_2 = 8$

16. $k(x) = \frac{3}{x}, x_1 = 1, x_2 = 5$

17. $f(x) = x^2 + 2x, x_1 = 0, x_2 = 6$

18. $g(x) = -x^2 + 4x, x_1 = -4, x_2 = 0$

19. $r(x) = \frac{1}{2}x^2 + \frac{1}{4}x, x_1 = 3, x_2 = 5$

20. $s(x) = \frac{1}{10}x^2 + \frac{1}{2}x, x_1 = 4, x_2 = 7$

For each function in Exercises 21–36, (a) *find the simplified form of the difference quotient and then* (b) *complete the following table.*

x	h	$\frac{f(x+h) - f(x)}{h}$
5	2	
5	1	
5	0.1	
5	0.01	

21. $f(x) = 5x^2$

22. $f(x) = 4x^2$

23. $f(x) = -5x^2$

24. $f(x) = -4x^2$

25. $f(x) = x^2 - x$

26. $f(x) = x^2 + x$

27. $f(x) = \frac{9}{x}$

28. $f(x) = \frac{2}{x}$

29. $f(x) = 2x + 3$

30. $f(x) = -2x + 5$

31. $f(x) = 12x^3$

32. $f(x) = 1 - x^3$

33. $f(x) = x^2 - 4x$

34. $f(x) = x^2 - 3x$

35. $f(x) = x^2 - 3x + 5$

36. $f(x) = x^2 + 4x - 3$

APPLICATIONS

Business and Economics

For Exercises 37–44, use each graph to estimate the average rate of change of the percentage of new employees in that type of employment from 2008 to 2012, from 2012 to 2017, and from 2008 to 2017. (Source: Bureau of Labor Statistics.)

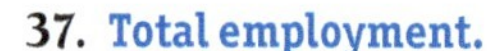

37. Total employment.

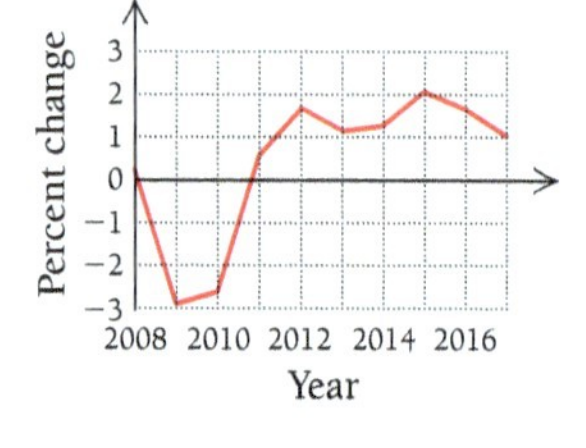

38. Construction.

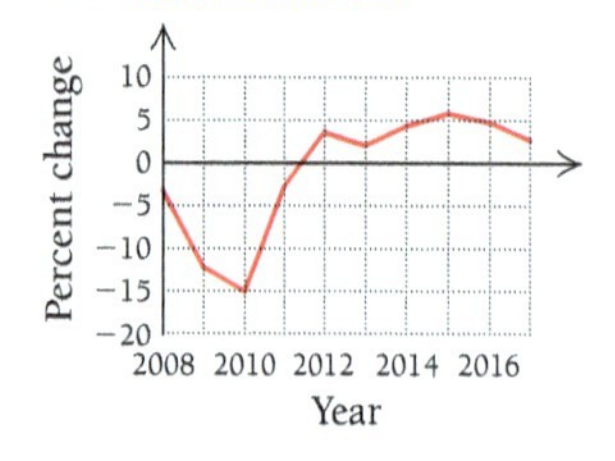

39. Professional services.

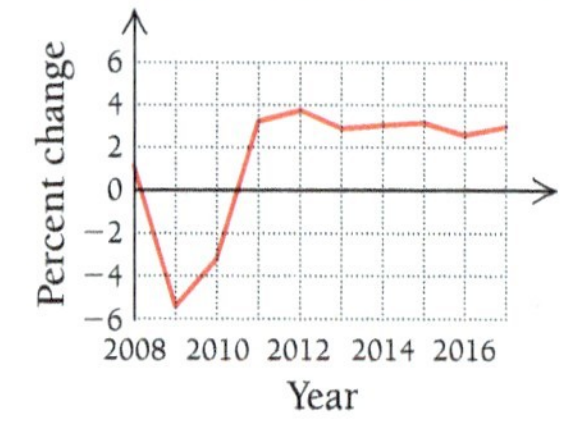

40. Health care.

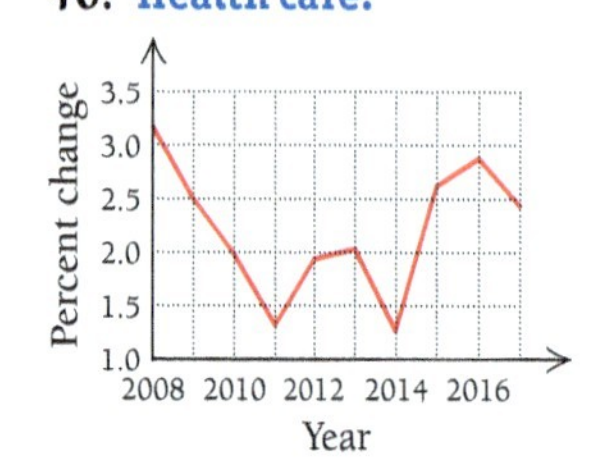

41. Education.

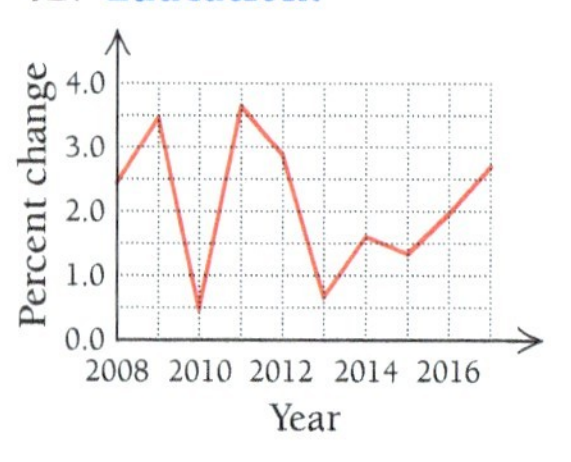

42. Government.

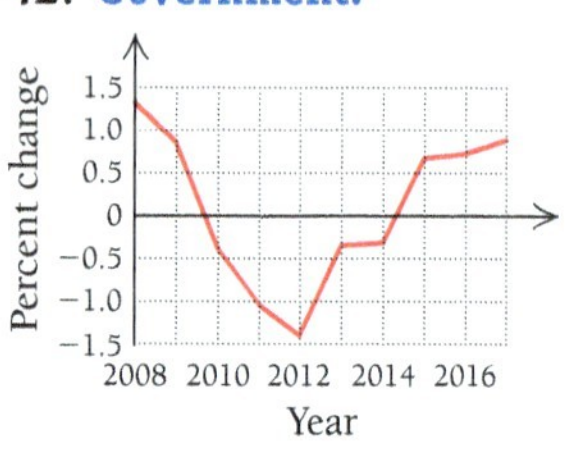

43. Mining and logging.

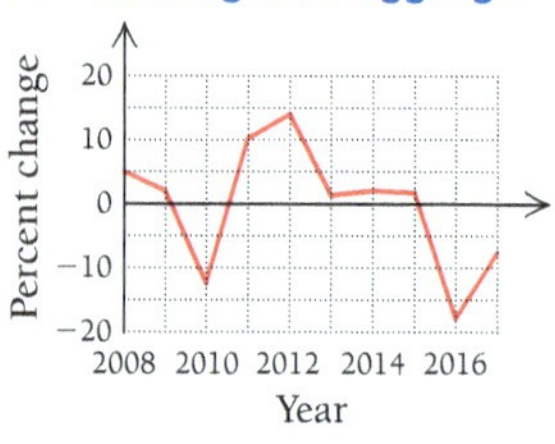

44. Manufacturing.

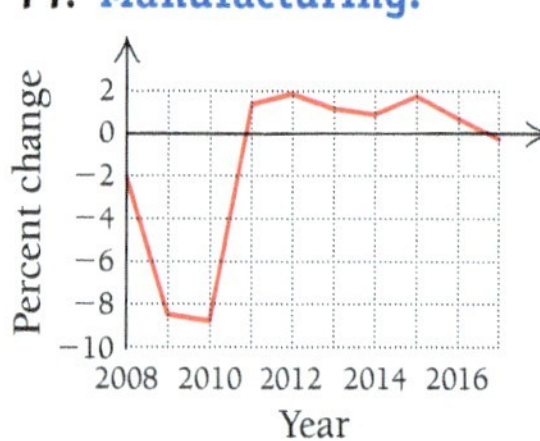

45. Use the following graph to find the average rate of change in U.S. median household income from 2010 to 2012, from 2012 to 2015, and from 2010 to 2015.

MEDIAN HOUSEHOLD INCOME IN THE UNITED STATES

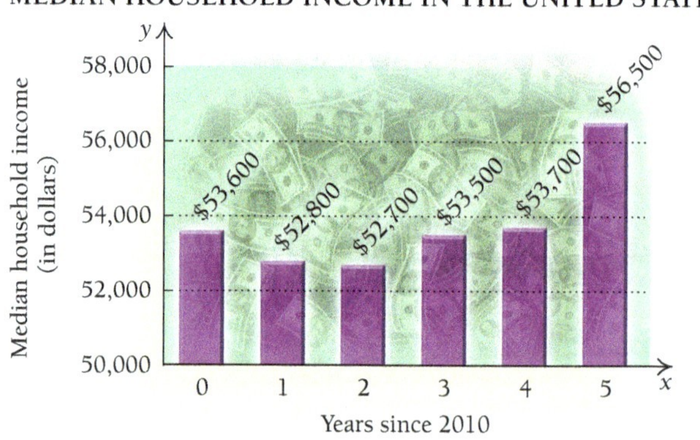

(*Source*: census.gov.)

46. Use the following graph to find the average rate of change of the U.S. trade deficit with Japan from 2011 to 2014, from 2014 to 2017, and from 2011 to 2017.

U.S. TRADE DEFICIT WITH JAPAN

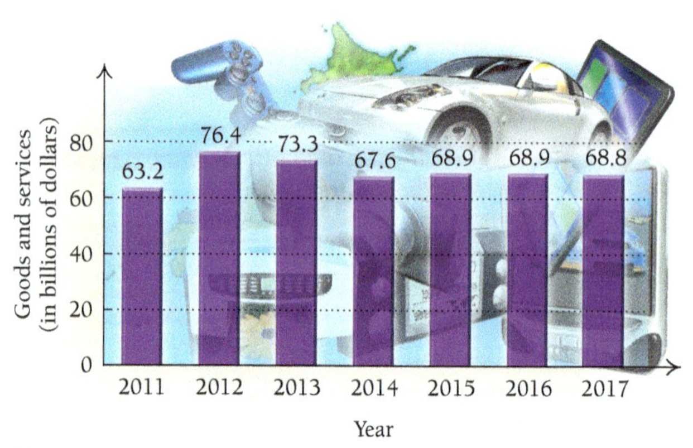

(*Source*: U.S. Census Bureau, Foreign Trade Statistics.)

47. Utility. Utility is a type of function that occurs in economics. When a consumer receives x units of a product, a certain amount of pleasure, or utility U, is gained. The following represents a typical utility function.

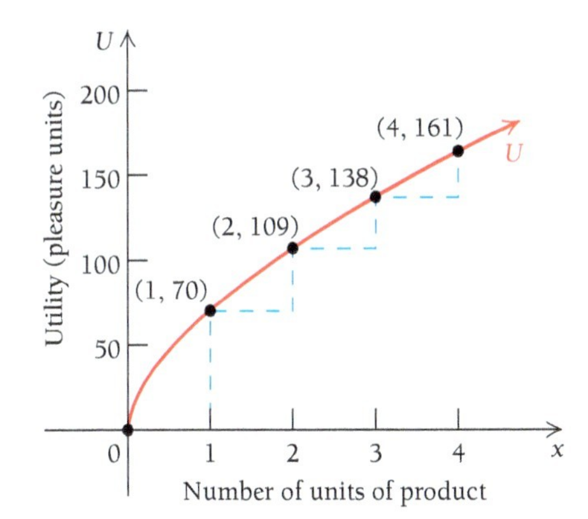

a) Find the average rate of change of U as x changes from 0 to 1; from 1 to 2; from 2 to 3; from 3 to 4.

b) Why do the average rates of change decrease as x increases?

48. Advertising results. The following graph shows a typical response to advertising. When amount a is spent on advertising, N units of a product are sold.

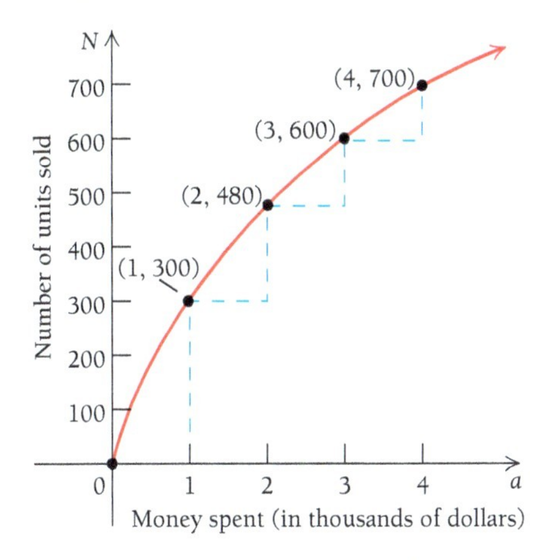

a) Find the average rate of change of N as a changes from 0 to 1; from 1 to 2; from 2 to 3; from 3 to 4.

b) Why do the average rates of change decrease as x increases?

49. Baseball ticket prices. The average price of a ticket to a major league game can be approximated by

$$p(x) = 0.0278x^3 - 0.436x^2 + 2.524x + 21.716,$$

where x is the number of years after 2006 and $p(x)$ is in dollars. (*Source*: Based on data from Major League Baseball.)

a) Find $p(4)$.
b) Find $p(10)$.
c) Find $p(10) - p(4)$.
d) Find $\dfrac{p(10) - p(4)}{10 - 4}$, and interpret this value.

50. Compound interest. The amount of money, $A(t)$, in a savings account that pays 6% interest, compounded quarterly for t years, when an initial investment of \$2000 is made, is given by

$$A(t) = 2000(1.015)^{4t}.$$

a) Find $A(3)$.
b) Find $A(5)$.
c) Find $A(5) - A(3)$.
d) Find $\dfrac{A(5) - A(3)}{5 - 3}$, and interpret this value.

51. Total cost. Suppose Fast Trends determines that the cost, in dollars, of producing x iPod holders is given by

$$C(x) = -0.05x^2 + 50x.$$

Find $\dfrac{C(305) - C(300)}{305 - 300}$, and interpret the significance of this result to the company.

52. Total revenue. Suppose Fast Trends determines that the revenue, in dollars, from the sale of x iPod holders is given by

$$R(x) = -0.001x^2 + 150x.$$

Find $\dfrac{R(305) - R(300)}{305 - 300}$, and interpret the significance of this result to the company.

53. Annual revenue. Since 2013, the annual revenue earned by Amazon can be modeled by

$$R(x) = 1.2x^2 + 11.62x + 61.22,$$

where x is the number of years since 2013 and $R(x)$ is the annual revenue, in billions of dollars. (*Source*: revenuesandprofits.com.) Find $\dfrac{R(4) - R(1)}{4 - 1}$, and interpret the significance of this result to the company.

54. Gross income. Since 2012, the gross annual income of Panera Bread Co. can be modeled by

$$m(x) = 7.34x^3 - 44.68x^2 + 67.85x + 409.88,$$

where x is the number of years since 2012 and $m(x)$ is the gross annual income, in millions of dollars. (*Source*: marketwatch.com.) Find $\dfrac{m(5) - m(2)}{5 - 2}$, and interpret the significance of this result to the company.

Life and Physical Sciences

55. Home range. It has been shown that the home range, in hectares, of a carnivorous mammal weighing w grams can be approximated by

$$H(w) = 0.11w^{1.36}.$$

(*Source*: Based on information in Emlen, J. M., *Ecology: An Evolutionary Approach*, p. 200, Reading, MA: Addison-Wesley, 1973; and Harestad, A. S., and Bunnel, F. L., "Home Range and Body Weight—A Reevaluation," *Ecology*, Vol. 60, No. 2, pp. 389–402.)

a) Find the average rate at which a carnivorous mammal's home range increases as the animal's weight grows from 500 g to 700 g.

b) Find $\dfrac{H(300) - H(200)}{300 - 200}$. What does this rate represent?

56. **Condor population.** The condor population in the Grand Canyon in Arizona can be approximated by $P(t) = 2.8t^{1.87}$, where t is the number of years since 2000. (*Source*: Based on data from www.nps.gov.)

a) Find the average rate of change in this population between 2010 and 2017.

b) Find $\dfrac{P(15) - P(7)}{15 - 7}$. What does this number represent?

57. **Memory.** Suppose that the total number of words, $M(t)$, a person can memorize in t minutes is shown in the following graph.

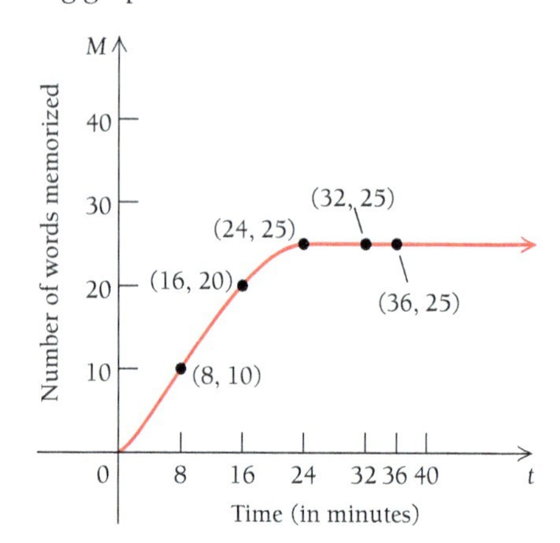

a) Find the average rate of change of M as t changes from 0 to 8; from 8 to 16; from 16 to 24; from 24 to 32; from 32 to 36.

b) Why do the average rates of change become 0 when t exceeds 24 min?

58. **Gas mileage.** At the beginning of a trip, the odometer on a car reads 30,680, and the car has a full tank of gas. At the end of the trip, the odometer reads 31,077. It takes 13.5 gal of gas to refill the tank.

a) What is the average rate of fuel efficiency, in miles per gallon?

b) What is the average rate of gas consumption in gallons per mile?

59. **Average velocity.** In t seconds, an object dropped from a certain height will fall $s(t)$ feet, where

$$s(t) = 16t^2.$$

a) Find $s(5) - s(3)$.

b) What is the average rate of change of distance with respect to time during the period from 3 to 5 sec? This is known as **average velocity**, or **speed**.

60. **Average velocity.** Suppose that in t hours, a truck travels $s(t)$ miles, where

$$s(t) = 40t^{1.2}.$$

a) Find $s(5) - s(2)$. What does this represent?

b) Find the average rate of change of distance with respect to time as t changes from $t_1 = 2$ to $t_2 = 5$. This is the *average velocity* over those hours.

Social Sciences

61. **Population growth.** The two curves below describe the population growth in two countries over t years.

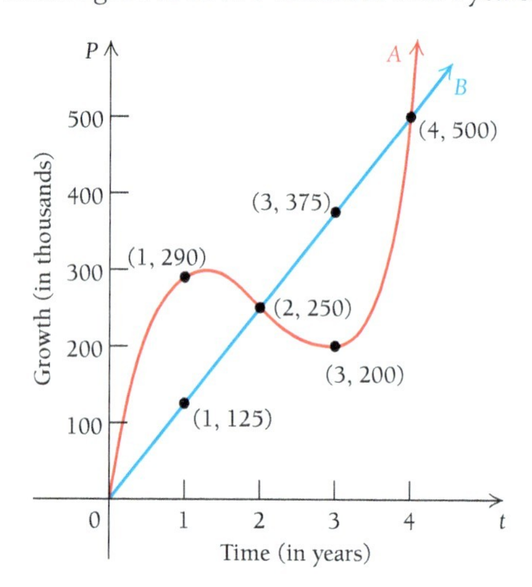

a) Find the average rate of change of each population with respect to time t as t changes from 0 to 4. This is the **average growth rate** over those years.

b) If the calculations in part (a) were the only ones made, would we detect the fact that the populations were growing differently? Why or why not?

c) Find the average rates of change of each population as t changes from 0 to 1; from 1 to 2; from 2 to 3; from 3 to 4.

d) For which population does the statement "the population grew consistently at a rate of 125 thousand per year" convey accurate information? Why?

62. **Population change.** The population of Payton County was 5400 at the last census and decreasing at the rate of 2.5% per year. The total population of the county after t years, $P(t)$, is given by

$$P(t) = 5400(0.975)^t.$$

Find $\dfrac{P(8) - P(5)}{8 - 5}$. What rate of change does this represent?

63. **Population change.** The undergraduate population at Harbor University was 17,000 and increasing at the rate of 4.2% per year. The undergraduate population after t years, $P(t)$, is given by

$$P(t) = 17{,}000(1.042)^t.$$

Find $\dfrac{P(6) - P(2)}{6 - 2}$. What rate of change does this represent?

SYNTHESIS

Find the simplified difference quotient for each function listed.

64. $f(x) = mx + b$

65. $f(x) = ax^2 + bx + c$

66. $f(x) = ax^3 + bx^2$

67. $f(x) = x^4$

68. $f(x) = x^5$

69. $f(x) = ax^5 + bx^4$

70. $f(x) = \frac{1}{x^2}$

71. $f(x) = \frac{1}{1 - x}$

72. Below are the steps in the simplification of the difference quotient for $f(x) = \sqrt{x}$ (see Example 8). Provide a brief justification for each step.

$$\frac{f(x+h) - f(x)}{h} = \frac{\sqrt{x+h} - \sqrt{x}}{h}$$

a) $= \frac{\sqrt{x+h} - \sqrt{x}}{h} \cdot \left(\frac{\sqrt{x+h} + \sqrt{x}}{\sqrt{x+h} + \sqrt{x}}\right)$

b) $= \frac{x + h + \sqrt{x}\sqrt{x+h} - \sqrt{x}\sqrt{x+h} - x}{h(\sqrt{x+h} + \sqrt{x})}$

c) $= \frac{h}{h(\sqrt{x+h} + \sqrt{x})}$

d) $= \frac{1}{\sqrt{x+h} + \sqrt{x}}$

For Exercises 73 and 74, find the simplified difference quotient.

73. $f(x) = \sqrt{2x + 1}$

74. $f(x) = \frac{1}{\sqrt{x}}$

Answers to Quick Checks

1. (a) It rained 1/2 in. per hour. **(b)** Your car gets 25 mi per gallon. **(c)** The temperature dropped 2 degrees per hour. **2.** \$122.5 million/yr **3. (a)** 21; **(b)** 7 **4.** 12.61, 12.0601

1.4 Differentiation Using Limits of Difference Quotients

- Find derivatives and values of derivatives.
- Find equations of tangent lines.

Recall from Section 1.3 that a *secant line* passes through two points on the graph of a function $y = f(x)$. If the two points are $(x, f(x))$ and $(x + h, f(x + h))$, then the slope of the secant line is given by the difference quotient:

$$\frac{f(x+h) - f(x)}{h}, \quad h \neq 0.$$

This is the *average rate of change* of f over the interval $[x, x + h]$. Although h cannot equal 0, we can let h approach 0 as a limit. When we do this, the two points forming the secant line become so close together that they appear to be a single point, and the rate of change of f over this interval is nearly instantaneous. In this section, we will investigate and develop an understanding of instantaneous rate of change by studying the slope of a *tangent line.*

Tangent Lines

A *tangent line* is a line that touches a curve at exactly one point. Using a circle, we can see the difference between a tangent line and a secant line:

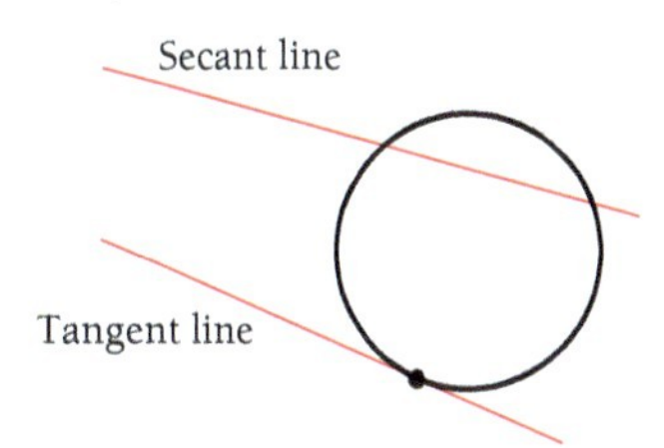

These ideas extend to any smooth curve: A tangent line touches a curve at a single point, just as for the circle in the above figure. In the figure below, the line L touches the curve at P, the *point of tangency*. Here L passes through the curve elsewhere, but it is still considered a tangent line to the curve at point P.

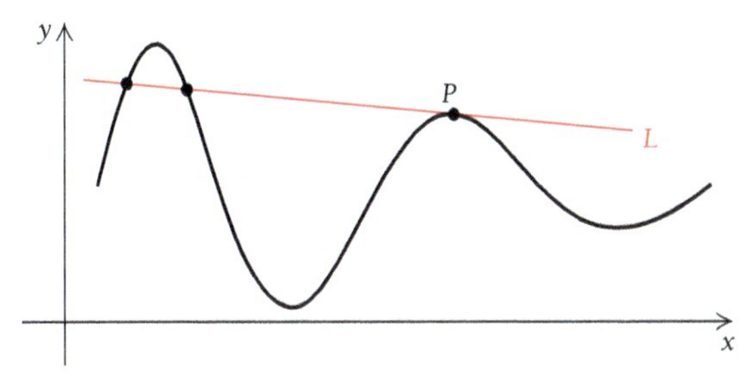

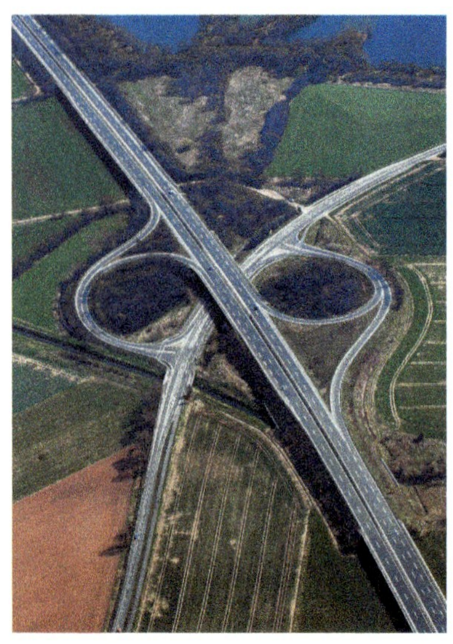

The four-lane highway is tangent to the access loops.

Technology Connection 

Exploratory

Graph $y_1 = 3x^5 - 20x^3$ with the viewing window $[-3, 3, -80, 80]$, with Xscl = 1 and Yscl = 10. Then graph $y_2 = -7x - 10$, $y_3 = -30x + 13$, and $y_4 = -45x + 28$. Which line appears to be tangent to the graph of y_1 at $(1, -17)$? If necessary, zoom in several times near $(1, -17)$ to confirm your answer.

In the next figure, the line M crosses the curve only at point P, but is not tangent to the curve; it does not touch the curve in the required manner.

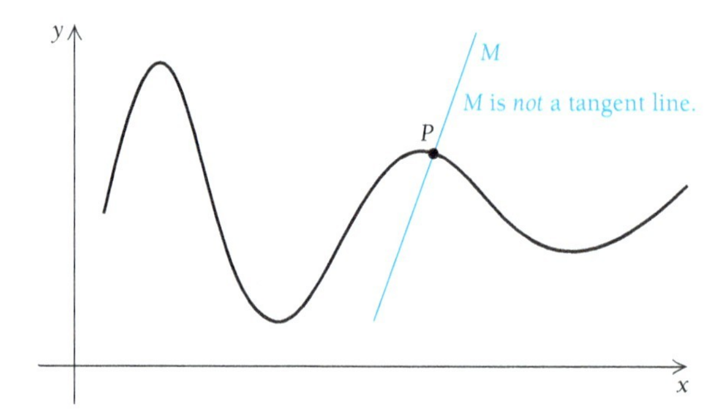

In the following figure, all of the lines except for L_1 and L_2 are tangent lines.

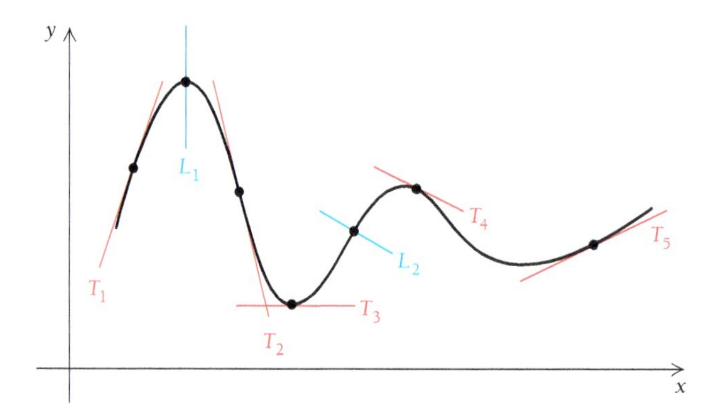

If a curve is smooth (has no corners or discontinuities), then each point on the curve has a *unique* tangent line; that is, exactly one tangent line can be drawn at any given point.

Differentiation Using Limits

We now define *tangent line* so that it makes sense for *any* curve. To do this, we use the notion of limit.

To obtain the line tangent to a curve at point P, we start with a sequence of secant lines through P and neighboring points Q_1, Q_2, and so on. As the Q's approach P, the secant lines approach line T. The slopes m_1, m_2, m_3, and so on, of the secant lines approach the slope m of line T. We *define* line T as the **tangent line**, the line that contains point P and has slope m, where m is the limit of the slopes of the secant lines as point Q (shown in the figure as $Q_1, Q_2, Q_3, Q_4, \ldots$) approaches P.

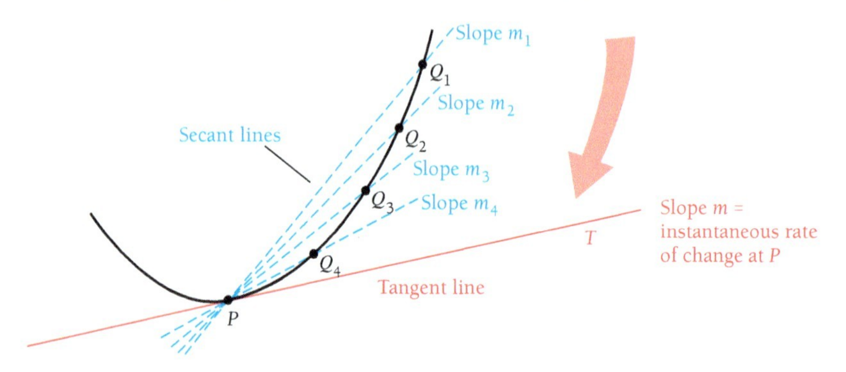

Visualize the sequence of secant lines as an animation: As the point Q moves closer to P, the resulting secant lines "lie down" on the tangent line.

How might we calculate the limit m? Suppose P has coordinates $(x, f(x))$. Then the first coordinate of Q is x plus some number h, or $x + h$. The coordinates of Q are $(x + h, f(x + h))$, as shown in the figure on the left below.

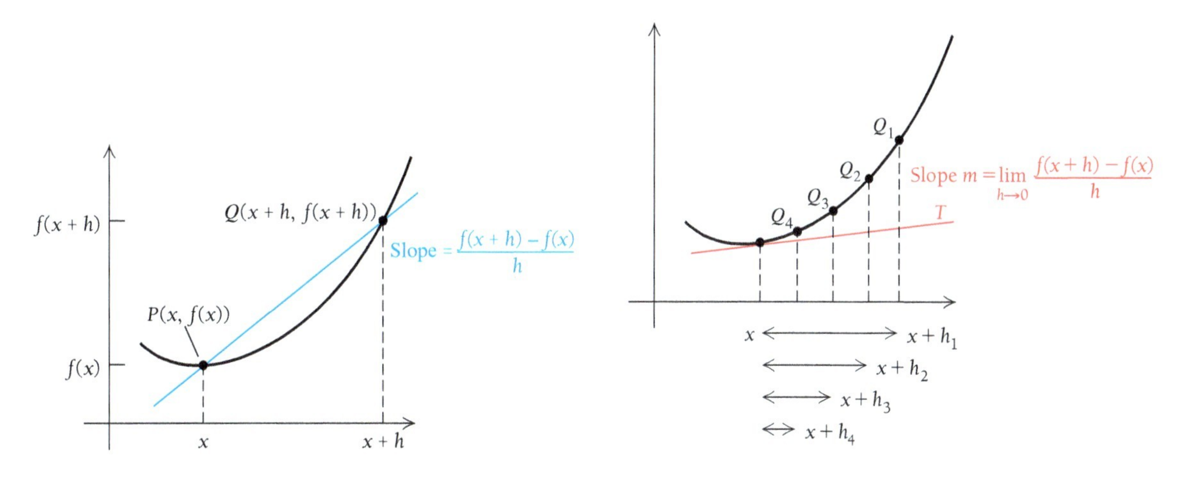

From Section 1.3, we know that the slope of secant line $\overleftrightarrow{PQ}$ is given by

$$\frac{f(x+h)-f(x)}{h}.$$

Now, as shown in the figure on the right above, as the Q's approach P, the values of $x + h$ approach x. That is, h approaches 0. Thus, we have the following.

> The slope of the tangent line at $(x, f(x))$ is $m = \lim_{h \to 0} \frac{f(x+h)-f(x)}{h}$.
>
> This limit is also the **instantaneous rate of change** of $f(x)$ at x.

The formal definition of the *derivative of a function* f can now be given. We will designate the derivative at x as $f'(x)$, rather than m. The notation $f'(x)$ is read "the derivative of f at x," "f prime at x," or "f prime of x."

"Nothing in this world is so powerful as an idea whose time has come."

Victor Hugo

DEFINITION

For a function f, given by $y = f(x)$, its **derivative** at x is the function f', where

$$f'(x) = \lim_{h \to 0} \frac{f(x+h)-f(x)}{h},$$

provided that the limit exists. If $f'(x)$ exists, then we say that f is **differentiable** at x.

Let's now find some formulas for calculating derivatives. That is, given a formula for a function f, we will attempt to find a formula for f'. The formula for f' can then be used to find the slope of a line tangent to $y = f(x)$ at a given x-value.

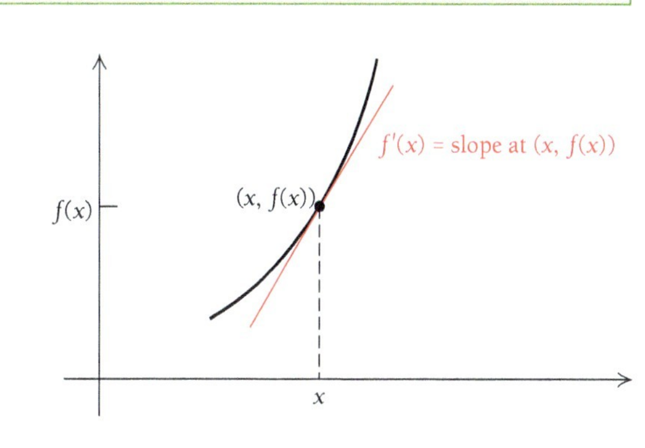

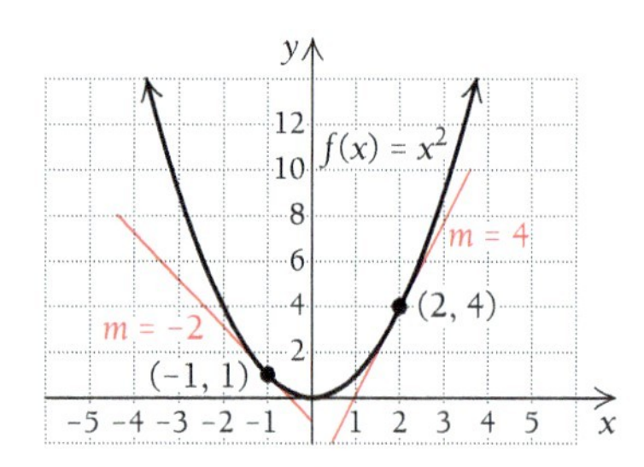

A visualization of Example 1

EXAMPLE 1 For $f(x) = x^2$, find $f'(x)$. Then find $f'(-1)$ and $f'(2)$.

Solution We first find the difference quotient:

$$\frac{f(x+h)-f(x)}{h} = \frac{(x+h)^2 - x^2}{h} \quad \text{Evaluating } f(x+h) \text{ and } f(x)$$

$$= \frac{x^2 + 2xh + h^2 - x^2}{h}$$

$$= \frac{2xh + h^2}{h} = \frac{h(2x+h)}{h} \quad \text{Simplifying}$$

$$= 2x + h, \quad h \neq 0.$$

Next, we take the limit:

$$f'(x) = \lim_{h\to 0} \frac{f(x+h)-f(x)}{h} = \lim_{h\to 0}(2x+h) = 2x.$$

Therefore, the derivative of $f(x) = x^2$ is given by

$$f'(x) = 2x.$$

Using the fact that $f'(x) = 2x$, it follows that

$$f'(-1) = 2\cdot(-1) = -2, \quad \text{and} \quad f'(2) = 2\cdot 2 = 4.$$

Thus, at $x = -1$, the tangent line has slope

$$f'(-1) = -2,$$

and at $x = 2$, the tangent line has slope

$$f'(2) = 4.$$

To summarize:

- The tangent line to the curve at the point $(-1, 1)$ has slope -2.
- The tangent line to the curve at the point $(2, 4)$ has slope 4.
- The instantaneous rate of change at $x = -1$ is -2.
- The instantaneous rate of change at $x = 2$ is 4.

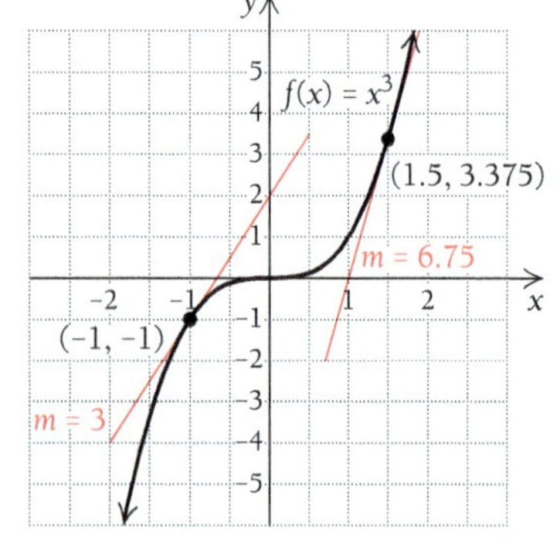

A visualization of Example 2

EXAMPLE 2 For $f(x) = x^3$, find $f'(x)$. Then find $f'(-1)$ and $f'(1.5)$.

Solution We have

$$\frac{f(x+h)-f(x)}{h} = \frac{(x+h)^3 - x^3}{h}.$$

In Example 6 of Section 1.3, we showed that this expression simplifies to

$$3x^2 + 3xh + h^2, \quad h \neq 0.$$

We then take the limit to find the derivative:

$$f'(x) = \lim_{h\to 0} \frac{f(x+h)-f(x)}{h} = \lim_{h\to 0}(3x^2 + 3xh + h^2) = 3x^2.$$

Thus,

$$f'(-1) = 3(-1)^2 = 3 \quad \text{and} \quad f'(1.5) = 3(1.5)^2 = 6.75.$$

1 ✓

Quick Check 1 ✓

Use the results from Examples 1 and 2 to find the derivative of $f(x) = x^3 + x^2$, and then calculate $f'(-2)$ and $f'(4)$. Interpret these results.

A visualization of Example 3

EXAMPLE 3 For $f(x) = 3x - 4$, find $f'(x)$ and $f'(2)$.

Solution We have

$$\frac{f(x+h) - f(x)}{h} = \frac{3(x+h) - 4 - (3x - 4)}{h}$$ The parentheses are important.

$$= \frac{3x + 3h - 4 - 3x + 4}{h}$$ Using the distributive law

$$= \frac{3h}{h} = 3, \quad h \neq 0.$$ Simplifying

To find the derivative, we take the limit:

$$f'(x) = \lim_{h \to 0} \frac{f(x+h) - f(x)}{h} = \lim_{h \to 0} 3 = 3, \text{ since 3 is a constant.}$$

Thus, if $f(x) = 3x - 4$, then $f'(x) = 3$ and $f'(2) = 3$.

The result of Example 3 suggests that, for the graph of any linear function, the slope of a tangent line is the slope of the line itself. That is, the derivative of

$$f(x) = mx + b$$

is

$$f'(x) = m.$$

This formula can be verified in a manner similar to that used in Example 3.

EXAMPLE 4 For $f(x) = \dfrac{1}{x}$:

a) Find $f'(x)$.

b) Find $f'(2)$.

c) Find an equation of the line tangent to the graph of f at $x = 2$.

Solution

a) We have

$$\frac{f(x+h) - f(x)}{h} = \frac{[1/(x+h)] - (1/x)}{h}.$$

In Example 7 of Section 1.3, we showed that this expression simplifies to

$$\frac{-1}{x(x+h)}, \quad h \neq 0.$$

As $h \to 0$, we have

$$f'(x) = \lim_{h \to 0} \frac{-1}{x(x+h)} = \frac{-1}{x \cdot x} = -\frac{1}{x^2}.$$

b) Since $f'(x) = -1/x^2$, we have

$$f'(2) = -\frac{1}{2^2} = -\frac{1}{4}.$$ This is the slope of the tangent line at $x = 2$.

c) To find an equation of the tangent line at $x = 2$, we need to know the line's slope and a point on the line. In part (b), we found that the slope at $x = 2$ is $-\frac{1}{4}$. To find a point on the line, we compute $f(2)$:

$$f(2) = \frac{1}{2}.$$ CAUTION! Be careful to use f when computing y-values and f' when computing slope.

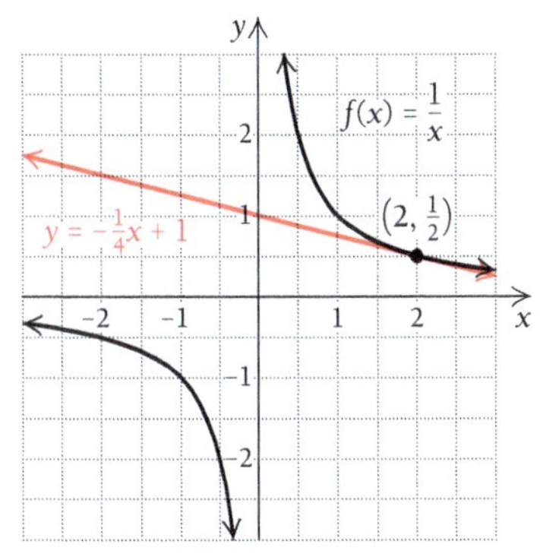

A visualization of Example 4(c)

To find the equation of the line passing through $(2, \frac{1}{2})$ and having a slope of $-\frac{1}{4}$, we substitute into the point–slope equation (see Section R.4):

$$y - y_1 = m(x - x_1)$$

$$y - \tfrac{1}{2} = -\tfrac{1}{4}(x - 2)$$

$$\left.\begin{aligned} y &= -\tfrac{1}{4}x + \tfrac{1}{2} + \tfrac{1}{2} \\ &= -\tfrac{1}{4}x + 1. \end{aligned}\right\} \text{Rewriting in slope–intercept form}$$

Quick Check 2✓

Repeat Example 4(a) for $f(x) = -\frac{2}{x}$. What are the similarities between this solution and that obtained for $f(x) = \frac{1}{x}$?

The equation of the line tangent to the graph of f at $x = 2$ is

$$y = -\tfrac{1}{4}x + 1.$$

2✓

In Example 4, note that since 0 is not in the domain of $f(x) = 1/x$, we cannot evaluate $f(0)$ or the difference quotient,

$$\frac{f(0 + h) - f(0)}{h}.$$

Thus, $f'(0)$ does not exist. We say that "f is not differentiable at 0."

> When a function is not defined at a point, it is not differentiable at that point. In general, if a function is discontinuous at a point, it is not differentiable at that point.

Sometimes a function f is continuous at a point, but f' still does not exist at this point. The function $f(x) = |x|$ is one example.

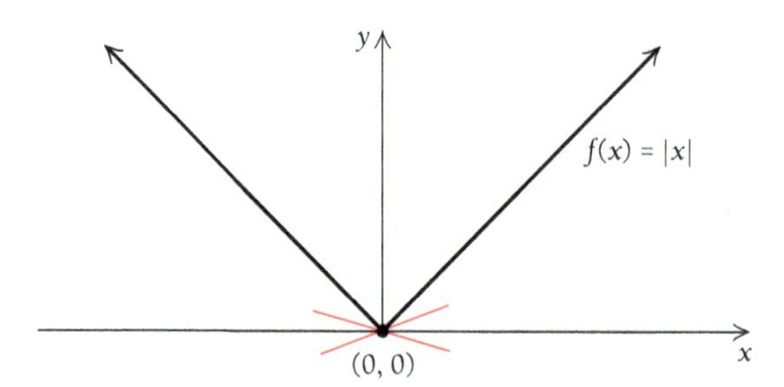

Suppose we try to draw a tangent line at $(0, 0)$. A function like this with a corner seems to have many tangent lines at $(0, 0)$. The derivative at such a point would not be unique. If we try to calculate the derivative at 0, using

$$f(x) = |x| = \begin{cases} x, & \text{for } x \geq 0, \\ -x, & \text{for } x < 0, \end{cases}$$

it follows that

$$f'(x) = \begin{cases} 1, & \text{for } x > 0, \\ -1, & \text{for } x < 0. \end{cases}$$

Since

$$\lim_{x \to 0^+} f'(x) \neq \lim_{x \to 0^-} f'(x),$$

that is, the left-hand limit does not equal the right-hand limit, it follows that $f'(0)$ does not exist.

In general, a function is not differentiable at any corners on its graph.

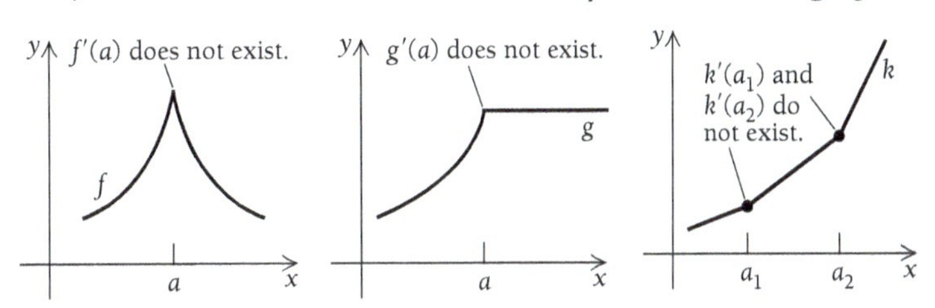

A function is also not differentiable at a point if it has a vertical tangent at that point. For example, the function shown to the right has a vertical tangent at point a. Since the slope of a vertical line is undefined, there is no derivative at such a point.

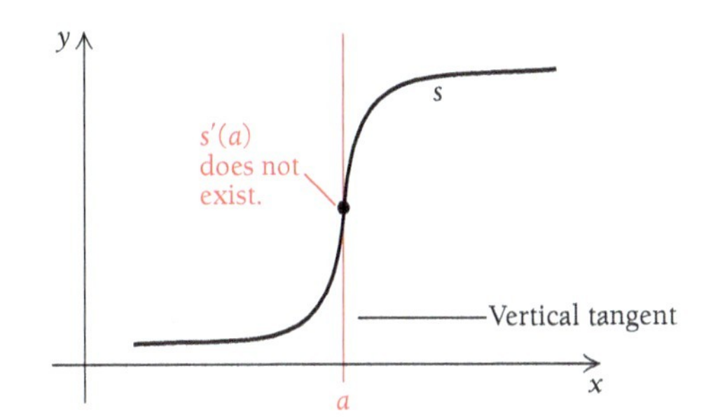

The function given by $f(x) = |x|$ illustrates the fact that although a function may be continuous over an interval I, it may not be differentiable at every point in I. That is, continuity at a point does not imply differentiability at that point. However, differentiability at a point *does* guarantee continuity at that point. That is, if $f'(a)$ exists, then f is continuous at a. The function $f(x) = x^2$ is an example of a function that is differentiable over $(-\infty, \infty)$ and is therefore continuous everywhere. Thus, when a function is differentiable over an interval, it is not just continuous, but is also *smooth* in the sense that there are no corners in its graph.

EXAMPLE 5 Below is the graph of $y = t(x)$. List all x-values for which t is not differentiable.

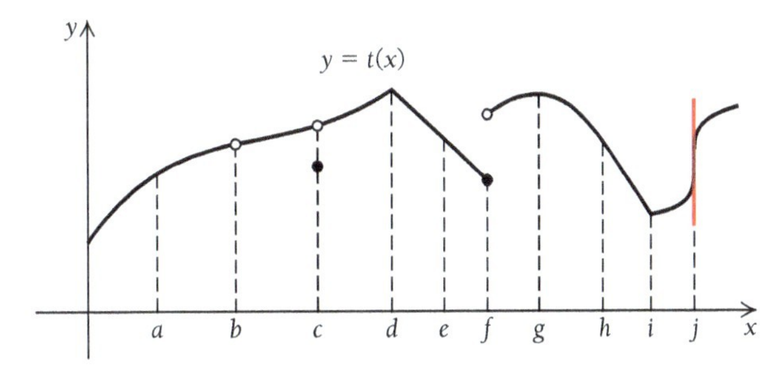

Solution A function is not differentiable where there is a discontinuity, a corner, or a vertical tangent. Therefore, t is not differentiable at the x-value b, c, or f since the function is discontinuous at these points; it is not differentiable at d or i since there are corners at these points; and it is not differentiable at j since there is a vertical tangent line (the slope is undefined) at $(j, t(j))$. **3 ✓**

Quick Check 3 ✓

Where is $f(x) = |x + 6|$ not differentiable? Why?

Section Summary

- A *tangent line* is a line that touches a smooth curve at a single point, the *point of tangency*. See the figure in the middle of p. 138 for examples of tangent lines and lines that are not tangent lines.
- The *derivative* of $f(x)$ is defined by

$$f'(x) = \lim_{h \to 0} \frac{f(x+h) - f(x)}{h}.$$

- The *slope* of the line tangent to the graph of $y = f(x)$ at $x = a$ is the value of the derivative at $x = a$; that is, the slope of the tangent line at $x = a$ is $f'(a)$.
- Slopes of tangent lines are interpreted as *instantaneous rates of change*.
- The equation of a tangent line at $x = a$ is

$$y - f(a) = f'(a)(x - a).$$

- If a function is differentiable at $x = a$, then it is *continuous* at $x = a$. That is, differentiability implies continuity at an x-value.
- However, continuity at $x = a$ does *not* guarantee differentiability at $x = a$. An example is the absolute-value function, $f(x) = |x|$, for which, at $x = 0$, the graph has a corner. Continuity alone is not sufficient to guarantee differentiability.
- A function is not differentiable at $x = a$ if:
  (1) there is a discontinuity at $x = a$,
  (2) there is a corner at $x = a$, or
  (3) there is a vertical tangent at $x = a$.

1.4 Exercise Set

In Exercises 1–16:

a) *Graph the function.*

b) *Draw lines tangent to the graph at the points with x-coordinates* -2, 0, *and* 1.

c) *Find* $f'(x)$ *by determining* $\lim_{h \to 0} \frac{f(x + h) - f(x)}{h}$.

d) *Find* $f'(-2)$, $f'(0)$, *and* $f'(1)$. *These slopes should match those of the lines you drew in part* (b).

1. $f(x) = \frac{3}{2}x^2$

2. $f(x) = \frac{1}{2}x^2$

3. $f(x) = -3x^2$

4. $f(x) = -2x^2$

5. $f(x) = x^3$

6. $f(x) = -x^3$

7. $f(x) = -2x + 5$

8. $f(x) = 2x + 3$

9. $f(x) = \frac{1}{2}x - 3$

10. $f(x) = \frac{3}{4}x - 2$

11. $f(x) = x^2 - x$

12. $f(x) = x^2 + x$

13. $f(x) = 2x^2 + 3x - 2$

14. $f(x) = 5x^2 - 2x + 7$

15. $f(x) = \frac{2}{x}$

16. $f(x) = \frac{1}{x}$

17. Find an equation of the line tangent to the graph of $f(x) = x^3$ at **(a)** $(-2, -8)$; **(b)** $(0, 0)$; **(c)** $(4, 64)$.

18. Find an equation of the line tangent to the graph of $f(x) = x^2$ at **(a)** $(3, 9)$; **(b)** $(-1, 1)$; **(c)** $(10, 100)$.

19. Find an equation of the line tangent to the graph of $f(x) = 2/x$ at **(a)** $(1, 2)$; **(b)** $(-1, -2)$; **(c)** $(100, 0.02)$.

20. Find an equation of the line tangent to the graph of $f(x) = -1/x$ at **(a)** $(-1, 1)$; **(b)** $(2, -\frac{1}{2})$; **(c)** $(-5, \frac{1}{5})$.

21. Find an equation of the line tangent to the graph of $f(x) = x^2 - 2x$ at **(a)** $(-2, 8)$; **(b)** $(1, -1)$; **(c)** $(4, 8)$.

22. Find an equation of the line tangent to the graph of $f(x) = 4 - x^2$ at **(a)** $(-1, 3)$; **(b)** $(0, 4)$; **(c)** $(5, -21)$.

23. Find $f'(x)$ for $f(x) = mx + b$.

24. Find $f'(x)$ for $f(x) = ax^2 + bx$.

For each graph in Exercises 25–30, list all x-values for which the function is not differentiable.

25.

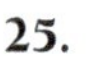

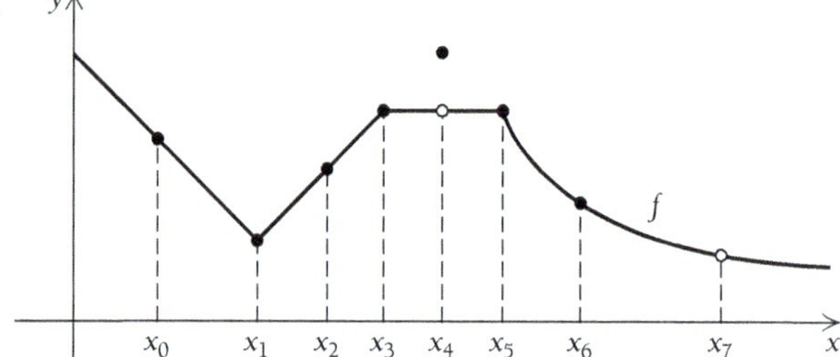

26.

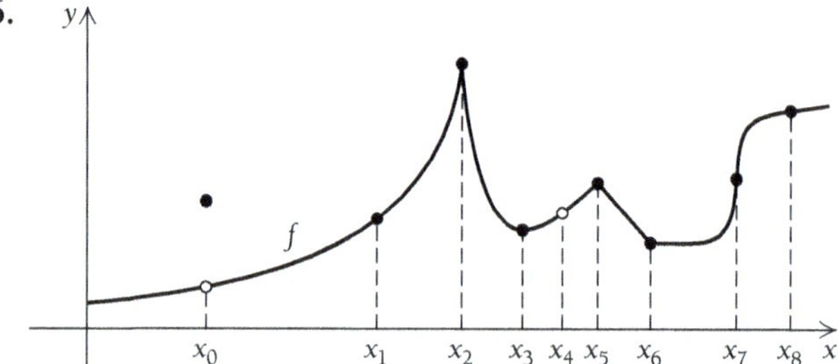

27.

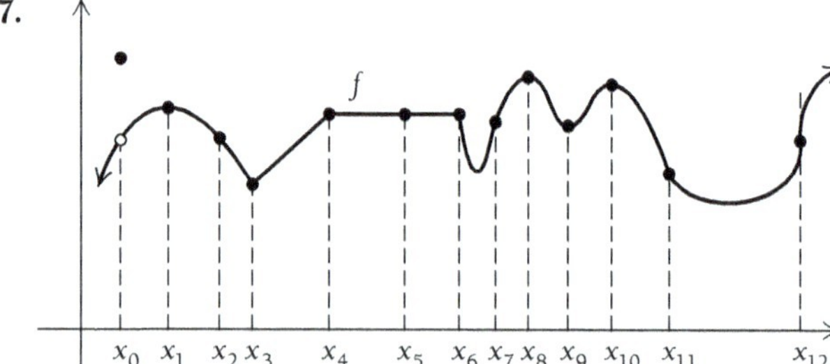

28.

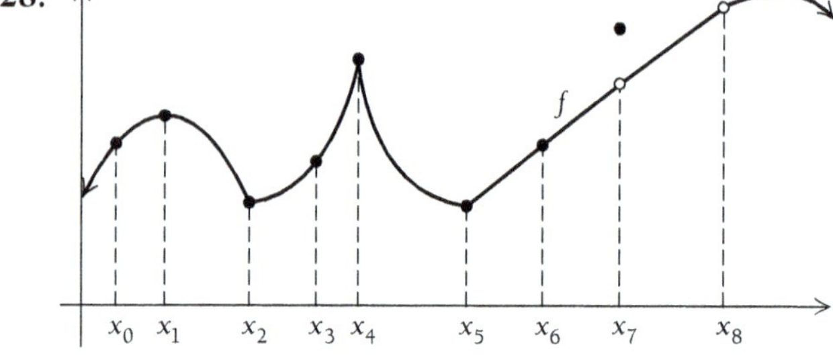

29.

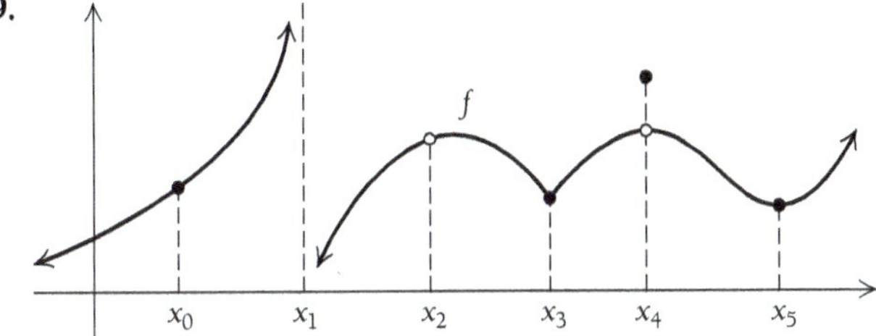

30.

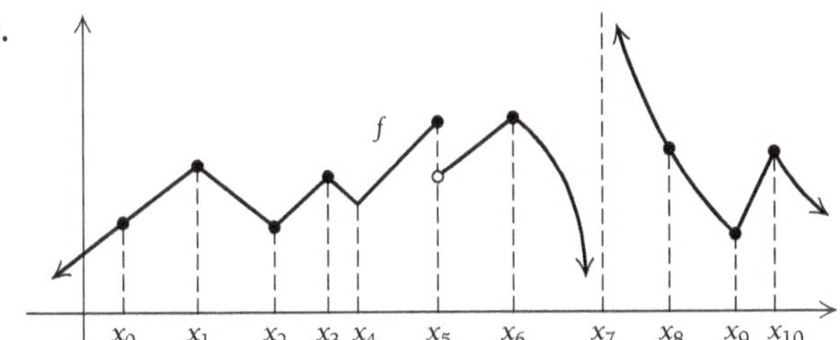

31. Draw a graph that is continuous, but not differentiable, at $x = 3$.

32. Draw a graph that is continuous, with no corners, but not differentiable, at $x = 1$.

33. Draw a graph that has a horizontal tangent line at $x = 5$.

34. Draw a graph that is differentiable and has horizontal tangent lines at $x = 0$, $x = 2$, and $x = 4$.

35. Draw a graph that has horizontal tangent lines at $x = 2$ and $x = 5$ and is continuous, but not differentiable, at $x = 3$.

36. Draw a graph that is continuous for all x, with no corners, but not differentiable at $x = -1$ and $x = 2$.

37. Draw a graph that is continuous, but not differentiable at $x = 1, 2, 3, 4, \ldots$.

38. Draw a graph that is smooth and continuous, but not differentiable at $x = 1, 2, 3, 4, \ldots$.

In Exercises 39–42, classify each statement as true or false.

39. If a graph is smooth at $x = a$, then it is differentiable at $x = a$.

40. If a graph is differentiable at $x = a$, then it is smooth at $x = a$.

41. If a graph is not differentiable at $x = a$, then there is a corner at $x = a$.

42. If a graph is horizontal at $x = a$, then it is not differentiable at $x = a$.

SYNTHESIS

43. Consider the following graph:

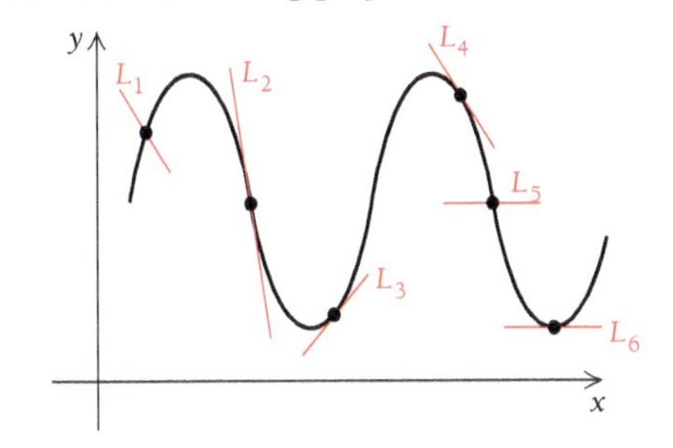

Which of the lines in the graph appear to be tangent lines? Why or why not?

44. On the following graph, use a colored pencil to draw each secant line from point P to the points Q_1, Q_2, Q_3, Q_4, and Q_5. Then use a different colored pencil to draw a tangent line to the curve at P. How do the slopes of the secant lines compare to the slopes of the tangent lines?

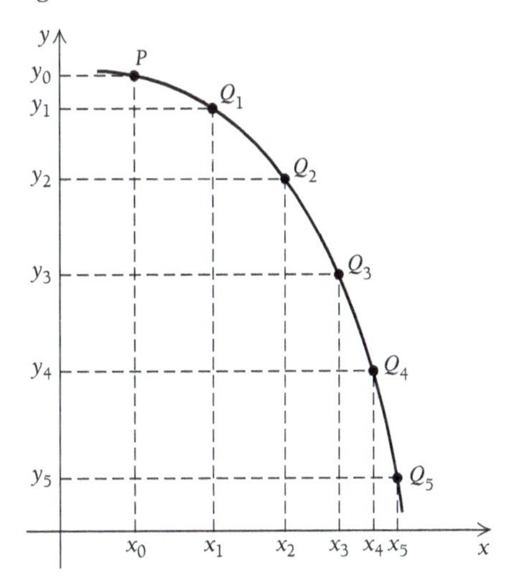

For Exercises 45–51, find $f'(x)$ for the given function.

45. $f(x) = \dfrac{1}{1 - x}$ (See Exercise 71 in Section 1.3.)

46. $f(x) = x^5$ (See Exercise 68 in Section 1.3.)

47. $f(x) = \dfrac{1}{x^2}$ (See Exercise 70 in Section 1.3.)

48. $f(x) = \sqrt{x}$ (See Example 8 in Section 1.3.)

49. $f(x) = \sqrt{2x + 1}$ (See Exercise 73 in Section 1.3.)

50. $f(x) = \dfrac{1}{\sqrt{x}}$ (See Exercise 74 in Section 1.3.)

51. $f(x) = ax^2 + bx + c$

52. Let $f(x) = \dfrac{x^2 + 4x + 3}{x + 1}$. A student recognizes that this function can be simplified as

$$f(x) = \frac{x^2 + 4x + 3}{x + 1} = \frac{(x + 1)(x + 3)}{x + 1} = x + 3.$$

Since $y = x + 3$ is a line with slope 1, the student makes the following conclusions: $f'(-2) = 1$, $f'(-1) = 1$, $f'(0) = 1$, $f'(1) = 1$. Where did the student make an error?

53. Consider the function f given by

$$f(x) = \frac{x^2 - 9}{x + 3}.$$

a) For what x-value(s) is the function not differentiable?

b) Are there any x-values in the function's domain where the function is not differentiable? Why or why not?

c) Find $f'(4)$.

54. Consider the function g given by $g(x) = \frac{x^2 + x}{2x}$.

a) For what x-value(s) is the function not differentiable?

b) Are there any x-values in the function's domain where the function is not differentiable? Why or why not?

c) What is $g'(3)$? Describe the simplest way to determine this.

55. Consider the function k given by $k(x) = |x - 3| + 2$.

a) For what x-value(s) is the function not differentiable?

b) Are there any x-values in the function's domain where the function is not differentiable? Why or why not?

c) Evaluate $k'(0)$, $k'(1)$, $k'(4)$, and $k'(10)$.

56. Consider the function k given by $k(x) = 2|x + 5|$.

a) For what x-value(s) is the function not differentiable?

b) Are there any x-values in the function's domain where the function is not differentiable? Why or why not?

c) Evaluate $k'(-10)$, $k'(-7)$, $k'(-2)$, and $k'(0)$.

57. Let $g(x) = \sqrt[3]{x}$. A student graphs this function, and the graph appears to be continuous for all real numbers x. The student concludes that g is differentiable for all x, which is false. Explain why the conclusion is false. What is the correct conclusion about the differentiability of g?

58. Let F be a function given by

$$F(x) = \begin{cases} x^2 + 1, & \text{for } x \leq 2, \\ 2x + 1, & \text{for } x > 2. \end{cases}$$

a) Verify that F is continuous at $x = 2$.

b) Is F differentiable at $x = 2$? Why or why not?

59. Let G be a function given by

$$G(x) = \begin{cases} x^3, & \text{for } x \leq 1, \\ 3x - 2, & \text{for } x > 1. \end{cases}$$

a) Verify that G is continuous at $x = 1$.

b) Is G differentiable at $x = 1$? Why or why not?

60. Let H be a function given by

$$H(x) = \begin{cases} 2x^2 - x, & \text{for } x \leq 3, \\ mx + b, & \text{for } x > 3. \end{cases}$$

Determine the values of m and b that make H differentiable at $x = 3$.

The Mean Value Theorem. *If f is defined over $[a, b]$ and differentiable over (a, b), then there exists at least one value c, where $a < c < b$, such that*

$$f'(c) = \frac{f(b) - f(a)}{b - a}.$$

Graphically, this means that there exists at least one point $(c, f(c))$ where the tangent line is parallel to the secant line connecting $(a, f(a))$ and $(b, f(b))$.

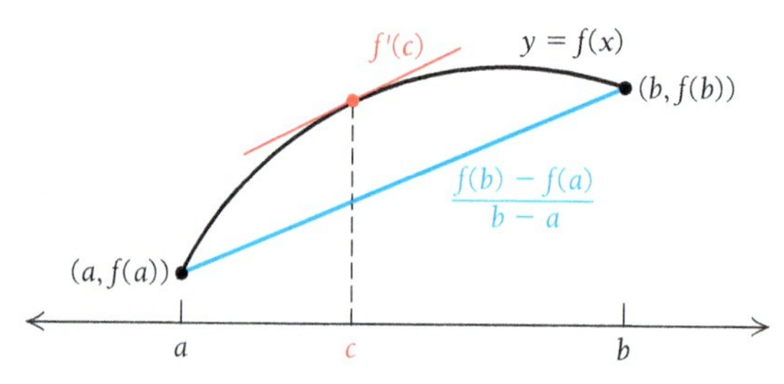

61. Let $f(x) = x^2$ over $[-1, 4]$. Find c such that $-1 < c < 4$, where $f'(c) = \frac{f(4) - f(-1)}{4 - (-1)}$.

62. Let $f(x) = -x^3$ over $[0, 5]$. Find c such that $0 < c < 5$, where $f'(c) = \frac{f(5) - f(0)}{5 - 0}$.

63. A trucker drives from Las Vegas to Phoenix (a distance of 290 mi) in 4 hr, but claims to have never exceeded a speed of 70 mi/hr. Use the Mean Value Theorem to prove that this claim is impossible.

64. Explain why the Mean Value Theorem does not apply for $g(x) = |x|$ over the interval $[-2, 3]$.

Answers to Quick Checks

1. $f'(x) = 3x^2 + 2x$; $f'(-2) = 8$, $f'(4) = 56$, meaning that the slope at $x = -2$ is 8 and the slope at $x = 4$ is 56. **2.** $f'(x) = \frac{2}{x^2}$, which is $-2 \cdot \frac{d}{dx}\left(\frac{1}{x}\right)$ **3.** At $x = -6$, the graph has a corner.

1.5 Leibniz Notation and the Power and Sum–Difference Rules

- Differentiate using the Power Rule or the Sum–Difference Rule.
- Differentiate a constant function or a constant times a function.
- Determine points at which a tangent line has a specified slope.

In this and several of the sections that follow, we develop ways to find derivatives of certain functions quickly. We begin with a discussion of derivative notation.

Leibniz Notation

Let $y = f(x)$. In Section 1.4, we used prime notation to express the derivative of f:

$$f'(x) = \lim_{h \to 0} \frac{f(x + h) - f(x)}{h}.$$

Often, we write y', read "y-prime," to denote the derivative $f'(x)$.

Historical Note: The German mathematician and philosopher Gottfried Wilhelm von Leibniz (1646–1716) and the English mathematician, philosopher, and physicist Sir Isaac Newton (1642–1727) are both credited with the invention of calculus, though each worked independently. Newton used the dot notation $\dot{y}$ for dy/dt, where y is a function of time; this notation is still used, though it is not as common as Leibniz notation.

Another common way to express "the derivative of y with respect to x" is to write

$$\frac{dy}{dx}.$$

This notation is called *Leibniz notation*, after German mathematician Gottfried von Leibniz. Leibniz notation, read by sounding out each letter "d y, d x," reminds us that the derivative of $y = f(x)$ is a ratio of two small quantities: dy, representing a small change in y, and dx, representing a small change in x. Using this notation, we often write the derivative as

$$\frac{dy}{dx} = f'(x).$$

It is important to note that the d's are not variables and that

$$\frac{dy}{dx} \neq \frac{y}{x}.$$

We can also express the derivative of f as

$$\frac{d}{dx}f(x).$$

The above expression is read as "d, d x, of $f(x)$," or "d f, d x." When placed next to an expression, the notation $\frac{d}{dx}$ acts as a command (called an *operator*) to find the derivative of the expression. For example,

$$\frac{d}{dx}(x^2) = 2x, \quad \frac{d}{dx}(x^3) = 3x^2, \quad \text{and} \quad \frac{d}{dx}\left(\frac{1}{x}\right) = -\frac{1}{x^2}.$$

We use these forms often, and with practice, their use becomes natural.

Leibniz notation is also useful when determining the units of a derivative. For example, if $y = f(x)$, where y is measured in feet and x is measured in seconds, then $\frac{dy}{dx} = f'(x)$ is measured in feet per second, or ft/sec.

EXAMPLE 1 For the function given by $Q = g(t)$, write four different ways to represent the derivative of Q with respect to t.

Solution Using prime notation, we write:

The derivative of Q with respect to t is $g'(t)$,

or the derivative of Q with respect to t is Q'.

Using Leibniz notation, we write:

The derivative of Q with respect to t is $\frac{dQ}{dt}$,

or the derivative of Q with respect to t is $\frac{d}{dt}g(t)$. **1✓**

Quick Check 1✓

For the function given by $A = P(r)$, write four different ways to represent the derivative of A with respect to r.

The Power Rule

The following list summarizes some of our work from Section 1.4. Do you see a pattern?

$$\frac{d}{dx}x^2 = 2x;$$

$$\frac{d}{dx}x^3 = 3x^2;$$

$$\frac{d}{dx}x^4 = 4x^3;$$

$$\frac{d}{dx}x^{-1} = -1x^{-2};$$

$$\frac{d}{dx}x^{1/2} = \frac{1}{2}x^{-1/2}.$$

The pattern can be described as follows: "To find the derivative of a power function, bring the exponent to the front of the variable as a coefficient and make the new exponent 1 less than the original exponent."

$$\frac{d}{dx}x^k = k \cdot x^{k-1}$$

Write the exponent as the coefficient.

Subtract 1 from the exponent.

This rule is summarized as the following theorem.

THEOREM 3 The Power Rule

For any real number k, if $y = x^k$, then

$$\frac{d}{dx}x^k = k \cdot x^{k-1}.$$

A proof of this theorem for a positive integer k is given below. Let $f(x) = x^k$. We first note a pattern when $(x + h)^k$ is raised to a power k, a positive integer:

$$\text{for } k = 1, \quad (x + h)^1 = x + h;$$

$$\text{for } k = 2, \quad (x + h)^2 = x^2 + 2xh + h^2;$$

$$\text{for } k = 3, \quad (x + h)^3 = x^3 + 3x^2h + 3xh^2 + h^3;$$

$$\text{for } k = 4, \quad (x + h)^4 = x^4 + 4x^3h + 6x^2h^2 + 4xh^3 + h^4.$$

In general, for k a positive integer, we have

$$f(x + k) = (x + h)^k = x^k + kx^{k-1}h + (h^2 \text{ and higher terms}),$$

where "h^2 and higher terms" are terms that all contain h raised to a power of 2 or greater.

Proof: We have

$$\frac{d}{dx}x^k = \lim_{h \to 0}\frac{(x + h)^k - x^k}{h} \qquad \text{Using the definition of the derivative}$$

$$= \lim_{h \to 0}\frac{x^k + kx^{k-1}h + (h^2 \text{ and higher terms}) - x^k}{h} \qquad \text{Substituting}$$

$$= \lim_{h \to 0}\frac{kx^{k-1}h + (h^2 \text{ and higher terms})}{h} \qquad \text{Simplifying: } x^k - x^k = 0$$

$$= \lim_{h \to 0}\frac{h \cdot (kx^{k-1} + (h \text{ and higher terms}))}{h} \qquad \text{Factoring}$$

$$= \lim_{h \to 0}(kx^{k-1} + (h \text{ and higher terms})) \qquad \text{Simplifying: } \frac{h}{h} = 1 \text{ for } h \neq 0$$

All the terms after kx^{k-1} contain h, and when the limit is taken, these terms approach 0. Thus,

$$\frac{d}{dx}x^k = kx^{k-1}.$$

■

EXAMPLE 2 Differentiate each of the following with respect to x:

a) $y = x^5$; **b)** $y = x$; **c)** $y = x^{-4}$.

Solution

a) $\frac{d}{dx}x^5 = 5 \cdot x^{5-1} = 5x^4$ Using the Power Rule

b) $\frac{d}{dx}x = 1 \cdot x^{1-1} = 1 \cdot x^0 = 1$

c) $\frac{d}{dx}x^{-4} = -4 \cdot x^{-4-1} = -4x^{-5}$, or $-4 \cdot \frac{1}{x^5}$, or $-\frac{4}{x^5}$ **2 ✓**

Quick Check 2 ✓
Differentiate with respect to x:
a) $y = x^{15}$;
b) $y = x^{-7}$.

The Power Rule also allows us to differentiate expressions with rational exponents.

EXAMPLE 3 Differentiate:

a) $y = \sqrt[5]{x}$; **b)** $y = x^{0.7}$.

Solution

a) $\frac{d}{dx}\sqrt[5]{x} = \frac{d}{dx}x^{1/5} = \frac{1}{5} \cdot x^{(1/5)-1} = \frac{1}{5}x^{-4/5}$, or $\frac{1}{5\sqrt[5]{x^4}}$

b) $\frac{d}{dx}x^{0.7} = 0.7x^{(0.7)-1} = 0.7x^{-0.3}$, or $\frac{7}{10x^{0.3}}$ **3 ✓**

Quick Check 3 ✓
Differentiate with respect to x:
a) $y = \sqrt[4]{x}$;
b) $y = x^{-1.25}$.

The Derivative of a Constant Function

Consider the constant function given by $f(x) = c$. Note that the slope of the tangent line at each point on its graph is 0.

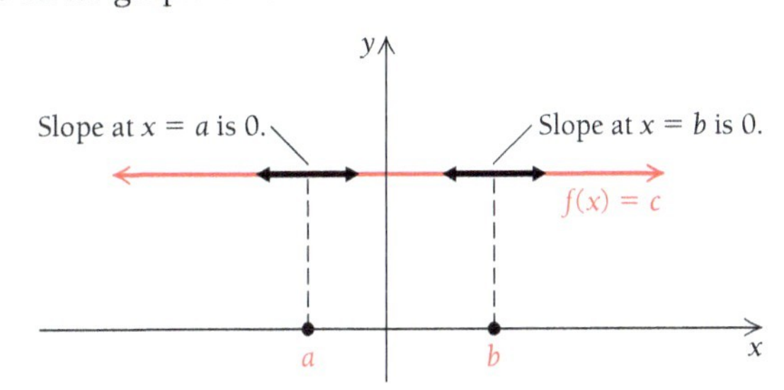

This suggests the following theorem.

> **THEOREM 4**
>
> The derivative of a constant function is 0. That is, $\frac{d}{dx}c = 0$.

Proof: Let f be the function given by $f(x) = c$. Then

$$\frac{d}{dx}c = \lim_{h \to 0}\frac{f(x+h) - f(x)}{h} \quad \text{Using the definition of the derivative}$$

$$= \lim_{h \to 0}\frac{c - c}{h} \quad f(x+h) = c \text{ and } f(x) = c$$

$$= \lim_{h \to 0}\frac{0}{h}$$

$$= 0. \quad \text{Using Limit Property L1}$$

■

EXAMPLE 4 Differentiate with respect to x:

a) $y = 7$; **b)** $y = \pi^2$.

Solution

a) $\frac{d}{dx}(7) = 0$ Using Theorem 4

b) $\frac{d}{dx}(\pi^2) = 0$ Note that π^2 is a constant.

4 ✓

Quick Check 4 ✓
Differentiate with respect to x:
$y = 100^{\sqrt{7}}$.

The Derivative of a Constant Times a Function

In Exercise 3 of Section 1.4, we found that $\frac{d}{dx}(-3x^2) = -6x$. Note that $-6x = -3 \cdot 2x = -3 \cdot \frac{d}{dx}x^2$. This suggests the following theorem.

THEOREM 5

The derivative of a constant times a function is the constant times the derivative of the function. Using derivative notation, we can write this as

$$\frac{d}{dx}[c \cdot f(x)] = c \cdot \frac{d}{dx}f(x).$$

Proof: Our proof makes use of the Limit Properties presented in Section 1.2.

$$\frac{d}{dx}[c \cdot f(x)] = \lim_{h \to 0} \frac{c \cdot f(x+h) - c \cdot f(x)}{h}$$ Using the definition of the derivative

$$= \lim_{h \to 0} \frac{c(f(x+h) - f(x))}{h}$$ Factoring

$$= c \cdot \lim_{h \to 0} \frac{f(x+h) - f(x)}{h}$$ Using Limit Property L6

$$= c \cdot \frac{d}{dx}f(x)$$ Using the definition of the derivative

■

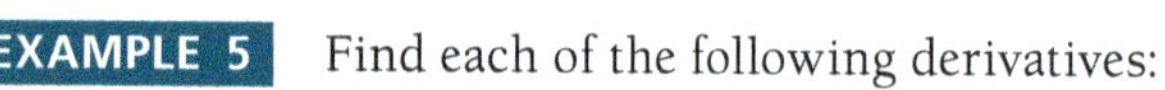

EXAMPLE 5 Find each of the following derivatives:

a) $\frac{d}{dx}7x^4$; **b)** $\frac{d}{dx}(-5\sqrt{x})$; **c)** $\frac{d}{dx}\left(\frac{1}{5x^2}\right)$.

Solution

a) $\frac{d}{dx}7x^4 = 7\frac{d}{dx}x^4 = 7 \cdot 4 \cdot x^{4-1} = 28x^3$ Using Theorem 3; with practice, this may be done in one step.

b) $\frac{d}{dx}(-5\sqrt{x}) = -5\frac{d}{dx}x^{1/2} = -5\left(\frac{1}{2}x^{-1/2}\right) = -\frac{5}{2}x^{-1/2}$

c) $\frac{d}{dx}\left(\frac{1}{5x^2}\right) = \frac{d}{dx}\left(\frac{1}{5}x^{-2}\right) = \frac{1}{5} \cdot \frac{d}{dx}x^{-2}$ Rewriting with a negative exponent

$$= \frac{1}{5}(-2)x^{-2-1}$$

$$= -\frac{2}{5}x^{-3}, \text{ or } -\frac{2}{5x^3}$$

5 ✓

Quick Check 5 ✓
Differentiate each of the following:
a) $y = 10x^9$;
b) $y = \pi x^3$;
c) $y = \frac{2}{3x^4}$.

Technology Connection 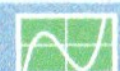

Exploratory

Let $y_1 = x(100 - x)$, and $y_2 = x\sqrt{100 - x^2}$. Using the Y-VARS option from the VARS menu, enter Y3 as Y1+ Y2. Find the derivative of each of the three functions at $x = 8$ using the numerical differentiation feature.

Compare your answers. How do you think you can find the derivative of a sum?

The Derivative of a Sum or a Difference

In Exercise 12 of Exercise Set 1.4, we found that the derivative of

$$f(x) = x^2 + x$$

is $$f'(x) = 2x + 1.$$

Note that the derivative of x^2 is $2x$, the derivative of x is 1, and the sum of these derivatives is $f'(x)$. This illustrates the following theorem.

THEOREM 6 The Sum–Difference Rule

Sum. The derivative of a sum is the sum of the derivatives:

$$\frac{d}{dx}[f(x) + g(x)] = \frac{d}{dx}f(x) + \frac{d}{dx}g(x).$$

Difference. The derivative of a difference is the difference of the derivatives:

$$\frac{d}{dx}[f(x) - g(x)] = \frac{d}{dx}f(x) - \frac{d}{dx}g(x).$$

We prove the Sum Rule and leave the proof of the Difference Rule as Exercise 112.

Proof: We have

$$\frac{d}{dx}[f(x) + g(x)] = \lim_{h\to 0}\frac{f(x+h) + g(x+h) - (f(x) + g(x))}{h}$$ Using the definition of the derivative

$$= \lim_{h\to 0}\frac{f(x+h) + g(x+h) - f(x) - g(x)}{h}$$ Distributing

$$= \lim_{h\to 0}\frac{f(x+h) - f(x) + g(x+h) - g(x)}{h}$$ Grouping terms

$$= \lim_{h\to 0}\left(\frac{f(x+h) - f(x)}{h} + \frac{g(x+h) - g(x)}{h}\right)$$

$$= \lim_{h\to 0}\frac{f(x+h) - f(x)}{h} + \lim_{h\to 0}\frac{g(x+h) - g(x)}{h}$$ Using Limit Property L3

$$= \frac{d}{dx}f(x) + \frac{d}{dx}g(x).$$ Using the definition of the derivative

■

EXAMPLE 6 Find each of the following derivatives:

a) $\frac{d}{dx}(5x^3 - 7)$;

b) $\frac{d}{dx}\left(24x - \sqrt{x} + \frac{5}{x}\right)$.

Solution

a) $$\frac{d}{dx}(5x^3 - 7) = \frac{d}{dx}(5x^3) - \frac{d}{dx}(7)$$
$$= 5\frac{d}{dx}x^3 - 0$$
$$= 5 \cdot 3x^2$$
$$= 15x^2$$

b) $$\frac{d}{dx}\left(24x - \sqrt{x} + \frac{5}{x}\right) = \frac{d}{dx}(24x) - \frac{d}{dx}(\sqrt{x}) + \frac{d}{dx}\left(\frac{5}{x}\right)$$
$$= 24 \cdot \frac{d}{dx}x - \frac{d}{dx}x^{1/2} + 5 \cdot \frac{d}{dx}x^{-1}$$
$$= 24 \cdot 1 - \frac{1}{2}x^{(1/2)-1} + 5(-1)x^{-1-1}$$
$$= 24 - \frac{1}{2}x^{-1/2} - 5x^{-2}$$
$$= 24 - \frac{1}{2\sqrt{x}} - \frac{5}{x^2}$$

Quick Check 6 ✓
Differentiate:

$$y = 3x^5 + 2\sqrt[3]{x} + \frac{1}{3x^2} + \sqrt{5}.$$

6 ✓

EXAMPLE 7 **Physical Science.** Akemi drives all afternoon to visit her family. Her distance traveled, in miles, t hours after starting out, is given by

$$f(t) = 1.85t^3 - 18.17t^2 + 82.51t, \qquad 0 \le t \le 5.$$

a) Find the distance Akemi has traveled at $t = 3$ hr.

b) Find the instantaneous rate of change (her velocity) at $t = 3$ hr.

Solution

a) After 3 hr, Akemi has traveled

$$f(3) = 1.85(3)^3 - 18.17(3)^2 + 82.51(3) \approx 134 \text{ mi}.$$

b) To find Akemi's velocity at any time t, we first find the derivative, $f'(t)$:

$$f'(t) = \frac{d}{dt}(1.85t^3 - 18.17t^2 + 82.51t)$$
$$= \frac{d}{dt}(1.85t^3) - \frac{d}{dt}(18.17t^2) + \frac{d}{dt}(82.51t) \qquad \text{Using Theorem 6}$$
$$= 1.85\frac{d}{dt}(t^3) - 18.17\frac{d}{dt}(t^2) + 82.51\frac{d}{dt}(t) \qquad \text{Using Theorem 5}$$
$$= 1.85(3t^2) - 18.17(2t) + 82.51(1) \qquad \text{Using Theorem 3}$$
$$= 5.55t^2 - 36.34t + 82.51.$$

Thus, $f'(t) = 5.55t^2 - 36.34t + 82.51$. When she has been driving for exactly 3 hr, Akemi's velocity is

$$f'(3) = 5.55(3)^2 - 36.34(3) + 82.51 \approx 23.4 \frac{\text{mi}}{\text{hr}}.$$

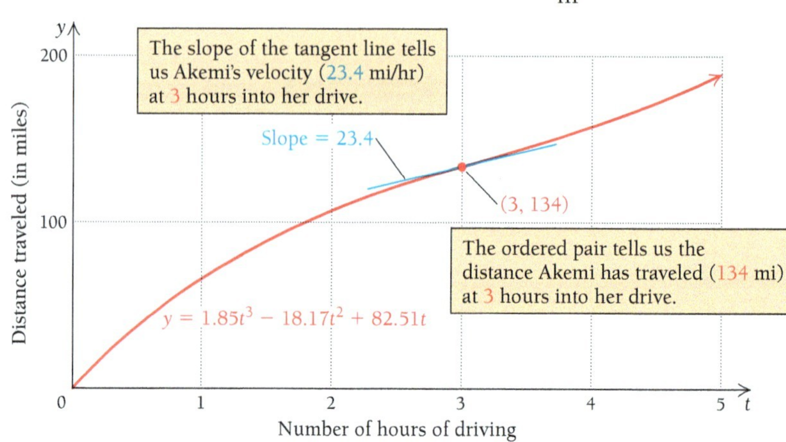

Quick Check 7 ✓
A bicyclist's distance traveled (in miles) t hours after starting a ride is given by $g(t) = 14\sqrt{t} + \frac{t}{3}$. Find the distance traveled and the velocity at $t = 2$ hr.

7 ✓

Slopes of Tangent Lines

It is important to be able to determine points at which the tangent line to a curve has a certain slope, that is, points at which the derivative, or rate of change, has a certain value.

EXAMPLE 8 Find any points on the graph of $f(x) = -x^3 + 6x^2$ at which **(a)** the tangent line is horizontal; **(b)** the tangent line has slope 9.

Solution

a) The derivative is used to find the slope of a tangent line. Since a horizontal tangent line has slope 0, we want to find all x for which $f'(x) = 0$:

$$f'(x) = 0 \qquad \text{Setting the derivative equal to 0}$$

$$\frac{d}{dx}(-x^3 + 6x^2) = 0$$

$$-3x^2 + 12x = 0. \qquad \text{Differentiating}$$

We factor and solve:

$$-3x(x - 4) = 0$$

$$-3x = 0 \quad or \quad x - 4 = 0$$

$$x = 0 \quad or \quad x = 4. \qquad \text{Using the Principle of Zero Products}$$

We are to find points *on the graph*, so we must determine the second coordinates from the original equation, $f(x) = -x^3 + 6x^2$.

$$f(0) = -0^3 + 6 \cdot 0^2 = 0.$$

$$f(4) = -4^3 + 6 \cdot 4^2 = -64 + 96 = 32.$$

Thus, the points we are seeking are (0, 0) and (4, 32), as shown on the following graph.

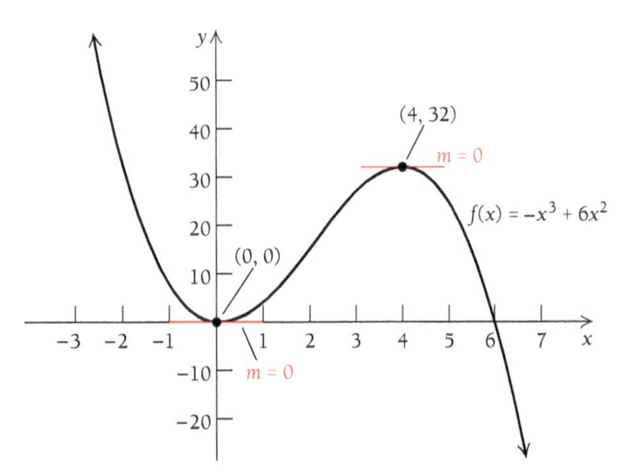

b) The tangent line has slope 9 when $f'(x) = 9$. Thus, we want to find x such that

$$-3x^2 + 12x = 9. \qquad \text{As in part (a), } \frac{d}{dx}(-x^3 + 6x^2) = -3x^2 + 12x.$$

To solve, we add -9 on both sides and get

$$-3x^2 + 12x - 9 = 0.$$

We then multiply both sides of the equation by $-\frac{1}{3}$, giving

$$x^2 - 4x + 3 = 0$$

$$(x - 3)(x - 1) = 0. \qquad \text{Factoring}$$

We have two solutions: $x = 1$ or $x = 3$. To find ordered pairs, we note that $f(1) = -(1)^3 + 6(1)^2 = 5$. Therefore, at the point $(1, 5)$, the tangent line has a slope of 9. Since $f(3) = -(3)^3 + 6(3)^2 = 27$, the tangent line at $(3, 27)$ has a slope of 9 as well. All of this is illustrated in the following graph.

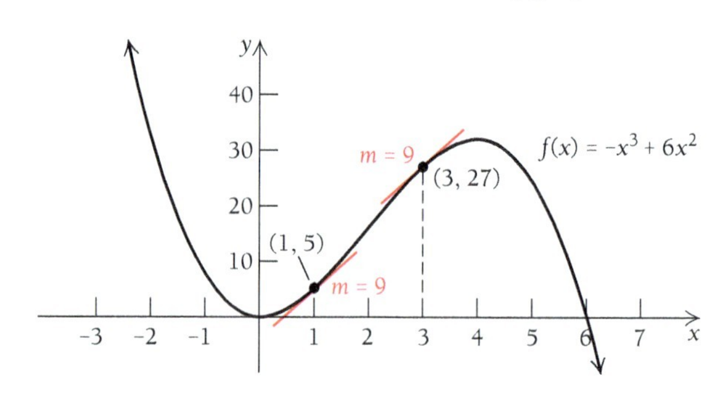

Quick Check 8 ✓

For the function in Example 8, find the points for which $f'(x) = -15$.

8 ✓

Section Summary

- Common forms of notation representing the derivative of a function are y', $f'(x)$, $\frac{dy}{dx}$, and $\frac{d}{dx}f(x)$.
- The *Power Rule* for differentiation is $\frac{d}{dx}[x^k] = kx^{k-1}$, for all real numbers k.
- The derivative of a constant is zero: $\frac{d}{dx}c = 0$.
- The derivative of a constant times a function is the constant times the derivative of the function:
$$\frac{d}{dx}[c \cdot f(x)] = c \cdot \frac{d}{dx}f(x).$$
- The derivative of a sum (or difference) is the sum (or difference) of the derivatives of the terms:
$$\frac{d}{dx}[f(x) \pm g(x)] = \frac{d}{dx}f(x) \pm \frac{d}{dx}g(x).$$

1.5 Exercise Set

1. For the function given by $u = f(v)$, write four different ways to represent the derivative of u with respect to v.
2. For the function given by $s = g(t)$, write four different ways to represent the derivative of s with respect to t.
3. For the function given by $p = R(q)$, write four different ways to represent the derivative of p with respect to q.
4. For the function given by $m = G(n)$, write four different ways to represent the derivative of m with respect to n.
5. For the function given by $h = m(k)$, write four different ways to represent the derivative of h with respect to k.
6. For the function given by $C = T(z)$, write four different ways to represent the derivative of C with respect to z.

Find $\frac{dy}{dx}$.

7. $y = x^7$
8. $y = x^8$
9. $y = -3x$
10. $y = -0.5x$
11. $y = 12$
12. $y = 7$
13. $y = 2x^{15}$
14. $y = 3x^{10}$
15. $y = x^{-6}$
16. $y = x^{-8}$
17. $y = 4x^{-2}$
18. $y = 3x^{-5}$
19. $y = x^3 + 3x^2$
20. $y = x^4 - 7x$
21. $y = 8\sqrt{x}$
22. $y = 4\sqrt{x}$
23. $y = x^{0.9}$
24. $y = x^{1.7}$
25. $y = \frac{1}{2}x^{4/5}$
26. $y = -4.8x^{1/3}$
27. $y = \frac{7}{x^3}$
28. $y = \frac{6}{x^4}$

Find each derivative.

29. $\frac{d}{dx}\left(\sqrt[4]{x} - \frac{3}{x}\right)$
30. $\frac{d}{dx}\left(\sqrt[3]{x} + \frac{4}{\sqrt{x}}\right)$
31. $\frac{d}{dx}(-2\sqrt[3]{x^5})$
32. $\frac{d}{dx}(-\sqrt[4]{x^3})$
33. $f(x) = \frac{5x}{11}$
34. $f(x) = \frac{2x}{3}$
35. $f(x) = \frac{2}{5x^6}$
36. $f(x) = \frac{4}{7x^3}$
37. $f(x) = \frac{4}{x} - x^{3/5}$
38. $f(x) = \frac{5}{x} - x^{2/3}$

Find $g'(x)$.

39. $g(x) = 7x - 14$
40. $g(x) = 4x - 7$
41. $g(x) = \frac{x^{3/2}}{3}$
42. $g(x) = \frac{x^{4/3}}{4}$

43. $g(x) = -0.01x^2 + 0.4x + 50$

44. $g(x) = -0.01x^2 - 0.5x + 70$

Find y'.

45. $y = x^{-3/4} - 3x^{2/3} + x^{5/4} + \frac{2}{x^4}$

46. $y = 3x^{-2/3} + x^{3/4} + x^{6/5} + \frac{8}{x^3}$

47. $y = \frac{x}{7} + \frac{7}{x}$

48. $y = \frac{2}{x} - \frac{x}{2}$

49. If $f(x) = \sqrt{x}$, find $f'(4)$.

50. If $f(x) = x^2 + 4x - 5$, find $f'(10)$.

51. If $y = x + \frac{2}{x^3}$, find $\frac{dy}{dx}$ at $x = 1$.

52. If $y = \frac{4}{x^2}$, find $\frac{dy}{dx}$ at $x = -2$.

53. If $y = \sqrt[3]{x} + \sqrt{x}$, find $\frac{dy}{dx}$ at $x = 64$.

54. If $y = x^3 + 2x - 5$, find $\frac{dy}{dx}$ at $x = -2$.

55. If $y = \frac{2}{5x^3}$, find $\frac{dy}{dx}$ at $x = 4$.

56. If $y = \frac{1}{3x^4}$, find $\frac{dy}{dx}$ at $x = -1$.

57. Find an equation of the line tangent to the graph of $f(x) = x^2 - \sqrt{x}$
 a) at $(1, 0)$;
 b) at $(4, 14)$;
 c) at $(9, 78)$.

58. Find an equation of the line tangent to the graph of $f(x) = x^3 - 2x + 1$
 a) at $(2, 5)$;
 b) at $(-1, 2)$;
 c) at $(0, 1)$.

59. Find the equation of the line tangent to the graph of $g(x) = \sqrt[3]{x^2}$
 a) at $(-1, 1)$;
 b) at $(1, 1)$;
 c) at $(8, 4)$.

60. Find an equation of the line tangent to the graph of $f(x) = \frac{1}{x^2}$
 a) at $(1, 1)$;
 b) at $(3, \frac{1}{9})$;
 c) at $(-2, \frac{1}{4})$.

For each function, find the points on the graph at which the tangent line is horizontal. If none exist, state that fact.

61. $y = -x^2 + 4$

62. $y = x^2 - 3$

63. $y = x^3 - 2$

64. $y = -x^3 + 1$

65. $y = 5x^2 - 3x + 8$

66. $y = 3x^2 - 5x + 4$

67. $y = -0.01x^2 + 0.4x + 50$

68. $y = -0.01x^2 - 0.5x + 70$

69. $y = -2x + 5$

70. $y = 2x + 4$

71. $y = -3$

72. $y = 4$

73. $y = -\frac{1}{3}x^3 + 6x^2 - 11x - 50$

74. $y = -x^3 + x^2 + 5x - 1$

75. $y = x^3 - 6x + 1$

76. $y = \frac{1}{3}x^3 - 3x + 2$

77. $f(x) = \frac{1}{3}x^3 - 3x^2 + 9x - 9$

78. $f(x) = \frac{1}{3}x^3 + \frac{1}{2}x^2 - 2$

For each function, find the points on the graph at which the tangent line has slope 1.

79. $y = 6x - x^2$

80. $y = 20x - x^2$

81. $y = -0.01x^2 + 2x$

82. $y = -0.025x^2 + 4x$

83. $y = \frac{1}{3}x^3 - x^2 - 4x + 1$

84. $y = \frac{1}{3}x^3 + 2x^2 + 2x$

85. $y = \sqrt[3]{x} - \frac{1}{3}x$

86. $y = \sqrt{x} + \frac{1}{2}x$

APPLICATIONS

Life Sciences

87. **Growth of a child.** The median weight of a boy whose age is between 0 and 36 months is approximated by

$$w(t) = 8.15 + 1.82t - 0.0596t^2 + 0.000758t^3,$$

where t is in months and w is in pounds.

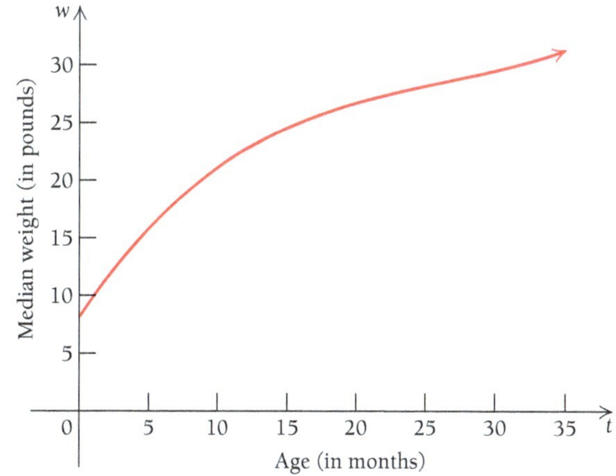

(*Source*: Centers for Disease Control. Developed by the National Center for Health Statistics in collaboration with the National Center for Chronic Disease Prevention and Health Promotion, 2000, reverified 2017.)

Use this model to approximate the following:
 a) The rate of change of weight with respect to time
 b) The weight of a boy at age 10 months
 c) The rate of change of a boy's weight with respect to time at age 10 months

88. Temperature during an illness. The temperature T of a person during a certain illness is given by

$$T(t) = -0.1t^2 + 1.2t + 98.6,$$

where T is the temperature, in degrees Fahrenheit, at time t, in days.

a) Find the rate of change of the person's temperature with respect to time.
b) Find the temperature at $t = 1.5$ days.
c) Find the rate of change at $t = 1.5$ days.

89. Heart rate. The equation

$$R(v) = \frac{6000}{v}$$

can be used to determine the heart rate, R, of a person whose heart pumps 6000 milliliters (mL) of blood per minute and v milliliters of blood per beat. (*Source*: *Mathematics Teacher*, Vol. 99, No. 4, November 2005.)

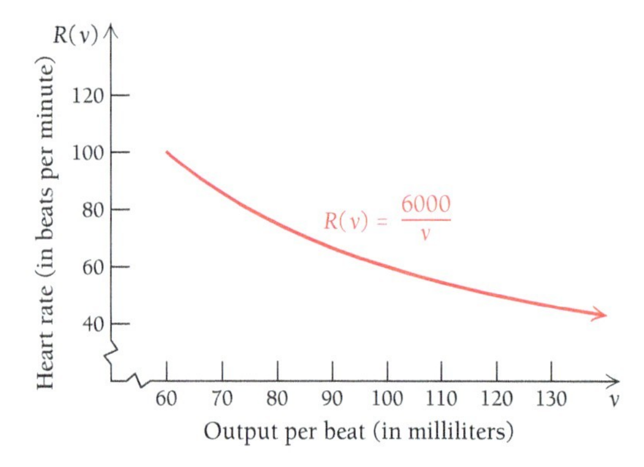

a) Find the rate of change of heart rate with respect to v, the output per beat.
b) Find the heart rate at $v = 80$ mL per beat.
c) Find the rate of change at $v = 80$ mL per beat.

90. Blood flow resistance. The equation

$$S(r) = \frac{1}{r^4}$$

can be used to determine the resistance to blood flow, S, of a blood vessel that has radius r, in millimeters (mm). (*Source*: *Mathematics Teacher*, Vol. 99, No. 4, November 2005.)

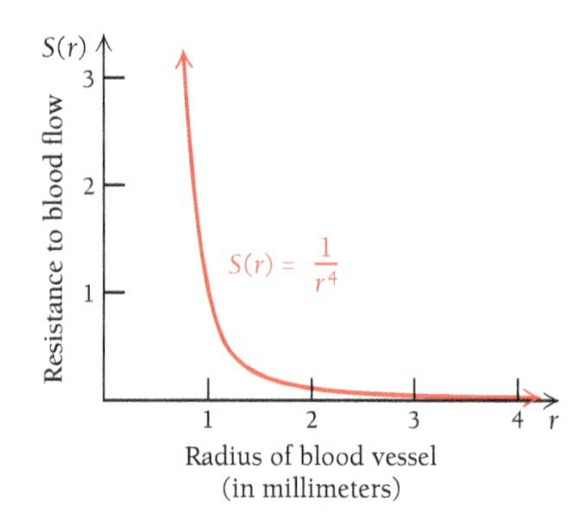

a) Find the rate of change of resistance with respect to r, the radius of the blood vessel.
b) Find the resistance at $r = 1.2$ mm.
c) Find the rate of change of S with respect to r when $r = 0.8$ mm.

Social Sciences

91. Population growth rate. In t years, the population of Kingsville grows from 100,000 to a size P given by

$$P(t) = 100{,}000 + 2000t^2.$$

a) Find the growth rate, dP/dt.
b) Find the population after 10 yr.
c) Find the growth rate at $t = 10$.
d) Explain the meaning of your answer to part (c).

92. Median age of women at first marriage. In the United States, median age of women at first marriage is approximated by

$$A(t) = 0.08t + 19.7,$$

where $A(t)$ is the median age of women marrying for the first time t years after 1950.

a) Find the rate of change of the median age A with respect to time t.
b) Explain the meaning of your answer to part (a).

General Interest

93. View to the horizon. The view V, or distance in miles, that one can see to the horizon from a height h, in feet, is given by

$$V = 1.22\sqrt{h}.$$

a) Find the rate of change of V with respect to h.
b) How far can one see to the horizon from an airplane window at a height of 40,000 ft?

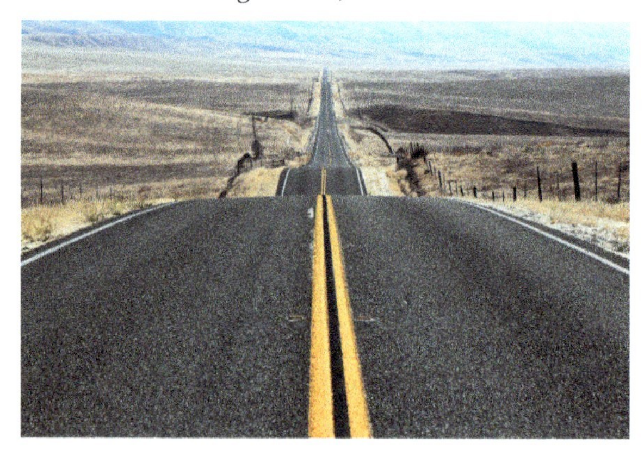

c) Find the rate of change at $h = 40{,}000$.
d) Explain the meaning of your answer to part (c).

94. Wave speed. The speed of a wave in shallow water is given by $s = 3.1\sqrt{d}$, where s is the speed, in meters per second, and d is the depth of the water, in meters. (*Source*: http://hyperphysics.phy-astr.gsu.edu/hbase/Waves/watwav2.html.)

a) Find the rate of change of s with respect to d.
b) What is the speed of a wave when the depth of the water is 10 m?
c) What is the rate of change in the wave's speed when the depth of the water is 10 m?

95. Super Bowl ticket prices. The price of a ticket to the Super Bowl t years after 1967 can be estimated by

$$p(t) = 0.858t^2 - 18.864t + 78.354.$$

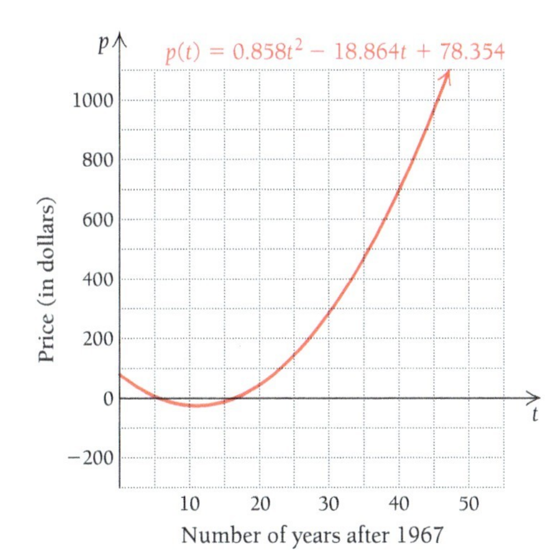

(*Source*: Based on data from extramustard.si.com.)

a) Use the function to predict the price of a Super Bowl ticket in 2020.

b) Find the rate of change of the ticket price with respect to the year, dp/dt.

c) At what rate will ticket prices be changing in 2020?

SYNTHESIS

For Exercises 96 and 97, find the interval(s) for which $f'(x)$ is positive.

96. $f(x) = x^2 - 4x + 1$

97. $f(x) = \frac{1}{3}x^3 - x^2 - 3x + 5$

98. Find the points on the graph of

$$y = x^4 - \tfrac{4}{3}x^2 - 4$$

at which the tangent line is horizontal.

99. Find the points on the graph of

$$y = 2x^6 - x^4 - 2$$

at which the tangent line is horizontal.

100. Use the derivative to help explain why $f(x) = x^5 + x^3$ is increasing for all x in $(-\infty, \infty)$.

101. Use the derivative to help explain why $g(x) = -2x - x^3$ is decreasing for all x in $(-\infty, \infty)$.

102. Use the derivative to help explain why $k(x) = \dfrac{1}{x^2}$ is decreasing for all x in $(0, \infty)$.

103. Use the derivative to help explain why $f(x) = x^3 + ax$ increases for all x in $(-\infty, \infty)$ when $a \geq 0$ but not when $a < 0$.

Find dy/dx. Each function can be differentiated using theorems developed in this section, if some algebra is performed beforehand.

104. $y = (x + 3)(x - 2)$

105. $y = (x - 1)(x + 1)$

106. $y = \dfrac{x^5 - x^3}{x^2}$

107. $y = \dfrac{x^5 + x}{x^2}$

108. $y = \sqrt{7x}$

109. $y = \sqrt[3]{8x}$

110. $y = \left(\sqrt{x} - \dfrac{1}{\sqrt{x}}\right)^2$

111. $y = (x + 1)^3$

112. Prove the Difference Rule:

$$\frac{d}{dx}[f(x) - g(x)] = \frac{d}{dx}f(x) - \frac{d}{dx}g(x).$$

Technology Connection

Graph each of the following. Then estimate the x-values at which tangent lines are horizontal.

113. $g(x) = x^4 - 3x^2 + 1$

114. $g(x) = \dfrac{5x^2 + 8x - 3}{3x^2 + 2}$

115. Let $f(x) = \sqrt{x} + \dfrac{1}{\sqrt{x}}$. Approximate the point(s) at which the slope of the line tangent to the graph of f is -1.

For each of the following, graph f and f' and then determine $f'(1)$.

116. $f(x) = x^4 - x^3$

117. $f(x) = \dfrac{4x}{x^2 + 1}$

118. $f(x) = \dfrac{5x^2 + 8x - 3}{3x^2 + 2}$

Answers to Quick Checks

1. The derivative of A with respect to r can be written as $P'(r)$; the derivative of A with respect to r can be written as A'; the derivative of A with respect to r can be written as $\dfrac{dA}{dr}$; the derivative of A with respect to r can be written as $\dfrac{d}{dr}P(r)$. **2. (a)** $y' = 15x^{14}$; **(b)** $y' = -7x^{-8} = -\dfrac{7}{x^8}$ **3. (a)** $y' = \frac{1}{4}x^{-3/4} = \dfrac{1}{4\sqrt[4]{x^3}}$; **(b)** $y' = -1.25x^{-2.25} = -\dfrac{1.25}{x^{2.25}}$ **4.** $y' = 0$ **5. (a)** $y' = 90x^8$; **(b)** $y' = 3\pi x^2$; **(c)** $y' = -\dfrac{8}{3x^5}$ **6.** $y' = 15x^4 + \dfrac{2}{3\sqrt[3]{x^2}} - \dfrac{2}{3x^3}$ **7.** 20.47 mi; 5.28 mi/hr **8.** $(-1, 7)$ and $(5, 25)$

1.6 The Product and Quotient Rules

- Differentiate using the Product and Quotient Rules.
- Use the Quotient Rule to differentiate the average cost, revenue, and profit functions.

The Product Rule

Some functions are easily viewed as the product of two other functions. For example, $F(x) = (x^2 + 3x)\sqrt{x}$ is the product of $f(x) = x^2 + 3x$ and $g(x) = \sqrt{x}$. However, as a rule, the derivative of a product is *not* the product of the derivatives.

THEOREM 7 The Product Rule

Let $F(x) = f(x) \cdot g(x)$. Then

$$F'(x) = \frac{d}{dx}[f(x) \cdot g(x)]$$
$$= f(x) \cdot \left[\frac{d}{dx}g(x)\right] + g(x) \cdot \left[\frac{d}{dx}f(x)\right].$$

The derivative of a product is the first factor times the derivative of the second factor, plus the second factor times the derivative of the first factor.

The proof of the Product Rule is outlined in Exercise 74 at the end of this section.

Usually we write the derivative of a product in simplified form. In Example 1, we do not simplify in order to better emphasize the steps being performed.

EXAMPLE 1 Find: **(a)** $\frac{d}{dx}[(x^4 - 2x^3 - 7)(3x^2 - 5x)]$ and

(b) $\frac{d}{dx}[(x^2 + 4x - 11)(7x^3 - \sqrt{x})]$. Do not simplify.

Solution

a) We let $f(x) = x^4 - 2x^3 - 7$ and $g(x) = 3x^2 - 5x$. By the Product Rule, the derivative of the given function is then

$$\frac{d}{dx}[\underbrace{(x^4 - 2x^3 - 7)}_{f(x)}\underbrace{(3x^2 - 5x)}_{g(x)}] = \underbrace{(x^4 - 2x^3 - 7)}_{f(x)} \cdot \underbrace{(6x - 5)}_{g'(x)} + \underbrace{(3x^2 - 5x)}_{g(x)} \cdot \underbrace{(4x^3 - 6x^2)}_{f'(x)}$$

b) We let $f(x) = x^2 + 4x - 11$ and $g(x) = 7x^3 - \sqrt{x}$.

$$\frac{d}{dx}[(x^2 + 4x - 11)(7x^3 - \sqrt{x})]$$
$$= (x^2 + 4x - 11)\left(21x^2 - \frac{1}{2}x^{-1/2}\right) + (7x^3 - x^{1/2})(2x + 4)$$

1 ✓

Quick Check 1 ✓

Use the Product Rule to find $\frac{dy}{dx}$. Do not simplify.

a) $y = (2x^5 + x - 1)(3x - 2)$

b) $y = (\sqrt{x} + 1)(\sqrt[5]{x} - x)$

EXAMPLE 2 Let $F(x) = (2x + 1)(x^2 - 3)$. Find $F'(x)$ two ways: first by multiplying the two binomials and differentiating the product, then by using the Product Rule. Verify that both methods give the same result.

Solution Multiplying the binomials, we have

$$F(x) = (2x + 1)(x^2 - 3) = 2x^3 + x^2 - 6x - 3.$$

Now, using the Sum–Difference Rule, we have

$$F'(x) = \frac{d}{dx}(2x^3) + \frac{d}{dx}(x^2) - \frac{d}{dx}(6x) - \frac{d}{dx}(3)$$
$$= 6x^2 + 2x - 6.$$

Quick Check 2✓

Let $G(x) = x^7$. Find $G'(x)$ by first using the Power Rule and then using the Product Rule, where $x^7 = x^5 \cdot x^2$ (or where $x^7 = x^3 \cdot x^4$). Verify that both methods give the same result.

Using the Product Rule, where the two factors are $f(x) = 2x + 1$ and $g(x) = x^2 - 3$, we have

$$F'(x) = \overbrace{(2x + 1)}^{f(x)}\overbrace{(2x)}^{g'(x)} + \overbrace{(x^2 - 3)}^{g(x)}\overbrace{(2)}^{f'(x)}$$

$$= 4x^2 + 2x + 2x^2 - 6 \quad \text{Using the distributive law}$$

$$= 6x^2 + 2x - 6.$$

We see that both methods give the same result. **2✓**

The Quotient Rule

The derivative of a quotient is *not* the quotient of the derivatives. To see why, consider x^5 and x^2 and assume $x \neq 0$. The quotient x^5/x^2 is x^3, and the derivative of this quotient is $3x^2$. The derivatives of the numerator and denominator are $5x^4$ and $2x$, respectively, and the quotient of these derivatives, $5x^4/(2x)$, is $(5/2)x^3$, which is not $3x^2$.

The rule for differentiating quotients is as follows.

THEOREM 8 The Quotient Rule

Let $F(x) = \dfrac{f(x)}{g(x)}$. Then $F'(x) = \dfrac{g(x) \cdot f'(x) - f(x) \cdot g'(x)}{[g(x)]^2}$.

The derivative of a quotient is the denominator times the derivative of the numerator, minus the numerator times the derivative of the denominator, all divided by the square of the denominator.

A proof of the Quotient Rule is outlined in Exercise 82 of Section 1.7.

EXAMPLE 3 Differentiate: $f(x) = \dfrac{1 + x^2}{x^3 + 1}$.

Solution We let $f(x) = 1 + x^2$ and $g(x) = x^3 + 1$. We have

$$\frac{dy}{dx} = \frac{\overbrace{(x^3 + 1)}^{g(x)}\overbrace{(2x)}^{f'(x)} - \overbrace{(1 + x^2)}^{f(x)}\overbrace{(3x^2)}^{g'(x)}}{\underbrace{(x^3 + 1)^2}_{(g(x))^2}} \quad \text{Using the Quotient Rule}$$

$$= \frac{2x^4 + 2x - 3x^2 - 3x^4}{(x^3 + 1)^2} \quad \text{Using the distributive law}$$

$$= \frac{-x^4 - 3x^2 + 2x}{(x^3 + 1)^2}. \quad \text{Simplifying}$$

3✓

Quick Check 3✓

Differentiate: $f(x) = \dfrac{1 - 3x}{x^2 + 2}$.

Simplify your result.

EXAMPLE 4 Let $G(x) = \dfrac{x^2 - 9}{x - 3}$. Find $G'(x)$ two ways: first by using the Quotient Rule and simplifying, then by first simplifying and then differentiating.

Solution Note that $x \neq 3$. This restriction will also apply to the derivative. Using the Quotient Rule, we have

Technology Connection

Checking Derivatives Graphically

To check Example 3, first enter the function:

$$y_1 = \frac{1 + x^2}{x^3 + 1}.$$

Then enter the possible derivative:

$$y_2 = \frac{-x^4 - 3x^2 + 2x}{(x^3 + 1)^2}.$$

As a third function, enter

$$y_3 = \text{nDeriv}(y_1, x, x).$$

Next, deselect y_1 and graph y_2 and y_3. Use different graph styles and the **Sequential** mode to see each graph as it appears on the screen.

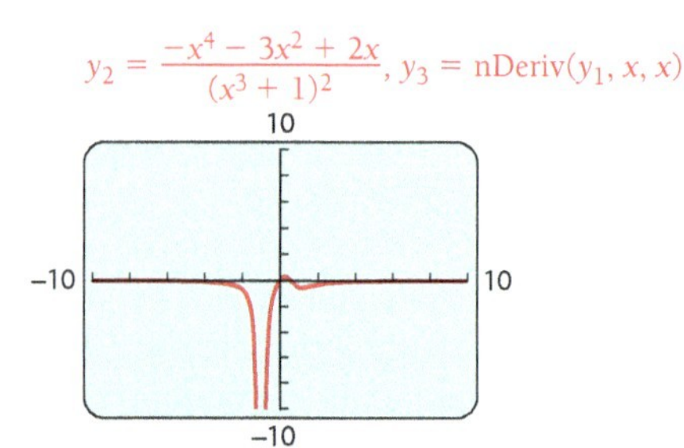

Since the graphs appear to coincide, it appears that $y_2 = y_3$ and we have a check. This is considered a partial check, however, because the graphs might not coincide with a different viewing window.

We can also use a table to check that $y_2 = y_3$.

X	Y2	Y3
-3	-.1686	-.1686
-2	-.6531	-.6531
-1	ERROR	ERROR
0	0	0
1	-.5	-.5
2	-.2963	-.2963
3	-.1301	-.1301

X = -3

EXERCISES

1. For the function

$$f(x) = \frac{x^2 - 4x}{x + 2},$$

use graphs and tables to determine which of the following seems to be the correct derivative.

a) $f'(x) = \frac{-x^2 - 4x - 8}{(x + 2)^2}$

b) $f'(x) = \frac{x^2 - 4x + 8}{(x + 2)^2}$

c) $f'(x) = \frac{x^2 + 4x - 8}{(x + 2)^2}$

2–4. Graphically check the results of Examples 1–3.

$$G'(x) = \frac{(x - 3)(2x) - (x^2 - 9)(1)}{(x - 3)^2}$$ Using the Quotient Rule: $\frac{dG}{dx} = \frac{g(x)f'(x) - f(x)g'(x)}{(g(x))^2}$

$$= \frac{2x^2 - 6x - x^2 + 9}{(x - 3)^2}$$ Using the distributive law

$$= \frac{x^2 - 6x + 9}{(x - 3)^2}$$ Simplifying

$$= \frac{(x - 3)^2}{(x - 3)^2}$$ Factoring the numerator

$$= 1, \quad x \neq 3.$$

Simplifying the function first, we have

$$G(x) = \frac{x^2 - 9}{x - 3} = \frac{(x + 3)(x - 3)}{x - 3} = x + 3, \quad \text{where } x \neq 3.$$

Differentiating, we have

$$G'(x) = 1, \quad x \neq 3.$$

Both methods give the same result. In general, it is easier to simplify the function before differentiating. 4 ✓

Quick Check 4 ✓

Let $y = \frac{x^2 + 4x + 3}{x + 1}$. Find $\frac{dy}{dx}$ first by using the Quotient Rule and simplifying, and then by simplifying the function before differentiating.

Application of the Quotient Rule

The total cost, total revenue, and total profit functions, discussed in Section R.4, pertain to the accumulated cost, revenue, and profit when x items are produced. Because of economies of scale and other factors, it is common for the cost, revenue (price), and profit for, say, the 10th item to differ from those for the 1000th item. For this reason, businesses often focus on *average* cost, revenue, and profit.

> **DEFINITION**
>
> If $C(x)$ is the cost of producing x items, then the **average cost** of producing x items is $\dfrac{C(x)}{x}$.
>
> If $R(x)$ is the revenue from the sale of x items, then the **average revenue** from selling x items is $\dfrac{R(x)}{x}$.
>
> If $P(x)$ is the profit from the sale of x items, then the **average profit** from selling x items is $\dfrac{P(x)}{x}$.

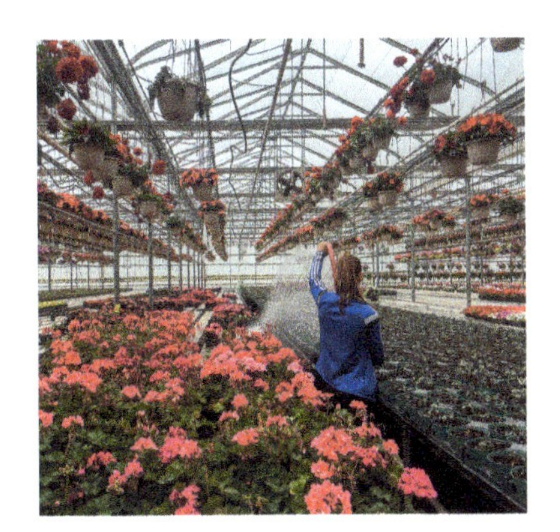

EXAMPLE 5 **Business.** Paulsen's Greenhouse finds that the cost, in dollars, of growing x hundred geraniums is modeled by

$$C(x) = 200 + 100\sqrt[4]{x}.$$

If revenue from the sale of x hundred geraniums is modeled by

$$R(x) = 120 + 90\sqrt{x},$$

find each of the following.

a) The average cost, average revenue, and average profit when 300 geraniums are grown and sold

b) The rate at which the average profit is changing when 300 geraniums are grown and sold

Solution

a) We let $\overline{C}$, $\overline{R}$, and $\overline{P}$ represent average cost, average revenue, and average profit, respectively. Thus,

$$\overline{C}(x) = \frac{C(x)}{x} = \frac{200 + 100\sqrt[4]{x}}{x};$$

$$\overline{R}(x) = \frac{R(x)}{x} = \frac{120 + 90\sqrt{x}}{x};$$

$$\overline{P}(x) = \frac{R(x) - C(x)}{x} = \frac{-80 + 90\sqrt{x} - 100\sqrt[4]{x}}{x}.$$

To find the average cost, average revenue, and average profit when 300 geraniums are grown and sold, we evaluate each function at $x = 3$:

$$\overline{C}(3) = \frac{200 + 100\sqrt[4]{3}}{3} \approx \$110.54 \text{ per hundred geraniums;}$$

$$\overline{R}(3) = \frac{120 + 90\sqrt{3}}{3} \approx \$91.96 \text{ per hundred geraniums;}$$

$$\overline{P}(3) = \frac{-80 + 90\sqrt{3} - 100\sqrt[4]{3}}{3} \approx -\$18.57 \text{ per hundred geraniums.}$$

b) To find the rate at which average profit is changing when 300 geraniums are grown and sold, we calculate $\overline{P}'(3)$:

$$\overline{P}'(x) = \frac{d}{dx}\left[\frac{-80 + 90x^{1/2} - 100x^{1/4}}{x}\right]$$

$$= \frac{x\left(\frac{1}{2}\cdot 90x^{1/2-1} - \frac{1}{4}\cdot 100x^{1/4-1}\right) - \left(-80 + 90x^{1/2} - 100x^{1/4}\right)\cdot 1}{x^2}$$

$$= \frac{45x^{1/2} - 25x^{1/4} + 80 - 90x^{1/2} + 100x^{1/4}}{x^2} = \frac{75x^{1/4} - 45x^{1/2} + 80}{x^2};$$

$$\overline{P}'(3) = \frac{75\sqrt[4]{3} - 45\sqrt{3} + 80}{3^2} \approx 11.20.$$

When 300 geraniums have been grown and sold, the average profit is increasing by \$11.20 per hundred geraniums for each additional 100 geraniums sold.

Section Summary

- The *Product Rule* is

$$\frac{d}{dx}[f(x)\cdot g(x)] = f(x)\cdot\frac{d}{dx}[g(x)] + g(x)\cdot\frac{d}{dx}[f(x)].$$

- The *Quotient Rule* is

$$\frac{d}{dx}\left[\frac{f(x)}{g(x)}\right] = \frac{g(x)\cdot f'(x) - f(x)\cdot g'(x)}{[g(x)]^2}.$$

- Be careful to note the order in which the factors are written when using the Quotient Rule. Because the Quotient Rule involves subtraction, the order in which the operations are performed is important.

1.6 Exercise Set

Differentiate each function two ways: first, by using the Product Rule; then, by multiplying the expressions before differentiating. Compare your results as a check. Use a graphing calculator to check your results.

1. $y = x^5 \cdot x^6$

2. $y = x^9 \cdot x^4$

3. $f(x) = (2x + 5)(3x - 4)$

4. $g(x) = (3x - 2)(4x + 1)$

5. $G(x) = 4x^2(x^3 + 5x)$

6. $F(x) = 3x^4(x^2 - 4x)$

7. $y = (3\sqrt{x} + 2)x^2$

8. $y = (4\sqrt{x} + 3)x^3$

9. $g(x) = (4x - 3)(2x^2 + 3x + 5)$

10. $f(x) = (2x + 5)(3x^2 - 4x + 1)$

11. $F(t) = (\sqrt{t} + 2)(3t - 4\sqrt{t} + 7)$

12. $G(t) = (2t + 3\sqrt{t} + 5)(\sqrt{t} + 4)$

Differentiate each function two ways: first, by using the Quotient Rule; then, by dividing the expressions before differentiating. Compare your results as a check. Use a graphing calculator to check your results.

13. $y = \frac{x^7}{x^3}$

14. $y = \frac{x^6}{x^4}$

15. $g(x) = \frac{3x^7 - x^3}{x}$

16. $f(x) = \frac{2x^5 + x^2}{x}$

17. $F(x) = \frac{x^3 + 27}{x + 3}$

18. $G(x) = \frac{8x^3 - 1}{2x - 1}$

19. $y = \frac{t^2 - 16}{t + 4}$

20. $y = \frac{t^2 - 25}{t - 5}$

Differentiate each function.

21. $f(x) = (3x^2 - 2x + 5)(4x^2 + 3x - 1)$

22. $g(x) = (5x^2 + 4x - 3)(2x^2 - 3x + 1)$

23. $y = \frac{5x^2 - 1}{2x^3 + 3}$

24. $y = \frac{3x^4 + 2x}{x^3 - 1}$

25. $G(x) = (8x + \sqrt{x})(5x^2 + 3)$

26. $F(x) = (-3x^2 + 4x)(7\sqrt{x} + 1)$

27. $g(t) = \dfrac{t}{3 - t} + 5t^3$

28. $f(t) = \dfrac{t}{5 + 2t} - 2t^4$

29. $F(x) = (x + 3)^2$

30. $G(x) = (5x - 4)^2$

31. $y = (x^3 - 4x)^2$

32. $y = (3x^2 - 4x + 5)^2$

33. $g(x) = 5x^{-3}(x^4 - 5x^3 + 10x - 2)$

34. $f(x) = 6x^{-4}(6x^3 + 10x^2 - 8x + 3)$

35. $F(t) = \left(t + \dfrac{2}{t}\right)(t^2 - 3)$

36. $G(t) = (3t^5 - t^2)\left(t - \dfrac{5}{t}\right)$

37. $y = \dfrac{x^2 + 1}{x^3 - 1} - 5x^2$

38. $y = \dfrac{x^3 - 1}{x^2 + 1} + 4x^3$

39. $y = \dfrac{\sqrt[3]{x} - 7}{\sqrt{x} + 3}$

40. $y = \dfrac{\sqrt{x} + 4}{\sqrt[3]{x} - 5}$

41. $f(x) = \dfrac{x}{x^{-1} + 1}$

42. $f(x) = \dfrac{x^{-1}}{x + x^{-1}}$

43. $F(t) = \dfrac{1}{t - 4}$

44. $G(t) = \dfrac{1}{t + 2}$

45. $f(x) = \dfrac{3x^2 + 2x}{x^2 + 1}$

46. $f(x) = \dfrac{3x^2 - 5x}{x^2 - 1}$

47. $g(t) = \dfrac{-t^2 + 3t + 5}{t^2 - 2t + 4}$

48. $f(t) = \dfrac{3t^2 + 2t - 1}{-t^2 + 4t + 1}$

49. Find an equation of the line tangent to the graph of $y = \sqrt{x}/(x + 1)$ at **(a)** $x = 1$; **(b)** $x = \frac{1}{4}$.

50. Find an equation of the line tangent to the graph of $y = 8/(x^2 + 4)$ at **(a)** $(0, 2)$; **(b)** $(-2, 1)$.

51. Find an equation of the line tangent to the graph of $y = 4x/(1 + x^2)$ at **(a)** $(0, 0)$; **(b)** $(-1, -2)$.

52. Find an equation of the line tangent to the graph of $y = x^2 + 3/(x - 1)$ at **(a)** $x = 2$; **(b)** $x = 3$.

APPLICATIONS

Business and Economics

53. **Average cost.** Preston's Leatherworks finds that the cost, in dollars, of producing x belts is given by $C(x) = 750 + 34x - 0.068x^2$. Find the rate at which average cost is changing when 175 belts have been produced.

54. **Average cost.** Tongue-Tied Sauces, Inc., finds that the cost, in dollars, of producing x bottles of barbecue sauce is given by $C(x) = 375 + 0.75x^{3/4}$. Find the rate at which average cost is changing when 81 bottles of barbecue sauce have been produced.

55. **Average revenue.** Preston's Leatherworks finds that the revenue, in dollars, from the sale of x belts is given by $R(x) = 45x^{9/10}$. Find the rate at which average revenue is changing when 175 belts have been produced and sold.

56. **Average revenue.** Tongue-Tied Sauces, Inc., finds that the revenue, in dollars, from the sale of x bottles of barbecue sauce is given by $R(x) = 7.5x^{0.7}$. Find the rate at which average revenue is changing when 81 bottles of barbecue sauce have been produced and sold.

57. **Average profit.** Use the information in Exercises 53 and 55 to determine the rate at which Preston's Leatherworks' average profit per belt is changing when 175 belts have been produced and sold.

58. **Average profit.** Use the information in Exercises 54 and 56 to determine the rate at which Tongue-Tied Sauces' average profit per bottle of barbecue sauce is changing when 81 bottles have been produced and sold.

59. **Average profit.** Sparkle Pottery has determined that the cost, in dollars, of producing x vases is given by

$$C(x) = 4300 + 2.1x^{0.6}.$$

If the revenue from the sale of x vases is given by $R(x) = 65x^{0.9}$, find the rate at which average profit per vase is changing when 50 vases have been made and sold.

60. **Average profit.** Cruzin' Boards has found that the cost, in dollars, of producing x skateboards is given by

$$C(x) = 900 + 18x^{0.7}.$$

If the revenue from the sale of x skateboards is given by $R(x) = 75x^{0.8}$, find the rate at which average profit per skateboard is changing when 20 skateboards have been built and sold.

Social Sciences

61. **Population growth.** The population P, in thousands, of the town of Coyote Wells is given by

$$P(t) = 75 + \frac{500t}{2t^2 + 9},$$

where t is the time, in years.

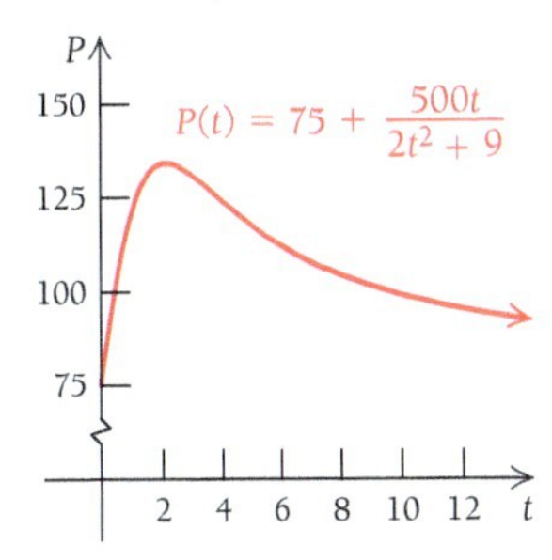

a) Find the growth rate.
b) Find the population after 2 yr.
c) Find the growth rate at $t = 2$ yr.
d) Find the population after 12 yr.
e) Find the growth rate at $t = 12$ yr.

Life and Physical Sciences

62. Temperature during an illness. Gina's temperature T during a recent illness is given by

$$T(t) = \frac{4t}{t^2 + 1} + 98.6,$$

where T is the temperature, in degrees Fahrenheit, at time t, in hours.

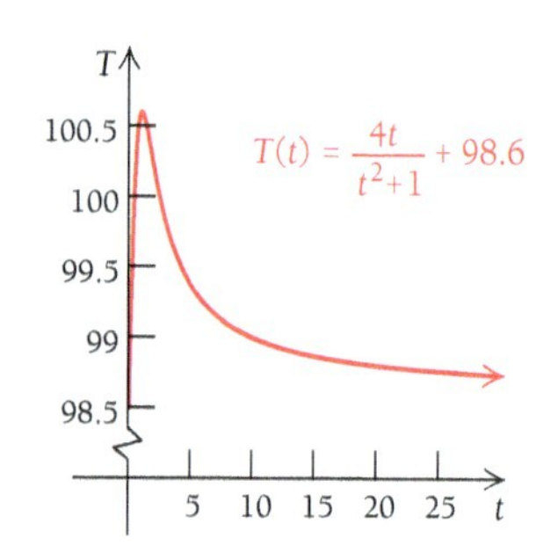

a) Find the rate of change of Gina's temperature with respect to time.
b) Find Gina's temperature at $t = 2$.
c) Find the rate of change of Gina's temperature at $t = 2$.
d) Find Gina's temperature after 1 day (at $t = 24$ hr).
e) Find the rate of change of Gina's temperature after 1 day.

SYNTHESIS

63. Use the graphs of f and g, shown below, to find the following.

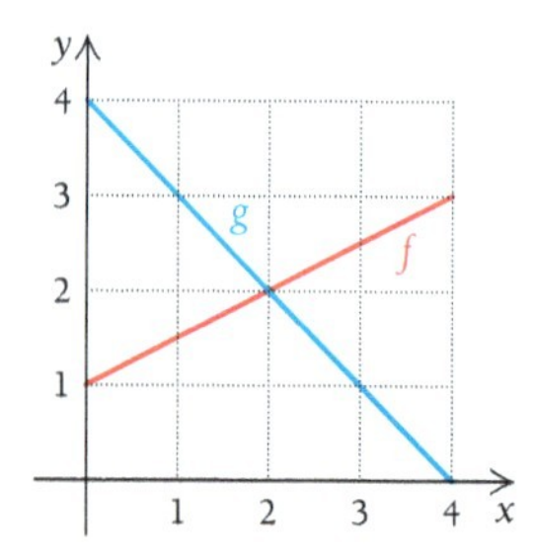

a) Find $(f \cdot g)'(1)$. (*Hint:* $(f \cdot g)(x) = f(x) \cdot g(x)$.)

b) Find $\left(\frac{f}{g}\right)'(2)$.

c) Find $(g \cdot f)'(3)$.

d) Find $\left(\frac{g}{f}\right)'(1)$.

64. Use the graphs of f and g, shown below, to find the following.

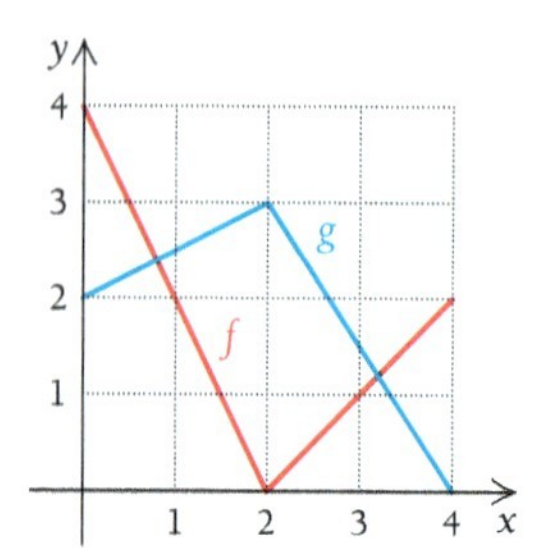

a) Find $(f \cdot g)'(3)$.

b) Find $\left(\frac{f}{g}\right)'(2)$.

c) Find $(f \cdot g)'(1)$.

d) Find $\left(\frac{g}{f}\right)'(1)$.

Differentiate each function.

65. $f(x) = \dfrac{7 - \dfrac{3}{2x}}{\dfrac{4}{x^2} + 5}$

66. $y(t) = 5t(t - 1)(2t + 3)$

67. $f(x) = x(3x^3 + 6x - 2)(3x^4 + 7)$

68. $g(x) = (x^3 - 8) \cdot \dfrac{x^2 + 1}{x^2 - 1}$

69. Let $f(x) = \dfrac{x}{x + 1}$ and $g(x) = \dfrac{-1}{x + 1}$.

a) Compute $f'(x)$.
b) Compute $g'(x)$.
c) What can you conclude about f and g on the basis of your results from parts (a) and (b)?

70. Let $f(x) = \dfrac{x^2}{x^2 - 1}$ and $g(x) = \dfrac{1}{x^2 - 1}$.

a) Compute $f'(x)$.
b) Compute $g'(x)$.
c) What can you conclude about the graphs of f and g on the basis of your results from parts (a) and (b)?

71. Write a rule for finding the derivative of $f(x) \cdot g(x) \cdot h(x)$. Describe the rule in as few words as possible.

72. Is the derivative of the reciprocal of $f(x)$ the reciprocal of the derivative of $f(x)$? Why or why not?

73. Sensitivity. The reaction R of the body to a dose Q of medication is often represented by the general function

$$R(Q) = Q^2\left(\frac{k}{2} - \frac{Q}{3}\right),$$

where k is a constant and R is in millimeters of mercury (mmHg) if the reaction is a change in blood pressure or in degrees Fahrenheit (°F) if the reaction is a change in temperature. The rate of change dR/dQ is defined to be the body's *sensitivity* to the medication.

a) Find a formula for the sensitivity.
b) Explain the meaning of your answer to part (a).

74. A proof of the Product Rule appears below. Provide a justification for each step.

a) $\frac{d}{dx}[f(x) \cdot g(x)] = \lim_{h \to 0} \frac{f(x+h)g(x+h) - f(x)g(x)}{h}$

b) $= \lim_{h \to 0} \frac{f(x+h)g(x+h) - f(x+h)g(x) + f(x+h)g(x) - f(x)g(x)}{h}$

c) $= \lim_{h \to 0} \frac{f(x+h)g(x+h) - f(x+h)g(x)}{h} + \lim_{h \to 0} \frac{f(x+h)g(x) - f(x)g(x)}{h}$

d) $= \lim_{h \to 0} \left[f(x+h) \cdot \frac{g(x+h) - g(x)}{h}\right] + \lim_{h \to 0} \left[g(x) \cdot \frac{f(x+h) - f(x)}{h}\right]$

e) $= f(x) \cdot \lim_{h \to 0} \frac{g(x+h) - g(x)}{h} + g(x) \cdot \lim_{h \to 0} \frac{f(x+h) - f(x)}{h}$

f) $= f(x) \cdot g'(x) + g(x) \cdot f'(x)$

g) $= f(x) \cdot \left[\frac{d}{dx} g(x)\right] + g(x) \cdot \left[\frac{d}{dx} f(x)\right]$

Technology Connection

75. Business. Refer to Exercises 54, 56, and 58. At what rate is Tongue-Tied Sauces' profit changing at the break-even point? At what rate is the average profit per bottle of barbecue sauce changing at that point?

76. Business. Refer to Exercises 53, 55, and 57. At what rate is Preston's Leatherworks' profit changing at the break-even point? At what rate is the average profit per belt changing at that point?

For each function in Exercises 77–80, graph f and f′. Then estimate the coordinates of the point where the tangent line to f is horizontal. If no such point exists, state that fact.

77. $f(x) = x^2(x-2)(x+2)$

78. $f(x) = \left(x + \frac{2}{x}\right)(x^2 - 3)$

79. $f(x) = \frac{x^3 - 1}{x^2 + 1}$

80. $f(x) = \frac{4x}{x^2 + 1}$

81. Use a graph to decide which of the following seems to be the correct derivative of the function in Exercise 80.

$y_1 = \frac{2}{x}$

$y_2 = \frac{4 - 4x}{x^2 + 1}$

$y_3 = \frac{4 - 4x^2}{(x^2 + 1)^2}$

$y_4 = \frac{4x^2 - 4}{(x^2 + 1)^2}$

Answers to Quick Checks

1. (a) $y' = (2x^5 + x - 1)(3) + (3x - 2)(10x^4 + 1)$; **(b)** $y' = (\sqrt{x} + 1)\left(\frac{1}{5\sqrt[5]{x^4}} - 1\right) + (\sqrt[5]{x} - x)\left(\frac{1}{2\sqrt{x}}\right)$

2. $\frac{d}{dx}(x^7) = 7x^6$; $\frac{d}{dx}(x^5 \cdot x^2) = x^5 \cdot 2x + x^2 \cdot 5x^4 = 2x^6 + 5x^6 = 7x^6$ **3.** $y' = \frac{3x^2 - 2x - 6}{(x^2 + 2)^2}$

4. $\frac{d}{dx}\left(\frac{x^2 + 4x + 3}{x + 1}\right) = \frac{(x+1)(2x+4) - (x^2 + 4x + 3)(1)}{(x+1)^2}$

$= \frac{2x^2 + 6x + 4 - x^2 - 4x - 3}{(x+1)^2} = \frac{x^2 + 2x + 1}{(x+1)^2} = \frac{(x+1)^2}{(x+1)^2} = 1, x \neq -1$

$\frac{x^2 + 4x + 3}{x + 1} = \frac{(x+3)(x+1)}{x+1} = x + 3, x \neq -1$. Thus, $\frac{d}{dx}(x + 3) = 1, x \neq -1$.

1.7

- Find the composition of two functions.
- Differentiate using the Chain Rule.

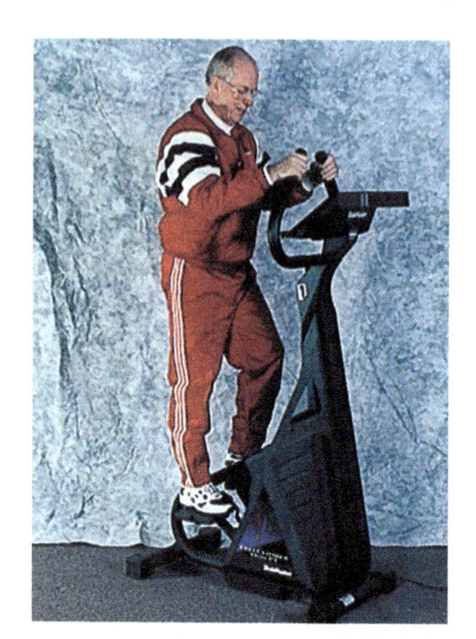

Author Marv Bittinger and his size-$11\frac{1}{2}$ running shoes

The Chain Rule

Composition of Functions

Before discussing the Chain Rule, let's consider *composition of functions.*

One author of this text exercises three times a week at a local YMCA. When he recently bought a pair of running shoes, the box indicated equivalent men's shoe sizes in five countries.

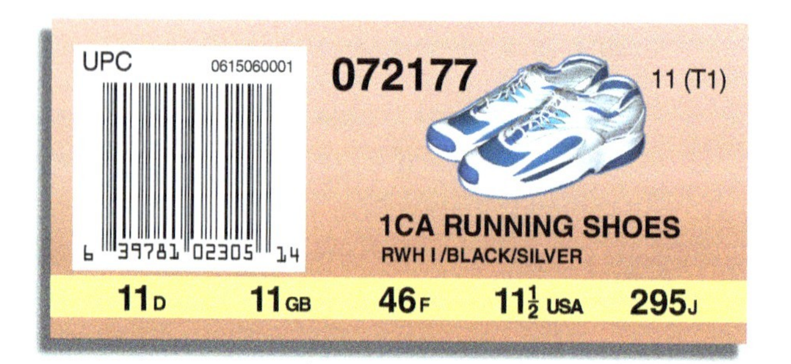

This suggests that there are functions that convert shoe sizes from those used in one country to those used in other countries. There is, indeed, a function g that gives a correspondence between men's shoe sizes in the United States and those in France:

$$g(x) = \frac{4x + 92}{3},$$

where x is the U.S. size and $g(x)$ is the French size. Thus, U.S. size $11\frac{1}{2}$ corresponds to French size

$$g(11\tfrac{1}{2}) = \frac{4 \cdot 11\frac{1}{2} + 92}{3}, \quad \text{or } 46.$$

There is also a function f that gives a correspondence between French and Japanese shoe sizes. That function is given by

$$f(x) = \frac{15x - 100}{2},$$

where x is the French size and $f(x)$ is the corresponding Japanese size. Thus, French size 46 corresponds to Japanese size

$$f(46) = \frac{15 \cdot 46 - 100}{2}, \quad \text{or } 295.$$

It seems reasonable to conclude that U.S. shoe size $11\frac{1}{2}$ corresponds to Japanese size 295 and that some function h describes this correspondence. Can we find a formula for h?

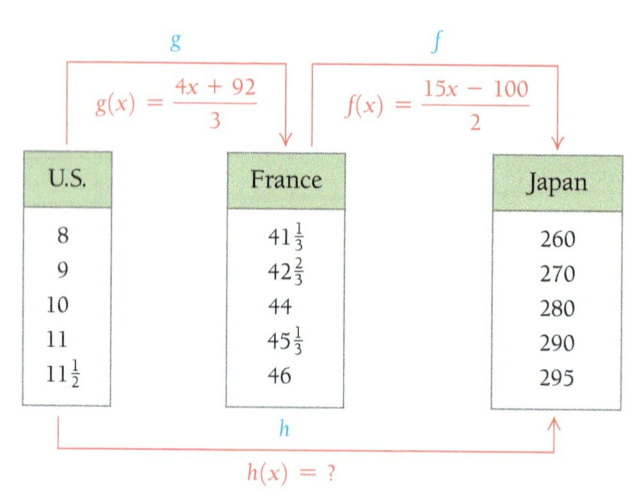

A U.S. size x corresponds to a French size $g(x) = (4x + 92)/3$. If we replace x in $f(x)$ with $(4x + 92)/3$, we can find the corresponding shoe size in Japan:

$$f(g(x)) = \frac{15[4x + 92]/3 - 100}{2}$$ This gives the Japanese shoe size corresponding to French size $g(x)$ and U.S. size x.

$$= \frac{5(4x + 92) - 100}{2} = \frac{20x + 460 - 100}{2}$$

$$= \frac{20x + 360}{2} = 10x + 180.$$ Simplifying

This gives a formula for h: $h(x) = 10x + 180$. As a check, U.S. size $11\frac{1}{2}$ corresponds to Japanese size $h(11\frac{1}{2}) = 10(11\frac{1}{2}) + 180 = 295$. The function h is the *composition* of f and g, symbolized by $f \circ g$ and read as "f composed with g."

DEFINITION

The **composed** function $f \circ g$, the **composition** of f and g, is defined as

$$(f \circ g)(x) = f(g(x)).$$

We can visualize the composition of functions as shown below.

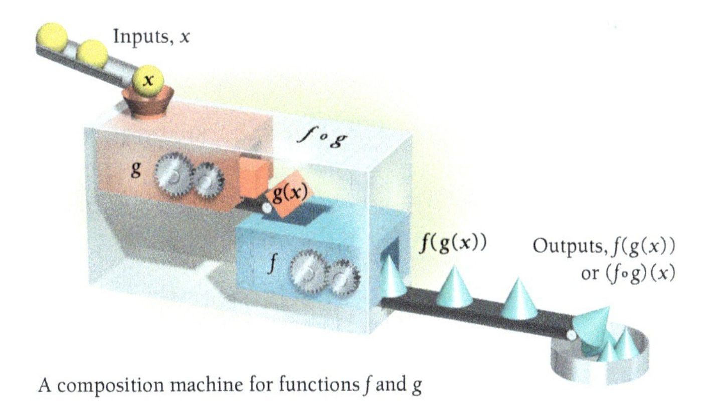

A composition machine for functions f and g

To find $(f \circ g)(x)$, we substitute $g(x)$ for x in $f(x)$. The function $g(x)$ is nested within $f(x)$.

EXAMPLE 1 For $f(x) = x^4$ and $g(x) = 2 + x^3$, find $(f \circ g)(x)$ and $(g \circ f)(x)$.

Solution Consider each function separately:

$$f(x) = x^4$$ This function raises each input to the 4th power.

and

$$g(x) = 2 + x^3.$$ This function adds 2 to the cube of each input.

We find $(f \circ g)(x) = f(g(x))$ by substituting $g(x)$ for x in $f(x)$:

$$(f \circ g)(x) = f(g(x)) = f(2 + x^3)$$

$$= (2 + x^3)^4$$ Using $g(x)$ as an input

$$= 16 + 32x^3 + 24x^6 + 8x^9 + x^{12}.$$

We find $(g \circ f)(x) = g(f(x))$ by substituting $f(x)$ for x in $g(x)$:

$$(g \circ f)(x) = g(f(x)) = g(x^4)$$

$$= 2 + (x^4)^3 = 2 + x^{12}.$$ Using $f(x)$ as an input **1 ✓**

Quick Check 1 ✓

Let $f(x) = x^2 + x$ and $g(x) = 3x + 2$.

Find:

a) $(f \circ g)(x)$;

b) $(g \circ f)(x)$.

Example 1 shows that, in general, $(f \circ g)(x) \neq (g \circ f)(x)$.

Using the Chain Rule to Differentiate a Composition of Functions

How do we differentiate a composition of functions? The following theorem tells us.

> **THEOREM 9 The Chain Rule**
>
> The derivative of the composition $f \circ g$ is given by
>
> $$\frac{d}{dx}[(f \circ g)(x)] = \frac{d}{dx}[f(g(x))] = f'(g(x)) \cdot g'(x).$$

To better understand the Chain Rule, suppose that a video game manufacturer wants to determine its rate of profit, in *dollars per day*. One way to find this rate is to multiply the rate of profit, in *dollars per unit*, by the production rate, in *units per day*. That is,

$$\text{Change in profit with respect to time} = \left[\begin{array}{c}\text{Change in profit with}\\ \text{respect to units produced}\end{array}\right] \cdot \left[\begin{array}{c}\text{Change in number of units}\\ \text{produced with respect to time}\end{array}\right],$$

or

$$\frac{\text{Profit in dollars}}{\text{day}} = \left[\frac{\text{Profit in dollars}}{\text{units}}\right] \cdot \left[\frac{\text{units}}{\text{day}}\right].$$

EXAMPLE 2 **Business: Rate of Profit.** GameBoss Video's profit, in dollars, is given by $y = f(u) = 0.1u^2 - 500$, where u is the number of units sold. Its sales are given by $u = g(x) = 125x + 40$, where x is the number of days after a new promotion begins. Find the rate at which profit is changing 5 days after the promotion begins.

Solution To find the rate of change in profit, y, on the xth day, we find dy/dx. Thus, we compose f and g, because $y = (f \circ g)(x)$ relates profit y to number of days x:

$$\begin{aligned} y &= (f \circ g)(x) = f(g(x)) \\ &= 0.1(125x + 40)^2 - 500. \quad \text{Substituting} \end{aligned}$$

Differentiating, we have

$$\begin{aligned} \frac{dy}{dx} = \frac{d}{dx}[(f \circ g)(x)] &= \frac{d}{dx}[0.1(125x + 40)^2 - 500] \\ &= 2 \cdot 0.1(125x + 40) \cdot 125 \quad \text{Using the Chain Rule} \\ &= 3125x + 1000. \quad \text{Simplifying} \end{aligned}$$

On the 5th day, profit is growing at a rate of $3125(5) + 1000 = \$16{,}625$ per day.

Note that we can also find dy/dx, the rate of change in profit per day, by finding the product of dy/du, the rate of change in profit per unit, and du/dx, the rate of change in units sold per day. We have

$$\frac{dy}{du} = \frac{d}{du}(0.1u^2 - 500) = 0.2u\,\frac{\text{dollars}}{\text{unit}}, \quad \text{and} \quad \frac{du}{dx} = \frac{d}{dx}(125x + 40) = 125\,\frac{\text{units}}{\text{day}}.$$

Thus,

$$\begin{aligned} \frac{dy}{dx} &= \frac{dy}{du} \cdot \frac{du}{dx} \\ &= (0.2u)(125) \\ &= 25u \\ &= 25(125x + 40). \quad \text{Substituting} \end{aligned}$$

Quick Check 2 ✓

GameBoss Video releases a special commemorative game. The company's profit, in thousands of dollars, from sales of this game is given by $y = u^2 + u$, where u is the number of units sold. If the number of units sold is given by $u = x^2 + x$, where x is the number of days since the game was released, find dy/dx and evaluate it at $x = 5$. Explain what this number represents.

For $x = 5$, we have $dy/dx = 25(125(5) + 40) = \$16{,}625$ per day.

Comparing units, we have

$$\frac{dy}{dx} = \frac{dy}{du} \cdot \frac{du}{dx}$$

or

$$\frac{\text{dollars}}{\text{day}} = \frac{\text{dollars}}{\text{unit}} \cdot \frac{\text{units}}{\text{day}}.$$

In a manner of speaking, the units "simplify," leaving dollars/day. 2 ✓

Note in Example 2 that the derivative of $y = 0.1(125x + 40)^2 - 500$ is

$$\frac{dy}{dx} = 0.1 \cdot 2(125x + 40)^1 \cdot 125.$$

This suggests a general rule.

THEOREM 10 The Extended Power Rule

Suppose that $g(x)$ is a differentiable function of x. Then, for any real number k,

$$\frac{d}{dx}[g(x)]^k = k[g(x)]^{k-1} \cdot \frac{d}{dx}g(x).$$

A justification of the Extended Power Rule, for k a positive integer, is outlined in Exercise 83. The proof for all real values of k is outside the scope of this text.

EXAMPLE 3 Differentiate:

a) $y = (x^2 + 3)^2$; **b)** $h(x) = 6(x^3 - 5x + 1)^{10}$.

Solution

a) Using the Extended Power Rule and letting $g(x) = x^2 + 3$, we have

$$\begin{aligned} \frac{dy}{dx} &= \frac{d}{dx}(x^2 + 3)^2 \\ &= 2(x^2 + 3)^1 \cdot (2x) && \text{Using the Extended Power Rule} \\ &= 4x(x^2 + 3) \\ &= 4x^3 + 12x. && \text{Simplifying} \end{aligned}$$

As a check, we rewrite $(x^2 + 3)^2$ as $x^4 + 6x^2 + 9$. Differentiating, we have

$$\frac{d}{dx}(x^4 + 6x^2 + 9) = 4x^3 + 12x. \quad \text{In this case, both methods work equally well.}$$

b) Letting $g(x) = x^3 - 5x + 1$, we have

$$\begin{aligned} h'(x) &= \frac{d}{dx}(6(x^3 - 5x + 1)^{10}) \\ &= 6 \cdot 10(x^3 - 5x + 1)^9 \cdot (3x^2 - 5) && \text{Using the Extended Power Rule} \\ &= 60(x^3 - 5x + 1)^9(3x^2 - 5). && \text{Simplifying} \end{aligned}$$

3 ✓

Quick Check 3 ✓

Differentiate:

a) $y = (3x + 7)^4$;

b) $y = -5(x^2 + 3x + 4)^7$.

EXAMPLE 4 Differentiate: **(a)** $y = (1 + x^3)^{1/2}$; **(b)** $y = \dfrac{5}{(1 - x^2)^3}$.

Solution

a) We have $\dfrac{dy}{dx} = \dfrac{1}{2}(1 + x^3)^{1/2-1} \cdot 3x^2$

$$= \frac{3x^2}{2}(1 + x^3)^{-1/2} = \frac{3x^2}{2\sqrt{1 + x^3}}.$$

b) Here we rewrite the function as $y = 5(1 - x^2)^{-3}$ and use the Extended Power Rule:

$$\frac{dy}{dx} = 5(-3(1 - x^2)^{-4}(-2x))$$

$$= \frac{30x}{(1 - x^2)^4}. \qquad \text{Simplifying}$$

4✓

Quick Check 4✓

a) Use the Extended Power Rule to differentiate $y = (x^4 + 2x^2 + 1)^3$.

b) Explain why

$$\frac{d}{dx}\left[(x^2 + 4x + 1)^4\right] = 4(x^2 + 4x + 1)^3 \cdot 2x + 4$$

is incorrect.

EXAMPLE 5 Differentiate: **(a)** $f(x) = (3x - 5)^4(7 - x)^{10}$; **(b)** $f(x) = \sqrt[4]{\dfrac{x + 3}{x - 2}}$.

Solution

a) Here we combine the Product Rule and the Extended Power Rule:

$$f'(x) = (3x - 5)^4 \cdot 10(7 - x)^9(-1) + (7 - x)^{10} \cdot 4(3x - 5)^3(3)$$
$$= -10(3x - 5)^4(7 - x)^9 + (7 - x)^{10}\left[12(3x - 5)^3\right]$$
$$= 2(3x - 5)^3(7 - x)^9[-5(3x - 5) + 6(7 - x)] \qquad \text{Factoring out } 2(3x - 5)^3(7 - x)^9$$
$$= 2(3x - 5)^3(7 - x)^9(-15x + 25 + 42 - 6x)$$
$$= 2(3x - 5)^3(7 - x)^9(67 - 21x).$$

b) Here we use the Quotient Rule to differentiate the inside function:

$$\frac{d}{dx}\sqrt[4]{\frac{x + 3}{x - 2}} = \frac{d}{dx}\left(\frac{x + 3}{x - 2}\right)^{1/4} = \frac{1}{4}\left(\frac{x + 3}{x - 2}\right)^{1/4-1}\left[\frac{(x - 2)1 - 1(x + 3)}{(x - 2)^2}\right]$$
$$= \frac{1}{4}\left(\frac{x + 3}{x - 2}\right)^{-3/4}\left[\frac{x - 2 - x - 3}{(x - 2)^2}\right]$$
$$= \frac{1}{4}\left(\frac{x + 3}{x - 2}\right)^{-3/4}\left[\frac{-5}{(x - 2)^2}\right], \quad \text{or} \quad \frac{-5}{4(x + 3)^{3/4}(x - 2)^{5/4}}.$$

5✓

Quick Check 5✓

Differentiate:

$$f(x) = \frac{2x^2 - 1}{(3x^4 + 2)^2}.$$

The Chain Rule may be required more than once when finding a derivative.

EXAMPLE 6 Differentiate $f(x) = (x^2 + (5 + 2x)^4)^7$.

Solution Let $g(x) = x^2 + (5 + 2x)^4$. Thus, $y = [g(x)]^7$, and by the Extended Power Rule, we have

$$\frac{dy}{dx} = 7[g(x)]^6 \cdot g'(x).$$

To find $g'(x)$, we use the Extended Power Rule again:

$$g'(x) = \frac{d}{dx}(x^2 + (5 + 2x)^4) = 2x + 4(5 + 2x)^3 \cdot 2 = 2x + 8(5 + 2x)^3.$$

Substituting, we have

$$f'(x) = 7[g(x)]^6 \cdot g'(x)$$
$$= 7(x^2 + (5 + 2x)^4)^6 \cdot (2x + 8(5 + 2x)^3).$$

6✓

Quick Check 6✓

Differentiate $y = (x^3 + (4x^2 + 2x + 1)^5)^{10}$.

Section Summary

- The *composition* of $f(x)$ with $g(x)$ is written $(f \circ g)(x)$ and is defined as $(f \circ g)(x) = f(g(x))$.
- In general, $(f \circ g)(x) \neq (g \circ f)(x)$.
- The *Chain Rule* is used to differentiate a composition of functions. If

$$F(x) = (f \circ g)(x) = f(g(x)),$$

then

$$F'(x) = \frac{d}{dx}[(f \circ g)(x)] = f'(g(x)) \cdot g'(x).$$

- The *Extended Power Rule* tells us that if $y = [f(x)]^k$, then

$$y' = \frac{d}{dx}[f(x)]^k = k[f(x)]^{k-1} \cdot f'(x).$$

1.7 Exercise Set

Differentiate each function using the Chain Rule.

1. $y = (3 - 2x)^2$
2. $y = (2x + 1)^2$

Check by expanding and then differentiating.

3. $y = (7 - x)^{55}$
4. $y = (8 - x)^{100}$
5. $y = \sqrt{3x^2 - 4}$
6. $y = \sqrt{4x^2 + 1}$
7. $y = \sqrt{1 - x}$
8. $y = \sqrt{1 + 8x}$
9. $y = (4x^2 + 1)^{-50}$
10. $y = (8x^2 - 6)^{-40}$
11. $y = (x - 4)^8(2x + 3)^6$
12. $y = (x + 5)^7(4x - 1)^{10}$
13. $y = \dfrac{1}{(4x + 5)^2}$
14. $y = \dfrac{1}{(3x + 8)^2}$
15. $y = \dfrac{4x^2}{(7 - 5x)^3}$
16. $y = \dfrac{7x^3}{(4 - 9x)^5}$
17. $f(x) = -5x(2x - 3)^4$
18. $f(x) = -3x(5x + 4)^6$
19. $F(x) = (5x + 2)^4(2x - 3)^8$
20. $g(x) = (3x - 1)^7(2x + 1)^5$
21. $f(x) = x^2\sqrt{4x - 1}$
22. $f(x) = x^3\sqrt{5x + 2}$
23. $F(x) = \sqrt[4]{x^2 - 5x + 2}$
24. $G(x) = \sqrt[3]{x^5 + 6x}$
25. $f(x) = \left(\dfrac{3x - 1}{5x + 2}\right)^4$
26. $f(x) = \left(\dfrac{2x}{x^2 + 1}\right)^3$
27. $h(x) = \left(\dfrac{1 - 3x}{2 - 7x}\right)^{-5}$
28. $g(x) = \left(\dfrac{2x + 3}{5x - 1}\right)^{-4}$
29. $f(x) = \dfrac{(5x - 4)^7}{(6x + 1)^3}$
30. $f(x) = \dfrac{(2x + 3)^4}{(3x - 2)^5}$
31. $g(x) = \sqrt{\dfrac{3 + 2x}{5 - x}}$
32. $g(x) = \sqrt{\dfrac{4 - x}{3 + x}}$

Find $\dfrac{dy}{du}$, $\dfrac{du}{dx}$, and $\dfrac{dy}{dx}$.

33. $y = \dfrac{15}{u^3}$ and $u = 2x + 1$
34. $y = \sqrt{u}$ and $u = x^2 - 1$
35. $y = u^{50}$ and $u = 4x^3 - 2x^2$
36. $y = \dfrac{u + 1}{u - 1}$ and $u = 1 + \sqrt{x}$

Find $\dfrac{dy}{dx}$ for each pair of functions.

37. $y = 5u^2 + 3u$, where $u = x^3 + 1$
38. $y = u^3 - 7u^2$, where $u = x^2 + 3$
39. Find $\dfrac{dy}{dt}$ if $y = \dfrac{1}{u^2 + u}$ and $u = 5 + 3t$.
40. Find $\dfrac{dy}{dt}$ if $y = \dfrac{1}{3u^5 - 7}$ and $u = 7t^2 + 1$.
41. Find an equation for the tangent line to the graph of $y = (x^3 - 4x)^{10}$ at the point $(2, 0)$.
42. Find an equation for the tangent line to the graph of $y = \sqrt{x^2 + 3x}$ at the point $(1, 2)$.

43. Find an equation for the tangent line to the graph of $y = x\sqrt{2x + 3}$ at the point $(3, 9)$.

44. Find an equation for the tangent line to the graph of $y = \left(\frac{2x + 3}{x - 1}\right)^3$ at the point $(2, 343)$.

45. Consider

$$g(x) = \left(\frac{6x + 1}{2x - 5}\right)^2.$$

a) Find $g'(x)$ using the Extended Power Rule.

b) Note that $g(x) = \frac{36x^2 + 12x + 1}{4x^2 - 20x + 25}$. Find $g'(x)$ using the Quotient Rule.

c) Compare your answers to parts (a) and (b). Which approach was easier, and why?

46. Consider

$$f(x) = \frac{x^2}{(1 + x)^5}.$$

a) Find $f'(x)$ using the Quotient Rule and the Extended Power Rule.

b) Note that $f(x) = x^2(1 + x)^{-5}$. Find $f'(x)$ using the Product Rule and the Extended Power Rule.

c) Compare your answers to parts (a) and (b).

47. Let $f(u) = u^3$ and $g(x) = u = 2x^4 + 1$. Find $(f \circ g)'(-1)$.

48. Let $f(u) = \frac{u + 1}{u - 1}$ and $g(x) = u = \sqrt{x}$. Find $(f \circ g)'(4)$.

49. Let $f(u) = \sqrt[3]{u}$ and $g(x) = u = 1 + 3x^2$. Find $(f \circ g)'(2)$.

50. Let $f(u) = 2u^5$ and $g(x) = u = \frac{3 - x}{4 + x}$. Find $(f \circ g)'(-10)$.

51. Let $h(x) = (3x^2 + 2x)^5$.

a) Find functions f and g such that $h(x) = (f \circ g)(x)$.

b) Find $(f \circ g)'(2)$.

52. Let $h(x) = \sqrt{1 + 5x^2}$.

a) Find functions f and g such that $h(x) = (f \circ g)(x)$.

b) Find $(f \circ g)'(4)$.

53. Let $h(x) = \frac{x^3 + 1}{x^3 + 4}$.

a) Find functions f and g such that $h(x) = (f \circ g)(x)$.

b) Find $(f \circ g)'(1)$.

54. Let $h(x) = \frac{1}{x^2 + 2x}$.

a) Find functions f and g such that $h(x) = (f \circ g)(x)$.

b) Find $(f \circ g)'(-3)$.

Differentiate each function.

55. $f(x) = (2x^3 + (4x - 5)^2)^6$

56. $f(x) = \left(-x^5 + 4x + \sqrt{2x + 1}\right)^3$

57. $f(x) = \sqrt{x^2 + \sqrt{1 - 3x}}$

58. $f(x) = \sqrt[3]{2x + (x^2 + x)^4}$

APPLICATIONS

Business and Economics

59. Total revenue. A total-revenue function is given by

$$R(x) = 1000\sqrt{x^2 - 0.1x},$$

where $R(x)$ is the total revenue, in thousands of dollars, from the sale of x airplanes. Find the rate at which total revenue is changing when 20 airplanes have been sold.

60. Total cost. A total-cost function is given by

$$C(x) = 2000(x^2 + 2)^{1/3} + 700,$$

where $C(x)$ is the total cost, in thousands of dollars, of producing x airplanes. Find the rate at which total cost is changing when 20 airplanes have been produced.

61. Total profit. Use the total-cost and total-revenue functions in Exercises 59 and 60 to find the rate at which total profit is changing when 20 airplanes have been produced and sold.

62. Total cost. Solid Seats, Inc., determines that its total cost, in thousands of dollars, for producing x chairs is

$$C(x) = \sqrt{5x^2 + 60},$$

and it plans to boost production t months from now according to the function

$$x(t) = 20t + 40.$$

How fast will costs be rising 4 months from now?

63. Compound interest. If \$1000 is invested at interest rate r, compounded quarterly, in 5 yr it will grow to an amount A, given by (see Section R.1)

$$A = \$1000\left(1 + \frac{r}{4}\right)^{20}.$$

a) Find the rate of change, dA/dr, and give its units.

b) Explain what dA/dr represents.

64. Compound interest. If \$1000 is invested at interest rate r, compounded monthly, in 3 yr it will grow to an amount A given by (see Section R.1)

$$A = \$1000\left(1 + \frac{r}{12}\right)^{36}.$$

a) Find the rate of change, dA/dr, and give its units.

b) Explain what dA/dr represents.

65. Business profit. Lightning Electronics is selling laptop computers. Its total profit, in dollars, is given by

$$P(x) = 0.08x^2 + 80x,$$

where x is the number of units produced and sold. Suppose that x is a function of time, in months, where $x = 5t + 1$.

a) Find the total profit as a function of time t.
b) Find the rate of change of total profit when $t = 48$ months.

66. **Consumer demand.** Suppose the demand function for a new autobiography is given by

$$D(p) = \frac{80{,}000}{p},$$

and that price p is a function of time, given by $p = 1.6t + 9$, where t is in days.

a) Find the demand as a function of time t.
b) Find the rate of change of the quantity demanded when $t = 100$ days.

Life and Physical Sciences

67. **Chemotherapy.** The dosage for Carboplatin chemotherapy drugs depends on several parameters for the particular drug as well as the age, weight, and sex of the patient. For female patients, the formulas giving the dosage for such drugs are

$$D = 0.85A(c + 25) \quad \text{and} \quad c = (140 - y)\frac{w}{72x},$$

where A and x depend on which drug is used, D is the dosage in milligrams (mg), c is called the creatine clearance, y is the patient's age in years, and w is the patient's weight in kilograms (kg). (*Source*: *U.S. Oncology*.)

a) Suppose a patient is a 45-year-old woman and the drug has parameters $A = 5$ and $x = 0.6$. Use this information to write formulas for D and c that express D as a function of c and c as a function of w.
b) Use your formulas from part (a) to compute dD/dc.
c) Use your formulas from part (a) to compute dc/dw.
d) Compute dD/dw.
e) Explain what dD/dw represents.

68. **Weights.** An object that weighs x kilograms at sea level has an equivalent weight of p pounds, where $p(x) = 2.20462x$. The equivalent weight in stone (a British unit), s, is given by $s(p) = \frac{1}{14}p$.

a) Find $(s \circ p)(100)$, and explain what this value represents.
b) Evaluate $\frac{d}{dx}(s \circ p)(x)$ at $x = 100$, including the units, and explain what this value represents.

69. **Boiling point of water and altitude.** The boiling point of water, C, in degrees Celsius, m meters above sea level is given by $C(m) = -\frac{1}{225}m + 100$. The equivalent temperature in Fahrenheit degrees is given by

$$F(C) = \frac{9}{5}C + 32.$$

(*Source*: www.engineeringtoolbox.com.)

a) Find $(F \circ C)(3000)$, and explain what this value represents.
b) Evaluate $\frac{d}{dx}(F \circ C)(m)$ at $m = 3000$, including the units, and explain what this value represents.

70. **Women's shoe sizes.** If x is the length of a woman's foot, in inches, then her shoe size in the United States is given by $U(x) = 3x - 21$. If U is a woman's shoe size in the United States, then her equivalent shoe size in Europe is given by $E = 1.35U + 28.25$. (*Source*: Based on data from gemplers.com.)

a) Find $(E \circ U)(9)$, and explain what this value represents.
b) Evaluate $\frac{d}{dx}(E \circ U)(x)$ at $x = 9$, including the units, and explain what this value represents.

SYNTHESIS

If $f(x)$ is a function, then $(f \circ f)(x) = f(f(x))$ is the composition of f with itself. This is called an iterated function, and the composition can be repeated many times. For example, $(f \circ f \circ f)(x) = f(f(f(x)))$. Iterated functions are very useful in many areas, including finance (compound interest is a simple case) and the sciences (in weather forecasting, for example). In Exercises 71–74, find the given derivative.

71. If $f(x) = x^2 + 1$, find $\frac{d}{dx}[(f \circ f)(x)]$.

72. If $f(x) = x + \sqrt{x}$, find $\frac{d}{dx}[(f \circ f)(x)]$.

73. If $f(x) = x^2 + 1$, find $\frac{d}{dx}[(f \circ f \circ f)(x)]$.

74. If $f(x) = \sqrt[3]{x}$, find $\frac{d}{dx}[(f \circ f \circ f)(x)]$.

Do you see a shortcut?

Differentiate.

75. $y = \sqrt[3]{x^3 + 6x + 1} \cdot x^5$

76. $y = (x\sqrt{1 + x^2})^3$

77. $y = \frac{\sqrt{1 - x^2}}{1 - x}$

78. $y = \left(\frac{x^2 - x - 1}{x^2 + 1}\right)^3$

79. $g(x) = \sqrt{\frac{x^2 - 4x}{2x + 1}}$

80. $f(t) = \sqrt{3t + \sqrt{t}}$

81. $F(x) = [6x(3 - x)^5 + 2]^4$

82. **Proof of the Quotient Rule.** The following is a proof of the Quotient Rule for differentiation (Section 1.6) that uses the Chain Rule. Let $y = \frac{f(x)}{g(x)}$. Provide a justification for each step.

a) $y = f(x) \cdot [g(x)]^{-1}$ ____________________
b) $\frac{dy}{dx} = \frac{d}{dx}(f(x) \cdot [g(x)]^{-1})$ ____________________
c) $\frac{dy}{dx} = f(x) \cdot \frac{d}{dx}[g(x)]^{-1} + [g(x)]^{-1} \cdot \frac{d}{dx}f(x)$

____

d) $\frac{dy}{dx} = f(x) \cdot (-1[g(x)]^{-2} \cdot g'(x)) + [g(x)]^{-1} \cdot f'(x)$

____

e) $\frac{dy}{dx} = -\frac{f(x)\cdot g'(x)}{[g(x)]^2} + \frac{f'(x)}{g(x)}$ ____________

f) $\frac{dy}{dx} = -\frac{f(x)\cdot g'(x)}{[g(x)]^2} + \frac{f'(x)\cdot g(x)}{[g(x)]^2}$ ____________

g) $\frac{dy}{dx} = \frac{g(x)\cdot f'(x) - f(x)\cdot g'(x)}{[g(x)]^2}$ ____________

83. The Extended Power Rule (for positive integer powers) can be verified using the Product Rule. For example, if $y = [f(x)]^2$, then the Product Rule is applied by recognizing that $[f(x)]^2 = f(x)\cdot f(x)$. Therefore,

$$\begin{aligned}\frac{d}{dx}(f(x)\cdot f(x)) &= f(x)\cdot f'(x) + f'(x)\cdot f(x)\\ &= 2f(x)\cdot f'(x).\end{aligned}$$

a) Use the Product Rule to show that $\frac{d}{dx}[f(x)]^3 = 3[f(x)]^2\cdot f'(x)$.

b) Use the Product Rule to show that $\frac{d}{dx}[f(x)]^4 = 4[f(x)]^3\cdot f'(x)$.

c) Generalize the pattern established in parts (a) and (b).

Technology Connection

For the function in each of Exercises 84 and 85, graph f and f′ over the given interval. Then estimate points at which the line tangent to f is horizontal.

84. $f(x) = 1.68x\sqrt{9.2 - x^2}$; $[-3, 3]$

85. $f(x) = \sqrt{6x^3 - 3x^2 - 48x + 45}$; $[-5, 5]$

Answers to Quick Checks

1. (a) $f(g(x)) = 9x^2 + 15x + 6$;
(b) $g(f(x)) = 3x^2 + 3x + 2$

2. $\frac{dy}{dx} = \frac{dy}{du}\cdot\frac{du}{dx} = (2u + 1)(2x + 1) = (2(x^2 + x) + 1)(2x + 1) = (2x^2 + 2x + 1)(2x + 1)$

At $x = 5$, $dy/dx = 671$, which means that on the 5th day, GameBoss Video's profit is growing by 671 thousand dollars per day.

3. (a) $\frac{dy}{dx} = 12(3x + 7)^3$;
(b) $\frac{dy}{dx} = -35(x^2 + 3x + 4)^6(2x + 3)$

4. (a) $y' = 12x(x^4 + 2x^2 + 1)^2(x^2 + 1)$
(b) The result lacks parentheses around $2x + 4$. It should be written: $4(x^2 + 4x + 1)^3(2x + 4)$.

5. $y' = \frac{-36x^5 + 24x^3 + 8x}{(3x^4 + 2)^3}$

6. $\frac{dy}{dx} = 10(x^3 + (4x^2 + 2x + 1)^5)^9\cdot(3x^2 + 10(4x^2 + 2x + 1)^4(4x + 1))$

1.8 Higher-Order Derivatives

- Find derivatives of higher order.
- Given a formula for distance, find velocity and acceleration.

The derivative f' is itself a function that can be differentiated. For $y = f(x)$, the derivative of $y' = f'(x)$, with respect to x, is written

$$y'' = \frac{d}{dx}f'(x) = f''(x).$$

This is called the *second-order derivative*, or *second derivative*, of *f*. It expresses the rate at which $f'(x)$ is changing with respect to x.

For example, let $y = f(x) = x^5 - 3x^4 + x$. Its derivative f' is given by

$$y' = \frac{d}{dx}f(x) = f'(x) = 5x^4 - 12x^3 + 1.$$

Its second derivative is

$$y'' = \frac{d}{dx}f'(x) = f''(x) = 20x^3 - 36x^2.$$

For higher-order derivatives, we use the notation $y^{(n)} = f^{(n)}(x)$ to express the nth derivative of f. For the function above, we have

$$y^{(3)} = f^{(3)}(x) = 60x^2 - 72x; \quad \text{The third derivative of } f$$
$$y^{(4)} = f^{(4)}(x) = 120x - 72; \quad \text{The fourth derivative of } f$$
$$y^{(5)} = f^{(5)}(x) = 120; \quad \text{The fifth derivative of } f$$
$$y^{(6)} = f^{(6)}(x) = 0. \quad \text{The sixth derivative of } f$$

Leibniz notation for the second derivative of a function given by $y = f(x)$ is

$$\frac{d}{dx}\left(\frac{dy}{dx}\right), \quad \text{or} \quad \frac{d^2y}{dx^2}.$$

For higher-order derivatives, Leibniz notation is

$$\frac{d^3y}{dx^3}, \quad \frac{d^4y}{dx^4}, \quad \text{and so on.}$$

These are read as "the third derivative of y with respect to x," "the fourth derivative of y with respect to x," and so on. Note that the superscripts 3 and 4 are *not* exponents.

EXAMPLE 1 For $y = 1/x$, find d^2y/dx^2.

Solution We have $y = x^{-1}$, so

$$\frac{dy}{dx} = -1 \cdot x^{-1-1} = -x^{-2}, \quad \text{or} \quad -\frac{1}{x^2}.$$

Then

$$\frac{d^2y}{dx^2} = (-2)(-1)x^{-2-1} = 2x^{-3}, \quad \text{or} \quad \frac{2}{x^3}.$$

EXAMPLE 2 For $y = (x^2 + 2)^6$, find y' and y''.

Solution To find y', we use the Extended Power Rule:

$$\frac{dy}{dx} = 6(x^2 + 2)^5(2x)$$
$$= 12x(x^2 + 2)^5.$$

To find y'', we use the Product Rule and the Extended Power Rule:

$$y'' = \frac{d}{dx}[12x(x^2 + 2)^5]$$
$$= 12\frac{d}{dx}[x(x^2 + 2)^5] \quad \text{Using Theorem 5 from Section 1.5}$$
$$= 12\left(x \cdot \frac{d}{dx}(x^2 + 2)^5 + (x^2 + 2)^5 \cdot \frac{d}{dx}(x)\right) \quad \text{Using the Product Rule}$$
$$= 12(x \cdot (5(x^2 + 2)^4(2x)) + (x^2 + 2)^5 \cdot 1) \quad \text{Using the Extended Power Rule}$$
$$= 12(10x^2(x^2 + 2)^4 + (x^2 + 2)^5)$$
$$= 12(x^2 + 2)^4(10x^2 + (x^2 + 2)) \quad \text{Factoring}$$
$$= 12(x^2 + 2)^4(11x^2 + 2). \quad \text{Simplifying}$$

1 ✓

Quick Check 1 ✓

a) Find y'':

(i) $y = -6x^4 + 3x^2$;

(ii) $y = \dfrac{2}{x^3}$;

(iii) $y = (3x^2 + 1)^2$.

b) Find $\dfrac{d^4}{dx^4}\left[\dfrac{1}{x}\right]$.

Velocity and Acceleration

We have seen that a function's derivative represents an instantaneous rate of change. When the function relates distance traveled to time, the instantaneous rate of change is called *speed*, or *velocity*.* The letter v is generally used to stand for velocity.

> **DEFINITION**
>
> The **velocity** of an object that is $s(t)$ units from a starting point at time t is given by
>
> $$\text{Velocity} = v(t) = s'(t) = \lim_{h \to 0} \frac{s(t + h) - s(t)}{h}.$$

Often velocity is a function of time. When a jet takes off or a moving vehicle comes to a stop, the change in velocity is easily felt by passengers. The rate at which velocity changes is called *acceleration*. If a Prius requires 10 sec to reach 60 mi/hr and a Tesla requires 4 sec, then the Tesla has *faster acceleration*. We generally use a to represent acceleration, which we regard as the rate at which velocity is changing.

> **DEFINITION**
>
> **Acceleration** $= a(t) = v'(t) = s''(t)$.

It is important to use correct units in every real-world application. Since velocity is the change in distance per unit of time, it has units of miles/hour, feet/second, meters/second, and so on. Acceleration is the change in velocity per unit of time, and it is given in units such as (miles/hour)/hour, (feet/second)/second, and (meters/second)/second, or mi/hr^2, ft/sec^2, and m/sec^2.

EXAMPLE 3 **Free Fall.** From the point at which an object is dropped, the distance it falls in t seconds, assuming negligible air resistance, is approximately

$$s(t) = 4.9t^2,$$

where $s(t)$ is in meters (m). If a stone is dropped from a cliff, find each of the following, assuming that air resistance is negligible: **(a)** how far the stone has traveled 5 sec after being dropped, **(b)** how fast it is traveling 5 sec after being dropped, and **(c)** its acceleration after it has been falling for 5 sec.

Solution

a) After 5 sec, the stone has traveled approximately

$$s(5) = 4.9(5)^2 = 4.9(25) = 122.5 \text{ m}.$$

b) The velocity at which the stone is traveling is approximated using

$$v(t) = s'(t) = 9.8t.$$

Thus,

$$v(5) \approx 9.8 \cdot 5 \approx 49 \text{ m/sec}.$$

c) The stone's acceleration after t sec is constant:

$$a(t) = v'(t) = s''(t) \approx 9.8 \text{ m/sec}^2.$$

Thus, $s''(5) \approx 9.8 \text{ m/sec}^2$. 2✓

Quick Check 2✓

A pebble is dropped from a hot-air balloon. Approximate how far it has fallen, how fast it is falling, and its acceleration after 3.5 sec. Let $s(t) = 16t^2$, where t is in seconds and s is in feet.

*In this text, the words "speed" and "velocity" are used interchangeably. In physics and engineering, this is not done, since velocity requires direction and speed does not.

On Earth, objects fall at a constant acceleration of approximately 9.8 m/sec^2, or 32 ft/sec^2. This value is called the *gravitational constant* and is abbreviated g. Often, a frame of reference is assumed in which "up" is considered positive, so objects falling toward the ground have negative velocity and negative acceleration.

If the graph of $y = s(t)$ represents an object's distance traveled, then the object's velocity at any time is the slope of the tangent line at that point. If the object "speeds up" (accelerates) or "slows down" (decelerates), these changes in velocity will appear as upward and downward bends, respectively, in the graph.

EXAMPLE 4 **Analyzing Velocity and Acceleration Graphically.** Kimberly leaves her home (distance $= 0$) for a 1.2-hr bicycle ride. The graph of her distance traveled with respect to time t is shown below.

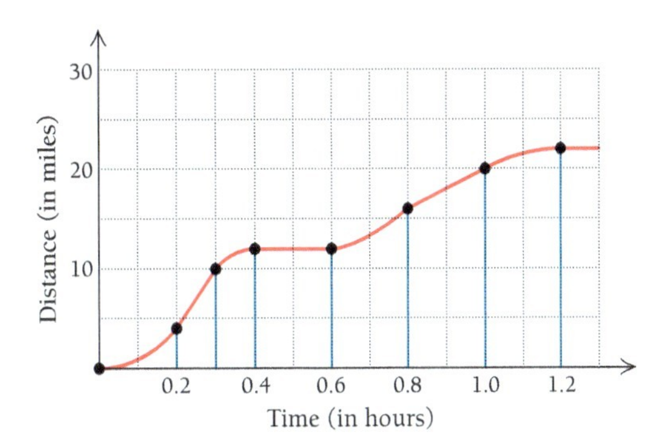

Find the interval(s) in which Kimberly is:

a) traveling at constant velocity;

b) accelerating (speeding up);

c) decelerating (slowing down).

Solution

a) Kimberly is traveling at constant velocity when the slopes of the tangent lines do not change, that is, when the graph is linear. Thus, she is traveling at a constant velocity in the intervals $(0.2, 0.3)$, $(0.4, 0.6)$, and $(0.8, 1.0)$. Since her velocity is constant in these intervals, the second derivative is zero; that is, she is neither accelerating nor decelerating during these intervals. Note that in the interval $(0.4, 0.6)$ the slopes of the tangent lines are zero, indicating that she has stopped.

b) Kimberly is speeding up (accelerating—the second derivative is positive) during the intervals $(0, 0.2)$ and $(0.6, 0.8)$. Acceleration appears as an upward bend in the graph.

c) Kimberly is slowing down (decelerating—the second derivative is negative) during the intervals $(0.3, 0.4)$ and $(1.0, 1.2)$. Deceleration (or negative acceleration) appears as a downward bend in the graph.

The upward and downward bends in the graph in Example 4 are examples of *concavities*, discussed in Chapter 3.

EXAMPLE 5 **Business: Tablet Sales.** The number of Apple iPads sold per year, in millions, t years after 2010, can be approximated by

$$N(t) = 0.106t^4 - 1.452t^3 + 5.659t^2 + 1.946t + 20.714.$$

(*Source*: Based on data from Apple, Inc.) Find $N(7)$, $N'(7)$, and $N''(7)$, and explain what these values represent.

Solution We have

$$N(7) = 0.106(7)^4 - 1.452(7)^3 + 5.659(7)^2 + 1.946(7) + 20.714 = 68.097.$$

In 2017, Apple sold approximately 68.097 million iPads.

The derivative is

$$N'(t) = \frac{d}{dt}(0.106t^4 - 1.452t^3 + 5.659t^2 + 1.946t + 20.714)$$
$$= 0.424t^3 - 4.356t^2 + 11.318t + 1.946.$$

Thus,

$$N'(7) = 0.424(7)^3 - 4.356(7)^2 + 11.318(7) + 1.946 = 13.16.$$

In 2017, Apple's yearly sales of iPads were increasing at the rate of about 13.16 million units/yr.

In the following graph, we see the sales during 2017 represented as a point on the graph of N at $t = 7$, and the rate of change of sales as the slope of the tangent line of the graph at $t = 7$.

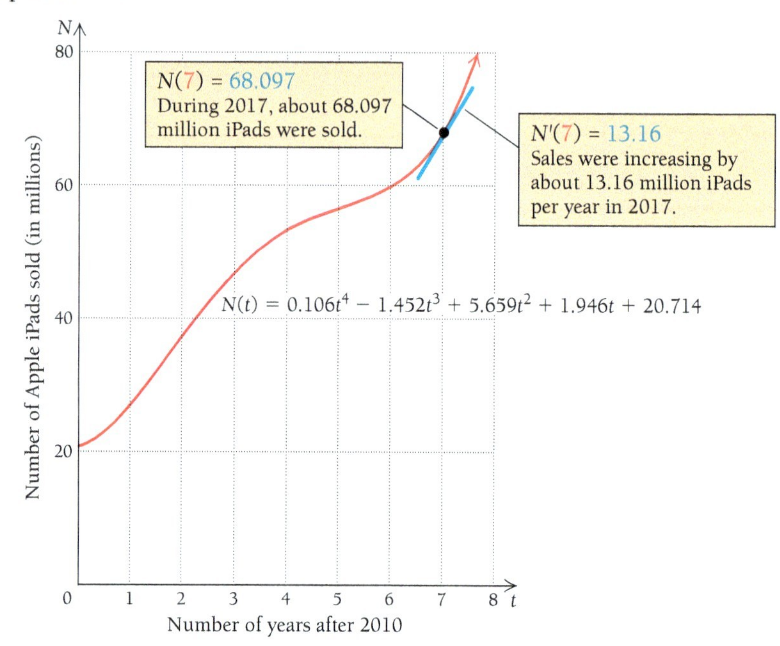

The second derivative is

$$N''(t) = \frac{d}{dt}(0.424t^3 - 4.356t^2 + 11.318t + 1.946)$$
$$= 1.272t^2 - 8.712t + 11.318.$$

Thus,

$$N''(7) = 1.272(7)^2 - 8.712(7) + 11.318 = 12.662.$$

In 2017, the rate of change is, itself, changing at a rate of 12.662 million units/year^2. Since the change in the rate of change of sales is positive, sales are accelerating. On the graph, we see this as an upward-turning bend in the graph of N at $t = 7$. **3 ✓**

Quick Check 3 ✓

Using the model in Example 5, find $N(4)$, $N'(4)$, and $N''(4)$, and explain what these values represent.

Section Summary

- The *second derivative* is the derivative of the first derivative of a function. In symbols, $f''(x) = \frac{d}{dx}[f'(x)]$.
- The second derivative represents the rate of change of the rate of change. In other words, it represents the rate of change of the first derivative.
- A real-world example of a second derivative is *acceleration*. If $s(t)$ represents distance traveled as a function of time for a moving object, then $v(t) = s'(t)$ represents speed (velocity). Any change in speed is the acceleration: $a(t) = v'(t) = s''(t)$.
- The common notation for the nth derivative of a function f is $f^{(n)}(x)$, or $\frac{d^n}{dx^n}f(x)$.

1.8 Exercise Set

Find d^2y/dx^2.

1. $y = x^5 + 9$
2. $y = x^4 - 7$
3. $y = 5x^3 + 4x$
4. $y = 2x^4 - 5x$
5. $y = 4x^2 + 3x - 1$
6. $y = 4x^2 - 5x + 7$
7. $y = 6x - 3$
8. $y = 7x + 2$
9. $y = \frac{1}{x^2}$
10. $y = \frac{1}{x^3}$
11. $y = \sqrt[4]{x}$
12. $y = \sqrt{x}$

Find $f''(x)$.

13. $f(x) = x^4 + \frac{3}{x}$
14. $f(x) = x^3 - \frac{5}{x}$
15. $f(x) = x^{1/3}$
16. $f(x) = x^{1/5}$
17. $f(x) = 4x^{-3}$
18. $f(x) = 2x^{-2}$
19. $f(x) = (x^3 + 2x)^6$
20. $f(x) = (x^2 + 3x)^7$
21. $f(x) = \sqrt[4]{(x^2 + 1)^3}$
22. $f(x) = \sqrt[3]{(x^2 - 1)^2}$

Find y''.

23. $y = x^{3/2} - 5x$
24. $y = x^{2/3} + 4x$
25. $y = (x^3 - x)^{3/4}$
26. $y = (x^4 + x)^{2/3}$
27. $y = \frac{3x + 1}{2x - 3}$
28. $y = \frac{2x + 3}{5x - 1}$
29. For $y = x^5$, find d^4y/dx^4.
30. For $y = x^4$, find d^4y/dx^4.
31. For $y = x^6 - x^3 + 2x$, find d^5y/dx^5.
32. For $y = x^7 - 8x^2 + 2$, find d^6y/dx^6.
33. For $f(x) = x^{-3} + 2x^{1/3}$, find $f^{(5)}(x)$.
34. For $f(x) = x^{-2} - x^{1/2}$, find $f^{(4)}(x)$.

APPLICATIONS

Life and Physical Sciences

35. Given
$$s(t) = t^3 + t,$$
where $s(t)$ is in feet and t is in seconds, find each of the following.
   a) $v(t)$
   b) $a(t)$
   c) The velocity and acceleration when $t = 4$ sec

36. Given
$$s(t) = -10t^2 + 2t + 5,$$
where $s(t)$ is in meters and t is in seconds, find each of the following.
   a) $v(t)$
   b) $a(t)$
   c) The velocity and acceleration when $t = 1$ sec

37. Given
$$s(t) = t^2 - \frac{1}{2}t + 3,$$
where $s(t)$ is in meters and t is in seconds, find each of the following.
   a) $v(t)$
   b) $a(t)$
   c) The velocity and acceleration when $t = 1$ sec

38. Given
$$s(t) = 3t + 10,$$
where $s(t)$ is in miles and t is in hours, find each of the following.
   a) $v(t)$
   b) $a(t)$
   c) The velocity and acceleration when $t = 2$ hr
   d) When the distance function is given by a linear function, we have *uniform motion*. What does uniform motion mean in terms of velocity and acceleration?

39. **Free fall.** When an object is dropped, the distance it falls in t seconds, assuming negligible air resistance, is given by
$$s(t) = 16t^2,$$
where $s(t)$ is in feet. Suppose a medic's reflex hammer falls from a hovering helicopter. Find **(a)** how far the hammer falls in 3 sec, **(b)** how fast the hammer is traveling 3 sec after being dropped, and **(c)** the hammer's acceleration after it has been falling for 3 sec.

40. **Free fall.** (See Exercise 39.) Suppose a worker drops a bolt from a bridge high above a river. Assuming negligible air resistance, find **(a)** how far the bolt falls in 2 sec, **(b)** how fast the bolt is traveling 2 sec after being dropped, and **(c)** the bolt's acceleration after it has been falling for 2 sec.

41. **Free fall.** Find the velocity and acceleration of the stone in Example 3 after it has been falling for 2 sec.

42. **Free fall.** Find the velocity and acceleration of the stone in Example 3 after it has been falling for 3 sec.

43. The following graph describes a bicycle racer's distance from a roadside television camera.

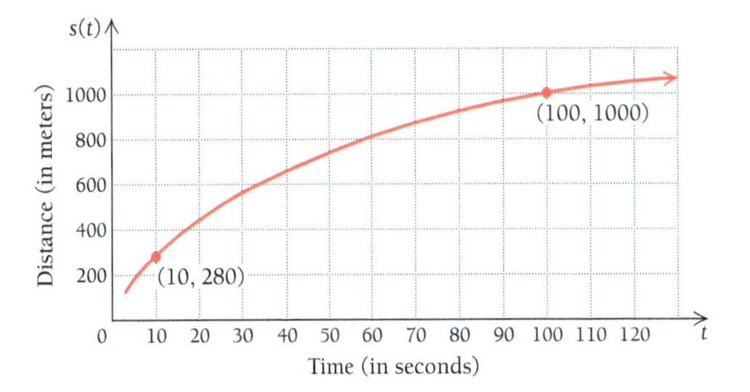

a) When is the bicyclist's velocity the greatest? How can you tell?
b) Is the bicyclist's acceleration positive or negative? How can you tell?

44. The following graph describes an airplane's distance from its last point of rest.

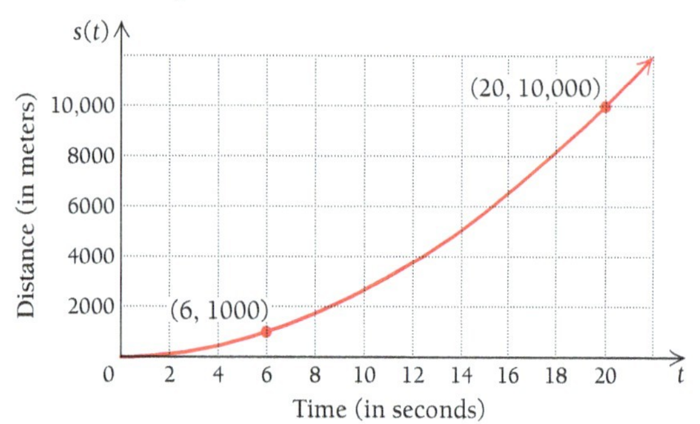

a) Is the plane's velocity greater at $t = 6$ sec or $t = 20$ sec? How can you tell?
b) Is the plane's acceleration positive or negative? How can you tell?

45. **Sales.** The following graph represents the sales, y, of a new video game after t weeks on the market.

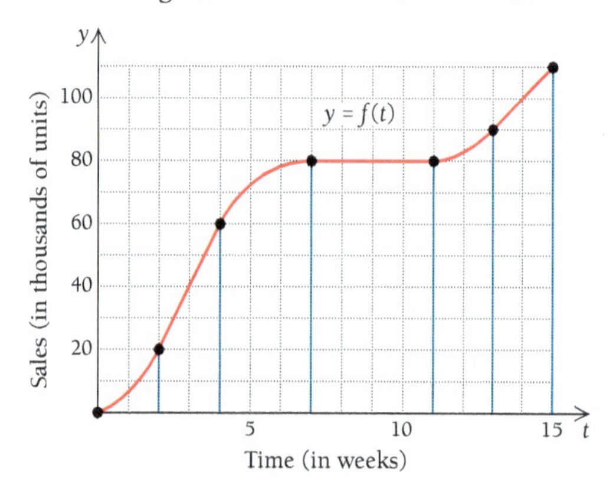

a) In what open interval(s) is $f'(t) = 0$?
b) In what open interval(s) is $f''(t) = 0$?
c) In what open interval(s) is $f''(t) > 0$?
d) In what open interval(s) is $f''(t) < 0$?
e) Describe in words and graphically the difference in meaning between "sales are increasing" and "the rate of sales is increasing."

46. **Velocity and acceleration.** The following graph describes the distance of Jesse's car from home as a function of time t.

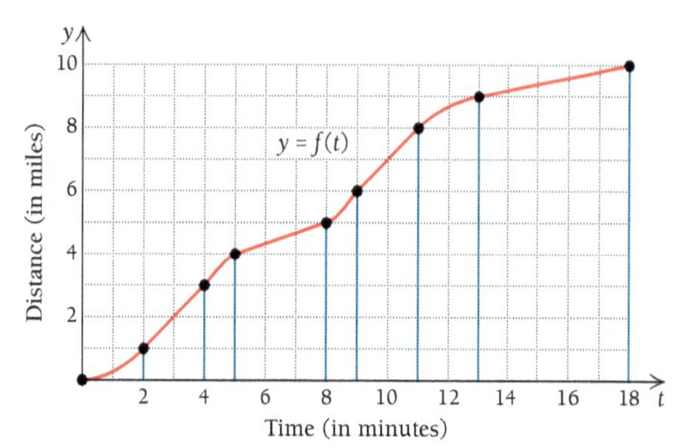

a) In what open interval(s) is Jesse's car accelerating?
b) In what open interval(s) is Jesse's car decelerating?
c) In what open interval(s) is Jesse's car maintaining a constant velocity?

47. **Sales.** A company determines that monthly sales $S(t)$, in thousands of dollars, after t months of marketing a product are given by

$$S(t) = 2t^3 - 40t^2 + 220t + 160.$$

a) Find $S'(1)$, $S'(2)$, and $S'(4)$.
b) Find $S''(1)$, $S''(2)$, and $S''(4)$.
c) Interpret the meaning of your answers to parts (a) and (b).

48. **Sales.** Nadia's Fashions discovers that the number of pendants sold t days after launching a new sales promotion is given by

$$N(t) = 2t^3 - 3t^2 + 2t.$$

a) Find $N'(1)$, $N'(2)$, and $N'(4)$.
b) Find $N''(1)$, $N''(2)$, and $N''(4)$.
c) Interpret the meaning of your answers to parts (a) and (b).

49. **Population.** The function $p(t) = \dfrac{2000t}{4t + 75}$ gives the population of deer in an area after t months.

a) Find $p'(10)$, $p'(50)$, and $p'(100)$.
b) Find $p''(10)$, $p''(50)$, and $p''(100)$.
c) Interpret the meaning of your answers to parts (a) and (b). What is happening to this population of deer in the long term?

50. **Medicine.** A medication is injected into the bloodstream, where it is quickly metabolized. The percent concentration p of the medication after t minutes in the bloodstream is modeled by the function $p(t) = \dfrac{2.5t}{t^2 + 1}$.

a) Find $p'(0.5)$, $p'(1)$, $p'(5)$, and $p'(30)$.
b) Find $p''(0.5)$, $p''(1)$, $p''(5)$, and $p''(30)$.
c) Interpret the meaning of your answers to parts (a) and (b). What is happening to the concentration of medication in the bloodstream in the long term?

Projectile motion. *An object that is launched follows a parabolic arc, assuming negligible air resistance. The equation $y(t) = -4.9t^2 + v_y t + h$ gives the height of the object in meters, t seconds after launch, where v_y is the object's initial velocity in the vertical direction and h is the object's initial height above the ground. The equation $x(t) = v_x t$ gives the object's distance in the horizontal direction in meters, t seconds after launch, where v_x is the object's initial velocity in the horizontal direction. In this situation, the positive vertical direction is considered "up."*

51. A rock is thrown from a building 50 meters above the ground. Its height above the ground is given by $y(t) = -4.9t^2 + 22.15t + 50$, and its horizontal distance is given by $x(t) = 27.25t$.

a) Find the rock's height above ground and horizontal distance 2 seconds after being released.

b) Find the rock's velocity in the vertical and the horizontal directions 2 seconds after being released.
c) Find the rock's acceleration in the vertical and horizontal directions 2 seconds after being released.
d) Is the rock moving upward or downward at $t = 2$ seconds? How can you tell?
e) Explain why acceleration in the vertical direction remains the same for the duration of the rock's flight.
f) Explain why there is no acceleration in the horizontal direction.

52. A ball moving 2 meters per second rolls off the edge of a flat roof 10 m above the ground. Its height above the ground is given by $y(t) = -4.9t^2 + 10$, and its horizontal distance is given by $x(t) = 2t$.

a) Find the ball's height above ground and horizontal distance 1 second after rolling off the roof.
b) Find the ball's velocity in the vertical and the horizontal directions 1 second after rolling off the roof.
c) Find the ball's acceleration in the vertical and horizontal directions 1 second after rolling off the roof.
d) Explain why the initial vertical velocity is 0.

A heavy ball rolls 10 meters in 1 minute. In Exercises 53–56, match a graph (I–IV) with each description.

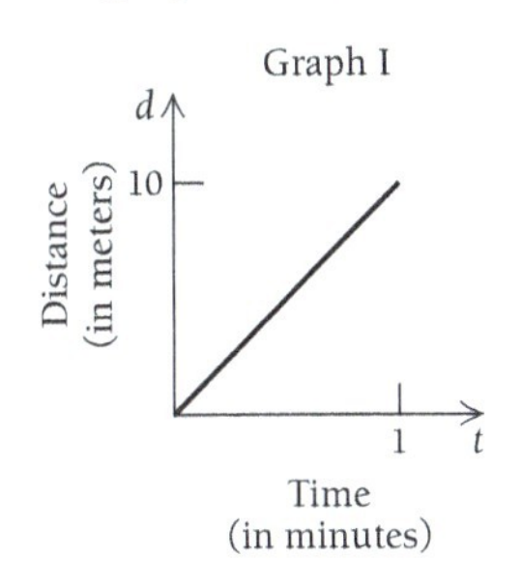

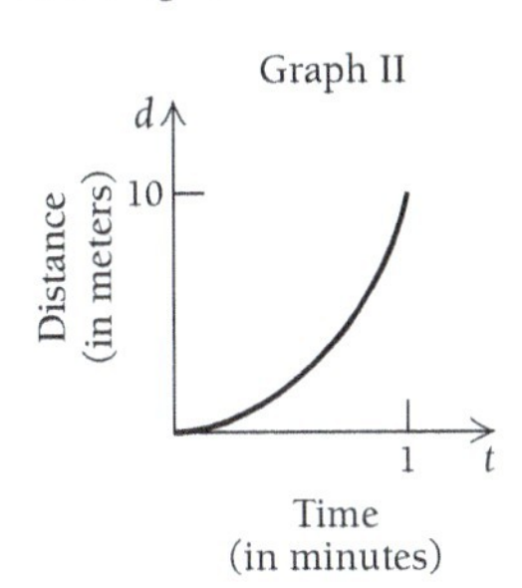

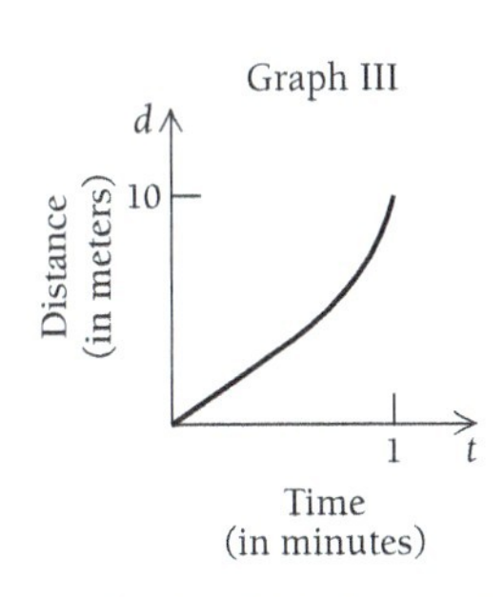

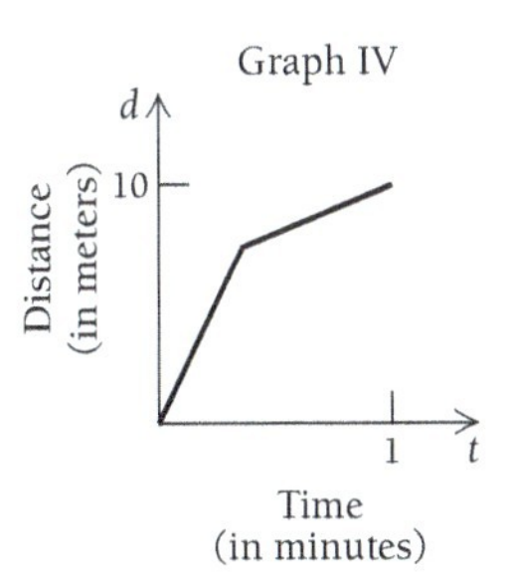

53. The ball rolled along a level sidewalk.

54. The ball rolled along a level sidewalk, then onto a level grassy lawn.

55. The ball rolled down an incline.

56. The ball rolled along a level sidewalk, then down an incline.

SYNTHESIS

In Exercises 57–59, classify each statement as true or false, and provide an example that supports your answer.

57. If an object's acceleration is 0, then the object is standing still.

58. If an object's velocity is 0 at an instant, then it can still be accelerating or decelerating.

59. If f is an nth-degree polynomial, then its nth derivative is 0.

60. Suppose $f(x) = \frac{1}{x}$. Find the first four derivatives of f, and use a pattern to find $f^{(12)}(x)$.

In Exercises 61 and 62, find the first through the fourth derivatives. Be sure to simplify each derivative before proceeding.

61. $f(x) = \dfrac{x - 1}{x + 2}$

62. $f(x) = \dfrac{x + 3}{x - 2}$

63. Free fall. On the moon, the free-fall distance function is given by $s(t) = 0.81t^2$, where t is in seconds and $s(t)$ is in meters. An object is dropped from a height of 200 meters above the moon. After $t = 2$ sec,

a) How far has the object fallen?
b) How fast is it traveling?
c) What is its acceleration?
d) Explain the meaning of the second derivative of this free-fall function.

64. Hang time. On Earth, an object travels 4.905 m after 1 sec of free fall. Thus, by symmetry, an athlete would require 1 sec to jump 4.905 m high, and another second to come back down. Is it possible for a person to stay in the air for (have a "hang time" of) 2 sec? Can a person have a hang time of 1.5 sec? 1 sec? What do you think is the longest possible hang time achievable by humans jumping from level ground?

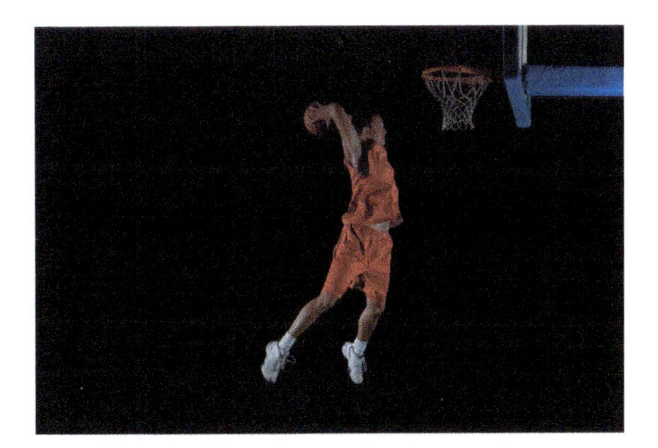

65. Free fall. Setting a world record, skateboarder Danny Way free-fell 28 ft from the Fender Stratocaster Guitar atop the Hard Rock Hotel & Casino in Las Vegas onto a ramp below. The distance $s(t)$, in feet, traveled by a body falling freely from rest in t seconds is approximated by $s(t) = 16t^2$. Estimate Way's velocity at the instant he touched down onto the ramp. (*Note*: Use the result from Exercise 30 in Section R.1.)

66. A bicyclist's distance from her starting point is given by $y = s(t)$. Suppose the graph of s has a corner. Give three situations in which a corner, rather than a smooth curve, can occur. What can you conclude about $s'(t)$ and $s''(t)$ at the corner of the graph of s?

67. The distance, in feet, of a self-operating vacuum cleaner from its base, t seconds after leaving the base, is shown in the graph below.

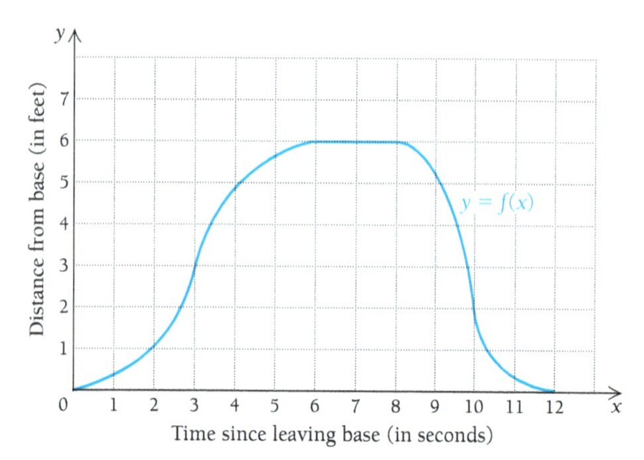

a) Over what interval of time is the vacuum cleaner stationary?
b) Over what interval of time is its velocity positive and its acceleration negative?
c) Over what interval of time is its velocity negative and its acceleration positive?
d) Over what interval of time is its velocity negative and its acceleration negative?
e) Over what interval of time is the vacuum cleaner returning to its base?
f) Visually, the vacuum cleaner would be "speeding up" between $t = 8$ and $t = 10$ seconds, yet the acceleration is negative. Explain why the observation that it is "speeding up" is still valid.

68. The vertical distance above the ground, in meters, of a drone, t seconds after it leaves the ground, is shown in the graph below.

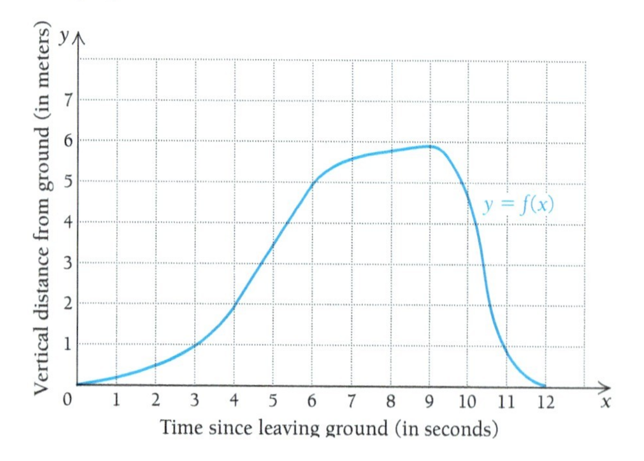

a) Over what interval of time is the drone moving upward?
b) Over what intervals of time is the drone's acceleration positive?
c) Over what interval of time is the drone's acceleration zero?
d) Over what interval of time is the drone's velocity negative?
e) The drone "slows" to a landing as x approaches 12 sec, yet its acceleration is positive. Explain why this observation is valid.

Technology Connection 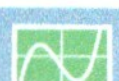

For the distance function in each of Exercises 69–72, graph s, v, and a over the given interval. Then use the graphs to determine the point(s) at which the velocity switches from increasing to decreasing or from decreasing to increasing.

69. $s(t) = 0.1t^4 - t^2 + 0.4;\quad [-5, 5]$
70. $s(t) = -t^3 + 3t;\quad [-3, 3]$
71. $s(t) = t^4 + t^3 - 4t^2 - 2t + 4;\quad [-3, 3]$
72. $s(t) = t^3 - 3t^2 + 2; [-2, 4]$

Answers to Quick Checks

1. (a) (i) $y'' = -72x^2 + 6$, **(ii)** $y'' = \dfrac{24}{x^5}$, **(iii)** $y'' = 108x^2 + 12$; **(b)** $y^{(4)} = \dfrac{24}{x^5}$
2. Distance $= s(3.5) = 196$ ft; velocity $= s'(3.5) = 112$ ft/sec; acceleration $= s''(3.5) = 32$ ft/sec^2
3. $N(4) = 53.25$; in 2014, Apple sold approximately 53.25 million iPads. $N'(4) = 4.658$; in 2014, Apple's sales of iPads were increasing by 4.658 million units per year. $N''(4) = -3.178$; in 2014, the rate at which iPad sales were changing was -3.178 million units per year^2. Sales were increasing but "slowing down."

Chapter 1 Summary

KEY TERMS AND CONCEPTS | **EXAMPLES**

SECTION 1.1

The notation $x \to a^-$ represents a sequence of numbers that approach a from the left.

- The sequence of numbers 0.69, 0.699, 0.6999, 0.6999, and so on, approaches 0.7 from the left, since the numbers in the sequence are all less than 0.7. This is represented as $x \to 0.7^-$.

The notation $x \to a^+$ represents a sequence of numbers that approach a from the right.

- The sequence of numbers 0.71, 0.701, 0.7001, 0.70001, and so on, approaches 0.7 from the right, since the numbers in the sequence are all greater than 0.7. This is represented as $x \to 0.7^+$.

As x approaches (but is not equal to) a, the **limit** of $f(x)$, if it exists, is L, which is written as

$$\lim_{x \to a} f(x) = L.$$

The limit L must be a unique real number.

$$\lim_{x \to 4} (2x + 3) = 11$$

Limit Numerically

	x	$2x + 3$
$x < 4$	3.9	10.8
	3.99	10.98
	3.999	10.998
$x > 4$	4.1	11.2
	4.01	11.02
	4.001	11.002

$$\lim_{x \to 1} \frac{x^2 - 1}{x - 1} = 2$$

Limit Graphically

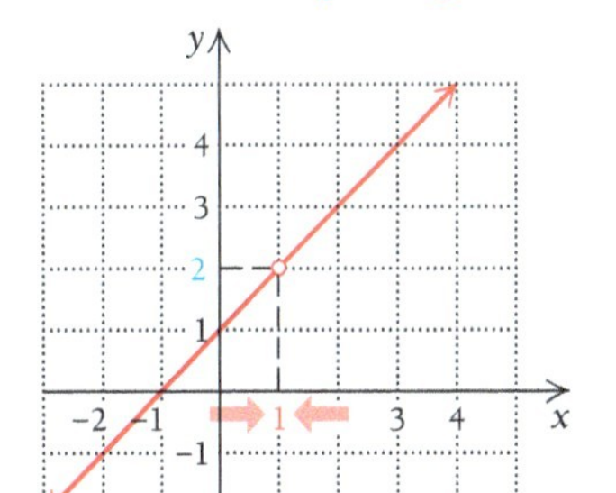

If x approaches a from the left $(x < a)$, and a **left-hand limit** exists, it is written as

$$\lim_{x \to a^-} f(x).$$

If x approaches a from the right $(x > a)$, and a **right-hand limit** exists, it is written as

$$\lim_{x \to a^+} f(x).$$

If the left-hand and right-hand limits are equal as x approaches a, then the limit as x approaches a exists.

If the left-hand and right-hand limits are *not* equal, then the limit as x approaches a does *not* exist.

Consider the function G given by

$$G(x) = \begin{cases} 4 - x, & \text{for } x < 3, \\ \sqrt{x - 2} + 1, & \text{for } x \geq 3. \end{cases}$$

Graph the function and find each limit, if it exists.

a) $\lim_{x \to 1} G(x)$ **b)** $\lim_{x \to 3} G(x)$

Check the limits from the left and from the right, both numerically and graphically.

a) *Limit Numerically*

$x \to 1^-$ $(x < 1)$	$G(x)$
0.9	3.1
0.99	3.01
0.999	3.001

$x \to 1^+$ $(x > 1)$	$G(x)$
1.1	2.9
1.01	2.99
1.001	2.999

These choices can vary.

Limit Graphically

$\lim_{x \to 1} G(x) = 3$

Both the tables and the graph show that as x gets closer to 1, the outputs $G(x)$ get closer to 3. Thus, $\lim_{x \to 1} G(x) = 3$.

KEY TERMS AND CONCEPTS	EXAMPLES

SECTION 1.1 (*continued*)

b) *Limit Numerically*

$x \to 3^-$ $(x < 3)$	$G(x)$
2.9	1.1
2.99	1.01
2.999	1.001

$x \to 3^+$ $(x > 3)$	$G(x)$
3.1	2.0489
3.01	2.0050
3.001	2.0005

These are approaching different values, so $\lim_{x \to 3} G(x)$ does not exist.

Limit Graphically

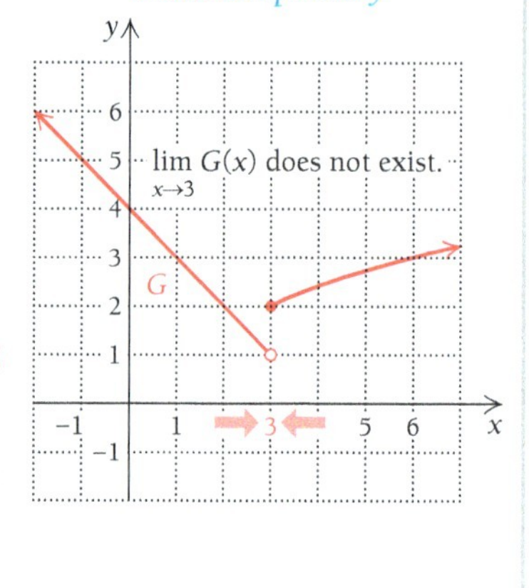

Both the tables and the graph indicate that $\lim_{x \to 3^-} G(x) \neq \lim_{x \to 3^+} G(x)$.

Since the left-hand and right-hand limits differ, $\lim_{x \to 3} G(x)$ does not exist.

SECTION 1.2

For any rational function F (see Section R.5) with a in its domain, we have

$$\lim_{x \to a} F(x) = F(a).$$

For $f(x) = 2x^2 + 3x - 1$ and $a = 2$, it follows that

$$\lim_{x \to 2} f(x) = f(2) = 2(2)^2 + 3(2) - 1 = 13.$$

For $g(x) = \dfrac{x^2 - 16}{x + 4}$ and $a = 6$, it follows that

$$\lim_{x \to 6} g(x) = \frac{(6)^2 - 16}{(6) + 4} = \frac{20}{10} = 2.$$

A function f is **continuous** at $x = a$ if the following three conditions are met:

1. $f(a)$ exists. (The output at a exists.)
2. $\lim_{x \to a} f(x)$ exists. (The limit as $x \to a$ exists.)
3. $\lim_{x \to a} f(x) = f(a)$. (The limit is the same as the output.)

If any one of these conditions is not fulfilled, the function is **discontinuous** at $x = a$.

Is the function g given by $g(x) = \dfrac{x^2 - 3x - 4}{x + 1}$ continuous over $(-\infty, \infty)$?

For g to be continuous over $(-\infty, \infty)$, it must be continuous at each point in $(-\infty, \infty)$. Note that

$$g(x) = \frac{x^2 - 3x - 4}{x + 1} = \frac{(x + 1)(x - 4)}{x + 1} = x - 4, \quad \text{provided } x \neq -1.$$

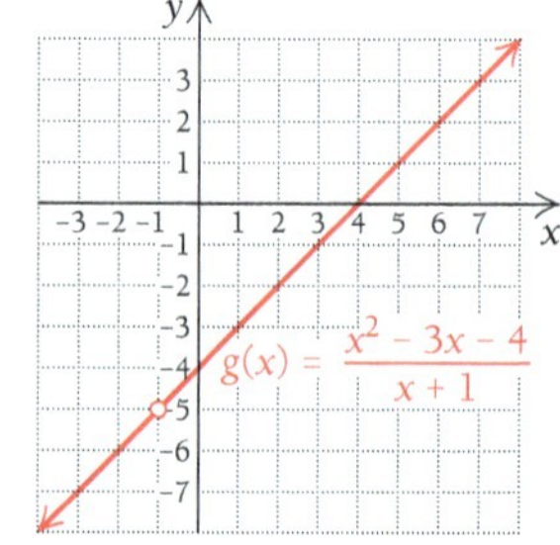

Since -1 is not in the domain of g, it follows that $g(-1)$ does not exist. Thus, g is not continuous over $(-\infty, \infty)$.

If f is a rational function in which the degrees of the numerator and the denominator are the same, then the limit of f, as x approaches positive or negative infinity, is the ratio of the leading coefficients. That is, if $f(x) = \dfrac{ax^n + \cdots}{bx^n + \cdots}$, then $\lim_{x \to \pm\infty} f(x) = \dfrac{a}{b}$.

- $\lim_{x \to \infty} \dfrac{3x^2 + 5x - 7}{4x^2 - 2x + 1} = \dfrac{3}{4}$
- $\lim_{x \to -\infty} \dfrac{3x^3 - x + 7}{x^3 + 6} = 3$

KEY TERMS AND CONCEPTS

EXAMPLES

SECTION 1.3

The **average rate of change** of y with respect to x between two points (x_1, y_1) and (x_2, y_2) is the slope of the line connecting the points:

$$\frac{y_2 - y_1}{x_2 - x_1}.$$

Business. At 1 p.m., Antiquarian Bookstore had revenue of \$570 for the day, and at 4 p.m., it had revenue of \$900 for the day. Therefore, the average rate of change of revenue with respect to time is

$$\frac{900 - 570}{4 - 1} = \frac{330}{3} = 110,$$

or \$110 per hour for the period of time between 1 p.m. and 4 p.m.

A line connecting two points on the graph of f is a **secant line**. Its slope is the average rate of change of f, which is given by the **difference quotient**:

$$\frac{f(x+h) - f(x)}{h},$$

where h is the difference between the two input x-values.

Let $f(x) = 3x^2$. Then

$$f(x+h) = 3(x+h)^2 = 3x^2 + 6xh + 3h^2.$$

The difference quotient for this function simplifies to

$$\frac{f(x+h) - f(x)}{h} = \frac{3x^2 + 6xh + 3h^2 - 3x^2}{h}$$
$$= 6x + 3h, \quad h \neq 0.$$

For example, when $x = 2$ and $h = 0.05$, the slope of the secant line between $x = 2$ and $x = 2.05$ is $6(2) + 3(0.05) = 12.15$.

SECTION 1.4

The **derivative** of a function f is

$$f'(x) = \lim_{h \to 0} \frac{f(x+h) - f(x)}{h}.$$

The derivative, if it exists, gives the slope of the line tangent to f at $x = a$, and that slope is the **instantaneous rate of change** of f at $x = a$. The process of finding a derivative is called **differentiation**.

If $f'(a)$ exists, then f is **differentiable** at $x = a$.

- Let $f(x) = 3x^2$. Its simplified difference quotient is $6x + 3h$, $h \neq 0$ (see above). Therefore, the derivative is

  $$f'(x) = \lim_{h \to 0} (6x + 3h) = 6x.$$

  The slope of the line tangent to f at $x = 2$ is

  $$f'(2) = 6(2) = 12.$$

- For $f(x) = -x^2 + 5$, find $f'(x)$ and $f'(2)$.

  The difference quotient is simplified first:

  $$\frac{f(x+h) - f(x)}{h} = \frac{-(x+h)^2 + 5 - (-x^2 + 5)}{h}$$
  $$= \frac{-(x^2 + 2xh + h^2) + 5 + x^2 - 5}{h}$$
  $$= \frac{-2xh - h^2}{h}$$
  $$= -2x - h, \quad h \neq 0.$$

  Thus,

  $$f'(x) = \lim_{h \to 0} \frac{f(x+h) - f(x)}{h} = \lim_{h \to 0} (-2x - h),$$

  and

  $$f'(x) = -2x.$$

  It follows that $f'(2) = -2 \cdot 2 = -4$ and f is differentiable at $x = 2$. In fact, f is differentiable for all real numbers x.

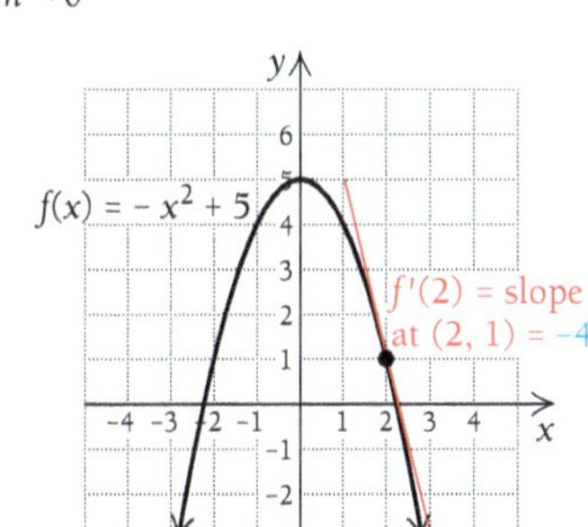

KEY TERMS AND CONCEPTS / EXAMPLES

SECTION 1.4 (continued)

Continuity (see Section 1.2):

If a function f is differentiable at $x = a$, then it is continuous at $x = a$. (Differentiability implies continuity.)

Continuity of a function f at $x = a$ does *not* necessarily mean that f is differentiable at $x = a$. Any function whose graph has a corner is continuous but not differentiable at the corner.

If a function f is discontinuous at $x = a$, then it is not differentiable at $x = a$.

Examples:

- Let $f(x) = 3x^2$. Since the derivative is $f'(x) = 6x$ and the derivative at $x = 2$ exists, it follows that $f(x)$ is continuous at $x = 2$.

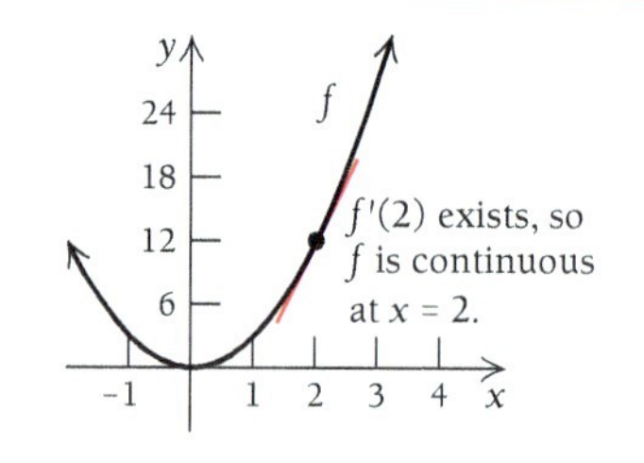

- The absolute-value function is continuous at $x = 0$ but not differentiable at $x = 0$, since there is a corner at $x = 0$.

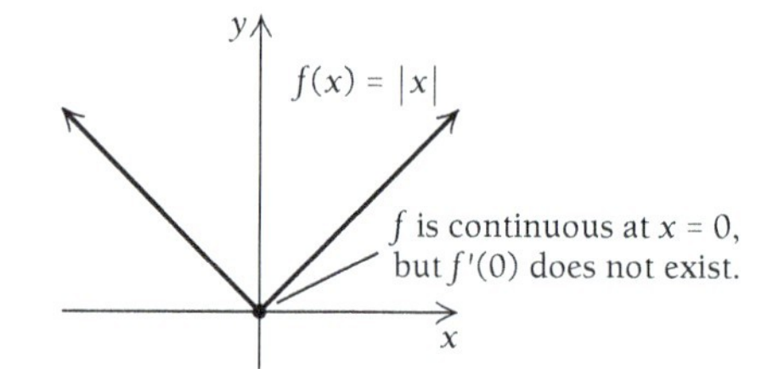

- The function $g(x) = \dfrac{x^2 - 16}{x + 4}$ is discontinuous at $x = -4$; therefore, g is not differentiable at $x = -4$. (Note that the derivative is defined at all other values of x.)

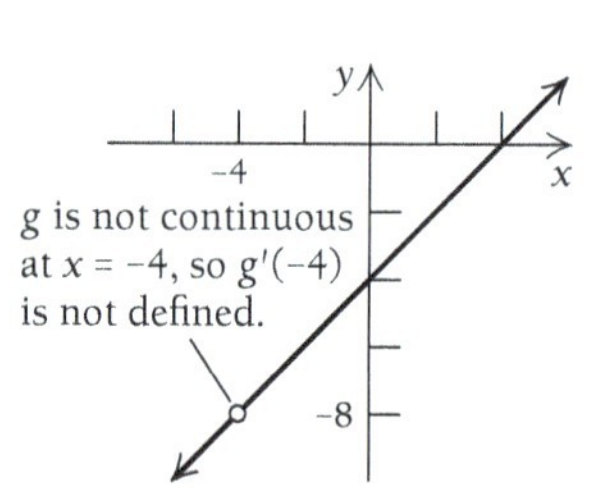

SECTION 1.5

If $y = f(x)$, the derivative in Leibniz notation is written $\dfrac{dy}{dx}$, or $\dfrac{d}{dx}f(x)$. Each has the same meaning as $f'(x)$.

Example: Let $y = x^3$. Then, in Leibniz notation, $\dfrac{dy}{dx} = 3x^2$.

The **Power Rule**:

For any real number k,

$$\frac{d}{dx}x^k = k \cdot x^{k-1}.$$

Examples:

- $\dfrac{d}{dx}x^7 = 7x^6$
- $\dfrac{d}{dx}\sqrt{x} = \dfrac{d}{dx}x^{1/2} = \dfrac{1}{2}x^{-1/2} = \dfrac{1}{2\sqrt{x}}$
- $\dfrac{d}{dx}\left(\dfrac{1}{x}\right) = \dfrac{d}{dx}x^{-1} = -1 \cdot x^{-2} = -\dfrac{1}{x^2}$

The derivative of a constant is

$$\frac{d}{dx}c = 0.$$

Examples:

- $\dfrac{d}{dx}34 = 0$
- $\dfrac{d}{dx}\sqrt{2} = 0$

The derivative of a constant times a function is

$$\frac{d}{dx}[c \cdot f(x)] = c \cdot \frac{d}{dx}f(x).$$

Examples:

- $\dfrac{d}{dx}3x^8 = 3 \cdot \dfrac{d}{dx}x^8 = 3 \cdot 8x^7 = 24x^7$
- $\dfrac{d}{dx}\left(\dfrac{2}{3x^2}\right) = \dfrac{2}{3} \cdot \dfrac{d}{dx}\left(\dfrac{1}{x^2}\right) = \dfrac{2}{3} \cdot (-2x^{-3}) = -\dfrac{4}{3x^3}$

KEY TERMS AND CONCEPTS	EXAMPLES
SECTION 1.5 (*continued*)	
The **Sum–Difference Rule**: $$\frac{d}{dx}[f(x) \pm g(x)] = \frac{d}{dx}f(x) \pm \frac{d}{dx}g(x).$$	• $\frac{d}{dx}(x^7 + 3x) = \frac{d}{dx}(x^7) + \frac{d}{dx}(3x) = 7x^6 + 3$ • $\frac{d}{dx}(5x - x^4) = 5 - 4x^3$
SECTION 1.6	
The **Product Rule**: $$\frac{d}{dx}[f(x) \cdot g(x)] = f(x) \cdot g'(x) + g(x) \cdot f'(x).$$	$\frac{d}{dx}[(2x+3)\sqrt{x}] = (2x+3)\frac{1}{2}x^{-1/2} + \sqrt{x} \cdot 2$ $= \frac{2x+3}{2\sqrt{x}} + 2\sqrt{x}$
The **Quotient Rule**: $$\frac{d}{dx}\left[\frac{f(x)}{g(x)}\right] = \frac{g(x) \cdot f'(x) - f(x) \cdot g'(x)}{[g(x)]^2}.$$	$\frac{d}{dx}\left(\frac{3x-1}{2x+5}\right) = \frac{(2x+5) \cdot 3 - (3x-1) \cdot 2}{(2x+5)^2} = \frac{17}{(2x+5)^2}$
SECTION 1.7	
The **Chain Rule**: $$\frac{d}{dx}[(f \circ g)(x)] = \frac{d}{dx}[f(g(x))] = f'(g(x)) \cdot g'(x).$$	• $\frac{d}{dx}\sqrt{3x^2+4} = \frac{d}{dx}(3x^2+4)^{1/2} = \frac{1}{2}(3x^2+4)^{-1/2}(6x)$ $= \frac{3x}{\sqrt{3x^2+4}}$ • $\frac{d}{dx}\left(\frac{1}{8x+1}\right) = \frac{d}{dx}(8x+1)^{-1} = -1(8x+1)^{-2}(8) = -\frac{8}{(8x+1)^2}$
The **Extended Power Rule**: $$\frac{d}{dx}[g(x)]^k = k[g(x)]^{k-1} \cdot \frac{d}{dx}g(x).$$	$\frac{d}{dx}(2x^5 + 4x)^7 = 7(2x^5+4x)^6(10x^4+4)$ $= 14(2x^5+4x)^6(5x^4+2)$
SECTION 1.8	
The **second derivative** is the derivative of the first derivative: $$\frac{d}{dx}[f'(x)] = [f'(x)]' = f''(x).$$ The second derivative indicates the rate of change of the derivative.	Let $f(x) = 2x^5 + 20x$. Then $$\frac{d}{dx}f(x) = f'(x) = 10x^4 + 20,$$ and therefore, $$\frac{d^2}{dx^2}f(x) = f''(x) = 40x^3.$$
Higher-order derivatives include second, third, fourth, and so on, derivatives of a function. The ***n*th derivative** of a function is written as $$\frac{d^ny}{dx^n} = f^{(n)}(x).$$	For $y = 2x^5 + 20$, it follows that $$\frac{d^3y}{dx^3} = f^{(3)}(x) = 120x^2,$$ $$\frac{d^4y}{dx^4} = f^{(4)}(x) = 240x,$$ $$\frac{d^5y}{dx^5} = f^{(5)}(x) = 240.$$

KEY TERMS AND CONCEPTS	EXAMPLES
SECTION 1.8 *(continued)*	
A real-world application of the second derivative is **acceleration**. If $s(t)$ represents distance as a function of time, then velocity is $v(t) = s'(t)$ and acceleration is the change in velocity: $a(t) = v'(t) = s''(t)$.	**Physical Science.** A particle moves according to the distance function $s(t) = 5t^3$, where t is in seconds and $s(t)$ in feet. Therefore, the particle's velocity is given by $v(t) = s'(t) = 15t^2$ and its acceleration by $a(t) = v'(t) = s''(t) = 30t$. At $t = 2$ sec, the particle is $s(2) = 40$ ft from the starting point, traveling at $v(2) = 60$ ft/sec and accelerating at $a(2) = 60$ ft/sec^2 (it's speeding up).

Chapter 1 Review Exercises

These review exercises are for test preparation. They can also be used as a practice test. Answers are at the back of the book. The red bracketed section references indicate the section(s) to restudy if your answer is incorrect.

CONCEPT REINFORCEMENT

Classify each statement as either true or false.

1. If $\lim_{x \to 5} f(x)$ exists, then $f(5)$ must exist. [1.1]

2. If $\lim_{x \to 2} f(x) = L$, then L must equal $f(2)$. [1.1]

3. If f is continuous at $x = 3$, then $\lim_{x \to 3} f(x) = f(3)$. [1.2]

4. A function's average rate of change over the interval $[2, 8]$ is the same as its instantaneous rate of change at $x = 5$. [1.3, 1.4]

5. A function's derivative at a point, if it exists, can be found as the limit of a difference quotient. [1.4]

6. For $f'(5)$ to exist, f must be continuous at 5. [1.4]

7. If f is continuous at 5, then $f'(5)$ must exist. [1.4]

8. The acceleration function is the derivative of the velocity function. [1.8]

Match each function in column A with the most appropriate rule to use for differentiating the function. [1.5, 1.6]

Column A

9. $f(x) = x^7$

10. $g(x) = x + 9$

11. $F(x) = (5x - 3)^4$

12. $G(x) = \dfrac{2x + 1}{3x - 4}$

13. $H(x) = f(x) \cdot g(x)$

14. $f(x) = 2x - 7$

Column B

a) Extended Power Rule

b) Product Rule

c) Sum Rule

d) Difference Rule

e) Power Rule

f) Quotient Rule

For Exercises 15–17, consider

$$\lim_{x \to -7} f(x), \text{ where } f(x) = \frac{x^2 + 4x - 21}{x + 7}.$$

15. Limit numerically. [1.1]

a) Find the limit by completing the following input–output tables.

$x \to -7^-$	$f(x)$
-7.1	
-7.01	
-7.001	

$x \to -7^+$	$f(x)$
-6.9	
-6.99	
-6.999	

b) Find $\lim_{x \to -7^-} f(x)$, $\lim_{x \to -7^+} f(x)$, and $\lim_{x \to -7} f(x)$, if each exists.

16. Limit graphically. Find the limit by graphing the function. [1.1]

17. Limit algebraically. Find the limit algebraically. Show your work. [1.2]

Find each limit, if it exists. If a limit does not exist, state that fact. [1.1, 1.2]

18. $\lim_{x \to -2} \dfrac{8}{x}$

19. $\lim_{x \to 1} (4x^3 - x^2 + 7x)$

20. $\lim_{x \to -7} \dfrac{x^2 + 2x - 35}{x + 7}$

21. $\lim_{x \to \infty} \dfrac{1}{x} + 3$

22. $\lim_{x \to \infty} \dfrac{4x^2 + 2x - 9}{x^2 + 16}$

23. $\lim_{x \to 5} \dfrac{x^2 + 25}{x - 5}$

For Exercises 24–33, consider the function g graphed below.

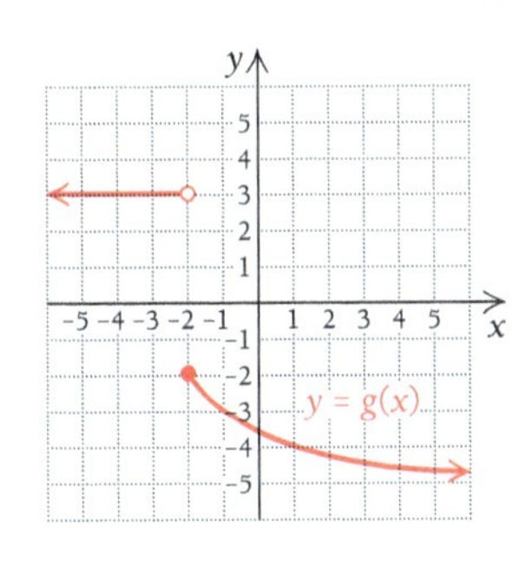

24. Find $\lim_{x \to 1} g(x)$. [1.1]

25. Find $g(1)$. [1.1]

26. Is g continuous at 1? Why or why not? [1.2]

27. Find $\lim_{x \to -2} g(x)$. [1.1]

28. Find $g(-2)$. [1.1]

29. Is g continuous at -2? Why or why not? [1.2]

30. Is g continuous over its domain? [1.2]

31. Find the average rate of change between $x = -2$ and $x = 1$. [1.3]

32. Find $g'(-4)$. [1.4]

33. For which value(s) is $g'(x)$ not defined? Why? [1.4]

For Exercises 34–38, consider the function f graphed below.

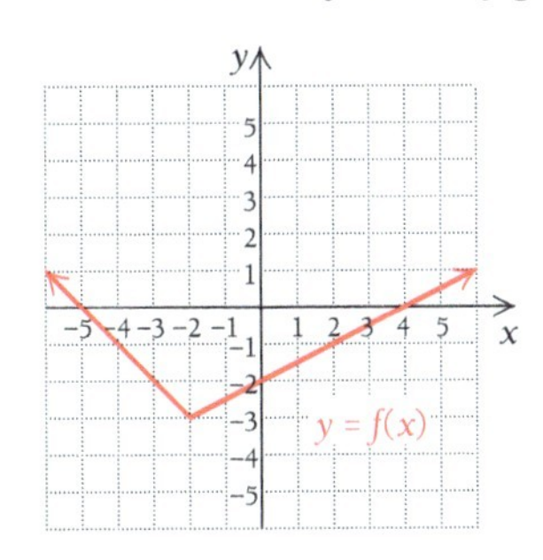

34. For which value(s) is $f'(x)$ not defined? Why? [1.4]

35. Find $\lim_{x \to 0} f(x)$. [1.1]

36. Find $\lim_{x \to -2} f(x)$. [1.1]

37. Is f continuous at $x = -2$? [1.4]

38. Is f continuous over its domain? [1.2]

39. For $f(x) = x^3 + x^2 - 2x$, find the average rate of change as x changes from -1 to 2. [1.3]

40. Find a simplified difference quotient for $g(x) = -3x^2 + 2$. [1.3]

41. Find an equation of the line tangent to the graph of $y = x^2 + 3x$ at the point $(-1, -2)$. [1.4]

42. Find the point(s) on the graph of $y = -x^2 + 8x - 11$ at which the tangent line is horizontal. [1.5]

Differentiate.

43. $y = 9x^5$ [1.5]

44. $y = 8\sqrt[3]{x}$ [1.5]

45. $y = -\frac{3}{x^8}$ [1.5]

46. $y = 15x^{2/5}$ [1.5]

47. $y = 0.1x^7 - 3x^4 - x^3 + 6$ [1.5]

48. $f(x) = \frac{5}{12}x^6 + 8x^4 - 2x$ [1.5]

49. $y = (x^3 - 5)(\sqrt{x} + 4x)$ [1.5, 1.6]

50. $y = \frac{x^2 + 8}{8 - x}$ [1.6]

51. $g(x) = (5 - x)^2(2x - 1)^5$ [1.6]

52. $f(x) = (x^5 - 3)^7$ [1.7]

53. $f(x) = x^2(4x + 2)^{3/4}$ [1.7]

54. For $y = x^3 - \frac{2}{x}$, find $\frac{d^4y}{dx^4}$. [1.8]

55. For $y = \frac{3}{42}x^7 - 10x^3 + 13x^2 + 28x - 2$, find y''. [1.8]

56. Social science: growth rate. The population of Lawton grows from an initial size of 10,000 to a size P, given by $P(t) = 10{,}000 + 50t^2$, where t is in years. [1.5]

a) Find the growth rate.

b) Find the population of Lawton after 20 yr.

c) Find the growth rate after 20 yr.

For Exercises 57–60, consider the graph of $y = s(t)$, the distance a jogger has run after t minutes. [1.8]

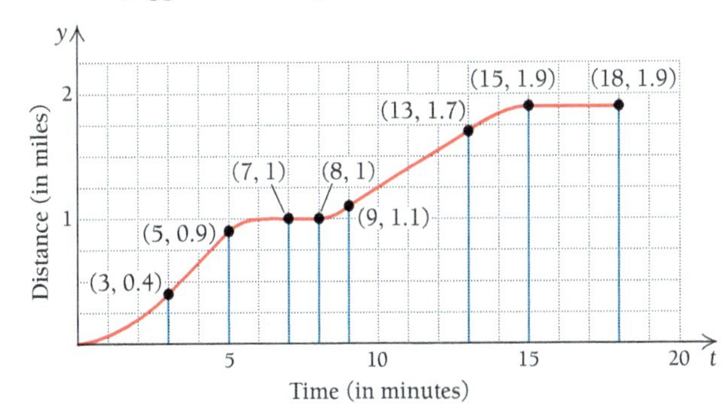

57. In what open interval(s) is the jogger running at a constant speed?

58. In what open interval(s) is she stopped?

59. In what open interval(s) is she accelerating?

60. In what open interval(s) is she decelerating?

61. Physical science: falling object. A rock is dropped from Navajo Bridge, which is 800 feet above the Colorado

River (near Page, Arizona). The rock's height h above the river t seconds after being released is given by

$$h(t) = 800 - 16t^2. \quad [1.8]$$

a) Find the rock's height above the river at $t = 3$ sec.
b) Find the rock's velocity at $t = 3$ sec.
c) Find the rock's acceleration at $t = 3$ sec.
d) Find the velocity at which the rock hits the water.
e) Explain why the rock's acceleration is the same for all values of t.

62. **Business: average revenue, cost, and profit.** Given revenue and cost functions $R(x) = 40x$ and $C(x) = 5\sqrt{x} + 100$, find each of the following. Assume $R(x)$ and $C(x)$ are in dollars and x is the number of lamps produced. [1.6]
a) The average cost, the average revenue, and the average profit when x lamps are produced and sold
b) The rate at which average cost is changing when 9 lamps are produced

63. Find $\frac{d}{dx}(f \circ g)(x)$ and $\frac{d}{dx}(g \circ f)(x)$, given $f(x) = x^2 + 5$ and $g(x) = 1 - 2x$. [1.7]

SYNTHESIS

64. Differentiate $y = \frac{x\sqrt{1 + 3x}}{1 + x^3}$. [1.7]

65. Find $\frac{d}{dx}(f \circ f \circ f \circ f \circ f)(x)$, where $f(x) = \sqrt[3]{x}$. [1.7]

Technology Connection

Create an input–output table to determine each of the following limits. Start with ΔTbl $= 0.1$ and then go to 0.01, 0.001, and 0.0001. When you think you know the limit, graph the functions, and use TRACE *to verify your assertion.*

66. $\lim_{x \to 1} \frac{2 - \sqrt{x + 3}}{x - 1}$ [1.1, 1.5]

67. $\lim_{x \to 11} \frac{\sqrt{x - 2} - 3}{x - 11}$ [1.1, 1.5]

68. Graph f and f' over the given interval. Then estimate points at which the tangent line to f is horizontal. [1.5]

$$f(x) = 3.8x^5 - 18.6x^3; \quad [-3, 3]$$

Chapter 1 Test

For Exercises 1–3, consider

$$\lim_{x \to 6} f(x), \text{ where } f(x) = \frac{x^2 - 36}{x - 6}.$$

1. **Numerical limits.**
a) Find the limit by completing the following input–output tables.

$x \to 6^-$	$f(x)$
5.9	
5.99	
5.999	

$x \to 6^+$	$f(x)$
6.1	
6.01	
6.001	

b) Find $\lim_{x \to 6^-} f(x)$, $\lim_{x \to 6^+} f(x)$, and $\lim_{x \to 6} f(x)$, if each exists.

2. **Graphical limits.** Find the limit by graphing the function.

3. **Algebraic limits.** Find the limit algebraically. Show your work.

Graphical limits. *For Exercises 4–15, consider the function f graphed below. Find each limit, if it exists.*

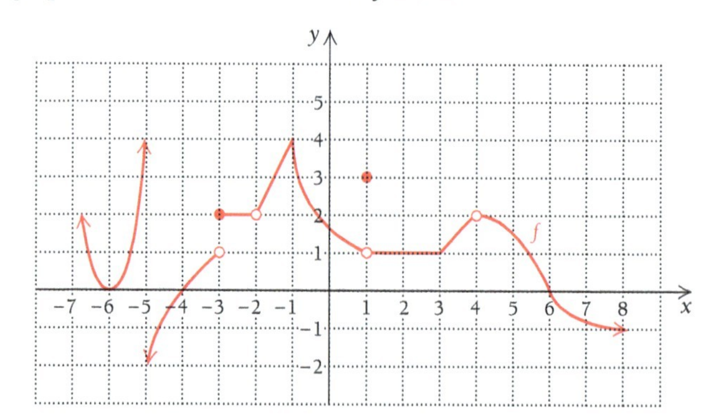

4. $\lim_{x \to -5} f(x)$
5. $\lim_{x \to -4} f(x)$
6. $\lim_{x \to -3} f(x)$
7. $\lim_{x \to -2} f(x)$
8. $\lim_{x \to -1} f(x)$
9. $\lim_{x \to 1} f(x)$
10. $\lim_{x \to 2} f(x)$
11. $\lim_{x \to 4} f(x)$
12. Find $f'(2)$.
13. Find $f'(-6)$.
14. State the value(s) of x at which f is not continuous.
15. State the value(s) of x for which $f'(x)$ is not defined.

Determine whether each function is continuous. If a function is not continuous, state why.

16.

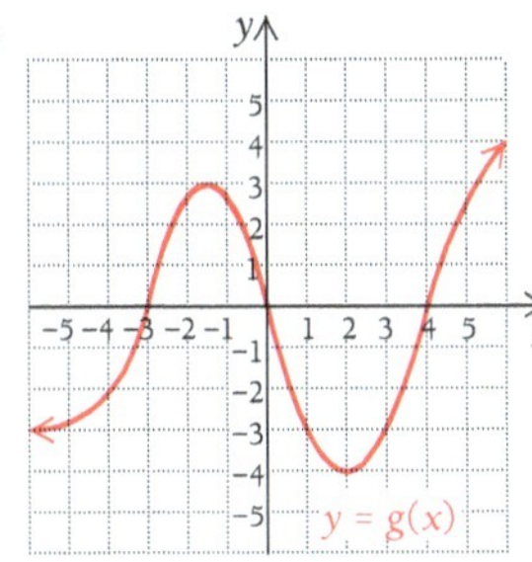

17.

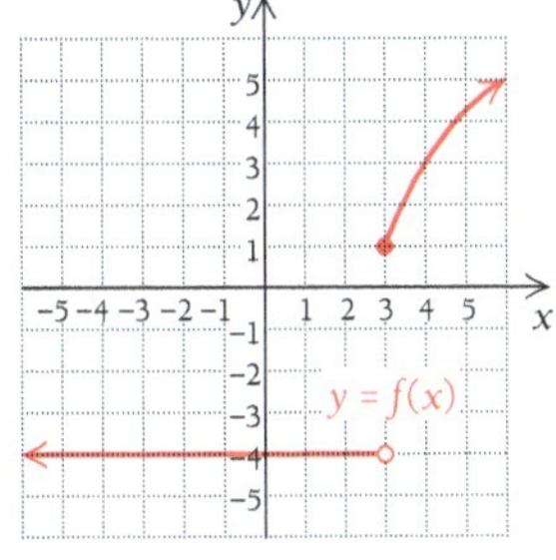

For Exercises 18 and 19, consider the function shown in Exercise 17.

18. a) Find $\lim_{x\to 3} f(x)$.

b) Find $f(3)$.

c) Is f continuous at 3?

19. Find $\lim_{x\to 4} f(x)$.

Find each limit, if it exists. If a limit does not exist, state why.

20. $\lim_{x\to 1} (3x^4 - 2x^2 + 5)$

21. $\lim_{x\to 2^+} \dfrac{x-2}{x(x^2-4)}$

22. $\lim_{x\to 0} \dfrac{7}{x}$

23. Find the simplified difference quotient for $f(x) = 2x^2 + 3x - 9$.

24. Find an equation of the line tangent to $y = x + (4/x)$ at the point $(4, 5)$.

25. Find the point(s) on the graph of $y = x^3 - 3x^2$ at which the tangent line is horizontal.

Find dy/dx.

26. $y = x^{23}$

27. $y = 4\sqrt[3]{x} + 5\sqrt{x}$

28. $y = \dfrac{-10}{x}$

29. $y = x^{5/4}$

30. $y = -0.5x^2 + 0.61x + 90$

31. $y = \dfrac{1}{3}x^3 - x^2 + 2x + 4$

32. $y = (3\sqrt{x} + 1)(x^2 - x)$

33. $f(x) = \dfrac{x}{5-x}$

34. $f(x) = (x+3)^4(7-x)^5$

35. $y = (x^5 - 4x^3 + x)^{-5}$

36. $f(x) = x\sqrt{x^2+5}$

37. For $y = x^4 - 3x^2$, find $\dfrac{d^3y}{dx^3}$.

38. Social sciences: memory. In a certain memory experiment, a person is able to memorize M words after t minutes, where $M = -0.001t^3 + 0.1t^2$.

a) Find the rate of change of the number of words memorized with respect to time.

b) How many words are memorized during the first 10 min (at $t = 10$)?

c) At what rate are words being memorized after 10 min (at $t = 10$)?

39. Business: average revenue, cost, and profit. Given revenue and cost functions

$$R(x) = 50x \quad \text{and} \quad C(x) = x^{2/3} + 750,$$

where x is the number of Bluetooth speakers produced and $R(x)$ and $C(x)$ are in dollars, find the following:

a) the average revenue, the average cost, and the average profit when x speakers are produced;

b) the rate at which average cost is changing when 8 speakers are produced.

For Exercises 40 and 41, let $f(x) = x^2 - x$ and $g(x) = 2x^3$.

40. Find $\dfrac{d}{dx}(f \circ g)(x)$.

41. Find $\dfrac{d}{dx}(g \circ f)(x)$.

42. A ball is placed on an inclined plane and, due to gravity alone, accelerates down the plane. Let $y = s(t)$ represent the ball's distance t seconds after starting to roll. Which graph below best represents s?

A. 

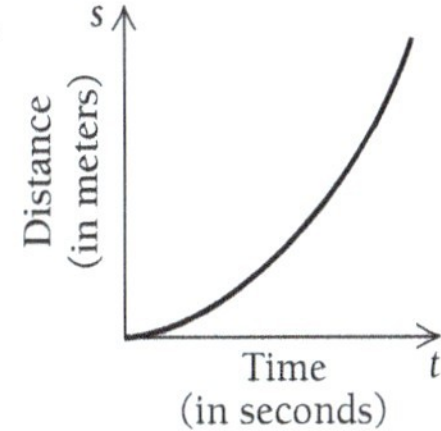

B. 

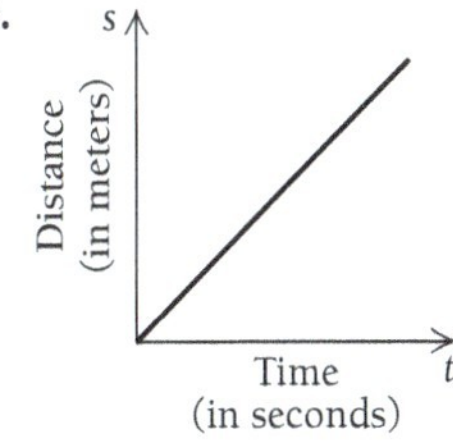

C.

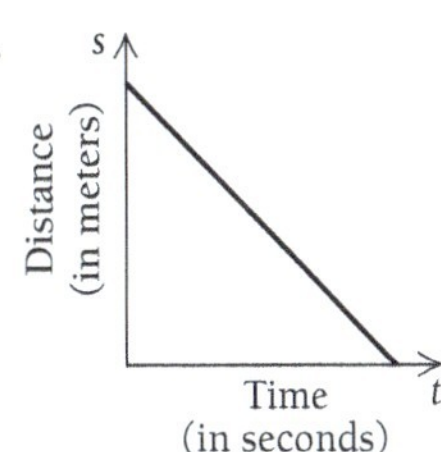

D.

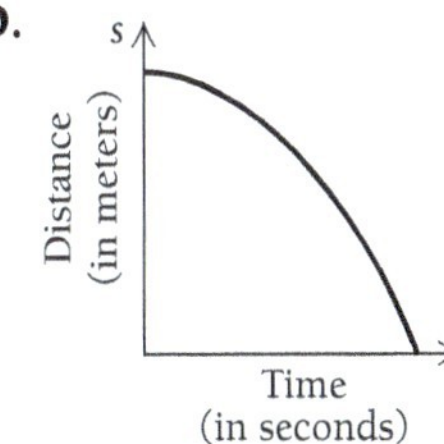

SYNTHESIS

43. Differentiate $y = \sqrt{(1-3x)^{2/3}(1+3x)^{1/3}}$.

44. Find $\lim_{x\to 3} \dfrac{x^3 - 27}{x - 3}$.

Technology Connection

45. Graph f and f' over the interval $[0, 5]$. Then estimate points at which the line tangent to f is horizontal.

$$f(x) = 5x^3 - 30x^2 + 45x + 5\sqrt{x}; \quad [0, 5]$$

46. Find the following limit by creating a table of values:

$$\lim_{x\to 0} \frac{\sqrt{5x+25} - 5}{x}.$$

Start with ΔTbl = 0.1 and then go to 0.01 and 0.001. When you think you know the limit, graph

$$y = \frac{\sqrt{5x+25} - 5}{x},$$

and use TRACE to verify your assertion.

EXTENDED TECHNOLOGY APPLICATION 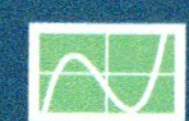

Path of a Baseball: The Tale of the Tape

Suppose a well-hit baseball hits a billboard 60 ft above the ground and 400 ft from home plate. A message on the scoreboard might proclaim, "According to the tale of the tape, the ball would have traveled 442 ft." How is such a calculation made? The answer is related to the curve formed by the path of a baseball.

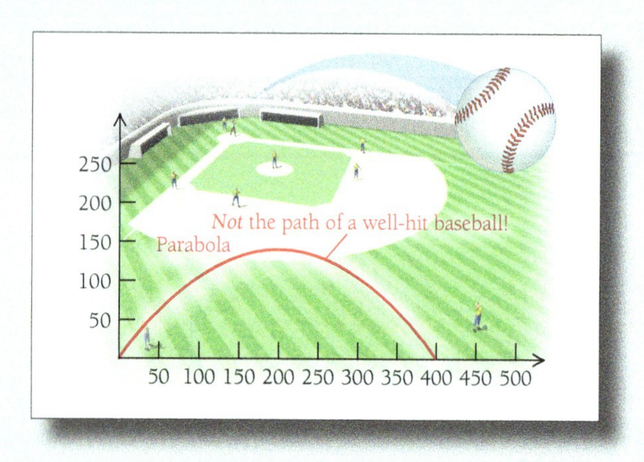

The path of a well-hit baseball is *not* the graph of a parabola,

$$f(x) = ax^2 + bx + c.$$

A well-hit baseball follows the path of a "skewed" curve, as shown below. One reason that the ball's flight is not parabolic is that it has backspin. This fact, combined with the frictional force generated as the ball's stitches interact with the air, skews the path of the ball in the direction of its landing.

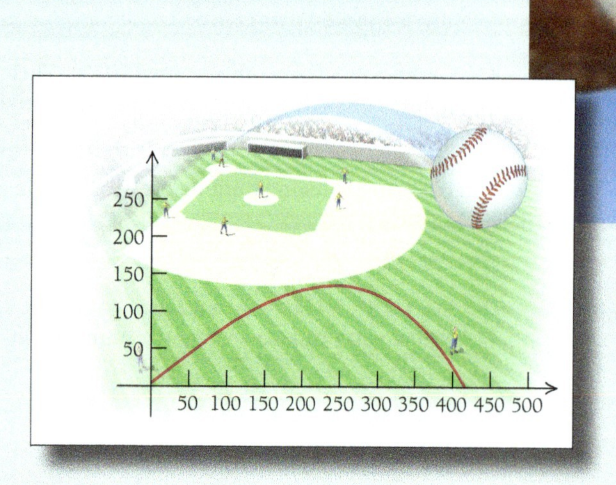

Let's see if we can model the path of a baseball. Consider the following data.

Horizontal Distance, x (in feet)	Vertical Distance, y (in feet)
0	4.5
50	43
100	82
200	130
285	142
300	134
360	100
400	60

Assume for the given data that $(0, 4.5)$ is the point at home plate at which the ball is hit, roughly 4.5 ft above the ground. Also, assume that the ball hits a billboard 60 ft above the ground and 400 ft from home plate.

Exercises

1. Plot the points and connect them with line segments. This can be done on many calculators by pressing STAT PLOT, turning on PLOT, and selecting the appropriate TYPE.

2. a) Use REGRESSION to find a cubic function

$$y = ax^3 + bx^2 + cx + d$$

that fits the data.

b) Graph the function over the interval $[0, 500]$.

c) Does the function closely model the given data?

d) Predict the horizontal distance from home plate at which the ball would have hit the ground had it not hit the billboard.

e) Find the rate of change of the ball's height with respect to its horizontal distance from home plate.

f) Find the point(s) at which the graph has a horizontal tangent line. Explain the significance of the point(s).

3. a) Use REGRESSION to find a quartic function

$$y = ax^4 + bx^3 + cx^2 + dx + e$$

that fits the data.

b) Graph the function over the interval $[0, 500]$.

c) Does the function closely model the given data?

d) Predict the horizontal distance from home plate at which the ball would have hit the ground had it not hit the billboard.

e) Find the rate of change of the ball's height with respect to its horizontal distance from home plate.

f) Find the point(s) at which the graph has a horizontal tangent line. Explain the significance of the point(s).

4. a) Although most calculators cannot fit such a function to the data, assume that the equation

$$y = 0.0015x\sqrt{202{,}500 - x^2}$$

has been found using a curve-fitting technique. Graph the function over the interval $[0, 500]$.

b) Predict the horizontal distance from home plate at which the ball would have hit the ground had it not hit the billboard.

c) Find the rate of change of the ball's height with respect to its horizontal distance from home plate.

d) Find the point(s) at which the graph has a horizontal tangent line. Explain the significance of the point(s).

5. Look at the answers in Exercises 2(d), 3(d), and 4(b). Compare the merits of the quartic model in Exercise 3 to those of the model in Exercise 4.

Tale of the tape. Actually, scoreboard operators in the major leagues use different models to predict the distance that a home run ball would have traveled. The models are linear and are related to the trajectory of the ball, that is, how high the ball is hit. See the following graph.

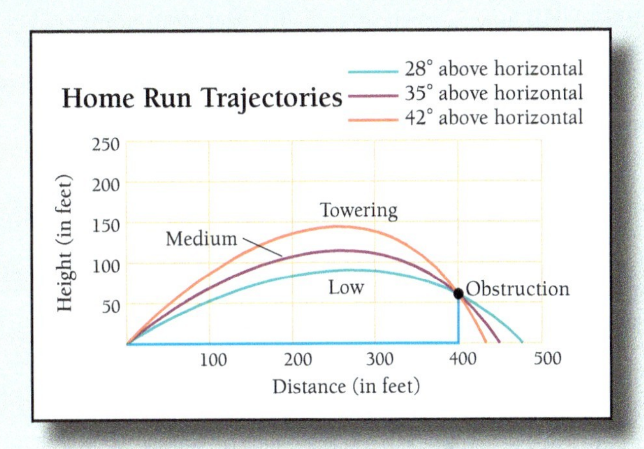

Suppose a ball hits an obstruction d feet horizontally from home plate at a height of H feet. Then the estimated horizontal distance D that the ball would have traveled, depending on its trajectory type, is

Low trajectory:	$D = 1.1H + d$,
Medium trajectory:	$D = 0.7H + d$,
Towering trajectory:	$D = 0.5H + d$.

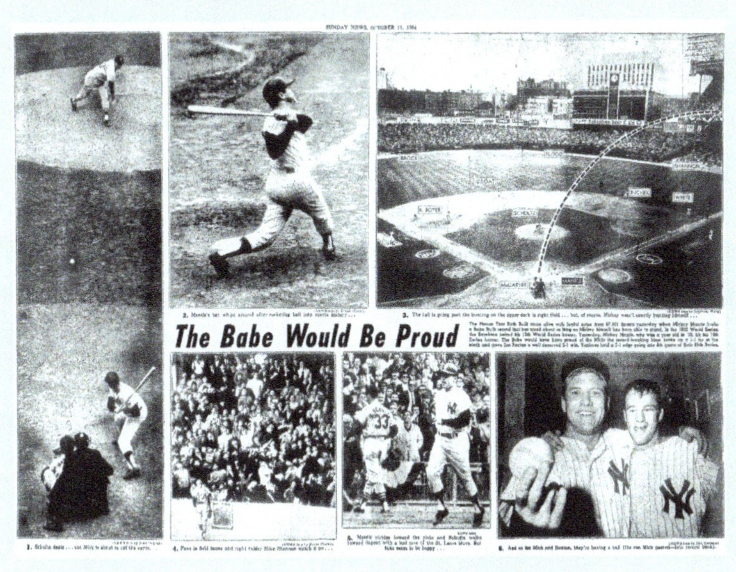

The Babe Would Be Proud

Exercises

6. For a ball striking an obstacle at $d = 400$ ft and $H = 60$ ft, estimate how far the ball would have traveled if it were following a low trajectory, a medium trajectory, or a towering trajectory.

7. In 1953, Mickey Mantle (New York Yankees) hit a towering home run in old Griffith Stadium in Washington, D.C., that hit an obstruction 60 ft high and 460 ft from home plate. Reporters asserted at the time that the ball would have traveled 565 ft. Is this estimate valid?

8. Use the appropriate formula to estimate the distance D for each of the following famous long home runs.

a) Ted Williams (Boston Red Sox, June 9, 1946): Purportedly the longest home run ball ever hit to right field at Boston's Fenway Park, Williams's ball landed in the stands 502 feet from home plate, 30 feet above the ground. Assume a medium trajectory.

b) Reggie Jackson (Oakland Athletics, July 13, 1971): Jackson's mighty blast hit an electrical transformer on top of the right-field roof at old Tiger Stadium in the 1971 All-Star Game. The transformer was 380 feet from home plate, 100 feet up. Find the distance the ball would have traveled, assuming a low trajectory and then a medium trajectory. (Jackson's home-run ball left the bat at an estimated 31.5° angle, about halfway between the low and medium range.)

c) Aaron Judge (New York Yankees, June 11, 2017): Judge's home run, the longest hit during the 2017 season, landed 496 feet from home plate in the right-center-field seats, approximately 50 feet above ground level. Assume a low trajectory. (According to hittracker.com, Judge's home run left the bat at a low angle of 26.4°, but with a speed of nearly 120 mi/hr.)

Many thanks to Robert K. Adair, professor of physics at Yale University, for many of the ideas presented in this application.

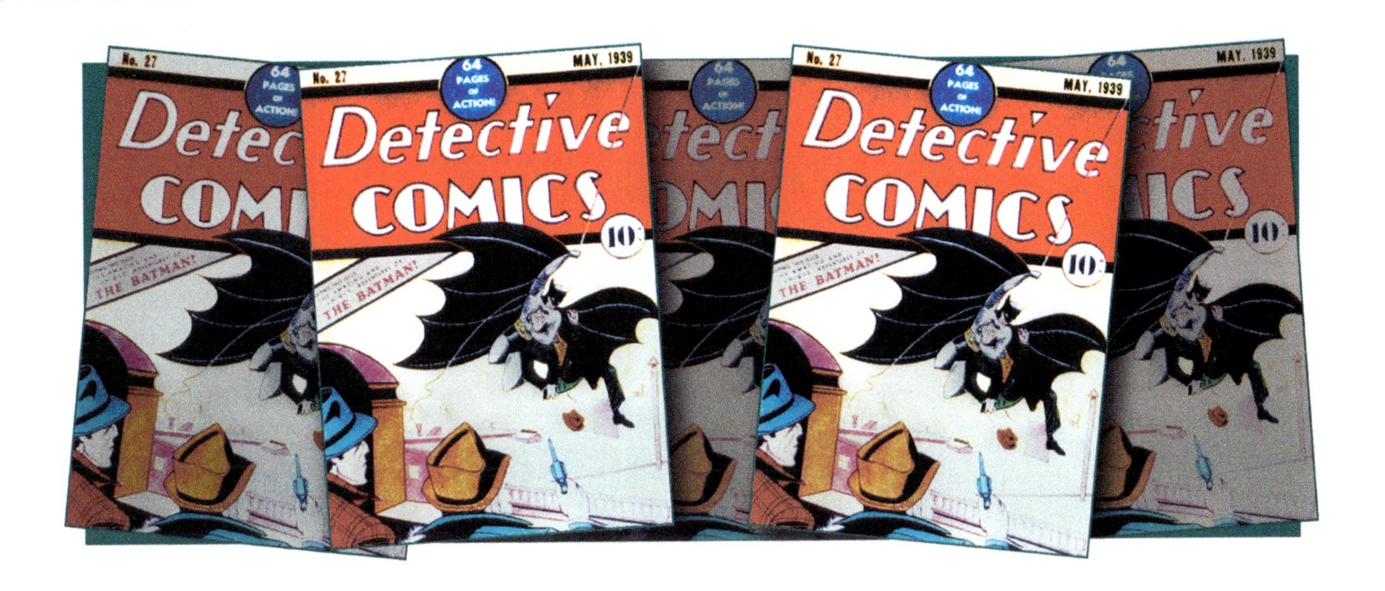

2 Exponential and Logarithmic Functions

What You'll Learn

Why It's Important

In this chapter, we consider two types of functions that are closely related: *exponential functions* and *logarithmic functions*. After learning to find derivatives of such functions, we will study applications in the areas of population growth and decay, continuously compounded interest, the spread of disease, and carbon dating.

Where It's Used

Value of a Comic Book: A 1939 comic book with the first appearance of Batman sold at auction in 2010 for \$1.075 million. The comic book originally sold for \$0.10. Assuming that the value of the comic book increases exponentially, estimate the value in 2025 and the rate, in dollars per year, at which the value is increasing in 2025.

(*This problem appears as Example 5 in Section 2.4.*)

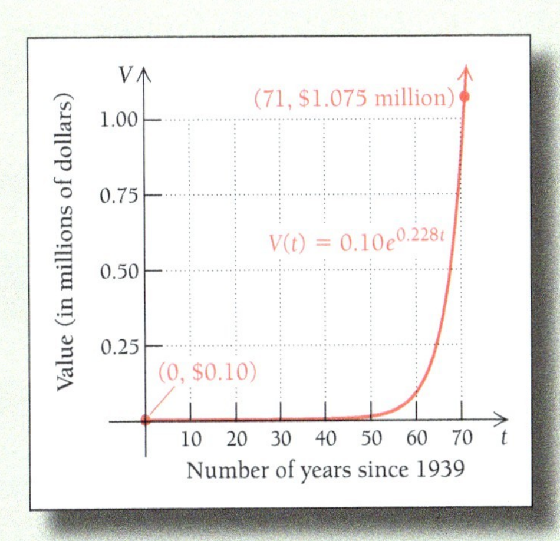

2.1 Exponential and Logarithmic Functions of the Natural Base, e

- Graph and solve exponential functions of the natural base, *e*.
- Graph and solve logarithmic functions of the natural base, *e*.

Consider the following graph. The rapid rise of the graph indicates that it approximates an *exponential function*. In this chapter, we consider such functions and many of their applications.

CUMULATIVE CAPACITY OF INSTALLED RENEWABLE POWER (ALL SOURCES)

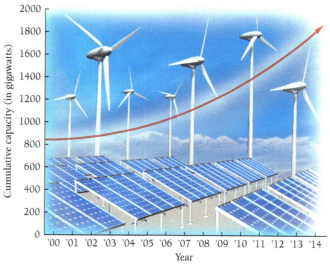

(*Source*: IRENA.)

As we saw in Section R.6, exponential functions are used to model real-world problems that involve heating/cooling, population growth and decay, compound interest, and much more.

The Natural Base, *e*

Recall from Section R.6 that an **exponential function** is given by $f(x) = a_0 \cdot a^x$, where $a > 0$ and $a \neq 1$. The number a is the **base**, the y-intercept is $(0, a_0)$, there are no x-intercepts, and the function is continuous for all real numbers. While the base of an exponential function may be any positive number except 1, we find that, in calculus, a special number called the *natural base* is useful. This number, denoted e, is approximately 2.718.

To appreciate the usefulness of e, consider calculating the future value of an investment that earns compound interest. If P dollars is invested at an annual percentage interest rate r (expressed as a decimal), then the *future value* of the investment after t years, $A(t)$, is given by

$$A(t) = P(1 + r)^t.$$

Here, interest is calculated (compounded) once per year. If n, called the *compounding frequency*, is the number of times that interest is calculated and added to the amount in an account each year, then the future value is given by

$$A = P\left(1 + \frac{r}{n}\right)^{nt}.$$

EXAMPLE 1 **Compound Interest: Future Value.** Luis invests \$5000 in an account that earns interest at an annual rate of 3.25%. Find the future value of Luis's account after 5 yr if interest is compounded **(a)** annually; **(b)** quarterly; **(c)** monthly; and **(d)** daily.

Solution We have $P = \$5000$, $r = 0.0325$ and $t = 5$.

a) If interest is compounded annually, then $n = 1$. Thus, after 5 yr, the value of Luis's account will be

$$A(5) = 5000\left(1 + \frac{0.0325}{1}\right)^{1 \cdot 5} = \$5867.06.$$

b) If interest is compounded quarterly (every 3 months), then $n = 4$. After 5 yr, the value of Luis's account will be

$$A(5) = 5000\left(1 + \frac{0.0325}{4}\right)^{4 \cdot 5} = \$5878.38.$$

c) If interest is compounded monthly, then $n = 12$. After 5 yr, the value of Luis's account will be

$$A(5) = 5000\left(1 + \frac{0.0325}{12}\right)^{12 \cdot 5} = \$5880.95.$$

d) If interest is compounded daily, then $n = 365$. Thus, after 5 yr, the value of Luis's account will be

$$A(5) = 5000\left(1 + \frac{0.0325}{365}\right)^{365 \cdot 5} = \$5882.20.$$

We see that as n increases, the value of Luis's account increases, but not significantly. The increase in value occurs because the interest on the account increases when it is compounded more frequently for the same value of r. 1 ✓

Quick Check 1 ✓

Rachel invests \$20,000 in an account that earns interest at an annual rate of 4%. Find the future value of her account after 3 yr if interest is compounded (a) annually; (b) semiannually ($n = 2$); and (c) weekly.

Let's consider the expression $\left(1 + \frac{1}{n}\right)^n$ and explore its value as n increases:

n	$\left(1 + \frac{1}{n}\right)^n$
10	$\left(1 + \frac{1}{10}\right)^{10} = 2.59374246\ldots$
100	$\left(1 + \frac{1}{100}\right)^{100} = 2.704813829\ldots$
1000	$\left(1 + \frac{1}{1000}\right)^{1000} = 2.716923932\ldots$
10,000	$\left(1 + \frac{1}{10{,}000}\right)^{10{,}000} = 2.718145926\ldots$
100,000	$\left(1 + \frac{1}{100{,}000}\right)^{100{,}000} = 2.718268237\ldots$

As n approaches ∞, growth occurs continuously, and $\left(1 + \frac{1}{n}\right)^n$ gets closer to a number approximated by 2.718 . . . . We call this number the *natural base*, denoted e.

DEFINITION

The **natural base**, denoted e, is the value given by

$$e = \lim_{n \to \infty}\left(1 + \frac{1}{n}\right)^n = 2.71828182845\ldots.$$

Now, consider

$$P\left(1 + \frac{r}{n}\right)^{nt},$$

and let $m = \frac{n}{r}$ so that $n = mr$. Substituting, we have

$$P\left(1 + \frac{r}{n}\right)^{nt} = P\left(1 + \frac{r}{mr}\right)^{mrt} = P\left(1 + \frac{1}{m}\right)^{mrt}.$$

As $n \to \infty$, then $m \to \infty$ also. Thus,

$$\lim_{n\to\infty}\left[P\left(1+\frac{r}{n}\right)^{nt}\right] = \lim_{m\to\infty}\left[P\left(1+\frac{1}{m}\right)^{mrt}\right]$$

$$= P\lim_{m\to\infty}\left[\left(1+\frac{1}{m}\right)^{m}\right]^{rt} \quad \text{Using properties of limits and exponents}$$

$$= Pe^{rt}. \quad \text{Using the definition of } e$$

At this point, the variable m is no longer needed, and we have the following result.

THEOREM 1 Continuous Exponential Growth

A quantity P, growing continuously at annual percentage rate r, expressed as a decimal, has a future value after t years given by Pe^{rt}.

Quick Check 2 ✓

Rachel invests $20,000 in an account that earns interest at an annual rate of 4%. Find the future value of her account after 3 yr if interest is compounded continuously.

EXAMPLE 2 **Continuous Growth.** Luis invests $5000 in an account that earns interest at an annual rate of 3.25%. Find the future value of Luis's account after 5 yr if interest is compounded continuously.

Solution We have $P = \$5000$, $r = 0.0325$, and $t = 5$. Since interest is compounded continuously, after 5 yr, Luis's account will be worth

$$A = 5000e^{0.0325(5)} \quad \text{Substituting}$$

$$= \$5882.24.$$

2 ✓

The graphs of $f(x) = e^x$ and $g(x) = e^{-x}$ are shown below. Both functions have the domain $(-\infty, \infty)$, the range $(0, \infty)$, the y-intercept $(0, 1)$, and no x-intercepts. As x increases in value, e^x increases in value without bound, but e^{-x} decreases toward 0 as a limit. That is, $\lim_{x\to\infty} e^{-x} = 0$.

x	$f(x)$
−2	0.135
−1	0.368
0	1
1	2.718
2	7.389

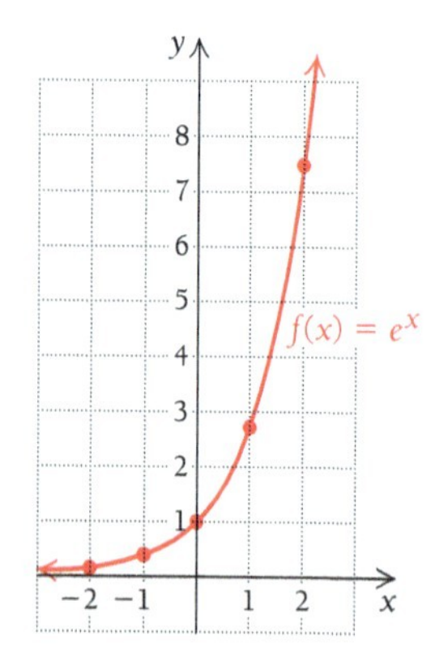

x	$g(x)$
−2	7.389
−1	2.718
0	1
1	0.368
2	0.135

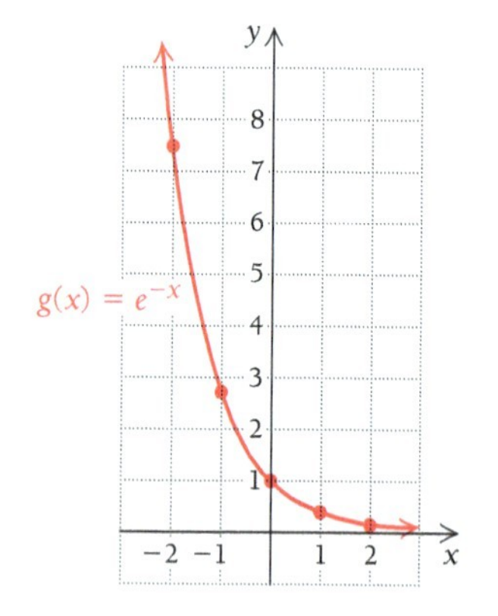

In general, the graph of a function of the form $y = Pe^{rt}$, with $P > 0$, is increasing for $r > 0$ and decreasing for $r < 0$ and has a y-intercept of $(0, P)$. Such functions, and their graphs, are examples of *exponential growth* and *exponential decay*, respectively.

The Natural Logarithm

Recall from Section R.6 that a logarithm is an exponent. When we write

$$\log_a x = y,$$

we are representing a value y such that

$$a^y = x. \quad \text{Recall that } a > 0 \text{ and } a \neq 1.$$

We now introduce the logarithm, base e, called the *natural logarithm* and denoted ln.

DEFINITION The Natural Logarithm

For any positive number x, the **natural logarithm**, or **logarithm, base e**, of x, is given by

$$\ln x = \log_e x.$$

The equation $y = \ln x$ is equivalent to $e^y = x$.

Using a calculator with an LN key, we can find natural logarithms directly.

EXAMPLE 3 Find each of the following. If necessary, use a calculator to approximate values to three decimal places.

a) $\ln e^3$ **b)** $\ln 1$ **c)** $\ln 5$ **d)** $\ln 0.01$

Solution

a) The equation $y = \ln e^3$ is equivalent to $e^y = e^3$, which implies that $y = 3$.

Check: $e^3 = e^3$

b) The equation $y = \ln 1$ is equivalent to $e^y = 1$. We want to find the power of e that gives 1. Thus, $y = \ln 1 = 0$.

Check: $e^0 = 1$

c) To find ln 5, we use a calculator, which gives $\ln 5 = 1.609$, rounded to three decimal places.

Check: $e^{1.609} = 4.9978\ldots \approx 5$

d) Using a calculator, we find $\ln 0.01 = -4.605$, rounded to three decimal places.

Check: $e^{-4.605} = 0.010001702\ldots \approx 0.01$ 3✓

Quick Check 3✓

Find each of the following. Round to three decimal places, if necessary.

a) $\ln e^{-1}$

b) $\ln e^2$

c) $\ln 14$

The following properties of natural logarithms mirror those given in Section R.6 for general logarithms.

THEOREM 2 Properties of Natural Logarithms

P1. $\ln(MN) = \ln M + \ln N$

P2. $\ln\left(\frac{M}{N}\right) = \ln M - \ln N$

P3. $\ln M^k = k \cdot \ln M$

P4. $\ln e = 1$

P5. $\ln 1 = 0$

P6. $\log_b M = \frac{\ln M}{\ln b}$ and $\ln M = \frac{\log M}{\log e}$

P7. $\ln e^x = x$, for all real numbers x

P8. $e^{\ln x} = x$, for all $x > 0$

EXAMPLE 4 Given

$$\ln 2 = 0.6931 \quad \text{and} \quad \ln 3 = 1.0986,$$

use the properties of natural logarithms to find each of the following:

a) $\ln 6$; **b)** $\ln 81$; **c)** $\ln \frac{1}{3}$; **d)** $\ln(2e^5)$; **e)** $\log_2 3$.

Solution

a) $\ln 6 = \ln(2\cdot3) = \ln 2 + \ln 3$ Using Property P1 of natural logarithms

$$= 0.6931 + 1.0986$$

$$= 1.7917$$

Quick Check 4 ✓

Given $\ln 2 = 0.6931$ and $\ln 5 = 1.6094$, use the properties of natural logarithms to find each of the following:

a) $\ln 10$;

b) $\ln \frac{5}{2}$;

c) $\ln \frac{2}{5}$;

d) $\ln 32$;

e) $\ln 5e^2$;

f) $\log_5 2$.

b) $\ln 81 = \ln(3^4)$
$= 4 \ln 3$ — Using Property P3
$= 4(1.0986)$
$= 4.3944$

c) $\ln \frac{1}{3} = \ln 1 - \ln 3$ — Using Property P2
$= 0 - 1.0986$ — Using Property P5
$= -1.0986$

d) $\ln(2e^5) = \ln 2 + \ln(e^5)$ — Using Property P1
$= 0.6931 + 5$ — Using Property P7
$= 5.6931$

e) $\log_2 3 = \dfrac{\ln 3}{\ln 2} = \dfrac{1.0986}{0.6931} \approx 1.5851$ — Using Property P6 **4 ✓**

There are two ways in which we might graph $y = f(x) = \ln x$. One is to graph the equivalent equation $x = e^y$ by selecting values for y and calculating the corresponding values of e^y. We then plot points, remembering that x is still the first coordinate.

x, or e^y	y
0.1	−2
0.4	−1
1.0	0
2.7	1
7.4	2
20.1	3

① Select y.
② Compute x.

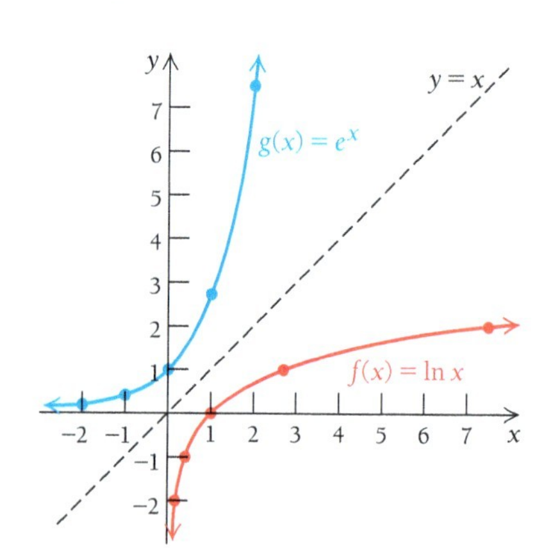

The graph above shows the graph of $g(x) = e^x$ for comparison with that of $f(x) = \ln x$. Note that the functions are inverses of each other. That is, the graph of $y = \ln x$, or $x = e^y$, is a reflection across the line $y = x$ of the graph of $y = e^x$. Any ordered pair (a, b) on the graph of g yields an ordered pair (b, a) on f.

A second method of graphing $y = \ln x$ is to use a calculator to find function values. For example, when $x = 2$, then $y = \ln 2 \approx 0.6931$. This gives the pair $(2, 0.6931)$ shown on the graph.

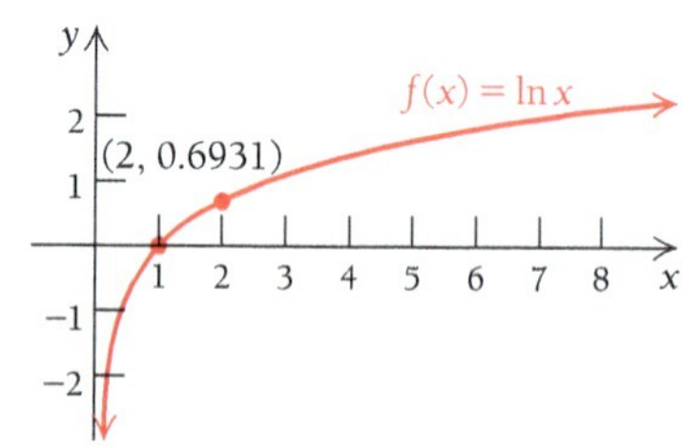

The following properties can be observed from the graph.

THEOREM 3

$\ln x$ exists only for positive numbers x. The domain is $(0, \infty)$.

$\ln x < 0$, for $0 < x < 1$;

$\ln x = 0$, for $x = 1$;

$\ln x > 0$, for $x > 1$.

The function given by $f(x) = \ln x$ is always increasing. The range is the entire real line, $(-\infty, \infty)$, or the set of real numbers, $\mathbb{R}$.

Note that for an expression such as $\ln(x - 2)$, we require that $x - 2 > 0$ or, equivalently, $x > 2$. Thus, the domain of $y = \ln(x - 2)$ is $(2, \infty)$.

EXAMPLE 5 Find the domain of $f(x) = \ln(5 - 2x)$.

Solution We require that $5 - 2x$ be positive. That is, we must have

$$5 - 2x > 0$$
$$-2x > -5$$
$$x < \frac{5}{2}.$$

Thus, the domain of f is $\left(-\infty, \frac{5}{2}\right)$. 5 ✓

Quick Check 5 ✓
Find the domain of $d(x) = \ln(7 - 3x)$.

Solving Exponential and Logarithmic Equations, Base *e*

A common method for solving exponential equations is to find the natural logarithm of both sides. We first isolate the exponential term, then write the equivalent logarithmic form of the equation:

$$e^x = b$$
$$\ln e^x = \ln b \quad \text{Finding the natural logarithm of both sides}$$
$$x = \ln b \quad \text{Using Property P7 of natural logarithms}$$

EXAMPLE 6 Solve the following exponential equations using logarithms. Round answers to three decimal places.

a) $e^{3x} = 2$ **b)** $250e^{0.015t} = 750$

Solution

a) We have

$$e^{3x} = 2 \quad \text{The exponential term is already isolated.}$$
$$\ln e^{3x} = \ln 2 \quad \text{Finding the natural logarithm of both sides}$$
$$3x = \ln 2 \quad \text{Using Property P7}$$
$$x = \frac{\ln 2}{3} \approx 0.231. \quad \text{Using a calculator}$$

Check: $e^{3(0.231)} = 1.999705\ldots \approx 2$

The solution is approximately 0.231.

b) We have

$$250e^{0.015t} = 750$$
$$e^{0.015t} = 3 \quad \text{Dividing both sides by 250 to isolate } e^{0.015t}$$
$$\ln e^{0.015t} = \ln 3 \quad \text{Finding the natural logarithm of both sides}$$
$$0.015t = \ln 3$$
$$t = \frac{\ln 3}{0.015} \approx 73.24. \quad \text{Using a calculator}$$

Check: $250e^{0.015(73.241)} = 750.002\ldots \approx 750$

The solution is approximately 73.24. 6 ✓

Quick Check 6 ✓
Solve each equation. Round answers to three decimal places.

a) $e^t = 80$
b) $e^{-0.08t} = 0.25$
c) $67e^{0.45t} = 500$

EXAMPLE 7 **Business: Growth of an Account.** Marisa invests \$12,000 in an account that earns 2.8% annual interest, compounded continuously. When will Marisa's account double in value?

Solution The value of Marisa's account after t years is given by

$$A(t) = 12{,}000e^{0.028t}.$$

To find the time needed for her original investment of \$12,000 to double in value, we substitute 24,000 for A and solve for t:

$$24{,}000 = 12{,}000e^{0.028t} \quad \text{Substituting 24,000 for } A$$
$$2 = e^{0.028t} \quad \text{Dividing both sides by 12,000}$$
$$\ln 2 = \ln e^{0.028t} \quad \text{Finding the natural logarithm of both sides}$$
$$\ln 2 = 0.028t \quad \text{Using Property P7}$$
$$t = \frac{\ln 2}{0.028} \approx 24.8 \text{ yr.} \quad \text{Dividing and using a calculator}$$

Thus, Marisa's account will double in value in approximately 24.8 yr. This "doubling time" is the same for any initial deposit. Had she invested \$50, it would take 24.8 yr for that amount to grow to \$100. 7 ✓

Quick Check 7 ✓

Rachel invests \$20,000 in an account that earns 4% annual interest, compounded continuously. When will her account be worth three times her initial deposit?

Example 7 suggests a general formula for finding the time needed for an initial quantity P to double in size. Letting T represent the doubling time, we have

$$2P = Pe^{rT}$$
$$2 = e^{rT} \quad \text{Dividing by } P$$
$$\ln 2 = \ln e^{rT} \quad \text{Finding the natural logarithm of both sides}$$
$$\ln 2 = rT.$$

Note that this relationship between r and T does not depend on P. It takes as long for \$1 to double as it does for \$10,000 to double. We have the following theorem.

THEOREM 4

The **exponential growth rate** r (expressed as a decimal) and the **doubling time** T are related by

$$rT = \ln 2, \quad \text{or} \quad r = \frac{\ln 2}{T}, \quad \text{and} \quad T = \frac{\ln 2}{r}.$$

Quick Check 8 ✓

Business: Growth of Digital Revenue. Revenue from sales of digital content by the *New York Times* doubled over the 6-yr period between 2011 and 2017. (*Source:* www.recode.net.) Assuming exponential growth of the digital revenue during this period, what was the exponential growth rate?

EXAMPLE 8 **Business: Facebook Membership.** Facebook connects people with other members they designate as friends. During its period of heaviest growth, membership in Facebook was doubling every 6 months. What was the exponential growth rate of Facebook membership, as a percentage?

Solution We have

$$r = \frac{\ln 2}{6} \approx 0.116 \cdot \frac{1}{\text{month}}.$$

The exponential growth rate of Facebook membership was 11.6% per month. 8 ✓

To solve a logarithmic equation, we isolate the logarithm on one side of the equation, then rewrite the equation in its equivalent exponential form and solve. Solutions must be checked to ensure that they are in the domain of the related logarithmic function.

EXAMPLE 9 Solve:

$$2 + 3\ln(x - 1) = 8.$$

Solution We first isolate the natural logarithm:

$$\begin{aligned} 2 + 3\ln(x - 1) &= 8 \\ 3\ln(x - 1) &= 6 && \text{Adding } -2 \text{ to both sides} \\ \ln(x - 1) &= 2 && \text{Dividing both sides by 3} \\ x - 1 &= e^2 && \text{Writing the equivalent exponential equation} \\ x &= e^2 + 1 \approx 8.389. && \text{Isolating } x \text{ and using a calculator} \end{aligned}$$

The domain of $\ln(x - 1)$ is $(1, \infty)$. Thus, 8.389 is in the domain and is a valid solution.

9 ✓

Quick Check 9 ✓

Solve: $\ln(4 - 2x) = 7$.

Section Summary

- The *natural base*, denoted e, is defined by

$$e = \lim_{n\to\infty}\left(1 + \frac{1}{n}\right)^n = 2.71828182845\ldots.$$

- *Continuous Exponential Growth:* A quantity P, with continuous compounding at an annual percentage rate r, has a future value after t years given by $A = Pe^{rt}$.
- The function given by $y = Pe^{rt}$, where $P > 0$, is increasing for $r > 0$ and decreasing for $r < 0$ and has a y-intercept of $(0, P)$. The domain is the set of all real numbers, and the range is $y > 0$.
- For any positive number x, the logarithm, base e, of x is given by $\ln x = \log_e x$. The equation $y = \ln x$ is equivalent to $e^y = x$. The expression $\ln x$ is defined for $x > 0$.
- *Properties of Natural Logarithms:*
  - **P1.** $\ln(MN) = \ln M + \ln N$
  - **P2.** $\ln\left(\frac{M}{N}\right) = \ln M - \ln N$
  - **P3.** $\ln M^k = k \cdot \ln M$
  - **P4.** $\ln e = 1$
  - **P5.** $\ln 1 = 0$
  - **P6.** $\log_b M = \frac{\ln M}{\ln b}$ and $\ln M = \frac{\log M}{\log e}$
  - **P7.** $\ln e^x = x$, for all real numbers x
  - **P8.** $e^{\ln x} = x$, for all $x > 0$
- The function $f(x) = \ln x$ has the domain $(0, \infty)$, the range $(-\infty, \infty)$, the x-intercept $(1, 0)$, and no y-intercept.
- The exponential growth rate r and the doubling time T are related by $rT = \ln 2$, so $T = \frac{\ln 2}{r}$ and $r = \frac{\ln 2}{T}$.

2.1 Exercise Set

Graph each function. Then identify the domain, range, and y-intercept and state whether the function is increasing or decreasing.

1. $g(x) = e^{-2x}$
2. $f(x) = e^{2x}$
3. $f(x) = e^{(1/3)x}$
4. $g(x) = e^{(1/2)x}$
5. $f(x) = \frac{1}{2}e^{-x}$
6. $g(x) = \frac{1}{3}e^{-x}$
7. $F(x) = -e^{(1/3)x}$
8. $G(x) = -e^{(1/2)x}$

For Exercises 9–16, an initial investment amount P, an annual interest rate r, and a time t are given. Find the future value of the investment when interest is compounded (a) annually, (b) monthly, (c) daily, and (d) continuously. Then find (e) the doubling time T for the given interest rate.

9. $P = \$1500$, $r = 3.15\%$, $t = 4$ yr
10. $P = \$2500$, $r = 2.75\%$, $t = 6$ yr
11. $P = \$75{,}000$, $r = 4.5\%$, $t = 3$ yr
12. $P = \$100{,}000$, $r = 2.29\%$, $t = 7$ yr
13. $P = \$250$, $r = 1.99\%$, $t = 10$ yr
14. $P = \$1500$, $r = 2.08\%$, $t = 12$ yr
15. $P = \$10{,}000$, $r = 4.1\%$, $t = 18$ months
16. $P = \$12{,}000$, $r = 3.7\%$, $t = 9$ months

For Exercises 17–26, use a calculator to find each logarithm, rounded to three decimal places when appropriate. Verify each result by showing that it solves the corresponding exponential equation.

17. $\ln 2$
18. $\ln 9$
19. $\ln 4.5$
20. $\ln 3.33$
21. $\ln 0.052$
22. $\ln 0.103$

23. $\ln\left(\frac{3}{4}\right)$
24. $\ln\left(\frac{6}{5}\right)$
25. $\ln e^5$
26. $\ln e^8$

Given $\ln 4 = 1.3863$ *and* $\ln 5 = 1.6094$, *use properties of natural logarithms to find each value. Do not use a calculator.*

27. $\ln 80$
28. $\ln 20$
29. $\ln \frac{1}{5}$
30. $\ln \frac{5}{4}$
31. $\ln(4e)$
32. $\ln(5e)$
33. $\ln \sqrt{e^8}$
34. $\ln \sqrt{e^6}$
35. $\ln \frac{4}{5}$
36. $\ln \frac{1}{4}$
37. $\ln\left(\frac{4}{e}\right)$
38. $\ln\left(\frac{e}{5}\right)$

Solve for t. Round the answer to three decimal places.

39. $e^t = 8$
40. $e^t = 10$
41. $e^{3t} = 900$
42. $e^{2t} = 1000$
43. $e^{-t} = 0.01$
44. $e^{-t} = 0.1$
45. $e^{-0.02t} = 0.06$
46. $e^{-0.07t} = 2$
47. $5e^{2t} = 15$
48. $8e^{3t} = 25$
49. $200e^{0.045t} = 600$
50. $3500e^{0.05t} = 10{,}000$

Find the domain of each logarithmic function and then graph the function.

51. $y = \ln(3x + 4)$
52. $y = \ln(5x - 2)$
53. $f(x) = \ln(4 - x)$
54. $f(x) = \ln(8 - 4x)$
55. $y = \ln(x + 3) + \ln(5 - x)$
56. $y = \ln(2 - x) + \ln(x + 1)$
57. $g(x) = \ln(x + 2) + \ln x$
58. $g(x) = \ln(x + 6) + \ln x$
59. $y = \ln(x^2 + 1)$
60. $y = \ln(x^2 + 2x + 4)$

Solve each logarithmic equation. Round the answer to three decimal places

61. $\ln x = 10$
62. $\ln x = 6.5$
63. $2 \ln x = 9$
64. $3 \ln x = 5$
65. $1 + 4\ln(2x + 1) = 7$
66. $3 - 5\ln(3x - 2) = 10$
67. $\ln(x + 3) + \ln(x - 3) = \ln 7$
68. $\ln(x + 2) + \ln x = \ln 24$

APPLICATIONS

Business and Economics

69. U.S. travel exports. U.S. travel exports (goods and services that international travelers buy while visiting the United States) are increasing exponentially. The value of such exports, t years after 2011, can be approximated by

$$V(t) = 115.32e^{0.094t},$$

where V is in billions of dollars. (*Source:* www.census.gov/foreign-trade/data/index.html.)

a) Estimate the value of U.S. travel exports in 2018 and 2020.
b) When will the value of U.S. travel exports reach \$150 billion?
c) When will the value of U.S. travel exports be double their value in 2011?

70. Organic food. More and more Americans are buying organic fruit and vegetables and products made with organic ingredients. The amount $A(t)$, in billions of dollars, spent on organic food and beverages t years after 2014 can be approximated by

$$A(t) = 35.8e^{0.104t}.$$

(*Source:* www.ota.com.)

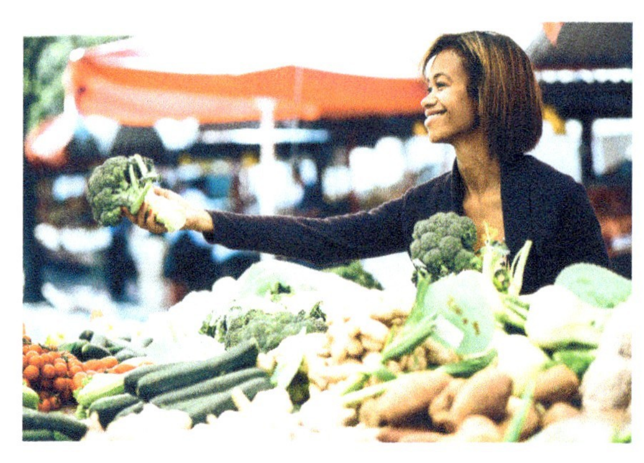

a) Estimate the amount that Americans spent on organic food and beverages in 2017.
b) When will the amount that Americans spend on organic food and beverages exceed \$50 billion?
c) When will the amount that Americans spend on organic food and beverages be double the amount spent in 2014?

71. Compound interest: future value. Dennis deposits \$10,000 in a savings account that earns 2.88% annual interest, compounded continuously.

a) Write a function of the form $A(t) = Pe^{rt}$ that gives the value of Dennis's account after t years.
b) How much will be in Dennis's account after 5 yr?
c) When will Dennis's account be worth \$15,000?
d) When will the value of Dennis's account be double the original value?

72. Compound interest: future value. Belinda invests \$25,000 in a retirement fund that earns 4.03% annual interest, compounded continuously.

a) Write a function of the form $A(t) = Pe^{rt}$ that gives the value of Belinda's account after t years.
b) How much will be in Belinda's account after 10 yr?
c) When will Belinda's account be worth \$40,000?
d) When will the value of Belinda's account be double the original value?

73. Value of a stock. The value of a share of Danube, Inc., stock, t weeks after being purchased, is given by

$$V(t) = 75 - 50e^{-0.04t}.$$

a) What is the value of the share after 20 weeks?
b) What was the original purchase price of the share?
c) When will the share of stock be worth \$60?

74. Value of a stock. The value of a share of St. Lawrence Corporation stock, t weeks after being purchased, is given by

$$V(t) = 140 - 80e^{-0.0225t}.$$

a) What is the value of the share after 35 weeks?
b) What was the original purchase price of the share?
c) When will the share of stock be worth \$125?

75. **Demand.** The price, in dollars per unit, that consumers are willing to pay for a popular high-end digital camera is given by

$$p(x) = 1450 - 150 \ln x,$$

where x is in thousands of units.

a) What price corresponds to a demand of 300,000 units?
b) How many units will consumers buy at a price of $300 per camera?

76. **Demand.** The price, in dollars per unit, that consumers are willing to pay for the Trailmaster mountain bike is given by

$$p(x) = 980 - 90 \ln x,$$

where x is in thousands of units.

a) What price corresponds to a demand of 150,000 units?
b) How many units will consumers buy at a price of $400 per bicycle?

General Interest

77. **Population.** The city of San Estaban had a population of 45,000 in 2015 ($t = 0$) and was growing continuously at an annual percentage rate of 3% per year.

a) Write a function of the form $A(t) = Pe^{rt}$ that gives the population of San Estaban t years after 2015.
b) What will the population be in 2025?
c) When will the population reach 55,000?
d) When will the population double in size?

78. **Student enrollment.** The student enrollment at Marina College was 2500 in 2016 ($t = 0$) and was growing continuously at an annual percentage rate of 2.5% per year.

a) Write a function of the form $A(t) = Pe^{rt}$ that gives the enrollment at Marina College t years after 2016.
b) What will the enrollment be in 2022?
c) When will the enrollment reach 4000?
d) When will the enrollment be double what it was in 2016?

79. **Bacterial growth.** A biologist swabs a sample of bacteria onto a petri dish, and this original colony covers an area of 2 mm^2. Every hour, the colony's area increases by 4.5%.

a) Write a function of the form $A(t) = Pe^{rt}$ that gives the area of the colony of bacteria after t hours.
b) What is the area of the colony after 10 hr?
c) When will the colony's area reach 50 mm^2?
d) When will the colony's area be double the original area?

80. **Population growth.** A fishing boat with an initial population of 50 quagga mussels on its hull is lowered into a pristine lake. A field biologist determines that the population of quagga mussels in the lake then grows by 55% every week.

a) Write a function of the form $Q(t) = Pe^{rt}$ that gives the population of quagga mussels in the lake after t weeks.
b) What is the population of quagga mussels in the lake after 15 weeks?
c) When will the population of quagga mussels reach 1,000,000?
d) When will the population of quagga mussels be double its original size?

81. **Cooling liquid.** A cup of hot coffee is placed on a counter and allowed to cool. The temperature T (in degrees Celsius) of the coffee t minutes after being placed on the counter is given by

$$T(t) = 30 + 45e^{-0.023t}.$$

a) What was the original temperature of the hot coffee?
b) What is the coffee's temperature after 20 min?
c) When will the coffee's temperature be 35°C?
d) Find $\lim_{t \to \infty} T(t)$, and explain what this number represents.

82. **Cooling liquid.** A boiling pot of water is removed from a stovetop and allowed to cool. The temperature T (in degrees Celsius) of the water t minutes after being removed from the stovetop is given by

$$T(t) = 22 + 78e^{-0.041t}.$$

a) What was the original temperature of the boiling water?
b) What is the water temperature after 15 min?
c) When will the water temperature be 40°C?
d) Find $\lim_{t \to \infty} T(t)$, and explain what this number represents.

83. **Decaying isotope.** A sample of 5 mg of the isotope gold-198 decays naturally. The amount A, in milligrams, of the sample still remaining after t days is given by

$$A(t) = 5e^{-0.257t}.$$

a) How much of the 5-mg sample remains after 1 day?
b) After how many days will 1 mg of gold-198 remain?
c) After how many days will half of the original sample remain?
d) Find $\lim_{t \to \infty} A(t)$, and explain what this number represents.

84. **Decaying population.** The population, P, of Cottonwood Cove, t years after 2017, is given by

$$P(t) = 17{,}250e^{-0.0512t}.$$

a) What will the population of Cottonwood Cove be in 2024?
b) When will the population of Cottonwood Cove first drop below 14,000?
c) When will the population of Cottonwood Cove be half of the 2017 value?
d) Find $\lim_{t \to \infty} P(t)$, and explain what this number represents.

SYNTHESIS

In Exercises 85–94, solve for x.

85. $e^{2x} - 5e^x + 4 = 0$. (*Hint*: Factor as a quadratic equation in e^x.)

86. $e^{2x} - 10e^x + 21 = 0$

87. $e^{2x} - 12e^x = -32$

88. $e^{2x} - 7e^x = -12$

89. $e^{2x} - e^x - 12 = 0$

90. $e^{2x} - 3e^x - 10 = 0$

91. $\ln(1 + \ln x) = 2$

92. $\ln(2 + 3 \ln x) = -1$

93. $(\ln x)^2 - 4 \ln x + 3 = 0$

94. $(\ln x)^2 - 2 \ln x - 15 = 0$

95. Jim deposited $1500 in a savings account that grows continuously, and 3 yr later the value of his account is $1800. Find the continuous annual growth rate, r, and the doubling time, T.

96. Biologists noted that an initial population of 250 quagga mussels in a lake had grown to 500,000 mussels after 6 months. Assuming exponential growth, find the continuous annual growth rate, r, and the doubling time, T.

97. A biologist noted that a colony of bacteria in a petri dish had grown to 5 times its original size in 8 hours. What is the doubling time of this colony of bacteria?

98. The time t (in years) required for Sharon's savings account to be worth \$$A$ is given by $t(A) = 35 \ln(A/7500)$.

a) Solve for A in terms of t. That is, find $A(t)$, the value of Sharon's account after t years.

b) What is the continuous annual growth rate of Sharon's account?

99. Explain why the domains of $y = \ln\left(\frac{x-1}{x+4}\right)$ and $y = \ln(x-1) - \ln(x+4)$ are different, even though the two expressions $\ln\left(\frac{x-1}{x+4}\right)$ and $\ln(x-1) - \ln(x+4)$ are equivalent.

The Rule of 70. *The relationship between doubling time T and growth rate r is the basis of the Rule of 70. Since*

$$T = \frac{\ln 2}{r} = \frac{0.693147}{r} = \frac{69.3147}{100r} \approx \frac{70}{100r},$$

we can estimate the length of time needed for a quantity to double by dividing the growth rate r (expressed as a percentage) into 70.

100. Estimate the time needed for an amount of money to double, if the interest rate is 7%, compounded continuously.

101. Estimate the time needed for the population in a city to double, if the growth rate is 3.5%, compounded continuously.

102. Using a calculator, find the exact doubling times for the amount of money in Exercise 100 and the population in Exercise 101.

103. Explain why a "Rule of 110" would be useful for finding the tripling time for a given growth rate r.

Technology Connection 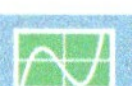

Solve for x. Round to three decimal places when appropriate.

104. $e^x - 3x = 0$

105. $e^{2x} + e^x - 9 = 0$

106. $\ln x = 2 - x^2$

107. $e^x + \ln x = 0$

Answers to Quick Checks

1. **(a)** \$22,497.28; **(b)** \$22,523.25; **(c)** \$22,548.90
2. \$22,549.94 **3.** **(a)** -1; **(b)** 2; **(c)** 2.639
4. **(a)** 2.3025; **(b)** 0.9163; **(c)** -0.9163; **(d)** 3.4655; **(e)** 3.6094; **(f)** 0.4307 **5.** $\left(-\infty, \frac{7}{3}\right)$
6. **(a)** 4.382; **(b)** 17.329; **(c)** 4.466 **7.** In 27.47 yr
8. 11.6% per year **9.** $x = \frac{4 - e^7}{2} \approx -546.32$

2.2 Derivatives of Exponential (Base-e) Functions

- Differentiate exponential (base-e) functions.
- Solve applied problems involving exponential (base-e) functions and their derivatives.

To find the derivative of the exponential function

$$f(x) = e^x,$$

we use the definition of the derivative given by

$$f'(x) = \lim_{h \to 0} \frac{f(x+h) - f(x)}{h} \qquad \text{Definition of the derivative}$$

$$= \lim_{h \to 0} \frac{e^{x+h} - e^x}{h} \qquad \text{Substituting } e^{x+h} \text{ for } f(x+h) \text{ and } e^x \text{ for } f(x)$$

$$= \lim_{h \to 0} \frac{e^x \cdot e^h - e^x \cdot 1}{h} \qquad \text{Using the laws for exponents}$$

$$= \lim_{h \to 0} \left(e^x \cdot \frac{e^h - 1}{h}\right) \qquad \text{Factoring}$$

$$= e^x \cdot \lim_{h \to 0} \frac{e^h - 1}{h}. \qquad \text{Noting that } e^x \text{ is constant with respect to } h \text{ and using a limit theorem}$$

Thus, $$f'(x) = e^x \cdot \lim_{h \to 0} \frac{e^h - 1}{h}.$$

Using a calculator, we find that $\lim_{h \to 0} \frac{e^h - 1}{h} = 1$ (see Exercise 75). Thus, if $f(x) = e^x$, then its derivative is $f'(x) = e^x$. This remarkable result is summarized in the following theorem.

THEOREM 5

The derivative of the function f given by $f(x) = e^x$ is the function itself:

$$f'(x) = f(x), \qquad \text{or} \qquad \frac{d}{dx} e^x = e^x.$$

Theorem 5 says that for $f(x) = e^x$, the derivative at x (the slope of the tangent line) is the same as the function value at x. That is, on the graph of $f(x) = e^x$, at the point $(0, 1)$, the slope is $m = 1$; at the point $(1, e)$, the slope is $m = e$; at the point $(2, e^2)$, the slope is $m = e^2$, and so on. The function given by $f(x) = e^x$ is the *only* nonzero function for which $f(x) = f'(x)$ is always true.

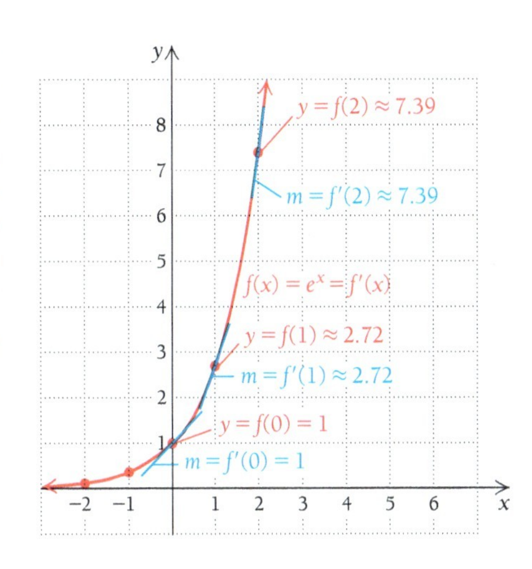

Finding Derivatives of Functions Involving *e*

We can combine Theorem 5 with earlier theorems to differentiate a variety of functions.

EXAMPLE 1 Find dy/dx:

a) $y = 3e^x$; **b)** $y = x^2e^x$; **c)** $y = \frac{e^x}{x^3}$.

Solution

a) $\frac{d}{dx}(3e^x) = 3\frac{d}{dx}e^x$ Recall that $\frac{d}{dx}[c \cdot f(x)] = c \cdot f'(x)$.

$= 3e^x$ Using Theorem 5

b) $\frac{d}{dx}(x^2e^x) = x^2 \cdot e^x + e^x \cdot 2x$ Using the Product Rule

$= xe^x(x + 2)$ Factoring

c) $\frac{d}{dx}\left(\frac{e^x}{x^3}\right) = \frac{x^3 \cdot e^x - e^x \cdot 3x^2}{x^6}$ Using the Quotient Rule

$= \frac{x^2e^x(x - 3)}{x^6}$ Factoring

$= \frac{e^x(x - 3)}{x^4}$ Simplifying

1 ✓

Quick Check 1 ✓

Find dy/dx:

a) $y = 6e^x$;

b) $y = x^3e^x$;

c) $y = \frac{e^x}{x^2}$.

The Chain Rule is needed when differentiating functions of the form $g(x) = e^{f(x)}$. Note that if we let $h(x) = e^x$, then we have $g(x) = (h \circ f)(x) = h(f(x))$. Thus,

$$\begin{aligned}\frac{d}{dx}g(x) &= \frac{d}{dx}h(f(x))\\ &= \frac{d}{dx}e^{f(x)} \cdot f'(x)\\ &= e^{f(x)} \cdot f'(x).\end{aligned}$$

We have the following theorem.

THEOREM 6

For a differentiable function f,

$$\frac{d}{dx}e^{f(x)} = e^{f(x)} \cdot f'(x), \quad \text{or} \quad \frac{d}{dx}e^u = e^u \cdot \frac{du}{dx}.$$

EXAMPLE 2 Differentiate each of the following with respect to x:

a) $y = e^{8x}$; **b)** $y = e^{-x^2+4x-7}$; **c)** $e^{\sqrt{x^2-3}}$.

Solution

a) $\frac{d}{dx}e^{8x} = e^{8x} \cdot 8$ Using the Chain Rule; the derivative is the original function times the derivative of the exponent.

$= 8e^{8x}$

b) $\frac{d}{dx}e^{-x^2+4x-7} = e^{-x^2+4x-7}(-2x + 4)$ Using the Chain Rule

$= -2(x - 2)e^{-x^2+4x-7}$

c) $\frac{d}{dx}e^{\sqrt{x^2-3}} = \frac{d}{dx}e^{(x^2-3)^{1/2}}$

$= e^{(x^2-3)^{1/2}} \cdot \frac{1}{2}(x^2 - 3)^{-1/2} \cdot 2x$ Using the Chain Rule twice

$= e^{\sqrt{x^2-3}} \cdot x \cdot (x^2 - 3)^{-1/2}$

$= \dfrac{e^{\sqrt{x^2-3}} \cdot x}{\sqrt{x^2 - 3}}$, or $\dfrac{xe^{\sqrt{x^2-3}}}{\sqrt{x^2 - 3}}$ 2 ✓

Quick Check 2 ✓

Differentiate:

a) $f(x) = e^{-4x}$;

b) $g(x) = e^{x^3+8x}$;

c) $h(x) = e^{\sqrt{x^2+5}}$.

For higher-order derivatives, we again need to use the rules for differentiation.

EXAMPLE 3 Find $\frac{d^2y}{dx^2}$ for $y = e^{-5x^2}$.

Solution Using the Chain Rule, we find the first derivative, dy/dx. We have

$$\begin{aligned}\frac{dy}{dx} &= \frac{d}{dx}\left(e^{-5x^2}\right)\\ &= e^{-5x^2}(-10x)\\ &= -10xe^{-5x^2}.\end{aligned}$$

Thus,

$$\frac{d^2y}{dx^2} = \frac{d}{dx}\left(-10xe^{-5x^2}\right)$$

$= (-10x) \cdot \left(-10xe^{-5x^2}\right) + \left(e^{-5x^2}\right) \cdot (-10)$ Using the Product and Chain Rules

$= 10e^{-5x^2}\left(10x^2 - 1\right).$ Factoring. 3 ✓

Quick Check 3 ✓

Find $\frac{d^2y}{dx^2}$ for $y = e^{1/x^2}$.

Application: Business and Economics

EXAMPLE 4 **Business: Growth of an Account.** Franco's Fishing Emporium invested \$50,000 in an account that earns 1.25% annual interest, compounded continuously. The value of the account after t years is given by

$$A(t) = 50{,}000e^{0.0125t}.$$

Find $A(5)$ and $A'(5)$, and interpret the meaning of each of these values.

Solution After $t = 5$ yr, the value of the account will be

$$A(5) = 50{,}000e^{0.0125(5)} \approx \$53{,}224.72. \quad \text{Rounding to two decimal places}$$

To find $A'(5)$, we first find $\frac{d}{dt}A(t)$:

$$\begin{aligned} \frac{d}{dt}A(t) &= \frac{d}{dt}(50{,}000e^{0.0125t}) \\ &= 50{,}000 \cdot \frac{d}{dt}(e^{0.0125t}) \\ &= 50{,}000e^{0.0125t}(0.0125) && \text{Using the Chain Rule} \\ &= 625e^{0.0125t}. && \text{Simplifying} \end{aligned}$$

Thus, we have

$$A'(5) = 625e^{0.0125(5)} \approx 665.31. \quad \text{Rounding to two decimal places}$$

After exactly 5 yr, the value of Franco's Fishing Emporium's account is \$53,224.72, and at that instant, the value is growing at the rate of \$665.31 per year. 4 ✓

Quick Check 4 ✓

Rachel deposits \$20,000 in a savings account that earns 4% annual interest, compounded continuously. The value of her account after t years is given by $A(t) = 20{,}000e^{0.04t}$. Find $A(10)$ and $A'(10)$, and interpret the meaning of each of these values.

EXAMPLE 5 **Business: Worker Output.** It is reasonable for a manufacturer to expect the daily output of a new worker to be low at first, increase over time, and then level off. A manufacturer of LED flashlights determines that after t workdays, the number of flashlights produced per day by the average worker can be modeled by

$$N = 80 - 70e^{-0.13t}.$$

a) Find N for $t = 1, 5, 10, 20$, and 30.

b) Graph $N(t)$.

c) Find $N'(t)$, and interpret this result as a rate of change.

d) What number of flashlights seems to be the number at which worker output levels off?

Solution

a) We make a table of input–output values.

t	1	5	10	20	30
$N(t)$	18.5	43.5	60.9	74.8	78.6

b) Using these values and/or a graphing calculator, we obtain the graph.

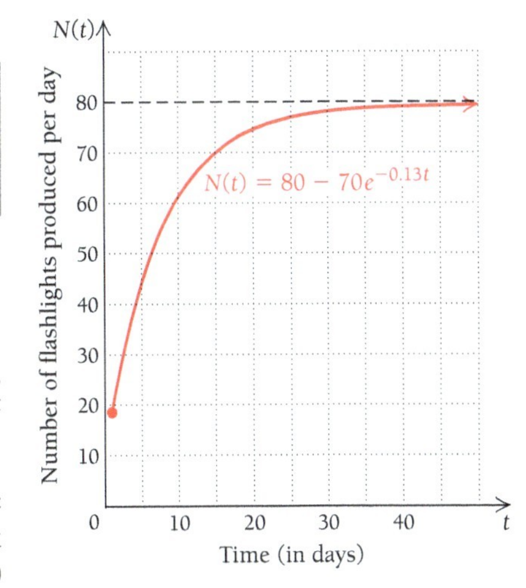

c) We have $N'(t) = -70e^{-0.13t}(-0.13) = 9.1e^{-0.13t}$; after t days, the average worker is producing flashlights at a rate of $9.1e^{-0.13t}$ flashlights per day.

d) Examining the graph and expanding the table of function values, it seems that worker output levels off at no more than 80 flashlights produced per day. 5 ✓

Quick Check 5 ✓

Business: Worker Output. Repeat Example 5 for the output function

$$N(t) = 80 - 60e^{-0.12t}.$$

In general, for $k > 0$, the graph of $h(x) = 1 - e^{-kx}$ is increasing, which we expect since $h'(x) = ke^{-kx}$ is always positive. Note that $h(x)$ approaches 1 as x approaches ∞.

Section Summary

- $\frac{d}{dx}(e^x) = e^x$
- For functions of the form $y = e^{f(x)}$, the Chain Rule gives $y' = \frac{dy}{dx} = e^{f(x)} \cdot f'(x)$.

2.2 Exercise Set

Differentiate.

1. $g(x) = e^{2x}$
2. $g(x) = e^{3x}$
3. $g(x) = 3e^{5x}$
4. $G(x) = 2e^{4x}$
5. $G(x) = x^3 - 5e^{2x}$
6. $f(x) = x^5 - 2e^{6x}$
7. $g(x) = x^5e^{2x}$
8. $f(x) = x^7e^{4x}$
9. $F(x) = \frac{e^{2x}}{x^4}$
10. $g(x) = \frac{e^{3x}}{x^6}$
11. $f(x) = (x^2 - 2x + 2)e^x$
12. $f(x) = (x^2 + 3x - 9)e^x$
13. $f(x) = e^{-x^2+8x}$
14. $f(x) = e^{-x^2+7x}$
15. $y = \sqrt{e^x - 1}$
16. $y = \sqrt{e^x + 1}$
17. $y = e^x + x^3 - xe^x$
18. $y = xe^{-2x} + e^{-x} + x^3$
19. $g(x) = (4x^2 + 3x)e^{x^2-7x}$
20. $g(x) = (5x^2 - 8x)e^{x^2-4x}$
21. $k(t) = \frac{t}{e^{2t}}$
22. $s(t) = \frac{t^2}{e^{3t}}$
23. $r(t) = \frac{t^2 + 2t}{e^{t^2}}$
24. $f(t) = \frac{t^3 - 5t}{e^{4t^3}}$

Find the second derivative.

25. $f(x) = e^{2x}$
26. $g(x) = e^{-3x}$
27. $h(x) = e^{(-1/2)x}$
28. $m(x) = e^{(2/3)x}$
29. $F(x) = e^{x^2}$
30. $C(x) = e^{x^3}$
31. $d(x) = e^{2x+1}$
32. $t(x) = e^{3-4x}$
33. $u(x) = e^{\sqrt{x}}$
34. $v(t) = e^{\sqrt[3]{t}}$
35. $w(x) = xe^x$
36. $y(x) = x^2e^x$
37. $f(t) = (2t + 3)e^{3t}$
38. $R(t) = (5t - 4)e^{-2t}$
39. $z(x) = (e^{2x} + 1)^2$
40. $u(x) = (3e^{4x} + 2)^3$
41. $w(t) = (t^2 + 2t + 3)e^{5t}$
42. $y(t) = (4t^3 - t)e^{1-2t}$
43. $z(x) = \frac{e^{3x}}{x^2}$
44. $m(x) = \frac{e^{8x}}{3x^4}$
45. $f(t) = \sqrt{e^{3t} - 1}$
46. $g(t) = \sqrt{1 - 5e^{-4t}}$

47. **Marginal cost.** The total cost, in millions of dollars, for Greenleaf Construction is given by

$$C(x) = 100 - 50e^{-x},$$

where x is the number of houses built.

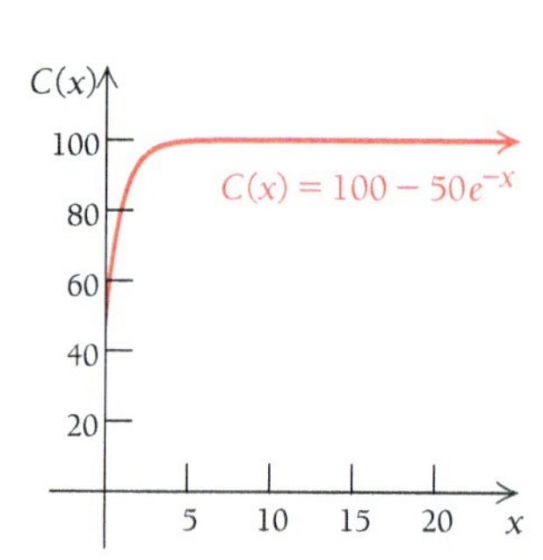

Find each of the following.

a) The marginal cost, $C'(x)$
b) $C'(0)$
c) $C'(4)$ (Round to the nearest thousand.)
d) Find $\lim_{x\to\infty} C(x)$ and $\lim_{x\to\infty} C'(x)$.

48. **Marginal cost.** The total cost, in millions of dollars, for Marcotte Industries is given by

$$C(x) = 200 - 40e^{-x},$$

where x is the time in years since the start-up date.

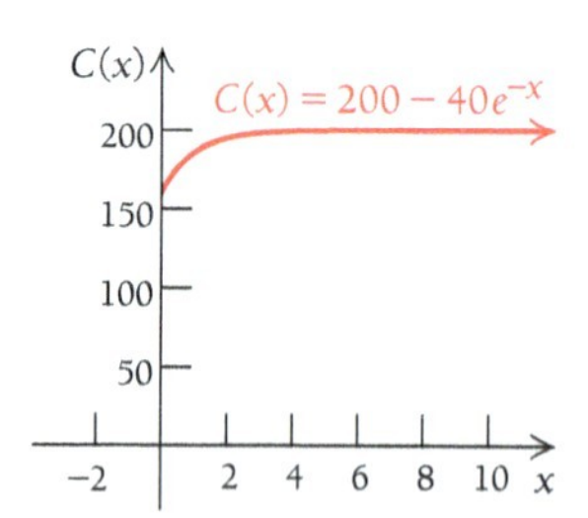

Find each of the following.

a) The marginal cost $C'(x)$
b) $C'(1)$
c) $C'(5)$ (Round to the nearest thousand.)
d) Find $\lim_{x\to\infty} C(x)$ and $\lim_{x\to\infty} C'(x)$.

49. **Growth of a retirement fund.** Maria invests \$20,000 in an IRA account whose value after t years is modeled by

$$V(t) = 20{,}000e^{0.0545t}.$$

a) Use the model to estimate the value of Maria's IRA account after 7 yr.
b) What is the rate of change in the value of the IRA account at the end of 7 yr?

50. Depreciation. Pelican Fabrics purchases a new video surveillance system. The value of the system is modeled by

$$V(t) = 17{,}500e^{-0.0834t},$$

where $V(t)$ is the value of the system, in dollars, t years after its purchase.

a) Use the model to estimate the value of the system 5 yr after it was purchased.
b) What is the rate of change in the value of the system at the end of 5 yr?

51. Depreciation. Perriot's Restaurant purchased kitchen equipment on January 1, 2017. On January 1, 2019, the value of the equipment was \$14,450. The value after that date is modeled by

$$V(t) = 14{,}450e^{-0.163t}.$$

a) What is the rate of change in the value of the equipment on January 1, 2019?
b) What was the original value of the equipment on January 1, 2017?

52. Stock prices. The value (price) of a share of stock in Barrington Gold was \$90 on June 15, 2018, and its value t weeks after that date is given by

$$V(t) = 90e^{0.0296t}.$$

a) What was the rate of change in the value of a share of the stock on June 15, 2018?
b) Use the model to estimate the value of a share of the stock 6 weeks prior to June 15, 2018.

Life and Physical Sciences

53. Medication concentration. The concentration C, in parts per million (ppm), of a medication in the body t hours after ingestion is given by the function

$$C(t) = 10t^2e^{-t}.$$

a) Find the concentration after 0 hr, 1 hr, 2 hr, 3 hr, and 10 hr.
b) Use a calculator to graph the function for $0 \le t \le 10$.
c) Find $C(5)$ and $C'(5)$, and explain what those values represent.

54. Medication concentration. The concentration C, in parts per million, of a medication in the body t minutes after ingestion is given by

$$C(t) = 250e^{-0.03t}.$$

a) Find the concentration after 1 min, 5 min, and 12 min.
b) Use a calculator to graph the function for $0 \le t \le 20$.
c) Find $C(8)$ and $C'(8)$, and explain what these numbers represent.

55. Antibiotic treatment. A biologist has a colony of a toxic strain of bacteria that covers 500 mm^2 in a petri dish. She observes that the area, in square millimeters, of the colony of bacteria t hours after an antibiotic is applied is given by

$$A(t) = 500e^{-0.06t}.$$

a) Find the area of the colony of bacteria after 2 hr, 5 hr, and 10 hr.
b) Use a calculator to graph the function for $0 \le t \le 40$.
c) Find $A(12)$ and $A'(12)$, and explain what these numbers represent.

56. Population control. A biologist determines that a lake contains 1200 of an invasive species of fish. A natural predator is introduced into the lake, and the population of the invasive species t weeks after that time is given by

$$P(t) = 1200e^{-0.079t}.$$

a) Find the population of the invasive species of fish at 2 weeks, 6 weeks, and 15 weeks after the introduction of the predator.
b) Use a calculator to graph the function for $0 \le t \le 40$.
c) Find $P(20)$ and $P'(20)$, and explain what these numbers represent.

Social Sciences

57. Ebbinghaus learning model. Suppose that you are given the task of learning 100% of a block of knowledge. Human nature is such that we retain only a percentage P of knowledge t weeks after we have learned it. The *Ebbinghaus learning model* asserts that P is given by

$$P(t) = Q + (100 - Q)e^{-kt},$$

where Q is the percentage that we would never forget and k is a constant that depends on the knowledge learned. Suppose that $Q = 40$ and $k = 0.7$.

a) Find the percentage retained after 0 weeks, 1 week, 2 weeks, 6 weeks, and 10 weeks.
b) Find $\lim_{t\to\infty} P(t)$.
c) Use a calculator to graph P.
d) Find the rate of change of $P(t)$ with respect to time t.
e) Interpret the meaning of the derivative.

58. Memory retention. A student memorized 120 vocabulary words for his Gaelic exam. After t days, the number of words, W, that he retained is given by

$$W(t) = 35 + 85e^{-0.08t}.$$

a) Find the number of words he retained after 4 days, 10 days, and 20 days.
b) Find $\lim_{t\to\infty} W(t)$.
c) Use a calculator to graph W for $0 \le t \le 30$.
d) Find $W(7)$ and $W'(7)$, and explain what these numbers represent.

SYNTHESIS

Differentiate.

59. $f(x) = e^{x/2} \cdot \sqrt{x - 1}$

60. $f(x) = \dfrac{xe^{-x}}{1 + x^2}$

61. $f(x) = \dfrac{e^x - e^{-x}}{e^x + e^{-x}}$

62. $f(x) = e^{e^x}$

63. $f(x) = x^e$

64. Let $f(x) = e^{-3x}$.

a) Find $f'(x)$, $f''(x)$, and $f'''(x)$.
b) Use the pattern in part (a) to find the 10th derivative of f.

65. Find the 7th derivative of $g(x) = e^{2x}$.

66. Find the equation of the line tangent to the graph of $f(x) = e^{3x}$ at $(0, 1)$.

67. Find the equation of the line tangent to the graph of $g(x) = 2e^{-4x}$ at $(0, 2)$.

68. Show that if $y = ae^{bx}$, then the equation of the tangent line at $x = 0$ is $y = abx + a$.

69. Find the point on the graph of $y = e^x$ where the tangent line at that point passes through the origin.

Technology Connection

For each of the functions in Exercises 70–73, graph f, f′, and f″.

70. $f(x) = e^x$

71. $f(x) = e^{-x}$

72. $f(x) = 2e^{0.3x}$

73. $f(x) = 1000e^{-0.08x}$

74. Graph

$$f(x) = \left(1 + \frac{1}{x}\right)^x.$$

Use the TABLE feature and very large values of x to confirm that e is approached as a limit.

75. Let $f(h) = \dfrac{e^h - 1}{h}$.

a) Complete the following table.

h	0.1	0.01	0.001	−0.1	−0.01	−0.001
$f(h)$						

b) Based on the table in part (a), find $\lim_{h \to 0} \dfrac{e^h - 1}{h}$.

Answers to Quick Checks

1. (a) $6e^x$; **(b)** $x^2e^x(x + 3)$; **(c)** $\dfrac{e^x(x-2)}{x^3}$
2. (a) $-4e^{-4x}$; **(b)** $e^{x^3+8x}(3x^2 + 8)$; **(c)** $\dfrac{xe^{\sqrt{x^2+5}}}{\sqrt{x^2+5}}$ **3.** $\dfrac{d^2y}{dx^2} = \dfrac{2e^{1/x^2}(3x^2+2)}{x^6}$
4. $A(10) = \$29{,}836.49$, which is the value of her account at $t = 10$ yr. At this time, her account is increasing in value at a rate given by $A'(10) = \$1193.46$ per year.
5. (a) 26.8, 47.1, 61.9, 74.6, 78.4
(b)

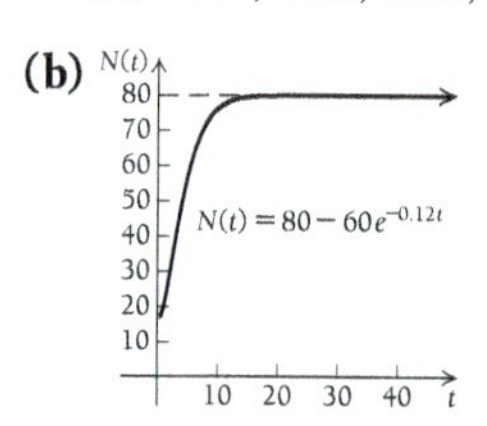

(c) $N'(t) = 7.2e^{-0.12t}$; after t days, the rate of change of the number of flashlights produced per day is given by $7.2e^{-0.12t}$. **(d)** 80 flashlights produced per day

2.3 Derivatives of Natural Logarithmic Functions

- Differentiate functions involving natural logarithms.
- Solve applied problems involving natural logarithmic functions and their derivatives.

To find the derivative of

$$f(x) = \ln x, \qquad (1)$$

we first write its equivalent exponential equation:

$$e^{f(x)} = x. \qquad \text{Recall that } y = \log_e x \text{ is equivalent to } e^y = x.$$

Now we differentiate both sides with respect to x:

$$\frac{d}{dx}e^{f(x)} = \frac{d}{dx}x$$

$$e^{f(x)} \cdot f'(x) = 1 \qquad \text{Using the Chain Rule}$$

$$x \cdot f'(x) = 1 \qquad \text{Substituting } x \text{ for } e^{f(x)} \text{ from equation (2)}$$

$$f'(x) = \frac{1}{x}.$$

Thus, we have the following.

THEOREM 7

For any positive number x,

$$\frac{d}{dx}\ln x = \frac{1}{x}.$$

Theorem 7 states that to find the slope of the tangent line at x for the function $f(x) = \ln x$, we need only take the reciprocal of x. This is true only for positive values of x, since $\ln x$ is defined only for positive numbers. Note that, for $cx > 0$,

$$\frac{d}{dx}\ln(cx) = \frac{1}{cx}\cdot c = \frac{1}{x},$$

and, for $x < 0$,

$$\frac{d}{dx}\ln(-x) = \frac{1}{(-x)}\cdot(-1) = \frac{1}{x}.$$

Thus, $y = \ln x$ is not the only function for which $dy/dx = 1/x$. Since

$$y = \ln|x| \quad \text{is equivalent to} \quad y = \begin{cases} \ln x, & \text{if } x > 0, \\ \ln(-x), & \text{if } x < 0, \end{cases}$$

it follows that

$$\frac{dy}{dx}\ln|x| = \frac{1}{x}, \quad \text{for all } x \neq 0.$$

This result will be important for our work in Chapter 4. In general, when we write $y = \ln x$, we assume that $x > 0$. For example, for the function given by $y = \ln(x^2 + 5x)$, we assume that x is chosen so that $x^2 + 5x > 0$.

Let's find some derivatives.

EXAMPLE 1 Differentiate:

a) $y = 3\ln x$; **b)** $y = x^2\ln x + 5x$; **c)** $y = \dfrac{\ln|2x|}{x^3}$.

Solution

a) $$\frac{d}{dx}(3\ln x) = 3\frac{d}{dx}\ln x = \frac{3}{x}$$

b) $$\frac{d}{dx}(x^2\ln x + 5x) = x^2\cdot\frac{1}{x} + 2x\cdot\ln x + 5 \qquad \text{Using the Product Rule on } x^2\ln x$$

$$= x + 2x\ln x + 5 \qquad \text{Simplifying}$$

c) $$\frac{d}{dx}\left(\frac{\ln|2x|}{x^3}\right) = \frac{x^3\cdot(1/2x)\cdot 2 - \ln|2x|(3x^2)}{(x^3)^2} \qquad \text{Using the Quotient Rule}$$

$$= \frac{x^2 - 3x^2\ln|2x|}{x^6}$$

$$= \frac{x^2(1 - 3\ln|2x|)}{x^6} \qquad \text{Factoring}$$

$$= \frac{1 - 3\ln|2x|}{x^4} \qquad \text{Simplifying}$$

1 ✓

Quick Check 1 ✓

Differentiate:

a) $y = 5\ln x$;

b) $y = x^3\ln x + 4x$;

c) $y = \dfrac{\ln|4x|}{x^2}$.

The following rule, which results directly from the Chain Rule, is used to find derivatives of functions of the form $h(x) = \ln f(x)$.

THEOREM 8

$$\frac{d}{dx}\ln f(x) = \frac{1}{f(x)}\cdot f'(x) = \frac{f'(x)}{f(x)}, \quad \text{or} \quad \frac{d}{dx}\ln u = \frac{1}{u}\cdot\frac{du}{dx}.$$

EXAMPLE 2 Differentiate:

a) $y = \ln(x^2 - 5)$; **b)** $f(x) = \ln\left(\frac{x^3 + 4}{x}\right)$.

Solution

a) If $y = \ln(x^2 - 5)$, then

$$\frac{dy}{dx} = \frac{1}{x^2 - 5}\cdot 2x \qquad \text{Using the Chain Rule}$$

$$= \frac{2x}{x^2 - 5}.$$

b) Often, using properties of logarithms simplifies the differentiation. For $f(x) = \ln\left(\frac{x^3 + 4}{x}\right)$, since $\ln\frac{M}{N} = \ln M - \ln N$, we have

$$f'(x) = \frac{d}{dx}[\ln(x^3 + 4) - \ln x] \qquad \text{Using Property P2 avoids use of the Quotient Rule.}$$

$$= \frac{3x^2}{x^3 + 4} - \frac{1}{x}.$$

2 ✓

Quick Check 2 ✓

Differentiate:

a) $y = \ln 5x$;

b) $y = \ln(3x^2 + 4)$;

c) $y = \ln\left(\frac{x^5 - 2}{x}\right)$.

Applications

EXAMPLE 3 **Social Science: Forgetting.** In a psychological experiment, students were shown a set of nonsense syllables, such as POK, RIZ, DEQ, and so on, and asked to recall them every minute thereafter. The percentage $R(t)$ who retained the syllables after t minutes was found to be given by the logarithmic learning model

$$R(t) = 80 - 27\ln t, \quad \text{for} \quad 1 \leq t \leq 15.$$

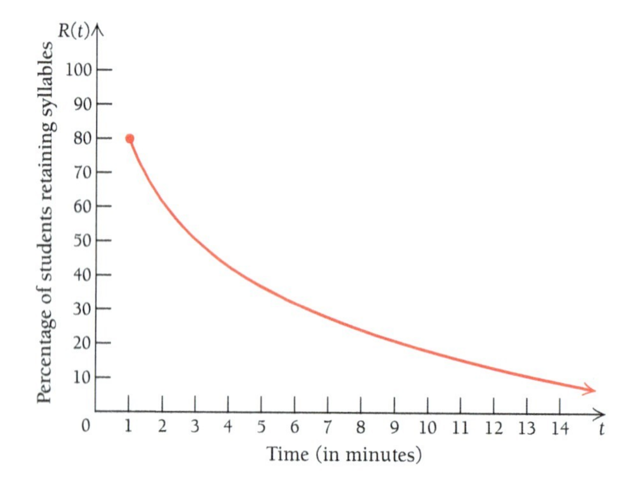

a) What percentage of students retained the syllables after 1 min?

b) Find $R'(2)$, and explain what it represents.

c) When will the percentage of students who retained the syllables drop to 20%?

Solution

a) $R(1) = 80 - 27 \cdot \ln 1 = 80 - 27 \cdot 0 = 80\%$

b) $\dfrac{d}{dt}(80 - 27 \ln t) = 0 - 27 \cdot \dfrac{1}{t} = -\dfrac{27}{t},$

so $R'(2) = -\dfrac{27}{2} = -13.5.$

This result indicates that 2 min after students have been shown the syllables, the percentage of them who retained the syllables is shrinking at the rate of 13.5% per minute.

c) To find when the percentage of students who retained the syllables drops to 20%, we set $R(t) = 20$ and solve for t:

$$20 = 80 - 27 \ln t$$
$$-60 = -27 \ln t$$
$$\frac{20}{9} = \ln t \qquad \text{Dividing both sides by } -27 \text{ and simplifying}$$
$$e^{20/9} = t \qquad \text{Writing as an equivalent exponential equation}$$
$$t \approx 9.23 \text{ min.} \qquad \text{Using a calculator}$$

The percentage of students who retained the syllables drops to 20% after about 9.23 min.

EXAMPLE 4 **Sales of a New Product.** The PhoneStare device is released into a test market of 1,000,000 potential customers. Initially, 500,000 free units are distributed in the market, with the intention of stimulating sales. After that, the number of weeks needed for the total number of units distributed or sold to reach n units is given by

$$t(n) = 28 \ln\left(\frac{500{,}000}{1{,}000{,}000 - n}\right), \quad \text{where } 500{,}000 \leq n < 1{,}000{,}000.$$

a) Find $t(900{,}000)$, and interpret its meaning.

b) Find $t'(900{,}000)$, and interpret its meaning.

c) How many units have been distributed or sold after 20 weeks?

Solution

a) We have

$$t(900{,}000) = 28 \ln\left(\frac{500{,}000}{1{,}000{,}000 - 900{,}000}\right) \qquad \text{Substituting}$$
$$= 28 \ln(5) \qquad \text{Simplifying}$$
$$\approx 45. \qquad \text{Using a calculator}$$

The time expected for the number of units distributed or sold to reach 900,000 units is about 45 weeks.

b) We first find $t'(n) = dt/dn$:

$$t'(n) = \frac{d}{dn}\left(28 \ln\left(\frac{500{,}000}{1{,}000{,}000 - n}\right)\right)$$
$$= 28 \cdot \frac{d}{dn}(\ln 500{,}000 - \ln(1{,}000{,}000 - n)) \qquad \text{Using Property P2}$$
$$= 28\left(0 - \frac{-1}{1{,}000{,}000 - n}\right) \qquad \text{Using the Chain Rule}$$
$$= \frac{28}{1{,}000{,}000 - n}. \qquad \text{Simplifying}$$

Thus,

$$t'(900{,}000) = \frac{28}{1{,}000{,}000 - 900{,}000} \quad \text{Substituting}$$
$$= \frac{28}{100{,}000}$$
$$= 0.00028 \, \frac{\text{week}}{\text{unit}}$$

When ownership has reached 900,000 units, the rate of change is about 0.00028 week per unit. This is equivalent to selling a new device every 2.8 minutes, approximately.

c) To find how many units have been distributed or sold after 20 weeks, we set $t = 20$, and solve for n:

$$20 = 28 \ln\left(\frac{500{,}000}{1{,}000{,}000 - n}\right) \quad \text{Substituting}$$
$$\frac{5}{7} = \ln\left(\frac{500{,}000}{1{,}000{,}000 - n}\right) \quad \text{Dividing both sides by 28 and simplifying}$$
$$e^{5/7} = \frac{500{,}000}{1{,}000{,}000 - n} \quad \text{Writing as an equivalent exponential equation}$$
$$(1{,}000{,}000 - n)e^{5/7} = 500{,}000$$
$$1{,}000{,}000e^{5/7} - ne^{5/7} = 500{,}000$$
$$-ne^{5/7} = 500{,}000 - 1{,}000{,}000e^{5/7}$$
$$n = \frac{500{,}000 - 1{,}000{,}000e^{5/7}}{-e^{5/7}}$$
$$\approx 755{,}229 \text{ units.} \quad \text{Solving for } n \text{ and using a calculator}$$

Thus, after 20 weeks, about 755,200 units have been distributed or sold. **3 ✓**

Quick Check 3 ✓

A new book, *Calculus Shortcuts Your Professor Never Told You*, is released, and the time t, in weeks, needed for sales to reach n units is given by

$$t(n) = 60 \ln\left(\frac{125{,}000}{400{,}000 - n}\right),$$

where $275{,}000 \le n < 400{,}000$. Find:

a) $t(325{,}000)$, and interpret its meaning;

b) $t'(325{,}000)$, and interpret its meaning;

c) the number of books sold after 30 weeks.

Section Summary

- $\dfrac{d}{dx}(\ln x) = \dfrac{1}{x}$, for all positive x
- For functions of the form $y = \ln f(x)$, the Chain Rule applies, and the derivative is $\dfrac{dy}{dx} = \dfrac{f'(x)}{f(x)}$.

2.3 Exercise Set

Differentiate.

1. $y = -9 \ln x$

2. $y = -8 \ln x$

3. $f(x) = \ln(9x)$

4. $f(x) = \ln(6x)$

5. $f(x) = \ln|10x|$

6. $f(x) = \ln|5x|$

7. $y = x^6 \ln x$

8. $y = x^4 \ln x$

9. $y = \dfrac{\ln x}{x^5}$

10. $y = \dfrac{\ln x}{x^4}$

11. $y = \ln \dfrac{x^2}{4}$ $\left(\textit{Hint}: \ln \dfrac{A}{B} = \ln A - \ln B.\right)$

12. $y = \ln \dfrac{x^4}{2}$

13. $y = \ln(3x^2 + 2x - 1)$

14. $y = \ln(7x^2 + 5x + 2)$

15. $f(x) = \ln\left(\dfrac{x^2 + 5}{x}\right)$

16. $f(x) = \ln\left(\dfrac{x^2 - 7}{x}\right)$

17. $g(x) = (\ln x)^4$ (*Hint*: Use the Extended Power Rule.)

18. $g(x) = (\ln x)^3$

19. $h(x) = \ln\left(\dfrac{x^2(x^3 + 1)}{e^{2x}}\right)$

20. $h(x) = \ln(2x^4 e^{3x}(x^2 + x + 1)^5)$

21. Find the equation of the line tangent to the graph of $y = (\ln x)^2$ at $x = 3$.

22. Find the equation of the line tangent to the graph of $y = \ln(4x^2 - 7)$ at $x = 2$.

23. Find the equation of the line tangent to the graph of $y = x \ln(x^2 - 1)$ at $x = 3$.

24. Find the equation of the line tangent to the graph of $y = x^2 \ln(5 + 3x^4)$ at $x = 1$.

APPLICATIONS

Business and Economics

25. **Advertising.** A model for consumers' response to advertising is given by

$$N(a) = 2000 + 500 \ln a, \quad a \geq 1,$$

where $N(a)$ is the number of units sold and a is the amount spent on advertising, in thousands of dollars.

a) How many units are sold when \$1000 is spent on advertising?
b) Find $N'(a)$ and $N'(10)$.
c) How much should be spent on advertising if 3000 units are to be sold?
d) Find $\lim_{a \to \infty} N'(a)$. Does it make sense to continue to spend more and more on advertising? Why or why not?

26. **Advertising.** A model for consumers' response to advertising is given by

$$N(a) = 1000 + 200 \ln a, \quad a \geq 1,$$

where $N(a)$ is the number of units sold and a is the amount spent on advertising, in thousands of dollars.

a) How many units are sold when \$1000 is spent on advertising?
b) Find $N'(a)$ and $N'(10)$.
c) How much should be spent on advertising if 1500 units are to be sold?
d) Discuss $\lim_{a \to \infty} N'(a)$. Does it make sense to spend more and more on advertising? Why or why not?

27. **Marginal revenue.** The demand for a new computer game can be modeled by

$$p(x) = 53.5 - 8 \ln x, \quad \text{for } 0 \leq x \leq 800,$$

where $p(x)$ is the price consumers will pay, in dollars, and x is the number of games sold, in thousands. Recall that total revenue is given by $R(x) = x \cdot p(x)$.

a) Find $R(x)$.
b) Find the marginal revenue, $R'(x)$.
c) How many units will be sold if the price that consumers are willing to pay is \$40?

28. **Marginal profit.** The profit, in thousands of dollars, from the sale of x thousand candles can be estimated by

$$P(x) = 2x - 0.3x \ln x.$$

a) Find the marginal profit, $P'(x)$.
b) Find $P'(150)$, and explain what this number represents.
c) How many candles (in thousands) should be sold in order to achieve a marginal profit of \$750 per thousand candles?

Social and Life Sciences

29. **Forgetting.** As part of a study, students in a psychology class took a final exam and then took equivalent forms of the exam at monthly intervals thereafter. After t months, the average score $S(t)$, as a percentage, was found to be given by

$$S(t) = 78 - 15 \ln(t + 1), \quad 0 \leq t \leq 80.$$

a) What was the average score when the students initially took the test?
b) What was the average score after 4 months?
c) What was the average score after 24 months?
d) Find $S'(t)$.
e) Find $S'(4)$ and $S'(24)$, and interpret the meaning of these numbers.

30. **Walking speed.** Bornstein and Bornstein found in a study that the average walking speed v, in feet per second, of a person living in a city of population p, in thousands, is

$$v(p) = 0.37 \ln p + 0.05.$$

(*Source:* M. H. Bornstein and H. G. Bornstein, "The Pace of Life," *Nature*, Vol. 259, pp. 557–559 (1976).)

a) The population of Seattle is 660,000 ($p = 660$). What is the average walking speed of a person living in Seattle?
b) The population of New York is 8,550,000. What is the average walking speed of a person living in New York?
c) Find $v'(660)$ and $v'(8550)$, and interpret the meaning of these numbers.
d) The average walking speed in a city is 2.31 ft/sec. What is this city's approximate population?

31. **Heating water.** The time t, in minutes, needed to allow a cup of cold water placed in a room to warm to T degrees Celsius is given by

$$t(T) = 50 \ln\left(\frac{15}{25 - T}\right), \quad 10 \leq T < 25.$$

a) Find $t(15)$ and $t'(15)$, and explain what each number represents.
b) What is the water's temperature after 1 hr?

32. **Warming a frozen package.** The time t, in minutes, needed to warm a frozen package of smoked salmon to T degrees Fahrenheit is given by

$$t(T) = 250 \ln\left(\frac{38}{76 - T}\right), \quad 38 \leq T < 76.$$

a) Find $t(60)$ and $t'(60)$, and explain what each number represents.
b) What is the package's temperature after 8 hr?

33. **Population.** The time t, in months, needed for the population of birds on an island to reach p individuals is given by

$$t(p) = 38 \ln\left(\frac{4500}{7500 - p}\right), \quad 4500 \leq T < 7500.$$

a) Find $t(5000)$ and $t'(5000)$, and explain what each number represents.
b) What is the population of birds after 5 yr?

34. **Population.** The time t, in weeks, needed for the population of fireflies in a field to reach p individuals is given by

$$t(p) = 60 \ln\left(\frac{10{,}000}{18{,}000 - p}\right), \quad 10{,}000 \leq T < 18{,}000.$$

a) Find $t(12{,}000)$ and $t'(12{,}000)$, and explain what each number represents.
b) What is the population of fireflies after 5 weeks?

SYNTHESIS

Find the second derivative.

35. $k(x) = x \ln x$

36. $r(t) = t^2 \ln(t + 1)$

37. $s(w) = \ln\left(\frac{w}{w - 1}\right)$

38. $t(x) = \ln(x^2(3x - 1))$

39. In Exercise 31, the time t, in minutes, needed to warm a cup of cold water to T degrees Celsius is given by

$t = 50 \ln\left(\frac{15}{25 - T}\right)$, for $10 \leq T < 25$.

a) Solve for T in terms of t.

b) Find $\lim_{t \to \infty} T(t)$, and explain what this number represents.

40. In Exercise 32, the time t, in minutes, needed to warm a frozen package of smoked salmon to T degrees Fahrenheit is given by $t = 250 \ln\left(\frac{38}{76 - T}\right)$, for $38 \leq T < 76$.

a) Solve for T in terms of t.

b) Find $\lim_{t \to \infty} T(t)$, and explain what this number represents.

41. In Exercise 33, the time t, in months, needed for the population of birds on an island to reach p individuals is given by $t = 38 \ln\left(\frac{4500}{7500 - p}\right)$, for $4500 \leq T < 7500$.

a) Solve for p in terms of t.

b) Find $\lim_{t \to \infty} p(t)$, and explain what this number represents.

42. In Exercise 34, the time t, in weeks, needed for the population of fireflies in a field to reach p individuals is given by $t = 60 \ln\left(\frac{10{,}000}{18{,}000 - p}\right)$, for $10{,}000 \leq T < 18{,}000$.

a) Solve for p in terms of t.

b) Find $\lim_{t \to \infty} p(t)$, and explain what this number represents.

Technology Connection

43. Find the intersection point(s) of $y_1 = 3 - 2x$ and $y_2 = \ln x$.

44. Find the intersection point(s) of $y_1 = x^2 - 4$ and $y_2 = \ln x$.

45. Let $y_1 = ax$ and $y_2 = \ln x$. Find a such that the graph of y_1 is tangent to the graph of y_2.

46. Let $y_1 = x + a$ and $y_2 = \ln x$. Find a such that the graph of y_1 is tangent to the graph of y_2.

Answers to Quick Checks

1. **(a)** $\frac{5}{x}$; **(b)** $x^2 + 3x^2 \ln x + 4$; **(c)** $\frac{1 - 2\ln|4x|}{x^3}$

2. **(a)** $\frac{1}{x}$; **(b)** $\frac{6x}{3x^2 + 4}$; **(c)** $\frac{4x^5 + 2}{x(x^5 - 2)}$

3. **(a)** 30.65, which is the number of weeks needed to sell 325,000 books; **(b)** 0.0008 week/unit, meaning that a book is sold about every 8 min; **(c)** about 324,200 books (rounded)

2.4 Applications: Uninhibited and Limited Growth Models

- Find functions that satisfy $dP/dt = kP$.
- Solve applied problems using exponential growth and limited growth models.

Exponential Growth

Consider the function given by

$$f(x) = 2e^{3x}.$$

Differentiating, we get

$$f'(x) = 2e^{3x} \cdot 3$$
$$= f(x) \cdot 3.$$

Graphically, this says that the derivative, or slope of the tangent line, is 3 times the function value.

Functions of the form $f(x) = ce^{kx}$ have the property that the derivative is a constant multiple k of the function.

THEOREM 9

A function $y = f(x)$ satisfies

$$\frac{dy}{dx} = ky \quad \text{or} \quad f'(x) = k \cdot f(x)$$

if and only if

$$y = ce^{kx} \quad \text{or} \quad f(x) = ce^{kx}.$$

The proof that functions of the form $f(x) = ce^{kx}$ are the only functions for which $f'(x) = k \cdot f(x)$ is beyond the scope of this text.

EXAMPLE 1 Find the function that satisfies each equation.

a) $\dfrac{dA}{dx} = 5A$ **b)** $\dfrac{dP}{dt} = kP$

Solution

a) From Theorem 9, we know that the desired function must be of the form $A(x) = ce^{kx}$. Since we have $k = 5$ in this case, the function is given by $A(x) = ce^{5x}$, where c is an arbitrary constant. As a check, note that

$$A'(x) = ce^{5x} \cdot 5 = 5 \cdot A(x).$$

b) The desired function is given by $P(t) = ce^{kt}$, where c is an arbitrary constant. As a check, note that

$$\frac{dP}{dt} = ce^{kt} \cdot k = kP.$$

1 ✓

Quick Check 1 ✓
Find the function that satisfies the equation

$$\frac{dN}{dt} = 0.005N.$$

The solutions of the equations in Example 1 are functions. An equation like $dP/dt = kP$, which includes a derivative and which has a function as a solution, is called a *differential equation*.

EXAMPLE 2 Solve the differential equation

$$f'(z) = 0.06 \cdot f(z).$$

Solution The solution is $f(z) = ce^{0.06z}$.

Check: $f'(z) = ce^{0.06z} \cdot 0.06 = f(z) \cdot 0.06$

2 ✓

Quick Check 2 ✓
Solve the differential equation

$$f'(t) = 0.25 \cdot f(t).$$

We study differential equations in more depth in Section 5.7.

Uninhibited Population Growth

The differential equation

$$\frac{dP}{dt} = kP \quad \text{or} \quad P'(t) = kP(t), \quad \text{with } k > 0,$$

is the model of uninhibited (unrestrained) population growth. In the absence of inhibiting or stimulating factors, a population normally reproduces at a rate proportional to its size, and this is exactly what $dP/dt = kP$ says. The only function that satisfies this differential equation is given by

$$P(t) = ce^{kt},$$

where t is time and k is the rate expressed in decimal notation. Note that

$$P(0) = ce^{k \cdot 0} = ce^0 = c \cdot 1 = c,$$

so c represents the initial population, which we denote as P_0:

$$P(t) = P_0e^{kt}.$$

The graph of $P(t) = P_0e^{kt}$, for $k > 0$, shows how uninhibited growth produces a "population explosion."

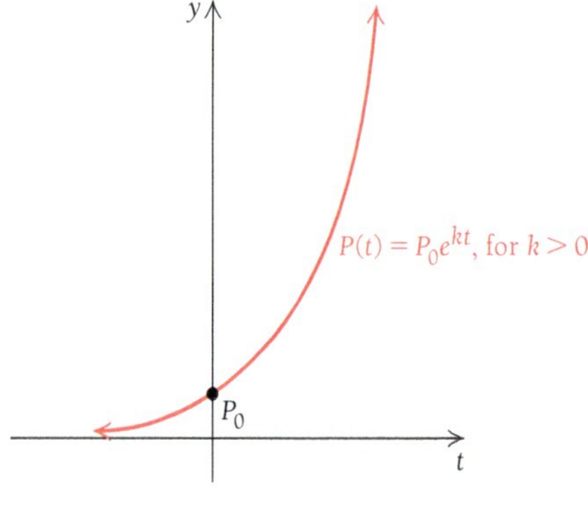

The constant k is the **rate of exponential growth**, or the **exponential growth rate.** This is *not* the instantaneous rate of change of the population size, which varies according to

$$\frac{dP}{dt} = kP,$$

but the constant by which P must be multiplied in order to get the instantaneous rate of change at any point in time. It is similar to the daily interest rate paid by a bank. When interest is compounded continuously, the interest rate is a true exponential growth rate.

EXAMPLE 3 **Business: Interest Compounded Continuously.** Suppose P_0, in dollars, is invested in the Von Neumann Hi-Yield Fund, with interest compounded continuously at 7% per year. That is, at any point in time after t years, the balance P, in dollars per year, is growing at the rate

$$\frac{dP}{dt} = 0.07P.$$

a) Find the function that satisfies the equation. Write it in terms of P_0 and 0.07.

b) Suppose that \$10,000 is invested. What is the balance after 1 yr?

c) If \$10,000 is invested, how fast is the balance growing at $t = 1$ yr?

Solution

a) $P(t) = P_0e^{0.07t}$ Note that $P(0) = P_0$.

b) Here, $P(t) = 10{,}000e^{0.07t}$, so

$$P(1) = 10{,}000e^{0.07(1)} = 10{,}000e^{0.07}$$
$$= \$10{,}725.08 \quad \text{Using a calculator and rounding}$$

c) We have $P(t) = 10{,}000e^{0.07t}$ and $P'(t) = 10{,}000(0.07)e^{0.07t} = 700e^{0.07t}$. Thus, $P'(1) = 700e^{0.07(1)} \approx 750.7557$. At $t = 1$ yr, the balance is growing at the rate of about \$750.76 per year. 3 ✓

Quick Check 3 ✓

Business: Interest Compounded Continuously. Repeat Example 3 for interest compounded continuously at 4% per year.

EXAMPLE 4 **Physical Science: Integrated Circuits.** In 1971, Intel Corporation released the Intel 4004 microprocessor, which held 2300 transistors. Since then, the number of transistors on a microprocessor has been growing exponentially at the rate of 0.35, or 35%, per year. (How was this estimate determined? The answer is in the model we develop in the following Technology Connection.) That is,

$$\frac{dP}{dt} = 0.35P,$$

where t is the number of years since 1971. (*Sources:* www.intel.com; www.motorola.com; www.microsoft.com.)

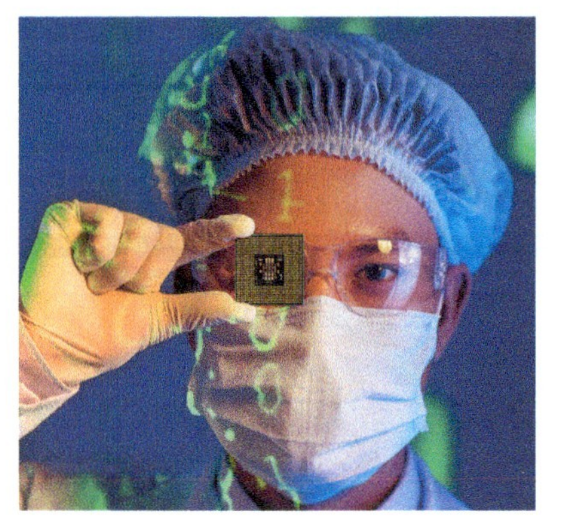

a) Find the function that satisfies this equation. Assume $P_0 = 2300$ and $k = 0.35$.

b) Estimate the number of transistors on a microprocessor in 2025.

c) Find the rate at which the number of transistors on a microprocessor is changing in 2025.

Technology Connection 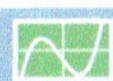

Exponential Model Using Regression

The table below shows data regarding the number of transistors on a microprocessor.

Year	Number of Transistors
1971 (Intel 4004)	2300
1979 (Intel 8088)	29,000
1984 (Motorola 68020)	200,000
1993 (Intel Pentium I)	3,100,000
2000 (Intel Pentium IV)	42,000,000
2010 (Intel Itanium Tukwila)	2,000,000,000
2013 (Microsoft Xbox One)	5,000,000,000
2015 (Oracle SPARC M7)	10,000,000,000

What is the projected number of transistors on a microprocessor in 2025? The graph of the data shows a rapidly growing transistor count that can be modeled with an exponential function. We carry out the regression procedure exactly as we did in Section R.7, but select ExpReg rather than LinReg.

```
EDIT CALC TESTS
7↑QuartReg
8:LinReg(a+bx)
9:LnReg
0:ExpReg
A:PwrReg
B:Logistic
C:SinReg
```

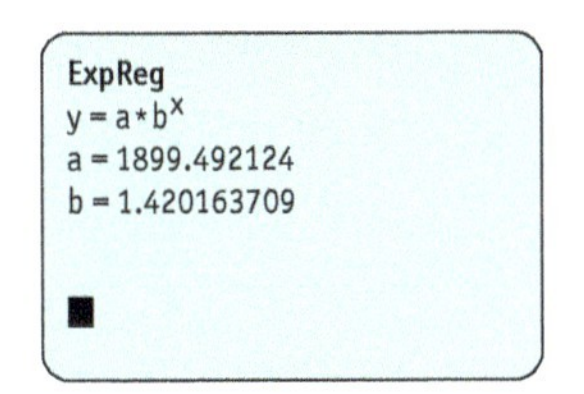

Note that this gives us an exponential model of the type $y = a \cdot b^x$, where y is the number of transistors x years after 1971:

$$y = 1899.492124 \cdot 1.420163709^x.$$

Since $b = e^{\ln b}$, we can write this function as an exponential function, with base e:

$$\begin{aligned} y &= 1899.492124 \cdot 1.420163709^x \\ &= 1899.492124(e^{\ln 1.420163709})^x \\ &= 1899.492124e^{0.350772153x}. \end{aligned}$$

Thus, in 2025 ($t = 54$), the number of transistors on a microprocessor is estimated to be

$$y = 1899.492124e^{0.350772153(54)} = 319.8 \text{ billion}.$$

EXERCISES

Estimate the number of transistors on a microprocessor in each of the following years.

1. 2030
2. 2050
3. 2100
4. Explain why this model differs slightly from the one used in Example 4. Do both models accurately estimate the number of transistors on a microprocessor over the years 1971–2025?

Solution

a) $P(t) = 2300e^{0.35t}$

b) Since 2025 is 54 yr after 1971, we have $P(54) = 2300e^{0.35(54)} \approx 3.714 \times 10^{11}$, or about 371.4 billion transistors.

c) Since $P(t) = 2300e^{0.35t}$, we have $P'(t) = 2300(0.35)e^{0.35t} = 805e^{0.35t}$. When $t = 54$, we have $P'(54) = 805e^{0.35(54)} \approx 1.3 \times 10^{11}$. Thus, in 2025, the rate of growth of the number of transistors on a microprocessor will be about 130 billion transistors per year. **4 ✓**

Quick Check 4 ✓

Life Science: Population Growth in China. In 2017, the population of China was 1.39 billion, and the exponential growth rate was 0.44% per year. Thus,

$$\frac{dP}{dt} = 0.0044P,$$

where t is the time, in years, after 2017. Assume uninhibited growth. (*Source:* www.worldometers.info2017.)

a) Find the function that satisfies the equation. Assume $P_0 = 1.39$ and $k = 0.0044$.

b) Estimate the population of China at the beginning of 2022.

c) Find the rate of change of China's population at the beginning of 2022.

It is possible to use two representative data points to determine P_0 and k in $P(t) = P_0e^{kt}$, as we will see next.

EXAMPLE 5 **Business: Value of a Batman Comic Book.** A 1939 comic book with the first appearance of the "Caped Crusader," Batman, sold at auction in Dallas in 2010 for a record \$1.075 million. The comic book originally cost 10¢ (or \$0.10). Using the data points (0, \$0.10) and (71, \$1,075,000), we can model the increasing value of the comic book. The modeling assumption is that the value V of the comic book grows exponentially, as given by

$$\frac{dV}{dt} = kV.$$

(*Source:* Heritage Auction Galleries; reverified in 2017.)

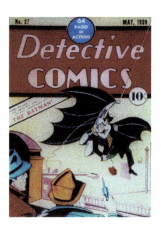

a) Find the function that satisfies this equation. Assume $V_0 = \$0.10$.

b) Estimate the value of the comic book at the start of 2025.

c) At what rate, in dollars per year, is the comic book increasing in value at the start of 2025?

Solution

a) Because of the modeling assumption, we have $V(t) = V_0 e^{kt}$. Since $V_0 = \$0.10$, it follows that

$$V(t) = 0.10e^{kt},$$

where $V(t)$ is the comic book's value, in dollars, t years after the start of 1939.

We have made use of the data point (0, \$0.10). Next, we use the data point (71, \$1,075,000) to determine k. We solve

$$V(t) = 0.10e^{kt}, \quad \text{or} \quad 1{,}075{,}000 = 0.10e^{k(71)}$$

for k, using natural logarithms:

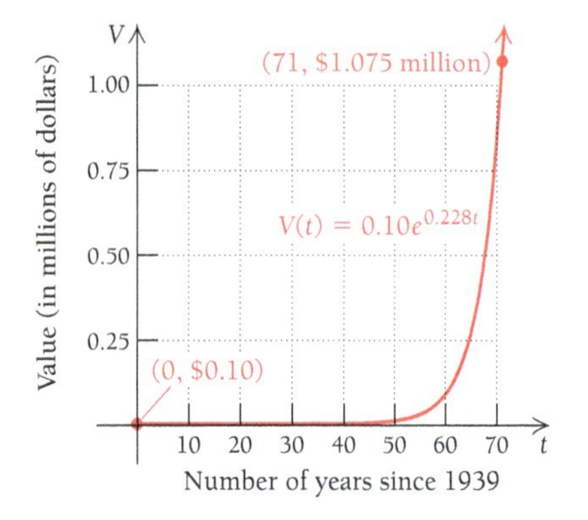

$$1{,}075{,}000 = 0.10e^{k(71)} = 0.10e^{71k}$$

$$\frac{1{,}075{,}000}{0.10} = e^{71k} \quad \text{Dividing to simplify}$$

$$10{,}750{,}000 = e^{71k}$$

$$\ln 10{,}750{,}000 = \ln e^{71k} \quad \text{Finding the logarithm of both sides}$$

$$\ln 10{,}750{,}000 = 71k \quad \text{Using Property P7}$$

$$\frac{\ln 10{,}750{,}000}{71} = k$$

$$0.228 \approx k. \quad \text{Using a calculator and rounding to the nearest thousandth}$$

The desired function is $V(t) = 0.10e^{0.228t}$.

b) To estimate the value of the comic book at the start of 2025, which is $2025 - 1939 = 86$ yr after the start of 1939, we substitute 86 for t in the equation:

$$V(t) = 0.10e^{0.228t}$$

$$V(86) = 0.10e^{0.228(86)} \approx 32{,}782{,}811.85.$$

Thus, at the start of 2025, the comic book's value will be about \$32.8 million.

c) Since $V(t) = 0.10e^{0.228t}$, we have $V'(t) = 0.10(0.228)e^{0.228t} = 0.0228e^{0.228t}$, and $V'(86) = 0.0228e^{0.228(86)} \approx 7{,}474{,}481.102$. Thus, at the start of 2025, the comic book's value is increasing by about \$7.47 million per year. 5 ✓

Quick Check 5 ✓

Business: Batman Comic Book. In Example 5, the consigner had purchased the comic book in the late 1960s for \$100. (*Source:* Heritage Auction Galleries.) Assume that the year of purchase was 1969 and that the value V of the comic book has since grown exponentially, as given by

$$\frac{dV}{dt} = kV,$$

where t is the number of years after 1969.

a) Use the data points (0, \$100) and (41, \$1,075,000) to find the function that satisfies the equation.

b) Estimate the value of the comic book at the start of 2025, and compare your answer to that of Example 5.

c) Estimate the rate of change of the value of the comic book at the start of 2025.

Models of Limited Growth

We have seen that the growth model $P(t) = P_0 e^{kt}$ applies to *unlimited*, or *unrestricted*, growth. However, there are often factors that prevent a quantity from exceeding some limiting value L. One model of such *limited*, or *restricted*, growth is

$$P(t) = \frac{L}{1 + Ce^{-Lkt}}, \quad \text{for } k > 0 \text{ and } L > 0,$$

which is called the *logistic equation*, or *logistic function*.

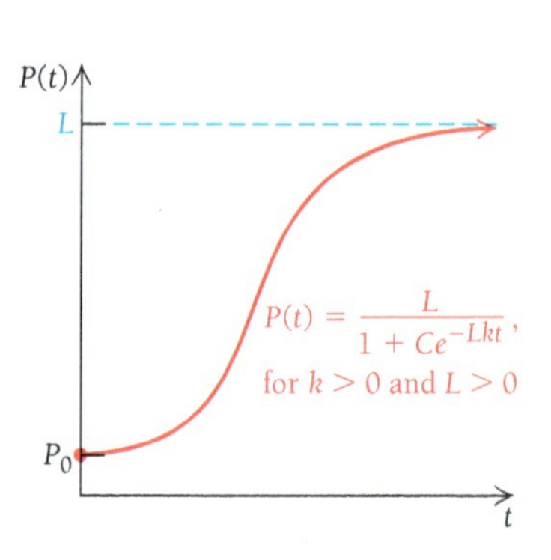

The differential equation

$$\frac{dP}{dt} = kP(L - P)$$

is the model for the **logistic function**, where L is the upper limit of the population P. The rate of change of the population is directly proportional to the population P and to the remaining room for population growth $L - P$. The function that solves this differential equation has the simplified form

$$P(t) = \frac{L}{1 + Ce^{-Lkt}}, \quad \text{or} \quad P(t) = \frac{L}{1 + Ce^{-rt}},$$

where $r = Lk$ and both $k > 0$ and $L > 0$.

The verification that $P(t) = \frac{L}{1 + Ce^{-Lkt}}$ solves $\frac{dP}{dt} = kP(L - P)$ is left as Exercise 50.

EXAMPLE 6 **Business: Revenue.** DISH Network's revenue, R, in billions of dollars, t years after 2008, can be modeled by the logistic equation

$$R(t) = \frac{31.95}{1 + 1.759e^{-0.0596t}}.$$

(*Source:* Investopedia, May 2017.)

a) Find the revenue in 2020 and 2023.

b) Find the rate at which the revenue was growing in 2015.

c) Graph the equation.

d) Explain why an unrestricted growth model is inappropriate but a logistic equation is appropriate to model this growth.

Solution

a) We use a calculator to find the function values:

$$R(12) = 17.2 \quad \text{and} \quad R(15) = 18.6.$$

After 12 yr, revenue will be about \$17.2 billion. After 15 yr, revenue will be about \$18.6 billion.

b) We find the rate of change using the Quotient Rule:

$$\frac{dR}{dt} = \frac{(1 + 1.759e^{-0.0596t}) \cdot 0 - 31.95 \cdot (1.759e^{-0.0596t})(-0.0596)}{(1 + 1.759e^{-0.0596t})^2}$$

$$= \frac{3.35e^{-0.0596t}}{(1 + 1.759e^{-0.0596t})^2}.$$

Next, we use a calculator to find the value of the derivative at $t = 7$:

$$R'(7) = \frac{3.35e^{-0.0596(7)}}{(1 + 1.759e^{-0.0596(7)})^2} \approx 0.474.$$

In 2015, the revenue was growing at a rate of \$0.474 billion, or \$474 million, per year.

Quick Check 6 ✓

Life Science: Spread of an Epidemic. In a town with a population of 3500, an epidemic of a disease occurs. The number of people, N, infected t days after the disease first appears is given by

$$N(t) = \frac{3500}{1 + 19.9e^{-0.6t}}.$$

a) How many people are initially infected with the disease ($t = 0$)?

b) Find the number of residents infected after 2 days, 8 days, and 18 days.

c) Graph the equation.

d) Find the rate at which the disease is spreading after 16 days.

e) Will all 3500 residents ever be infected? Why or why not?

c) Using a graphing utility, we obtain the following graph.

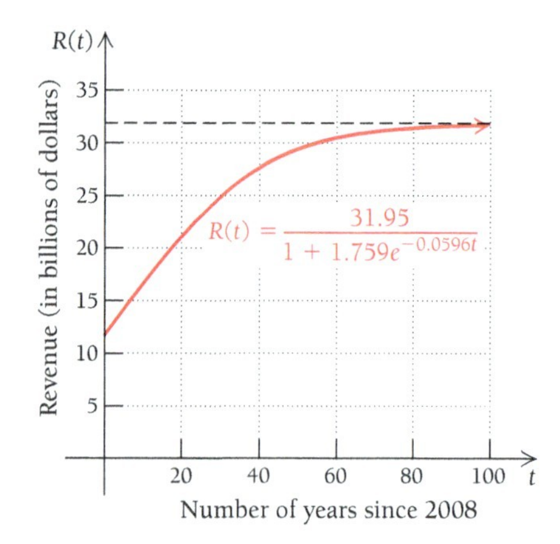

d) An unrestricted growth model is inappropriate because as more people subscribe to DISH, there will be fewer people remaining in the population who could become new customers. Thus, revenue growth is fast at first, but levels off in the long term. It appears that revenue will approach a limit of about \$32 billion, assuming that the logistic growth model remains valid for forecasting revenue into the future. Market trends, new technology, and other factors will likely require new models in the future. **6 ✓**

Another model of limited growth is given by

$$P(t) = L + Ce^{-kt}, \quad \text{for } k > 0 \text{ and } L > 0,$$

which is graphed below. This function increases over its domain, $[0, \infty)$, but increases most rapidly at the beginning, unlike a logistic function.

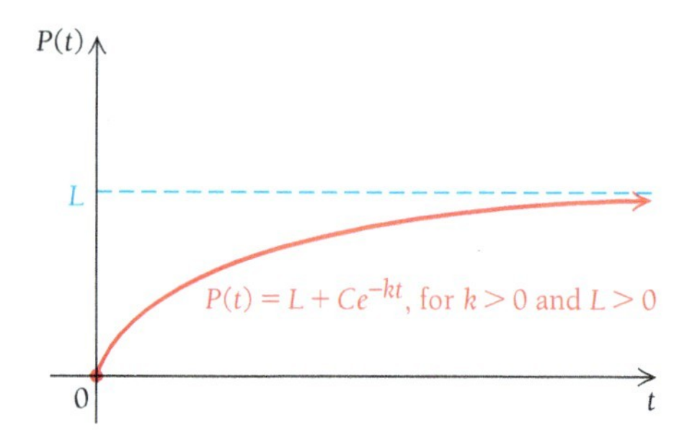

The differential equation

$$\frac{dP}{dt} = k(L - P)$$

models the **limited growth function**, in which L is the upper limit of the population, P, and the rate of change of P is directly proportional only to the remaining room for population growth, $L - P$. The solution of this differential equation is

$$P(t) = L + Ce^{-kt}, \quad \text{where} \quad k > 0 \text{ and } L > 0.$$

Verification that $P(t) = L + Ce^{-kt}$ solves $\frac{dP}{dt} = k(L - P)$ is left as Exercise 51.

EXAMPLE 7 **Business: Value of Headphones.** A new model of Bluetooth-capable headphones originally sells for \$45 per set and then, 5 weeks later, is selling for \$52. Market analysts expect that the headphones will eventually sell for \$70.

a) Use the limited growth model, $P(t) = L + Ce^{-kt}$, to find $P(t)$, the value of the headphones after t weeks.

b) Find $P'(15)$, and interpret the meaning of this number.

c) When will the value of the headphones be \$65?

Solution

a) We let $L = 70$, the upper limit of the value of the headphones, and use the ordered pair $(0, 45)$, representing the initial value, to find C:

$$\begin{aligned} 45 &= 70 + Ce^{-k(0)} && \text{Substituting} \\ -25 &= C(1) \\ C &= -25. \end{aligned}$$

Now we use the ordered pair $(5, 52)$, representing the value of the headphones after 5 weeks, to find k:

$$\begin{aligned} 52 &= 70 - 25e^{-k(5)} && \text{Substituting} \\ -18 &= -25e^{-5k} \\ \frac{18}{25} &= e^{-5k} \\ \ln\left(\frac{18}{25}\right) &= -5k && \text{Finding the natural logarithm of both sides and using a property of logarithms} \\ k &= \frac{\ln\left(\frac{18}{25}\right)}{-5} \approx 0.0657 && \text{Using a calculator} \end{aligned}$$

Thus, the function that models the value of the headphones after t weeks is given by

$$P(t) = 70 - 25e^{-0.0657t}.$$

b) To find $P'(15)$, we first find $P'(t)$:

$$\begin{aligned} \frac{d}{dt}P(t) &= \frac{d}{dt}(70 - 25e^{-0.0657t}) \\ P'(t) &= -25e^{-0.0657t}(-0.0657) && \text{Using the Chain Rule} \\ &= 1.6425e^{-0.0657t}. \end{aligned}$$

Thus,

$$P'(15) = 1.6425e^{-0.0657(15)} \approx 0.613.$$

After exactly 15 weeks, the value of the headphones is increasing by about \$0.61 per week.

c) To find the time at which the value reaches \$65, we substitute 65 for P, and solve for t:

$$\begin{aligned} 65 &= 70 - 25e^{-0.0657t} && \text{Substituting} \\ -5 &= -25e^{-0.0657t} \\ 0.2 &= e^{-0.0657t} && \text{Dividing both sides by } -25 \\ \ln(0.2) &= -0.0657t \\ t &= \frac{\ln(0.2)}{-0.0657} \approx 24.5 \text{ weeks.} && \text{Using a calculator} \end{aligned}$$

The value will reach \$65 after about 24.5 weeks.

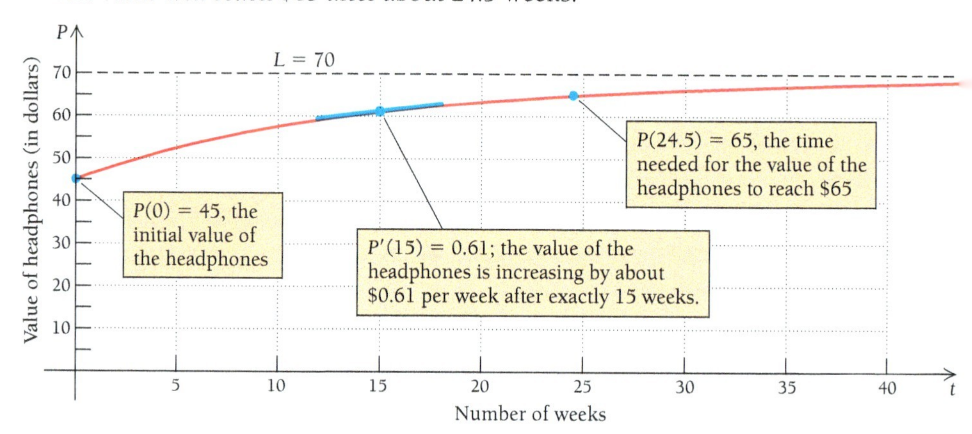

7 ✓

Quick Check 7 ✓

A bottle of soda with a temperature of 34°F is placed in a room in which the temperature is 75°F, and allowed to warm naturally. After 15 minutes, the soda's temperature is 45°F. Find:

a) $P(t)$, the soda's temperature after t minutes;

b) $P'(20)$, and interpret its meaning;

c) the time at which the soda's temperature will reach 70°F.

Section Summary

- Uninhibited growth can be modeled by a *differential equation* of the form $\frac{dP}{dt} = kP$, which has the solution $P(t) = P_0e^{kt}$.
- Certain kinds of limited growth can be modeled by equations such as $P(t) = \frac{L}{1 + Ce^{-Lkt}}$, called the *logistic function*, and $P(t) = L + Ce^{-kt}$, called the *limited growth function*. In both cases, $k > 0$ and $L > 0$.

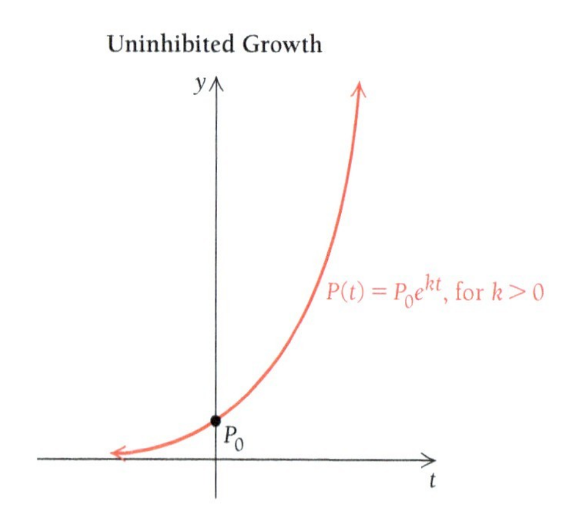

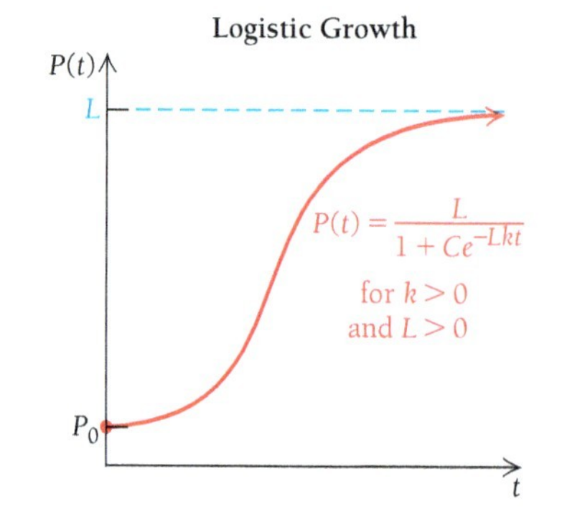

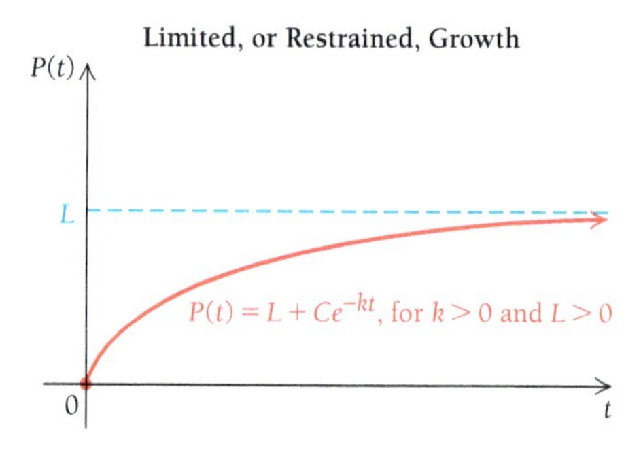

2.4 Exercise Set

1. Find f if $f'(x) = 4f(x)$.
2. Find g if $g'(x) = 6g(x)$.
3. Find the function that satisfies $dA/dt = -9A$.
4. Find the function that satisfies $dP/dt = -3P(t)$.
5. Find the function that satisfies $dQ/dt = kQ$.
6. Find the function that satisfies $dR/dt = kR$.

APPLICATIONS

Business and Economics

7. **U.S. patents.** Between 2006 and 2016, the number of applications for patents, N, grew by about 3.9% per year. That is, $N'(t) = 0.039N(t)$. (*Source:* www.uspto.gov.)

a) Find the function that satisfies this equation. Assume that $t = 0$ corresponds to 2006, when approximately 453,000 patent applications were received.
b) Estimate the number of patent applications in 2020.
c) Estimate the rate of change in the number of patent applications in 2020.

8. **Franchise expansion.** Pete Zah's, Inc., is selling franchises for pizza shops throughout the country. The marketing manager estimates that the number of franchises, N, will increase at the rate of 10% per year, that is,

$$\frac{dN}{dt} = 0.10N.$$

a) Find the function that satisfies this equation. Assume that the number of franchises at $t = 0$ is 50.
b) How many franchises will there be in 20 yr?
c) Estimate the rate of change in the number of franchises in 20 yr.

9. **Compound interest.** If an amount P_0 is invested in the Mandelbrot Bond Fund and interest is compounded continuously at 5.9% per year, the balance P grows at the rate given by

$$\frac{dP}{dt} = 0.059P.$$

a) Find the function that satisfies the equation. Write it in terms of P_0 and 0.059.
b) Suppose \$1000 is invested. What is the balance after 1 yr? After 2 yr?
c) What is the rate of change of the balance after 1 yr? After 2 yr?

10. **Compound interest.** If an amount P_0 is deposited in a savings account and interest is compounded continuously at 4.3% per year, the balance P grows at the rate given by

$$\frac{dP}{dt} = 0.043P.$$

a) Find the function that satisfies the equation. Write it in terms of P_0 and 0.043.
b) Suppose \$20,000 is deposited. What is the balance after 1 yr? After 2 yr?
c) What is the rate of change of the balance after 1 yr? After 2 yr?

11. **Bottled water sales.** The volume of bottled water sold, G, in billions of gallons, t years after 2015 is growing at the rate given by

$$\frac{dG}{dt} = 0.085G.$$

(*Source:* bottledwater.org.)

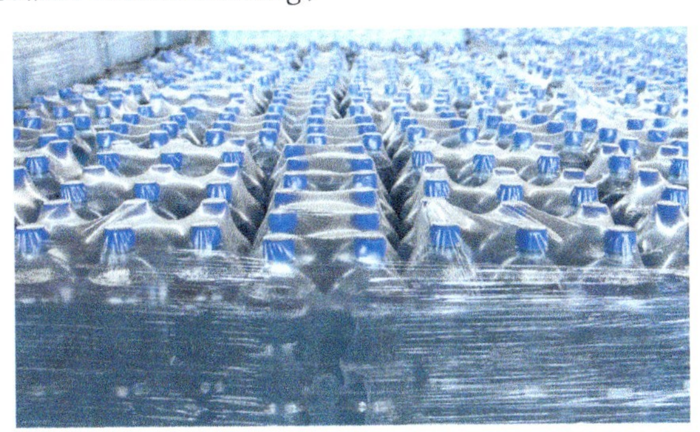

a) Find the function that satisfies the equation, given that approximately 11.8 billion gallons of bottled water were sold in 2015.
b) Predict the number of gallons of bottled water sold in 2025.
c) Estimate the rate of change of the number of gallons of bottled water sold in 2025.

12. **Apps downloads.** Since June 2014, the number of apps, in billions, downloaded from the Apple App Store has increased at the rate of approximately 29.2% per year. That is, the number of apps, A, in billions, downloaded t years after June 2014 is growing at the rate of

$$\frac{dA}{dt} = 0.292A.$$

(*Source:* Apple Inc.)

a) Find the function that satisfies this equation, given that approximately 75 billion apps were downloaded in June 2014.
b) Predict the number of apps that will be downloaded in June 2022.
c) Estimate the rate of change in the number of apps downloaded in June 2022.

13. **Art masterpieces.** In 2004, a collector paid \$104,168,000 for Pablo Picasso's "Garcon à la Pipe." The same painting sold for \$30,000 in 1950. (*Source:* BBC News, 5/6/04.)

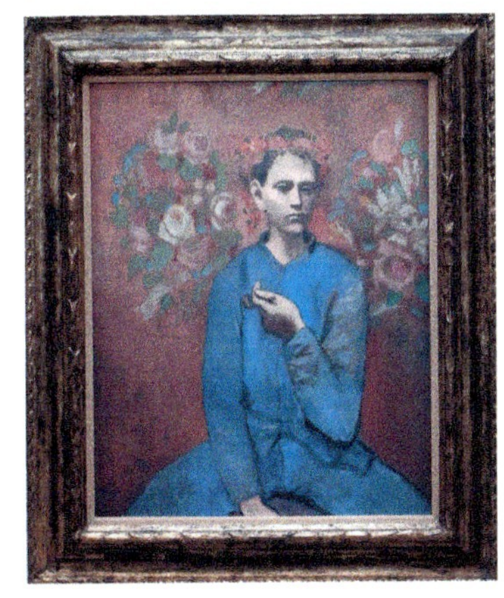

a) Find the exponential growth rate k, to three decimal places, and determine the exponential growth function V, for which $V(t)$ is the painting's value, in dollars, t years after 1950.
b) Predict the value of the painting in 2025, rounded to the nearest million dollars.
c) Estimate the rate of change of the painting's value, rounded to the nearest million dollars, in 2025.
d) How long after 1950 will the value of the painting be \$4 billion?

14. **Per capita income.** In 2012, U.S. per capita personal income, I, was \$52,840. In 2015, it was \$56,430. (*Source:* data.worldbank.org.) Assume that the growth of U.S. per capita personal income follows an exponential model.

a) Find the function that estimates U.S. per capita personal income, $I(t)$, in dollars, t years after 2012.
b) Predict what U.S. per capita personal income will be in 2025.
c) Estimate the rate of change of U.S. per capita personal income in 2025.

15. Federal receipts. In 2013, U.S. federal receipts (money taken in) totaled \$2.77 trillion. In 2016, total federal receipts were \$3.27 trillion. (*Source:* usgovernmentrevenue.com.) Assume that the growth of total federal receipts, F, can be modeled by an exponential function and use 2013 as the base year ($t = 0$).

a) Find the growth rate k to six decimal places, and write the exponential function $F(t)$, for total federal receipts in trillions of dollars.
b) Estimate total federal receipts in 2020.
c) When will total federal receipts be \$10 trillion?

16. Consumer price index. The *consumer price index* compares the costs, c, of goods and services over various years, where 1983 is used as a base ($t = 0$). The same goods and services that cost \$100 in 1983 cost \$243 in 2017. (*Source:* Bureau of Labor Statistics.)

a) Model c as an exponential function, rounding the growth rate k to six decimal places. Let t be the number of years after 1983.
b) Estimate what the goods and services costing \$100 in 1983 will cost in 2023.
c) Estimate the rate of change in 2023 of the cost of goods and services that cost \$100 in 1983.

Total mobile data traffic. *The following graph shows the predicted monthly mobile data traffic for the years 2016–2021. Use these data in Exercises 17 and 18.*

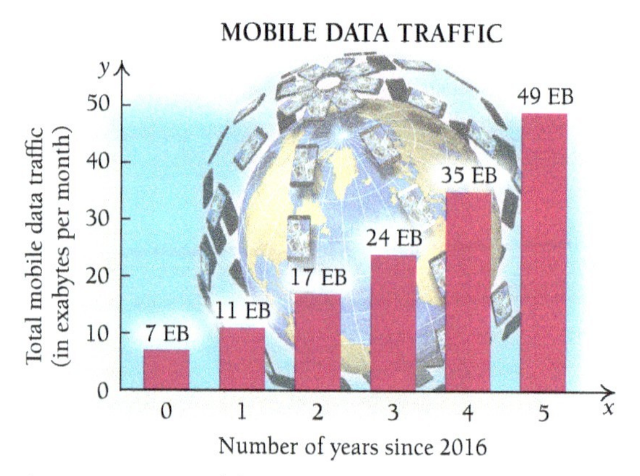

(*Source:* Cisco VNI Mobile, 2016.)

17. a) Use REGRESSION to fit an exponential function $y = a \cdot b^x$ to the data. Let y be the monthly mobile data traffic in exabytes (EB, 1 exabyte = 1 billion gigabytes) and x the number of years since 2016. Then convert the function to an exponential function, base e, using the fact that $b = e^{\ln b}$.
b) What is the exponential growth rate, as a percentage?
c) Estimate the total monthly mobile data traffic in 2024.
d) When will total monthly mobile data traffic exceed 200 exabytes?
e) Estimate the rate of change in mobile data traffic at the time found in part (d).

18. a) Find an exponential function, base e, that fits the data shown in the graph, using the points (0, 7) and (2, 17). Let x represent the number of years since 2016.
b) Estimate the total monthly mobile data traffic in 2022 and 2025.
c) When will total monthly mobile data traffic exceed 200 exabytes?
d) What is the doubling time for total monthly mobile traffic?
e) Compare your answer for part (c) with that of Exercise 17. Decide which exponential function seems to fit the data better, and explain why.

19. Value of Manhattan Island. Peter Minuit of the Dutch West India Company purchased Manhattan Island from the natives living there in 1626 for \$24 worth of merchandise. Assuming an exponential rate of inflation of 5%, how much will Manhattan be worth in 2025?

20. Total revenue. Intel, a computer chip manufacturer, reported \$1265 million in total revenue in 1986. In 2016, the total revenue was \$59.4 billion. (*Source:* intel.com.) Assuming an exponential model, find the growth rate k, to four decimal places, and determine the revenue function R, with $R(t)$ in billions of dollars, t years after 1986. Then predict the company's total revenue for 2025.

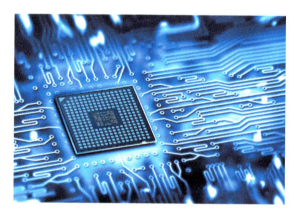

21. The U.S. Forever Stamp. The U.S. Postal Service sells the Forever Stamp, which is always valid as first-class postage on standard envelopes weighing 1 ounce or less, regardless of any subsequent increases in the first-class rate. (*Source:* U.S. Postal Service.)

a) The cost of a first-class postage stamp was 4¢ in 1962 and 50¢ in 2018. This increase represents exponential growth. Write the function S for the cost of a stamp t years after 1962 ($t = 0$).
b) What was the growth rate in the cost of a stamp?
c) Predict the cost of a first-class postage stamp in 2022 and 2024.
d) Red-Hot Promotions spent \$5000 on 10,000 first-class postage stamps at the beginning of 2018. Knowing it will need 10,000 first-class stamps in each of the years 2019–2028, it decides to try to save money by also buying enough stamps to cover those years at the time of the 2018 purchase. Assuming there is a postage increase in each of the years 2022 and 2024 to the cost predicted in part (c), how much money will the firm save by buying the Forever Stamps in 2018?
e) Discuss the pros and cons of the purchase decision described in part (d).

22. **Average salary of Major League baseball players.** In 1970, the average salary of Major League baseball players was \$29,303. In 2016, the average salary was \$4,400,000. (*Source:* mlb.com.) Assuming exponential growth occurred, what was the growth rate to the nearest hundredth of a percent? What will the average salary be in 2025? Round your answer to the nearest thousand dollars.

23. **Effect of advertising.** Suppose that SpryBorg Inc. introduces a new computer game in Houston using television advertisements. Surveys show that $P\%$ of the target audience buys the game after x ads are broadcast, satisfying

$$P(x) = \frac{100}{1 + 49e^{-0.13x}}.$$

a) What percentage of the target audience buys the game without seeing a TV ad $(x = 0)$?
b) What percentage buys the game after the ad is run 5 times? 10 times? 20 times? 30 times? 50 times? 60 times?
c) Find the rate of change, $P'(x)$.
d) Graph the function.

24. **Cost of a Hershey bar.** The cost of a Hershey bar in a supermarket was \$0.05 in 1962 and \$1.59 in 2016.

a) Find an exponential function c that fits the data, where $c(t)$ is the cost, in dollars, t years after 1962.
b) Predict the cost of a Hershey bar in 2025.
c) Estimate the rate of change of the cost of a Hershey bar in 2025.

25. **Superman comic book.** In August 2014, a 1938 comic book featuring the first appearance of Superman sold at auction for a record price of \$3.2 million. The comic book originally cost 10¢ (\$0.10). (*Sources:* eBay; money .cnn.com.) Use the two data points $(0, \$0.10)$ and $(76, \$3{,}200{,}000)$, and assume that the value V of the comic book has grown exponentially, as given by

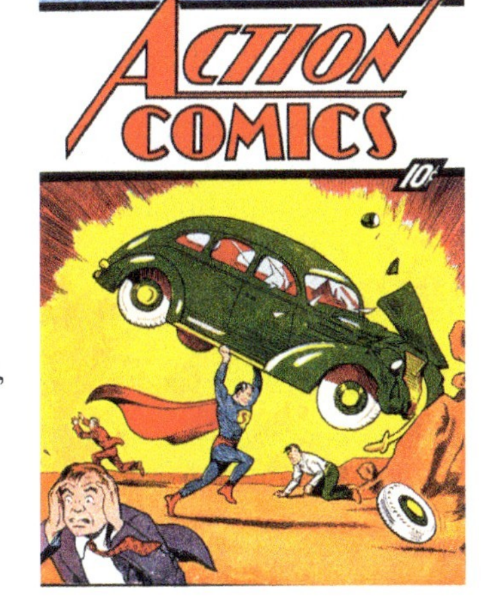

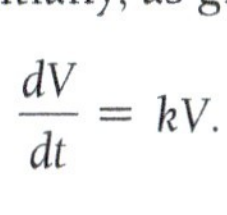

$$\frac{dV}{dt} = kV.$$

(In the summer of 2010, a family faced foreclosure on their mortgage. As they were packing, they came across some old comic books in the basement, and one of them was a copy of this first Superman comic. They sold it and saved their house.)

a) Find the function that satisfies this equation. Assume that $V_0 = \$0.10$ and t is the number of years after 1938.
b) Estimate the value of the comic book in 2020.
c) After what time will the value of the comic book be \$30 million, assuming there is no change in the growth rate?

26. **Batman comic book.** Refer to Example 5. In what year will the value of the comic book be \$5 million?

27. **Batman comic book.** Refer to Example 5. In what year will the value of the comic book be \$10 million?

Life and Physical Sciences

28. **Bicentennial growth of the United States.** The population of the United States in 1776 was about 2,508,000. In the country's bicentennial year, 1976, the population was about 216,000,000.

a) Assuming exponential growth for the t years after 1776, what was the growth rate of the population of the United States through its bicentennial year?
b) Is exponential growth a reasonable assumption? Why or why not?

29. **Limited population growth: human population.** Seventeen adults came ashore from the British ship *HMS Bounty* in 1790 to settle on the uninhabited South Pacific island Pitcairn. The population, $P(t)$, of the island t years after 1790 can be approximated by the logistic equation

$$P(t) = \frac{3400}{17 + 183e^{-0.0982t}}.$$

(*Source:* www.government.pn.)

a) Find the population of the island after 10 yr, 50 yr, and 75 yr.
b) Find the rate of change in the population, $P'(t)$.
c) Find the rate of change in the population after 10 yr, 50 yr, and 75 yr.
d) What is the limiting value for the population of Pitcairn? (The limiting value is the number that the population gets closer and closer to but never reaches.)

30. **Limited population growth: tortoise population.** The tortoise population, $P(t)$, in a square mile of the Mojave Desert after t years can be approximated by the logistic equation

$$P(t) = \frac{3000}{20 + 130e^{-0.214t}}.$$

(*Source:* www.deserttortoise.org.)

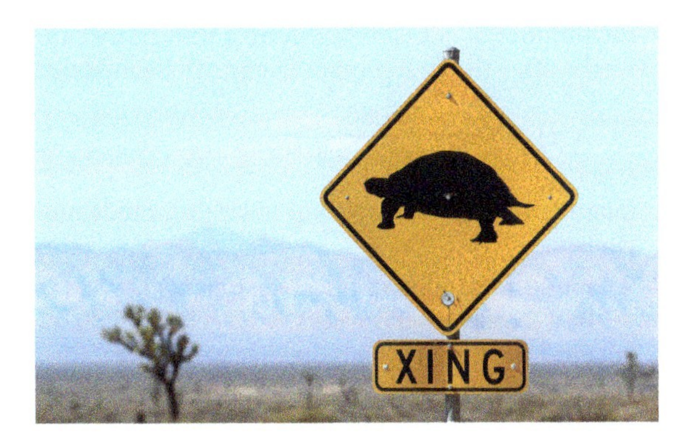

a) Find the tortoise population after 0 yr, 5 yr, 15 yr, and 25 yr.
b) Find the rate of change in the population, $P'(t)$.
c) Find the rate of change in the population after 0 yr, 5 yr, 15, yr, and 25 yr.
d) What is the limiting value for the population of tortoises in a square mile of the Mojave Desert?

31. Limited population growth. A lake is stocked with 400 rainbow trout. The size of the lake, the availability of food, and the number of other fish restrict population growth to a limiting value of 2500 trout. The population of trout in the lake after t months is approximated by

$$P(t) = \frac{2500}{1 + 5.25e^{-0.32t}}.$$

a) Find the population after 0 months, 1 month, 5 months, 10 months, 15 months, and 20 months.
b) Find the rate of change, $P'(t)$.
c) Graph the function.

Social Sciences

32. Women college graduates. The number of women earning a bachelor's degree from a 4-yr college in the United States grew from 48,869 in 1930 to approximately 1,082,000 in 2015. (*Source:* National Center for Education Statistics.) Find an exponential function that fits the data, and determine the exponential growth rate, rounded to the nearest hundredth of a percent. Let $N(t)$ be the number of women who earned a degree t years after 1930.

33. Hullian learning model. The Hullian learning model asserts that the probability p of mastering a task after t learning trials is approximated by

$$p(t) = 1 - e^{-kt},$$

where k is a constant that depends on the task to be learned. Suppose a new dance is taught to an aerobics class. For this particular dance, assume $k = 0.28$.

a) What is the probability of mastering the dance in 1 trial? 2 trials? 5 trials? 11 trials? 16 trials? 20 trials?
b) Find the rate of change, $p'(t)$.
c) Graph the function.

34. Spread of infection. Spread by skin-to-skin contact or via shared towels or clothing, methicillin-resistant *Staphylococcus aureus* (MRSA) can easily infect growing numbers of students at a university. Left unchecked, the number of cases of MRSA on a university campus t weeks after the first 9 cases occur can be modeled by

$$N(t) = \frac{568.803}{1 + 62.200e^{-0.092t}}.$$

(*Source:* Vermont Department of Health, Epidemiology Division.)

a) Find the number of infected students beyond the first 9 cases after 3 weeks, 40 weeks, and 80 weeks.
b) Find the rate at which the disease is spreading after 20 weeks.
c) Explain why an unrestricted growth model is inappropriate but a logistic equation *is* appropriate for this situation. Then use a calculator to graph the equation.

35. Acceptance of new medication. Pharmaceutical firms invest significantly in testing new medications. After a drug is approved by the Federal Drug Administration, it takes time for physicians to fully accept and start prescribing it. The acceptance by physicians approaches a *limiting value* of 100%, or 1, after t months. Suppose that the percentage P of physicians prescribing a new cancer medication after t months is approximated by

$$P(t) = 100(1 - e^{-0.4t}).$$

a) What percentage of doctors are prescribing the medication after 0 months? 1 month? 2 months? 3 months? 5 months? 12 months? 16 months?
b) Find $P'(7)$, and interpret its meaning.
c) Graph the function.

36. Spread of a rumor. The rumor "People who study math all get scholarships" spreads within a technical high school. Data in the following table show the number of students N who have heard the rumor after t days.

Time, t (in days)	Number, N, Who Have Heard the Rumor
1	1
2	2
3	4
4	7
5	12
6	18
7	24
8	26
9	28
10	28
11	29
12	30

a) Use REGRESSION to fit a logistic equation,

$$N(t) = \frac{c}{1 + ae^{-bt}},$$

to the data.
b) Estimate the limiting value of the function. At most, how many students will hear the rumor?
c) Graph the function.
d) Find the rate of change, $N'(t)$.
e) Find $\lim_{t \to \infty} N'(t)$, and explain its meaning.

SYNTHESIS

We have now studied models for linear, quadratic, exponential, and logistic growth. In the real world, understanding which is the most appropriate type of model for a given situation is an important skill. For each situation in Exercises 37–49, identify the most appropriate type of model and explain why you chose that model. List any restrictions you would place on the domain of the function.

37. The growth in value of a U.S. savings bond

38. The growth in the length of Zachary's hair following a haircut

39. The growth in sales of electric cars

40. The drop and rise of a lake's water level during and after a drought

41. The rapidly growing sales of organic foods

42. The number of manufacturing jobs that have left the United States since 1995

43. The life expectancy of the average American

44. The occupancy (number of apartments rented) of a newly opened apartment complex

45. The decrease in population of a city after its principal industry closes

46. The weight of a dog from birth to adulthood

47. The efficiency of an employee as a function of number of hours worked

48. The number of U.S. jobs related to solar or wind power

49. The number of driverless vehicles on U.S. roads

50. Use substitution to show that $P(t) = \dfrac{L}{1 + Ce^{-Lkt}}$ is a solution of the differential equation $\dfrac{dP}{dt} = kP(L - P)$.

51. Use substitution to show that $P(t) = L + Ce^{-kt}$ is a solution of the differential equation $\dfrac{dP}{dt} = k(L - P)$.

Answers to Quick Checks

1. $N(t) = ce^{0.005t}$ **2.** $f(t) = ce^{0.25t}$ **3.** **(a)** $P(t) = P_0e^{0.04t}$; **(b)** \$10,408.11; **(c)** \$416.32/yr **4.** **(a)** $P(t) = 1.39e^{0.0044t}$; **(b)** 1.42 billion; **(c)** 0.00625 billion people/yr, or about 6.25 million people/yr **5.** **(a)** $V(t) = 100e^{0.226t}$; **(b)** \$31,363,965.18; **(c)** \$7,088,256.13/yr **6.** **(a)** 167; **(b)** 500, 3007, 3499 **(c)**

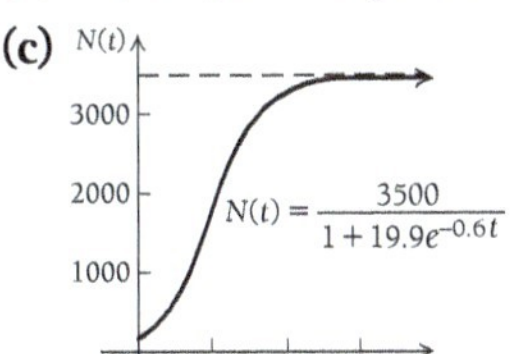

(d) After 16 days, the number of people infected is growing at the rate of about 2.8 people per day. **(e)** According to the model, $\lim_{t\to\infty} N(t) = 3500$, so virtually all of the town's residents will be affected. **7.** **(a)** $P(t) = 75 - 41e^{-0.0208t}$; **(b)** $P'(20) = 0.56$, meaning that the soda's temperature is increasing at a rate of about 0.56 °F/min; **(c)** 101.2 min

2.5 Applications: Exponential Decay

- Find a function that satisfies $dP/dt = -kP$.
- Convert between decay rate and half-life.
- Solve applied problems involving exponential decay.

In the equation of population growth, $dP/dt = kP$, the constant k is given by

$$k = (\text{Birth rate}) - (\text{Death rate}).$$

Thus, a population "grows" when the birth rate is greater than the death rate and decreases when the birth rate is less than the death rate. For convenience in our computations, we will express such a decreasing rate as $-k$, where $k > 0$. The equation

$$\frac{dP}{dt} = -kP, \quad \text{where } k > 0,$$

shows P to be *decreasing*, or decaying, as a function of time, and the solution

$$P(t) = P_0e^{-kt}$$

shows P to be decreasing exponentially. This is called **exponential decay.** The amount present initially at $t = 0$ is again P_0.

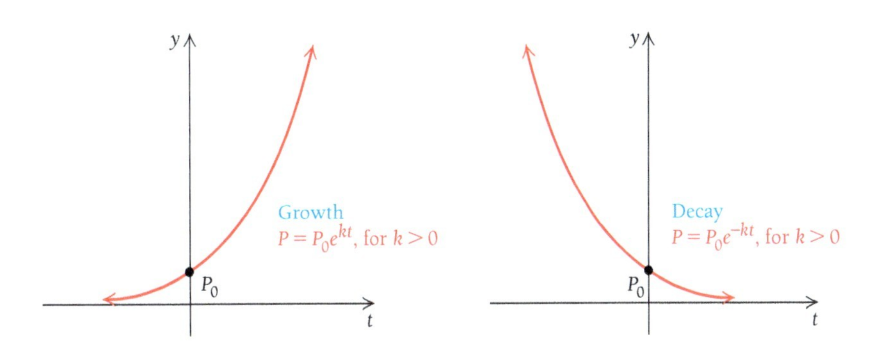

Radioactive Decay

Radioactive isotopes decay exponentially; that is, they are continuously decaying at a rate that is proportional to the amount present.

EXAMPLE 1 **Physical Science: Decay.** Strontium-90 has a continuous decay rate of 2.8% per year. The rate of change of an amount N of this radioactive isotope is given by

$$\frac{dN}{dt} = -0.028N.$$

a) Find the function that satisfies the equation. Let N_0 represent the amount present at $t = 0$.

b) Suppose that 1000 grams (g) of strontium-90 is present at $t = 0$. How much will remain after 70 yr?

c) Find the rate of change of the amount of strontium-90 after 70 yr.

d) After how long will exactly half of the original 1000 g remain?

Solution

a) $N(t) = N_0e^{-0.028t}$

b)
$$\begin{aligned} N(70) &= 1000e^{-0.028(70)} \\ &= 1000e^{-1.96} \\ &\approx 140.8584209. \quad \text{Using a calculator} \end{aligned}$$

After 70 yr, about 140.9 g of the strontium-90 remains.

c) We first find $N'(t)$ by observing that $dN/dt = -0.028N$:

$$\begin{aligned} \frac{dN}{dt} &= -0.028N && \text{Using the original equation} \\ &= -0.028(1000e^{-0.028t}) && \text{Substituting} \\ N'(t) &= -28e^{-0.028t}. && \text{Simplifying} \end{aligned}$$

At $t = 70$, we have

$$N'(70) = -28e^{-0.028(70)} \approx -3.944.$$

Thus, after 70 yr, the amount of strontium-90 is decreasing by about 3.944 g/yr.

d) We are asking, "At what time T will $N(T)$ be half of N_0, or $\frac{1}{2} \cdot 1000$?" The number T is called the **half-life** of strontium-90. To find T, we solve

$$\begin{aligned} 500 &= 1000e^{-0.028T} && \text{We use 500 because } 500 = \tfrac{1}{2} \cdot 1000. \\ \tfrac{1}{2} &= e^{-0.028T} && \text{Dividing both sides by 1000} \\ \ln \tfrac{1}{2} &= \ln e^{-0.028T} && \text{Finding the natural logarithm of both sides} \\ \ln 1 - \ln 2 &= -0.028T && \text{Using the properties of logarithms} \\ 0 - \ln 2 &= -0.028T \\ \frac{-\ln 2}{-0.028} &= T && \text{Dividing both sides by } -0.028 \\ \frac{\ln 2}{0.028} &= T \\ 25 &\approx T. && \text{Using a calculator} \end{aligned}$$

Thus, the half-life of strontium-90 is about 25 yr. **1 ✓**

Quick Check 1 ✓

Physical Science: Decay. Xenon-133 has a decay rate of 14% per day. The rate of change of an amount N of this radioactive isotope is given by

$$\frac{dN}{dt} = -0.14N.$$

a) Find the function that satisfies the equation. Let N_0 represent the amount present at $t = 0$.

b) Suppose 1000 g of xenon-133 is present at $t = 0$. How much will remain after 10 days?

c) Find the rate of change of the amount of xenon-133 after 10 days.

d) After how long will half of the original 1000 g remain?

To find a general expression relating decay rate k and half-life T, we solve

$$\begin{aligned} \tfrac{1}{2}P_0 &= P_0e^{-kT} \\ \tfrac{1}{2} &= e^{-kT} \\ \ln \tfrac{1}{2} &= \ln e^{-kT} \\ \ln 1 - \ln 2 &= -kT \\ 0 - \ln 2 &= -kT \\ -\ln 2 &= -kT \\ \ln 2 &= kT. \end{aligned}$$

How can scientists determine that the remains of an animal or plant have lost 30% of the carbon-14? The assumption is that the percentage of carbon-14 in the atmosphere and in living plants and animals is the same. When a plant or animal dies, its carbon-14 decays exponentially. A scientist burns the remains and uses a Geiger counter to determine the percentage of carbon-14 in the smoke. The amount by which this varies from the percentage in the atmosphere indicates how much carbon-14 was lost through decay.

The process of carbon-14 dating was developed by the American chemist Willard F. Libby in 1952. It is known that the radioactivity of a living plant measures 16 disintegrations per gram per minute. Since the half-life of carbon-14 is 5730 years, a dead plant with an activity of 8 disintegrations per gram per minute is 5730 years old, one with an activity of 4 disintegrations per gram per minute is about 11,500 years old, and so on. Carbon-14 dating can be used to determine the age of organic objects that are up to 40,000 years old. Beyond such an age, it is too difficult to measure the radioactivity, and other methods are used.

Therefore, we have the following theorem.

THEOREM 10

The **decay rate**, k, and the **half-life**, T, are related by

$$kT = \ln 2, \quad \text{or} \quad k = \frac{\ln 2}{T} \quad \text{and} \quad T = \frac{\ln 2}{k}.$$

Thus, half-life, T, depends only on decay rate, k, and is independent of the initial population size.

The effect of half-life is shown in the radioactive decay curve below. Note that the exponential function gets close to, but never reaches, 0 as t gets larger. Thus, in theory, a radioactive substance never completely decays.

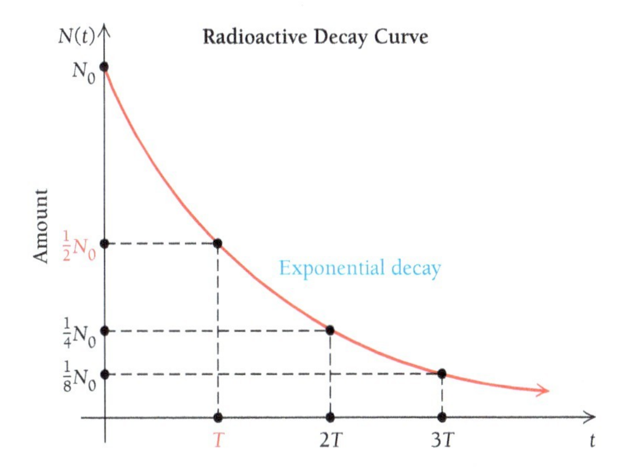

Quick Check 2 ✓

Physical Science: Half-life.

a) The decay rate of cesium-137 is 2.3% per year. What is its half-life?

b) The half-life of barium-140 is 13 days. What is its decay rate?

EXAMPLE 2 **Physical Science: Half-life.** Plutonium-239, a common product of a functioning nuclear reactor, can be deadly to people exposed to it. Its decay rate is about 0.0028% per year. What is its half-life?

Solution We have

$$\begin{aligned} T &= \frac{\ln 2}{k} \\ &= \frac{\ln 2}{0.000028} \qquad \text{Converting 0.0028\% to decimal notation} \\ &\approx 24{,}755. \end{aligned}$$

Thus, the half-life of plutonium-239 is about 24,755 yr. **2 ✓**

EXAMPLE 3 **Life Science: Carbon Dating.** The radioactive element carbon-14 has a half-life of 5730 yr. The percentage of carbon-14 present in the remains of plants and animals is used to determine age. Archaeologists found that the linen wrapping from one of the Dead Sea Scrolls had lost 22.3% of its carbon-14. How old was the linen wrapping?

Solution We need to find an exponential equation of the form $N(t) = N_0e^{-kt}$, replace $N(t)$ with $(1 - 0.223)N_0$, and solve for t. To do so, we first find the decay rate, k:

$$k = \frac{\ln 2}{T} = \frac{\ln 2}{5730} \approx 0.00012097, \quad \text{or} \quad 0.012097\% \text{ per year.}$$

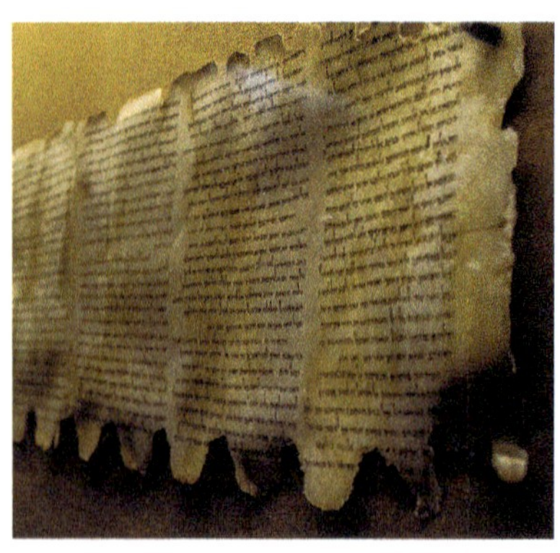

In 1947, a Bedouin youth looking for a stray goat climbed into a cave at Kirbet Qumran on the shores of the Dead Sea near Jericho and came upon earthenware jars containing an incalculably valuable treasure: ancient manuscripts that concern the Jewish books of the Bible. Shown here are fragments of those so-called Dead Sea Scrolls, a portion of some 600 or so texts found so far. Officials date them before A.D. 70, making them the oldest biblical manuscripts by 1000 years.

Thus, the amount $N(t)$ that remains from an initial amount N_0 after t years is given by

$$N(t) = N_0 e^{-0.00012097t}. \qquad \text{Remember: } k \text{ is positive, so } -k \text{ is negative.}$$

(*Note:* This equation can be used for all subsequent carbon-dating problems.)

If the linen wrapping from a Dead Sea Scroll lost 22.3% of its carbon-14 from an initial amount N_0, then $77.7\% \cdot N_0$ remains. To find the age t of the wrapping, we solve the following equation for t:

$$\begin{aligned}
77.7\% N_0 &= N_0 e^{-0.00012097t} \\
0.777 &= e^{-0.00012097t} \\
\ln 0.777 &= \ln e^{-0.00012097t} \\
\ln 0.777 &= -0.00012097t \\
\frac{\ln 0.777}{-0.00012097} &= t \\
2086 &\approx t.
\end{aligned}$$

Thus, the linen wrapping from the Dead Sea Scroll is about 2086 yr old. **3 ✓**

Quick Check 3 ✓

Life Science: Carbon Dating. How old is a skeleton found at an archaeological site if tests show that it has lost 60% of its carbon-14?

A Business Application: Present Value

Bankers and financial planners are often concerned with problems like the following.

EXAMPLE 4 **Business: Present Value.** Following the birth of their granddaughter, Doug and Andrea want to make an initial investment, P_0, that will grow to \$10,000 by the child's 20th birthday. Interest is compounded continuously at an annual rate of 4%. What should the initial investment be?

Solution Using $P = P_0 e^{kt}$, we find P_0 such that

$$10{,}000 = P_0 e^{0.04 \cdot 20},$$

or $$10{,}000 = P_0 e^{0.8}.$$

Now

$$\frac{10{,}000}{e^{0.8}} = P_0,$$

or $$10{,}000 e^{-0.8} = P_0,$$

and, using a calculator, we have

$$\begin{aligned}
P_0 &= 10{,}000 e^{-0.8} \\
&\approx 4493.29.
\end{aligned}$$

Thus, Doug and Andrea should make an initial investment of \$4493.29, which will grow to \$10,000 by the child's 20th birthday.

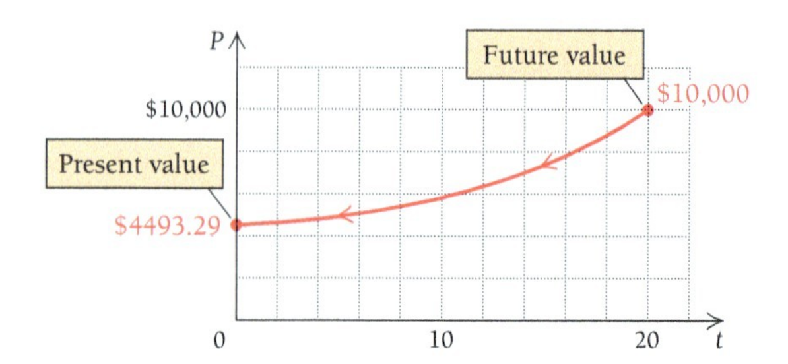

4 ✓

Quick Check 4 ✓

Business: Present Value. Repeat Example 4 using an interest rate of 6%.

Economists call \$4493.29 the *present value* of \$10,000 due 20 yr from now at 4% per year, compounded continuously. The process of computing present value is called **discounting.** Another way to pose this problem is to ask "What should I have invested

20 years ago, at 4% per year, compounded continuously, in order to have $10,000 today?" Thus, computing present value can be interpreted as exponential decay from the future back to the present.

In general, the present value P_0 of an amount P due t years later is found by solving the following equation for P_0:

$$P_0 e^{kt} = P$$
$$P_0 = \frac{P}{e^{kt}} = Pe^{-kt}.$$

THEOREM 11

The **present value** P_0 of an amount P due t years later, at interest rate k, compounded continuously, is given by

$$P_0 = Pe^{-kt}.$$

Newton's Law of Cooling

Consider the following situation. A hot cup of soup, at a temperature of 200°, is placed in a 70° room.* The temperature of the soup decreases over time t according to the model known as **Newton's Law of Cooling.**

Newton's Law of Cooling

The temperature T of a cooling object drops at a rate proportional to the difference $T - C$, where C is the constant temperature of the surrounding medium. Thus,

$$\frac{dT}{dt} = -k(T - C), \quad \text{for } k > 0. \qquad (1)$$

The function that satisfies equation (1) is

$$T = T(t) = ae^{-kt} + C. \qquad (2)$$

To check that $T(t) = ae^{-kt} + C$ is the solution, find dT/dt and substitute dT/dt and $T(t)$ into equation (1). This check is left to the student.

EXAMPLE 5 **Life Science: Scalding Coffee.** McDivett's Pie Shoppes, a national chain, finds that the temperature of its freshly brewed coffee is 130°. The company fears that if customers spill hot coffee on themselves, lawsuits might result. Room temperature in the restaurants is generally 72°. The temperature of the coffee cools to 120° after 4.3 min. McDivett's decides that it is safer to serve coffee at 105°. How long does it take a cup of coffee to cool to 105°?

Solution Note that C, the surrounding air temperature, is 72°. To find the value of a in equation (2) for Newton's Law of Cooling, we observe that at $t = 0$ min, we have $T(0) = 130°$. We solve for a as follows:

$$130 = ae^{-k \cdot 0} + 72$$
$$130 = a + 72$$
$$58 = a. \qquad \text{Noting that } a = 130 - 72\text{, the difference between the original temperatures}$$

*Assume throughout this section that all temperatures are in degrees Fahrenheit unless noted otherwise.

Next, we find k using the fact that $T(4.3) = 120$:

$$120 = 58e^{-k\cdot(4.3)} + 72$$
$$48 = 58e^{-4.3k}$$
$$\frac{48}{58} = e^{-4.3k}$$
$$\ln\left(\frac{48}{58}\right) = \ln e^{-4.3k} \quad \text{Finding the natural logarithm of both sides}$$
$$\ln\left(\frac{48}{58}\right) = -4.3k \quad \text{Using Property P7 of natural logarithms}$$
$$\frac{\ln\left(\frac{48}{58}\right)}{-4.3} = k$$
$$k \approx 0.044. \quad \text{Using a calculator}$$

We now have $T(t) = 58e^{-0.044t} + 72$, where t is the cooling time, in minutes. To see how long it will take the coffee to cool to 105°, we set $T(t) = 105$ and solve for t:

$$105 = 58e^{-0.044t} + 72$$
$$33 = 58e^{-0.044t}$$
$$\frac{33}{58} = e^{-0.044t}$$
$$\ln\left(\frac{33}{58}\right) = \ln e^{-0.044t}$$
$$\ln\left(\frac{33}{58}\right) = -0.044t \quad \text{Using Property P7}$$
$$\frac{\ln\left(\frac{33}{58}\right)}{-0.044} = t$$
$$t \approx 12.8 \text{ min.} \quad \text{Using a calculator}$$

To reach a temperature of 105°, the coffee should cool for about 13 min. **5 ✓**

Quick Check 5 ✓

Physical Science: Scalding Coffee. Repeat Example 5, but assume that the coffee is sold in an ice cream shop, where room temperature is 70°, and it cools to a temperature of 120° in 4 min.

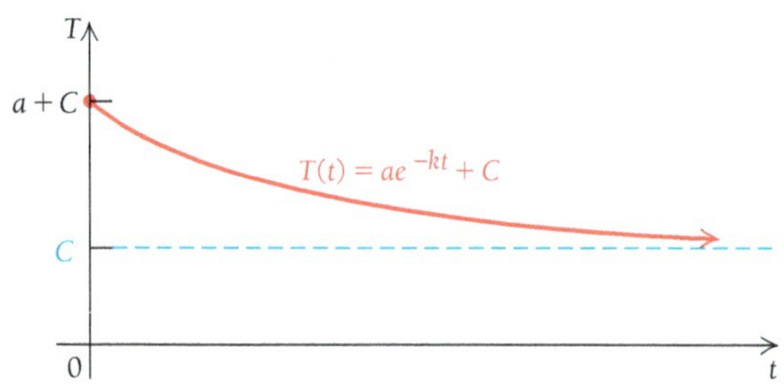

The graph of $T(t) = ae^{-kt} + C$ shows that $\lim_{t\to\infty} T(t) = C$. The temperature of the object decreases toward the temperature of the surrounding medium.

Mathematically, this model demonstrates that the object's temperature never quite reaches C. In practice, the temperature of the cooling object will get so close to that of the surrounding medium that no device could detect a difference. Let's now use Newton's Law of Cooling to solve a crime.

EXAMPLE 6 **Forensics: Determining Time of Death.** A body is found slumped over a desk in a study. The coroner arrives at noon, immediately takes the temperature of the body, and finds it to be 94.6°. She waits 1 hr, takes the temperature again, and finds it to be 93.4°. She also notes that the temperature of the room is 70°. What was the approximate time of death?

Solution Note that C, the surrounding air temperature, is 70°. We let t be the time elapsed, in hours, where $t = 0$ represents noon, when the coroner took the first reading. Thus, $T = 94.6°$ at $t = 0$, and we use this to find a:

$$94.6 = ae^{-k(0)} + 70$$
$$a = 24.6.$$

Thus, $T(t) = 24.6e^{-kt} + 70$.

To find k, we use the fact that at $t = 1$, the body's temperature was 93.4°:

$$93.4 = 24.6e^{-k(1)} + 70 \quad \text{Substituting}$$
$$23.4 = 24.6e^{-k}$$
$$\frac{23.4}{24.6} = e^{-k}$$
$$\ln\left(\frac{23.4}{24.6}\right) = -k$$
$$k = -\ln\left(\frac{23.4}{24.6}\right) \approx 0.05.$$

The function that models the body temperature t hours after the coroner's first reading is therefore given by

$$T(t) = 24.6e^{-0.05t} + 70.$$

To determine the approximate time of death, we assume that the individual had a normal body temperature, 98.6°, at the time of death. We substitute this value for T and solve for t:

$$98.6 = 24.6e^{-0.05t} + 70$$
$$28.6 = 24.6e^{-0.05t}$$
$$\frac{28.6}{24.6} = e^{-0.05t}$$
$$\ln\left(\frac{28.6}{24.6}\right) = -0.05t$$
$$t = \frac{\ln\left(\frac{28.6}{24.6}\right)}{-0.05} \approx -3.01.$$

Since $t = 0$ represents noon, the time of death was about 3 hours earlier, or at about 9:00 a.m. 6 ✓

Quick Check 6 ✓

Forensics. Repeat Example 6, assuming that the coroner arrives at 2 a.m., immediately takes the temperature of the body, and finds it to be 92.8°. She waits 1 hr, takes the temperature again, and finds it to be 90.6°. She also notes that the temperature of the room is 72°. What was the approximate time of death?

Section Summary

- The *decay rate*, k, and the *half-life*, T, are related by $kT = \ln 2$, or
$$k = \frac{\ln 2}{T} \quad \text{and} \quad T = \frac{\ln 2}{k}.$$
- The *present value* P_0 of an amount P due t years later, at an interest rate k, compounded continuously, is given by $P_0 = Pe^{-kt}$.
- According to *Newton's Law of Cooling*, the temperature T of a cooling object drops at a rate proportional to the difference $T - C$, when C is the constant temperature of the surrounding medium. Thus, we have
$$\frac{dT}{dt} = -k(T - C), \text{ for } k > 0, \quad \text{and} \quad T(t) = ae^{-kt} + C.$$

2.5 Exercise Set

APPLICATIONS

Physical and Social Sciences

1. **Radioactive decay.** Iodine-131 has a decay rate of 9.6% per day. The rate of change of an amount N of iodine-131 after t days is given by
$$\frac{dN}{dt} = -0.096N.$$
   a) Let N_0 represent the amount of iodine-131 present at $t = 0$. Find the exponential function that models the decay.
   b) Suppose 500 g of iodine-131 is present at $t = 0$. How much will remain after 4 days?
   c) What is the rate of change of the amount of iodine-131 after 4 days?
   d) After how many days will half of the original 500 g of iodine-131 remain?

2. Radioactive decay. Carbon-14 has a decay rate of 0.012097% per year. The rate of change of an amount N of carbon-14 after t years is given by

$$\frac{dN}{dt} = -0.00012097N.$$

a) Let N_0 represent the amount of carbon-14 present at $t = 0$. Find the exponential function that models the decay.
b) Suppose 200 g of carbon-14 is present at $t = 0$. How much will remain after 800 yr?
c) What is the rate of change of the amount of carbon-14 after 800 yr?
d) After how many years will half of the original 200 g of carbon-14 remain?

3. Radioactive decay. Curium-245 has a decay rate of 0.0081547% per year. The rate of change of an amount N of curium-245 after t years is given by

$$\frac{dN}{dt} = -0.000081547N.$$

a) Let N_0 represent the amount of curium-245 present at $t = 0$. Find an exponential function that models this situation.
b) Suppose 60 mg of curium-245 is present at $t = 0$. How much will remain after 1500 yr?
c) What is the rate of change of the amount of curium-245 after 1500 yr?
d) After how many years will half of the original 60 mg of curium-245 remain?

4. Radioactive decay. Oxygen-19 has a decay rate of 2.62% per second. The rate of change of an amount N of oxygen-19 after t seconds is given by

$$\frac{dN}{dt} = -0.0262N.$$

a) Let N_0 represent the amount of oxygen-19 present at $t = 0$. Find an exponential function that models this situation.
b) Suppose 250 mg of oxygen-19 is present at $t = 0$. How much will remain after 1 min?
c) What is the rate of change of the amount of oxygen-19 after 1 min?
d) After how many seconds will half of the original 250 mg of oxygen-19 remain?
e) After how many seconds will 99% of the oxygen-19 have decayed?

5. Radioactive decay. Gold-198 has a decay rate of 25.72% per day. The rate of change of an amount N of gold-198 after t days is given by

$$\frac{dN}{dt} = -0.2572N.$$

a) Let N_0 represent the amount of gold-198 present at $t = 0$. Find an exponential function that models this situation.
b) Suppose 10 mg of gold-198 is present at $t = 0$. How much will remain after 1 week?
c) What is the rate of change of the amount of gold-198 after 1 week?
d) After how many days will half of the original 10 mg of gold-198 remain?
e) After how many days will 85% of the gold-198 have decayed?

6. Radioactive decay. Chromium-51 has a decay rate of 2.5% per day. The rate of change of an amount N of chromium-51 after t days is given by

$$\frac{dN}{dt} = -0.025N.$$

a) Let N_0 represent the amount of chromium-51 present at $t = 0$. Find an exponential function that models this situation.
b) Suppose 20 mg of chromium-51 is present at $t = 0$. How much will remain after 30 days?
c) What is the rate of change of the amount of chromium-51 after 30 days?
d) After how many days will half of the original 20 mg of chromium-51 remain?
e) After how many days will 95% of the chromium-51 have decayed away?

7. Population decay. Since 1990, the population of Gary, Indiana, has been decreasing by 1.87% per year. The rate of change of the city's population P, t years after 1990, is given by

$$\frac{dP}{dt} = -0.0187P.$$

a) In 1990, the population of Gary was 116,646. (*Source:* U.S. Census Bureau.) Find an exponential function that models this situation.
b) Estimate the population of Gary in 2025.
c) What is the rate of change of the population of Gary in 2025?
d) After how many years will the population of Gary be half of what it was in 1990?

8. Population decay. Since 1980, the population of Trenton, New Jersey, has been decreasing by 2.72% per year. The rate of change of the city's population P, t years after 1980, is given by

$$\frac{dP}{dt} = -0.0272P.$$

a) In 1980, the population of Trenton was 92,124. (*Source:* U.S. Census Bureau.) Find an exponential function that models this situation.
b) Estimate the population of Trenton in 2030.
c) What is the rate of change of the population of Trenton in 2030?
d) After how many years will the population of Trenton be half of what it was in 1980?

9. Chemistry. Substance A decomposes at a rate proportional to the amount of A present.

a) Write an equation that gives the amount A left of an initial amount A_0 after t hours.
b) It is found that 10 lb of A will decrease to 5 lb in 3.3 hr. After how long will there be only 1 lb left?

10. Chemistry. Substance A decomposes at a rate proportional to the amount of A present.

a) Write an equation that gives the amount A left of an initial amount A_0 after t hours.
b) It is found that 8 g of A will decrease to 4 g in 3 hr. After how long will there be only 1 g left?

11. **Chemistry.** Carbon-11 decays at a rate proportional to the amount present.
   a) A lab technician has a 35-mg sample of carbon-11, and 20.3 min later, the mass of the sample has decreased to 17.5 mg. Write an equation that gives the amount, $A(t)$, of carbon-11 present after t minutes.
   b) After how long will only 20% of the original sample remain?

12. **Chemistry.** Erbium-165 decays at a rate proportional to the amount present.
   a) A lab technician has a 4-mg sample of erbium-165, and 10.4 hr later, the sample has reduced to 2 mg. Write an equation that gives the amount, $A(t)$, of erbium-165 present after t hours.
   b) After how long will only 10% of the original sample remain?

13. **Population decay.** The population of Cortez Breaks decreases at a rate proportional to the current size of the population.
   a) In 2012, the population was 5000; by 2018, the population was 2500. Write an equation that gives the population, $P(t)$, of Cortez Breaks t years after 2012.
   b) After how long will the population of Cortez Breaks be only 30% of the 2012 population?

14. **Population decay.** The student population at Silver Bell College decreases at a rate proportional to the current size of the population.
   a) In 2010, the student population was 10,000; by 2017, the student population was 5000. Write an equation that gives the student population, $P(t)$, of Silver Bell College after t years.
   b) After how long will the student population be only 40% of the 2010 population?

In Exercises 15–22, find the half-life for each situation.

15. An element loses 12% of its mass every year.
16. A population of bacteria decreases by 5.75% per month.
17. A vehicle loses 0.8% of its value every month.
18. A city loses 3.9% of its population every year.
19. The value of a dollar decreases by 3% every year.
20. An element loses 1.75% of its mass every day.
21. An investment loses 1.9% of its value every week.
22. A motor home loses 0.5% of its value every week.

Radioactive decay. *For Exercises 23–26, complete the following.*

Radioactive Substance	Decay Rate, k	Half-life, T
23. Polonium-218	________	3 min
24. Radium-226	________	1600 yr
25. Lead-210	3.15%/yr	________
26. Strontium-90	2.77%/yr	________

27. **Half-life.** Of an initial amount of 1000 g of lead-210, how much will remain after 100 yr? See Exercise 25 for the value of k.

28. **Half-life.** Of an initial amount of 1000 g of polonium-218, how much will remain after 20 min? See Exercise 23 for the value of k.

29. **Carbon dating.** How old is an ivory tusk that has lost 40% of its carbon-14? (See Exercise 2.)

30. **Carbon dating.** How old is a piece of wood that has lost 90% of its carbon-14? (See Exercise 2.)

31. **Cancer treatment.** Iodine-125 is often used to treat cancer and has a half-life of 60.1 days. In one sample, the amount of iodine-125 decreased by 25% while in storage. How long was the sample in storage?

32. **Carbon dating.** How old is a Chinese artifact that has lost 60% of its carbon-14? (See Exercise 2.)

33. **Carbon dating.** While digging in Chaco Canyon, New Mexico, archaeologists found corn pollen that had lost 38.1% of its carbon-14. (See Exercise 2.) The age of this corn pollen was evidence that Native Americans had been cultivating crops in the Southwest centuries earlier than previously thought. (*Source: American Anthropologist.*) What was the age of the pollen?

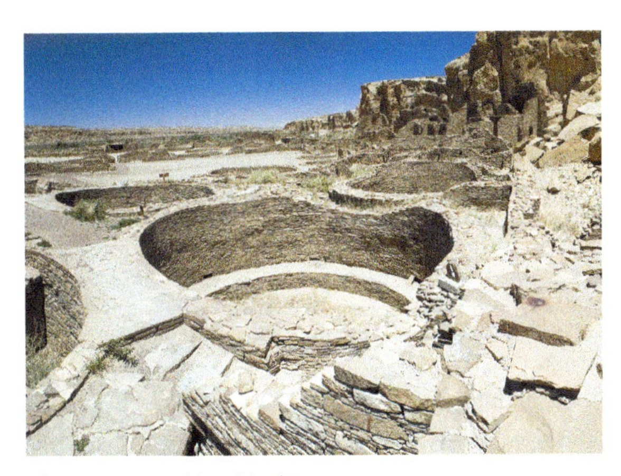

Chaco Canyon, New Mexico

Business and Economics

34. **Present value.** Following the birth of her child, Roxanne wants to make an initial investment P_0 that will grow to \$30,000 by the child's 20th birthday. Interest is compounded continuously at 6%. What should the initial investment be?

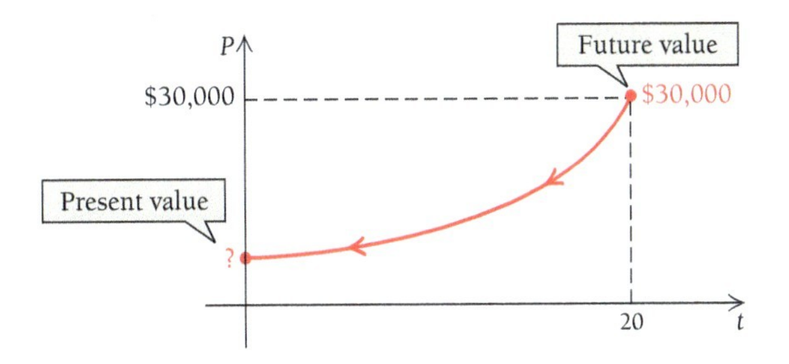

35. **Present value.** Following the birth of their child, the Irwins want to make an initial investment P_0 that will grow to \$40,000 by the child's 20th birthday. Interest is compounded continuously at 5.3%. What should the initial investment be?

36. Present value. Desmond wants to have \$15,000 available in 5 yr to pay for new siding. Interest is 4.3%, compounded continuously. How much money should be invested?

37. Sports salaries. An athlete signs a contract that guarantees a yearly salary of \$9 million 6 yr from now. Assuming that money is invested at 4.7%, with interest compounded continuously, what is the present value of that \$9-million salary?

38. Actors' salaries. An actor signs a film contract that will pay \$12 million when the film is completed 3 yr from now. Assuming that money is invested at 4.2%, with interest compounded continuously, what is the present value of that payment?

39. Estate planning. Shannon has a trust fund that will yield \$80,000 in 13 yr. An accountant preparing a financial statement for Shannon wants to find the present value of that trust fund in computing Shannon's net worth. Interest is compounded continuously at 4.8%. What is the present value of the trust fund?

40. Trust fund. Marisa just had her 12th birthday. Her grandmother sets up a trust fund that, when Marisa turns 21, will be worth \$50,000. Assuming that interest is compounded continuously at an annual rate of 3.75%, what is the present value of this trust fund?

41. Salvage value. Lucas Mining estimates that the salvage value $V(t)$, in dollars, of a piece of machinery after t years is given by

$$V(t) = 40{,}000e^{-t}.$$

a) What did the machinery cost initially?
b) What is the salvage value after 2 yr?
c) Find the rate of change of the salvage value, and explain its meaning.

42. Salvage value. Will's Taxi Service purchases a sedan and estimates that its salvage value $V(t)$, in dollars, after t years, is given by

$$V(t) = 18{,}000e^{-0.06t}.$$

a) What did the sedan cost originally?
b) What is the salvage value after 3 yr?
c) Find the rate of change of the salvage value, and explain its meaning.

43. Salvage value. The Barn Eatery purchases booths for seating and estimates that their salvage value $V(t)$, in dollars, after t years, is given by

$$V(t) = 23{,}500e^{-0.12t}.$$

a) What did the booths cost originally?
b) What is the salvage value after 4 yr?
c) Find the rate of change of the salvage value, and explain its meaning.

44. Depreciation. The Larsons purchase a motorboat and estimate that its value $V(t)$, in dollars, after t years, is given by

$$V(t) = 30{,}000e^{-0.27t}.$$

a) What did the motorboat cost originally?
b) What is the motorboat's value after 6 yr?
c) Find the rate of change of the motorboat's value after 6 yr, and explain its meaning.

45. Depreciation. Ed purchases a set of drums and estimates that its value $V(t)$, in dollars, after t years, is given by

$$V(t) = 2600e^{-0.09t}.$$

a) What did the drum set cost originally?
b) What is the drum set's value after 2 yr?
c) Find the rate of change of the drum set's value after 2 yr, and explain its meaning.

46. Salvage value. Suppose that Leonard Investments tracks the value of a main-frame computer over a period of years. The data in the table below show the value of the computer t years after the purchase date.

Time, t (in years)	Salvage Value
0	\$34,000
1	22,791
2	15,277
3	10,241
4	6,865
5	4,600
6	3,084

a) Use REGRESSION to fit an exponential function $y = a \cdot b^x$ to the data. Then convert that formula to $V(t) = V_0e^{-kt}$, where V_0 is the value when the computer is purchased and t is the number of years since the purchase date.
b) Estimate the salvage value of the computer after 7 yr and after 10 yr.
c) After what amount of time will the salvage value be \$1000?
d) After how long will the computer be worth half of its original value?
e) Find the rate of change of the salvage value, and interpret its meaning.

47. Actuarial science. An actuary calculates premiums for an insurance company. Given an actual mortality rate (probability of death) for a given age, actuaries sometimes need to project future expected mortality rates of people of that age. For example,

$$Q(t) = (Q_0 - 0.00055)e^{0.163t} + 0.00055,$$

where Q_0 is the mortality rate at $t = 0$ and $Q(t)$ is the future mortality rate t years into the future.

a) Suppose the actual mortality rate of a group of females aged 25 is 0.014 (14 deaths per 1000). What is the future expected mortality rate of this group of females 3, 5, and 10 yr in the future?
b) Sketch the graph of the mortality function $Q(t)$ for the group in part (a) for $0 \le t \le 10$.

48. Actuarial science. Use the formula from Exercise 47.

a) Suppose the actual mortality rate of a group of males aged 25 is 0.023 (23 deaths per 1000). What is the future expected mortality rate of this group of males 3, 5, and 10 yr in the future?
b) Sketch the graph of the mortality function $Q(t)$ for the group in part (a) for $0 \le t \le 10$.
c) What is the ratio of the mortality rate for 25-year-old males 10 yr in the future to that for 25-year-old females 10 yr in the future (Exercise 47a)?

49. U.S. farms. The number N of farms in the United States has declined continually since 1950. In 1950, there were 5,650,000 farms, and in 2016, that number had decreased to 2,060,000. (*Sources:* U.S. Department of Agriculture; National Agricultural Statistics Service.)

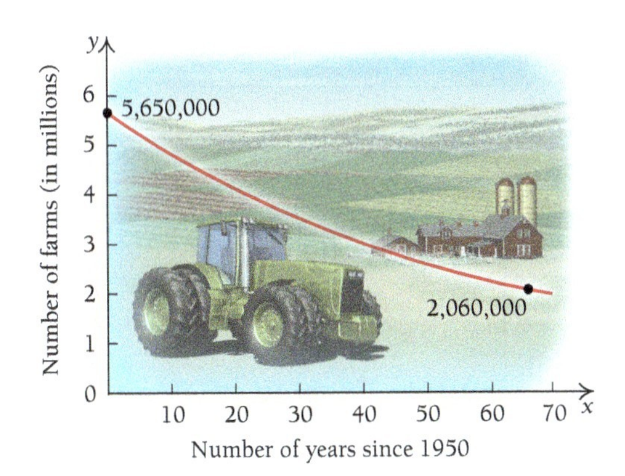

Assuming the number of farms decreased according to the exponential decay model:

a) Find the value of k, and write an exponential function that describes the number of farms after time t, where t is the number of years since 1950.
b) Estimate the number of U.S. farms in 2025.
c) At this decay rate, when will only 1,000,000 farms remain?

Social Sciences

50. Decline in beef consumption. Annual consumption of beef per person was about 64.6 lb in 2000 and about 61.2 lb in 2008. Assuming that $B(t)$, the annual beef consumption t years after 2000, is decreasing according to the exponential decay model:

a) Find the value of k, and write the equation.
b) Estimate the consumption of beef in 2015.
c) In what year (theoretically) will the consumption of beef be 20 lb per person?

51. Population decrease of Puerto Rico. The population of Puerto Rico dropped from 3.81 million in 2000 to 3.47 million in 2015. (*Source:* CIA–*The World Factbook.*) Assume that $P(t)$, the population, in millions, t years after 2000, is decreasing according to the exponential decay model.

a) Find the value of k, and write the equation.
b) Estimate the population of Puerto Rico in 2020.
c) When will the population of Puerto Rico be 3.2 million?

52. Population decrease of Latvia. The population of Latvia dropped from 2.37 million in 2000 to 1.98 million in 2015. (*Source:* CIA–*The World Factbook.*) Assume that $P(t)$, the population, in millions, t years after 2000, is decreasing according to the exponential decay model.

a) Find the value of k, and write the equation.
b) Estimate the population of Latvia in 2020.
c) In what year will the population of Latvia be 1.75 million, according to this model?

Life and Natural Sciences

53. Cooling. After warming the water in a hot tub to 100°, the heating element fails. The surrounding air temperature is 40°, and in 5 min the water temperature drops to 95°.

a) Find the value of the constant a in Newton's Law of Cooling.
b) Find the value of the constant k. Round to five decimal places.
c) What is the water temperature after 10 min?
d) How long does it take the water to cool to 41°?
e) Find the rate of change of the water temperature, and interpret its meaning.

54. Cooling. The temperature in a whirlpool bath is 102°, and the room temperature is 75°. The water cools to 90° in 10 min.

a) Find the value of the constant a in Newton's Law of Cooling.
b) Find the value of the constant k. Round to five decimal places.
c) What is the water temperature after 20 min?
d) How long does it take the water to cool to 80°?
e) Find the rate of change of the water temperature, and interpret its meaning.

55. Forensics. A coroner arrives at a murder scene at 2 a.m. He takes the temperature of the body and finds it to be 61.6°. He waits 1 hr, takes the temperature again, and finds it to be 57.2°. The body is in a freezer, where the temperature is 10°. When was the murder committed?

56. Forensics. A coroner arrives at a murder scene at 11 p.m. She finds the temperature of the body to be 85.9°. She waits 1 hr, takes the temperature again, and finds it to be 83.4°. She notes that the room temperature is 60°. When was the murder committed?

57. Prisoner-of-war protest. The initial weight of a prisoner of war is 140 lb. To protest the conditions of her imprisonment, she begins a fast. Her weight t days after her last meal is approximated by

$$W = 140e^{-0.009t}.$$

a) How much does the prisoner weigh after 25 days?
b) At what rate is the prisoner's weight changing after 25 days?

58. Political protest. A monk weighing 170 lb begins a fast to protest a war. His weight after t days is given by

$$W = 170e^{-0.008t}.$$

a) When the war ends 20 days later, how much does the monk weigh?
b) At what rate is the monk losing weight after 20 days (before any food is consumed)?

59. Atmospheric pressure. Atmospheric pressure P at an altitude of a feet is given by

$$P = P_0e^{-0.00005a},$$

where P_0 is the pressure at sea level. Assume that $P_0 = 14.7\ \text{lb/in}^2$ (pounds per square inch).

a) Find the pressure at an altitude of 1000 ft.
b) Find the pressure at an altitude of 20,000 ft.
c) At what altitude is the pressure $14.7\ \text{lb/in}^2$?
d) Find the rate of change of the pressure, and interpret its meaning.

60. **Satellite power.** The power supply of a satellite is a radioisotope (radioactive substance). The power output P, in watts (W), decreases at a rate proportional to the amount present and is given by

$$P = 50e^{-0.004t},$$

where t is the time, in days.

a) How much power will be available after 375 days?
b) What is the half-life of the power supply?
c) The satellite cannot operate on less than 10 W of power. How long can the satellite stay in operation?
d) How much power did the satellite have to begin with?
e) Find the rate of change of the power output, and interpret its meaning.

61. **Cases of tuberculosis.** The number of cases N of tuberculosis in the United States has decreased continually since 1956. In 1956, there were 69,895 cases. By 2016, this number had decreased by over 85%, to 9287 cases. (*Source:* www.cdc.gov.)

a) Find the value of k, and write an exponential function that describes the number of tuberculosis cases t years after 1956.
b) Estimate the number of cases in 2020 and in 2024.
c) At this decay rate, in what year will there be 5000 cases?

Modeling

For each of the scatterplots in Exercises 62–71, determine which, if any, of these functions might be used as a model for the data:

a) Quadratic: $f(x) = ax^2 + bx + c$
b) Polynomial, not quadratic
c) Exponential: $f(x) = ae^{kx}$, $k > 0$
d) Exponential: $f(x) = ae^{-kx}$, $k > 0$
e) Logarithmic: $f(x) = a + b \ln x$
f) Logistic: $f(x) = \dfrac{a}{1 + be^{-kx}}$

62.

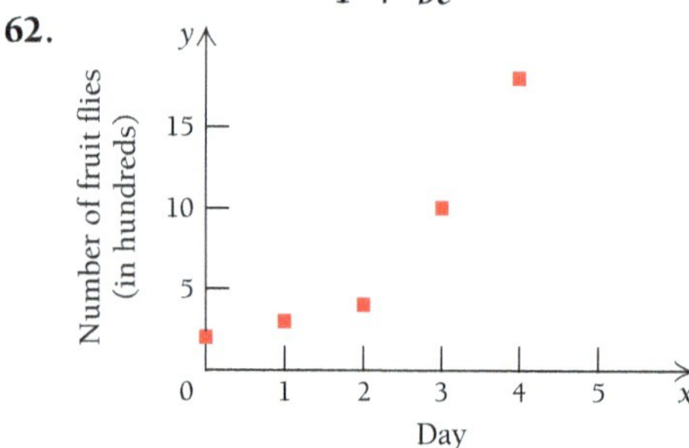

63.

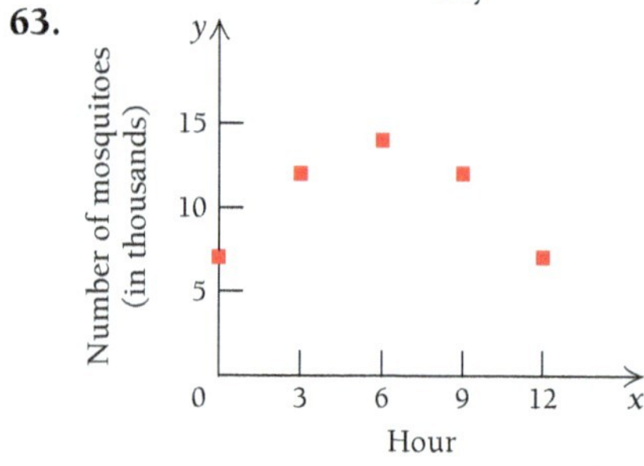

64. 65.

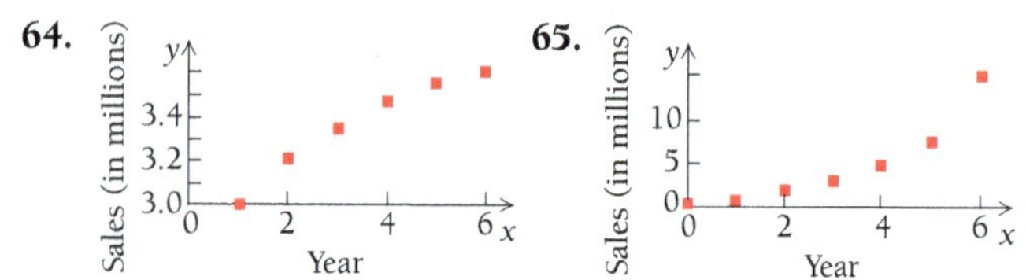

66.

67.

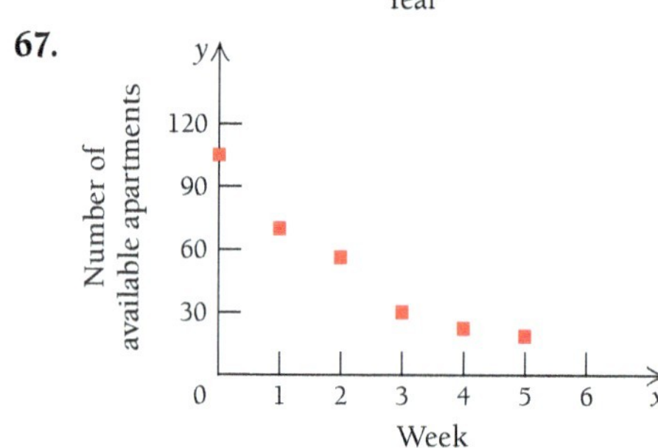

68. 69.

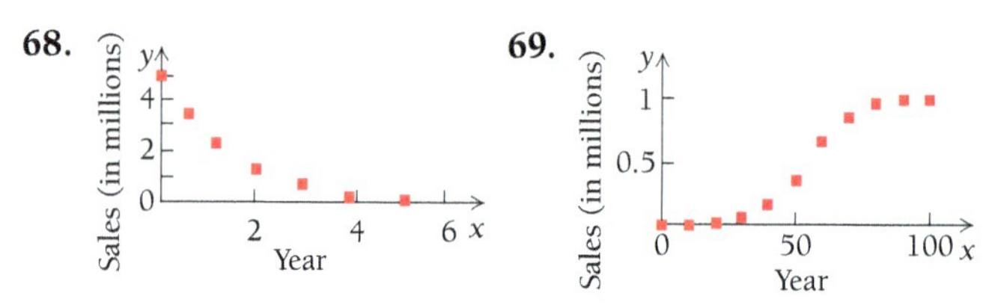

70. 71.

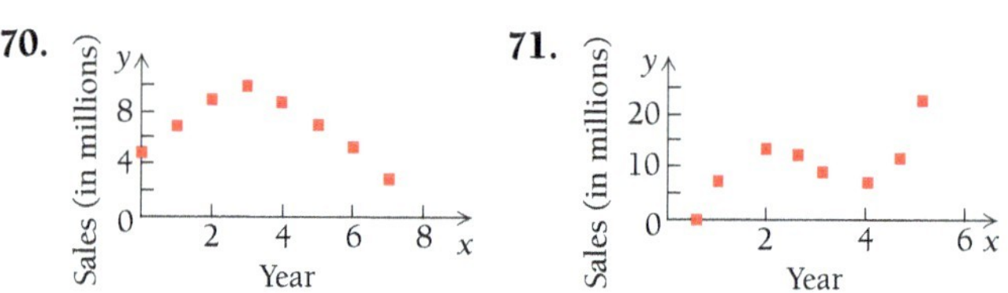

SYNTHESIS

72. A sample of an element lost 25% of its mass in 5 weeks.

a) Find the half-life.
b) After how many weeks will the sample have lost 75% of its mass?

73. A vehicle lost 15% of its value in 1 yr.

a) Find the half-life.
b) After how many years will the vehicle be worth 40% of its original value?

The Beer–Lambert Law. *A beam of light enters a medium such as water or smoky air with initial intensity I_0. Its intensity is decreased depending on the thickness (or concentration) of the medium. The intensity I at a depth (or concentration) of x units is given by*

$$I = I_0e^{-\mu x}.$$

The constant μ ("mu"), called the coefficient of absorption, varies with the medium. Use this law for Exercises 74 and 75.

74. **Light through smog.** Concentrations of particulates in the air due to pollution reduce sunlight. In a smoggy area, $\mu = 0.01$ and x is the concentration of particulates measured in micrograms per cubic meter (mcg/m^3). What change is more significant—dropping pollution levels from 100 mcg/m^3 to 90 mcg/m^3 or dropping them from 60 mcg/m^3 to 50 mcg/m^3? Why?

75. Light through sea water. Sea water has $\mu = 1.4$ and x is measured in meters. What would increase cloudiness more—dropping x from 2 m to 5 m or dropping x from 7 m to 10 m? Explain.

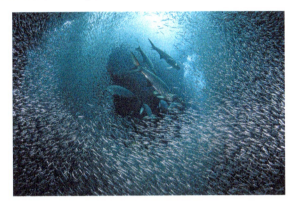

76. Newton's Law of Cooling. Consider the following exploratory situation. Fill a glass with hot tap water. Place a thermometer in the glass and measure the temperature. Check the temperature every 30 min thereafter. Plot your data on this graph, and connect the points with a smooth curve.

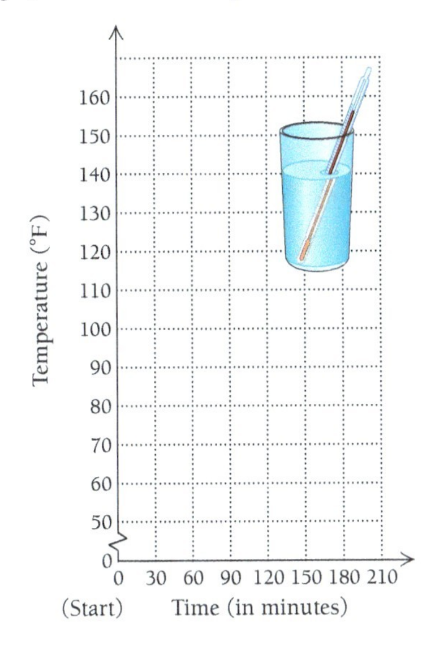

a) What was the temperature of the water when you began?
b) At what temperature does there seem to be a leveling off of the graph?
c) What is the difference between your answers to parts (a) and (b)?
d) How does the water temperature in part (b) compare with the room temperature?
e) Find an equation that fits the data. Use this equation to check values of other data points. How do they compare?
f) Is it ever "theoretically" possible for the temperature of the water to be the same as the room temperature? Explain.
g) Find the rate of change of the water temperature, and interpret its meaning.

77. An interest rate decreases from 8% to 7.2%. Explain why this increases the present value of an amount due 10 yr later.

78. The city of Rayburn loses half its population every 12 yr.
a) Explain why Rayburn's population will not be zero after 2 half-lives, or 24 yr.
b) What percentage of the original population remains after 2 half-lives?
c) What percentage of the original population remains after 4 half-lives?

Answers to Quick Checks

1. (a) $N(t) = N_0e^{-0.14t}$; (b) 246.6 g; (c) -34.52 g per day; (d) 4.95 days **2.** (a) 30.1 yr; (b) 5.3% per day **3.** About 7574 yr **4.** \$3011.94 **5.** 11.7 min **6.** $t = -2.2$ hr, so the time of death was about 2 hr and 12 min before the coroner arrived, at about 11:48 p.m. on the previous day.

2.6 The Derivatives of a^x and $\log_a x$

- Differentiate functions involving a^x.
- Differentiate functions involving $\log_a x$.

Using Bases Other than 10 or *e*

In many applications involving exponential growth or decay, bases other than 10 or e can be used. For example, in situations where a doubling time or tripling time is known, an exponential function in base 2 or base 3 can be used.

Suppose a sample of bacteria in a petri dish doubles in population every 7 hr. That means that in 7 hr an initial population of P_0 grows to $2P_0$, and in 14 hr the original population, P_0, has quadrupled and is now $4P_0$, or $2^2 \cdot P_0$. At 21 hr, the population after 14 hr has doubled, meaning that the population is now $8P_0$, or $2^3 \cdot P_0$. Generalizing, if a population or quantity doubles in T units of time, then after t units of time, the original population has doubled t/T times. Using an exponential function with base 2 to model this growth, the population, $P(t)$, after t hours is given by

$$P(t) = P_0 \cdot 2^{kt}, \qquad \text{where} \qquad k = \frac{1}{T}.$$

This suggests the following.

Base-n Exponential Growth

If a quantity increases n-fold over a fixed period of time T, then the quantity $P(t)$ at time t is given by

$$P(t) = P_0 \cdot n^{t/T},$$

where P_0 is the initial quantity.

Here, increasing a quantity "2-fold" is the same as doubling the quantity, increasing a quantity "3-fold" is the same as tripling the quantity.

Note that base-n exponential growth can be expressed in an equivalent form in base e, where $n = e^{\ln n}$. Both forms have their advantages, as the following two examples illustrate.

EXAMPLE 1 **Business: Growth of an App.** The number of user accounts for a new photo-sharing app doubles every 3 months. Assume that there were 1000 user accounts when the app became available to the general public ($t = 0$).

a) Find an exponential function with base 2 that gives the number $P(t)$ of user accounts after t months.

b) Find an exponential function with base e that gives the number $P(t)$ of user accounts after t months.

c) What is the number of user accounts after 12 months? Which form of the exponential function is easier to use to find this information?

Solution

a) Using the form $P(t) = P_0 \cdot n^{t/T}$, we have $n = 2$ and a doubling time of $T = 3$ hr. Thus, the exponential function, base 2, that models the population $P(t)$ of user accounts after t hours is given by

$$P(t) = 1000 \cdot 2^{t/3}.$$

b) To write the exponential function in the form $P(t) = P_0 e^{kt}$, we rewrite the base 2 as $e^{\ln 2}$:

$$\begin{aligned} P(t) &= 1000 \cdot 2^{t/3} \\ &= 1000 \cdot (e^{\ln 2})^{t/3} && \text{Recalling that } n = e^{\ln n} \\ &= 1000 \cdot (e^{0.69315})^{t/3} && \text{Using a calculator} \\ &= 1000e^{0.23105t} && \text{Multiplying exponents and simplifying} \end{aligned}$$

c) To find the number of user accounts after 12 months, we can use either form of the function P:

$$P(12) = 1000 \cdot 2^{12/3} = 1000 \cdot 2^4 = 16{,}000.$$
$$P(12) = 1000e^{0.23105(12)} = 16{,}000.2 \approx 16{,}000.$$

The exponential function with base 2 is easier to use, since in 12 months the number of user accounts has doubled 4 times. In this case, a calculator is not necessary to calculate $1000 \cdot 2 \cdot 2 \cdot 2 \cdot 2 = 16{,}000$. 1 ✓

Quick Check 1 ✓

The population of Big Horn doubles every 18 yr. Its population was 2500.

a) Find an exponential function using base 2 that gives the population $P(t)$ of Big Horn after t years.

b) Find an equivalent exponential function using base e.

c) Without using a calculator, find Big Horn's population after 36 yr.

EXAMPLE 2 Irma invested \$15,000 in a high-yield hedge fund, and after 14 yr, her original investment has tripled. Find exponential functions using base 3 and base e that give the value A of her account after t years. What is the yearly percentage growth rate of her fund? Which exponential function is easier to use to find this information?

Solution Using base 3 ($n = 3$) and a tripling time of $T = 14$, we have

$$A(t) = 15{,}000 \cdot 3^{t/14}.$$

Quick Check 2 ✓

In 6 days, the number of memberships at a new online shopping portal quadrupled. Originally, there were 50 members. Assume exponential growth for the immediate future.

a) Find an exponential function with base 4 that gives the number of memberships, $M(t)$, after t days.

b) What is the daily percentage growth rate?

Quick Check 3 ✓

A stock is losing 30% of its value every 7 weeks.

a) Find an exponential function that gives the value $V(t)$ of the stock after t weeks.

b) Find the percentage of the value lost over 14 weeks.

In base e, this is equivalent to

$$\begin{aligned} A(t) &= 15{,}000 \cdot (e^{\ln 3})^{t/14} \\ &= 15{,}000(e^{1.0986})^{t/14} \\ &= 15{,}000e^{0.0785t}. \quad \text{Multiplying exponents and simplifying} \end{aligned}$$

Irma's hedge fund has a yearly percentage growth rate of 7.85%. Using the function with base e, we can read this value directly from the exponent. **2 ✓**

EXAMPLE 3 After its salt mine closed, Nackleville lost 15% of its population every 4 yr.

a) Find an exponential function that gives the population P of Nackleville after t years.

b) What percentage of the population has been lost after 8 yr?

Solution

a) Since 15% of the population is lost every 4 yr, we use the base $n = 1 - 0.15 = 0.85$ (see Section R.6) and $T = 4$. Thus, using P_0 to represent the population at the time of the mine's closing, a function that models the population of Nackleville after t years is given by

$$P(t) = P_0(0.85)^{t/4}.$$

b) After 8 yr, we have $P(8) = P_0(0.85)^{8/4} = P_0(0.85)^2 = 0.7225P_0$. This means that 72.25% of the original population remains. Thus, $1 - 0.7225 = 0.2775$, or 27.75% of the population has been lost. **3 ✓**

The Derivative of a^x

To find the derivative of a^x, for $a > 0$, $a \neq 1$, we first express a^x as a power of e, using the property $a = e^{\ln a}$. Thus,

$$a^x = e^{\ln a^x}. \tag{1}$$

Now, we differentiate both sides:

$$\begin{aligned} \frac{d}{dx}a^x &= \frac{d}{dx}e^{\ln a^x} \\ &= \frac{d}{dx}e^{(\ln a)x} && \text{Using the property } \ln b^c = c \ln b \\ &= e^{(\ln a)x} \cdot \ln a && \text{Differentiating and using the Chain Rule} \\ &= e^{\ln a^x} \cdot \ln a && \text{Using the property } c \ln b = \ln b^c \\ &= a^x \cdot \ln a. && \text{Using equation (1)} \end{aligned}$$

Thus, we have the following theorem.

THEOREM 12

$$\frac{d}{dx}a^x = (\ln a)a^x$$

As a special case, note that

$$\frac{d}{dx}e^x = e^x \cdot \ln e = e^x \cdot 1 = e^x.$$

We see that finding derivatives is simpler when using base e, since $\ln e = 1$.

EXAMPLE 4 Differentiate: **a)** $y = 2^x$; **b)** $y = (1.4)^x$; **c)** $f(x) = 3^{2x+1}$.

Solution

a) $\frac{d}{dx}2^x = (\ln 2)2^x$ Using Theorem 12

Quick Check 4 ✓

Differentiate:

a) $y = 5^x$;

b) $f(x) = 4^x$;

c) $y = 7^{x^2}$.

b) $\frac{d}{dx}(1.4)^x = (\ln 1.4)(1.4)^x$ Using Theorem 12

c) Since $f(x) = 3^{2x+1}$ is of the form $f(x) = 3^{g(x)}$, the Chain Rule applies:

$$f'(x) = (\ln 3)3^{2x+1} \cdot \frac{d}{dx}(2x + 1)$$
$$= \ln 3 \cdot 3^{2x+1} \cdot 2 = 2 \ln 3 \cdot 3^{2x+1}.$$

4 ✓

EXAMPLE 5 Irma invested \$15,000 in a high-yield hedge fund, and after 14 yr, her original investment has tripled. Find the rate at which the value of her account was growing, in dollars per year, at the start of the 5th year.

Solution In Example 2, we found that the value $A(t)$ of her account after t years is given by

$$A(t) = 15{,}000 \cdot 3^{t/14}.$$

Differentiating, we have

$$A'(t) = \frac{d}{dt}(A(t)) = \frac{d}{dt}(15{,}000 \cdot 3^{t/14})$$
$$= 15{,}000 \cdot (\ln 3) \cdot 3^{t/14} \cdot \frac{1}{14} \quad \text{Using the Chain Rule}$$
$$= 1177.08 \cdot 3^{t/14}. \quad \text{Using a calculator}$$

Thus,

$$A'(5) = 1177.08 \cdot 3^{5/14} \approx 1742.63.$$

At the start of the 5th year, Irma's account was growing at a rate of about \$1742.63 per year.

5 ✓

Quick Check 5 ✓

In 6 days, the number of memberships at a new online shopping portal quadrupled. Using the result from Quick Check 2, find the rate at which the number of memberships is changing on the 10th day.

In Example 5, we have two rates of growth. The value of Irma's account is growing by 7.85% per year (from Example 2), and this rate stays constant from year to year. However, the actual monetary value of her account, $A(t)$, is changing as a function of time, given by $A'(t) = 1177.08 \cdot 3^{t/14}$, where the units of $A'(t)$ are dollars per year.

The Derivative of $\log_a x$

Just as the derivative of a^x is expressed in terms of $\ln a$, so too is the derivative of $\log_a x$. To find this derivative, we first express $\log_a x$ in terms of $\ln a$ using the change-of-base formula (P6 of Theorem 4 in Section R.6):

$$\frac{d}{dx}\log_a x = \frac{d}{dx}\left(\frac{\log_e x}{\log_e a}\right) \quad \text{Using the change-of-base formula}$$
$$= \frac{d}{dx}\left(\frac{\ln x}{\ln a}\right)$$
$$= \frac{1}{\ln a} \cdot \frac{d}{dx}(\ln x) \quad \frac{1}{\ln a} \text{ is a constant.}$$
$$= \frac{1}{\ln a} \cdot \frac{1}{x}.$$

THEOREM 13

$$\frac{d}{dx}\log_a x = \frac{1}{\ln a} \cdot \frac{1}{x} = \frac{1}{x \ln a}$$

As a special case, note that

$$\frac{d}{dx}(\log_e x) = \frac{1}{\ln e} \cdot \frac{1}{x} = \frac{1}{x}.$$

Again, finding derivatives is simpler when using base e, since $\frac{1}{\ln e} = \frac{1}{1} = 1$.

EXAMPLE 6 Differentiate:

a) $y = \log_8 x$; **b)** $y = \log x$; **c)** $f(x) = \log_3 (x^2 + 1)$; **d)** $f(x) = x^3 \log_5 x$.

Solution

a) $\frac{d}{dx} \log_8 x = \frac{1}{\ln 8} \cdot \frac{1}{x}$ Using Theorem 13

$= \frac{1}{x \ln 8}$ Simplifying

b) $\frac{d}{dx} \log x = \frac{1}{\ln 10} \cdot \frac{1}{x}$

$= \frac{1}{x \ln 10}$

c) Note that $f(x) = \log_3 (x^2 + 1)$ is of the form $f(x) = \log_3 (g(x))$, so the Chain Rule is required:

$$f'(x) = \frac{1}{\ln 3} \cdot \frac{1}{x^2 + 1} \cdot \frac{d}{dx}(x^2 + 1) \quad \text{Using the Chain Rule}$$

$$= \frac{1}{\ln 3} \cdot \frac{1}{x^2 + 1} \cdot 2x$$

$$= \frac{2x}{(\ln 3)(x^2 + 1)}.$$

d) Since $f(x) = x^3 \log_5 x$ is of the form $f(x) = g(x) \cdot h(x)$, we use the Product Rule:

$$f'(x) = x^3 \cdot \frac{d}{dx} \log_5 x + \log_5 x \cdot \frac{d}{dx} x^3 \quad \text{Using the Product Rule}$$

$$= x^3 \cdot \frac{1}{\ln 5} \cdot \frac{1}{x} + \log_5 x \cdot 3x^2 \quad \text{Differentiating}$$

$$= \frac{x^2}{\ln 5} + 3x^2 \log_5 x.$$

6 ✓

Quick Check 6 ✓

Differentiate:

a) $y = \log_2 x$;

b) $f(x) = -7 \log x$;

c) $g(x) = x^6 \log x$;

d) $y = \log_8 (x^3 - 7)$.

As the input variable increases, functions of the form $y = a^x$, where $a > 1$, increase more and more quickly. Conversely, logarithmic growth can be very slow. As the input variable increases, functions of the form $y = \log_a x$, where $a > 1$, increase, but more and more slowly, since $\lim_{x \to \infty} \frac{1}{x \cdot \ln a} = 0$.

Section Summary

- If a quantity increases n-fold over a fixed time period T, then the exponential function that gives the quantity, $P(t)$, at time t is given by $P(t) = P_0 \cdot n^{t/T}$, where $P_0 = P(0)$ is the initial quantity.
- The derivative of the general exponential function $f(x) = a^x$ is $f'(x) = (\ln a)a^x$.
- The derivative of the general logarithmic function $f(x) = \log_a x$ is $f'(x) = \frac{1}{\ln a} \cdot \frac{1}{x} = \frac{1}{x \ln a}$.

2.6 Exercise Set

In Exercises 1–12, find an exponential function of the form $P(t) = P_0 n^{t/T}$ that models the situation, and then find the equivalent exponential model of the form $P(t) = P_0 e^{rt}$.

1. Doubling time of 5 yr, initial population of 450
2. Doubling time of 25 weeks, initial population of 1300
3. Tripling time of 8 months, initial population of 5000
4. Tripling time of 9 hr, initial population of 6
5. Grows 7-fold in 12 yr, initial population of 100
6. Grows 5-fold in 20 months, initial population of 35,000
7. Decreases by 10% every 2 months, initial population of 1200
8. Decreases by 25% every 36 hr, initial population of 100,000
9. Decreases by 40% every 8 weeks, initial population of 60,000
10. Decreases by 7.5% every 9 yr, initial population of 25,000
11. Increases by 50% every 6 months, initial population of 6500
12. Increases by 125% every 2 yr, initial population of 75

Differentiate.

13. $y = 6^x$
14. $y = 7^x$
15. $g(t) = 15^t$
16. $g(t) = 20^t$
17. $y = 12.5^x$
18. $y = \left(\frac{3}{4}\right)^x$
19. $f(x) = 3 \cdot 5^x$
20. $f(x) = 24 \cdot 9^x$
21. $y = 7^{x^4+2}$
22. $y = 4^{x^2+5}$
23. $f(t) = 100 \cdot (0.52)^t$
24. $f(t) = 3500 \cdot (0.038)^t$
25. $y = \log_6 x$
26. $y = \log_{13} x$
27. $y = 3 \log_4 x$
28. $y = 7 \log_{11} x$
29. $f(x) = \log_2 (3x - 1)$
30. $f(x) = \log_3 (5 - 4x)$
31. $y = 5 \log_6 (x^2 + x)$
32. $y = 8 \log_3 (2x - x^3)$
33. $y = 4^x \cdot \log_5 x$
34. $y = 7^x \cdot \log_{12} x$
35. $f(x) = x^2 \cdot 3^x$
36. $f(x) = 2x^4 \cdot 5^x$
37. $g(x) = x^3 \log_7 x$
38. $g(x) = x^6 \log_4 x$
39. $y = \dfrac{9^x}{2x + 1}$
40. $y = \dfrac{3x + 2}{\log_6 x}$

APPLICATIONS

General Interest

41. The population of Nilam doubles in size every 9 yr. In 1990, its population was 10,000.
   a) Find an exponential function of the form $P(t) = P_0 n^{t/T}$ that models Nilam's population after t years.
   b) Find the equivalent exponential model of the form $P(t) = P_0 e^{rt}$.
   c) What is Nilam's yearly percentage growth rate?
   d) Without using a calculator, find Nilam's population in 2017.
   e) How fast was Nilam's population changing in 2008?
42. Justin's investment of $5000 doubles in size every 8 yr.
   a) Find an exponential function of the form $A(t) = A_0 n^{t/T}$ that models the value of Justin's account after t years.
   b) Find the equivalent exponential model of the form $A(t) = A_0 e^{rt}$.
   c) What is the account's yearly percentage growth rate?
   d) Without using a calculator, find the value of Justin's account after 16 yr.
   e) How fast is the value of Justin's account changing after 24 yr?
43. Beth originally had 50 followers of her blog. After she published her memoir, the number of followers tripled every 7 months.
   a) Find an exponential function of the form $F(t) = F_0 n^{t/T}$ that models the number of followers of Beth's blog after t months.
   b) Find the equivalent exponential model of the form $F(t) = F_0 e^{rt}$.
   c) What is the monthly percentage growth rate of the number of followers?
   d) Without using a calculator, find the number of followers of Beth's blog after 14 months.
   e) How fast is the number of followers changing after 21 months?
44. A strain of bacteria is grown in a laboratory. The original sample had a mass of 0.005 mg. The population quintuples every 36 hr.
   a) Find an exponential function of the form $M(t) = M_0 n^{t/T}$ that models the mass of the bacteria after t hours.
   b) Find the equivalent exponential model of the form $M(t) = M_0 e^{rt}$.
   c) What is the hourly percentage growth rate of the bacteria?
   d) Without using a calculator, find the mass of the bacteria after 72 hr.
   e) How fast is the mass changing after 108 hr?
45. A stock originally valued at $100 per share is losing 50% of its value every 5 days.
   a) Find an exponential function of the form $V(t) = V_0 n^{t/T}$ that models the value of a share of the stock after t days.
   b) Find the equivalent exponential model of the form $V(t) = V_0 e^{rt}$.
   c) What is the hourly percentage decay rate of the value of a share?
   d) Without using a calculator, find the value of a share of the stock after 15 days.
   e) How fast is the value changing after 10 days?

46. A 50-g mass of a radioactive substance is losing 20% of its mass every 2 weeks.
   a) Find an exponential function of the form $M(t) = M_0 n^{t/T}$ that models the mass of the substance after t weeks.
   b) Find the equivalent exponential model of the form $M(t) = M_0 e^{rt}$.
   c) What is the weekly percentage decay rate of the mass?
   d) Without using a calculator, find the mass of the substance after 4 weeks.
   e) How fast is the mass changing after 6 weeks?

47. Greta deposited \$50,000 in a savings account that increased in value by 20% every 4 yr.
   a) Find an exponential function of the form $A(t) = A_0 n^{t/T}$ that models the value of Greta's account after t years.
   b) Find $A(8)$, and explain its meaning.
   c) Find $A'(8)$, and explain its meaning.

48. Suppose that the value of a rare autograph increases by 35% every 10 yr, and the autograph was worth \$2500 in 2000.
   a) Find an exponential function of the form $V(t) = V_0 n^{t/T}$ that models the value of the autograph after t years.
   b) Find $V(20)$, and explain its meaning.
   c) Find $V'(20)$, and explain its meaning.

Business and Economics

49. **Double declining balance depreciation.** An office machine is purchased for \$5200. Assume that its salvage value, V, in dollars, depreciates, according to a method called *double declining balance*, by 20% each year and is given by

$$V(t) = 5200(0.80)^t,$$

where t is the time, in years, after purchase.
   a) Find $V(5)$, and explain its meaning.
   b) Find $V'(5)$, and explain its meaning.
   c) When will the salvage value of the office machine be half of the purchase price?

50. **Recycling aluminum cans.** It is known that 49.4% of all aluminum cans distributed are recycled each year. A beverage company uses 250,000 lb of aluminum cans. After recycling, the amount of aluminum, in pounds, still in use after t years is given by

$$N(t) = 250{,}000(0.494)^t.$$

(*Source:* aluminum.org, 2017.)
   a) Find $N(3)$, and explain its meaning.
   b) Find $N'(3)$, and explain its meaning.
   c) When will 10% of the original amount of aluminum still be in use?

51. **Recycling glass.** In 2012, 34.1% of all glass containers were recycled. A beverage company used 400,000 lb of glass containers per year. After recycling, the amount of glass, in pounds, still in use after t years is given by

$$N(t) = 400{,}000(0.341)^t.$$

(*Source:* www.gpi.org.)
   a) Find $N(4)$, and explain its meaning.
   b) Find $N'(4)$, and explain its meaning.
   c) When will 5% of the original amount of glass still be in use?

52. **Agriculture.** Farmers wishing to avoid the use of nonheirloom seeds are increasingly concerned about inadvertently growing nonheirloom plants as a result of pollen drifting from nearby farms. Assuming that these farmers raise their own seeds, the fractional portion of their crop that remains free of nonheirloom plants t years later can be approximated by

$$P(t) = (0.98)^t.$$

   a) Using this model, predict the fractional portion of the crop that will be nonheirloom 10 yr after a neighboring farm begins to use nonheirloom seeds.
   b) Find $P'(10)$, and explain its meaning.
   c) When will half of the crop be nonheirloom plants?

Physical Sciences

53. **Earthquake intensity.** The intensity of an earthquake is given by

$$I(R) = I_0 10^R,$$

where R is the magnitude on the Richter scale and I_0 is the minimum intensity, at which $R = 0$, used for comparison.
   a) Find I, in terms of I_0, for an earthquake of magnitude 7 on the Richter scale.
   b) Find I, in terms of I_0, for an earthquake of magnitude 8 on the Richter scale.
   c) Compare your answers to parts (a) and (b).
   d) Find the rate of change dI/dR.
   e) Interpret the meaning of dI/dR.

54. **Intensity of sound.** The intensity of a sound is given by

$$I(L) = I_0 10^{0.1L},$$

where L is the loudness of the sound measured in decibels and I_0 is the minimum intensity detectable by the human ear.
   a) Find I, in terms of I_0, for the loudness of a power mower, which is 100 decibels.
   b) Find I, in terms of I_0, for the loudness of a barely audible sound, which is 10 decibels.
   c) Compare your answers to parts (a) and (b).
   d) Find the rate of change dI/dL.
   e) Interpret the meaning of dI/dL.

55. **Earthquake magnitude.** The magnitude R (measured on the Richter scale) of an earthquake of intensity I is defined as

$$R = \log \frac{I}{I_0},$$

where I_0 is the minimum intensity (used for comparison).
   a) Find the rate of change dR/dI.
   b) Interpret the meaning of dR/dI.

56. Loudness of sound. The loudness L of a sound of intensity I is defined as

$$L = 10 \log \frac{I}{I_0},$$

where I_0 is the minimum intensity detectable by the human ear and L is the loudness measured in decibels.

a) Find the rate of change dL/dI.
b) Interpret the meaning of dL/dI.

SYNTHESIS

57. Population growth. Suppose $P(t) = 35{,}000e^{0.0427t}$ gives the population, $P(t)$, of Perryville t years after the last census.

a) Rewrite the function in the form $P(t) = 35{,}000 \cdot 2^{t/T}$.
b) Rewrite the function in the form $P(t) = 35{,}000 \cdot 4^{t/T}$.
c) How do the two T values in parts (a) and (b) compare?
d) Without using a calculator, find T if the model is written as $P(t) = 35{,}000 \cdot 8^{t/T}$.

58. Radioactive decay. Suppose $M(t) = 25e^{-0.109t}$ gives the mass, $M(t)$, of a sample of a radioactive substance t hours after observation started.

a) Rewrite the function in the form $M(t) = 25 \cdot \left(\frac{1}{2}\right)^{t/T}$.
b) Rewrite the function in the form $M(t) = 25 \cdot \left(\frac{1}{4}\right)^{t/T}$.
c) How do the two T values in parts (a) and (b) compare?
d) Without using a calculator, find T if the model is written as $M(t) = 25 \cdot \left(\frac{1}{8}\right)^{t/T}$.

59. Population decay. Suppose $P(t) = 100{,}000e^{-0.033t}$ gives the population, $P(t)$, of a city t years after its principal industry shuts down.

a) Rewrite the function in the form $P(t) = 100{,}000 \cdot \left(\frac{1}{3}\right)^{t/T}$.
b) Rewrite the function in the form $P(t) = 100{,}000 \cdot \left(\frac{1}{9}\right)^{t/T}$.
c) How do the two T values in parts (a) and (b) compare?
d) Without using a calculator, find T if the model is written as $P(t) = 100{,}000 \cdot \left(\frac{1}{27}\right)^{t/T}$.

60. Growth of an investment. Suppose $A(t) = 2500e^{0.0255t}$ gives the amount, $A(t)$, in Jerry's account t years after his original investment.

a) Rewrite the function in the form $P(t) = 2500 \cdot 3^{t/T}$.
b) Rewrite the function in the form $P(t) = 2500 \cdot 9^{t/T}$.
c) How do the two T values in parts (a) and (b) compare?
d) Without using a calculator, find T if the model is written as $P(t) = 2500 \cdot 27^{t/T}$.

61. A population P_0 doubles every 5 yr.

a) Find the tripling time of this population.
b) Find the percent increase of the population after two tripling periods.

62. A population P_0 triples every 7 months.

a) Find the doubling time of this population.
b) Find the percent increase of the population after two doubling periods.

63. The original mass M_0 of a sample of a radioactive substance decreases by a third in 22 hr.

a) Find the substance's half-life.
b) Find the percentage of the original mass that has decayed after two half-life periods.

64. The half-life of a radioactive substance is 6.2 yr.

a) Find the time needed for a sample of the substance to lose 20% of its original mass.
b) Find the percentage of the original mass still present after two periods of time of the length found in part (a).

Differentiating $f(x) = a^x$ using the definition of the derivative, we have

$$\frac{d}{dx}a^x = \lim_{h\to 0}\frac{a^{x+h} - a^x}{h} = \lim_{h\to 0}\frac{a^x a^h - a^x}{h}$$
$$= a^x \cdot \lim_{h\to 0}\frac{a^h - 1}{h}.$$

In this section, we showed that $\frac{d}{dx}a^x = (\ln a)a^x$.

65. What is $\lim_{h\to 0}\frac{a^h - 1}{h}$?

66. Find $\lim_{h\to 0}\frac{3^h - 1}{h}$ without using a calculator.

67. Find $\lim_{h\to 0}\frac{7^h - 1}{h}$ without using a calculator.

68. Find $\lim_{h\to 0}\frac{e^h - 1}{h}$ without using a calculator.

Answers to Quick Checks

1. (a) $P(t) = 2500 \cdot 2^{t/18}$; **(b)** $P(t) = 2500e^{0.03851t}$; **(c)** $2500 \cdot 2 \cdot 2 = 10{,}000$ people
2. (a) $M(t) = 50 \cdot 4^{t/6}$; **(b)** $\frac{\ln 4}{6} \approx 0.231$, or about 23.1% per day **3. (a)** $V(t) = V_0(0.7)^{t/7}$; **(b)** 51%
4. (a) $(\ln 5)5^x$; **(b)** $(\ln 4)4^x$; **(c)** $(\ln 7)(7^{x^2})(2x)$
5. About 116 memberships per day **6. (a)** $\frac{1}{x \ln 2}$;
(b) $-\frac{7}{x \ln 10}$; **(c)** $\frac{x^5}{\ln 10} + 6x^5 \log x$
(d) $\frac{3x^2}{(\ln 8)(x^3 - 7)}$

Chapter 2 Summary

KEY TERMS AND CONCEPTS	EXAMPLES
SECTION 2.1	
The **natural base**, denoted e, is defined by $e = \lim_{n\to\infty}\left(1 + \frac{1}{n}\right)^n = 2.71828182845\ldots$. *Continuous exponential growth:* With continuous compounding at an annual interest rate r, expressed as a percentage, a quantity P has a future value after t years given by $A = Pe^{rt}$. The function given by $y = Pe^{rt}$, where $P > 0$, is increasing for $r > 0$ and decreasing for $r < 0$ and has the y-intercept $(0, P)$. The domain is the set of all real numbers, $\{x \mid -\infty < x < \infty\}$, and the range is $\{y \mid y > 0\}$.	Kadi deposits \$25,000 in a savings account that earns 2.5% annual interest. • The amount in her account after t years is given by $A(t) = 25{,}000e^{0.025t}$. • The future value of her account after 6 yr is given by $A(6) = 25{,}000e^{0.025(6)} = \$29{,}045.86$.
For any positive number x, the logarithm, base e, of x, called the **natural logarithm**, is given by $\ln x = \log_e x$. The equation $y = \ln x$ is equivalent to $e^y = x$.	Using a calculator and rounding, $\ln 9 \approx 2.19722$. **Check:** Note that $e^{2.19722} \approx 9$.
The function given by $f(x) = \ln x$ has the domain $\{x \mid 0 < x < \infty\}$, the range $\{y \mid -\infty < y < \infty\}$, the x-intercept $(1, 0)$, and no y-intercept.	Consider $g(x) = \ln(2x + 5)$. • To assure that $2x + 5 > 0$, it follows that $x > -\frac{5}{2}$. Thus, the domain of g is $\{x \mid -\frac{5}{2} < x < \infty\}$. • For $x = 0$, it follows that $g(0) = \ln(2(0) + 5) = \ln 5 \approx 1.609$. Thus, the y-intercept is $(0, 1.609)$. • For $y = 0$, it is possible to solve for x: $0 = \ln(2x + 5)$; $e^0 = 2x + 5$ (Using Property P8 of natural logarithms); $x = -2$. (Solving for x) • Thus, the x-intercept is $(-2, 0)$. • The range of g is $\{y \mid -\infty < y < \infty\}$.
Properties of natural logarithms: **P1.** $\ln(MN) = \ln M + \ln N$ **P2.** $\ln\left(\frac{M}{N}\right) = \ln M - \ln N$ **P3.** $\ln M^k = k \cdot \ln M$ **P4.** $\ln e = 1$ **P5.** $\ln 1 = 0$ *(continued)*	Given $\ln 5 = 1.609$ and $\ln 7 = 1.946$, we can evaluate the following expressions: • $\ln 35 = \ln(5 \cdot 7)$ $= \ln 5 + \ln 7$ (Using Property P1) $= 1.609 + 1.946$ $= 3.555$

KEY TERMS AND CONCEPTS / EXAMPLES

SECTION 2.1 (*continued*)

P6. $\log_b M = \dfrac{\ln M}{\ln b}$ and $\ln M = \dfrac{\log M}{\log e}$

P7. $\ln e^x = x$, for all real numbers x

P8. $e^{\ln x} = x$, for all $x > 0$

- $\ln 25 = \ln 5^2$
  $= 2 \ln 5$ Using Property P3
  $= 2(1.609)$
  $= 3.218$

Logarithms can be used to solve certain exponential equations.

Solve: $5e^{2t} = 80$.

We have

$$\begin{aligned} 5e^{2t} &= 80 \\ e^{2t} &= 16 && \text{Dividing both sides by 5} \\ \ln e^{2t} &= \ln 16 && \text{Finding the natural logarithm of both sides} \\ 2t &= \ln 16 && \text{Using Property P7} \\ t &= \frac{\ln 16}{2} \\ t &\approx 1.386. \end{aligned}$$

The **exponential growth rate** r and the **doubling time** T are related by $rT = \ln 2$; thus, $T = \dfrac{\ln 2}{r}$ and $r = \dfrac{\ln 2}{T}$.

Kadi deposits $25,000 in a savings account that earns interest at an annual rate of 2.5%, compounded continuously. The time needed for the value of her account to double is

$$T = \frac{\ln 2}{0.025} = 27.7 \text{ yr}.$$

SECTION 2.2

The derivative of the function given by $y = e^x$ is the function itself:

$$y' = \frac{dy}{dx} = \frac{d}{dx}e^x = e^x.$$

More generally, for $y = e^{f(x)}$, it follows that

$$y' = \frac{dy}{dx} = e^{f(x)} \cdot f'(x).$$

- $\dfrac{d}{dx}e^{2x^3+x} = e^{2x^3+x} \cdot \dfrac{d}{dx}(2x^3 + x)$ Using the Chain Rule
  $= e^{2x^3+x} \cdot (6x^2 + 1)$
- $\dfrac{d}{dx}(xe^{3x}) = x \cdot \dfrac{d}{dx}e^{3x} + e^{3x} \cdot \dfrac{d}{dx}x$ Using the Product Rule
  $= x \cdot 3e^{3x} + e^{3x} \cdot 1$
  $= e^{3x}(3x + 1)$

SECTION 2.3

The derivative of the natural logarithm of x is the reciprocal of x:

$$\frac{d}{dx}\ln x = \frac{1}{x}, \text{ for } x > 0, \text{ and}$$

$$\frac{d}{dx}\ln|x| = \frac{1}{x}, \text{ for } x \neq 0.$$

The derivative of $y = \ln f(x)$ is

$$\frac{d}{dx}\ln f(x) = \frac{f'(x)}{f(x)}.$$

- $\dfrac{d}{dx}[\ln(x^2 + 8)] = \dfrac{1}{x^2 + 8} \cdot 2x = \dfrac{2x}{x^2 + 8}$
- $\dfrac{d}{dx}[\ln(5x) \cdot (x^3 - 7x)]$
  $= \ln(5x) \cdot \dfrac{d}{dx}(x^3 - 7x) + (x^3 - 7x) \cdot \dfrac{d}{dx}[\ln(5x)]$ Using the Product Rule
  $= \ln(5x) \cdot (3x^2 - 7) + (x^3 - 7x) \cdot \dfrac{1}{5x} \cdot 5$
  $= (3x^2 - 7)\ln(5x) + x^2 - 7$ Simplifying

KEY TERMS AND CONCEPTS	EXAMPLES
SECTION 2.4	

Because exponential functions have the property that the derivative (rate of change) is directly proportional to the function value for any input value, these functions can model many real-world situations involving uninhibited growth.

If $\frac{dP}{dt} = kP$, with $k > 0$, then $P(t) = P_0e^{kt}$, where P_0 is the initial quantity at $t = 0$.

Business. The balance P in an account with Turing Mutual Funds grows at a rate given by

$$\frac{dP}{dt} = 0.04P,$$

where t is time, in years. Find the function that satisfies the equation if the initial investment, P_0, is $25,000.

The function is given by

$$P = 25{,}000e^{0.04t}.$$

Check: $\frac{d}{dt}25{,}000e^{0.04t} = 25{,}000e^{0.04t} \cdot 0.04$ Using the Chain Rule

$= 0.04 \cdot 25{,}000e^{0.04t}$

$= 0.04P$

Two models for restricted growth are

$$P(t) = \frac{L}{1 + Ce^{-Lkt}},$$

called the **logistic function**, and

$$P(t) = L + Ce^{-kt},$$

called the **limited growth function.** For both models, $k > 0$ and the limiting value $L > 0$.

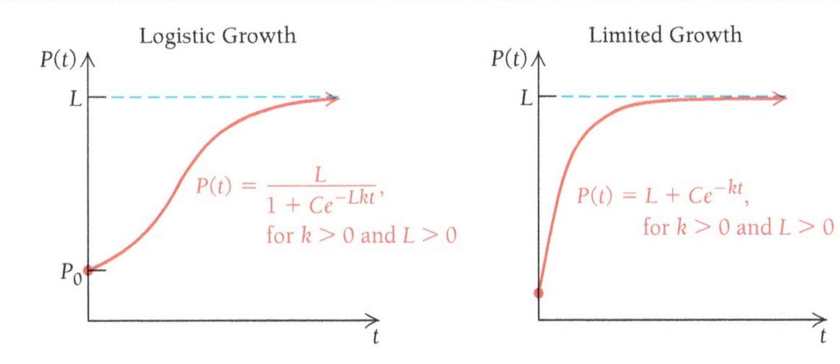

SECTION 2.5	

Exponential growth is modeled by $P(t) = P_0e^{kt}$, $k > 0$, and **exponential decay** is modeled by $P(t) = P_0e^{-kt}$, $k > 0$.

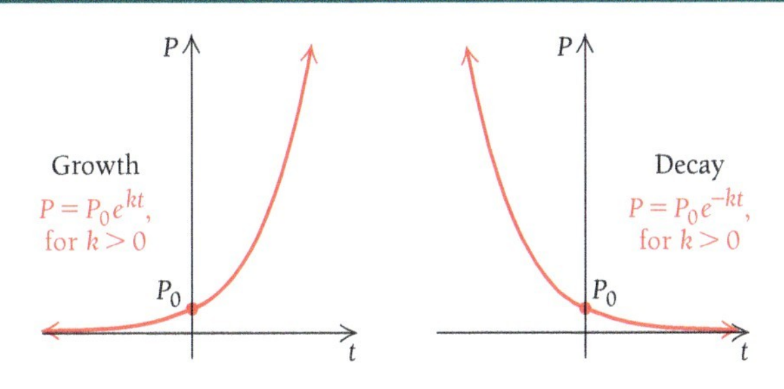

Exponential decay characterizes many real-world phenomena. One of the most common is *radioactive decay*.

Physical Science. Lead-210 has a decay rate of 3.15% per year. The rate of change of an amount N of lead-210 is given by

$$\frac{dN}{dt} = -0.0315N.$$

Find the function that satisfies the equation. How much of an 80-g sample of lead-210 remains after 20 yr? How quickly is the sample decaying after 20 yr?

The function is given by $N(t) = N_0e^{-0.0315t}$.

Check: $\frac{d}{dt}(N_0e^{-0.0315t}) = N_0e^{-0.0315t}(-0.0315)$

$= -0.0315 \cdot N(t)$

KEY TERMS AND CONCEPTS	EXAMPLES
SECTION 2.5 (*continued*)	
	The amount of an 80-g sample remaining after 20 yr is $N(20) = 80e^{-0.0315(20)} \approx 42.6$ g. Since $N'(t) = -0.0315N(t)$, the rate of change in the amount of lead-210 in the sample after 20 yr is $N'(20) = -0.0315 \cdot 80e^{-0.0315(20)} = -1.3421$ g/yr.
Half-life, T, and **decay rate**, k, are related by $k = \frac{\ln 2}{T}$ and $T = \frac{\ln 2}{k}$.	The half-life of a radioactive isotope is 38 days. The decay rate is $T = \frac{\ln 2}{38} \approx 0.0182 = 1.82\%$ per day. If N_0 represents the original amount of the isotope, then the amount $A(t)$ present after t days is given by the function $A(t) = N_0 e^{-0.0182t}$.
The **present value** P_0 of an amount P due t years later, at interest rate k, compounded continuously, is given by $P_0 = Pe^{-kt}$.	The present value of \$200,000 due 8 yr from now, at an annual interest rate of 4.6%, compounded continuously, is given by $P_0 = Pe^{-kt} = 200{,}000e^{-0.046 \cdot 8} = \$138{,}423.44$. This means that one would have to deposit \$138,423.44 now, at an annual interest rate of 4.6%, compounded continuously, to achieve a value of \$200,000 in 8 yr.
SECTION 2.6	
If a quantity increases n-fold over a fixed period of time T, then the quantity $P(t)$ at time t is given by the exponential function $P(t) = P_0 \cdot n^{t/T}$, where P_0 is the initial quantity.	The value of Beverley's mountain cottage doubles every 9 yr. She originally paid \$75,000 for the cottage. The value, $A(t)$, of the cottage after t years is given by $A(t) = 75{,}000 \cdot 2^{t/9}$. Using Property P8 of natural logarithms, we have $2 = e^{\ln 2}$. Thus, $A(t) = 75{,}000(e^{\ln 2})^{t/9}$. Since $\frac{1}{9}\ln 2 \approx 0.077$, the function A can be written in base e as follows: $A(t) = 75{,}000e^{0.077t}$. Beverley's cottage is increasing in value at a rate of approximately 7.7% per year.
If $y = a^x$, then $\frac{dy}{dx} = (\ln a)a^x$.	• $\frac{d}{dx}(7^x) = (\ln 7)7^x$ • $\frac{d}{dx}(3^{x^2+5x}) = (\ln 3)3^{x^2+5x}(2x + 5)$ Using the Chain Rule
If $y = \log_a x$, then $\frac{dy}{dx} = \frac{1}{\ln a} \cdot \frac{1}{x} = \frac{1}{x \cdot \ln a}$.	• $\frac{d}{dx}(\log_{13} x) = \frac{1}{x \ln 13}$ • $\frac{d}{dx}(\log_6 (x^2 + 1)) = \frac{2x}{(x^2 + 1)\ln 6}$ Using the Chain Rule

Chapter 2 Review Exercises

These review exercises are for test preparation. They can also be used as a practice test. Answers are at the back of the book. The red bracketed section references tell you what part(s) of the chapter to restudy if your answer is incorrect.

CONCEPT REINFORCEMENT

In Exercises 1–6, match each equation in column A with the most appropriate graph in column B. [2.1–2.5]

Column A / **Column B**

1. $P(t) = 50e^{0.03t}$

a)

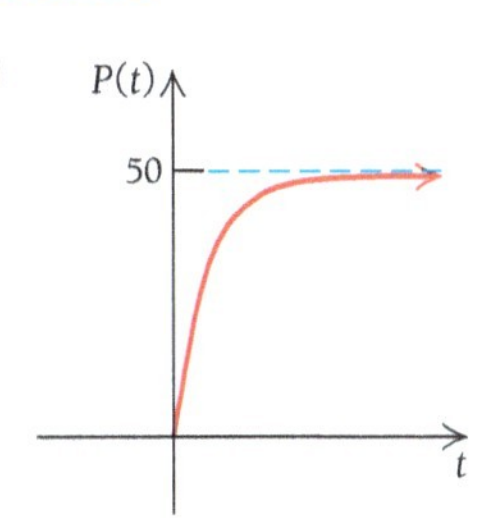

2. $P(t) = \dfrac{50}{1 + 2e^{-0.02t}}$

b)

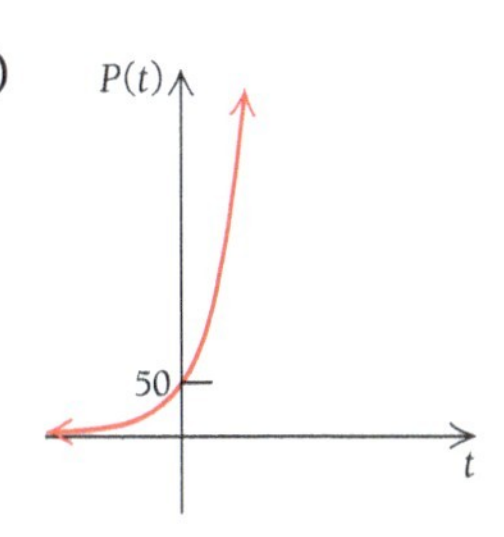

3. $P(t) = 50e^{-0.20t}$

c)

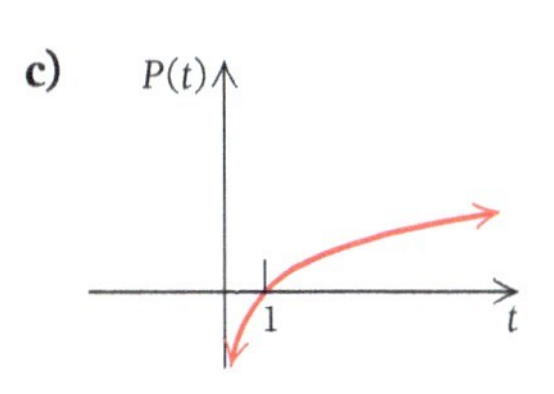

4. $P(t) = \ln t$

d)

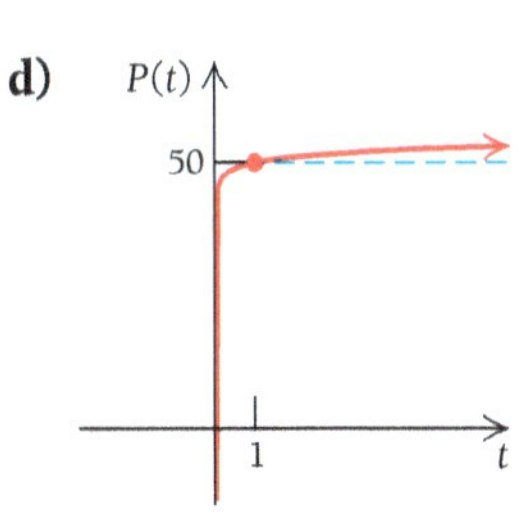

5. $P(t) = 50(1 - e^{-0.04t})$

e)

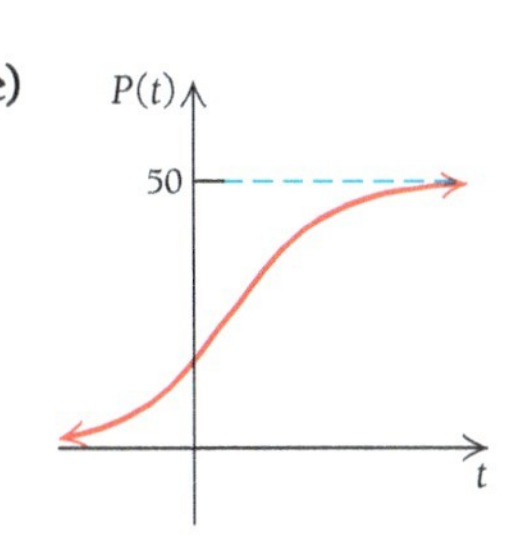

6. $P(t) = 50 + \ln t$

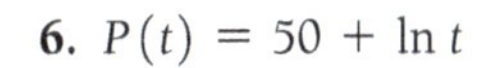

f)

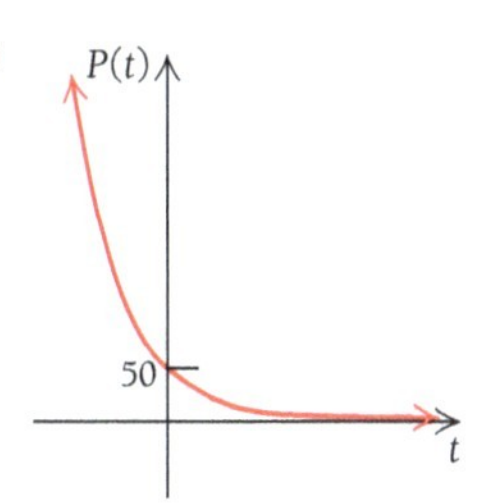

Classify each statement as either true or false.

7. The range of an exponential function of the form $y = Pe^{rt}$, for $P > 0$, is the set of all real numbers. [2.1]

8. Since $\ln(30) = \ln(6 \cdot 5)$, we have $\ln(30) = \ln(6) \cdot \ln(5)$. [2.1]

9. With exponential growth, the doubling time depends on the size of the original population. [2.1]

10. The derivative of $f(x) = e^{2x}$ is $f'(x) = e^{2x}$. [2.2]

11. If $f'(x) = c \cdot f(x)$ for $c \neq 0$ and $f(x) \neq 0$, then f must be an exponential function. [2.4]

12. A radioactive isotope's half-life can be used to determine the value of its decay constant. [2.5]

13. A radioactive isotope's half-life depends on how much of the isotope is initially present. [2.5]

14. For any exponential function of the form $f(x) = a^x$, it follows that $f'(x) = \ln a \cdot a^x$. [2.6]

15. For any logarithmic function of the form $g(x) = \log_a x$, it follows that $g'(x) = \dfrac{1}{a} \cdot \dfrac{1}{x}$. [2.6]

16. The function given by $f(t) = 50(5)^{t/2}$ models a population that doubles every 5 yr. [2.6]

REVIEW EXERCISES

Differentiate each function. [2.2], [2.3], [2.6]

17. $y = \ln x$

18. $y = e^x$

19. $y = \ln(x^4 + 5)$

20. $y = e^{2\sqrt{x}}$

21. $f(x) = \ln\sqrt{x}$

22. $f(x) = x^4 e^{3x}$

23. $f(x) = \dfrac{\ln x}{x^3}$

24. $f(x) = e^{x^2} \cdot \ln 4x$

25. $f(x) = e^{4x} - \ln \dfrac{x}{4}$

26. $y = \dfrac{\ln e^x}{e^x}$

27. $F(x) = 9^x$

28. $g(x) = \log_2 x$

29. $y = 3^x \cdot \log_4 (2x + 1)$

For Exercises 30 and 31, determine any x- or y-intercepts, state the domain and range, and then graph each function. [2.1]

30. $f(x) = e^{x-2}$

31. $g(x) = \ln(4 - 2x)$

Given $\ln 2 = 0.693$ *and* $\ln 7 = 1.946$, *find each logarithm.* [2.1]

32. $\ln 14$

33. $\ln \frac{2}{7}$

34. $\ln 28$

35. $\ln 3.5$

36. $\ln \sqrt{7}$

37. $\ln \frac{1}{4}$

38. Find the function Q that satisfies $dQ/dt = 7Q$, given that $Q = 25$ when $t = 0$. [2.4]

39. Life science: population growth. The population of Boomtown doubles every 16 yr. [2.1, 2.2, 2.4, 2.6]

a) Find r, the continuous yearly growth rate of the population of Boomtown.

b) Suppose that the population of Boomtown was 4000 in 2017 ($t = 0$). Find an exponential function that models Boomtown's population.

c) Estimate Boomtown's population in 2024.

d) Estimate the rate of change of Boomtown's population in 2024.

40. Business: interest compounded continuously. Suppose \$8300 is invested in Noether Bond Fund, for which the interest rate is 3.8%, compounded continuously. Find the rate of change, in dollars per year, of the value of the investment in 7 yr. [2.1, 2.4]

41. Business: price of a prime-rib dinner. Suppose the average price, C, of a prime-rib dinner was \$15.81 in 1986 and \$29.95 in 2017. Assume that the exponential growth model applies to price as a function of time, in years, since 1986. [2.4]

a) Find the exponential growth rate to three decimal places, and write the function that models the situation.

b) What will the price of a prime-rib dinner be in 2024?

c) Estimate the rate of change of the price of a prime-rib dinner in 2024.

42. Business: price of Oreo Cookies. The average price, C, of Oreo Cookies was \$2.69/lb in 1990 and \$3.00/lb in 2018. (*Source:* foodtimeline.org; walmart.org; target.org.) Assume that the exponential growth model applies. [2.4]

a) Find the exponential growth rate to four decimal places, and write the function that models the situation.

b) What will the price of 1 lb of Oreo Cookies be in 2030?

c) Estimate the rate of change of the price of 1 lb of Oreo Cookies in 2030.

43. Business: stock price. One share of Beskco stock was originally worth \$80, and the value was expected to never exceed \$120. After 4 weeks, the stock's value was \$86. [2.4]

a) Using the inhibited growth model, $P(t) = L + Ce^{-kt}$, find a function that models the price, $P(t)$, of a share of the stock after t weeks.

b) Find $P'(20)$, and interpret its meaning.

c) When will the value of a share of the stock reach \$110?

44. Life science: spread of a virus. A cruise ship carries 1000 people. Initially, 20 people become ill due to a viral infection, and after 24 hours, a total of 80 people are ill. [2.4]

a) Using the logistic model, $N(t) = \frac{L}{1 + Ce^{-rt}}$, find a function that models the number of sick people, $N(t)$, t hours after the viral infection began to spread.

b) When will half of the people on the cruise ship be ill?

45. Business: franchise growth. Fashionista Clothing is selling franchises throughout the United States and Canada. It is estimated that the number of franchises N will increase at the rate of 12% per year, that is,

$$\frac{dN}{dt} = 0.12N,$$

where t is the time, in years. [2.4]

a) Find the function that satisfies the equation, assuming that the number of franchises in 2014 ($t = 0$) was 60.

b) How many franchises will there be in 2022?

c) Estimate the rate of change of the number of franchises in 2022.

46. Business: franchise growth. The Coffee Casa is selling franchises throughout the southwestern United States. It is estimated that the number of franchises N will increase at the rate of 7% per year, that is,

$$\frac{dN}{dt} = 0.07N,$$

where t is the time, in years. [2.4]

a) Find the function that satisfies the equation, assuming that the number of franchises in 2010 ($t = 0$) was 24.

b) How many franchises will there be in 2026?

c) Estimate the rate of change of the number of franchises in 2026.

47. Physical science: decay rate. The decay rate of a certain radioactive substance is 13% per year. [2.1, 2.5]

a) A lab technician originally had 10 mg of this substance. Find the function $N(t)$ that models the amount of the substance remaining after t years.

b) Estimate how much of the substance remains after 3 yr.

c) Estimate the rate of change of the amount of the substance after 3 yr.

48. Physical science: half-life. The half-life of radon-222 is 3.8 days. [2.1, 2.5]

a) Find the decay rate, k.

b) Suppose that a sample of radon-222 has a mass of 50 mg. Find the function $N(t)$ that models the amount of the sample remaining after t days.

c) Estimate the rate of change of the amount of the sample after 6 days.

49. Physical science: decay rate. A certain radioactive isotope has a decay rate of 7% per day, that is,

$$\frac{dA}{dt} = -0.07A,$$

where A is the amount of isotope present after t days. [2.5]

a) Find a function that satisfies the equation if the amount of the isotope present at $t = 0$ is 800 g.

b) After 20 days, how much of the 800 g will remain? Round to the nearest gram.

c) Estimate the rate of change of the amount of the isotope after 20 days.

50. Social science: Hullian learning model. The probability $p(t)$ of mastering a certain assembly-line task after t learning trials is given by

$$p(t) = 1 - e^{-0.7t}. \quad [2.4]$$

a) What is the probability of learning the task after 1 trial? 2 trials? 5 trials? 10 trials?

b) Find the rate of change, $p'(t)$.

c) Interpret the meaning of $p'(t)$.

d) Sketch a graph of the function.

51. Business: present value. Find the present value of $1,000,000 due 40 yr later at 4.2%, compounded continuously. [2.5]

52. Business: growth of an investment. Patrice invests $2500 in a growth fund that doubles in value every 6.5 yr. [2.6]

a) Find an exponential function in base 2 that models the value, $P(t)$, of Patrice's investment after t years.

b) Rewrite the model in part (a) using base e.

c) What is the yearly percentage growth rate of the fund?

d) Without using a calculator, find the value of Patrice's investment after 13 yr.

53. Population growth. The population of Oak Fork was 15,000 in 1990 and was growing by 25% every 5 yr. [2.6]

a) Find an exponential function in base 1.25 that models the population, $P(t)$, of Oak Fork t years after 1990.

b) Find $P(10)$, and interpret its meaning.

c) Find $P'(10)$, and interpret its meaning.

SYNTHESIS

54. Let $y = 4^{x^3+2x+1}$. Find $\dfrac{d^2y}{dx^2}$. [2.6]

55. Suppose that the doubling time for a population is 12 yr. Find the population's tripling time. [2.6]

56. The half-life of a radioactive isotope is 45 yr. How long will it take for 25% of a sample of this isotope to decay? [2.6]

Technology Connection 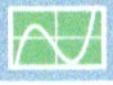

57. Find $\displaystyle\lim_{x \to 0} \frac{e^{1/x}}{(1 + e^{1/x})^2}$. [2.1]

58. Business: shopping online. Online sales of all types of consumer goods increased exponentially in recent years. Data in the following table show online retail sales in the United States, in billions of dollars. [2.3]

Years, t, after 2010	U.S. Online Retail Sales (in billions of dollars)
1	1005.0
2	1068.6
3	1107.8
4	1133.5
5	1160.7
6	1189.3
7	1250.0

(*Source:* www.census.gov.)

a) Use REGRESSION to fit an exponential function $y = a \cdot b^x$ to the data. Then rewrite that function as an equivalent exponential function, base e, where t is the number of years after 2010. Finally determine the exponential growth rate.

b) Estimate online sales in 2025.

c) When will online retail sales first reach $2 trillion?

d) What is the doubling time for online sales?

Chapter 2 Test

Differentiate.

1. $y = 2e^{3x}$

2. $y = (\ln x)^4$

3. $f(x) = e^{-x^2}$

4. $f(x) = \ln \dfrac{x}{7}$

5. $f(x) = e^x - 5x^3$

6. $f(x) = 3e^x \ln x$

7. $y = 7^x + 3^x$

8. $y = \log_{14} x$

9. Solve:

a) $\ln(2x + 1) = 3$;

b) $30e^{4x} = 90$.

Given $\ln 2 = 0.693$ *and* $\ln 5 = 1.609$, *find each of the following.*

10. $\ln 10$

11. $\ln 25$

12. $\ln 0.4$

13. Find the function that satisfies $dM/dt = 6M$, if $M = 2$ at $t = 0$.

APPLICATIONS

14. Life science: doubling time. The doubling time for a certain bacteria population is 3 hr. What is the growth rate? Round to the nearest tenth of a percent.

15. **Business: interest compounded continuously.** An investment of \$10,000 is made at 6.931% per year, compounded continuously.
    a) Find the function that models the value, $A(t)$, of the investment after t years.
    b) Estimate the value of the investment after 4 yr.
    c) Estimate the rate of change of the value of the investment after 4 yr.

16. **Business: price of milk.** The price, C, of a gallon of milk was \$3.22 in 2006. In 2017, it was \$3.32. (*Source:* U.S. Department of Labor, Bureau of Labor Statistics.) Assume that the exponential growth model applies.
    a) Find the exponential growth rate to the nearest hundredth of a percent, and write the equation.
    b) Estimate the price of a gallon of milk in 2024.
    c) Estimate the rate of change of the price of a gallon of milk in 2024.

17. **Life science: drug dosage.** A dose of a drug is injected into the body of a patient. The drug amount in the body decreases at the rate of 10% per hour, that is,

$$\frac{dA}{dt} = -0.1A,$$

where A is the amount in the body and t is the time, in hours.
    a) A dose of 3 cubic centimeters (cc) is administered. Assuming $A_0 = 3$, find the function that satisfies the equation.
    b) How much of the initial dose of 3 cc remains after 10 hr?
    c) Estimate the rate of change of the amount of the drug in the body after 10 hr.
    d) After how long does half of the original dose remain?

18. **Physical science: decay rate.** The decay rate of radium-226 is 4.209% per century. What is its half-life?

19. **Physical science: half-life.** The half-life of bohrium-267 is 17 sec.
    a) Suppose that a sample of bohrium-267 originally had a mass of 14 mg. Find the function that models the amount, $A(t)$, remaining after t seconds.
    b) Estimate the amount of the sample remaining after 1 min.
    c) Estimate the rate of change of the amount of the sample after 1 min.

20. **Business: effect of advertising.** Twin City Roasters introduced a new coffee in a trial run. The firm advertised the coffee on television and found that the percentage $P(t)$ of people who bought the coffee and viewed the ad t times was

$$P(t) = \frac{100}{1 + 24e^{-0.28t}}.$$

    a) What percentage of people who bought the coffee never viewed the ad ($t = 0$)?
    b) What percentage bought the coffee after viewing the ad 1 time? 5 times? 10 times? 20 times? 30 times?
    c) Find the rate of change, $P'(t)$.
    d) Interpret the meaning of $P'(t)$.
    e) Sketch a graph of the function.

21. **Business: savings account.** Andres deposited \$10,000 in a savings account. After 8.25 yr, the value of his account had doubled.
    a) Find the function in base 2 that models the value, $A(t)$, of Andres's account after t years.
    b) Rewrite the model from part (a) using base e.
    c) What is the yearly percentage growth rate of the account?
    d) Find $A'(12)$, and interpret its meaning.

22. **Population decay.** After a large manufacturing plant closed, Parsonville's population decreased by 20% every 3 yr. Assume that the population was 7500 when the plant closed.
    a) Find the function in base 0.8 that models the population, $P(t)$, of Parsonville t years after the plant closed.
    b) How much time is needed for Parsonville to lose half of the population it had when the plant closed?
    c) Find $P'(8)$, and interpret its meaning.

SYNTHESIS

23. Differentiate: $y = x(\ln x)^2 - 2x \ln x + 2x$.

24. Let $y = \log_3 (3x^2 + 4)$. Find $\frac{d^2y}{dx^2}$.

Technology Connection 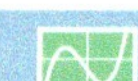

25. Find $\lim_{x \to 0} \frac{e^x - e^{-x}}{xe^x}$.

26. **Business: average price of a television commercial.** The cost of a 30-sec television commercial that runs during the Super Bowl was increasing exponentially from 1991 to 2018. Data in the table below show costs for those years.

Years, t, after 1990	Cost of Commercial
1	\$800,000
3	850,000
5	1,000,000
8	1,300,000
13	2,100,000
16	2,600,000
22	3,500,000
24	4,000,000
28	5,000,000

(*Source:* National Football League.)

    a) Use REGRESSION to fit an exponential function $y = a \cdot b^x$ to the data. Then rewrite that function as an equivalent exponential function, base e, where t is the number of years after 1990.
    b) Estimate the cost of a commercial run during the Super Bowl in 2022.
    c) After what amount of time will the cost first reach \$1 billion?
    d) What is the doubling time of the cost of a commercial run during the Super Bowl?

EXTENDED TECHNOLOGY APPLICATION 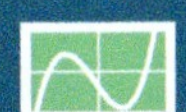

The Business of Motion Picture Revenue

People access movies on different platforms, including tablets and smart phones, as well as disc formats such as DVD and Blu-ray. The timing of release dates for films on these secondary platforms is a major concern for movie executives. There has been increasing pressure to narrow the gap between the theatrical release of a movie and the release to secondary platforms. Movie executives want to reduce marketing expenses, and a studio realizes greater profit from selling a disc than from providing the movie in streaming format. Theater owners, on the other hand, want to protect their revenue and fear that with a shorter time between theater release and disc release, more people will skip the theater presentation and wait. Timing of the disc release becomes important to maximize the potential for profit.

The table at the right gives t, the number of days between theater release and disc release, for 10 movies. Note that the average time lag is about 14 weeks, or a little over 3 months.

Movie	Release Dates	Number of Days Between Release Dates
Hidden Figures	Theater: January 6, 2017 Disc: April 11, 2017	95
Logan	Theater: March 3, 2017 Disc: May 23, 2017	81
Gifted	Theater: April 12, 2017 Disc: July 25, 2017	104
T2: Trainspotting	Theater: March 31, 2017 Disc: June 27, 2017	88
The Lost City of Z	Theater: April 21, 2017 Disc: July 11, 2017	81
Wonder Woman	Theater: June 2, 2017 Disc: September 19, 2017	110
Star Wars: The Last Jedi	Theater: December 15, 2017 Disc: March 27, 2018	103
Blade Runner 2049	Theater: October 6, 2017 Disc: January 16, 2018	103
The Post	Theater: January 12, 2018 Disc: April 17, 2018	96
Hostiles	Theater: January 26, 2018 Disc: April 24, 2018	88

(*Sources:* imdb.com; boxofficemojo.com; dvdreleasedates.com.)

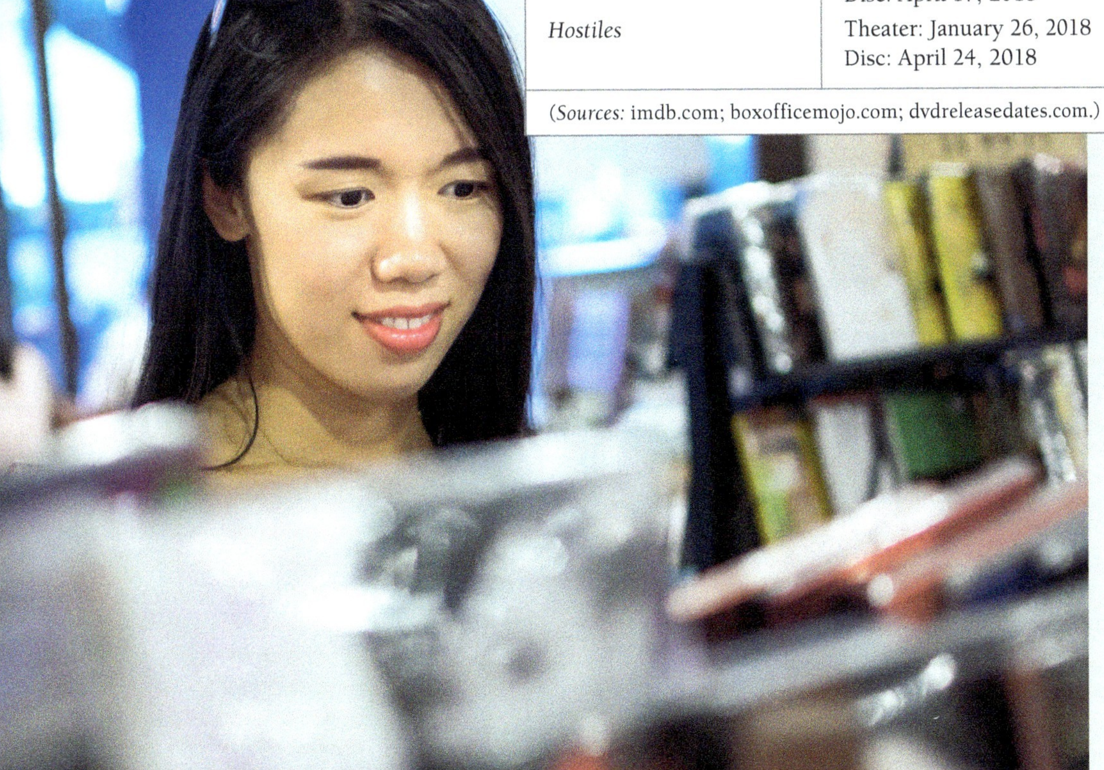

Let's examine data for *Gifted*. The table below presents weekly estimates of gross revenue, G, for that movie. Total revenue, R, is approximated by adding each week's gross revenue to the previous week's total revenue.

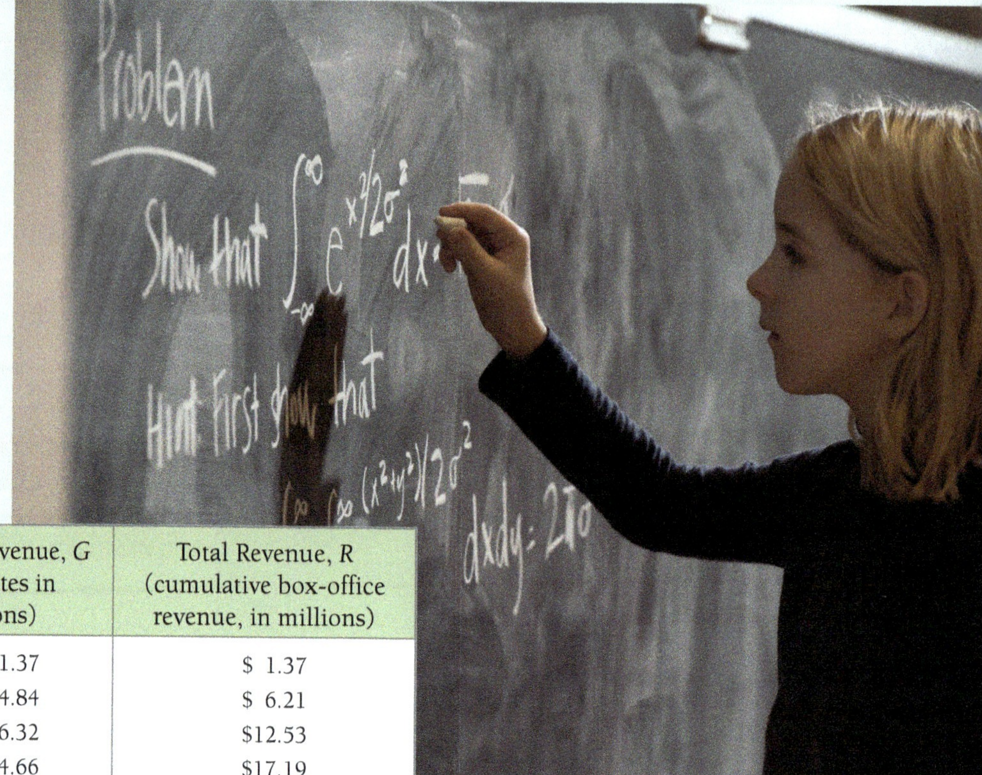

Revenue for *Gifted*

Week in Release, t (week 1 began 4/7/17)	Weekly Revenue, G (estimates in millions)	Total Revenue, R (cumulative box-office revenue, in millions)
1, April 7	$1.37	$ 1.37
2, April 14	$4.84	$ 6.21
3, April 21	$6.32	$12.53
4, April 28	$4.66	$17.19
5, May 5	$2.88	$20.07
6, May 12	$2.07	$22.14
7, May 19	$1.11	$23.25
8, May 26	$0.65	$23.90
9, June 2	?	?
10, June 9	?	?
11, June 16	?	?
12, June 23	?	?
13, June 30	?	?

(*Sources:* imdb.com; boxofficemojo.com; dvdreleasedates.com.)

Exercises

1. A movie executive wants to fit a function to the data for *Gifted*. Make a scatterplot of the data points (t, G); then use REGRESSION to fit linear, quadratic, cubic, and exponential functions to the data, and graph each equation with the scatterplot. Which function fits best? Why?

2. Use the exponential function to predict gross revenue, G, for weeks 9 through 13.

3. Use your predictions from Exercise 2 to compute total revenue, R, for weeks 9 through 13.

4. Use REGRESSION to fit a logistic function of the form $R(t) = c/(1 + ae^{-bt})$ to the data points (t, R) for weeks 1–8. Based on these results, what seems to be a limiting value for the total revenue from *Gifted*? Does the value seem reasonable?

5. Repeat Exercise 4, ignoring the first two data points (that is, consider only weeks 3 through 8, and the total revenue, R, during those weeks). Does this function seem to be a better predictor of future earnings for *Gifted*? Why or why not?

6. The disc release of *Gifted* occurred 15 weeks after its theatrical release. Based on the given data, do you think that this release date was appropriate? What factors might influence the release date of a movie onto disc format?

Now consider the revenue data for *Hidden Figures*, shown in the following table. This movie was released in selected theaters on December 25, 2016 and released nationwide (United States and Canada) on January 6, 2017.

Revenue for *Hidden Figures*

Week in Release, t (week 1 began 1/6/17)	Weekly Revenue, G (estimates in millions)	Total Revenue, R (cumulative box-office revenue, in millions)
1, Jan 6	$31.43	$ 31.43
2, Jan 13	$33.61	$ 65.04
3, Jan 20	$22.03	$ 87.07
4, Jan 27	$19.28	$106.35
5, Feb 3	$14.15	$120.50
6, Feb 10	$12.04	$132.54
7, Feb 17	$11.45	$143.99
8, Feb 24	$ 8.00	$151.99
9, Mar 3	?	?
10, Mar 10	?	?
11, Mar 17	?	?
12, Mar 24	?	?
13, Mar 31	?	?
14, Apr 7	?	?

(*Sources:* imdb.com; boxofficemojo.com; dvdreleasedates.com.)

Exercises

7. Make a scatterplot of the data points (t, G) for weeks 1 through 8, and fit linear, quadratic, cubic, and exponential functions to the data. Which function, if any, best estimates the weekly gross revenue for weeks 9 through 14?

8. Use the exponential model to predict the gross revenue, G, for *Hidden Figures* for weeks 9 through 14.

9. Use REGRESSION to fit a logistic function of the form $R(t) = c/(1 + ae^{-bt})$ to the data points (t, R) for *Hidden Figures* for weeks 1 through 8. Based on these results, what is the limiting value of the total revenue? Does this figure seem accurate, too high, or too low?

10. Repeat Exercise 9, but using only the data points for weeks 3 through 8. What is the limiting value of total revenue from *Hidden Figures*? Does this seem to be a better estimate? Why or why not?

11. A movie executive decides to release *Hidden Figures* to disc when the gross theatrical revenues reach $160 million. In what week should the executive plan to release *Hidden Figures* in disc format?

12. Why might it be wise to ignore the first two weeks of data when finding a logistic function that models the long-term behavior of a movie's total revenue?

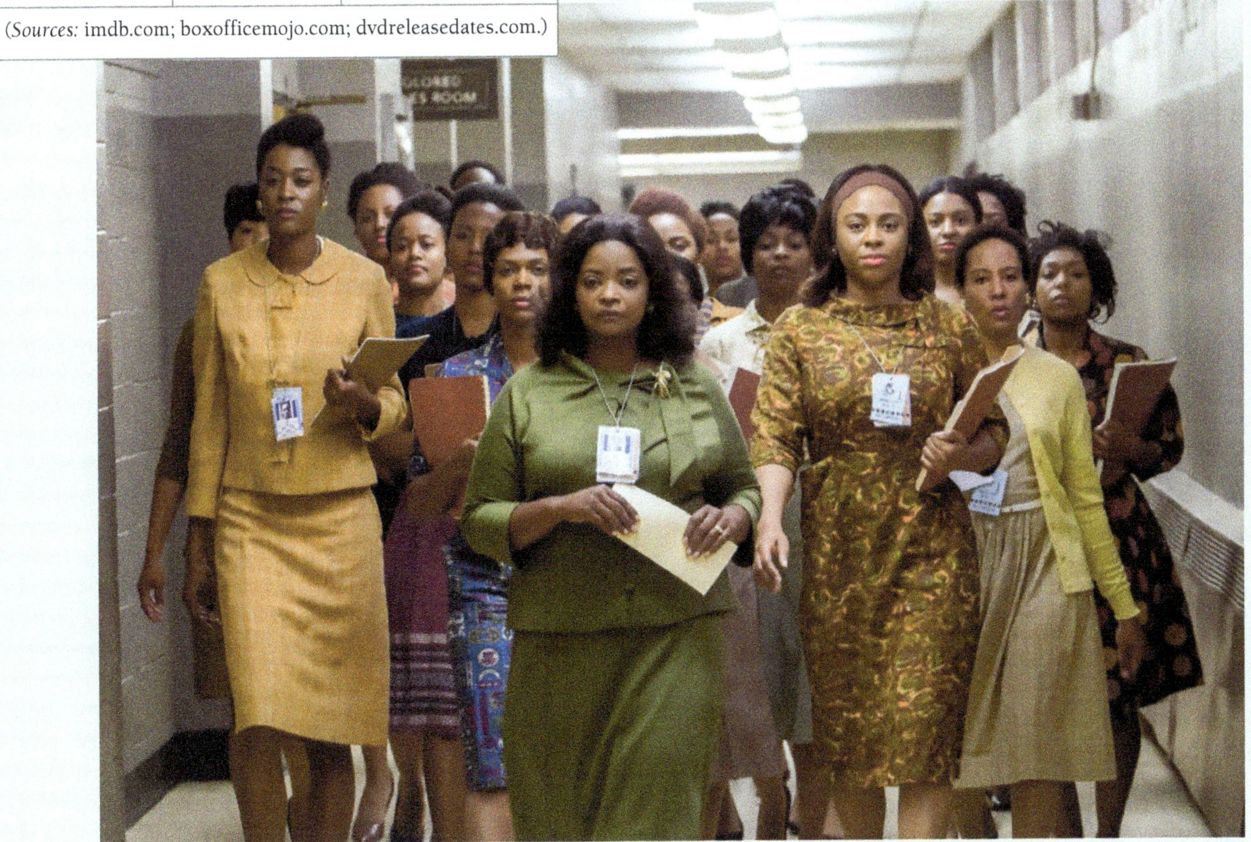

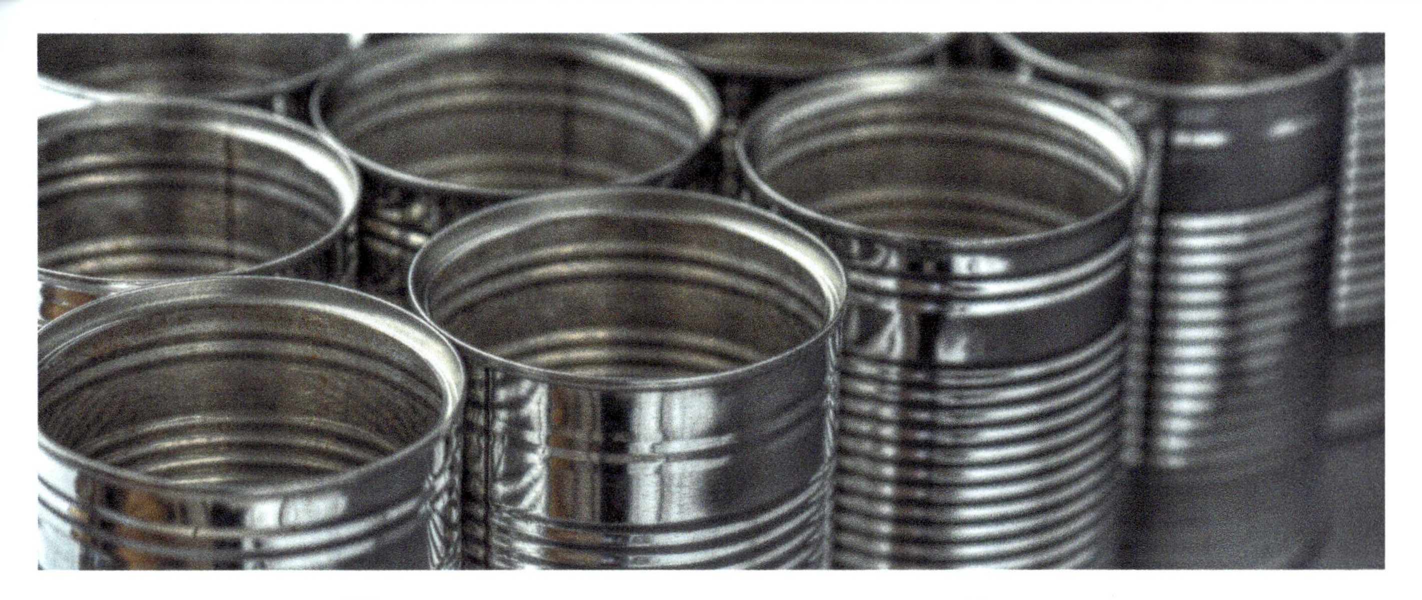

3 Applications of Differentiation

What You'll Learn

Why It's Important

In this chapter, we explore many applications of differentiation. We learn to find the maximum and minimum values of functions, and that skill allows us to solve many kinds of problems in which we need to optimize a value in a real-world situation. Our differentiation skills will be applied to graphing, and we will use differentials to approximate function values. We will also use differentiation to explore elasticity of demand and related rates.

Where It's Used

Minimizing Cost: Minimizing cost is a common goal in manufacturing. For example, cylindrical food cans come in a variety of sizes. Suppose a soup can is to have a volume of 250 cm^3. The cost of material for the two circular ends is $\$0.0008/\text{cm}^2$, and the cost of material for the side is $\$0.0015/\text{cm}^2$. What dimensions minimize the cost of material for the soup can?

(This problem appears as Example 3 in Section 3.5.)

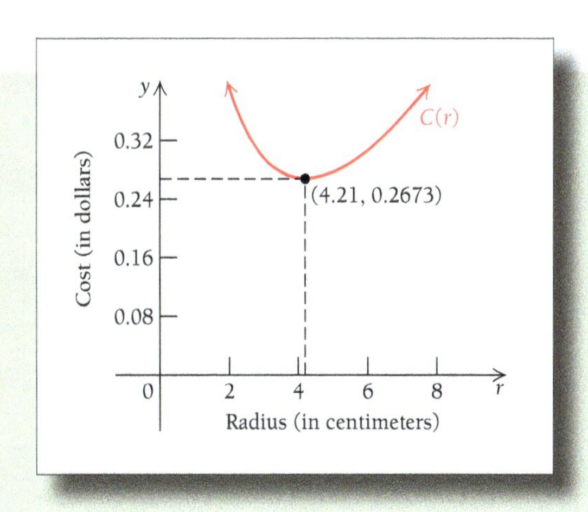

3.1 Using First Derivatives to Classify Maximum and Minimum Values and Sketch Graphs

- Find relative extrema of a continuous function using the First-Derivative Test.
- Sketch graphs of continuous functions.

The graph below shows sales revenue for vinyl long-playing (LP) records since 1973. Note that the number of sales varies with respect to time. Revenue increased to a point of maximum revenue in about 1978, then decreased in the 1980s as new technology (such as compact discs) entered the market. Revenue reached low points in the early 1990s and again in the mid-2000s as digital and online streaming options became available. In recent years, however, sales revenue for vinyl LP records has increased slightly due to factors such as improved technology, nostalgia, and so on.

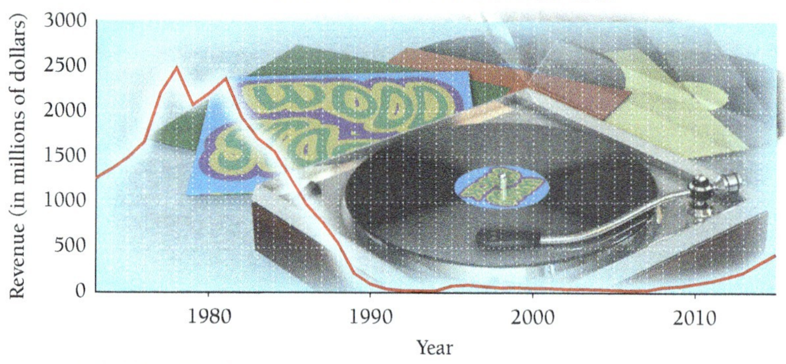

(Source: *Digital Music News*.)

Finding the largest and smallest values of a function—that is, the maximum and minimum values—has extensive applications in many fields. We use first and second derivatives to provide information about the graph of a function, to locate maximum and minimum points on the graph, and to identify intervals of increasing and decreasing values.

Increasing and Decreasing Functions

If the graph of a function rises from left to right over an interval I, the function is said to be **increasing** on, or over, I. If the graph drops from left to right, the function is said to be **decreasing** on, or over, I.

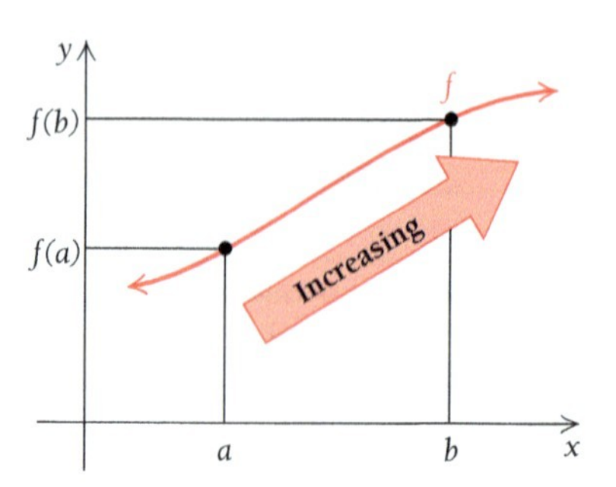

If the input a is less than the input b, then the output for a is less than the output for b.

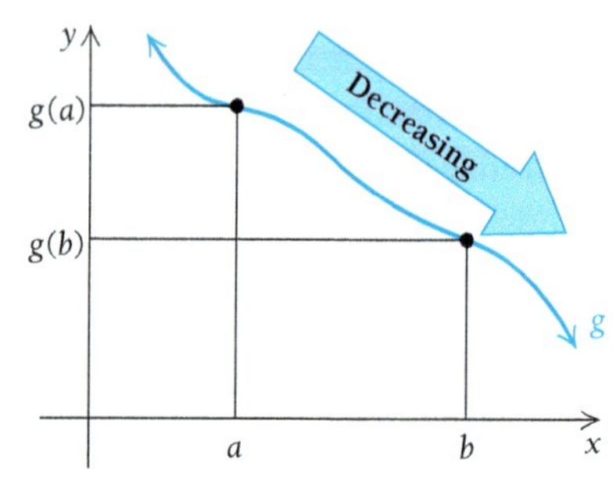

If the input a is less than the input b, then the output for a is greater than the output for b.

Technology Connection 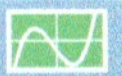

Exploratory

Using the window $[-10, 25, -100, 150]$, with Xscl $= 5$ and Yscl $= 25$, graph

$$f(x) = -\tfrac{1}{3}x^3 + 6x^2 - 11x - 50$$

and its derivative,

$$f'(x) = -x^2 + 12x - 11.$$

Next, TRACE from left to right along each graph. Moving the cursor from left to right, note that the x-coordinate always increases. If the function is increasing, the y-coordinate increases as well. If the function is decreasing, the y-coordinate will decrease.

Over what intervals is f increasing? Over what intervals is f decreasing? Over what intervals is $f'(x)$ positive? Over what intervals is $f'(x)$ negative? What rules might relate the sign of $f'(x)$ to the behavior of f?

We can define these concepts as follows.

DEFINITIONS

A function f is **increasing** over I if, for every a and b in I,

if $a < b$, then $f(a) < f(b)$.

A function f is **decreasing** over I if, for every a and b in I,

if $a < b$, then $f(a) > f(b)$.

The above definitions can be restated in terms of slopes of secant lines:

Increasing: $\dfrac{f(b) - f(a)}{b - a} > 0$. Decreasing: $\dfrac{f(b) - f(a)}{b - a} < 0$.

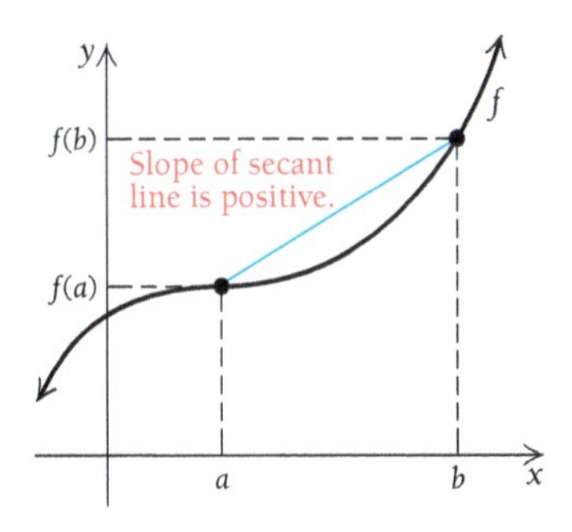

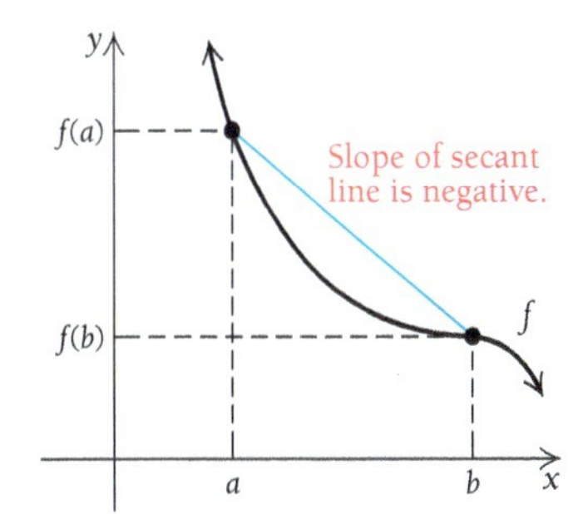

Since the derivative of a function f tells us the slope of the tangent line to f at any input x, we can also define an increasing or decreasing function using the derivative.

THEOREM 1

Let f be differentiable over an open interval I.
If $f'(x) > 0$ for all x in I, then f is increasing over I.
If $f'(x) < 0$ for all x in I, then f is decreasing over I.

Theorem 1 is illustrated in the following graph of $f(x) = \frac{1}{3}x^3 - x + \frac{2}{3}$.

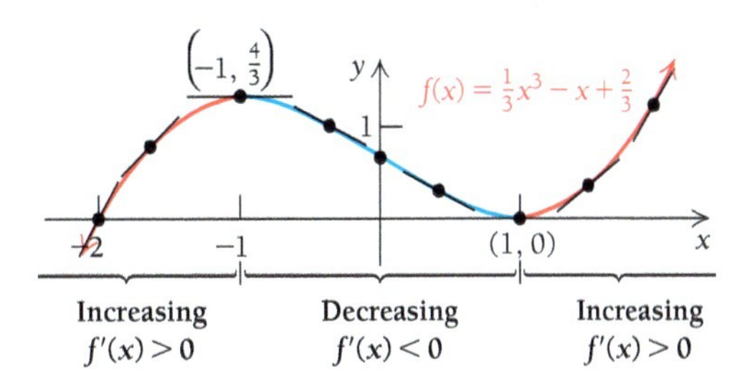

f is increasing over the intervals $(-\infty, -1)$ and $(1, \infty)$; slopes of tangent lines are positive.

f is decreasing over the interval $(-1, 1)$; slopes of tangent lines are negative.

Note in the graph above that $x = -1$ and $x = 1$ are not included in any interval over which the function is increasing or decreasing. These values are examples of *critical values*.

Critical Values

Consider the following graph of a continuous function f.

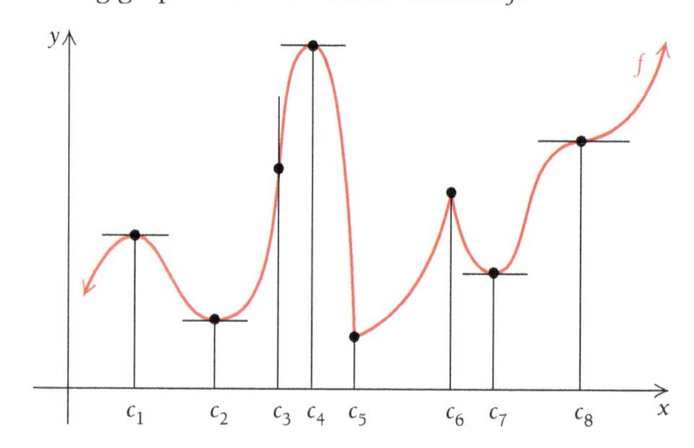

Note the following:

1. $f'(x) = 0$ for $x = c_1, c_2, c_4, c_7$, and c_8. That is, the tangent line to the graph is horizontal at these values.

2. $f'(x)$ does not exist for $x = c_3, c_5$, and c_6. The tangent line is vertical at c_3, and there are corners at both c_5 and c_6. (See also the discussion at the end of Section 1.4.)

> **DEFINITION**
>
> A **critical value** of a function f is any number c in the domain of f for which the tangent line at $(c, f(c))$ is horizontal or for which the derivative does not exist. That is, c is a critical value if $f(c)$ exists and
>
> $$f'(c) = 0 \quad \text{or} \quad f'(c) \text{ does not exist.}$$
>
> If c is a critical value of a function f, then $(c, f(c))$ is a **critical point**.

Thus, in the graph of f above:

- c_1, c_2, c_4, c_7, and c_8 are critical values because $f'(c) = 0$ for each value.
- c_3, c_5, and c_6 are critical values because $f'(c)$ does not exist for each value.

A continuous function can change from increasing to decreasing or from decreasing to increasing *only* at a critical value. In the above graph, c_1, c_2, c_4, c_5, c_6, and c_7 separate intervals in which the function f increases from those in which it decreases or intervals in which the function decreases from those in which it increases. Although c_3 and c_8 are critical values, they do not separate intervals over which the function changes from increasing to decreasing or from decreasing to increasing.

Finding Relative Maximum and Minimum Values

Now consider a graph with "peaks" and "valleys" at $x = c_1, c_2, c_3, c_4$, and c_5:

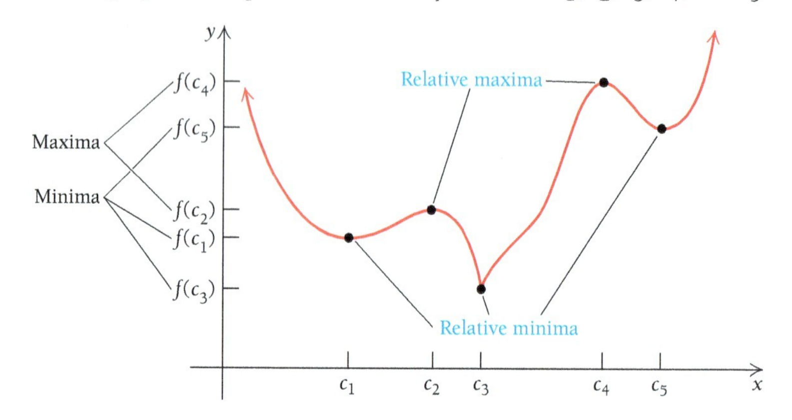

Here, $f(c_2)$ and $f(c_4)$ are each an example of a **relative, or local, maximum** (plural: **maxima**), and $f(c_1), f(c_3)$, and $f(c_5)$ are each an example of a **relative, or local, minimum** (plural: **minima**). Collectively, maximum and minimum values are called **extrema** (singular: **extremum**). Note that it is possible for a relative minimum to be greater than a relative maximum; for example, $f(c_5) > f(c_2)$ in the graph at the bottom of the preceding page.

Note that x-values at which a continuous function has relative extrema are those values for which the derivative is 0 or for which the derivative does not exist—the critical values.

THEOREM 2

If a function f has a relative extreme value $f(c)$ on an open interval, then c is a critical value, and

$$f'(c) = 0 \quad \text{or} \quad f'(c) \text{ does not exist.}$$

A *relative extreme point*, $(c, f(c))$, is higher or lower than all other points over an open interval containing c. A *relative minimum point*, $(c, f(c))$, is lower than all other points over an open interval containing c. A relative minimum point has a y-value that is *less* than those of a neighborhood of points to the left and right of c. Similarly, a *relative maximum point*, $(c, f(c))$, is higher than all other points over an open interval containing c. A relative maximum point has a y-value that is *greater* than those of a neighborhood of points to the left and right of c. In the preceding graph, $(c_1, f(c_1))$, $(c_3, f(c_3))$, and $(c_5, f(c_5))$ are all relative minimum points. Similarly, $(c_2, f(c_2))$ and $(c_4, f(c_4))$ are both relative maximum points.

Theorem 2 is useful and important to understand. It says that to find relative extrema, we need only consider inputs for which the derivative is 0 or for which the derivative does not exist. Each critical value is a *candidate* for a value where a relative extremum *might* occur. Theorem 2 does not guarantee that every critical value will yield a relative maximum or minimum. Consider, for example, the graph of

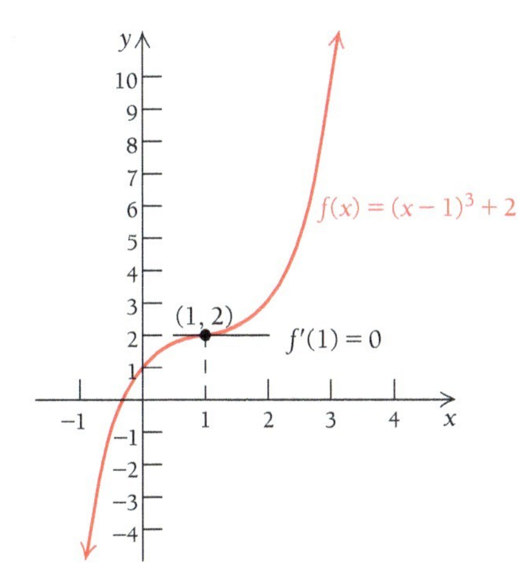

$$f(x) = (x - 1)^3 + 2,$$

shown at the left. Note that

$$f'(x) = 3(x - 1)^2, \quad \text{and} \quad f'(1) = 3(1 - 1)^2 = 0.$$

Thus, $c = 1$ is a critical value, but f has no relative maximum or minimum at that value. In fact, this function has no extrema anywhere.

Theorem 2 does guarantee that if a relative maximum or minimum occurs, then the first coordinate of that extremum is a critical value. How can we tell when the existence of a critical value indicates a relative extremum? The following graph leads us to a test.

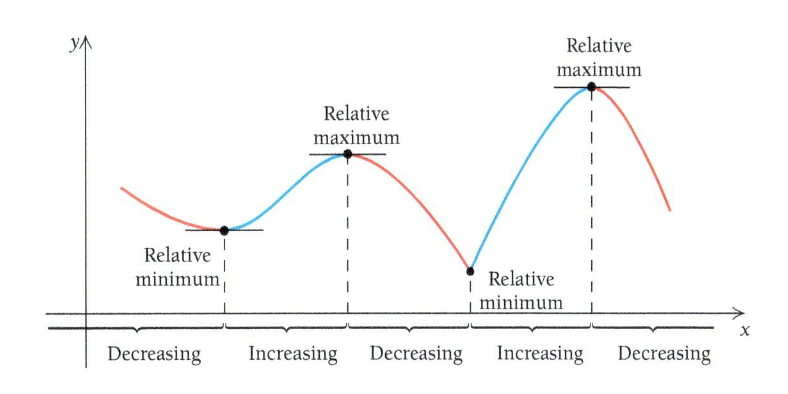

Note that at a critical value where there is a relative minimum, the function f is decreasing on the left of the critical value and increasing on the right. At a critical value where there is a relative maximum, the function f is increasing on the left of the critical value and decreasing on the right. In both cases, the derivative changes signs on either side of the critical value.

Graph over the interval (a, b)	$f(c)$	Sign of $f'(x)$ for x in (a, c)	Sign of $f'(x)$ for x in (c, b)	Increasing or decreasing
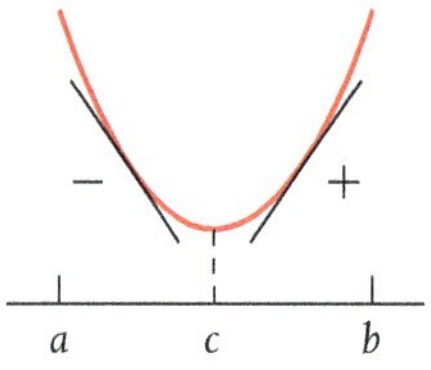	Relative minimum	$-$	$+$	Decreasing on (a, c); increasing on (c, b)
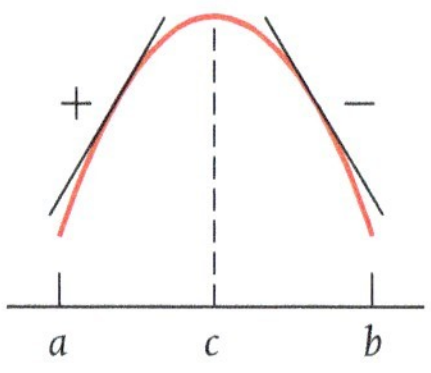	Relative maximum	$+$	$-$	Increasing on (a, c); decreasing on (c, b)
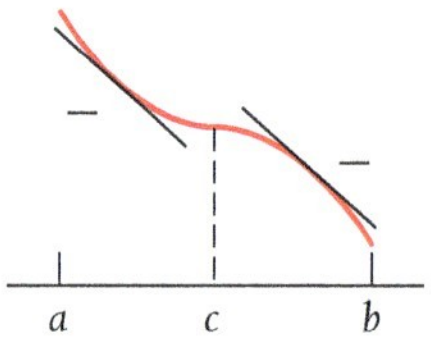	No relative maxima or minima	$-$	$-$	Decreasing on (a, b)
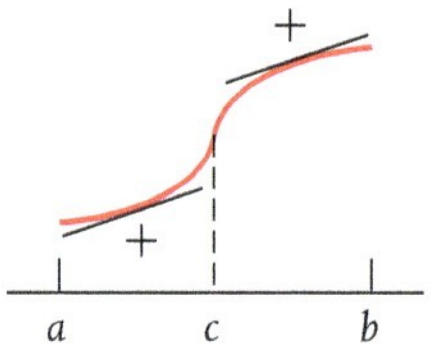	No relative maxima or minima	$+$	$+$	Increasing on (a, b)

Derivatives can tell us when a function is increasing or decreasing. This leads us to the First-Derivative Test.

THEOREM 3 The First-Derivative Test for Relative Extrema

For any continuous function f that has exactly one critical value c in an open interval (a, b):

F1. f has a relative minimum at c if $f'(x) < 0$ on (a, c) and $f'(x) > 0$ on (c, b). That is, f is decreasing to the left of c and increasing to the right of c.

F2. f has a relative maximum at c if $f'(x) > 0$ on (a, c) and $f'(x) < 0$ on (c, b). That is, f is increasing to the left of c and decreasing to the right of c.

F3. f has neither a relative maximum nor a relative minimum at c if $f'(x)$ has the same sign on (a, c) as on (c, b).

We can use the First-Derivative Test to find relative extrema.

EXAMPLE 1 Consider the function f given by

$$f(x) = 4x^3 - 9x^2 - 30x + 25.$$

Find any relative extrema.

Solution We begin by finding the critical values of f. To do so, we find its derivative, f':

$$f'(x) = 12x^2 - 18x - 30.$$

We next determine where $f'(x)$ does not exist or where $f'(x) = 0$. Here, $f'(x)$ is defined for all real numbers, so there is no value x for which $f'(x)$ does not exist. The only possibilities for critical values occur where $f'(x) = 0$. To find such values, we solve $f'(x) = 0$:

$$12x^2 - 18x - 30 = 0$$

$$2x^2 - 3x - 5 = 0 \qquad \text{Dividing both sides by 6}$$

$$(x + 1)(2x - 5) = 0 \qquad \text{Factoring}$$

$$x + 1 = 0 \quad \text{or} \quad 2x - 5 = 0 \qquad \text{Using the Principle of Zero Products}$$

$$x = -1 \quad \text{or} \quad x = \tfrac{5}{2}.$$

The critical values are -1 and $\frac{5}{2}$. Since it is at these values that a relative maximum or minimum might exist, we examine the sign of the derivative on the intervals $(-\infty, -1)$, $(-1, \frac{5}{2})$, and $(\frac{5}{2}, \infty)$.

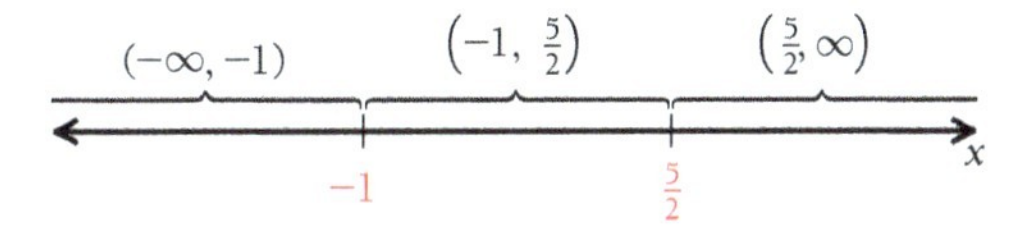

To do so, we select a convenient test value in each interval and evaluate $f'(x)$. Let's use the values -2, 0, and 4.

$$(-\infty, -1)\text{: Test } -2, \quad f'(-2) = 12(-2)^2 - 18(-2) - 30$$
$$= 48 + 36 - 30 = 54 > 0;$$
$$(-1, \tfrac{5}{2})\text{: Test } 0, \quad f'(0) = 12(0)^2 - 18(0) - 30 = -30 < 0;$$
$$(\tfrac{5}{2}, \infty)\text{: Test } 4, \quad f'(4) = 12(4)^2 - 18(4) - 30$$
$$= 192 - 72 - 30 = 90 > 0.$$

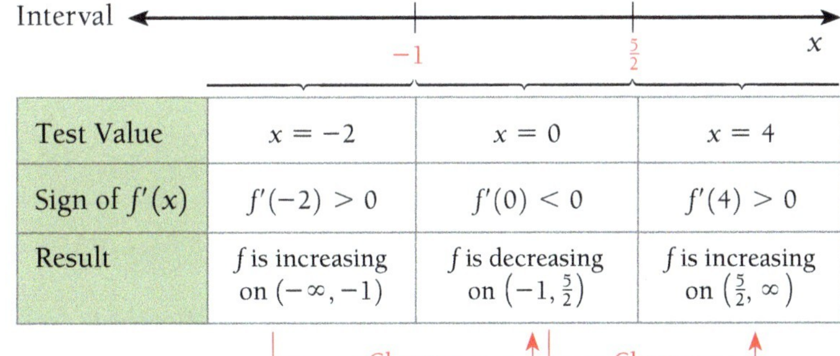

Interval: -1, $\frac{5}{2}$, x

Test Value	$x = -2$	$x = 0$	$x = 4$
Sign of $f'(x)$	$f'(-2) > 0$	$f'(0) < 0$	$f'(4) > 0$
Result	f is increasing on $(-\infty, -1)$	f is decreasing on $(-1, \frac{5}{2})$	f is increasing on $(\frac{5}{2}, \infty)$

Change indicates a relative maximum at $x = -1$.

Change indicates a relative minimum at $x = \frac{5}{2}$.

By the First-Derivative Test, f has a relative maximum at $x = -1$ and a relative minimum at $x = \frac{5}{2}$. The value of the relative maximum is given by

$$f(-1) = 4(-1)^3 - 9(-1)^2 - 30(-1) + 25 \qquad \text{Substituting } -1 \text{ for } x \text{ in the } \textit{original} \text{ function}$$

$$= 42 \qquad \text{This is a relative maximum.}$$

Quick Check 1 ✓

Graph the function g given by $g(x) = x^3 - 27x - 6$, and find any relative extrema.

The value of the relative minimum is given by

$$f\left(\tfrac{5}{2}\right) = 4\left(\tfrac{5}{2}\right)^3 - 9\left(\tfrac{5}{2}\right)^2 - 30\left(\tfrac{5}{2}\right) + 25 = -\tfrac{175}{4}.$$ This is a relative minimum.

Thus, there is a relative maximum point at $(-1, 42)$ and a relative minimum point at $\left(\tfrac{5}{2}, -\tfrac{175}{4}\right)$. 1 ✓

The information obtained in Example 1 from the first derivative is useful in graphing the function. We know where it is increasing, where it is decreasing, and where it has relative extrema. We draw the graph by plotting the relative maximum and minimum points and calculating additional function values, as shown in the table below. The graph of the function, shown below in red, is scaled to clearly show its important features.

x	$f(x)$
−3	−74
−2	17
−1	42
0	25
1	−10
2	−39
3	−38
4	17

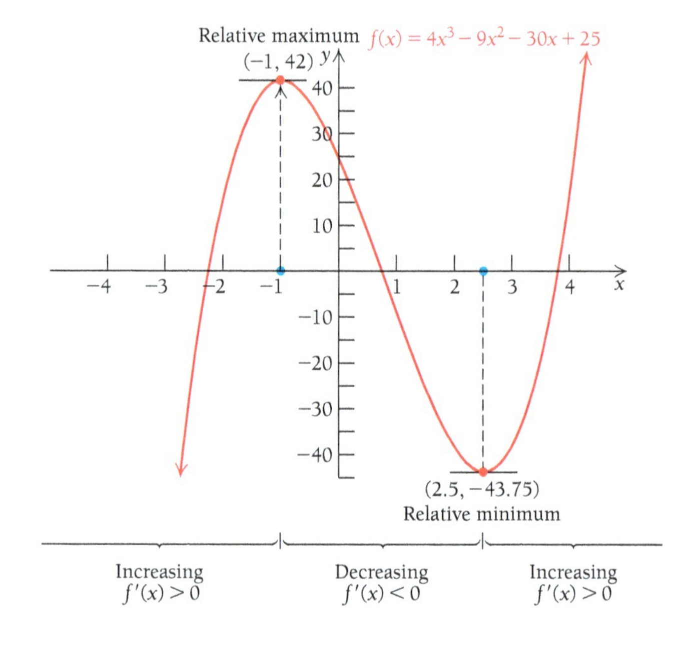

Technology Connection 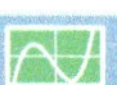

Exploratory

Consider the function f given by

$$f(x) = x^3 - 3x + 2.$$

Graph both f and f' using the same set of axes. Examine the graphs using the TABLE and TRACE features. Where do you think the relative extrema of f occur? Where is the derivative equal to 0? Where does f have critical values?

To better understand these concepts, let's examine the graph of the derivative of f, shown in blue below.

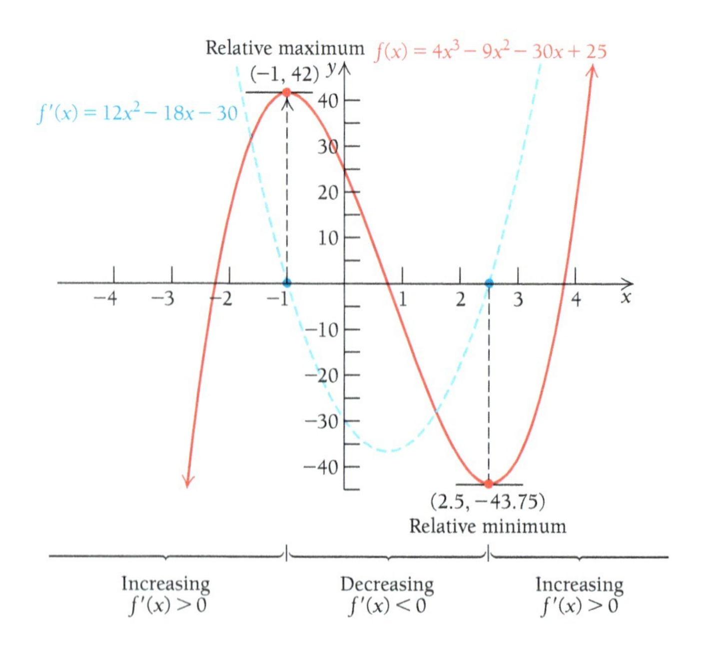

Note that $f'(x) = 0$ where $f(x)$ has relative extrema. We summarize the behavior of this function by noting where it is increasing or decreasing and by characterizing its critical points:

- f is increasing over the interval $(-\infty, -1)$.
- f has a relative maximum point at $(-1, 42)$.
- f is decreasing over the interval $\left(-1, \frac{5}{2}\right)$.
- f has a relative minimum point at $\left(\frac{5}{2}, -\frac{175}{4}\right)$.
- f is increasing over the interval $\left(\frac{5}{2}, \infty\right)$.

To use the first derivative for graphing a function f:

1. Find all critical values by determining where $f'(x)$ is 0 and where $f'(x)$ is undefined (but $f(x)$ is defined). Find $f(x)$ for each critical value.
2. Use the critical values to divide the x-axis into intervals and choose a test value in each interval.
3. Find the sign of $f'(x)$ for each test value chosen in step 2, and use this information to determine where f is increasing or decreasing and to classify any extrema as relative maxima or minima.
4. Plot some additional points and sketch the graph.

EXAMPLE 2 Find the relative extrema and sketch the graph of the function f given by

$$f(x) = 2x^3 - x^4.$$

Solution The derivative of f is

$$f'(x) = 6x^2 - 4x^3.$$

Since $f'(x)$ is defined for all real numbers x, the only critical values occur where $f'(x) = 0$:

$$6x^2 - 4x^3 = 0$$

$$2x^2(3 - 2x) = 0 \qquad \text{Factoring}$$

$$x = 0 \quad or \quad x = \tfrac{3}{2} \qquad \text{Using the Principle of Zero Products}$$

The critical values are 0 and $\frac{3}{2}$. We use these values to divide the x-axis into three intervals: $(-\infty, 0)$, $\left(0, \frac{3}{2}\right)$, and $\left(\frac{3}{2}, \infty\right)$.

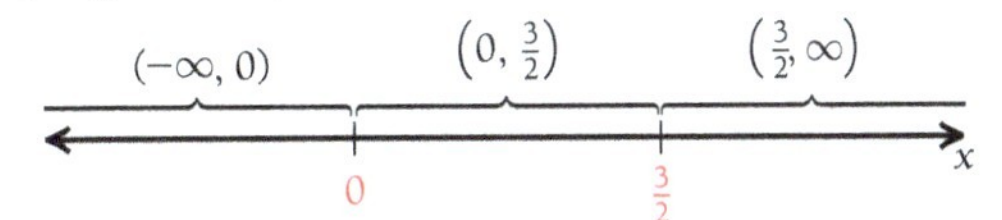

We next find the sign of $f'(x)$ on each interval, using a test value.

$(-\infty, 0)$: Test -1, $f'(-1) = 6(-1)^2 - 4(-1)^3 = 6 + 4 = 10 > 0$;

$\left(0, \frac{3}{2}\right)$: Test 1, $f'(1) = 6(1)^2 - 4(1)^3 = 6 - 4 = 2 > 0$;

$\left(\frac{3}{2}, \infty\right)$: Test 2, $f'(2) = 6(2)^2 - 4(2)^3 = 24 - 32 = -8 < 0$.

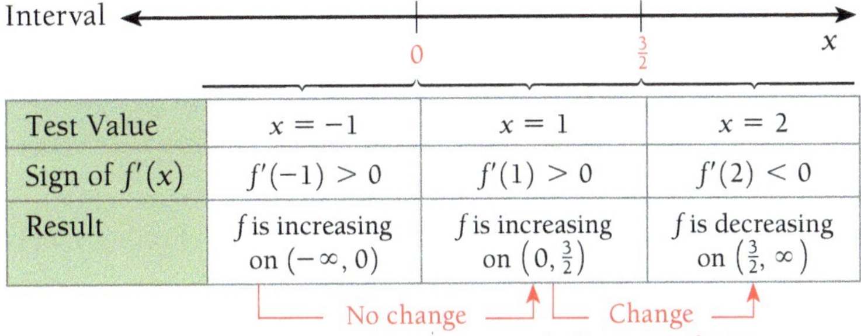

Test Value	$x = -1$	$x = 1$	$x = 2$
Sign of $f'(x)$	$f'(-1) > 0$	$f'(1) > 0$	$f'(2) < 0$
Result	f is increasing on $(-\infty, 0)$	f is increasing on $\left(0, \frac{3}{2}\right)$	f is decreasing on $\left(\frac{3}{2}, \infty\right)$

No change

Change indicates a relative maximum at $x = \frac{3}{2}$.

Therefore, by the First-Derivative Test, f has no extremum at $x = 0$ (since f is increasing on both sides of 0) and has a relative maximum at $x = \frac{3}{2}$. Thus,

$$f\left(\tfrac{3}{2}\right) = 2\left(\tfrac{3}{2}\right)^3 - \left(\tfrac{3}{2}\right)^4$$
$$= 2 \cdot \tfrac{27}{8} - \tfrac{81}{16}$$
$$= \tfrac{108}{16} - \tfrac{81}{16} = \tfrac{27}{16}$$

is a relative maximum.

We use the above information to sketch the graph below. Other function values are listed in the table.

x	$f(x)$, approximately
-1	-3
-0.5	-0.31
0	0
0.5	0.19
1	1
1.25	1.46
2	0

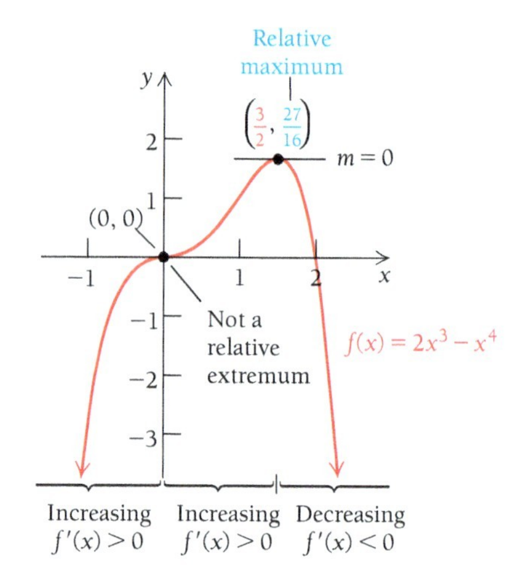

- f is increasing over the interval $(-\infty, 0)$.
- f has a critical value at $x = 0$, but the critical point $(0, 0)$ is neither a minimum nor a maximum.
- f is increasing over the interval $\left(0, \frac{3}{2}\right)$.
- f has a relative maximum at the point $\left(\frac{3}{2}, \frac{27}{16}\right)$.
- f is decreasing over the interval $\left(\frac{3}{2}, \infty\right)$.

Since f is increasing over $(-\infty, 0)$ and $\left(0, \frac{3}{2}\right)$, we can say that f is increasing over $\left(-\infty, \frac{3}{2}\right)$ despite the fact that $f'(0) = 0$ within this interval. Note that any secant line connecting two points within this interval has a positive slope. **2 ✓**

Quick Check 2 ✓

Find the relative extrema of the function h given by $h(x) = x^4 - \frac{8}{3}x^3$. Then sketch the graph.

EXAMPLE 3 Find any relative extrema and sketch the graph of the function g given by

$$g(x) = x^2 e^{-x}.$$

Solution First, we determine the critical values. To do so, we find $g'(x)$:

$$g'(x) = x^2(-e^{-x}) + 2xe^{-x} \quad \text{Using the Product Rule}$$
$$= -x^2e^{-x} + 2xe^{-x}. \quad \text{Simplifying}$$

Next, we find where g' does not exist or where $g'(x) = 0$. Since $g'(x)$ can be evaluated for any real number x, the only candidates for critical values are those where $g'(x) = 0$:

$$-x^2e^{-x} + 2xe^{-x} = 0 \quad \text{Setting } g'(x) \text{ equal to 0}$$
$$xe^{-x}(-x + 2) = 0. \quad \text{Factoring}$$

Since $e^{-x} > 0$ for all real numbers x, this factor will not provide any critical values. We use the Principle of Zero Products on the remaining factors, x and $(-x + 2)$:

$$xe^{-x}(-x + 2) = 0$$
$$x = 0 \quad or \quad -x + 2 = 0$$
$$x = 0 \quad or \quad x = 2.$$

The critical values are 0 and 2. We use these values to divide the x-axis into three intervals: $(-\infty, 0)$, $(0, 2)$, and $(2, \infty)$.

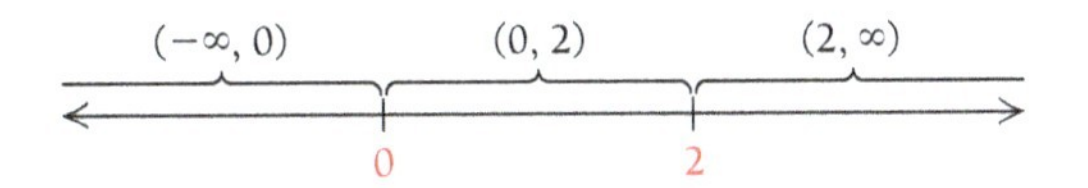

We next find the sign of $g'(x)$ on each interval, using a test value.

$(-\infty, 0)$: Test -1, $g'(-1) = (-1)e^{-(-1)}(-(-1) + 2) = -3e < 0$;

$(0, 2)$: Test 1, $g'(1) = (1)e^{-(1)}(-(1) + 2) = e^{-1} > 0$;

$(2, \infty)$: Test 3, $g'(3) = (3)e^{-(3)}(-(3) + 2) = -3e^{-3} < 0$.

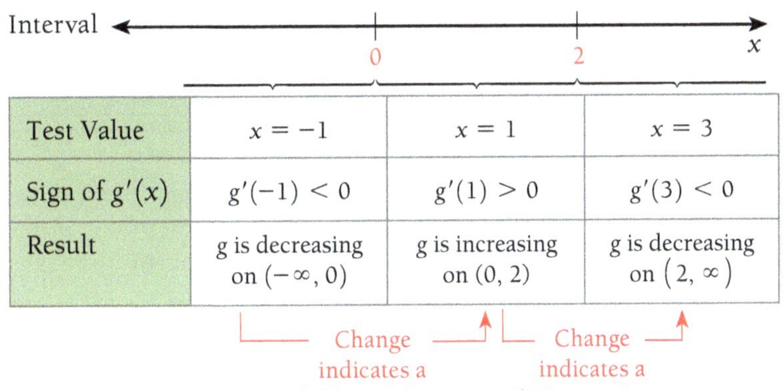

Test Value	$x = -1$	$x = 1$	$x = 3$
Sign of $g'(x)$	$g'(-1) < 0$	$g'(1) > 0$	$g'(3) < 0$
Result	g is decreasing on $(-\infty, 0)$	g is increasing on $(0, 2)$	g is decreasing on $(2, \infty)$

Therefore, by the First-Derivative Test, g has a relative minimum at $x = 0$ and a relative maximum at $x = 2$. Evaluating $g(x)$ at these x-values, we have

$g(0) = (0)^2e^{-(0)} = 0$, so $(0, 0)$ is a relative minimum point;

and $g(2) = (2)^2e^{-(2)} = 4e^{-2}$, so $(2, 4e^{-2})$ is a relative maximum point.

We use this information, with other points found using a calculator, to sketch the graph of g below.

x	$g(x)$, approximately
−2	29.556
−1	2.718
0	0 Relative minimum
1	0.368
2	0.541 Relative maximum
3	0.448
4	0.293

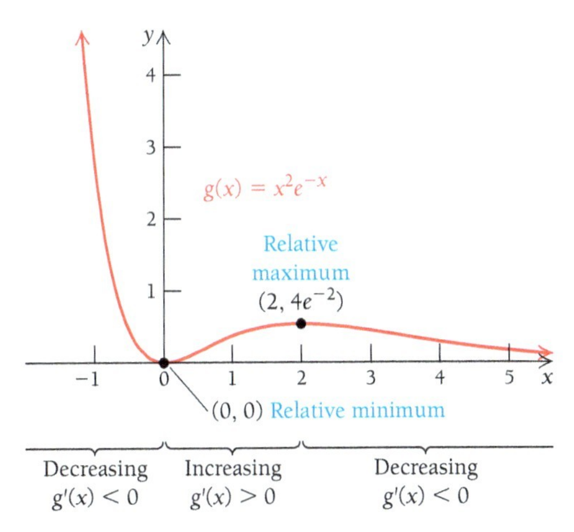

Summarizing,

- g is decreasing over the interval $(-\infty, 0)$.
- g has a relative minimum point at $(0, 0)$.
- g is increasing over the interval $(0, 2)$.
- g has a relative maximum point at $(2, 4e^{-2})$.
- g is decreasing over the interval $(2, \infty)$.

3 ✓

Quick Check 3 ✓

Find the relative extrema of the function k given by $k(x) = xe^{-x}$. Then sketch the graph.

Technology Connection 

EXERCISES

In Exercises 1 and 2, consider the function f given by

$$f(x) = 2 - (x - 1)^{2/3}.$$

1. Graph the function using the viewing window $[-4, 6, -2, 4]$.
2. Graph the first derivative. What happens to the graph of the derivative at the critical values?

EXAMPLE 4 Find the relative extrema and sketch the graph of the function f given by

$$f(x) = (x - 2)^{2/3} + 1.$$

Solution First, we find $f'(x)$ and determine any critical values:

$$f'(x) = \frac{2}{3}(x - 2)^{-1/3}$$

$$= \frac{2}{3\sqrt[3]{x - 2}}. \quad \text{Simplifying}$$

Next, we find where $f'(x)$ does not exist or where $f'(x) = 0$. Note that $f'(x)$ does not exist at 2, although $f(x)$ does. Thus, 2 is a critical value. Since the only way for a fraction to be 0 is if its numerator is 0, we see that $f'(x) = 0$ has no solution. Thus, 2 is the only critical value. We use 2 to divide the x-axis into the intervals $(-\infty, 2)$ and $(2, \infty)$.

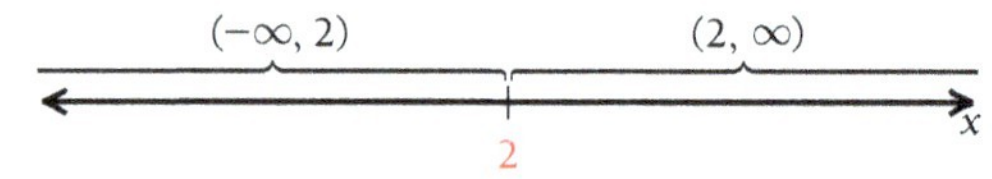

To determine the sign of $f'(x)$ we choose a test value in each interval. It is not necessary to find an exact value of the derivative; we need only determine the sign. Sometimes we can do this by just examining the formula for the derivative. We choose test values 0 and 3.

$(-\infty, 2)$: Test 0, $f'(0) = \dfrac{2}{3\sqrt[3]{0 - 2}} < 0$; Noting that the cube root of a negative number is negative

$(2, \infty)$: Test 3, $f'(3) = \dfrac{2}{3\sqrt[3]{3 - 2}} > 0$. Noting that the cube root of a positive number is positive

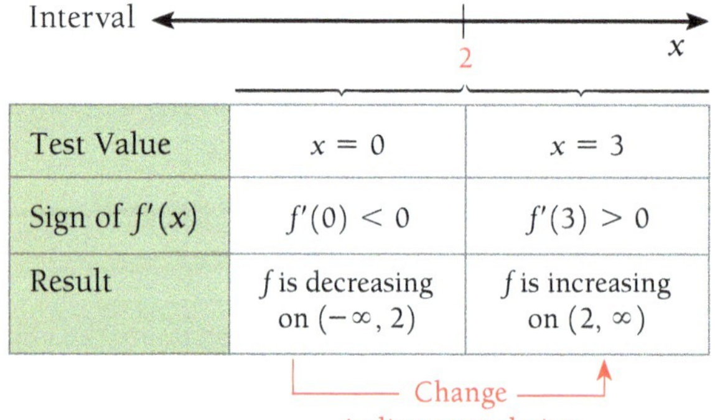

Test Value	$x = 0$	$x = 3$
Sign of $f'(x)$	$f'(0) < 0$	$f'(3) > 0$
Result	f is decreasing on $(-\infty, 2)$	f is increasing on $(2, \infty)$

Change indicates a relative minimum at $x = 2$.

Since we have a change from decreasing to increasing, we conclude from the First-Derivative Test that a relative minimum occurs at $(2, f(2))$, or $(2, 1)$. The graph has *no* tangent line at $(2, 1)$ since $f'(2)$ does not exist.

We use this information and some other function values to sketch the graph.

x	$f(x)$, approximately
−1	3.08
0	2.59
1	2
2	1
3	2
4	2.59

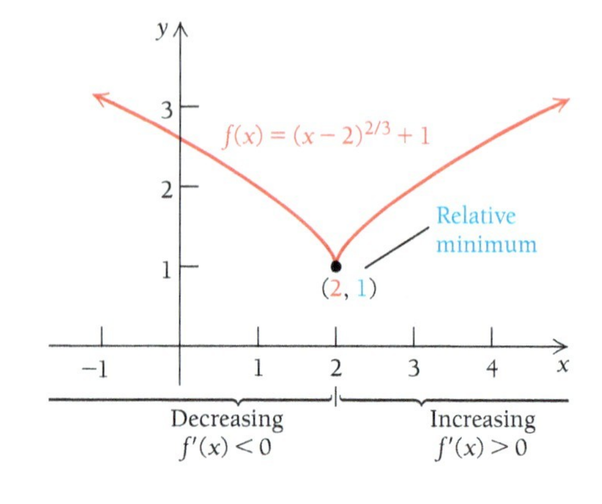

Quick Check 4 ✓

Find the relative extrema of the function g given by $g(x) = 3 - x^{1/3}$. Then sketch the graph.

- f is decreasing over the interval $(-\infty, 2)$.
- f has a relative minimum at the point $(2, 1)$.
- f is increasing over the interval $(2, \infty)$.

4 ✓

Technology Connection 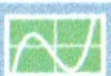

Finding Relative Extrema

To explore methods for approximating relative extrema, let's graph

$$f(x) = -0.4x^3 + 6.2x^2 - 11.3x - 54.8$$

using a window that reveals the curvature.

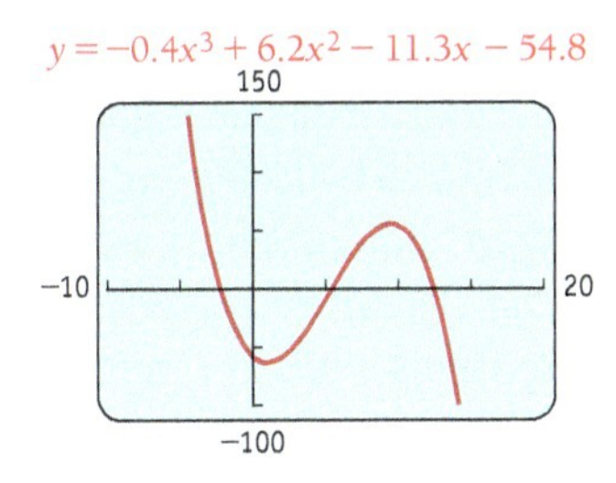

Method 1: TRACE

Using TRACE, we can move the cursor along the curve, noting where relative extrema might occur.

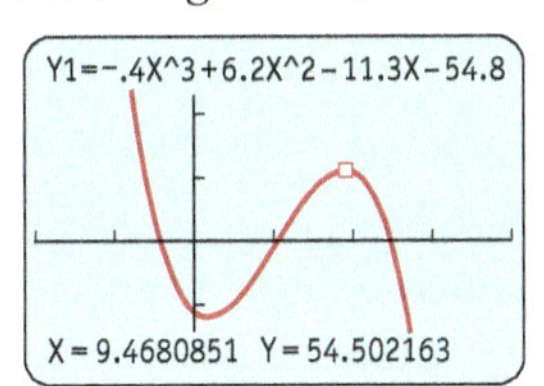

A relative maximum seems to be about $y = 54.5$ at $x = 9.47$. To refine the approximation, we zoom in, press TRACE, and move the cursor, again noting where the y-value is largest. The approximation is about $y = 54.61$ at $x = 9.31$.

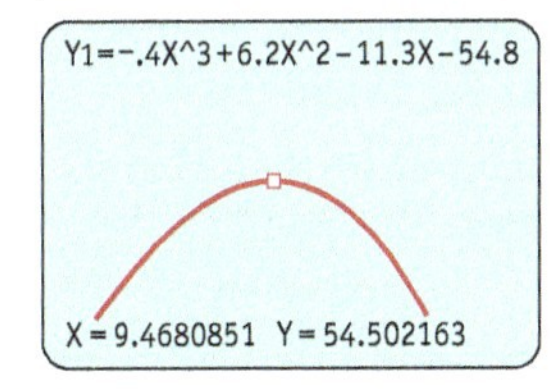

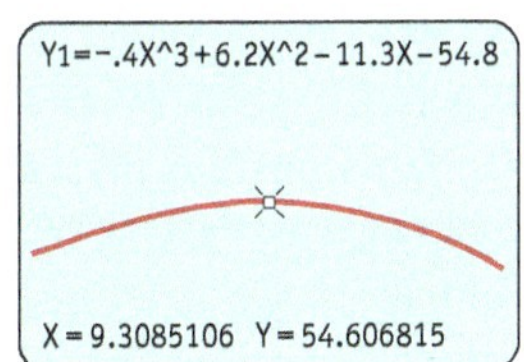

We can repeat to refine the accuracy.

Method 2: TABLE

We can also use the TABLE feature, adjusting starting points and step values to improve accuracy:

TblStart = 9.3 ΔTbl = .01

X	Y1	
9.3	54.605	
9.31	54.607	
9.32	54.608	
9.33	54.608	
9.34	54.607	
9.35	54.604	
9.36	54.601	

X=9.32

The relative maximum seems to be nearly $y = 54.61$ at an x-value between 9.32 and 9.33. We could next set up a new table showing function values between $f(9.32)$ and $f(9.33)$ to refine the approximation.

Method 3: MAXIMUM, MINIMUM

Using the MAXIMUM option from the CALC menu, we find that a relative maximum of about 54.61 occurs at $x \approx 9.32$.

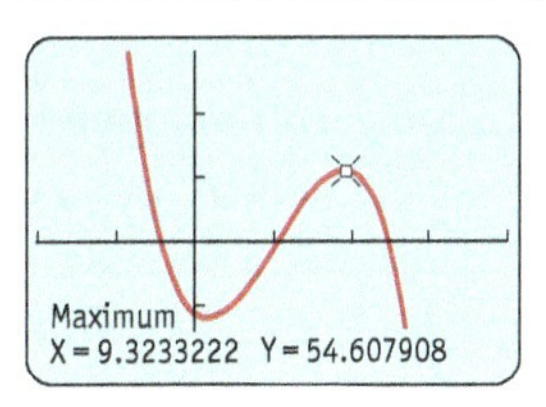

Method 4: fMax or fMin

The fMax or fMin feature calculates a relative maximum or minimum value over any closed interval. We see from the initial graph that a relative maximum occurs in $[-10, 20]$. Using the fMax option from the MATH menu, we see that a relative maximum occurs in $[-10, 20]$ when $x \approx 9.32$.

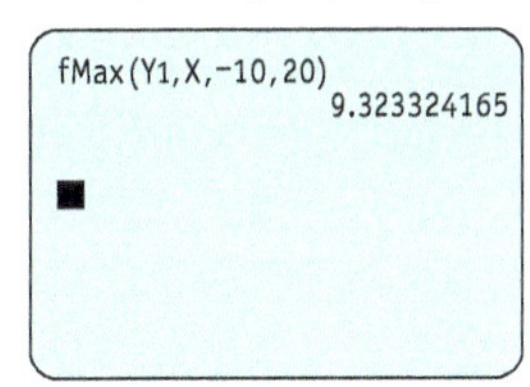

To obtain the maximum value, we evaluate the function at that x-value, obtaining the following.

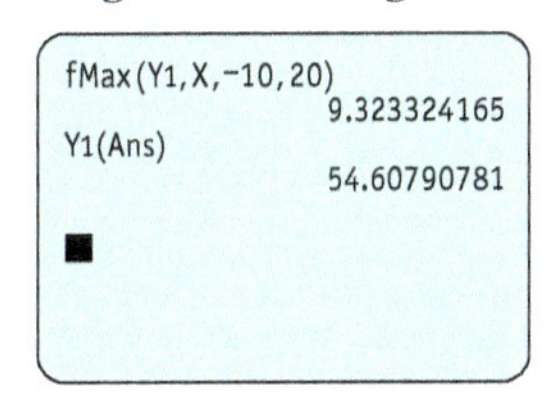

The approximation is about $y = 54.61$ at $x = 9.32$.

Using any of these methods, we find the relative minimum $y \approx -60.30$ at $x \approx 1.01$.

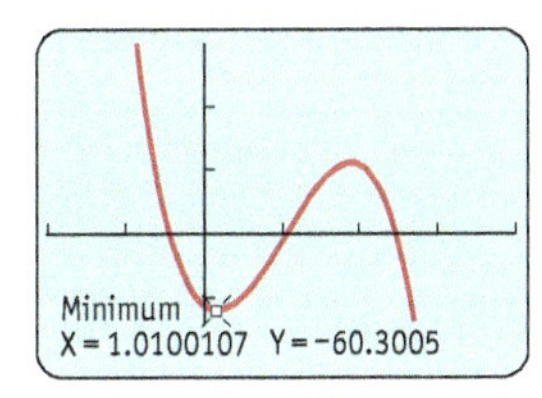

EXERCISE

1. Using at least one of the above methods, approximate the relative extrema of the function in Example 1.

Section Summary

- A function f is *increasing* over an interval I if, for all a and b in I such that $a < b$, we have $f(a) < f(b)$. Equivalently, the slope of the secant line connecting $(a, f(a))$ and $(b, f(b))$ is positive:

$$\frac{f(b) - f(a)}{b - a} > 0.$$

- A function f is *decreasing* over an interval I if, for all a and b in I such that $a < b$, we have $f(a) > f(b)$. Equivalently, the slope of the secant line connecting $(a, f(a))$ and $(b, f(b))$ is negative:

$$\frac{f(b) - f(a)}{b - a} < 0.$$

- A function f is *increasing* over an open interval I if, for all x in I, the slope of the tangent line at x is positive; that is, $f'(x) > 0$. Similarly, a function f is *decreasing* over an open interval I if, for all x in I, the slope of the tangent line is negative; that is, $f'(x) < 0$.
- A *critical value* is a number c in the domain of f such that $f'(c) = 0$ or $f'(c)$ does not exist. The point $(c, f(c))$ is called a *critical point*.
- Minimum and maximum values are collectively called *extrema*.
- A *relative extreme point*, $(c, f(c))$, is higher or lower than all other points over an open interval containing c. A *relative minimum point*, $(c, f(c))$, is lower than all other points over an open interval containing c. A relative minimum point has a y-value that is *less* than those of a neighborhood of points to the left and right of c. Similarly, a *relative maximum point*, $(c, f(c))$, is higher than all other points over an open interval containing c. A relative maximum point has a y-value that is *greater* than those of a neighborhood of points to the left and right of c.
- Critical points are candidates for possible relative extrema. The *First-Derivative Test* is used to determine if a critical value yields a relative minimum, a relative maximum, or neither.

3.1 Exercise Set

For each graph in Exercises 1–4, identify all (a) critical values, (b) relative minima, (c) relative maxima, (d) relative minimum points, and (e) relative maximum points.

1.

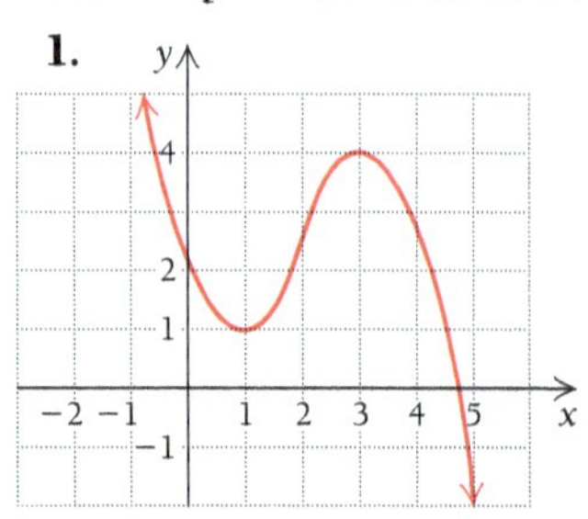

2.

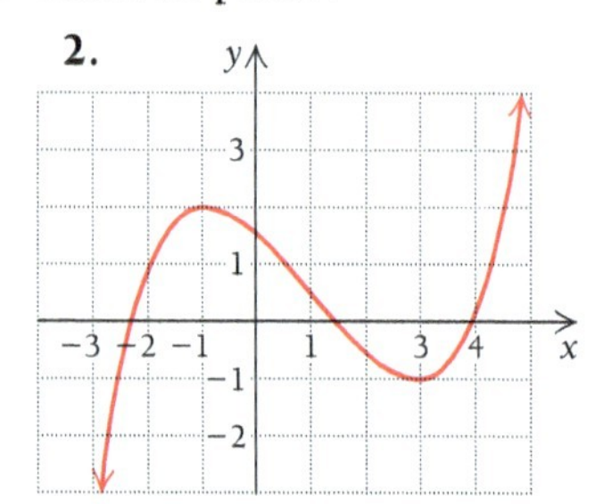

3.

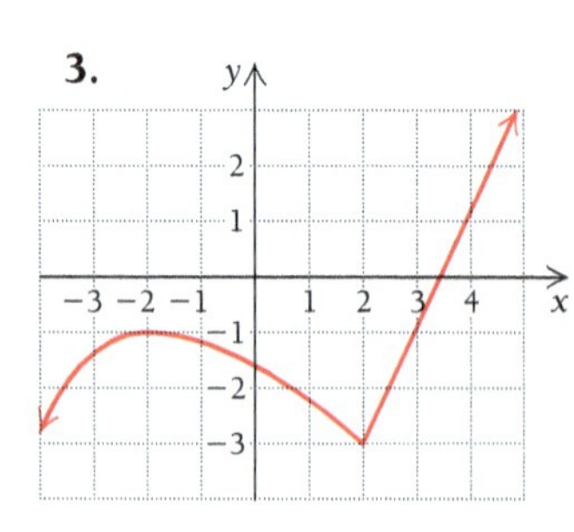

4.

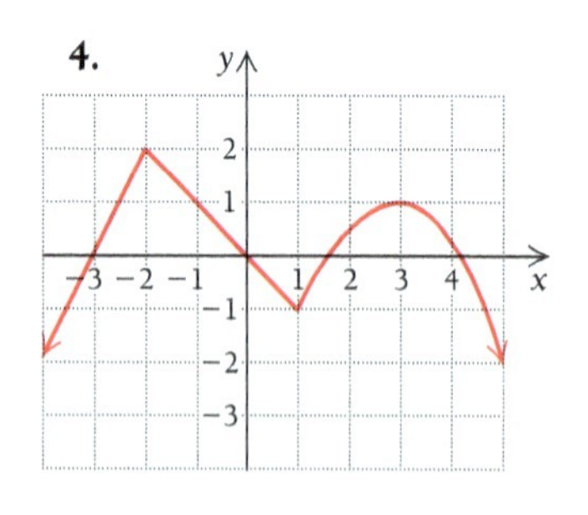

For Exercises 5–16, draw a graph to match the description given. Answers will vary.

5. $f(x)$ is increasing over $(-\infty, 2)$ and decreasing over $(2, \infty)$.

6. $g(x)$ is decreasing over $(-\infty, -3)$ and increasing over $(-3, \infty)$.

7. $G(x)$ is decreasing over $(-\infty, 4)$ and $(9, \infty)$ and increasing over $(4, 9)$.

8. $F(x)$ is increasing over $(-\infty, 5)$ and $(12, \infty)$ and decreasing over $(5, 12)$.

9. $g(x)$ has a positive derivative over $(-\infty, -3)$ and a negative derivative over $(-3, \infty)$.

10. $f(x)$ has a negative derivative over $(-\infty, 1)$ and a positive derivative over $(1, \infty)$.

11. $F(x)$ has a negative derivative over $(-\infty, 2)$ and $(5, 9)$ and a positive derivative over $(2, 5)$ and $(9, \infty)$.

12. $G(x)$ has a positive derivative over $(-\infty, -2)$ and $(4, 7)$ and a negative derivative over $(-2, 4)$ and $(7, \infty)$.

13. $g(x)$ has a negative derivative over $(-\infty, 5)$ and $(5, 8)$, a positive derivative over $(8, \infty)$, and a derivative equal to 0 at $x = 5$.

14. $G(x)$ has a positive derivative over $(-\infty, 0)$ and $(3, \infty)$ and a negative derivative over $(0, 3)$, but neither $G'(0)$ nor $G'(3)$ exists.

15. $g(x)$ has a positive derivative over $(-\infty, -3)$ and $(0, 3)$, a negative derivative over $(-3, 0)$ and $(3, \infty)$, and a derivative equal to 0 at $x = -3$ and $x = 3$, but $g'(0)$ does not exist.

16. $K(x)$ is decreasing over $(-\infty, \infty)$, but the derivative does not exist at $x = 0$ and $x = 2$.

For each function given in Exercises 17–32, find (a) any critical values and (b) any relative extrema.

17. $f(x) = x^2 + 2x + 2$

18. $f(x) = x^2 - 6x + 1$

19. $g(x) = x^3 - 12x + 5$
20. $g(x) = x^3 - 3x - 6$
21. $h(x) = x^3 - 6x^2 - 15x + 1$
22. $h(x) = x^3 + \frac{11}{2}x^2 + 6x + 1$
23. $k(x) = |x - 2|$
24. $k(x) = |1 - 3x| + 2$
25. $d(x) = (x - 2)^{2/3} + 5$
26. $d(x) = (3 - x)^{2/3} - 1$
27. $t(x) = x^3 + 4x - 2$
28. $t(x) = x^3 + x - 5$
29. $f(x) = xe^{4x}$
30. $f(x) = xe^{-6x}$
31. $g(x) = \ln(x^2 + 2x + 6)$
32. $g(x) = \ln(x^2 + 4x + 10)$

For Exercises 33–46, find any relative extrema of each function. List each extremum along with the x-value at which it occurs. Identify intervals over which the function is increasing and over which it is decreasing. Then sketch a graph of the function.

33. $f(x) = x^2 + 6x - 3$
34. $f(x) = 5 - x - x^2$
35. $F(x) = 0.5x^2 + 2x - 11$
36. $g(x) = 1 + 6x + 3x^2$
37. $g(x) = x^3 + \frac{1}{2}x^2 - 2x + 5$
38. $G(x) = x^3 - x^2 - x + 2$
39. $f(x) = x^3 - 3x^2$
40. $f(x) = 3x^2 + 2x^3$
41. $F(x) = 1 - x^3$
42. $g(x) = 2x^3 - 16$
43. $h(x) = xe^{2x}$
44. $k(x) = xe^{-3x}$
45. $f(x) = e^{2x} - e^x$
46. $m(x) = e^x - e^{4x}$

For Exercises 47–64, find all relative extrema and sketch the graph.

47. $G(x) = x^3 - 6x^2 + 10$
48. $f(x) = 12 + 9x - 3x^2 - x^3$
49. $g(x) = x^3 - x^4$
50. $f(x) = x^4 - 2x^3$
51. $G(x) = \sqrt[3]{x + 2}$
52. $F(x) = \sqrt[3]{x - 1}$
53. $f(x) = 1 - x^{2/3}$
54. $f(x) = (x + 3)^{2/3} - 5$
55. $G(x) = \dfrac{-8}{x^2 + 1}$
56. $F(x) = \dfrac{5}{x^2 + 1}$
57. $k(x) = e^x - 2x$
58. $g(x) = e^x - 4x$
59. $f(x) = e^{x^2-4x}$
60. $r(x) = e^{x^2+3x}$
61. $k(x) = x^3e^{3x}$
62. $g(x) = x^3e^{-2x}$
63. $F(x) = \ln(x^2 + x + 3)$
64. $G(x) = \ln(x^2 + 4x + 7)$
65. Consider this graph.

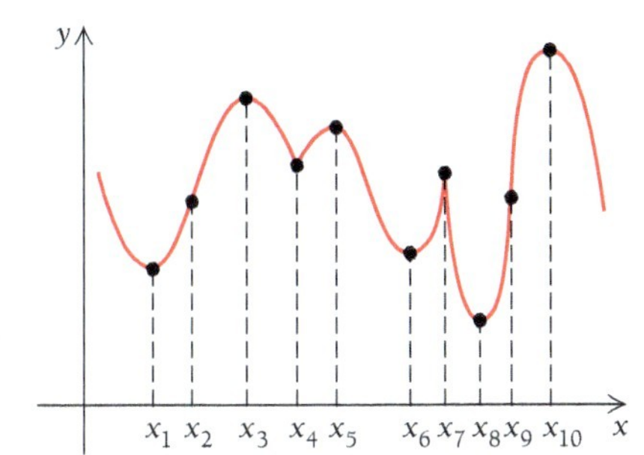

What makes an x-value a critical value? Which x-values shown on the graph are critical values, and why?

66. Consider this graph.

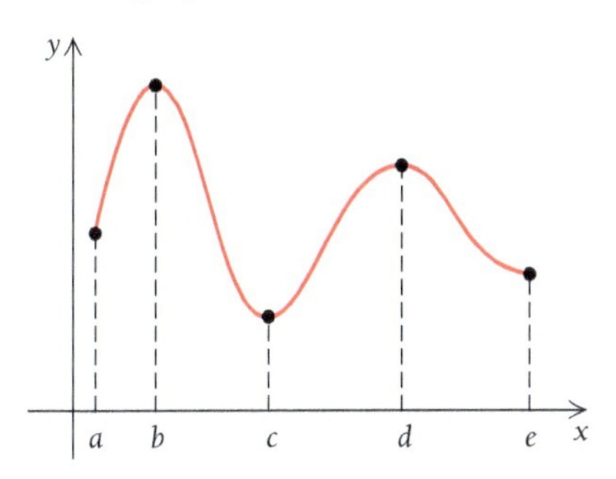

Using the graph and the intervals noted, explain how a function being increasing or decreasing relates to the first derivative.

APPLICATIONS

Business and Economics

67. **Optimizing revenue.** A hotel owner notices that she rents y rooms per night when the price is x dollars per room, with $y = 200 - 2x$.
    a) Find $R(x)$, the total revenue generated per night when the price of each room is x dollars.
    b) Find the relative extremum of R, and interpret this result.
68. **Optimizing revenue.** A software developer notices that the number y of downloads of an app (in thousands) is related to the price x (in dollars) of the app by $y = 2.6 - 0.4x$.
    a) Find $R(x)$, the total revenue generated when the price of the app is x dollars.
    b) Find the relative extremum of R, and interpret this result.
69. **Optimizing revenue.** An artist sells y sculptures when the price of each sculpture is x dollars, where $y = 500 - 5x$.
    a) Find $R(x)$, the total revenue generated when the price of each sculpture is x dollars.
    b) Find the relative extremum of R, and interpret this result.
70. **Optimizing yield.** Each apple tree yields y apples when there are x trees in an orchard, where $y = 300 - 6x$.
    a) Find $R(x)$, the total yield generated when there are x apple trees in the orchard.
    b) Find the relative extremum of R, and interpret this result.

Life and Physical Sciences

71. **Solar eclipse.** On July 2, 2019, a total solar eclipse was observable over the South Pacific Ocean and parts of South America. (*Source*: eclipse.gsfc.nasa.gov.) The path of the eclipse is modeled by

$$f(t) = 0.00259t^2 - 0.457t + 36.237,$$

where $f(t)$ is the latitude in degrees south of the equator at t minutes after the start of the total eclipse. What is the latitude closest to the equator, in degrees, at which the total eclipse was visible?

72. Temperature during an illness. The temperature (in °F) of a person during an intestinal illness is given by

$$T(t) = -0.1t^2 + 1.2t + 98.6, \quad 0 \le t \le 12,$$

where $T(t)$ is the temperature t days after the onset of the illness. Find the relative extrema and sketch a graph of the function.

SYNTHESIS

In Exercises 73–78, the graph of a derivative f' is shown. Use the information in each graph to determine where f is increasing or decreasing and the x-values of any extrema. Then sketch a possible graph of f.

73.

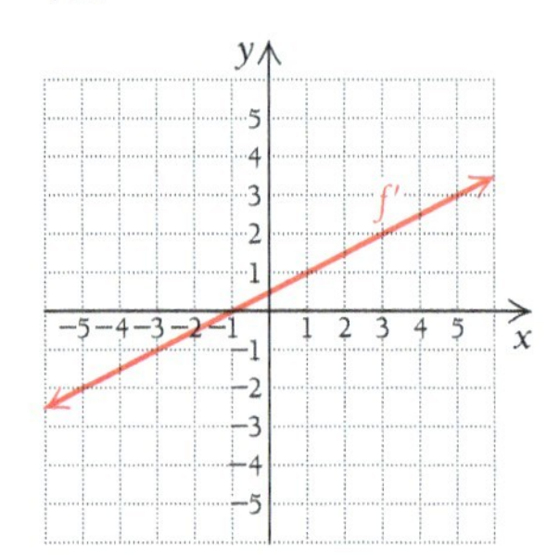

74.

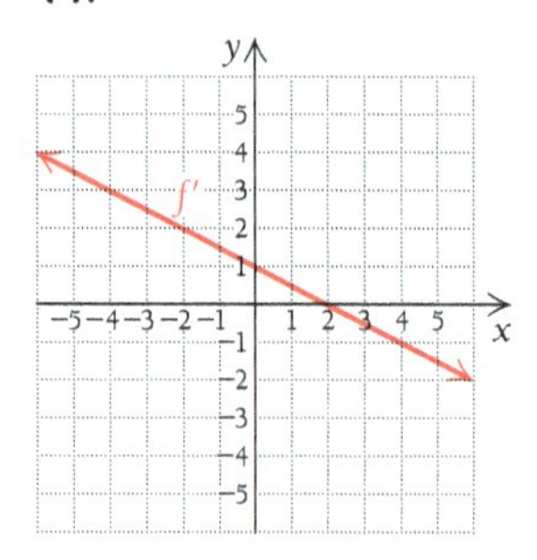

75.

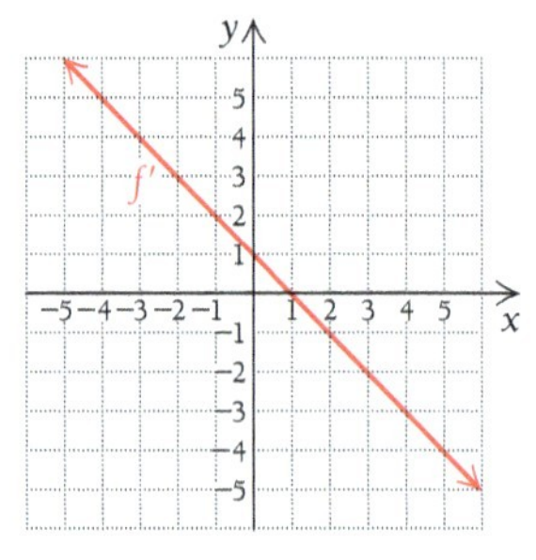

76.

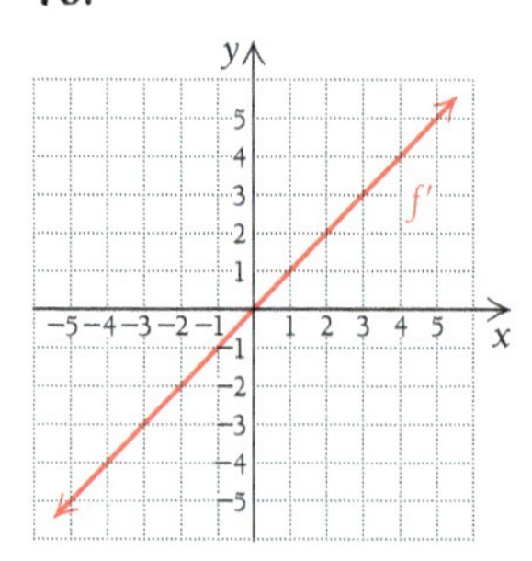

77.

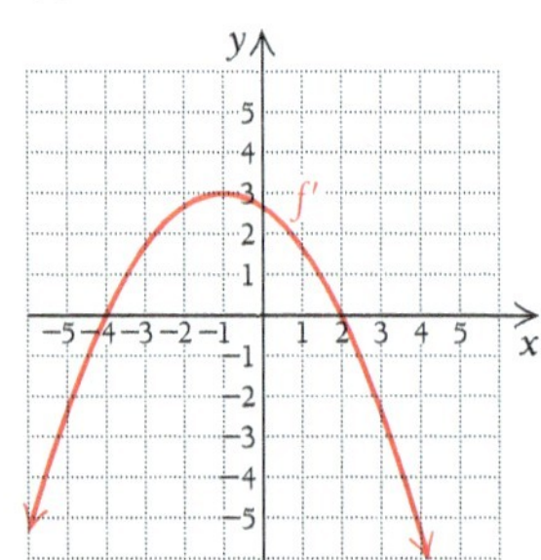

78.

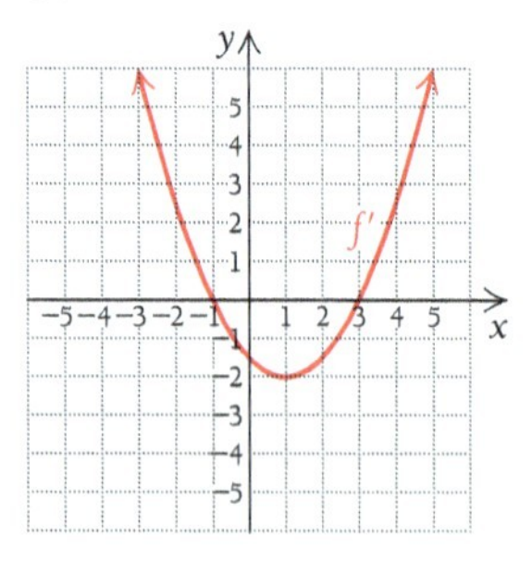

79. Find a function of the form $f(x) = x^2 + ax + b$ such that its minimum point is $(3, 7)$.

80. Find a function of the form $g(x) = -x^2 + ax + b$ such that its maximum point is $(-2, 5)$.

81. Find a function of the form $h(x) = xe^{ax}$ that has a relative maximum at $x = \frac{1}{5}$.

82. Find a function of the form $h(x) = -xe^{ax}$ that has a relative minimum at $x = 2$.

83. Let $f(x) = x^2 + ax + 4$.

a) Find a such that f has a critical value at $x = 5$.
b) Find $f(5)$, using the value for a found in part (a).
c) Classify $f(5)$ as a relative maximum, a relative minimum, or neither.

84. Let $g(x) = -x^2 + ax - 2$.

a) Find a such that g has a critical value at $x = -3$.
b) Find $g(-3)$, using the value for a found in part (a).
c) Classify $g(-3)$ as a relative maximum, a relative minimum, or neither.

85. Let $h(x) = e^{x^2+ax}$.

a) Find a such that h has a critical value at $x = -2$.
b) Find $h(-2)$, using the value for a found in part (a).
c) Classify $h(-2)$ as a relative maximum, a relative minimum, or neither.

86. Let $r(x) = e^{3x^2+ax}$.

a) Find a such that r has a critical value at $x = 1$.
b) Find $r(1)$, using the value for a found in part (a).
c) Classify $r(1)$ as a relative maximum, a relative minimum, or neither.

87. Let $F(x) = xe^{ax}$.

a) Find a such that F has a critical value at $x = \frac{1}{2}$.
b) Find $F\left(\frac{1}{2}\right)$, using the value for a found in part (a).
c) Classify $F\left(\frac{1}{2}\right)$ as a relative maximum, a relative minimum, or neither.

88. Let $G(x) = -xe^{ax}$.

a) Find a such that G has a critical value at $x = 1$.
b) Find $G(1)$, using the value for a found in part (a).
c) Classify $G(1)$ as a relative maximum, a relative minimum, or neither.

Technology Connection 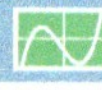

Graph each function. Then estimate any relative extrema.

89. $f(x) = -x^6 - 4x^5 + 54x^4 + 160x^3 - 641x^2 - 828x + 1200$

90. $f(x) = x\sqrt{9 - x^2}$

Use a calculator's absolute-value feature to graph each function and determine relative extrema and intervals over which the function is increasing or decreasing. State any x-values at which the derivative does not exist.

91. $f(x) = |x - 2|$

92. $f(x) = |x^2 - 3x + 2|$

93. $f(x) = |x^2 - 1|$

94. $f(x) = |x^3 - 1|$

95. $f(x) = |2 - e^x|$

96. $f(x) = |\ln(x - 3)|$

Life science: caloric intake and life expectancy. *The data in the following table give, for various countries for the period 2007–2014, daily caloric intake, projected life expectancy, and under-five mortality. Use the data for Exercises 97 and 98.*

Country	Daily Caloric Intake	Life Expectancy at Birth (in years)	Under-Five Mortality (number of deaths before age 5 per 1000 births)
Argentina	3030	76	14
Australia	3220	82	5
Bolivia	2100	66	51
Canada	3530	81	6
Dominican Republic	2270	73	25
Germany	3540	80	4
Haiti	1850	62	70
Mexico	3260	77	17
United States	3750	78	8
Venezuela	2650	74	16

(*Source: U.N. FAO Statistical Yearbook*, 2017.)

97. Life expectancy and daily caloric intake.

a) Use the regression procedures of Section R.7 to fit a cubic function $y = f(x)$ to the data in the table, where x is daily caloric intake and y is life expectancy. Then fit a quartic function and decide which fits best.

b) What is the domain of the function?

c) Does the function have any relative extrema?

98. Under-five mortality and daily caloric intake.

a) Use the regression procedures of Section R.7 to fit a cubic function $y = f(x)$ to the data in the table, where x is daily caloric intake and y is under-five mortality. Then fit a quartic function and decide which fits best.

b) What is the domain of the function?

c) Does the function have any relative extrema?

Answers to Quick Checks

1. Relative maximum at $(-3, 48)$, relative minimum at $(3, -60)$

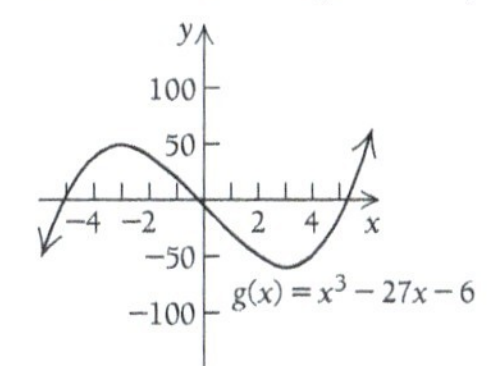

2. Relative minimum at $(2, -\frac{16}{3})$

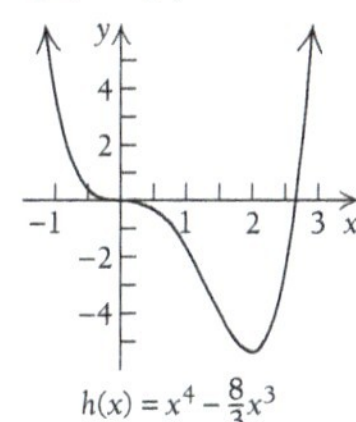

3. Relative maximum at $(1, e^{-1})$

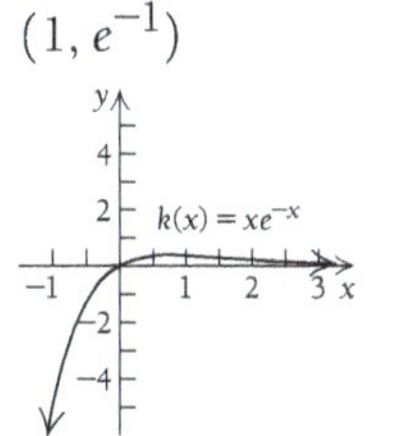

4. There are no extrema.

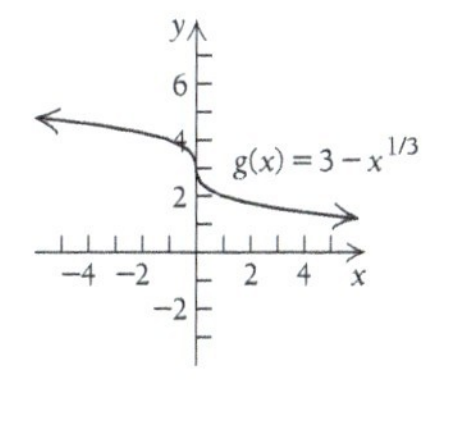

3.2 Using Second Derivatives to Classify Maximum and Minimum Values and Sketch Graphs

- Classify the relative extrema of a function using the Second-Derivative Test.
- Graph a continuous function in a manner that shows concavity.

The graphs of two continuous functions are shown at the top of the next page. The graph of f bends upward and the graph of g bends downward. Let's relate these observations to each function's derivative.

We draw tangent lines moving along the graph of f from left to right. What happens to the slopes of the tangent lines? We do the same for the graph of g. Is there a relationship between the changing slopes and the way the graph bends?

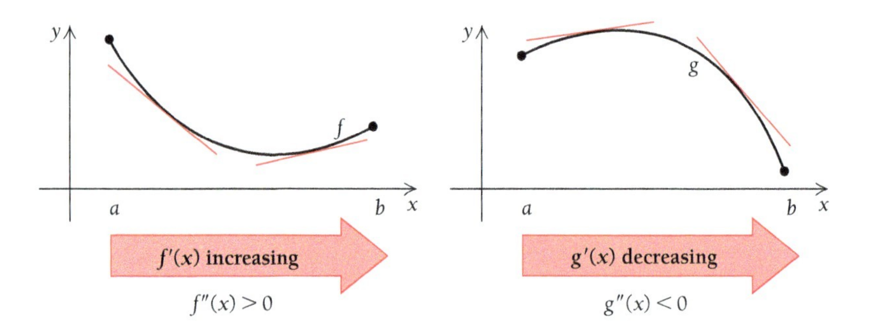

Concavity: Increasing and Decreasing Derivatives

For the graph of f, the slopes of the tangent lines are increasing. That is, f' is increasing over the interval. This can be determined by noting that $f''(x)$ is positive, since the relationship between f' and f'' is like the relationship between f and f'. For the graph of g, the slopes are decreasing. This can be determined by noting that g' is decreasing whenever $g''(x)$ is negative. The bending of each curve is called the graph's *concavity*.

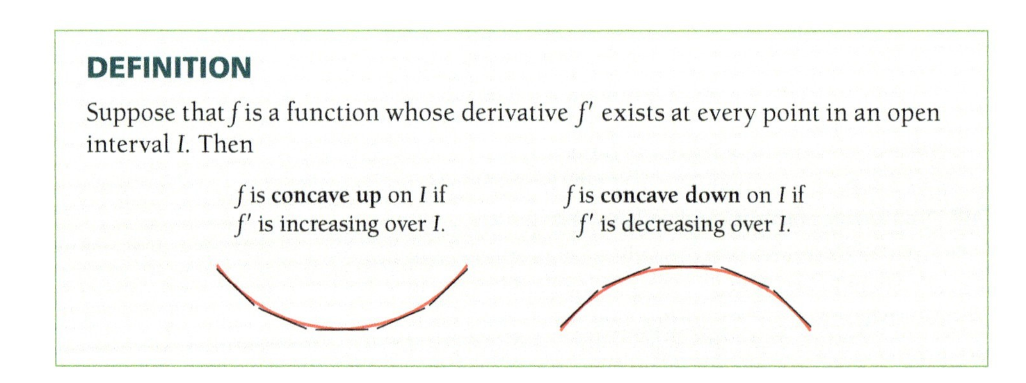

DEFINITION

Suppose that f is a function whose derivative f' exists at every point in an open interval I. Then

f is **concave up** on I if f' is increasing over I.

f is **concave down** on I if f' is decreasing over I.

The following theorem states how concavity and the second derivative are related.

THEOREM 4 A Test for Concavity

1. If $f''(x) > 0$ for all x on an open interval I, then the graph of f is concave up on I.

2. If $f''(x) < 0$ for all x on an open interval I, then the graph of f is concave down on I.

A function can be decreasing and concave up, decreasing and concave down, increasing and concave up, or increasing and concave down. That is, *concavity* and *increasing/decreasing* are separate concepts. It is the increasing or decreasing aspect of the *derivative* that tells us about the function's concavity. The following table summarizes these relationships.

Technology Connection 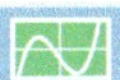

Exploratory

Graph

$$f(x) = -\tfrac{1}{3}x^3 + 6x^2 - 11x - 50$$

and its second derivative,

$$f''(x) = -2x + 12,$$

using the viewing window $[-10, 25, -100, 150]$, with Xscl = 5 and Yscl = 25.

Over what intervals is the graph of f concave up? Over what intervals is the graph of f concave down? Over what intervals is the graph of f'' positive? Over what intervals is the graph of f'' negative? How do you think the sign of $f''(x)$ relates to the concavity of f?

Now graph the first derivative,

$$f'(x) = -x^2 + 12x - 11,$$

and the second derivative,

$$f''(x) = -2x + 12,$$

using $[-10, 25, -200, 50]$, with Xscl = 5 and Yscl = 25.

Over what intervals is the first derivative f' increasing? Over what intervals is the first derivative f' decreasing? Over what intervals is $f''(x)$ positive? Over what intervals is $f''(x)$ negative? How does the sign of $f''(x)$ relate to the concavity of f?

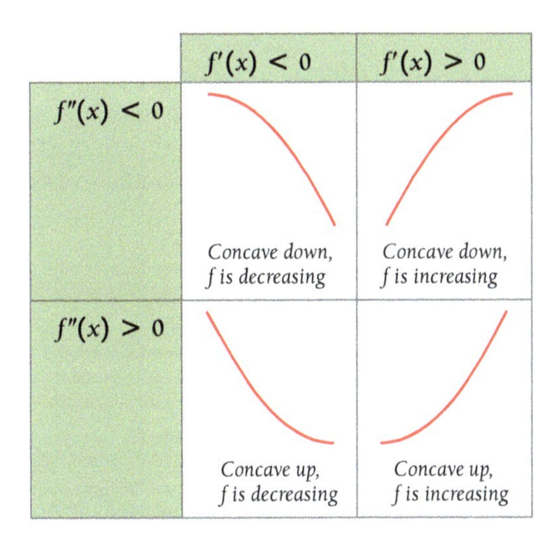

Classifying Relative Extrema Using Second Derivatives

Let's see how we can use second derivatives to determine whether a function has a relative extremum on an open interval.

The following graphs show both types of concavity at a critical value, where $f'(c) = 0$. When the second derivative is positive (graph is concave up) at the critical value, the critical point is a relative minimum point, and when the second derivative is negative (graph is concave down), the critical point is a relative maximum point.

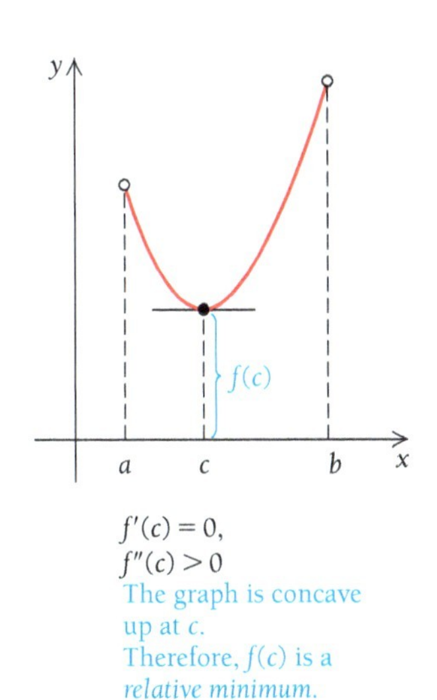

$f'(c) = 0$,
$f''(c) > 0$
The graph is concave up at c.
Therefore, $f(c)$ is a *relative minimum*.

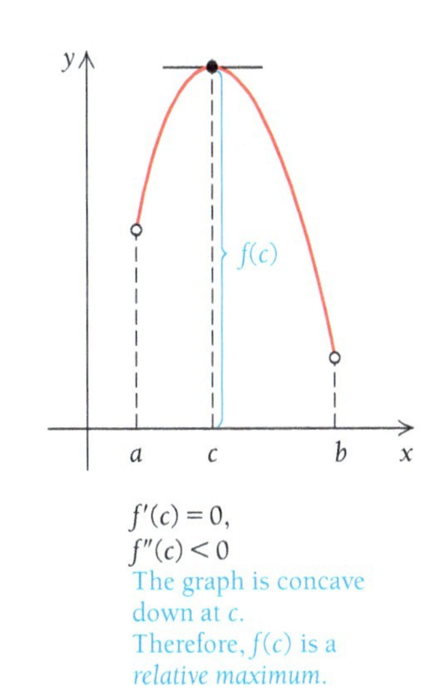

$f'(c) = 0$,
$f''(c) < 0$
The graph is concave down at c.
Therefore, $f(c)$ is a *relative maximum*.

This analysis is summarized in Theorem 5:

THEOREM 5 The Second-Derivative Test for Relative Extrema

Suppose that f is differentiable for every x in an open interval (a, b) and that there is a critical value c in (a, b) for which $f'(c) = 0$. Then:

1. $f(c)$ is a relative minimum if $f''(c) > 0$.

2. $f(c)$ is a relative maximum if $f''(c) < 0$.

For $f''(c) = 0$, the First-Derivative Test can be used to determine whether $f(x)$ is a relative extremum.

When c is a critical value and $f''(c) = 0$, an extremum may or may not exist at c. Consider the following graphs. In each one, $f'(x)$ and $f''(x)$ are both 0 at $c = 2$, but the function in the graph on the left has an extremum and the other function does not. An approach other than the Second-Derivative Test must be used to determine whether $f(c)$ is an extremum in cases like this.

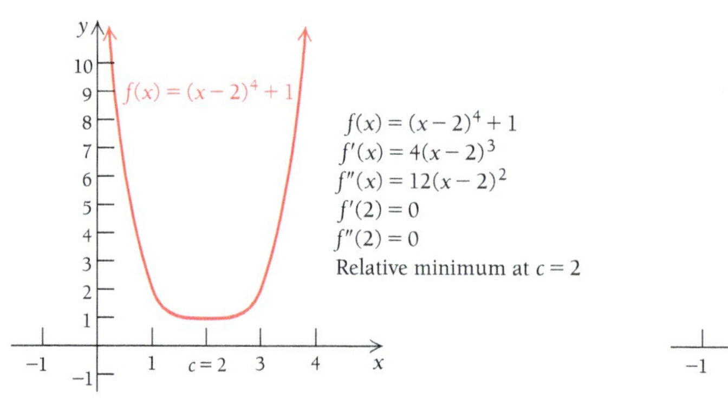

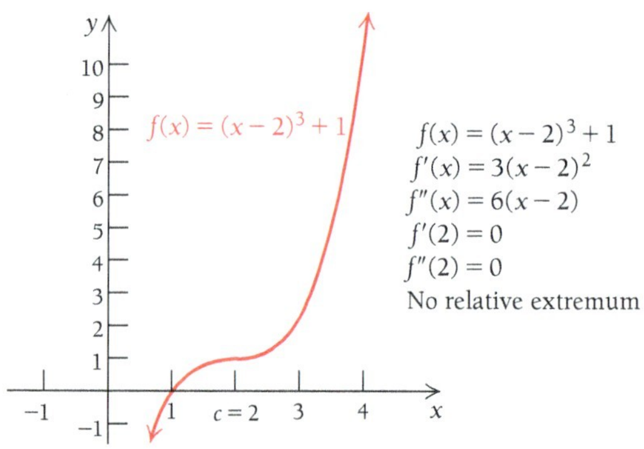

The second derivative is used to help identify extrema and determine the overall behavior of a graph, as we see in the following examples.

EXAMPLE 1 Find any relative extrema and graph the function f given by

$$f(x) = x^3 + 3x^2 - 9x - 13.$$

Solution We find the first derivative:

$$f'(x) = 3x^2 + 6x - 9.$$

To find any critical values, we solve $f'(x) = 0$:

$$3x^2 + 6x - 9 = 0$$

$$x^2 + 2x - 3 = 0 \quad \text{Dividing both sides by 3}$$

$$(x + 3)(x - 1) = 0 \quad \text{Factoring}$$

$$x + 3 = 0 \quad or \quad x - 1 = 0 \quad \text{Using the Principle of Zero Products}$$

$$x = -3 \quad or \quad x = 1. \quad \text{The critical values are } -3 \text{ and } 1.$$

We next find second coordinates by substituting the critical values in the original function, f:

$$f(-3) = (-3)^3 + 3(-3)^2 - 9(-3) - 13 = 14;$$

$$f(1) = (1)^3 + 3(1)^2 - 9(1) - 13 = -18.$$

The critical points are $(-3, 14)$ and $(1, -18)$.

Next, we find the second derivative:

$$f''(x) = 6x + 6.$$

We use the Second-Derivative Test with the critical values -3 and 1:

$$f''(-3) = 6(-3) + 6 = -12 < 0; \longrightarrow \text{Relative maximum and concave down at } x = -3$$

and

$$f''(1) = 6(1) + 6 = 12 > 0. \longrightarrow \text{Relative minimum and concave up at } x = 1$$

Thus, $f(-3) = 14$ is a relative maximum and $f(1) = -18$ is a relative minimum. We plot both $(-3, 14)$ and $(1, -18)$, including short arcs at each point to indicate the concavity, as shown in the graph on the left at the top of the next page. By plotting more points, we can make a sketch, as shown in the graph on the right.

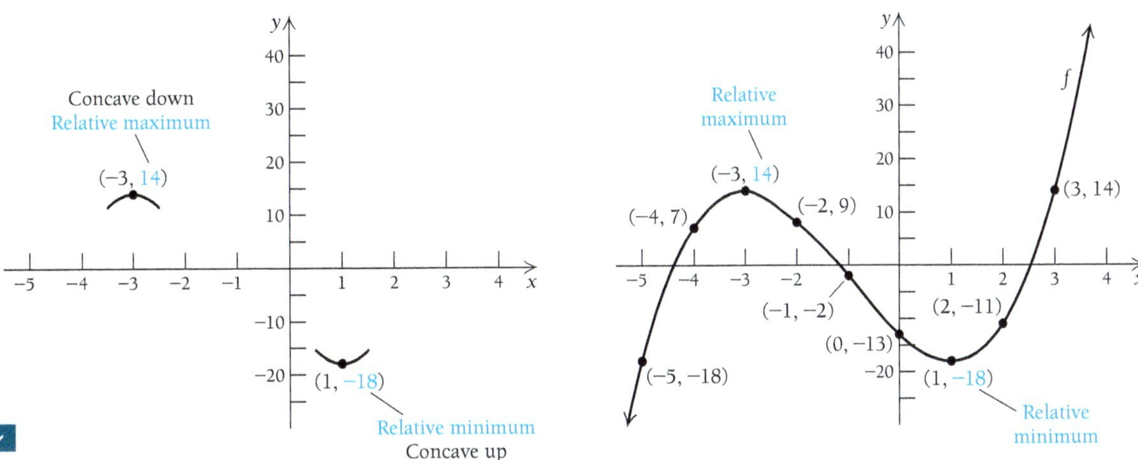

Quick Check 1 ✓

Find any relative extrema and graph $g(x) = x^3 - 12x$.

1 ✓

EXAMPLE 2 Find any relative extrema and graph the function k given by

$$k(x) = e^{2x} - e^x.$$

Solution We find the first derivative:

$$k'(x) = 2e^{2x} - e^x.$$

To find any critical values, we solve $k'(x) = 0$:

$$2e^{2x} - e^x = 0$$

$$e^x(2e^x - 1) = 0 \quad \text{Factoring by recalling that } e^x \cdot e^x = e^{x+x} = e^{2x}$$

$$2e^x - 1 = 0 \quad \text{Since } e^x > 0, \text{ only the factor } 2e^x - 1 \text{ can yield a solution.}$$

$$e^x = \frac{1}{2} = 0.5$$

$$x = \ln 0.5 \quad \text{Using the definition of logarithm}$$

The critical value is ln 0.5, or, using a calculator, about -0.693.

We next find the second coordinate by substituting the critical value in the original function k:

$$\begin{aligned} k(\ln 0.5) &= e^{2(\ln 0.5)} - e^{\ln 0.5} \\ &= e^{\ln 0.5^2} - e^{\ln 0.5} && \text{Using the property } b \ln x = \ln x^b \\ &= 0.5^2 - 0.5 && \text{Using the property } e^{\ln x} = x \\ &= 0.25 - 0.5 \\ &= -0.25. \end{aligned}$$

Next, we find the second derivative:

$$k''(x) = 4e^{2x} - e^x.$$

We use the Second-Derivative Test with the critical value ln 0.5:

$$\begin{aligned} k''(\ln 0.5) &= 4e^{2(\ln 0.5)} - e^{\ln 0.5} \\ &= 4e^{\ln 0.5^2} - e^{\ln 0.5} \\ &= 4(0.25) - 0.5 && \text{Using the property } e^{\ln x} = x \\ &= 0.5 > 0. && \longrightarrow \text{Relative minimum and concave up at } x = \ln 0.5 \end{aligned}$$

Since the second derivative is positive at ln 0.5, we conclude that $k(\ln 0.5) = -0.25$ is a relative minimum. We plot $(\ln 0.5, -0.25)$ and complete the graph (shown on the next page) by plotting other points as needed.

(ln 0.5, −0.25)
Relative minimum
Concave up

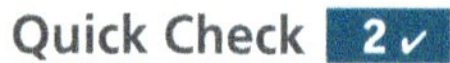

Find any relative extrema and graph $h(x) = xe^{-x}$.

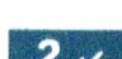

Points of Inflection

A point at which concavity changes from down to up or from up to down is called a **point of inflection**, or an **inflection point**. In the figures below, point P is an inflection point. The figures display the sign of $f''(x)$ to indicate the concavity on either side of P.

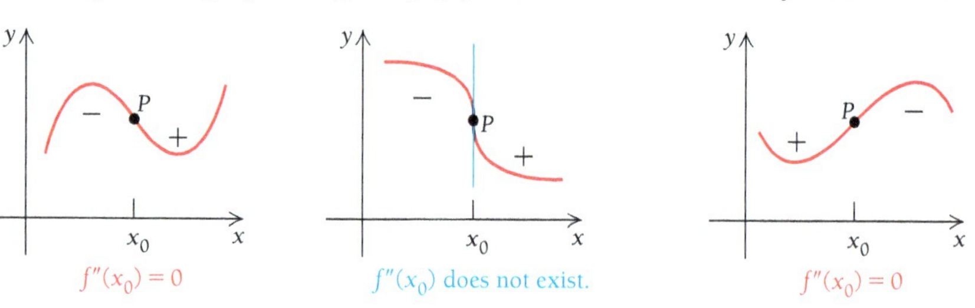

As we move along each curve, the concavity changes at P. Since the sign of $f''(x)$ changes, the value of $f''(x_0)$ at P either must be 0 or must not exist.

THEOREM 6 Finding Points of Inflection

If f has a point of inflection, it must occur at a value x_0, in the domain of f, where

$$f''(x_0) = 0 \quad \text{or} \quad f''(x_0) \text{ does not exist.}$$

The converse of Theorem 6 is not necessarily true. That is, if $f''(x_0)$ is 0 or does not exist, then there is not necessarily a point of inflection at x_0. There must be a change in concavity on either side of x_0 for $(x_0, f(x_0))$ to be a point of inflection. For example, for $f(x) = (x - 2)^4 + 1$ (see the graph on p. 282), we have $f''(2) = 0$, but $(2, f(2))$ is not a point of inflection since the graph of f is concave up on both sides of $x = 2$.

To find *candidates* for points of inflection, we look for x-values at which $f''(x) = 0$ or $f''(x)$ does not exist. If $f''(x)$ changes sign on either side of the x-value, we have a point of inflection.

EXAMPLE 3 Find the points of inflection on the graphs of

a) $f(x) = x^3 + 3x^2 - 9x - 13$ (see Example 1);

b) $k(x) = e^{2x} - e^x$ (see Example 2).

Solution

a) In Example 1, the second derivative of $f(x) = x^3 + 3x^2 - 9x - 13$ is $f''(x) = 6x + 6$. We set $f''(x) = 0$ to find x-values of possible points of inflection:

$$6x + 6 = 0 \qquad \text{Setting } f''(x) \text{ equal to } 0$$
$$x = -1.$$

We now check to see if the sign of $f''(x)$ changes at $x = -1$:

Interval $(-\infty, -1)$: Test -2: $f''(-2) = 6(-2) + 6 = -6 < 0$
f is concave down on $(-\infty, -1)$.

Interval $(-1, \infty)$: Test 0: $f''(0) = 6(0) + 6 = 6 > 0$
f is concave up on $(-1, \infty)$.

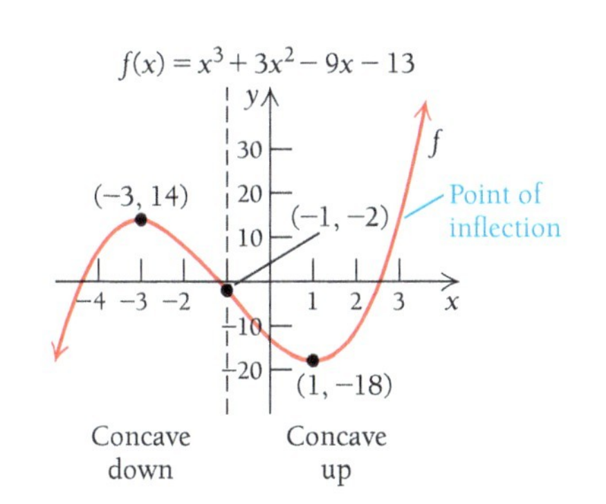

The second coordinate at $x = -1$ is $f(-1) = -2$. The sign of $f''(x)$ changes on either side of $x = -1$, so $(-1, -2)$ is a point of inflection, as shown in the graph at the left.

b) In Example 2, the second derivative of $k(x) = e^{2x} - e^x$ is $k''(x) = 4e^{2x} - e^x$. We set $k''(x) = 0$ and solve:

$$4e^{2x} - e^x = 0 \qquad \text{Setting } k''(x) \text{ equal to } 0$$
$$e^x(4e^x - 1) = 0 \qquad \text{Factoring}$$
$$4e^x - 1 = 0 \qquad \text{Only the factor } 4e^x - 1 \text{ can provide a solution since } e^x \text{ is never } 0.$$
$$e^x = 0.25$$
$$x = \ln 0.25.$$

We now check that the sign of $k''(x)$ changes at $x = \ln 0.25 \approx -1.386$:

Interval $(-\infty, -1.386)$: Test -2: $k''(-2) = 4e^{2(-2)} - e^{-2}$
$= 4e^{-4} - e^{-2} \approx -0.06 < 0.$
k is concave down on $(-\infty, -1.386)$.

Interval $(-1.386, \infty)$: Test 0: $k''(0) = 4e^{2(0)} - e^0 = 3 > 0.$
k is concave up on $(-1.386, \infty)$.

The second coordinate at $x = \ln 0.25$ is

$$\begin{aligned} k(\ln 0.25) &= e^{2(\ln 0.25)} - e^{\ln 0.25} \\ &= e^{\ln 0.25^2} - e^{\ln 0.25} \\ &= 0.25^2 - 0.25 \\ &= \tfrac{1}{16} - \tfrac{1}{4} = -\tfrac{3}{16}. \end{aligned}$$

The sign of $k''(x)$ changes on either side of $x = \ln 0.25$, so $\left(\ln 0.25, -\frac{3}{16}\right)$ is a point of inflection, as shown in the graph below:

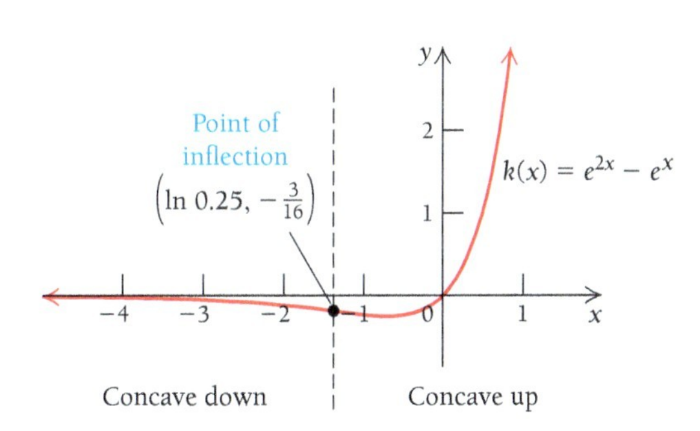

3 ✓

Quick Check 3 ✓

Find any points of inflection on the graph of $h(x) = xe^{-x}$.

Curve Sketching

The first and second derivatives enhance our ability to sketch curves. We use the following strategy:

Strategy for Sketching Graphs*

a) *Derivatives and domain.* Find $f'(x)$ and $f''(x)$. Note the domain of f.

b) *Critical values of f.* Find the critical values by solving $f'(x) = 0$ and by finding where $f'(x)$ does not exist. These numbers yield candidates for relative maxima or minima. Find the function values at these points.

c) *Increasing and/or decreasing; relative extrema.* Substitute each critical value, x_0, from step (b) into $f''(x)$. If $f''(x_0) < 0$, then $f(x_0)$ is a relative maximum and f is increasing on the left of x_0 and decreasing on the right. If $f''(x_0) > 0$, then $f(x_0)$ is a relative minimum and f is decreasing on the left of x_0 and increasing on the right.

d) *Inflection points.* Determine candidates for inflection points by finding where $f''(x) = 0$ or where $f''(x)$ does not exist. Find the function values at any such points.

e) *Concavity.* Use any candidates for inflection points from step (d) to define intervals. Substitute test values into $f''(x)$ to determine where the graph is concave up ($f''(x) > 0$) and where it is concave down ($f''(x) < 0$). Step (c) may have provided some of this information.

f) *Sketch the graph.* Sketch the graph using the information from steps (a)–(e), plotting extra points as needed.

The examples that follow apply this step-by-step strategy.

EXAMPLE 4 Find any relative extrema and inflection points and graph

$$f(x) = x^4 - 2x^2.$$

Solution

a) *Derivatives and domain.* Find $f'(x)$ and $f''(x)$:

$$f'(x) = 4x^3 - 4x,$$
$$f''(x) = 12x^2 - 4.$$

The domain of f, f', and f'' is $\mathbb{R}$.

b) *Critical values.* Since the domain of f' is $\mathbb{R}$, the only critical values are where $f'(x) = 0$:

$$4x^3 - 4x = 0 \quad \text{Setting } f'(x) \text{ equal to 0}$$
$$4x(x^2 - 1) = 0$$
$$4x = 0 \quad or \quad x^2 - 1 = 0$$
$$x = 0 \quad or \quad x^2 = 1$$
$$x = \pm 1. \quad \text{Using the Principle of Square Roots}$$

y, 2, 1, (0, 0), −2, −1, 1, 2, x, −1, (−1, −1), (1, −1), −2

We have $f(0) = 0, f(-1) = -1$, and $f(1) = -1$, so $(0, 0)$, $(-1, -1)$, and $(1, -1)$ are on the graph.

*This strategy is refined further, for rational functions, in Section 3.3.

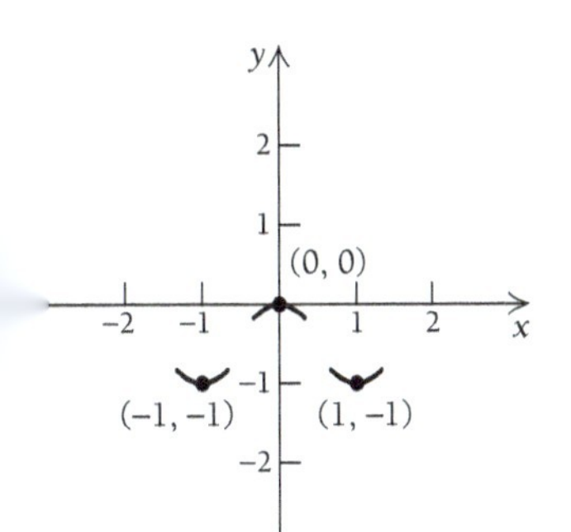

c) *Increasing and/or decreasing; relative extrema.* Substitute each critical value into $f''(x)$ to determine if the point is a relative maximum, a relative minimum, or neither. This information will also be useful in step (e). For $x = -1$, we have

$$f''(-1) = 12(-1)^2 - 4 = 8 > 0,$$

so $f(-1) = -1$ is a relative minimum, with f decreasing on $(-\infty, -1)$ and increasing on $(-1, 0)$. For $x = 0$, we have

$$f''(0) = 12 \cdot 0^2 - 4 = -4 < 0,$$

so $f(0) = 0$ is a relative maximum, with f increasing on $(-1, 0)$ and decreasing on $(0, 1)$. For $x = 1$, we have

$$f''(1) = 12 \cdot 1^2 - 4 = 8 > 0,$$

so $f(1) = -1$ is also a relative minimum, with f decreasing on $(0, 1)$ and increasing on $(1, \infty)$.

d) *Inflection points.* Find where $f''(x)$ does not exist and where $f''(x) = 0$. Since the domain of f'' is $\mathbb{R}$, we need only find points where $f''(x) = 0$:

$$\begin{aligned} 12x^2 - 4 &= 0 && \text{Setting } f''(x) \text{ equal to 0} \\ 4(3x^2 - 1) &= 0 \\ 3x^2 - 1 &= 0 && \text{Dividing both sides by 4} \\ 3x^2 &= 1 \\ x^2 &= \frac{1}{3} \\ x &= \pm\frac{1}{\sqrt{3}}. && \text{Using the Principle of Square Roots} \end{aligned}$$

We have

$$f\left(\frac{1}{\sqrt{3}}\right) = \left(\frac{1}{\sqrt{3}}\right)^4 - 2\left(\frac{1}{\sqrt{3}}\right)^2 = \frac{1}{9} - \frac{2}{3} = -\frac{5}{9}$$

and

$$f\left(-\frac{1}{\sqrt{3}}\right) = -\frac{5}{9}.$$

Thus, $\left(-\frac{1}{\sqrt{3}}, -\frac{5}{9}\right)$ and $\left(\frac{1}{\sqrt{3}}, -\frac{5}{9}\right)$ are possible inflection points.

e) *Concavity.* Find the intervals on which f is concave up or concave down. From step (c), we can conclude that f is concave up over the intervals $(-\infty, -1/\sqrt{3})$ and $(1/\sqrt{3}, \infty)$ and concave down over the interval $(-1/\sqrt{3}, 1/\sqrt{3})$.

Interval (number line in x with points $-1/\sqrt{3}$ and $1/\sqrt{3}$)

Test Value	$x = -1$	$x = 0$	$x = 1$
Sign of $f''(x)$	$f''(-1) > 0$	$f''(0) < 0$	$f''(1) > 0$
Result	f' is increasing; f is concave up on $(-\infty, -1/\sqrt{3})$	f' is decreasing; f is concave down on $(-1/\sqrt{3}, 1/\sqrt{3})$	f' is increasing; f is concave up on $(1/\sqrt{3}, \infty)$

Change indicates a point of inflection at $x = -1/\sqrt{3}$.

Change indicates a point of inflection at $x = 1/\sqrt{3}$.

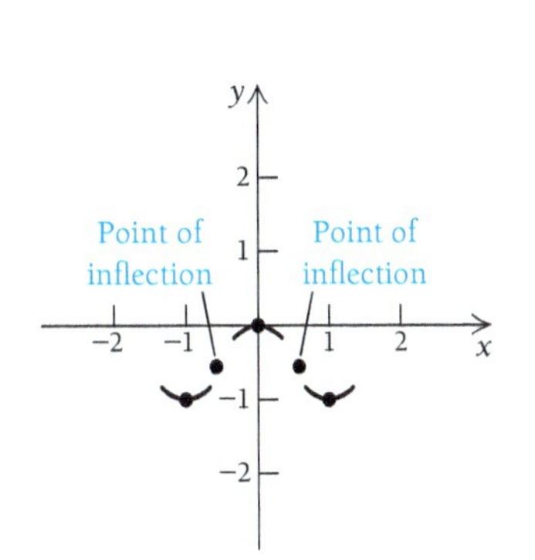

f) *Sketch the graph.* Sketch the graph using the information in steps (a)–(e). By solving $x^4 - 2x^2 = 0$, we can find the x-intercepts easily. They are $(-\sqrt{2}, 0)$, $(0, 0)$, and $(\sqrt{2}, 0)$. Other function values can also be calculated.

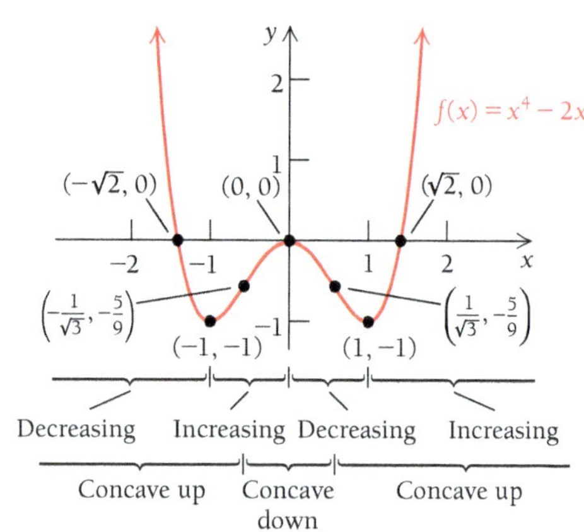

Quick Check 4 ✓

Find any relative extrema and inflection points and graph the function f given by $f(x) = 1 + 8x^2 - x^4$.

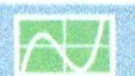

For the next example, recall that the domain of $y = \ln x$ is $\{x|x > 0\}$. However, given a function of the form $h(x) = \ln f(x)$, if $f(x) > 0$ for all x, then the domain of h is $\mathbb{R}$.

Technology Connection

EXERCISE

1. Consider

$$f(x) = x^3(x - 2)^3.$$

How many relative extrema do you anticipate finding? Where do you think they will be?

Graph f, f', and f'' using $[-1, 3, -2, 6]$ as a viewing window. Estimate any relative extrema and any inflection points for f. Then check your work using the method of Examples 4 and 5.

EXAMPLE 5 Find any relative extrema and inflection points, and graph

$$h(x) = \ln(x^2 + 6).$$

Solution

a) *Derivatives and domain.* Find $h'(x)$ and $h''(x)$:

$$h'(x) = \frac{2x}{x^2 + 6},$$

$$h''(x) = \frac{(x^2 + 6) \cdot 2 - (2x) \cdot 2x}{(x^2 + 6)^2} \quad \text{Using the Quotient Rule}$$

$$= \frac{-2x^2 + 12}{(x^2 + 6)^2}. \quad \text{Simplifying}$$

The expression $x^2 + 6$ has the domain $\mathbb{R}$, and since $x^2 \geq 0$ for all x, we have $x^2 + 6 > 0$. Thus, the domain of $h(x) = \ln(x^2 + 6)$ is $\mathbb{R}$. The domains of h' and h'' are also $\mathbb{R}$.

b) *Critical values.* Since the domain of h' is $\mathbb{R}$, the only critical values will be found by solving $h'(x) = 0$. This is true when the numerator, $2x$, equals 0. Thus, $x = 0$ is a critical value. Using a calculator, we find the second coordinate of this critical point:

$$h(0) = \ln((0)^2 + 6) \approx 1.792.$$

c) *Increasing and/or decreasing; relative extrema.* Using the Second-Derivative Test, we evaluate $h''(x)$ at the critical value $x = 0$:

$$h''(0) = \frac{-2(0)^2 + 12}{((0)^2 + 6)^2} = \frac{1}{3} > 0.$$

Since the second derivative is positive, the critical point $(0, 1.792)$ is a relative minimum point. Thus, h is decreasing on the interval $(-\infty, 0)$ and increasing on $(0, \infty)$.

d) *Inflection points.* Since the domain of h'' is $\mathbb{R}$, any inflection point will be found by solving $h''(x) = 0$. This is true when the numerator, $-2x^2 + 12$, is 0. Solving for x, we have

$$x = \pm\sqrt{6}, \quad \text{or} \quad x \approx -2.449, 2.449.$$

Using a calculator, we find $h(-2.449) = \ln 12 \approx 2.485$ and $h(2.449) = \ln 12 \approx 2.485$. Thus, we have two possible points of inflection, $(-2.449, 2.485)$ and $(2.449, 2.485)$.

e) *Concavity.* We check the concavity of h on the intervals $(-\infty, -2.449)$, $(-2.449, 2.449)$, and $(2.449, \infty)$:

Interval $(-\infty, -2.449)$: Test -3: $h''(-3) = \dfrac{-2(-3)^2 + 12}{((-3)^2 + 6)^2} = -0.027 < 0$,

Interval $(-2.449, 2.449)$: Test 0: $h''(0) = \dfrac{-2(0)^2 + 12}{((0)^2 + 6)^2} = \dfrac{1}{3} > 0$,

Interval $(2.449, \infty)$: Test 3: $h''(3) = \dfrac{-2(3)^2 + 12}{((3)^2 + 6)^2} = -0.027 < 0$.

Since the sign of $h''(x)$ changes at $x \approx -2.449$ and again at $x \approx 2.449$, we conclude that $(-2.449, 2.485)$ and $(2.449, 2.485)$ are points of inflection. The graph of h is concave down on the intervals $(-\infty, -2.449)$ and $(2.449, \infty)$ and concave up on the interval $(-2.449, 2.449)$.

f) *Sketch the graph.* We use the information found in steps (a)–(e). By letting $x = 0$, we find that the graph has a y-intercept at $(0, \ln 6)$, or approximately $(0, 1.792)$. The graph has no x-intercepts. Other points may be found using a calculator.

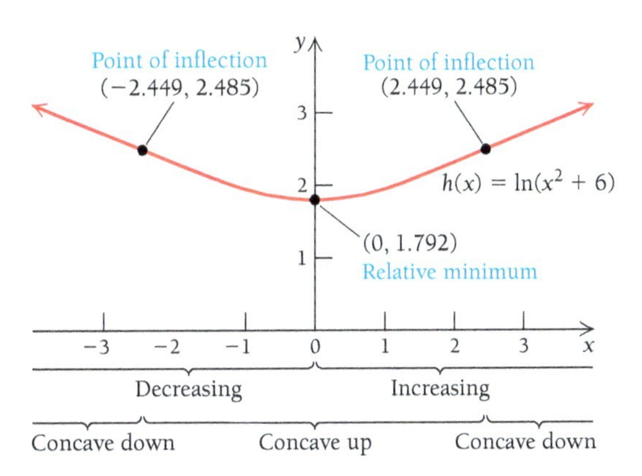

Quick Check 5 ✓

Find any relative extrema and points of inflection, and graph the function m given by

$$m(x) = \ln(x^2 + 4).$$

5 ✓

The following figures illustrate some information that can be found from first and second derivatives. Note that the x-coordinates of the x-intercepts of f' are the critical values of f. Note that the intervals over which f is increasing or decreasing are those intervals for which $f'(x)$ is positive or negative, respectively.

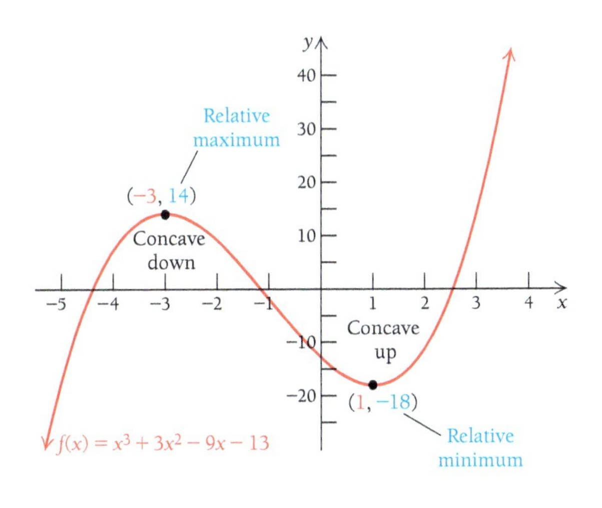

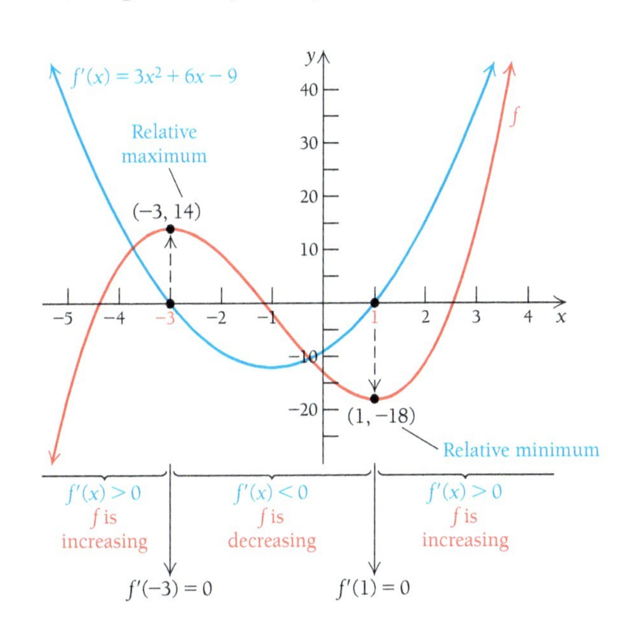

In the figures below, note that the intervals over which f' is increasing or decreasing are, respectively, those intervals over which $f''(x)$ is positive (the graph is concave up) or negative (the graph is concave down).

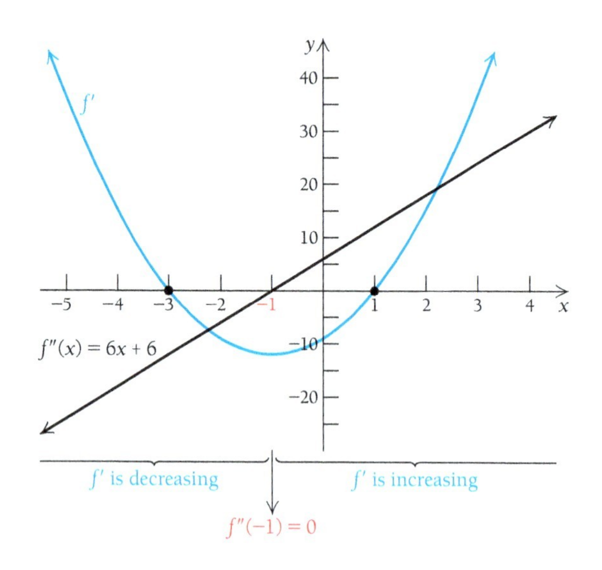

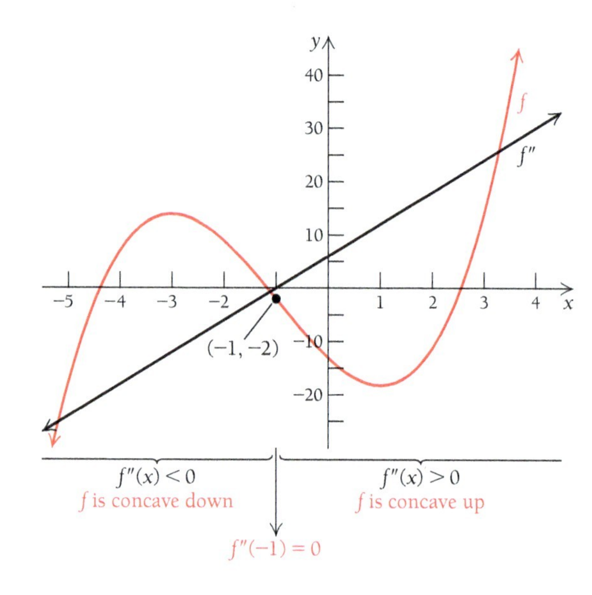

Section Summary

- The second derivative f'' is used to determine the *concavity* of the graph of f.
- If $f''(x_0) > 0$, then the graph of f is concave up at $(x_0, f(x_0))$.
- If $f''(x_0) < 0$, then the graph of f is concave down at $(x_0, f(x_0))$.
- If c is a critical value and $f''(c) > 0$, then $f(c)$ is a relative minimum.
- If c is a critical value and $f''(c) < 0$, then $f(c)$ is a relative maximum.
- If c is a critical value and $f''(c) = 0$, the First-Derivative Test must be used to determine whether $f(c)$ is a relative extremum.
- If $f''(x_0) = 0$ or $f''(x_0)$ does not exist, and there is a change in concavity on the left and on the right of x_0, then the point $(x_0, f(x_0))$ is called a *point of inflection*.
- Finding relative extrema, intervals over which a function is increasing or decreasing, intervals of upward or downward concavity, and points of inflection is a strategy for accurate curve sketching.

3.2 Exercise Set

In Exercises 1–6, identify (a) the point(s) of inflection and (b) the intervals where the function is concave up or concave down.

1.

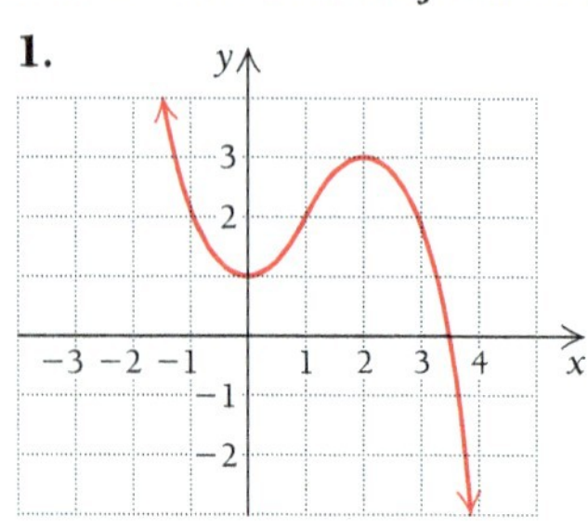

2.

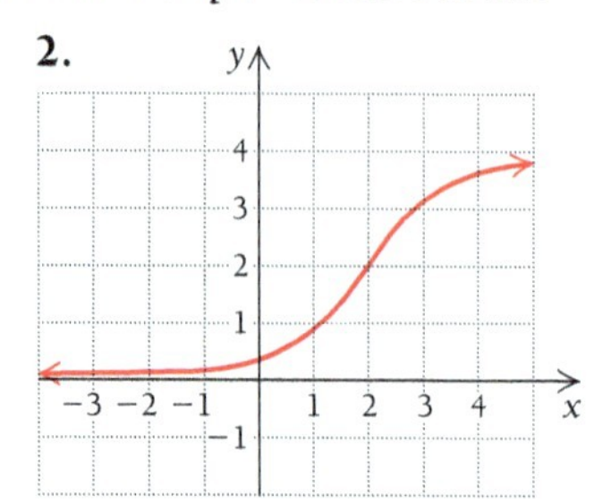

3.

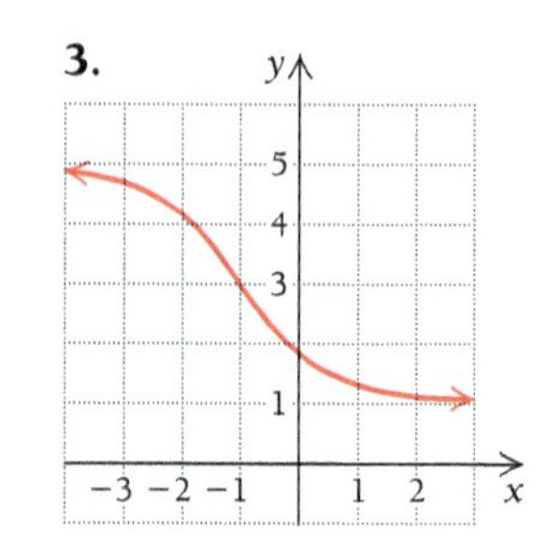

4.

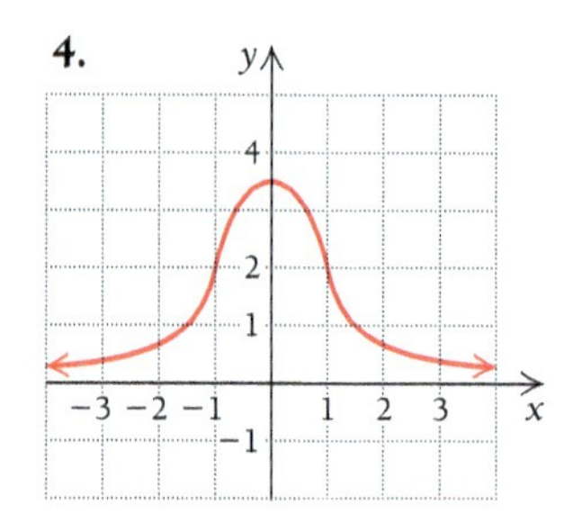

5.

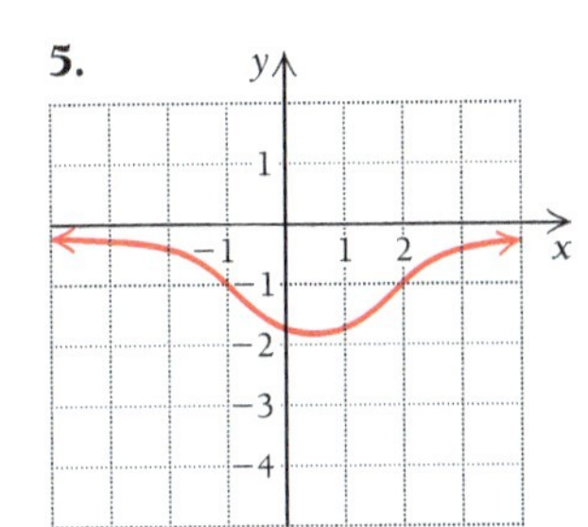

6.

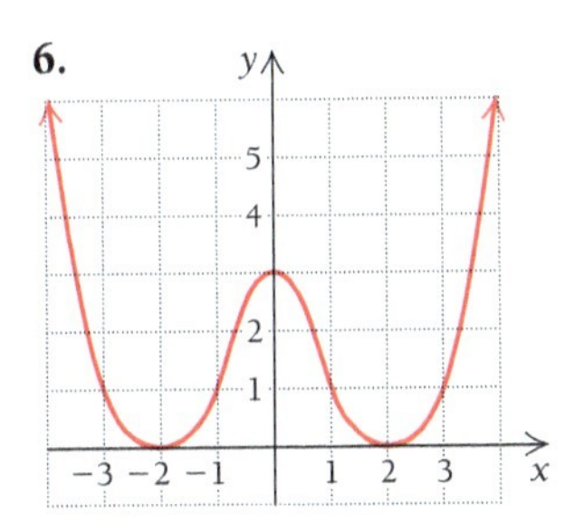

For each function in Exercises 7–28, (a) give the coordinates of any critical points and classify each point as a relative maximum, a relative minimum, or neither; (b) identify intervals where the function is increasing or decreasing; (c) give the coordinates of any points of inflection; (d) identify intervals where the function is concave up or concave down, and (e) sketch the graph.

7. $f(x) = x^2 - 10x + 2$

8. $g(x) = x^2 + 12x - 4$

9. $t(x) = -x^2 + 6x + 7$

10. $y(x) = -x^2 - 8x + 1$

11. $F(x) = 3x^2 + 4x + 2$

12. $G(x) = 5x^2 - 2x - 3$

13. $h(x) = x^3 - 27x$

14. $g(x) = x^3 - 48x - 1$

15. $f(x) = xe^{3x}$

16. $b(x) = xe^{-4x}$

17. $a(x) = \ln(x^2 + 9)$

18. $c(x) = \ln(x^2 + 16)$

19. $g(x) = x^3 - 6x^2 + 9x + 1$

20. $h(x) = x^3 - 2x^2 - 4x + 3$

21. $k(x) = x^4 - 2x^3$

22. $j(x) = 3x^4 + 4x^3$

23. $f(x) = e^{3x} - e^x$

24. $k(x) = e^{2x} - e^{4x}$

25. $q(x) = \dfrac{8x}{x^2 + 1}$

26. $r(x) = -\dfrac{4}{x^2 + 1}$

27. $g(x) = x^2 \ln x$

28. $k(x) = 2x^3 \ln x$

For Exercises 29–38, sketch a graph that possesses the characteristics listed. Answers may vary.

29. f is decreasing and concave up on $(-\infty, 2)$, f is decreasing and concave down on $(2, \infty)$.

30. f is increasing and concave up on $(-\infty, 4)$, f is increasing and concave down on $(4, \infty)$.

31. f is decreasing and concave down on $(-\infty, 3)$, f is decreasing and concave up on $(3, \infty)$.

32. f is increasing and concave down on $(-\infty, 1)$, f is increasing and concave up on $(1, \infty)$.

33. f is concave up at $(1, -3)$, concave down at $(8, 7)$, and has an inflection point at $(5, 4)$.

34. f is concave down at $(1, 5)$, concave up at $(7, -2)$, and has an inflection point at $(4, 1)$.

35. $f'(-3) = 0, f''(-3) < 0, f(-3) = 8; f'(9) = 0, f''(9) > 0, f(9) = -6; f''(2) = 0$, and $f(2) = 1$

36. $f'(-1) = 0, f''(-1) > 0, f(-1) = -5; f'(7) = 0, f''(7) < 0, f(7) = 10; f''(3) = 0$, and $f(3) = 2$

37. $f'(0) = 0, f''(0) < 0, f(0) = 5; f'(2) = 0, f''(2) > 0, f(2) = 2; f'(4) = 0, f''(4) < 0$, and $f(4) = 3$

38. $f'(-1) = 0, f''(-1) > 0, f(-1) = -2; f'(1) = 0, f''(1) > 0, f(1) = -2; f'(0) = 0, f''(0) < 0$, and $f(0) = 0$

APPLICATIONS

Business and Economics

39. Labor force. The percentage of the U.S. civilian labor force aged 45–54 can be modeled by the function f given by

$$f(x) = -0.0115x^2 + 0.125x + 81.7,$$

where x is the number of years after 1994. (*Source*: Based on data from www.bls.gov.) Sketch the graph of this function for $0 \le x \le 25$, and find the year in which the percentage of the labor force aged 45–54 was highest.

40. Labor force. The size of the U.S. civilian labor force aged 16–24 can be modeled by the function g given by

$$g(x) = -8.145x^2 + 147.05x + 21{,}612,$$

where $g(x)$ is the size of the civilian labor force, in thousands, x years after 1994. (*Source*: Based on data from www.bls.gov.) Graph this function for $0 \le x \le 25$, and find the year in which the size of the civilian labor force aged 16–24 was highest.

41. Sales saturation. The Gottahavit device is introduced in a market with 150,000,000 potential buyers. The unit sales are modeled by the function s given by

$$s(x) = -0.0131x^3 + 0.661x^2 - 2.021x + 6.865,$$

where s is total sales, in millions of units, x months after the device was released.

a) Find the point of inflection, and interpret its meaning in terms of the rate of change in sales.

b) Graph $y = s(x)$ for $0 \le x \le 30$.

42. Investing. Jeff owns two properties. The combined value, $A(t)$, of the two properties, t years after Jeff's initial investment in them, is given by

$$A(t) = 10{,}000e^{0.025t} + 15{,}000e^{-0.04t}.$$

a) After how many years will the combined value of the two properties be a minimum, and what will the combined value be at that time?

b) Graph $y = A(t)$ for $0 \le t \le 20$.

Life and Physical Sciences

43. Rainfall in Reno. The average monthly rainfall in Reno, Nevada, for the period between January 1 and July 1 is approximated by

$$R(t) = -0.006t^4 + 0.213t^3 - 1.702t^2 + 0.615t + 27.745,$$

where $R(t)$ is the amount of rainfall in millimeters at t months after January 1. (*Source*: Based on data from weather.com.)

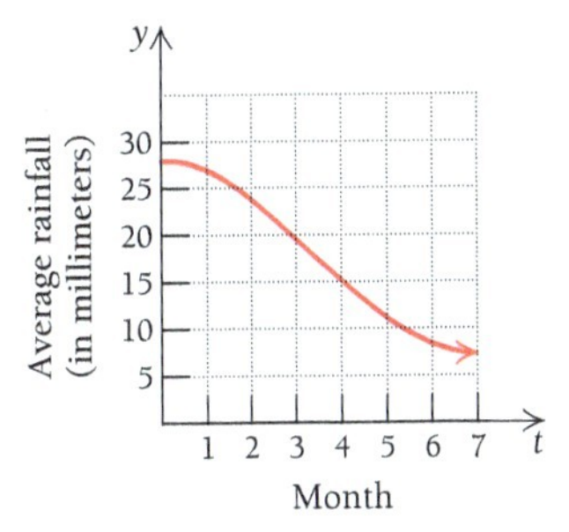

Find the point(s) of inflection for R. What is the significance of the point(s)?

44. Coughing velocity. A person coughs when a foreign object is in the windpipe. The velocity of the cough depends on the size of the object. Suppose a person has a windpipe with a 20-mm radius. If a foreign object has a radius r, in millimeters, then the coughing velocity $V(r)$, in millimeters per second, needed to remove the object is given by

$$V(r) = k(20r^2 - r^3), \quad 0 \le r \le 20,$$

where k is some positive constant. What size object requires the maximum coughing velocity to be removed?

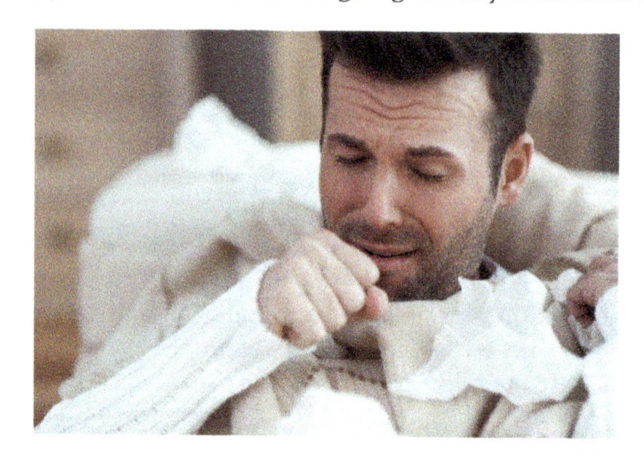

45. Population. The population of Red Rock t years after 2010 is given by $y = 35{,}000e^{0.05t}$, while the population of a neighboring town, Curwood Village, t years after 2010 is given by $y = 50{,}000e^{-0.07t}$.

a) Write the function $P(t)$ that gives the combined population of Red Rock and Curwood Village t years after 2010.

b) Over what interval of time is the combined population decreasing?

c) Over what interval of time is the combined population increasing?

d) Find the critical point, and interpret its meaning.

46. Internet traffic. The number of visitors P to a website in a given week over a 1-yr period is given by $P(t) = 120 + (t - 85)e^{0.02t}$, where t is the week and $1 \le t \le 52$.

a) Over what interval of time during the 1-yr period is the number of visitors decreasing?

b) Over what interval of time during the 1-yr period is the number of visitors increasing?

c) Find the critical point, and interpret its meaning.

SYNTHESIS

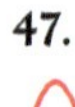

In each of Exercises 47 and 48, determine which graph is the derivative of the other and explain why.

47.

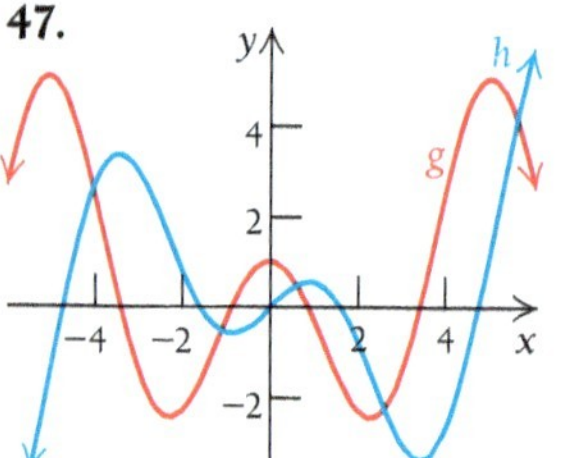

48.

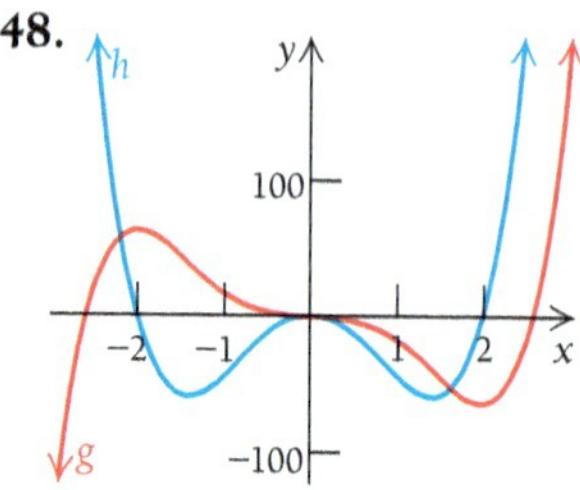

49. Use calculus to prove that the relative minimum or maximum for any function f for which

$$f(x) = ax^2 + bx + c, \quad a \neq 0,$$

occurs at $x = -b/(2a)$.

50. Use calculus to prove that the point of inflection for any function g given by

$$g(x) = ax^3 + bx^2 + cx + d, \quad a \neq 0,$$

occurs at $x = -b/(3a)$.

51. Use calculus to prove that a relative extremum for the function given by $f(x) = xe^{ax}$ occurs at $x = -\frac{1}{a}$.

52. Use calculus to prove that a point of inflection for the function given by $f(x) = xe^{ax}$ occurs at $x = -\frac{2}{a}$.

For Exercises 53–59, assume that f is differentiable over $(-\infty, \infty)$. Classify each of the following statements as either true or false. If a statement is false, explain why.

53. If f has exactly two critical values at $x = a$ and $x = b$, where $a < b$, then there must exist exactly one point of inflection at $x = c$ such that $a < c < b$. In other words, exactly one point of inflection must exist between any two critical points.

54. If f has exactly two critical values at $x = a$ and $x = b$, where $a < b$, then there must exist at least one point of inflection at $x = c$ such that $a < c < b$. In other words, at least one point of inflection must exist between any two critical points.

55. A function f can have no extrema but still have at least one point of inflection.

56. If f has two points of inflection, then there is a critical value located between those points of inflection.

57. The function f can have a point of inflection at a critical value.

58. The function f can have a point of inflection at an extreme value.

59. A function f can have exactly one extreme value but no points of inflection.

60. Hours of daylight. The number of hours of daylight in Chicago is represented in the graph below. On what dates is the number of hours of daylight changing most rapidly? How can you tell?

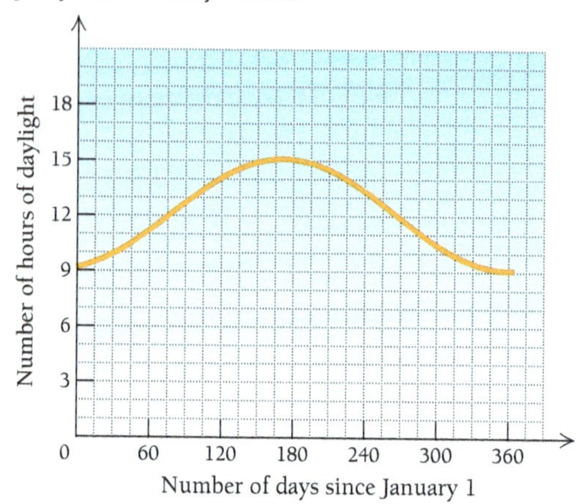

(*Source*: Astronomical Applications Dept., U.S. Naval Observatory.)

61. The table below shows the distance traveled, in meters, by a walker over a 10-min interval. Estimate the time at which a point of inflection occurs. Explain your reasoning.

Time (in minutes)	1	2	3	4	5	6	7	8	9	10
Distance (in meters)	40	100	150	185	205	220	245	300	360	460

Technology Connection 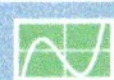

Graph each function. Then estimate any relative extrema. Where appropriate, round to three decimal places.

62. $f(x) = 4x - 6x^{2/3}$

63. $f(x) = 3x^{2/3} - 2x$

64. $f(x) = x^2(1 - x)^3$

65. $f(x) = x^2(x - 2)^3$

66. $f(x) = (x - 1)^{2/3} - (x + 1)^{2/3}$

67. $f(x) = x - \sqrt{x}$

68. $f(x) = x^3e^{2x}$

69. $f(x) = x^2 + e^{-x}$

70. Earnings for holders of a bachelor's degree. The data in the graph below show the mean earnings from 2005 to 2015 for individuals in the United States who have a bachelor's degree but no higher degree.

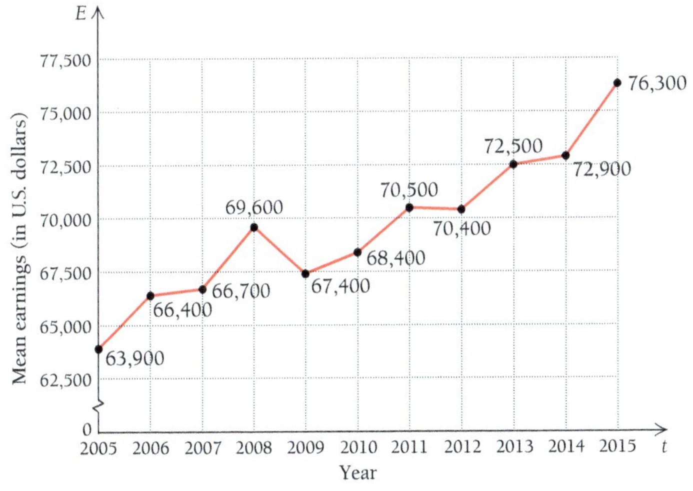

(*Source*: U.S. Census Bureau.)

a) Use regression (see Section R.7) to fit linear, cubic, and quartic functions, $E = f(t)$, to the data, where t is the number of years since 2005 and E is the mean earnings of individuals with a bachelor's degree. Which function best fits the data?

b) What is the domain of E?

c) Does E have any relative extrema? How can you tell?

Filling a vase with water. *Water is poured at a constant rate into each of the 8-inch-tall vases shown in Exercises 71–74. Let $h(t)$ be the depth of the water, in inches, in a vase after t seconds. For each vase, (a) sketch a graph of h, and (b) identify the depth(s) at which the graph has a point of inflection and explain why.*

71.

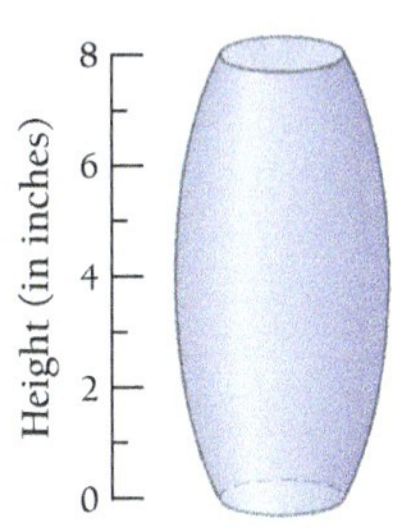

72.

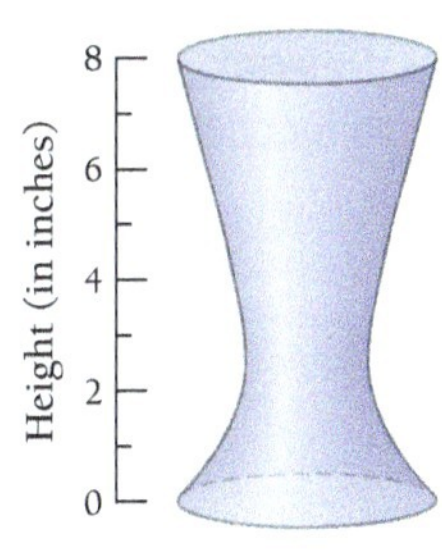

73.

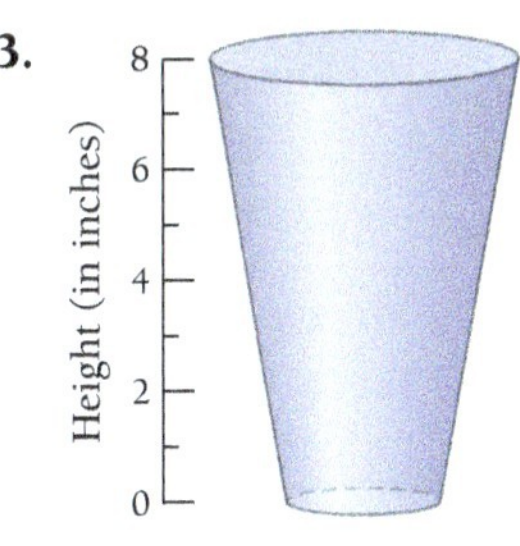

74.

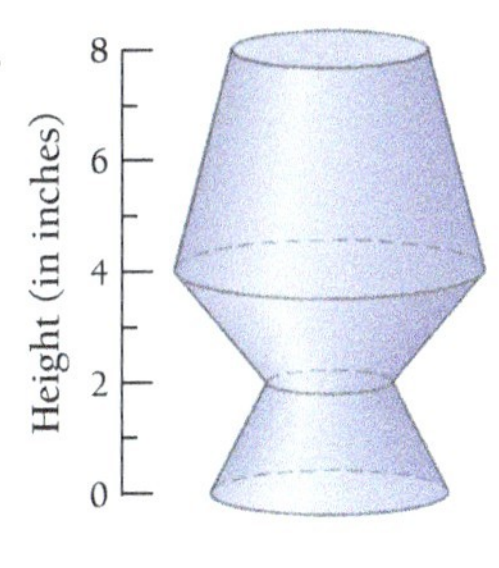

Answers to Quick Checks

1. Relative maximum of 16 at $x = -2$; relative minimum of -16 at $x = 2$

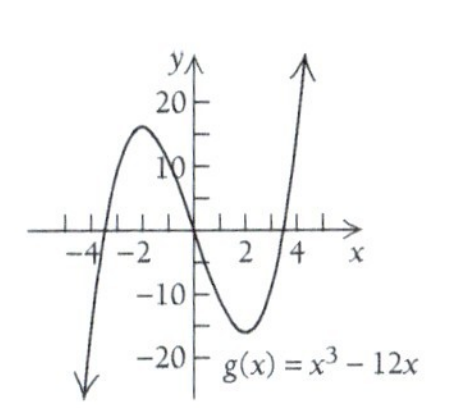

2. Relative maximum of $e^{-1} \approx 0.368$ at $x = 1$

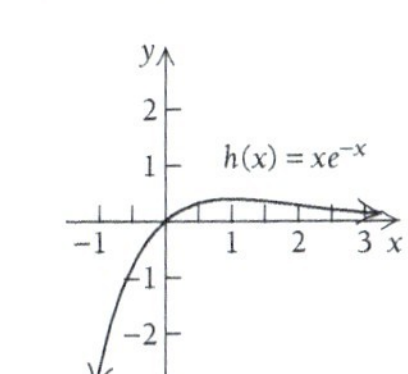

3. Inflection point at $(2, 2e^{-2})$

4. Relative maxima: 17 at $x = -2$ and $x = 2$; relative minimum: 1 at $x = 0$; inflection points at $\left(-\frac{2}{\sqrt{3}}, \frac{89}{9}\right)$ and $\left(\frac{2}{\sqrt{3}}, \frac{89}{9}\right)$

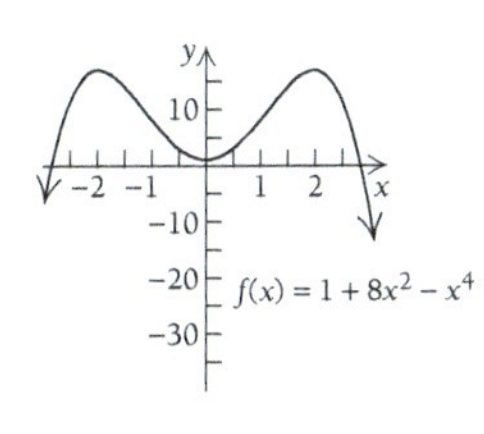

5. Relative minimum of ln 4 at $x = 0$; inflection points at $(-2, \ln 8)$ and $(2, \ln 8)$

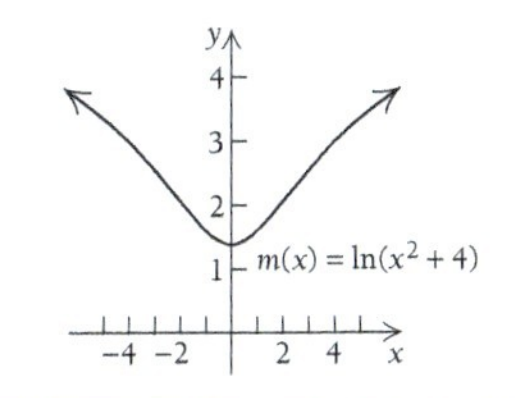

3.3 Graph Sketching: Asymptotes and Rational Functions

- Find limits involving infinity.
- Determine the asymptotes of a function's graph.
- Graph rational functions.

In this section, we consider discontinuous functions, many of which are rational functions.

Recall the definition of a rational function:

> **DEFINITION**
>
> A **rational function** is a function f that can be described by
>
> $$f(x) = \frac{P(x)}{Q(x)},$$
>
> where $P(x)$ and $Q(x)$ are polynomials, with $Q(x)$ not the zero polynomial. The domain of f consists of all x for which $Q(x) \neq 0$.

We wish to graph rational functions in which the denominator is not a constant. Before doing so, we need to review vertical and horizontal asymptotes.

Vertical Asymptotes

The graph of $f(x) = \dfrac{x^2 - 1}{x^2 + x - 6} = \dfrac{(x - 1)(x + 1)}{(x - 2)(x + 3)}$ is shown below.

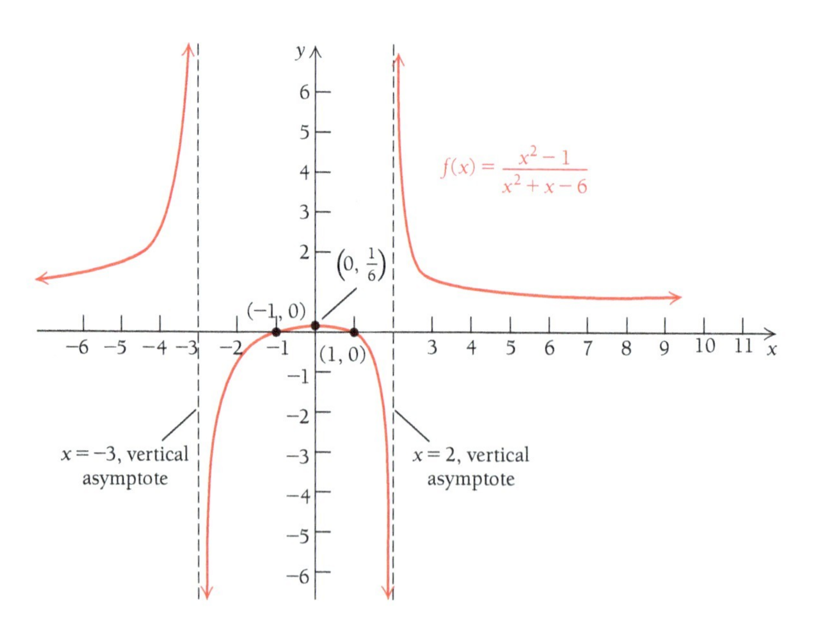

Note that as x gets closer to 2 from the left, the function values approach $-\infty$. As x gets closer to 2 from the right, the function values approach ∞. Thus,

$$\lim_{x \to 2^-} f(x) = -\infty \quad \text{and} \quad \lim_{x \to 2^+} f(x) = \infty.$$

For this graph, we regard the line $x = 2$ as a "limiting line" called a *vertical asymptote*. The line $x = -3$ is another vertical asymptote.

Technology Connection 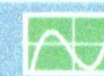

Vertical Asymptotes

Graph $f(x) = 8/(x^2 - 4)$ in CONNECTED mode, using the window $[-6, 6, -8, 8]$. Vertical asymptotes occur at $x = -2$ and $x = 2$. These lines are not part of the graph.

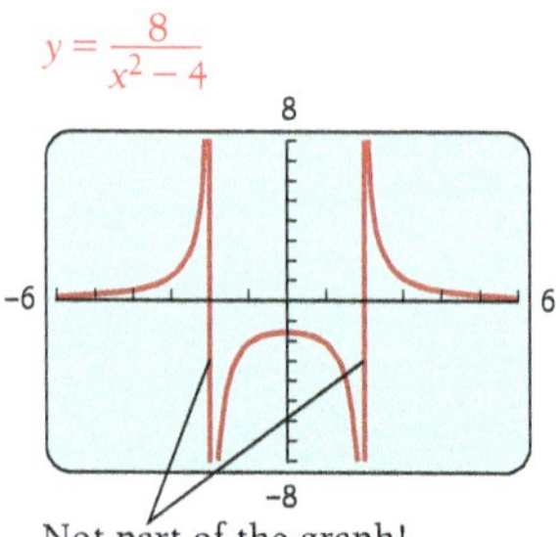

EXERCISES

Graph each of the following in both DOT and CONNECTED modes. Try to locate the vertical asymptotes visually. Then verify your results using the method of Examples 1 and 2. You may need to vary the viewing windows.

1. $f(x) = \dfrac{x^2 + 7x + 10}{x^2 + 3x - 28}$
2. $f(x) = \dfrac{3x - 4}{x}$

DEFINITION

The line $x = a$ is a **vertical asymptote** of $f(x)$ if any of these statements is true:

$$\lim_{x \to a^-} f(x) = \infty, \quad \lim_{x \to a^-} f(x) = -\infty, \quad \lim_{x \to a^+} f(x) = \infty, \quad \text{or} \quad \lim_{x \to a^+} f(x) = -\infty.$$

If a rational function f is simplified, meaning that the numerator and denominator have no common factor other than -1 or 1, then if a makes the denominator 0, the line $x = a$ is a vertical asymptote. For example,

$$f(x) = \frac{x^2 - 9}{x - 3} = \frac{(x - 3)(x + 3)}{x - 3}$$

does not have a vertical asymptote at $x = 3$ because $(x - 3)$ is a common factor of the numerator and the denominator. In contrast,

$$g(x) = \frac{x^2 - 4}{x^2 + x - 12} = \frac{(x + 2)(x - 2)}{(x - 3)(x + 4)}$$

has $x = 3$ and $x = -4$ as vertical asymptotes since neither $(x - 3)$ nor $(x + 4)$ is a factor of the numerator.

The figures below show four ways in which a vertical asymptote can occur. The dashed lines represent the asymptotes. They are shown for visual assistance only; they are not part of the graphs of the functions.

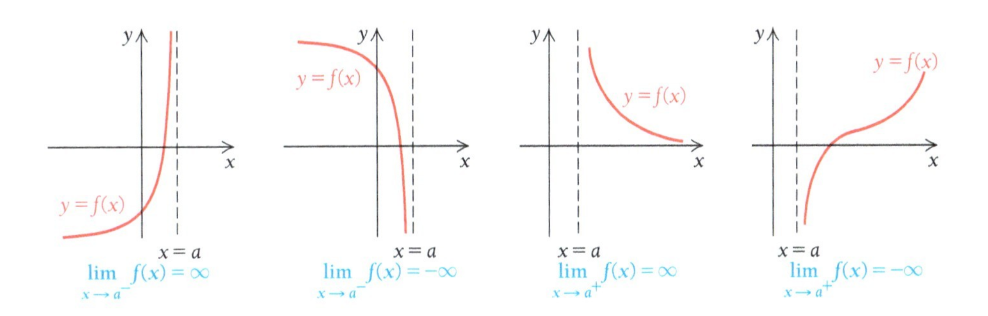

Quick Check 1 Determine the vertical asymptotes of

$$f(x) = \frac{1}{x(x^2 - 16)}.$$

EXAMPLE 1 Determine the vertical asymptotes of $f(x) = \dfrac{3x - 2}{x(x - 5)(x + 3)}$.

Solution The expression is simplified. Thus, the vertical asymptotes are the lines $x = 0$, $x = 5$, and $x = -3$. **1 ✓**

Quick Check 2 Determine the vertical asymptotes of

$$g(x) = \frac{x - 2}{x^3 - x^2 - 2x}.$$

EXAMPLE 2 Determine the vertical asymptotes of $f(x) = \dfrac{x^2 - 2x}{x^3 - x}$.

Solution We first simplify the expression:

$$f(x) = \frac{x^2 - 2x}{x^3 - x} = \frac{x(x - 2)}{x(x - 1)(x + 1)}$$

$$= \frac{x - 2}{(x - 1)(x + 1)}, \quad x \neq 0.$$

We now see that the vertical asymptotes are the lines $x = -1$ and $x = 1$. **2 ✓**

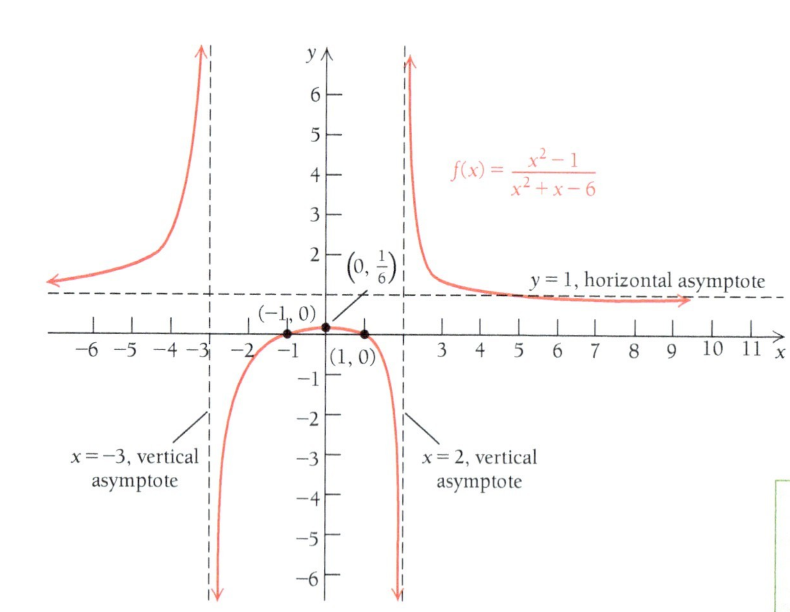

Horizontal Asymptotes

Look again at the graph of $f(x) = \frac{x^2 - 1}{x^2 + x - 6}$, shown at the left. Note that function values approach 1 as x approaches $-\infty$, meaning that $f(x) \to 1$ as $x \to -\infty$. Also, function values approach 1 as x approaches ∞, meaning that $f(x) \to 1$ as $x \to \infty$. Thus,

$$\lim_{x \to -\infty} f(x) = 1 \quad \text{and} \quad \lim_{x \to \infty} f(x) = 1.$$

The line $y = 1$ is called a *horizontal asymptote*.

DEFINITION

The line $y = b$ is a **horizontal asymptote** of $f(x)$ if either or both of the following statements are true:

$$\lim_{x \to -\infty} f(x) = b \quad \text{or} \quad \lim_{x \to \infty} f(x) = b.$$

Horizontal asymptotes of a rational function occur when the degree of the numerator is less than or equal to the degree of the denominator. Recall that the degree of a polynomial in one variable is the highest power of that variable. The following figures show three ways in which horizontal asymptotes can occur.

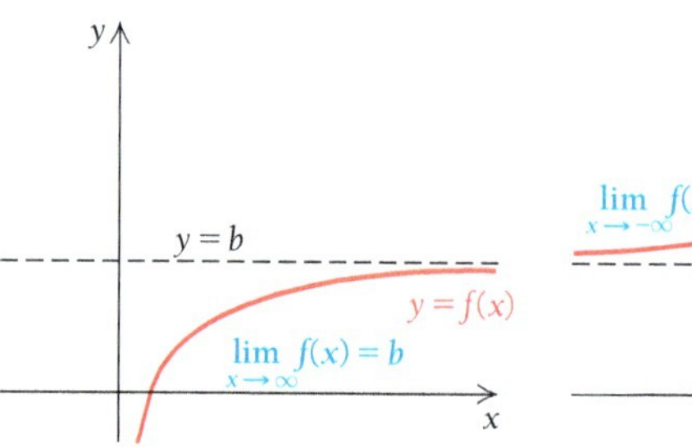

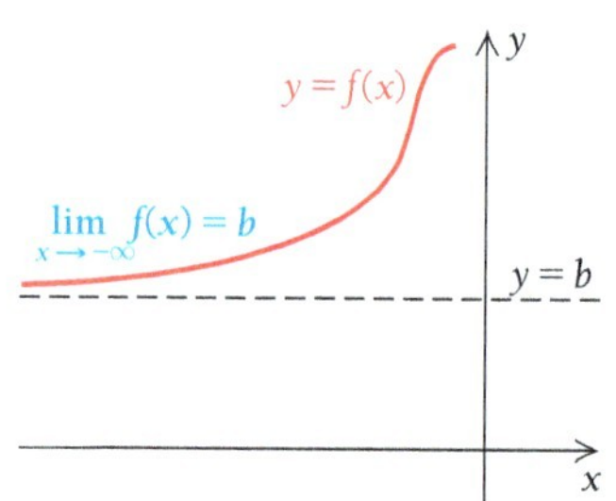

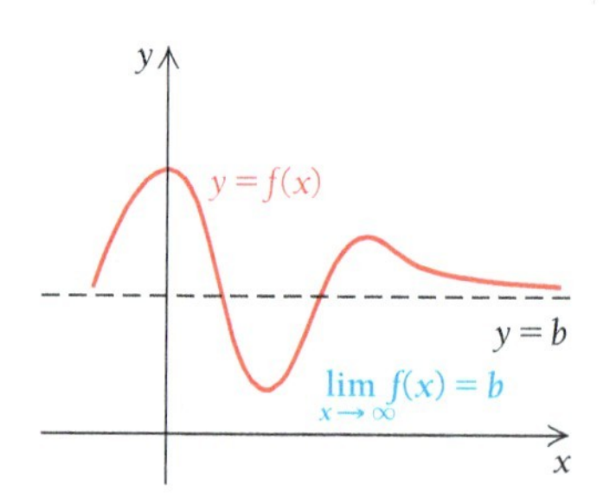

A horizontal asymptote is the limit of a rational function as inputs approach $-\infty$ or ∞.

In Section 1.2, we showed that if f is a rational function given by

$$f(x) = \frac{ax^m + \cdots}{bx^n + \cdots},$$

where $m = n$, then its limit as x approaches ∞ or $-\infty$ is

$$\lim_{x \to \pm\infty} f(x) = \frac{a}{b}.$$

If $n > m$, then

$$\lim_{x \to \pm\infty} f(x) = 0.$$

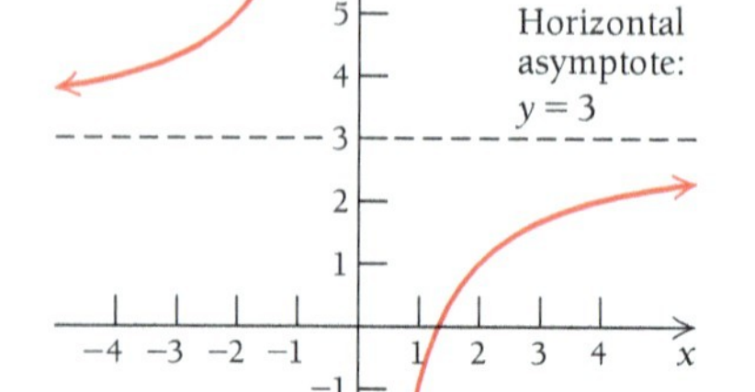

A visualization of Example 3

EXAMPLE 3 Determine the horizontal asymptote of $f(x) = \frac{3x - 4}{x}$.

Solution To find the horizontal asymptote, we consider

$$\lim_{x \to \infty} f(x) = \lim_{x \to \infty} \frac{3x - 4}{x}.$$

Since the degree of the numerator and the degree of the denominator are equal, we have

$$\lim_{x\to\infty} \frac{3x - 4}{1x} = \frac{3}{1} = 3.$$

In a similar manner, it can be shown that

$$\lim_{x\to-\infty} f(x) = 3.$$

The horizontal asymptote is the line $y = 3$. 3 ✓

Quick Check 3 ✓

Determine the horizontal asymptote of

$$f(x) = \frac{(2x - 1)(x + 1)}{(3x + 2)(5x + 6)}.$$

EXAMPLE 4 Determine the horizontal asymptote of $f(x) = \dfrac{2x + 3}{x^3 - 2x^2 + 4}$.

Solution Since the degree of the denominator is greater than the degree of the numerator, we have

$$\lim_{x\to\infty} \frac{2x + 3}{x^3 - 2x^2 + 4} = 0.$$

Thus, the line $y = 0$ (the x-axis) is a horizontal asymptote.

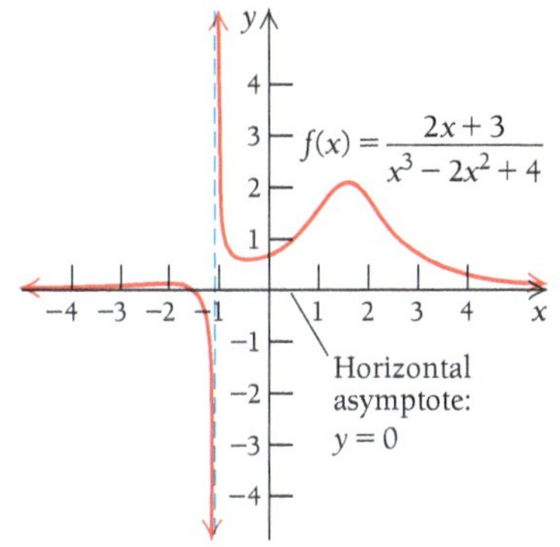

A visualization of Example 4

4 ✓

Quick Check 4 ✓

Determine the horizontal asymptote of

$$g(x) = \frac{10{,}000x}{x^2 + 1}.$$

Slant Asymptotes

Some asymptotes are neither vertical nor horizontal. For example, in the graph of

$$f(x) = \frac{x^2 - 4}{x - 1},$$

shown at left, as $|x|$ approaches ∞, the curve approaches the line $y = x + 1$. The line $y = x + 1$ is called a *slant asymptote*, or *oblique asymptote*. In Example 5, we will see how the line $y = x + 1$ is determined.

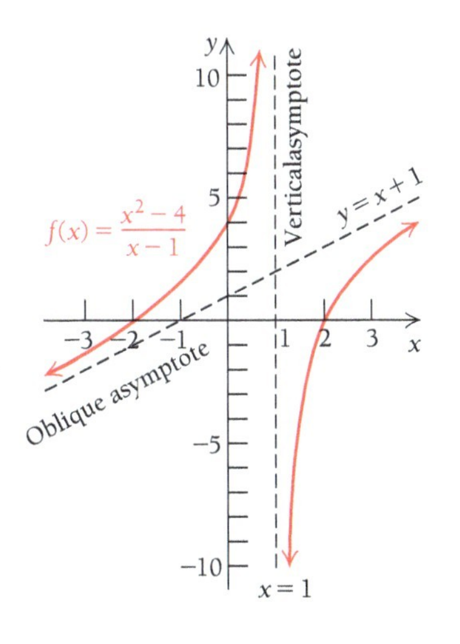

DEFINITION

A linear asymptote that is neither vertical nor horizontal is called a **slant asymptote**, or an **oblique asymptote**. For any rational function of the form $f(x) = P(x)/Q(x)$, a slant asymptote occurs when the degree of $P(x)$ is exactly 1 more than the degree of $Q(x)$.

We find a slant asymptote by division.

EXAMPLE 5 Find the slant asymptote of $f(x) = \dfrac{x^2 - 4}{x - 1}$.

Solution When we divide the numerator by the denominator, we obtain a quotient of $x + 1$ and a remainder of -3:

$$\begin{array}{r|l} & x + 1 \\ x - 1 & x^2 \quad - 4 \\ & \underline{x^2 - x} \\ & x - 4 \\ & \underline{x - 1} \\ & -3 \end{array}$$

$$f(x) = \frac{x^2 - 4}{x - 1} = (x + 1) + \frac{-3}{x - 1}.$$

Technology Connection

EXERCISES

Graph each of the following. Try to determine the horizontal asymptotes using the TABLE and TRACE features. Verify your results using the method of Examples 3 and 4.

1. $f(x) = \dfrac{9x^4 - 7x^2 - 9}{3x^4 + 7x^2 + 9}$

2. $f(x) = \dfrac{135x^5 - x^2}{x^7}$

Quick Check 5

Find the slant asymptote of

$$g(x) = \frac{2x^2 + x - 1}{x - 3}.$$

Note that as $|x|$ approaches ∞, $-3/(x - 1)$ approaches 0. Thus, $y = x + 1$ is the slant asymptote. **5 ✓**

Asymptotes of Exponential and Logarithmic Functions

In Section R.6 and in Chapter 2, we saw many examples of exponential and logarithmic functions. Both types of functions have asymptotes, which we summarize below:

- An exponential function of the form $f(x) = ae^{bx}$, for $b > 0$, has a horizontal asymptote of $y = 0$ (the x-axis) as $x \to -\infty$.

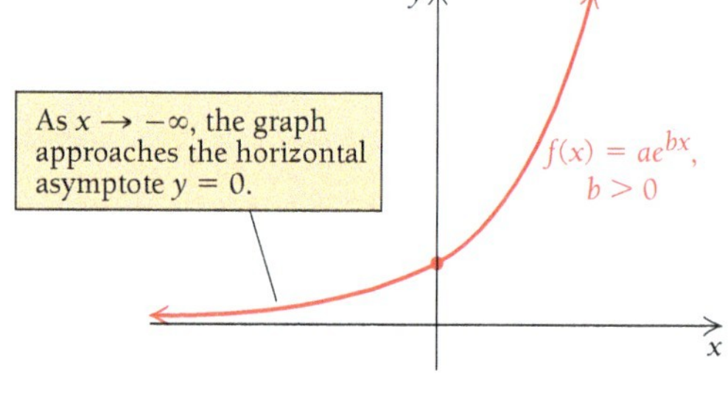

- An exponential function of the form $f(x) = ae^{bx}$, for $b < 0$, has a horizontal asymptote of $y = 0$ (the x-axis) as $x \to \infty$.

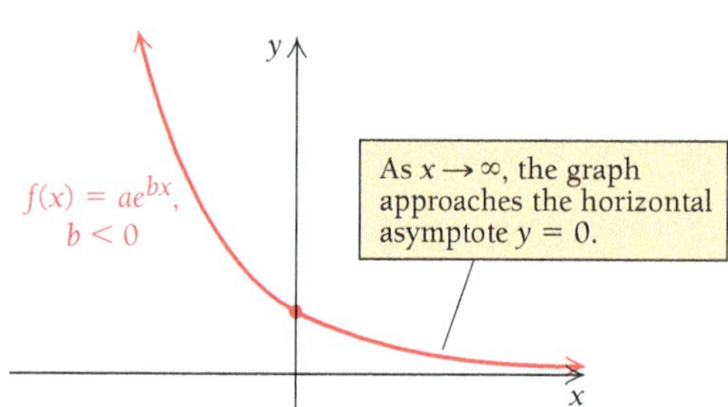

- A logarithmic function of the form $f(x) = \ln(x - a)$ has a vertical asymptote at $x = a$ as $x \to a^+$.

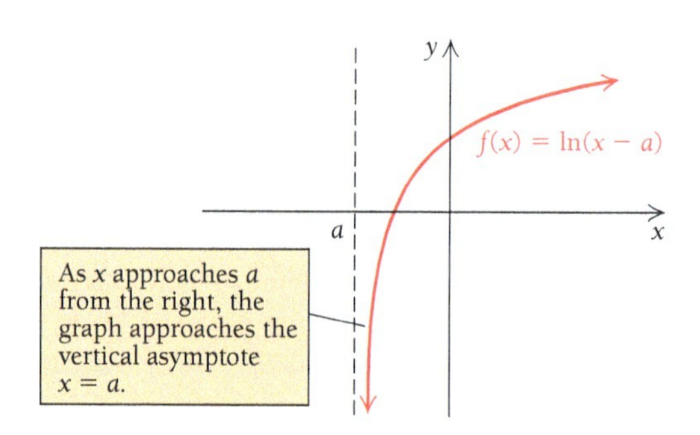

- A logarithmic function of the form $f(x) = \ln(a - x)$ has a vertical asymptote at $x = a$ as $x \to a^-$.

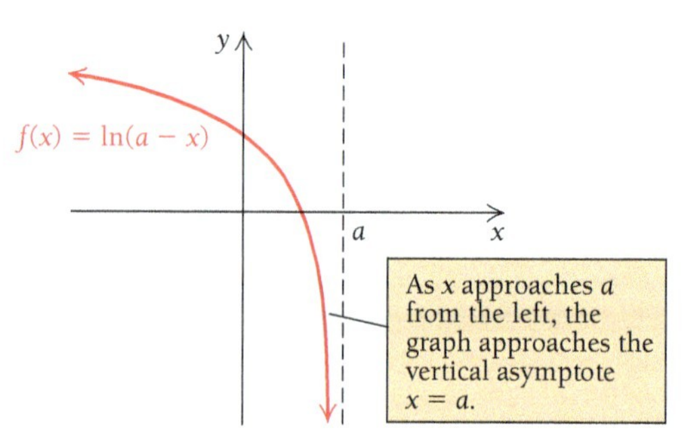

We use these properties to find limits of functions containing exponential or logarithmic terms, as the following example illustrates.

EXAMPLE 6 Find the horizontal asymptotes of $f(x) = \dfrac{200}{1 + 25e^{-0.04x}}$.

Solution As $x \to \infty$, the expression $25e^{-0.04x}$ approaches 0. That is,

$$\lim_{x\to\infty} 25e^{-0.04x} = 0.$$

Thus,

$$\lim_{x\to\infty} \frac{200}{1 + 25e^{-0.04x}} = \frac{200}{1 + 0} \qquad \text{Using the above result}$$

$$= 200.$$

The line $y = 200$ is a horizontal asymptote. Now, as $x \to -\infty$, the expression $25e^{-0.04x}$ approaches ∞. That is,

$$\lim_{x \to -\infty} 25e^{-0.04x} = \infty.$$

Thus, we have

$$\lim_{x \to -\infty} \frac{200}{1 + 25e^{-0.04x}} = \frac{200}{1 + \infty} \quad \text{Using the preceding result; the denominator approaches } \infty \text{ as a limit.}$$
$$= 0.$$

The line $y = 0$ is a second horizontal asymptote of f. The graph of f is shown below, with the two horizontal asymptotes included.

Quick Check 6 ✓

Find the horizontal asymptotes of

$$p(x) = \frac{55}{3 + 2e^{-0.07x}}.$$

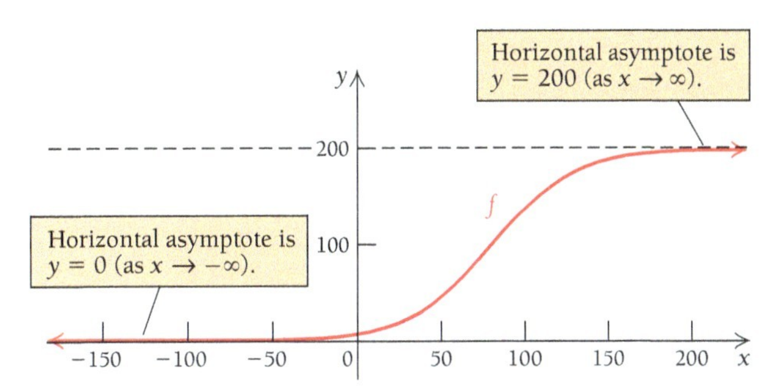

6 ✓

Intercepts

If they exist, **x-intercepts** occur at values of x for which $y = f(x) = 0$ and are points at which the graph crosses (or touches) the x-axis. If it exists, the **y-intercept** occurs at the value of y for which $x = 0$ and is the point at which the graph crosses (or touches) the y-axis.

EXAMPLE 7 Find the intercepts of the function given by

$$f(x) = \frac{x^3 - x^2 - 6x}{x^2 - 3x + 2}.$$

Solution We factor the numerator and the denominator:

$$f(x) = \frac{x(x + 2)(x - 3)}{(x - 1)(x - 2)}.$$

To find the x-intercepts, we solve $f(x) = 0$. Such values occur when the numerator is 0 and the denominator is nonzero. Thus, we solve

$$x(x + 2)(x - 3) = 0.$$

The x-values that make the numerator 0 are 0, −2, and 3. Since none of these make the denominator 0, they yield the x-intercepts: (0, 0), (−2, 0), and (3, 0).

To find the y-intercept, we let $x = 0$:

$$f(0) = \frac{0^3 - 0^2 - 6(0)}{0^2 - 3(0) + 2} = 0.$$

In this case, the y-intercept is also an x-intercept, (0, 0).

7 ✓

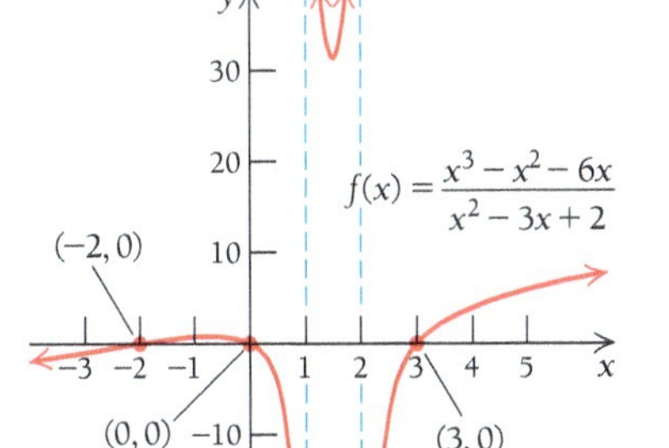

A visualization of Example 7

Quick Check 7 ✓

Find the intercepts of the function given by

$$h(x) = \frac{x^3 - x}{x^2 - 4}.$$

EXAMPLE 8 Find all asymptotes and intercepts of $g(x) = -2 + e^{0.5x}$.

Solution Since g is defined for all x, there are no vertical asymptotes. As $x \to -\infty$, the expression $e^{0.5x}$ approaches 0, and we have

$$\lim_{x \to -\infty} (-2 + e^{0.5x}) = -2 + 0 = -2.$$

Thus, the line $y = -2$ is a horizontal asymptote.

To find the y-intercept, we set $x = 0$:

$$g(0) = -2 + e^{0.5(0)} = -2 + 1 = -1.$$

The point $(0, -1)$ is the y-intercept. To find any x-intercepts, we set $y = 0$, and solve for x:

$$\begin{aligned} -2 + e^{0.5x} &= 0 \\ e^{0.5x} &= 2 \\ 0.5x &= \ln 2 && \text{Finding the natural logarithm of both sides} \\ x &= \frac{\ln 2}{0.5} \approx 1.386. \end{aligned}$$

The point $(1.386, 0)$ is the x-intercept. The graph of g is shown below.

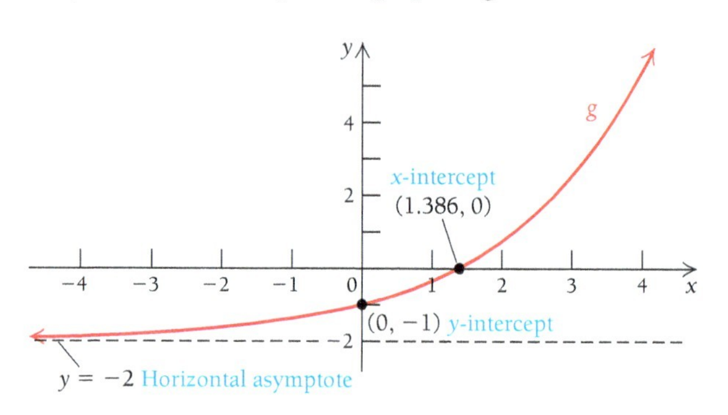

Quick Check 8 ✓

Find all asymptotes and intercepts of $h(x) = \ln(x + 5)$.

8 ✓

Sketching Graphs

We can now refine our strategy for graphing.

Strategy for Sketching Graphs

a) *Intercepts.* Find any x- and y-intercepts.

b) *Asymptotes.* Find any vertical, horizontal, or slant asymptotes.

c) *Derivatives and domain.* Find $f'(x)$ and $f''(x)$. Find the domain of f.

d) *Critical values of f.* Find any inputs for which $f'(x)$ is not defined or for which $f'(x) = 0$.

e) *Increasing and/or decreasing; relative extrema.* Substitute each critical value, x_0, from step (d) into $f''(x)$. If $f''(x_0) < 0$, then x_0 yields a relative maximum and f is increasing on the left of x_0 and decreasing on the right. If $f''(x_0) > 0$, then x_0 yields a relative minimum and f is decreasing on the left of x_0 and increasing on the right. If $f''(x_0) = 0$ or on intervals where no critical value exists, use f' and test values to find where f is increasing or decreasing and to classify any extrema not found by using f''.

f) *Inflection points.* Determine candidates for inflection points by finding x-values for which $f''(x)$ does not exist or for which $f''(x) = 0$. Find the function values at these points. If a function value $f(x)$ does not exist, then the function does not have an inflection point at x.

g) *Concavity.* Use the values from step (f) as endpoints of intervals. Determine the concavity over each interval by checking to see where f' is increasing—that is, where $f''(x) > 0$—and where f' is decreasing—that is, where $f''(x) < 0$. Do this by substituting a test value from each interval into $f''(x)$.

h) *Sketch the graph.* Use the information from steps (a)–(g) to sketch the graph, plotting extra points as needed.

EXAMPLE 9 Sketch the graph of $f(x) = \frac{8}{x^2 - 4}$.

Solution

a) *Intercepts.* Any x-intercepts occur at values for which the numerator is 0 but the denominator is not. Here, the numerator is a constant, so there are no x-intercepts. To find the y-intercept, we compute $f(0)$:

$$f(0) = \frac{8}{0^2 - 4} = \frac{8}{-4} = -2.$$

This gives us one point on the graph, $(0, -2)$.

b) *Asymptotes.*

Vertical: The denominator, $x^2 - 4 = (x + 2)(x - 2)$, is 0 for x-values of -2 and 2. Thus, the lines $x = -2$ and $x = 2$ are vertical asymptotes. We draw them as dashed lines (they are guidelines, *not* part of the actual graph).

Horizontal: The degree of the numerator is less than the degree of the denominator, so the x-axis, $y = 0$, is the horizontal asymptote.

Slant: There is no slant asymptote since the degree of the numerator is not 1 more than the degree of the denominator.

c) *Derivatives and domain.* The student can confirm, using the Quotient Rule, that

$$f'(x) = \frac{-16x}{(x^2 - 4)^2} \quad \text{and} \quad f''(x) = \frac{16(3x^2 + 4)}{(x^2 - 4)^3}.$$

The domain of f, f', and f'' is $(-\infty, -2) \cup (-2, 2) \cup (2, \infty)$, as determined in step (b).

d) *Critical values of f.* We look for values of x for which $f'(x) = 0$ or for which $f'(x)$ does not exist. From step (c), we see that $f'(x) = 0$ for values of x for which $-16x = 0$ and the denominator is not 0. The only such number is 0 itself. The derivative $f'(x)$ does not exist at -2 and 2, but neither value is in the domain of f. Thus, the only critical value is 0.

e) *Increasing and/or decreasing; relative extrema.* We use the undefined values and the critical values to determine the intervals over which f is increasing and the intervals over which f is decreasing. The values to consider are -2, 0, and 2. Since

$$f''(0) = \frac{16(3 \cdot 0^2 + 4)}{(0^2 - 4)^3} = \frac{64}{-64} < 0,$$

we know that a relative maximum exists at $(0, f(0))$, or $(0, -2)$. Thus, f is increasing over the interval $(-2, 0)$ and decreasing over $(0, 2)$.

Since $f''(x)$ does not exist for the x-values -2 and 2, we use $f'(x)$ and test values to see if f is increasing or decreasing on $(-\infty, -2)$ and $(2, \infty)$.

Test -3: $f'(-3) = \frac{-16(-3)}{[(-3)^2 - 4]^2} = \frac{48}{25} > 0$, so f is increasing on $(-\infty, -2)$.

Test 3: $f'(3) = \frac{-16(3)}{[(3)^2 - 4]^2} = \frac{-48}{25} < 0$, so f is decreasing on $(2, \infty)$.

f) *Inflection points.* We determine candidates for inflection points by finding where $f''(x)$ does not exist and where $f''(x) = 0$. The only values for which $f''(x)$ does not exist are where $x^2 - 4 = 0$, or -2 and 2. Neither value is in the domain of f, so we focus solely on where $f''(x) = 0$, or

$$16(3x^2 + 4) = 0.$$

Since $16(3x^2 + 4) > 0$ for all real numbers x, there are no points of inflection.

g) *Concavity.* Since no values were found in step (f), the only place where concavity could change is on either side of the vertical asymptotes, $x = -2$ and $x = 2$. To check, we see where $f''(x)$ is positive or negative. The numbers -2 and 2 divide the x-axis into three intervals. We choose a test value in each interval and substitute into $f''(x)$.

Test -3: $\quad f''(-3) = \dfrac{16[3(-3)^2 + 4]}{[(-3)^2 - 4]^3} > 0.$

Test 0: $\quad f''(0) = \dfrac{16[3(0)^2 + 4]}{[(0)^2 - 4]^3} < 0.$ We already knew this from step (e).

Test 3: $\quad f''(3) = \dfrac{16[3(3)^2 + 4]}{[(3)^2 - 4]^3} > 0.$

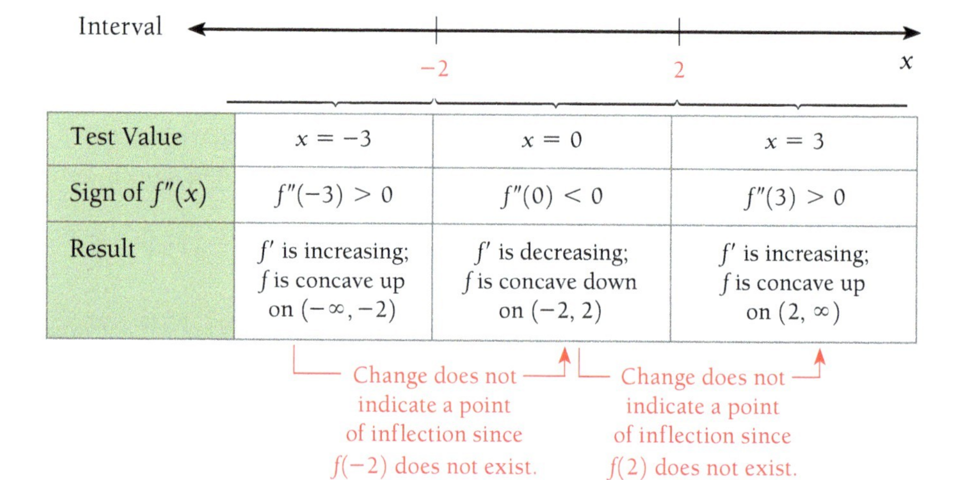

Test Value	$x = -3$	$x = 0$	$x = 3$
Sign of $f''(x)$	$f''(-3) > 0$	$f''(0) < 0$	$f''(3) > 0$
Result	f' is increasing; f is concave up on $(-\infty, -2)$	f' is decreasing; f is concave down on $(-2, 2)$	f' is increasing; f is concave up on $(2, \infty)$

Change does not indicate a point of inflection since $f(-2)$ does not exist.

Change does not indicate a point of inflection since $f(2)$ does not exist.

The function is concave up over the intervals $(-\infty, -2)$ and $(2, \infty)$. The function is concave down over $(-2, 2)$.

h) *Sketch the graph.* We sketch the graph using the information in the following table, plotting extra points as needed. The graph is shown below.

x	$f(x)$
-4	$\frac{2}{3}$
-3	1.6
-1	$-2\frac{2}{3}$
0	-2
1	$-2\frac{2}{3}$
3	1.6
4	$\frac{2}{3}$

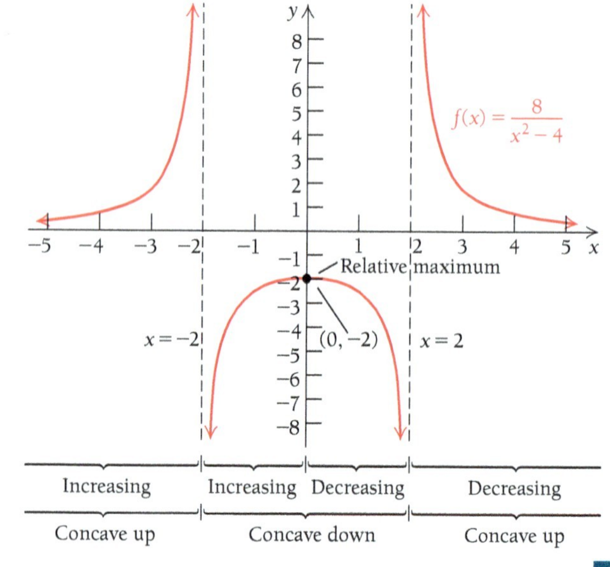

9 ✓

Quick Check 9 ✓

Sketch the graph of

$$f(x) = \frac{x^2 + 4}{x}.$$

Determine the intercepts, intervals where the function is increasing or decreasing, relative extrema, intervals where it is concave up or down, any points of inflection, and any asymptotes.

EXAMPLE 10 Sketch the graph of $g(x) = e^{-x^2}$.

Solution

a) *Intercepts.* Since $g(0) = e^{-0^2} = 1$, we see that $(0, 1)$ is the y-intercept. There are no x-intercepts since $e^{-x^2} > 0$ for all x.

b) *Asymptotes.* As $x \to \infty$, we have

$$\lim_{x\to\infty} e^{-x^2} = \lim_{x\to\infty}\left(\frac{1}{e^{x^2}}\right) = 0.$$

Similarly, as $x \to -\infty$, we have the same limit:

$$\lim_{x\to-\infty}\left(\frac{1}{e^{x^2}}\right) = 0.$$

Thus, $y = 0$ (the x-axis) is the horizontal asymptote as $x \to \infty$ and as $x \to -\infty$.

c) *Derivatives and domain.* The domain of $g(x) = e^{-x^2}$ is $\mathbb{R}$. The derivatives are

$$g'(x) = -2xe^{-x^2},$$

and $$g''(x) = 4x^2e^{-x^2} - 2e^{-x^2}.$$ Using the Product Rule

The domains of both g' and g'' are also $\mathbb{R}$.

d) *Critical values of g.* Since g' is defined for all x, the only critical values are where $g'(x) = 0$. We have

$$-2xe^{-x^2} = 0$$
$$x = 0.$$

The only critical value is $x = 0$, which is the y-intercept, $(0, 1)$.

e) *Increasing and/or decreasing; relative extrema.* The critical value $x = 0$ creates two intervals, $(-\infty, 0)$ and $(0, \infty)$. We use the first derivative and evaluate a test point from each interval:

Interval $(-\infty, 0)$: Test -1: $g'(-1) = -2(-1)e^{-(-1)^2} = 2e^{-1} > 0$;

Interval $(0, \infty)$: Test 1: $g'(1) = -2(1)e^{-(1)^2} = -2e^{-1} < 0$.

Thus, g is increasing on the interval $(-\infty, 0)$ and decreasing on the interval $(0, \infty)$. The point $(0, 1)$ is thus a relative maximum.

f) *Inflection points.* Since g'' is defined for all x, the only inflection points are where $g''(x) = 0$. We have

$$4x^2e^{-x^2} - 2e^{-x^2} = 0$$
$$2e^{-x^2}(2x^2 - 1) = 0 \quad \text{Factoring}$$
$$2x^2 - 1 = 0 \quad \text{Using the Principle of Zero Products; } e^{x^2} \text{ is never 0.}$$
$$2x^2 = 1$$
$$x^2 = \frac{1}{2}$$
$$x = \pm\sqrt{\frac{1}{2}} = \pm\frac{\sqrt{2}}{2}.$$

Evaluating $g(x)$ at these x-values gives us the second coordinates: $g\left(-\frac{\sqrt{2}}{2}\right) = e^{-(-\sqrt{1/2})^2} = e^{-1/2}$ and $g\left(\frac{\sqrt{2}}{2}\right) = e^{-(\sqrt{1/2})^2} = e^{-1/2}$. Thus, possible inflection points are $\left(-\frac{\sqrt{2}}{2}, e^{-1/2}\right)$ and $\left(\frac{\sqrt{2}}{2}, e^{-1/2}\right)$. Using a calculator, we find that these points are approximately $(-0.707, 0.607)$ and $(0.707, 0.607)$.

g) *Concavity.* We next check the concavity of g over the intervals $\left(-\infty, -\frac{\sqrt{2}}{2}\right)$, $\left(-\frac{\sqrt{2}}{2}, \frac{\sqrt{2}}{2}\right)$, and $\left(\frac{\sqrt{2}}{2}, \infty\right)$.

Interval $\left(-\infty, -\frac{\sqrt{2}}{2}\right)$: Test -1: $g''(-1) = 4(-1)^2e^{-(-1)^2} - 2e^{-(-1)^2} = 2e^{-1} > 0$;

Interval $\left(-\frac{\sqrt{2}}{2}, \frac{\sqrt{2}}{2}\right)$: Test 0: $g''(0) = 4(0)^2e^{-(0)^2} - 2e^{-(0)^2} = -2 < 0$;

Interval $\left(\frac{\sqrt{2}}{2}, \infty\right)$: Test 1: $g''(1) = 4(1)^2e^{-(1)^2} - 2e^{-(1)^2} = 2e^{-1} > 0$.

Thus, g is concave up over the intervals $\left(-\infty, -\frac{\sqrt{2}}{2}\right)$ and $\left(\frac{\sqrt{2}}{2}, \infty\right)$, and concave down over the interval $\left(-\frac{\sqrt{2}}{2}, \frac{\sqrt{2}}{2}\right)$. Since there is a change in concavity at both $x = \pm\frac{\sqrt{2}}{2}$, the points $\left(-\frac{\sqrt{2}}{2}, e^{-1/2}\right)$ and $\left(\frac{\sqrt{2}}{2}, e^{-1/2}\right)$ are both points of inflection.

h) *Sketch the graph.* We use the information from steps (a)–(g) to sketch the graph, plotting extra points as needed.

x	$g(x)$
-2	0.0183
-1	0.3679
0	1
1	0.3679
2	0.0183

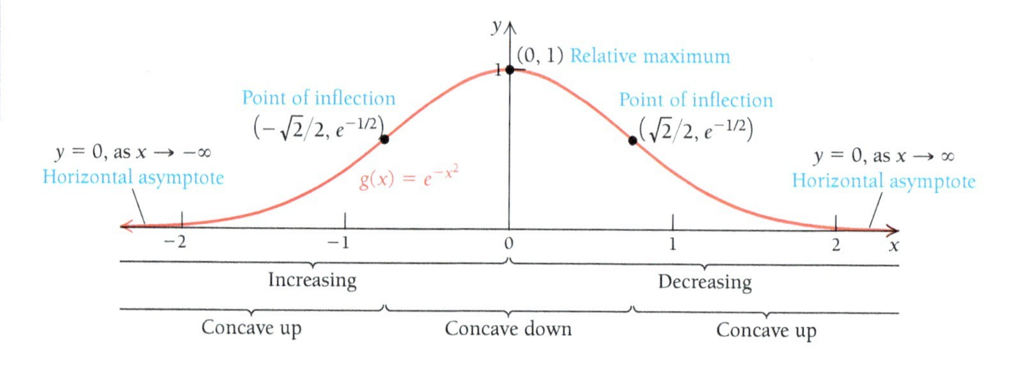

This graph, called a *bell curve*, or *normal curve*, is used often in statistics. **10 ✓**

Quick Check 10 ✓

Sketch the graph of $h(x) = xe^{-x^2}$. Determine the intercepts, intervals in which the function is increasing or decreasing, any relative extrema, intervals in which it is concave up or down, any points of inflection, and any asymptotes.

Section Summary

- A line $x = a$ is a *vertical asymptote* of the graph of f if $\lim_{x\to a^-} f(x) = \infty$ or $\lim_{x\to a^+} f(x) = \infty$ or $\lim_{x\to a^-} f(x) = -\infty$ or $\lim_{x\to a^+} f(x) = -\infty$.
- A line $y = b$ is a *horizontal asymptote* of the graph of f if $\lim_{x\to\infty} f(x) = b$ or $\lim_{x\to-\infty} f(x) = b$.
- A *slant asymptote* occurs when graphing a rational function if the degree of the numerator is 1 greater than the degree of the denominator. Division of polynomials can be used to determine the equation of the slant asymptote.
- Vertical, horizontal, and slant asymptotes can be used as guides for accurate curve sketching. Asymptotes are not a part of a graph but are visual guides only.

3.3 Exercise Set

Determine the vertical asymptote(s) of each function. If none exists, state that fact.

1. $f(x) = \dfrac{x+4}{x-2}$
2. $f(x) = \dfrac{2x-3}{x-5}$
3. $f(x) = \dfrac{5x}{x^2-25}$
4. $f(x) = \dfrac{3x}{x^2-9}$
5. $f(x) = \dfrac{x+3}{x^3-x}$
6. $f(x) = \dfrac{x+2}{x^3-6x^2+8x}$
7. $f(x) = \dfrac{x+2}{x^2+6x+8}$
8. $f(x) = \dfrac{x+6}{x^2+7x+6}$
9. $f(x) = \dfrac{7}{x^2+49}$
10. $f(x) = \dfrac{6}{x^2+36}$
11. $f(x) = \ln(x+7)$
12. $f(x) = \ln(x-3)$
13. $f(x) = \ln(x^2+6)$
14. $f(x) = \ln(e^x+1)$
15. $f(x) = e^{-2x}$
16. $f(x) = 15 + 4e^{5x}$

Determine the horizontal asymptote of each function. If none exists, state that fact.

17. $f(x) = \dfrac{6x}{8x+3}$
18. $f(x) = \dfrac{3x^2}{6x^2+x}$
19. $f(x) = \dfrac{4x}{x^2-3x}$
20. $f(x) = \dfrac{2x}{3x^3-x^2}$
21. $f(x) = 4 + \dfrac{2}{x}$
22. $f(x) = 5 - \dfrac{3}{x}$
23. $f(x) = \dfrac{6x^3+4x}{3x^2-x}$
24. $f(x) = \dfrac{8x^4-5x^2}{2x^3+x^2}$
25. $f(x) = \dfrac{4x^3-3x+2}{x^3+2x-4}$
26. $f(x) = \dfrac{6x^4+4x^2-7}{2x^5-x+3}$
27. $f(x) = \dfrac{2x^3-4x+1}{4x^3+2x-3}$
28. $f(x) = \dfrac{5x^4-2x^3+x}{x^5-x^3+8}$
29. $f(x) = e^{8x}$
30. $f(x) = e^{1.25x}$
31. $f(x) = \dfrac{25}{1+3e^{-0.25x}}$
32. $f(x) = \dfrac{10}{1+4.5e^{0.7x}}$
33. $f(x) = \dfrac{6000}{1+12e^{0.025x}}$
34. $f(x) = \dfrac{7500}{1+25e^{-0.88x}}$

Sketch the graph of each function. Indicate where each function is increasing or decreasing, where any relative extrema occur, where asymptotes occur, where the graph is concave up or concave down, where any points of inflection occur, and where any intercepts occur.

35. $f(x) = \dfrac{-2}{x-5}$
36. $f(x) = \dfrac{1}{x+2}$
37. $f(x) = \dfrac{2x+1}{x}$
38. $f(x) = \dfrac{3x-1}{x}$
39. $f(x) = x + \dfrac{2}{x}$
40. $f(x) = x + \dfrac{9}{x}$
41. $f(x) = \dfrac{x^2-9}{x+1}$
42. $f(x) = \dfrac{x^2-4}{x+3}$
43. $f(x) = \dfrac{x-3}{x^2+2x-15}$
44. $f(x) = \dfrac{x+1}{x^2-2x-3}$
45. $f(x) = \dfrac{1}{1+e^{-x}}$
46. $f(x) = \dfrac{3}{1+2e^{-x}}$
47. $f(x) = x^2e^{5x}$
48. $f(x) = x^2e^{-3x}$
49. $f(x) = 5 + \ln(2x-3)$
50. $f(x) = -2 + \ln(4-3x)$
51. $f(x) = -1 - \ln(5+2x)$
52. $f(x) = 8 - \ln(4+x)$

APPLICATIONS

Business and Economics

53. **Average cost.** The total cost, in thousands of dollars, for Blueblaze, Inc., to produce x computer cases is given by

$$C(x) = 3x^2 + 80.$$

a) The *average cost* is given by $\overline{C}(x) = C(x)/x$. Find $\overline{C}(x)$.
b) Graph the average cost.
c) Find the slant asymptote for the graph of $y = \overline{C}(x)$, and interpret its significance.

54. **Depreciation.** Suppose that the value V of the inventory at Fido's Pet Supply, in thousands of dollars, decreases (depreciates) after t months, where

$$V(t) = 50 - \frac{25t^2}{(t+2)^2}.$$

a) Find $V(0)$, $V(5)$, $V(10)$, and $V(70)$.
b) Find the maximum value of the inventory over the interval $[0, \infty)$.
c) Graph V.
d) Does there seem to be a value below which $V(t)$ will never fall? Explain.

55. **Total cost and revenue.** The total cost and total revenue, in dollars, from producing x couches are given by

$$C(x) = 5000 + 600x \quad \text{and} \quad R(x) = -\tfrac{1}{2}x^2 + 1000x.$$

a) Find the total-profit function, $P(x)$.
b) The *average profit* is given by $\overline{P}(x) = P(x)/x$. Find $\overline{P}(x)$.
c) Find the slant asymptote for the graph of $y = \overline{P}(x)$.
d) Graph the average profit.

56. **Cost of pollution control.** Cities and companies find that the cost of pollution control increases along with the percentage of pollutants being removed. Suppose the cost C, in dollars, of removing $p\%$ of the pollutants from a chemical spill is given by

$$C(p) = \frac{48{,}000}{100 - p}.$$

a) Find $C(0)$, $C(20)$, $C(80)$, and $C(90)$.
b) Find the domain of C.
c) Graph C.
d) Can the company or city afford to remove 100% of the pollutants due to this spill? Explain.

57. **Value of a stock.** The value, in dollars, of one share of stock of Hanrahan Corporation, t weeks after it was bought, is given by

$$V(t) = 50 - 15e^{-0.035t}.$$

a) Find any asymptotes, and explain their significance.
b) List any intervals where the graph of V is concave up or concave down, and explain their significance.
c) Find the domain and range of V, in the context of the problem.
d) Graph V.

58. **Sales saturation.** The sales of a new cookbook are given by

$$S(t) = \frac{20{,}000}{1 + 9e^{-0.1t}},$$

where t is the number of months since the book was released.

a) Find any asymptotes, and explain their significance.
b) List any intervals where the graph of S is concave up or concave down, and explain their significance.
c) Find any points of inflection, and explain their significance.
d) Find the domain and range of S, in the context of the problem.
e) Graph S.

Life and Physical Sciences

59. **Medication in the bloodstream.** After an injection, the amount of a medication A, in cubic centimeters (cc), in the bloodstream decreases with time t, in hours. Suppose that under certain conditions A is given by

$$A(t) = \frac{A_0}{t^2 + 1},$$

where A_0 is the initial amount of the medication. Assume that an initial amount of 100 cc is injected.

a) Find $A(0)$, $A(1)$, $A(2)$, $A(7)$, and $A(10)$.
b) Find the maximum amount of medication in the bloodstream over the interval $[0, \infty)$.
c) Graph the function.
d) According to this function, does the medication ever completely leave the bloodstream? Explain your answer.

60. **Newton's Law of Cooling.** A bowl of soup with an initial temperature of 165°F is placed in a 72°F room. The temperature of the soup after t minutes is given by

$$T(t) = 72 + 93e^{-0.08t}.$$

a) Find $T(0)$, $T(5)$, $T(15)$, and $T(30)$.
b) Find any asymptotes, and explain their significance.
c) List any intervals where the graph of T is concave up or down, and explain their significance.
d) Find the domain and range of T in the context of the problem.
e) Graph T.

General Interest

61. **Baseball: earned-run average.** A pitcher's *earned-run average* (the average number of runs given up per 9 innings, or 1 complete game) is given by

$$E = 9 \cdot \frac{r}{n},$$

where r is the number of earned runs allowed in n innings. If we set the number of earned runs allowed at 4 and let n vary, we get a function given by

$$E(n) = 9 \cdot \frac{4}{n}.$$

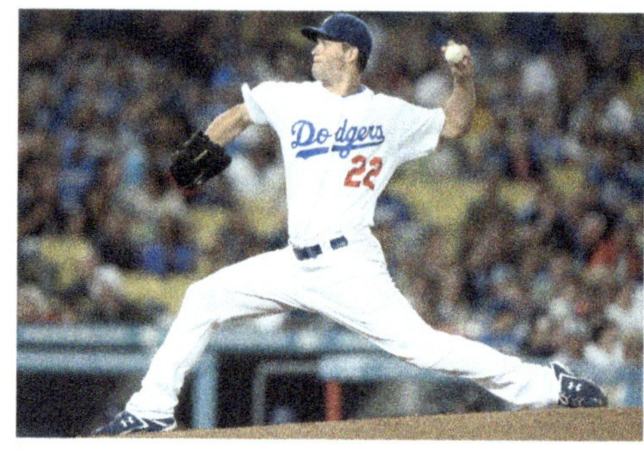

As of 2018, Clayton Kershaw of the Los Angeles Dodgers had the lowest earned-run average in the National League in five different years.

a) Complete the following table, rounding to two decimal places (note that $\frac{1}{3}$ of an inning pitched means that the pitcher recorded just 1 out):

Innings Pitched, n	9	6	3	1	$\frac{2}{3}$	$\frac{1}{3}$
Earned-Run Average, E						

b) Complete the table in part (a) assuming that a pitcher has given up $n = 6$ earned runs.
c) Based on the trends in parts (a) and (b), is it possible for a pitcher to have an "infinite" earned-run average? Give an example of how this may occur.

62. **Purchasing power.** The purchasing power of the U.S. dollar t years after 1990 can be modeled by the function

$$P(x) = \frac{1}{1 + 0.0362x}.$$

(*Source*: Based on data from the Consumer Price Index.)

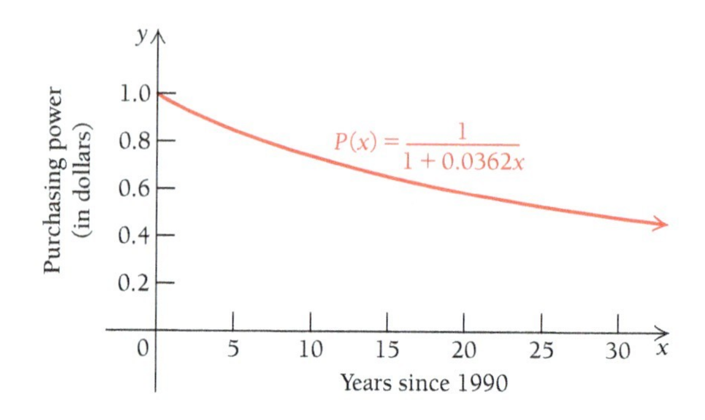

a) Find $P(5)$, $P(10)$, and $P(25)$.
b) When was the purchasing power \$0.50?
c) Find $\lim_{x \to \infty} P(x)$.

SYNTHESIS

63. Explain why a function can have one or two horizontal asymptotes, but not three or more.

64. Explain why it is possible for the graph of a function to cross a horizontal or slant asymptote, but not a vertical asymptote.

65. Explain why a vertical asymptote is only a guide and is not part of the graph of a function.

66. Using graphs and limits, explain how three types of asymptotes are used when graphing rational functions.

In Exercises 67–70, use the fact that $\sqrt{ax^2 + bx + c} \approx \sqrt{ax^2}$ as $x \to \infty$ to find each limit.

67. $\lim_{x \to \infty} \frac{\sqrt{4x^2 + 1}}{3x}$

68. $\lim_{x \to \infty} \frac{\sqrt{9x^2 + x - 2}}{6x + 1}$

69. $\lim_{x \to \infty} \frac{4x + 7}{\sqrt{9x^2 + 5x + 2}}$

70. $\lim_{x \to \infty} \frac{-2x + 5}{\sqrt{3x^2 + 1}}$

Find each limit, if it exists.

71. $\lim_{x \to -\infty} \frac{-3x^2 + 5}{2 - x}$

72. $\lim_{x \to 0} \frac{|x|}{x}$

73. $\lim_{x \to -2} \frac{x^3 + 8}{x^2 - 4}$

74. $\lim_{x \to -\infty} \frac{-6x^3 + 7x}{2x^2 - 3x - 10}$

75. $\lim_{x \to 1} \frac{x^3 - 1}{x^2 - 1}$

Technology Connection 

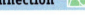

Graph each function using a graphing utility.

76. $f(x) = \frac{x^3 + 4x^2 + x - 6}{x^2 - x - 2}$

77. $f(x) = \frac{x^3 + 2x^2 - 15x}{x^2 - 5x - 14}$

78. $f(x) = \frac{x^3 + 2x^2 - 3x}{x^2 - 25}$

79. $f(x) = \left|\frac{1}{x} - 2\right|$

80. Refer to the graph on p. 294. The function is given by

$$f(x) = \frac{x^2 - 1}{x^2 + x - 6}.$$

a) Inspect the graph and estimate the coordinates of any extrema.
b) Find f' and use it to determine the critical values. (*Hint*: You will need the quadratic formula.) Round the x-values to the nearest hundredth.
c) Graph f in the window $[0, 0.2, 0.16, 0.17]$. Use TRACE or MAXIMUM to confirm your results from part (b).
d) Graph f in the window $[9.8, 10, 0.9519, 0.95195]$. Use TRACE or MINIMUM to confirm your results from part (b).
e) How close were your estimates of part (a)? Would you have been able to identify the relative minimum point without calculus?

In Exercises 81–85, determine a rational function that meets the given conditions, and sketch its graph. Answers may vary.

81. The function f has a vertical asymptote at $x = 0$, a horizontal asymptote at $y = 3$, and $f(1) = 2$.

82. The function g has vertical asymptotes at $x = -1$ and $x = 1$, a horizontal asymptote at $y = 1$, and $g(0) = 2$.

83. The function g has vertical asymptotes at $x = -2$ and $x = 0$, a horizontal asymptote at $y = -3$, and $g(1) = 4$.

84. The function h has vertical asymptotes at $x = -3$ and $x = 2$, a horizontal asymptote at $y = 0$, and $h(1) = 2$.

85. The function h has vertical asymptotes at $x = -\frac{1}{2}$ and $x = \frac{1}{2}$, a horizontal asymptote at $y = 0$, and $h(0) = -3$.

Answers to Quick Checks

1. The lines $x = 0$, $x = 4$, and $x = -4$ are vertical asymptotes. **2.** The lines $x = -1$ and $x = 0$ are vertical asymptotes. **3.** The line $y = \frac{2}{15}$ is a horizontal asymptote. **4.** The line $y = 0$ is a horizontal asymptote. **5.** The line $y = 2x + 7$ is a slant asymptote. **6.** The lines $y = \frac{55}{3}$ (as $x \to \infty$) and $y = 0$ (as $x \to -\infty$) are horizontal asymptotes. **7.** x-intercepts: $(1, 0)$, $(-1, 0)$, $(0, 0)$; y-intercept: $(0, 0)$ **8.** The x-intercept is $(-4, 0)$, the y-intercept is $(0, \ln 5)$, and the vertical asymptote is $x = -5$. **9.** No x-intercepts, no y-intercepts, relative maximum at $(-2, -4)$, relative minimum at $(2, 4)$, increasing on $(-\infty, -2)$ and on $(2, \infty)$, decreasing on $(-2, 0)$ and on $(0, 2)$, concave down on $(-\infty, 0)$, concave up on $(0, \infty)$, no inflection points, slant asymptote is $y = x$, vertical asymptote at $x = 0$.

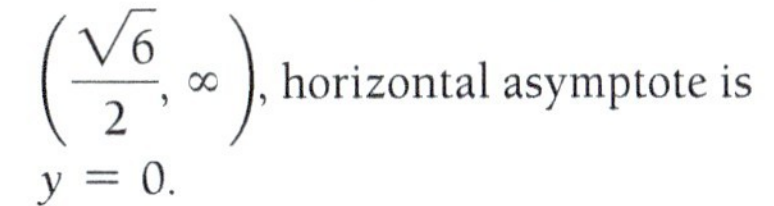

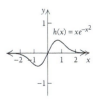

10. The x-intercept and y-intercept are both $(0, 0)$, relative maximum at $\left(\frac{\sqrt{2}}{2}, \frac{\sqrt{2}e^{-1/2}}{2}\right)$, relative minimum at $\left(-\frac{\sqrt{2}}{2}, -\frac{\sqrt{2}e^{-1/2}}{2}\right)$, increasing on $\left(-\frac{\sqrt{2}}{2}, \frac{\sqrt{2}}{2}\right)$, decreasing on $\left(-\infty, -\frac{\sqrt{2}}{2}\right)$ and on $\left(\frac{\sqrt{2}}{2}, \infty\right)$, inflection points at $\left(-\frac{\sqrt{6}}{2}, -\frac{\sqrt{6}e^{-3/2}}{2}\right)$, $(0, 0)$, and $\left(\frac{\sqrt{6}}{2}, \frac{\sqrt{6}e^{-3/2}}{2}\right)$, concave down on $\left(-\infty, -\frac{\sqrt{6}}{2}\right)$ and on $\left(0, \frac{\sqrt{6}}{2}\right)$, concave up on $\left(-\frac{\sqrt{6}}{2}, 0\right)$ and on $\left(\frac{\sqrt{6}}{2}, \infty\right)$, horizontal asymptote is $y = 0$.

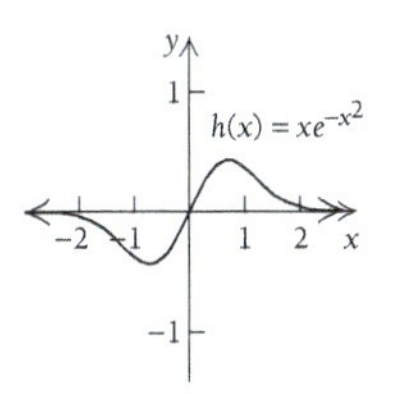

3.4 Optimization: Finding Absolute Maximum and Minimum Values

- Find absolute extrema using Maximum–Minimum Principle 1.
- Find absolute extrema using Maximum–Minimum Principle 2.

An extremum that is the highest or lowest value over a function's entire domain is called an *absolute extremum*. For example, the parabola given by $f(x) = x^2 + 1$ has a relative minimum at $(0, 1)$. This is also the lowest point for the *entire* graph of f, so it is also the absolute minimum. In applications, we often want to determine absolute extrema, a process called *optimization*.

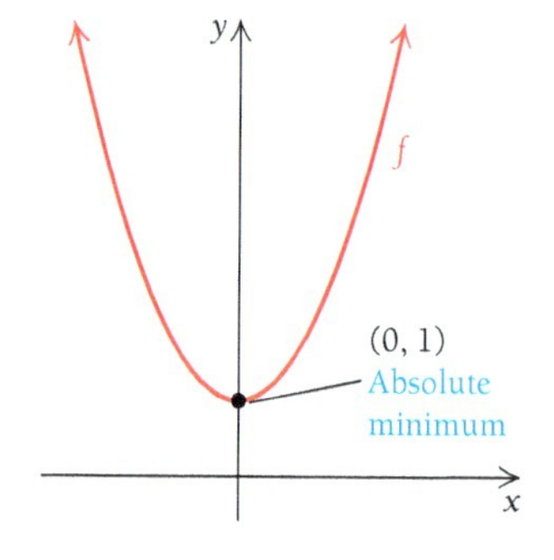

Absolute Maximum and Minimum Values

A relative minimum may or may not be an *absolute minimum*, meaning the smallest value of the function over its entire domain. Similarly, a relative maximum may or may not be an *absolute maximum*, meaning the largest value of a function over its entire domain.

The function in the following graph has relative minima at c_1 and c_3. Note that the function's domain is the closed interval $[a, b]$.

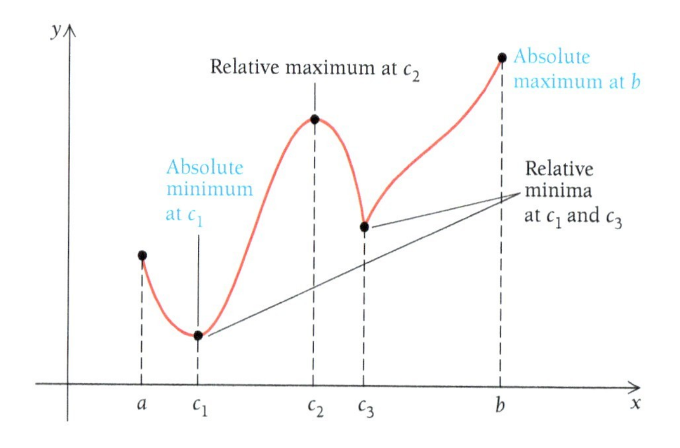

The relative minimum at c_1 is also the absolute minimum. On the other hand, the relative maximum at c_2 is *not* the absolute maximum. The absolute maximum occurs at b. Absolute maximum and absolute minimum points may occur at the endpoints of a closed interval. However, relative maximum and relative minimum points cannot occur at the endpoints of a closed interval, since they are always defined over an open interval.

DEFINITION

Suppose that f is a function with domain I.
$f(c)$ is an **absolute minimum** if $f(c) \leq f(x)$ for all x in I.
$f(c)$ is an **absolute maximum** if $f(c) \geq f(x)$ for all x in I.

Finding Absolute Maximum and Minimum Values over Closed Intervals

Let's consider continuous functions for which the domain is a closed interval. Look at the following graphs of f and g, and determine visually where the absolute extrema occur for each function.

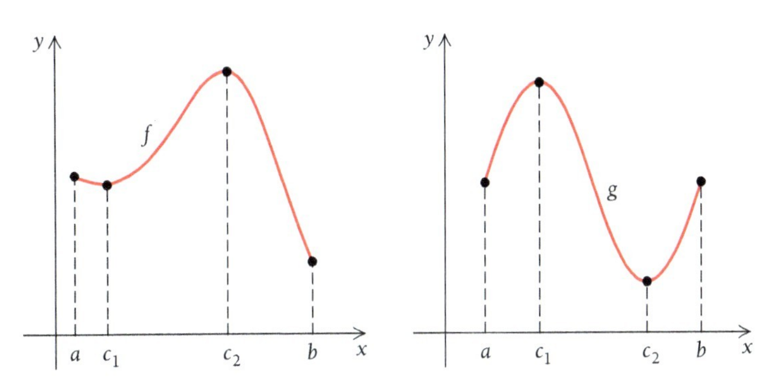

The function f has absolute extrema at c_2 and b, and the function g has absolute extrema at c_1 and c_2. This leads us to the following theorem.

THEOREM 7 The Extreme-Value Theorem

A continuous function f defined over a closed interval $[a, b]$ must have an absolute maximum value and an absolute minimum value over $[a, b]$.

Look again at f and g in the preceding figure and consider the critical values and the endpoints. It seems reasonable that whatever the maximum and minimum values are, they occur at a critical value or an endpoint.

THEOREM 8 Maximum–Minimum Principle 1

Suppose f is a continuous function defined over a closed interval $[a, b]$. To find the absolute maximum and minimum values over $[a, b]$:

a) Find $f'(x)$.

b) Determine all critical values in $[a, b]$. That is, find all c in $[a, b]$ for which

$$f'(c) = 0 \quad \text{or} \quad f'(c) \text{ does not exist.}$$

c) List the values from step (b) and the endpoints of the interval:

$$a, c_1, c_2, \ldots, c_n, b.$$

d) Evaluate $f(x)$ for each value in step (c):

$$f(a), f(c_1), f(c_2), \ldots, f(c_n), f(b).$$

The largest of these is the **absolute maximum of f over $[a, b]$**. The smallest of these is the **absolute minimum of f over $[a, b]$**.

EXAMPLE 1 Find the absolute maximum and absolute minimum values of

$$f(x) = x^3 - 3x + 2$$

over the interval $\left[-2, \frac{3}{2}\right]$.

Solution Keep in mind that we are considering only the interval $\left[-2, \frac{3}{2}\right]$.

a) Find $f'(x)$: $f'(x) = 3x^2 - 3$.

b) Determine the critical values. The derivative exists for all real numbers in $\left[-2, \frac{3}{2}\right]$. Thus, we solve $f'(x) = 0$:

$$\begin{aligned} 3x^2 - 3 &= 0 \\ 3x^2 &= 3 \\ x^2 &= 1 \\ x &= \pm 1. \end{aligned}$$

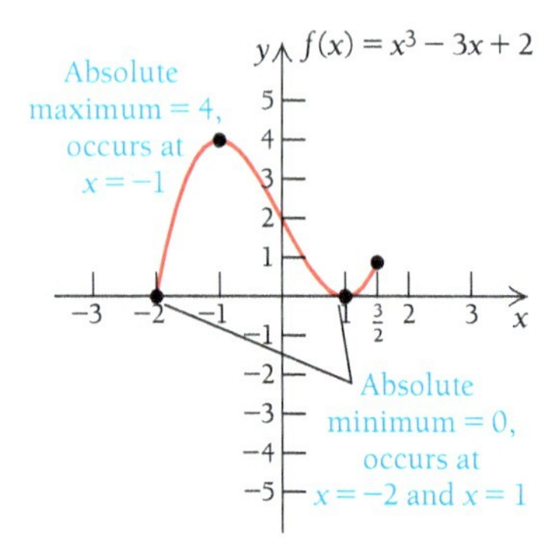

A visualization of Example 1

Quick Check 1 ✓

Find the absolute maximum and absolute minimum values of $g(x) = x^2 - 2$ over the interval $[-3, 3]$.

c) List the critical values and the endpoints: $-2, -1, 1,$ and $\frac{3}{2}$.

d) Evaluate $f(x)$ at each value in step (c):

$$f(-2) = (-2)^3 - 3(-2) + 2 = -8 + 6 + 2 = 0;$$
$$f(-1) = (-1)^3 - 3(-1) + 2 = -1 + 3 + 2 = 4;$$
$$f(1) = (1)^3 - 3(1) + 2 = 1 - 3 + 2 = 0;$$
$$f(\tfrac{3}{2}) = (\tfrac{3}{2})^3 - 3(\tfrac{3}{2}) + 2 = \tfrac{27}{8} - \tfrac{9}{2} + 2 = \tfrac{7}{8}$$

The largest of these values, 4, is the maximum. It occurs at $x = -1$. The smallest of these values is 0. It occurs twice: at $x = -2$ and $x = 1$. Thus, over the interval $\left[-2, \frac{3}{2}\right]$, the

absolute maximum $= 4$ at $x = -1$

and the

absolute minimum $= 0$ at $x = -2$ and $x = 1$. **1 ✓**

As we see in Example 1, an absolute maximum or minimum value can occur at more than one point.

EXAMPLE 2 Find the absolute maximum and absolute minimum values of $f(x) = 2e^{3x}$ over $\left[-2, \frac{1}{2}\right]$.

Solution The derivative of f is $f'(x) = 6e^{3x}$. Note that $f'(x)$ exists for all x in $\left[-2, \frac{1}{2}\right]$ and $f'(x) = 0$ has no solutions. Thus, there are no critical values and the absolute extrema must occur at the endpoints of the interval:

$$f(-2) = 2e^{3(-2)} = 2e^{-6} \approx 0.005,$$
$$f(\tfrac{1}{2}) = 2e^{3(1/2)} = 2e^{1.5} \approx 8.963.$$

The absolute maximum of $f(x) = 2e^{3x}$ over $\left[-2, \frac{1}{2}\right]$ is $2e^{1.5}$, or about 8.963, which occurs at $x = \frac{1}{2}$, and the absolute minimum is $2e^{-6}$, or about 0.005, which occurs at $x = -2$.

Quick Check 2 ✓

Find the absolute maximum and absolute minimum values of $f(x) = \ln x$ over the interval $[1, 5]$.

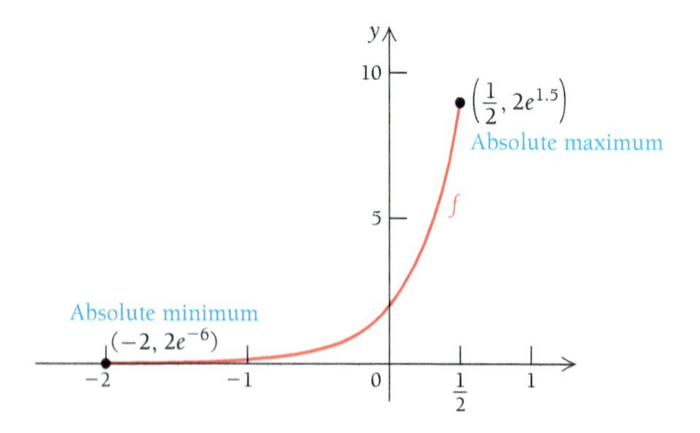

2 ✓

Finding Absolute Maximum and Minimum Values over Other Intervals

When there is only one critical value c in I, we may not need to check endpoint values to determine whether the function has an absolute maximum or minimum value at that point.

THEOREM 9 Maximum–Minimum Principle 2

Suppose f is a function such that $f'(x)$ exists for every x in an interval I and there is *exactly one* (critical) value c in I, for which $f'(c) = 0$. Then

$f(c)$ is the absolute maximum value over I if $f''(c) < 0$

or

$f(c)$ is the absolute minimum value over I if $f''(c) > 0$.

Theorem 9 holds no matter what the interval I is—whether open, closed, or infinite in length. If $f''(c) = 0$, either we must use Maximum–Minimum Principle 1 or we must know more about the behavior of the function over the given interval.

If the requirements for Maximum–Minimum Principle 1 or Principle 2 are not met, then we can use a combination of graphing and the First-Derivative or Second-Derivative Test to determine absolute extrema.

EXAMPLE 3 Find the absolute extrema of $f(x) = 4x - x^2$ over each interval:
a) $(-\infty, \infty)$; **b)** $[1, 4]$.

Solution

a) In this case, the domain is the set of all real numbers. We find $f'(x)$:

$$f'(x) = 4 - 2x.$$

Now we determine any critical values. The derivative exists for all real numbers. Thus, we need only solve $f'(x) = 0$:

$$4 - 2x = 0$$
$$-2x = -4$$
$$x = 2.$$

Since there is only one critical value, we apply Maximum–Minimum Principle 2 using the second derivative:

$$f''(x) = -2.$$

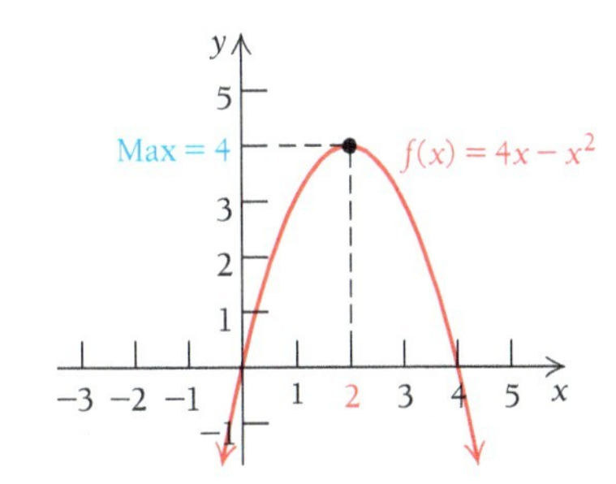

The second derivative is constant. Thus, $f''(2) = -2$, and since this is negative, we have the absolute maximum:

$$f(2) = 4 \cdot 2 - 2^2,$$
$$= 8 - 4 = 4.$$

The function has no minimum, as the graph at left indicates.

b) From part (a), we know that the absolute maximum of f on $(-\infty, \infty)$ is $f(2)$, or 4. Since 2 is in $[1, 4]$, we know that the absolute maximum of f over $[1, 4]$ will occur at 2. To find the absolute minimum, we need to check the endpoints:

$$f(1) = 4 \cdot 1 - 1^2 = 3$$

and

$$f(4) = 4 \cdot 4 - 4^2 = 0.$$

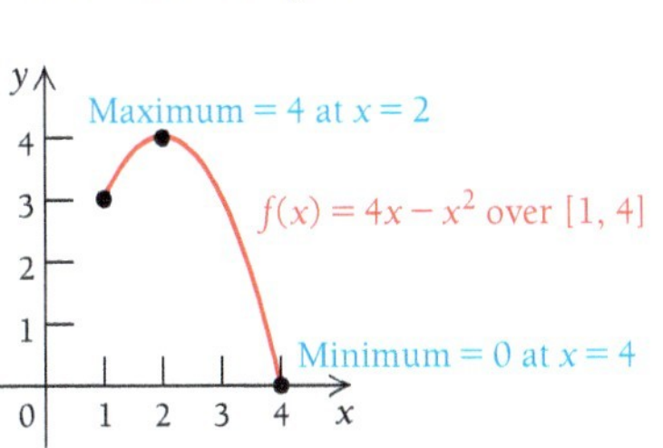

We also see from the graph that the minimum is 0. It occurs at $x = 4$. Thus, the

absolute maximum = 4 at $x = 2$,

and the

absolute minimum = 0 at $x = 4$.

3 ✓

Quick Check 3 ✓

Find the absolute extrema of $f(x) = x^2 - 10x$ over each interval:

a) $(-\infty, \infty)$; **b)** $[4, 10]$.

EXAMPLE 4 Find the absolute maximum and absolute minimum values of

$$f(x) = (x - 2)^3 + 1.$$

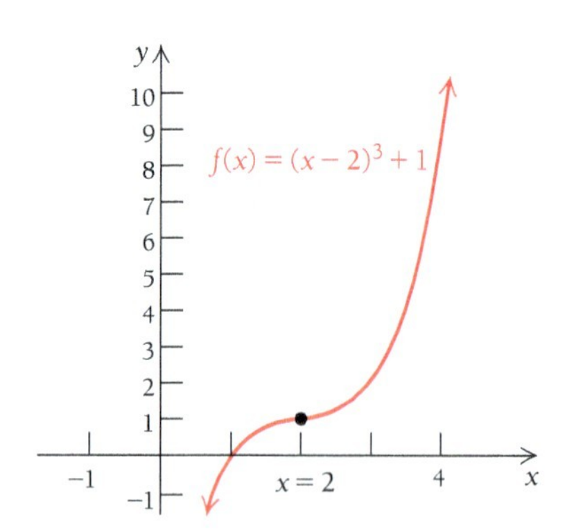

A visualization of Example 4

Quick Check 4 ✓

Let $f(x) = x^n$, where n is a positive odd integer. Explain why functions of this form never have an absolute minimum or maximum.

Solution We find $f'(x)$.

$$f'(x) = 3(x - 2)^2.$$

Next, we determine any critical values. The derivative exists for all real numbers. Thus, we solve $f'(x) = 0$:

$$\begin{aligned} 3(x - 2)^2 &= 0 \\ (x - 2)^2 &= 0 \\ x - 2 &= 0 \\ x &= 2. \end{aligned}$$

Since there is only one critical value and there are no endpoints, we can try to apply Maximum–Minimum Principle 2 using the second derivative:

$$f''(x) = 6(x - 2).$$

We have

$$f''(2) = 6(2 - 2) = 0,$$

so Maximum–Minimum Principle 2 does not apply. We cannot use Maximum–Minimum Principle 1 because there are no endpoints. Using the First-Derivative Test, we can see that $f'(x) = 3(x - 2)^2$ is never negative. Thus, $f(x)$ is increasing everywhere except at $x = 2$, so there is no maximum and no minimum. 4 ✓

EXAMPLE 5 **Business: Minimizing Average Cost.** The cost of materials, C, in dollars, to produce x dozen birthday cakes at Yum's Bakery is given by $C(x) = 0.5x^2 + 40x + 200$.

a) Find the average cost, $\overline{C}(x) = \dfrac{C(x)}{x}$.

b) Find the minimum average cost, and interpret the result.

Solution

a) The average cost is given by

$$\overline{C}(x) = \frac{0.5x^2 + 40x + 200}{x} = 0.5x + 40 + \frac{200}{x}.$$

Since x must be positive, the practical domain is $(0, \infty)$.

b) We note that $\overline{C}$ is defined for all x in the interval $(0, \infty)$. Thus, any critical values are found by solving $\overline{C}'(x) = 0$. The student can verify that the derivative is

$$\overline{C}'(x) = 0.5 - \frac{200}{x^2}.$$

We now set $\overline{C}'(x) = 0$, and solve:

$$\begin{aligned} 0.5 - \frac{200}{x^2} &= 0 \\ 0.5 &= \frac{200}{x^2} && \text{Adding } \frac{200}{x^2} \text{ to both sides} \\ 0.5x^2 &= 200 && \text{Multiplying both sides by } x^2 \\ x^2 &= \frac{200}{0.5} = 400 \\ x &= \sqrt{400} = 20. && \text{Using only the positive square root } (x > 0) \end{aligned}$$

Since there is only one critical value and no endpoints, we can apply Maximum–Minimum Principle 2 using the second derivative. The student can confirm that

$$\overline{C}''(x) = \frac{400}{x^3}.$$

Evaluating the second derivative at $x = 20$, we have

$$\overline{C}''(20) = \frac{400}{20^3} > 0.$$

Thus, $\overline{C}$ is concave up over the interval $(0, \infty)$, indicating that the point $(20, \overline{C}(20))$ is the absolute minimum point. Evaluating $\overline{C}(20)$, we have

$$\overline{C}(20) = 0.5(20) + 40 + \frac{200}{20} = 60.$$

When Yum's Bakery produces 20 dozen birthday cakes, the average cost of materials is \$60 per dozen. This is the most efficient use of materials. For any value of x below or above 20, the average cost is higher.

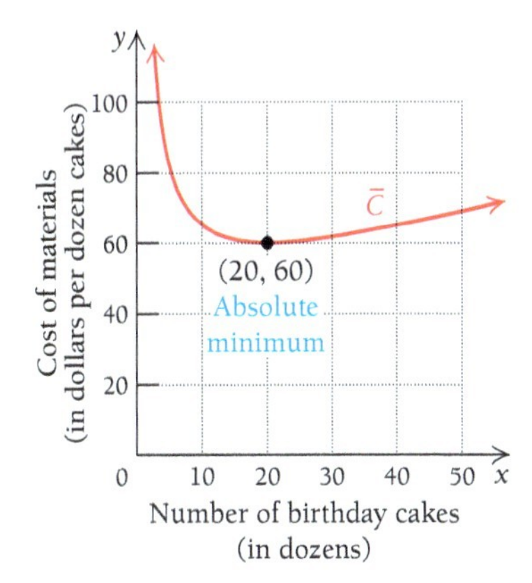

5 ✓

Quick Check 5 ✓

Find the absolute maximum and absolute minimum values of

$$g(x) = \frac{2x^2 + 18}{x}$$

over the interval $(0, \infty)$.

Section Summary

- An *absolute minimum* of f is a value $f(c)$ such that $f(c) \le f(x)$ for all x in the domain of f.
- An *absolute maximum* of f is a value $f(c)$ such that $f(c) \ge f(x)$ for all x in the domain of f.
- If the domain of f is a closed interval and f is continuous over that domain, then the *Extreme-Value Theorem* guarantees the existence of both an absolute minimum and an absolute maximum.
- Endpoints of a closed interval may be absolute extrema, but not relative extrema.
- If f is continuous over a closed interval, then use Maximum–Minimum Principle 1 to find absolute extrema.
- If there is exactly one critical value c in the domain of f such that $f'(c) = 0$ and if the domain is an open interval, then use Maximum–Minimum Principle 2 to determine extrema.
- In all other cases, use a combination of graphing and the First-Derivative and Second-Derivative Tests to determine extrema.

3.4 Exercise Set

1. **Fuel economy.** According to the U.S. Department of Energy, a vehicle's fuel economy, in miles per gallon (mpg), decreases significantly at speeds over 60 mph.
   a) Estimate the speed at which the absolute maximum fuel economy is obtained.
   b) Estimate the speed at which the absolute minimum fuel economy is obtained.
   c) What is the fuel economy obtained at 70 mph?
2. **Fuel economy.** Using the graph in Exercise 1, estimate the absolute maximum and the absolute minimum fuel economy over the interval $[30, 70]$.

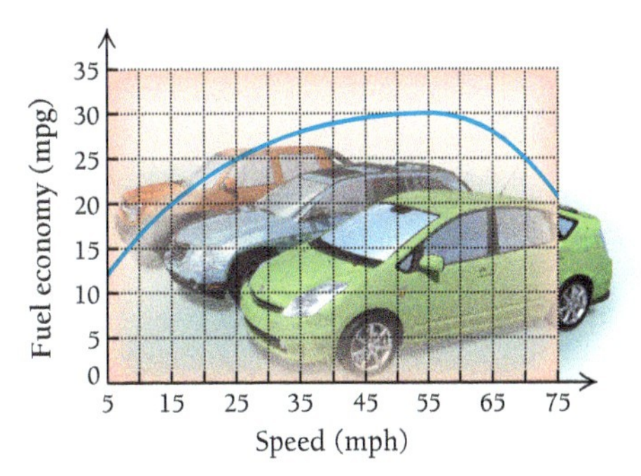

(*Sources*: U.S. Dept. of Energy; a study by West, B.H., McGill, R.N., Hodgson, J.W., Sluder, S.S., and Smith, D.E., Oak Ridge National Laboratory, 1999; www.mpgforspeed.com, 2017.)

Find the absolute maximum and minimum values of each function over the indicated interval, and indicate the x-values at which they occur.

3. $f(x) = 5 + x - x^2$; $[0, 2]$

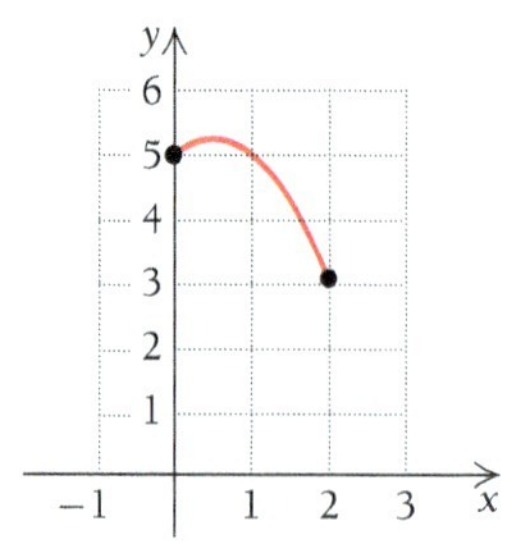

4. $f(x) = 4 + x - x^2$; $[0, 2]$

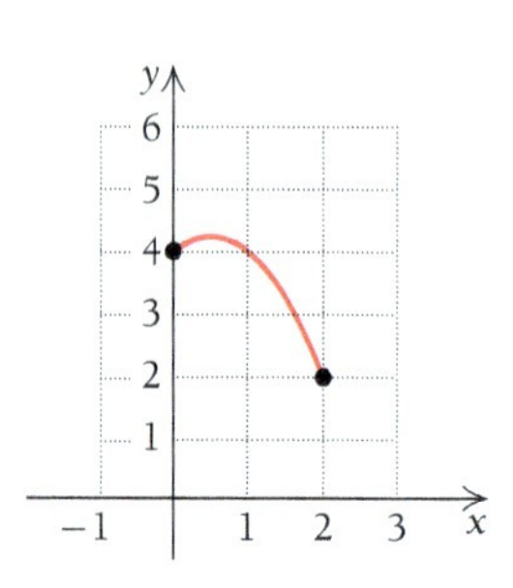

5. $f(x) = x^3 + \frac{1}{2}x^2 - 2x + 5$; $[-2, 1]$

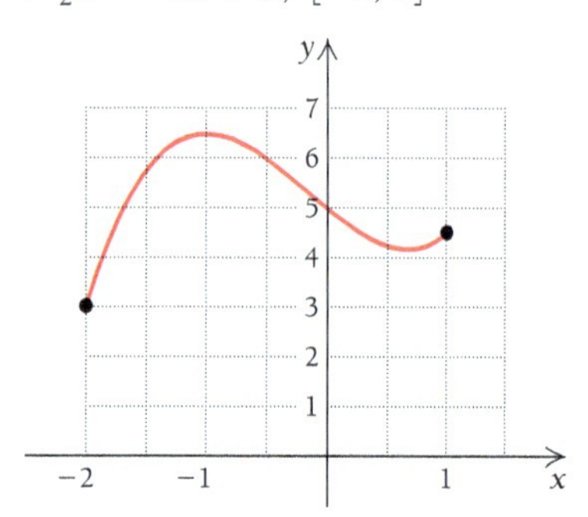

6. $f(x) = x^3 - x^2 - x + 2$; $[-1, 2]$

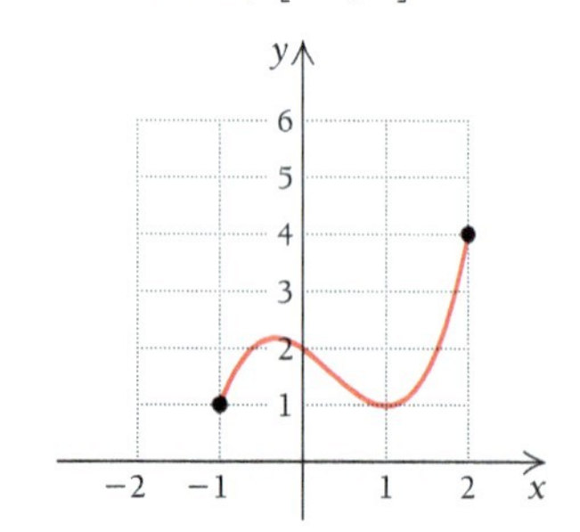

7. $f(x) = 2x + 4$; $[-1, 1]$

8. $f(x) = 5x - 7$; $[-2, 3]$

9. $f(x) = x^2 - 6x - 3$; $[-1, 5]$

10. $f(x) = 3 - 2x - 5x^2$; $[-3, 3]$

11. $f(x) = x^3 + \frac{1}{2}x^2 - 2x + 4$; $[-2, 0]$

12. $f(x) = x^3 - x^2 - x + 3$; $[-1, 0]$

13. $f(x) = 1 + 6x - 3x^2$; $[0, 4]$

14. $f(x) = x^3 - 3x + 6$; $[-1, 3]$

15. $f(x) = x^3 - x^4$; $[-1, 1]$

16. $f(x) = x^4 - 2x^3$; $[-2, 2]$

17. $f(x) = 1 - x^{2/3}$; $[-8, 8]$

18. $f(x) = (x + 3)^{2/3} - 5$; $[-4, 5]$

19. $f(x) = x + \frac{4}{x}$; $[-8, -1]$

20. $f(x) = x + \frac{1}{x}$; $[1, 20]$

21. $f(x) = \frac{x^2}{x^2 + 1}$; $[-2, 2]$

22. $f(x) = \frac{4x}{x^2 + 1}$; $[-3, 3]$

23. $f(x) = e^{3x} - e^{2x}$; $[-2, 1]$

24. $f(x) = e^x - e^{4x}$; $[-1, 1]$

25. $f(x) = \ln(x^3 - 3x + 4)$; $\left[-\frac{3}{2}, \frac{3}{2}\right]$

26. $f(x) = \ln(x^2 + 4)$; $[-3, 1]$

27. $f(x) = xe^{-(1/4)x}$; $[-1, 10]$

28. $f(x) = xe^{0.5x}$; $[-4, 2]$

Find the absolute extrema of each function, if they exist, over the indicated interval. Also indicate the x-value at which each extremum occurs. When no interval is specified, use the real numbers, $(-\infty, \infty)$.

29. $f(x) = 16x - \frac{4}{3}x^3$; $(0, \infty)$

30. $f(x) = x - \frac{4}{3}x^3$; $(0, \infty)$

31. $f(x) = -0.001x^2 + 4.8x - 60$

32. $f(x) = -0.01x^2 + 1.4x - 30$

33. $f(x) = x^2 + \frac{432}{x}$; $(0, \infty)$

34. $f(x) = x^2 + \frac{250}{x}$; $(0, \infty)$

35. $f(x) = \sqrt[3]{x}$; $[0, 8]$

36. $f(x) = \sqrt{x}$; $[0, 4]$

37. $f(x) = 2xe^{-6x}$

38. $f(x) = 3xe^{-x}$

39. $f(x) = 75 - 15e^{-0.05x}$; $[0, \infty)$

40. $f(x) = 50 + 25e^{-0.4x}$; $[0, \infty)$

41. $f(x) = e^{4x} - e^{3x}$

42. $f(x) = e^{5x} - e^{2x}$

43. $f(x) = 500e^{0.05x} + 700e^{-0.07x}$; $[0, \infty)$

44. $f(x) = 15{,}000e^{0.04x} + 20{,}000e^{-0.05x}$; $[0, \infty)$

45. $f(x) = \ln x$; $[1, \infty)$

46. $f(x) = 3 + 2\ln x$; $[2, \infty)$

47. $f(x) = 30e^{0.01x}$; $[-10, 20]$

48. $f(x) = -15e^{-0.2x}$; $[-5, 7]$

APPLICATIONS

Business and Economics

49. Monthly productivity. An employee's monthly productivity M, in number of units produced, is found to be a function of t, the number of years of employment. For a certain product, a productivity function is given by

$$M(t) = -2t^2 + 100t + 180, \quad 0 \leq t \leq 40.$$

Find the maximum productivity and the year in which it is achieved.

50. Advertising. Sound Software estimates that it will sell N units of a program after spending a thousands of dollars on advertising, where

$$N(a) = -a^2 + 300a + 6, \quad 0 \le a \le 300.$$

Find the maximum number of units that can be sold and the amount that must be spent on advertising in order to achieve that maximum.

51. Investing. Gina has just invested in two funds. The combined value V, in dollars, of the two investments after t years is given by

$$V(t) = 20{,}000e^{0.033t} + 25{,}000e^{-0.052t}.$$

Find the absolute minimum and absolute maximum combined value of the two investments if Gina keeps her money in both funds for 20 yr.

52. Investing. Goldsmith Investments has two properties that it invested in for speculative purposes. The combined value of the two properties, in dollars, is given by

$$V(t) = 250{,}000e^{0.04t} + 300{,}000e^{-0.06t},$$

where t is the number of years since the original investment was made. Find the absolute minimum and absolute maximum combined value of the properties if Goldsmith holds onto them for 30 yr.

53. Average cost. Kennedy's Brickyard calculates that the cost, in dollars, C to produce x tons of paver bricks is given by

$$C(x) = 0.2x^2 + 125x + 3500.$$

a) Find the average cost $\overline{C}$ per ton of paver bricks produced.
b) How many tons should be produced to minimize the average cost per ton, and what is the average cost at this point?

54. Average cost. The LaChance Candy Company determines that the cost, in dollars per case, to produce its choco-nutty bar is given by

$$C(x) = 0.035x^2 + 500x + 12{,}500.$$

a) Find the average cost $\overline{C}$ per case of choco-nutty bars produced.
b) How many cases should be produced to minimize the average cost per case, and what is the average cost at this point?

General Interest

55. Ideal dimensions. The amount of material used to construct a certain box is given by

$$A(x) = 2x^2 + \frac{4000}{x^2},$$

where x is the length of one side of the square base of the box, in inches, and A is the amount of material used, in square inches.

a) Find the value x for which the amount of material is minimized.
b) What amount of material is used at the point found in part (a)?

56. Ideal dimensions. The amount of material used to construct a certain box is given by

$$A(x) = 4x^2 + \frac{6000}{x^2},$$

where x is the length of one side of the square base of the box, in inches, and A is the amount of material used, in square inches.

a) Find the value x for which the amount of material is minimized.
b) What amount of material is used at the point found in part (a)?

57. Minimizing cost of materials. The cost C, in dollars, to build a fence around a rectangular field with an area of 1000 m^2 is given by

$$C(x) = 8x + \frac{12{,}000}{x},$$

where x is the length of one side of the field.

a) Find the value x for which the cost to build the fence is minimized.
b) What is the cost at the value of x found in part (a)?

Life Science

58. Blood pressure. With a dosage of x cubic centimeters (cc) of a certain drug, the resulting blood pressure B, in millimeters of mercury (mmHg), is approximated by

$$B(x) = 50 + 30{,}500x^2 - 183{,}000x^3, \quad 0 \le x \le 0.16.$$

Find the maximum blood pressure and the dosage at which it occurs.

SYNTHESIS

59. The function $f(x) = e^{-x}$ is always positive and has a horizontal asymptote $y = 0$ as $x \to \infty$. Explain why 0 is not considered a minimum value of f.

60. The function $g(x) = 2x$ over the interval $[1, 3]$ has an absolute minimum at the point $(1, 2)$ and an absolute maximum at the point $(3, 6)$. Explain why there are no absolute extrema for $g(x) = 2x$ when the interval is open, that is, over $(1, 3)$.

For Exercises 61–64, find the absolute maximum and absolute minimum points for each function, and sketch the graph.

61. $f(x) = \begin{cases} 2x + 1, & \text{for } -3 \le x \le 1, \\ 4 - x^2, & \text{for } 1 < x \le 2 \end{cases}$

62. $g(x) = \begin{cases} x^2, & \text{for } -2 \le x \le 0, \\ 5x, & \text{for } 0 < x \le 2 \end{cases}$

63. $h(x) = \begin{cases} 1 - x^2, & \text{for } -4 \le x < 0, \\ 1 - x, & \text{for } 0 \le x < 1, \\ x - 1, & \text{for } 1 \le x \le 2 \end{cases}$

64. $F(x) = \begin{cases} x^2 + 4, & \text{for } -2 \le x < 0, \\ 4 - x, & \text{for } 0 \le x < 3, \\ \sqrt{x - 2}, & \text{for } 3 \le x \le 67 \end{cases}$

Technology Connection 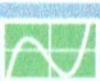

For Exercises 65–68, use a graphing utility to graph each function. Identify an interval over which any extremum occurs, and give the extremum.

65. $f(x) = |x| + |x - 2|$
66. $f(x) = |x - 1| + |x + 3|$
67. $f(x) = |2x + 1| + |2x + 10|$
68. $f(x) = |1 - 4x| + |6 - 4x|$

In Exercises 69–74, use a graphing utility to find the absolute extrema, if they exist, for each function. If no interval is stated, use $(-\infty, \infty)$.

69. $y = x^4 - 5x^3 + 6x^2 + 2x - 1$
70. $y = x^4 + 3x^3 - 8x^2 + x - 5$
71. $y = x^6 + 2x^5 + 2x, \quad [-2, 1]$
72. $y = x^6 - 4x^3 + x, \quad [0, 2]$
73. $y = \dfrac{x + 2}{x^4 + x^2 + 1}$
74. $y = \dfrac{x^2 + x + 1}{x^2 + 4}$

75. Explain why $f(x) = \begin{cases} 1 + x, & x < 2 \\ 4 - x, & x \geq 2 \end{cases}$ does not have an absolute maximum value.

Answers to Quick Checks

1. Absolute maximum is 7 at $x = -3$ and $x = 3$; absolute minimum is -2 at $x = 0$. **2.** Absolute minimum is 0 at $x = 1$; absolute maximum is ln 5 (or approximately 1.609) at $x = 5$. **3. (a)** Absolute minimum is -25 at $x = 5$; no absolute maximum. **(b)** Absolute minimum is -25 at $x = 5$; absolute maximum is 0 at $x = 10$. **4.** The derivative is $f'(x) = nx^{n-1}$. If n is odd, then $n - 1$ is even. Thus, nx^{n-1} is 0 or positive, but never negative. **5.** Absolute minimum is 12 at $x = 3$; no absolute maximum.

3.5 Optimization: Business, Economics, and General Applications

- Solve optimization (maximum–minimum) problems using calculus.

An important use of calculus is in solving real-world *optimization* problems. An optimization problem involves an *objective function* that models the specific quantity being maximized or minimized and often has more than one input variable. A *constraint* may be imposed that relates the input variables in an equation. Through substitution that makes use of the constraint equation, we can often write the objective function as a function of just one input variable.

For example, a manufacturer of aluminum cans may want to use as little material per can as possible, to save on manufacturing costs. Here, the objective function will be a cost function related to the amount of material used in each can, where the radius r and the height h are the two variables that describe the dimensions of the can. If the can is required to contain a certain volume, r and h will be related in a single equation, which is a constraint that can be used to express one variable in terms of the other. We can then use substitution to write the cost function in terms of a single variable. We discuss this function in Example 3.

EXAMPLE 1 **Maximizing Area.** The Hobby Farm has 20 ft of fencing to fence off a rectangular area for an electric train in one corner of its display room. The two sides up against the wall require no fence. What dimensions of the rectangle will maximize the area? What is the maximum area?

Solution We let x be the length of one side of the rectangle and y the length of the other side. The area A of the rectangle formed by the fencing is given by the objective function

$$A = xy. \qquad \text{This represents length} \cdot \text{width.}$$

We are limited in the amount of fencing available: This is the constraint. Since 20 ft of fencing is available, the two side lengths x and y are related by the equation

$$x + y = 20, \quad \text{or} \quad y = 20 - x.$$

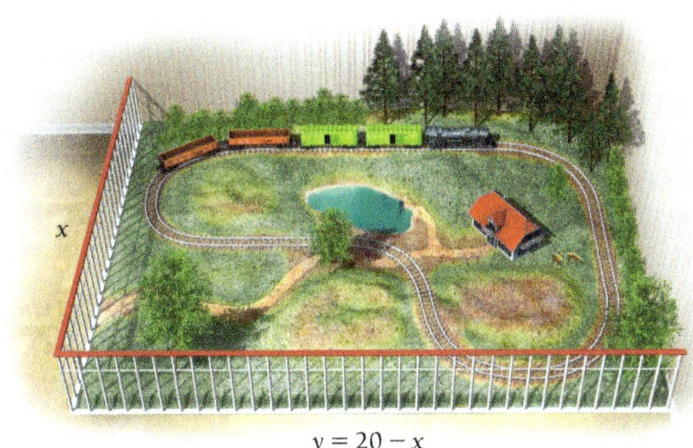

The practical domain is $0 \leq x \leq 20$, since the amount of fencing used for one side cannot be negative or greater than 20 ft.

Let's try choosing values for x, and see if we can estimate the maximum area:

Length of one side: x	Length of other side: $y = 20 - x$	Area: $A = xy$
8 ft	12 ft	$8 \cdot 12 = 96$ ft^2
9 ft	11 ft	$9 \cdot 11 = 99$ ft^2
10 ft	10 ft	$10 \cdot 10 = 100$ ft^2
11 ft	9 ft	$11 \cdot 9 = 99$ ft^2
12 ft	8 ft	$12 \cdot 8 = 96$ ft^2

Based on the table, it appears that letting $x = 10$ ft will result in a maximum area of 100 ft^2. To be sure, we use calculus. Substituting the constraint $y = 20 - x$ into the formula for area, we have

$$A = xy \quad \text{The objective function is expressed using two variables.}$$

$$A = x(20 - x) \quad \text{Substituting } y = 20 - x$$

$$A(x) = 20x - x^2 \quad \text{This is the objective function in one variable.}$$

Thus, we want to maximize $A(x) = 20x - x^2$ over $[0, 20]$.

We find $A'(x)$:

$$A'(x) = 20 - 2x.$$

This derivative exists for all x in $(0, 20)$. The only critical values are where $A'(x) = 0$:

$$20 - 2x = 0$$
$$20 = 2x$$
$$x = 10.$$

Evaluating the objective function at the critical value, $x = 10$, we have

$$A(10) = 20(10) - (10)^2 = 200 - 100 = 100.$$

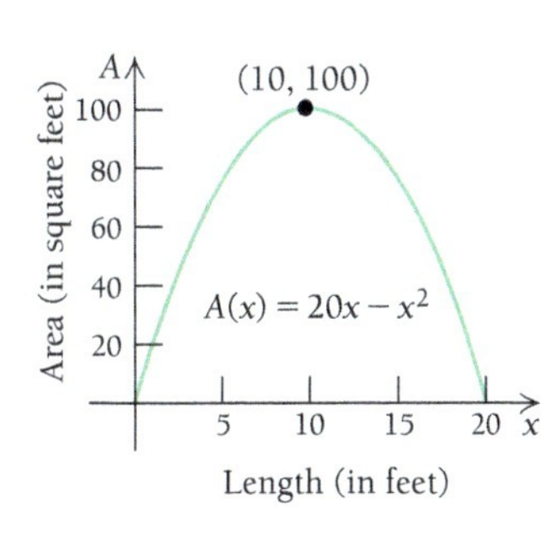

Thus, the point $(10, 100)$ is a critical point on the graph of A. The student can confirm that the endpoints $x = 0$ and $x = 20$ both result in a minimum area of 0 ft^2. We use the Second-Derivative Test to classify $(10, 100)$ as a relative maximum or a relative minimum. The second derivative is

$$A''(x) = -2.$$

This means that the graph of A is concave down for all x, so $(10, 100)$ is a relative maximum point. By Maximum–Minimum Principle 1, we conclude that the *absolute* maximum value of A over the interval $[0, 20]$ occurs at $x = 10$.

Quick Check 1 ✓

Repeat Example 1 with 100 ft of fencing. If you had n feet of fencing, what would be the dimensions of the maximum area (in terms of n)?

The Hobby Farm should use 10 ft of fencing on one side and 10 ft on the other, to achieve the largest possible area of 100 ft^2. Using calculus has shown that this time our original intuition of using 10 feet of fencing to a side was correct. **1 ✓**

Here is a general strategy for solving maximum–minimum problems.

A Strategy for Solving Maximum–Minimum Problems

1. Read the problem carefully. Make a drawing, and label any dimensions, if possible.
2. Make a list of appropriate variables and constraints, noting what varies, what stays fixed, and what units are being used. Label the measurements on your drawing.
3. Translate the problem to an objective function f that expresses the quantity to be maximized or minimized. Represent f in terms of the variables of step 2.
4. Use algebra and substitution as needed to express f as a function of one variable.
5. Use the procedures developed in Sections 3.1–3.4 to determine the maximum or minimum values and the points at which they occur.

EXAMPLE 2 **Maximizing Volume.** From a sheet of cardboard, 8 in. by 11 in., squares are cut out at the corners so that the sides can be folded up to make a box. What dimensions will yield a box of maximum volume? What is the maximum volume?

Solution We make a drawing in which x is the length, in inches, of each square to be cut out. It is important to note that since the original rectangle is 8 in. by 11 in., after the squares are removed, the lengths of the sides of the box will be $(8 - 2x)$ in. and $(11 - 2x)$ in.

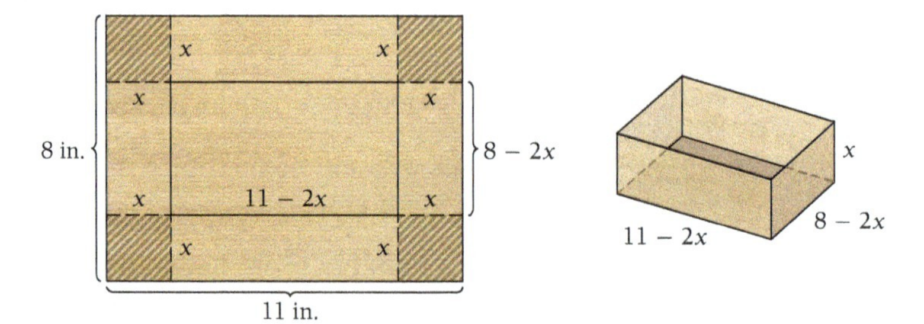

After the four squares are removed and the sides are folded up, the volume V of the resulting box is

$$V = l \cdot w \cdot h = (11 - 2x) \cdot (8 - 2x) \cdot x.$$

Let's choose values for x and calculate the box's volume to gain a sense of how much should be cut out at each corner to maximize the box's volume:

Height of box: $h = x$	Length of base: $l = 11 - 2x$	Width of base: $w = 8 - 2x$	Volume of box: $V = l \cdot w \cdot h$
0.5	$11 - 2(0.5) = 10$	$8 - 2(0.5) = 7$	$10 \cdot 7 \cdot 0.5 = 35$ in^3
1	$11 - 2(1) = 9$	$8 - 2(1) = 6$	$9 \cdot 6 \cdot 1 = 54$ in^3
1.5	$11 - 2(1.5) = 8$	$8 - 2(1.5) = 5$	$8 \cdot 5 \cdot 1.5 = 60$ in^3
2	$11 - 2(2) = 7$	$8 - 2(2) = 4$	$7 \cdot 4 \cdot 2 = 56$ in^3
2.5	$11 - 2(2.5) = 6$	$8 - 2(2.5) = 3$	$6 \cdot 3 \cdot 2.5 = 45$ in^3

Based on the table, it appears that if we cut a 1.5-in. square from each corner, the resulting box will have a volume of 60 in^3. Is this the largest possible volume? We will use calculus to answer this question. However, our work so far indicates that the optimal volume should occur when x is close to 1.5 in.

We have $V = l \cdot w \cdot h = (11 - 2x) \cdot (8 - 2x) \cdot x$. Multiplying gives us the objective function:

$$V(x) = 4x^3 - 38x^2 + 88x.$$

The amount cut out at each corner cannot be negative, nor can it be more than half of the 8-in. side length. Thus, the domain is $0 \le x \le 4$. Note that for $x = 0$ or $x = 4$, the volume is 0: In the first case, the box has no height, and in the second case, the box has no width.

To determine critical values, we find $V'(x)$:

$$V'(x) = 12x^2 - 76x + 88.$$

Since $V'(x)$ is defined for all x in the interval $(0, 4)$, we set $V'(x) = 0$ to find any critical values. Using the quadratic formula with $a = 12, b = -76$, and $c = 88$, we have

$$x = \frac{-(-76) \pm \sqrt{(-76)^2 - 4(12)(88)}}{2(12)} = \frac{76 \pm \sqrt{1552}}{24}.$$

Using a calculator and rounding to three decimal places, we have $x = \frac{76 - \sqrt{1552}}{24} \approx 1.525$ and $x = \frac{76 + \sqrt{1552}}{24} \approx 4.808$. However, the second value is not within the domain of the objective function, so the only critical value is 1.525. Thus, the point $(1.525, V(1.525))$ is a critical point. To classify this critical point, we use the Second-Derivative Test. The second derivative is

$$V''(x) = 24x - 76.$$

Evaluating at $x = 1.525$, we obtain

$$V''(1.525) = 24(1.525) - 76 = -39.4 < 0.$$

Since $V''(1.525)$ is negative, the graph of V is concave down, indicating that $(1.525, V(1.525))$ is a relative maximum point over the interval $[0, 4]$. Since we have already determined that both $x = 0$ and $x = 4$ (the endpoints) give zero volume, by Maximum–Minimum Principle 1, we conclude that $(1.525, V(1.525))$ must also be the *absolute* maximum point over $[0, 4]$.

Thus, to maximize the volume of the box, we should cut a square of side length $x = 1.525$ in. from each corner, then fold up the flaps. The box will have a maximum volume of

$$V(1.525) = 4(1.525)^3 - 38(1.525)^2 + 88(1.525) = 60.0126 \text{ in}^3.$$

This answer agrees well with our initial estimation based on the table. **2 ✓**

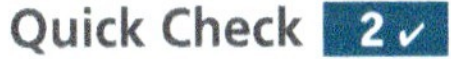

Quick Check 2 ✓

Repeat Example 2 starting with a sheet of cardboard measuring 10 in. by 10 in.

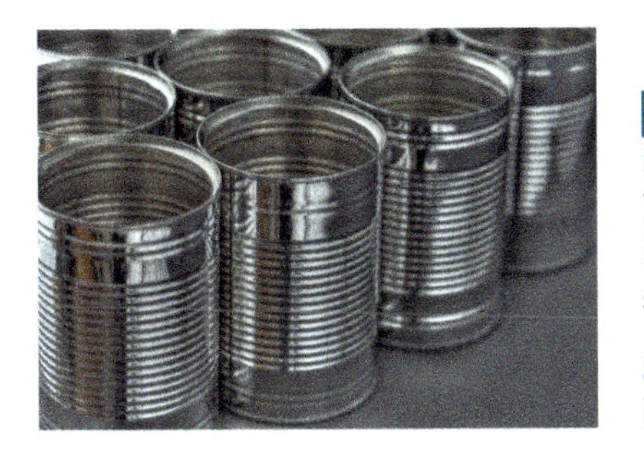

EXAMPLE 3 **Minimizing Cost of Material.** Mendoza Manufacturers specializes in food-storage containers and makes a cylindrical soup can with a volume of 250 cm^3. The cost of material for the two circular ends is $\$0.0008/\text{cm}^2$, and the cost of material for the side is $\$0.0015/\text{cm}^2$. What dimensions minimize the cost of material for the soup can? What is the minimum cost?

Solution Recall from Section R.1 that we estimated the dimensions that give the lowest cost using a spreadsheet, as shown on the following page.

	A	B
1	radius	cost
2	r, in cm	C, in dollars
38	4	0.267924772
39	4.1	0.267423105
40	4.2	0.26723974
41	4.3	0.267359482
42	4.4	0.267768519
43	4.5	0.268454269

← Possible lowest cost (row 40)

The spreadsheet suggests that a radius of about 4.2 cm gives a minimal cost of \$0.26723974 per can.

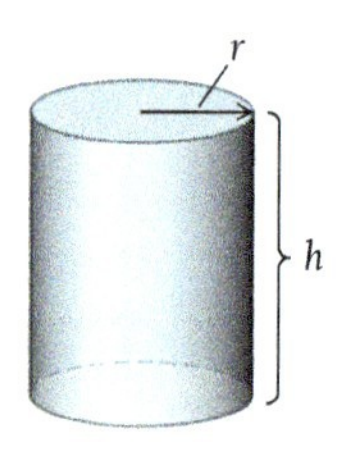

Let's use calculus to find the *exact* dimensions that minimize production costs. We let $r =$ the radius of the base and $h =$ the height of the can, both measured in centimeters. The can has two circular ends, each with an area of πr^2. Thus, the cost of material for the two circular ends is $2(0.0008)\pi r^2 = 0.0016\pi r^2$.

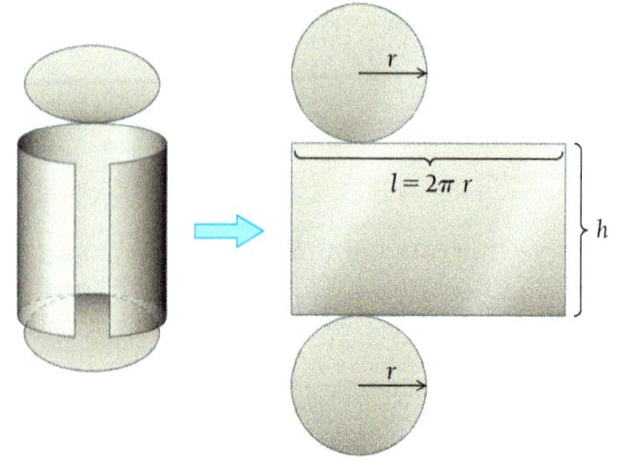

Each of the circular ends of the disassembled can has an area of πr^2, and the side has an area of $2\pi rh$.

The side of the can, when disassembled, is a rectangle of area $2\pi rh$, as shown at left. The cost of material for the side is $2(0.0015)\pi rh = 0.003\pi rh$.

Thus, the total cost of material for one can is given by

$$C = 0.0016\pi r^2 + 0.003\pi rh.$$

This is the objective function, but it contains two input variables, h and r. These two variables are related to one another by the fixed volume of the can. The formula for the volume of a cylinder is

$$V = \pi r^2 h.$$

Since we know that the volume of the can is 250 cm^3, this formula allows us to relate h and r, expressing one in terms of the other. We solve for h in terms of r:

$$\pi r^2 h = 250$$

$$h = \frac{250}{\pi r^2}.$$

This equation constrains h and r: Once one is known, the other can be determined. We substitute this expression for h into the cost function, making it a function in a single variable, r:

$$C = 0.0016\pi r^2 + 0.003\pi rh$$

$$= 0.0016\pi r^2 + 0.003\pi r\left(\frac{250}{\pi r^2}\right). \quad \text{Substituting}$$

Simplifying this, we see that the total cost of material for one can is given by

$$C(r) = 0.0016\pi r^2 + \frac{0.75}{r}, \text{ where } r > 0.$$

Differentiating, we have

$$C'(r) = 0.0032\pi r - \frac{0.75}{r^2}.$$

We set the derivative equal to zero and solve to find any critical value(s):

$$0.0032\pi r - \frac{0.75}{r^2} = 0$$

$$0.0032\pi r = \frac{0.75}{r^2}$$

$$0.0032\pi r^3 = 0.75 \quad \text{Multiplying both sides by } r^2$$

$$r^3 = \frac{0.75}{0.0032\pi}$$

$$r = \sqrt[3]{\frac{0.75}{0.0032\pi}}$$

$$r \approx 4.21 \quad \text{Using a calculator}$$

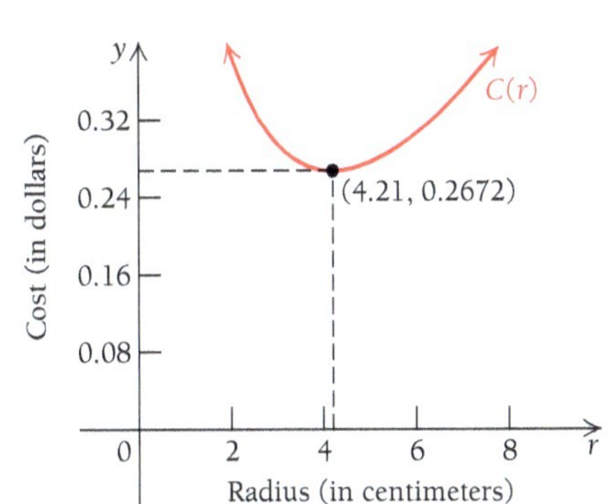

Note that the critical value $r \approx 4.21$ is the only critical value in the interval $(0, \infty)$. To determine whether this yields a minimum or maximum value of C, we use the Second-Derivative Test:

$$C''(r) = 0.0032\pi + \frac{1.5}{r^3}$$

$$C''(4.21) = 0.0032\pi + \frac{1.5}{(4.21)^3} > 0.$$

The second derivative is positive, so the critical value yields a minimum point. Thus, the cost of material for one can is minimized when $r = 4.21$ cm. The can will have a height of $h = 250/[\pi(4.21)^2] \approx 4.49$ cm, and the cost of material will be $C(4.21) = \$0.2672$ per can.

We rounded our answer above. If we do not, we find that a radius of 4.209725752 . . . cm will give a minimal cost of \$0.26723831 . . . per can. A manufacturer who produces millions of cans may be interested in carrying the precision of the calculations to six or seven decimal places. **3 ✓**

Quick Check 3 ✓

Repeat Example 3, assuming that the can has an open top. That is, it consists of one circular end and the side.

EXAMPLE 4 **Life Science: Concentration of a Drug in the Bloodstream.** A drug is administered into the bloodstream of a patient. Let $C(t) = 25te^{-0.04t}$ represent the concentration, $C(t)$, in nanograms per milliliter (ng/mL), of the drug t minutes after it is administered. What is the peak concentration of the drug in the bloodstream, and when does this peak occur?

Solution We differentiate C:

$$C'(t) = \frac{dC}{dt} = 25t(-0.04e^{-0.04t}) + 25e^{-0.04t} \quad \text{Using the Product Rule}$$

$$= -te^{-0.04t} + 25e^{-0.04t}. \quad \text{Simplifying}$$

We then solve $C'(t) = 0$ to determine any critical values:

$$-te^{-0.04t} + 25e^{-0.04t} = 0$$

$$e^{-0.04t}(-t + 25) = 0$$

$$t = 25.$$

Evaluating C at the critical value $t = 25$, we have

$$C(25) = 25(25)e^{-0.04(25)} \quad \text{Substituting}$$

$$= 625e^{-1}$$

$$\approx 229.92\,\frac{\text{ng}}{\text{mL}}. \quad \text{Using a calculator}$$

We use the second derivative to classify the critical point:

$$C''(t) = -t(-0.04e^{-0.04t}) - e^{-0.04t} + 25(-0.04e^{-0.04t})$$
$$= 0.04te^{-0.04t} - 2e^{-0.04t} \quad \text{Simplifying}$$

When $t = 25$, we have

$$C''(25) = 0.04(25)e^{-0.04(25)} - 2e^{-0.04(25)} \quad \text{Substituting}$$
$$= e^{-1} - 2e^{-1}$$
$$= -e^{-1} < 0.$$

Since $C''(25) < 0$, the graph is concave down, and the critical point $(25, 229.92)$ is a local maximum point. The drug reaches its highest concentration of 229.92 ng/mL 25 min after it was administered.

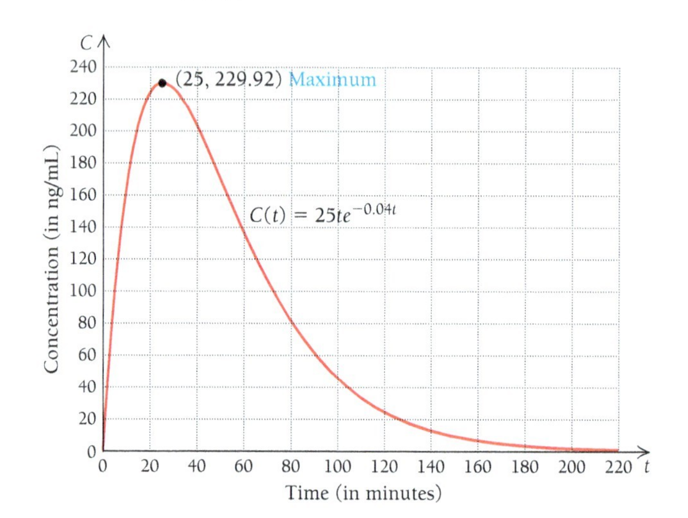

4 ✓

Quick Check 4 ✓

Let $C(t) = 50te^{-0.01t}$ represent the concentration, $C(t)$, in nanograms per milliliter (ng/mL), of a drug t minutes after being administered into a patient's bloodstream. What is the peak concentration of the drug in the bloodstream, and when does this peak occur?

EXAMPLE 5 **Business: Maximizing Revenue.** Cruzing Tunes determines that in order to sell x units of a new car audio receiver, the price per unit, in dollars, must be

$$p(x) = 1000 - x.$$

It also determines that the total cost of producing x units is given by

$$C(x) = 3000 + 20x.$$

a) Find the total revenue, $R(x)$.

b) Find the total profit, $P(x)$.

c) How many units must be made and sold in order to maximize profit?

d) What is the maximum profit?

e) What price per unit yields this maximum profit?

Solution

a) $R(x)$ = Total revenue
= (Number of units) · (Price per unit)
$= x \cdot p$
$= x \cdot (1000 - x)$ Substituting
$= 1000x - x^2.$

b) $P(x)$ = Total revenue − Total cost
$= R(x) - C(x)$
$= (1000x - x^2) - (3000 + 20x)$
$= -x^2 + 980x - 3000$

c) To find the maximum value of $P(x)$, we first find $P'(x)$:

$$P'(x) = -2x + 980.$$

Note that $x \geq 0$. Any critical value(s) are found by solving $P'(x) = 0$:

$$P'(x) = -2x + 980 = 0$$
$$-2x = -980$$
$$x = 490.$$

There is only one critical value. We can therefore try to use the second derivative to determine whether we have an absolute maximum. Note that

$$P''(x) = -2, \text{ a constant.}$$

Since $P''(490)$ is negative, profit is maximized when 490 units are produced and sold.

d) The maximum profit is given by

$$P(490) = -(490)^2 + 980 \cdot 490 - 3000 = \$237{,}100.$$

Thus, Cruzing Tunes makes a maximum profit of \$237,100 by producing and selling 490 units.

e) The price per unit needed to maximize profit is

$$p = 1000 - 490 = \$510.$$

5 ✓

Quick Check 5 ✓

Repeat Example 5 with the price function

$$p(x) = 1750 - 2x$$

and the total cost function

$$C(x) = 2250 + 15x.$$

Round your answers when necessary.

Let's take a general look at profit, cost, and revenue.

Figure 1 shows an example of total-cost and total-revenue functions. We can estimate what the maximum profit is by looking for the widest gap between $R(x)$ and $C(x)$, with $R(x) > C(x)$. Points B_0 and B_2 are break-even points.

Figure 2 shows the related total-profit function. Note that when production is too low ($< x_0$), there is a loss, perhaps due to high fixed or initial costs and low revenue. When production is too high ($> x_2$), there is also a loss, perhaps due to the increased cost of overtime pay or expansion.

The business operates at a profit everywhere between x_0 and x_2. Note that maximum profit occurs at a critical value x_1. Assuming that $P'(x)$ exists for all x in some interval, usually $[0, \infty)$, the critical value x_1 occurs at some number x such that

$$P'(x) = 0 \quad \text{and} \quad P''(x) < 0.$$

Since $P(x) = R(x) - C(x)$, it follows that

$$P'(x) = R'(x) - C'(x) \quad \text{and} \quad P''(x) = R''(x) - C''(x).$$

Thus, maximum profit occurs at some number x such that

$$P'(x) = R'(x) - C'(x) = 0 \quad \text{and} \quad P''(x) = R''(x) - C''(x) < 0,$$

or $$R'(x) = C'(x) \quad \text{and} \quad R''(x) < C''(x).$$

In summary, we have the following theorem.

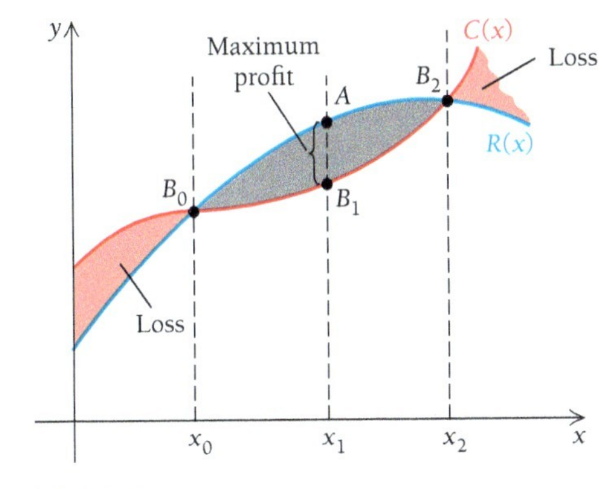

FIGURE 1

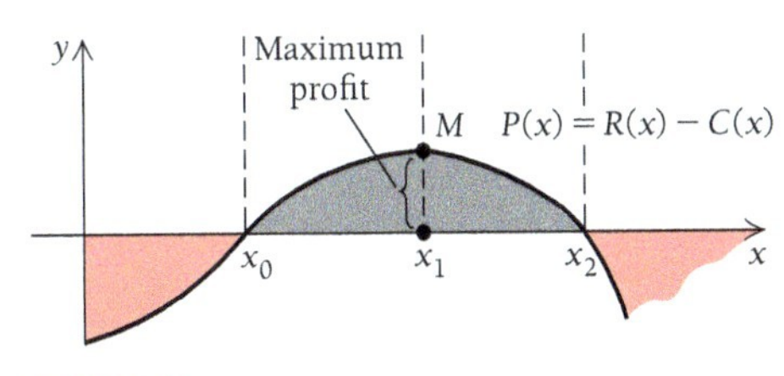

FIGURE 2

THEOREM 10

Maximum profit occurs at those x-values for which

$$R'(x) = C'(x) \quad \text{and} \quad R''(x) < C''(x),^*$$

where $R(x)$ is the total revenue and $C(x)$ is the total cost when x units are produced.

---

* In Section 3.6, the concepts of *marginal revenue* and *marginal cost* are introduced, allowing $R'(x) = C'(x)$ to be regarded as Marginal revenue = Marginal cost.

The results in parts (c) and (d) of Example 5 can be easily confirmed using Theorem 10.

EXAMPLE 6 **Business: Determining Ticket Price.** By keeping records, a theater determines that at a ticket price of \$26, it averages 1000 people in attendance. For every drop in price of \$1, it gains 50 customers. Each customer spends an average of \$4 on concessions. What ticket price should the theater charge in order to maximize total revenue?

Solution Let x be the number of dollars by which the ticket price of \$26 should be decreased. (If x is negative, the price is increased.) We first express the total revenue R as a function of x. Note that the increase in ticket sales is $50x$ when the price drops x dollars:

$$\begin{aligned} R(x) &= (\text{Revenue from tickets}) + (\text{Revenue from concessions}) \\ &= (\text{Number of people}) \cdot (\text{Ticket price}) + (\text{Number of people}) \cdot 4 \\ &= (1000 + 50x)(26 - x) + (1000 + 50x) \cdot 4 \\ &= -50x^2 + 500x + 30{,}000. \end{aligned}$$

To find x such that $R(x)$ is a maximum, we first find $R'(x)$:

$$R'(x) = -100x + 500.$$

This derivative exists for all real numbers x. Thus, the only critical values are where $R'(x) = 0$; so we solve that equation:

$$\begin{aligned} -100x + 500 &= 0 \\ -100x &= -500 \\ x &= 5 \qquad \text{This corresponds to lowering the price by \$5.} \end{aligned}$$

Quick Check 6 ✓

A baseball team charges \$30 per ticket and averages 20,000 people in attendance per game. Each person spends an average of \$8 on concessions. For every drop of \$1 in the ticket price, the attendance rises by 800 people. What ticket price will maximize total revenue?

Since this is the only critical value, we can use the second derivative,

$$R''(x) = -100,$$

to determine whether we have a maximum. Since $R''(5)$ is negative, $R(5)$ is a maximum. Therefore, in order to maximize revenue, the theater should charge

$$\$26 - \$5, \quad \text{or} \quad \$21 \text{ per ticket.}$$

6 ✓

Minimizing Inventory Costs

Most retail businesses need to be concerned about inventory costs. Suppose, for example, that a home electronics store sells 2500 televisions per year. It *could* operate by ordering all the TVs at once. But then the owners would face the carrying costs (insurance, building space, and so on) of storing them all. Thus, they might make several smaller orders, so that they would never store more than 500. However, each time they reorder, there are costs for paperwork, delivery charges, labor, and so on. It seems that there must be some balance between storage costs and reorder costs. Let's use calculus to help determine what that balance might be. We are trying to minimize the following function:

$$\text{Total inventory costs} = (\text{Yearly storage costs}) + (\text{Yearly reorder costs}).$$

The *lot size* x is the largest number ordered each reordering period. If x units are ordered each period, then during that time somewhere between 0 and x units are in stock. To represent the amount in stock at any time in the period, we can use the average, $x/2$. This represents the average amount held in stock over the course of each time period.

Refer to the following graphs. If the lot size is 2500, then, on average, there are $2500/2$, or 1250 units in stock. If the lot size is 1250, then, on average, there are $1250/2$, or 625 units in stock, but twice as many orders are placed.

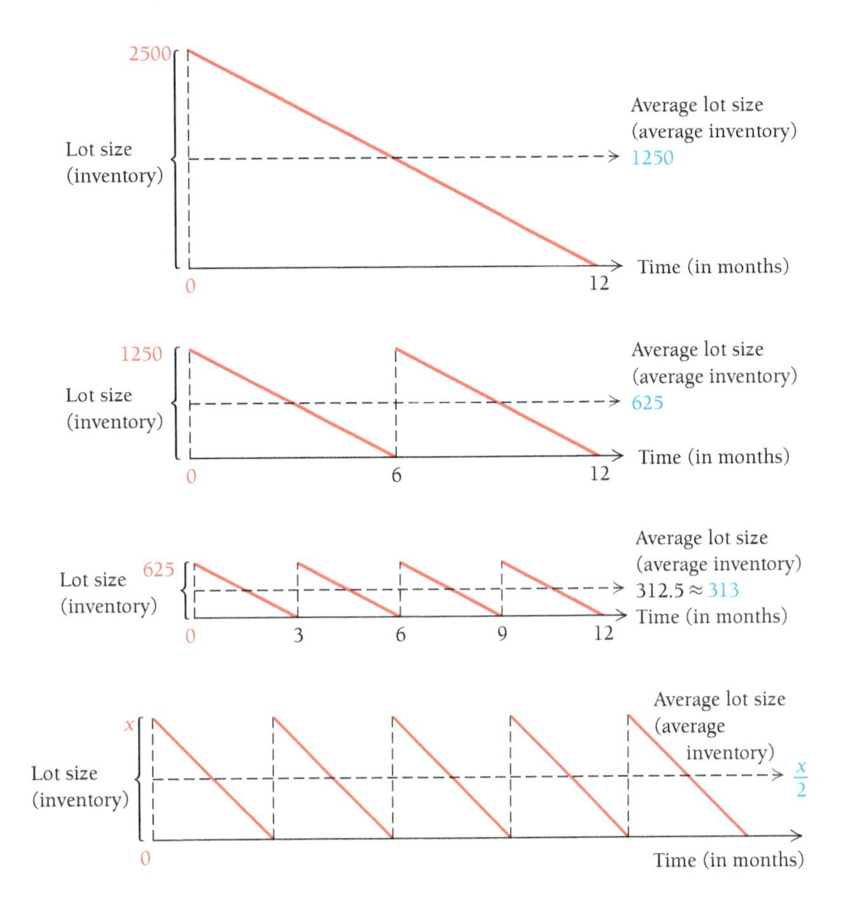

EXAMPLE 7 **Business: Minimizing Inventory Costs.** Fred's Electronics sells 2500 televisions per year. It costs \$20 to store one TV for a year. To reorder, there is a fixed cost of \$20 for the order, plus a fee of \$9 per TV. How many times per year should the store reorder, and in what lot size, to minimize inventory costs?

Solution Let $x =$ the lot size. Inventory costs are given by

$$C(x) = (\text{Yearly storage costs}) + (\text{Yearly reorder costs}).$$

We consider each component of inventory costs separately.

a) *Yearly storage costs.* The average amount held in stock is $x/2$, and it costs \$20 per set for storage. Thus,

$$\begin{aligned}\text{Yearly storage costs} &= \begin{pmatrix}\text{Yearly cost}\\ \text{per item}\end{pmatrix}\cdot\begin{pmatrix}\text{Average number}\\ \text{of items}\end{pmatrix}\\ &= 20\cdot\frac{x}{2}.\end{aligned}$$

b) *Yearly reorder costs.* We know that x is the lot size, and we let N be the number of reorders each year. Then $x = 2500/N$, and $N = 2500/x$. Thus,

$$\begin{aligned}\text{Yearly reorder costs} &= \begin{pmatrix}\text{Cost of each}\\ \text{order}\end{pmatrix}\cdot\begin{pmatrix}\text{Number of}\\ \text{reorders}\end{pmatrix}\\ &= (20 + 9x)\frac{2500}{x}.\end{aligned}$$

c) Thus, we have

$$\begin{aligned}C(x) &= 20\cdot\frac{x}{2} + (20 + 9x)\frac{2500}{x}\\ &= 10x + \frac{50{,}000}{x} + 22{,}500 = 10x + 50{,}000x^{-1} + 22{,}500.\end{aligned}$$

d) To minimize $C(x)$ over $[1, 2500]$, we first find $C'(x)$:

$$C'(x) = 10 - \frac{50{,}000}{x^2}.$$

e) Since $C'(x)$ exists for all x in $[1, 2500]$, the only critical values are x-values for which $C'(x) = 0$. We solve $C'(x) = 0$:

$$\begin{aligned} 10 - \frac{50{,}000}{x^2} &= 0 \\ 10 &= \frac{50{,}000}{x^2} \\ 10x^2 &= 50{,}000 \\ x^2 &= 5000 \\ x &= \sqrt{5000} \approx 70.7. \end{aligned}$$

Since 70.7 is the only critical value in $[1, 2500]$, we can try to use the second derivative to see whether that value yields a maximum or a minimum:

$$C''(x) = \frac{100{,}000}{x^3}.$$

$C''(x)$ is positive for all x in $[1, 2500]$, so we have a minimum at $x \approx 70.7$.

Because it is impossible to reorder 70.7 TVs each time, we consider the two whole numbers closest to 70.7, which are 70 and 71. Since

$$C(70) \approx \$23{,}914.29 \quad \text{and} \quad C(71) \approx \$23{,}914.23,$$

it follows that the lot size that minimizes cost is 71. (*Note*: Such a procedure will not work for all functions but will work for the type we are considering here.) The number of times an order should be placed is $2500/71 = 35$, with a remainder of 15, indicating that 35 orders should be placed. Of those, $35 - 15 = 20$ will be for 71 items and 15 will be for 72 items.

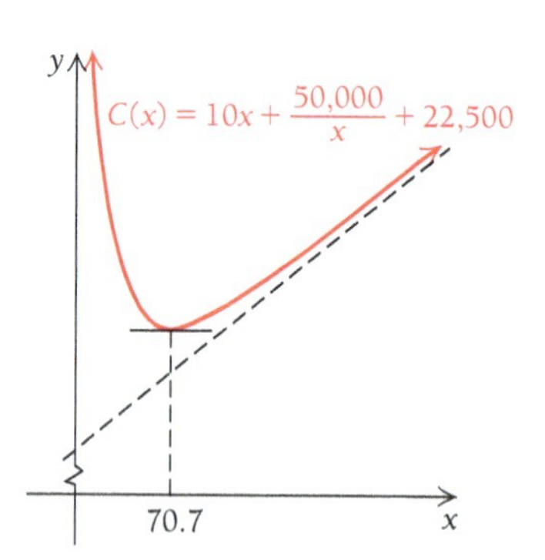

Quick Check 7 ✓

Repeat Example 7 with a storage cost of \$30 per TV and assuming that the store sells 3000 TVs per year.

7 ✓

The lot size that minimizes total inventory costs is often referred to as the *economic ordering quantity*. Three assumptions are made in using the preceding method to determine the economic ordering quantity. First, the demand for the product is the same year round. For computers, this may be reasonable, but for bathing suits, this assumption is unrealistic. Second, the time between placing an order and receiving the product remains consistent year-round. Finally, the costs involved, such as storage, shipping charges, and so on, do not vary. Variation in these costs can be allowed for by anticipating what they might be and using average costs.

Technology Connection 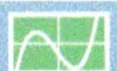

Using Excel Spreadsheets to Numerically Estimate Minimum and Maximum Values

An Excel spreadsheet can numerically estimate absolute extrema. For example, to estimate the values for Example 2, we open a blank spreadsheet and enter text in the cells as shown to the right.

	A	B	C	D
1	Starting value			
2	Step size:			
3				
4	Height	Length	Width	Volume
5	H=x	L=11-2x	W=8-2x	V=H*L*W

In cell A6, we enter =B1; in cell B6, we enter 11-2*A6; in cell C6, we enter =8-2*A6; and in cell D6, we enter =A6*B6*C6. In cell A7, we enter =A6+B2. We copy cells B6, C6, and D6 and paste them into cells B7, C7, and D7, then copy cells A7 through D7 and paste them into cells A8 through D14. This creates nine active rows. More rows can be added if necessary.

In cell B1, we enter a starting x-value, and in cell B2, a step size. For example, if we enter 0 into cell B1 and 0.25 into cell B2, the values in cells A6–A19 will be $x = 0, 0.25, 0.5, 0.75, 1,$ and so on. The result is the table at the right.

We see that a possible maximum volume of 60 in^3 occurs when $x = 1.5$ in.

	A	B	C	
1	Starting value	0		
2	Step size:	0.25		
3				
4	Height	Length	Width	Volume
5	H=x	L=11-2x	W=8-2x	V=H*L*W
6	0	11	8	0
7	0.25	10.5	7.5	19.6875
8	0.5	10	7	35
9	0.75	9.5	6.5	46.3125
10	1	9	6	54
11	1.25	8.5	5.5	58.4375
12	1.5	8	5	60
13	1.75	7.5	4.5	59.0625
14	2	7	4	56
15	2.25	6.5	3.5	51.1875
16	2.5	6	3	45
17	2.75	5.5	2.5	37.8125
18	3	5	2	30
19	3.25	4.5	1.5	21.9375

Possible largest volume (row 12)

To refine our estimate, we enter 1.45 into cell B1 and 0.02 into cell B2, giving the table at the right.

By reducing the step size, we obtain a new possible maximum volume of 60.012108 in^3 when $x = 1.53$ in. Although we could further reduce the step size, we now have an estimate of the maximum volume and the x-value at which it occurs. We use calculus to determine these values exactly.

	A	B	C	
1	Starting value	1.45		
2	Step size:	0.02		
3				
4	Height	Length	Width	Volume
5	H=x	L=11-2x	W=8-2x	V=H*L*W
6	1.45	8.1	5.1	59.8995
7	1.47	8.06	5.06	59.951892
8	1.49	8.02	5.02	59.987996
9	1.51	7.98	4.98	60.008004
10	1.53	7.94	4.94	60.012108
11	1.55	7.9	4.9	60.0005
12	1.57	7.86	4.86	59.973372

Possible largest volume (row 10)

EXERCISES

1. Use a spreadsheet to verify the results of Example 1.
2. Use a spreadsheet to verify the results of Example 3.
3. Use a spreadsheet to verify the results of Example 4.
4. Use a spreadsheet to verify the results of Example 5.

Section Summary

- In many real-world applications, we need to determine the minimum or maximum value of a function modeling a situation.
- Maximum profit occurs at those x-values for which $R'(x) = C'(x)$ and $R''(x) < C''(x)$, where $R(x)$ is the total revenue and $C(x)$ is the total cost when x units are produced.

3.5 Exercise Set

1. Of all the numbers that add to 70, find the pair that has the maximum product. That is, maximize the objective function $Q = xy$ subject to the constraint $x + y = 70$.
2. Of all the numbers that add to 50, find the pair that has the maximum product. That is, maximize the objective function $P = xy$ subject to the constraint $x + y = 50$.
3. Of all the numbers whose difference is 6, find the pair that has the minimum product. That is, minimize the objective function $M = xy$ subject to the constraint $x - y = 6$.
4. Of all the numbers whose difference is 4, find the pair that has the minimum product. That is, minimize the objective function $N = xy$ subject to the constraint $y = x - 4$.
5. Maximize $B = xy^2$, where x and y are positive numbers such that $x + y^2 = 4$.
6. Maximize $C = xy^2$, where x and y are positive numbers such that $x + y^2 = 1$.
7. Minimize $E = x^2 + 2y^2$, where $x + y = 3$.
8. Minimize $F = 2x^2 + 3y^2$, where $x + y = 5$.
9. Maximize $A = xy$, where x and y are positive numbers such that $x + \frac{4}{3}y^2 = 1$.
10. Maximize $Z = xy$, where x and y are positive numbers such that $\frac{4}{3}x^2 + y = 16$.
11. Minimize $V = e^x + e^y$, where $x + y = 1$.
12. Minimize $W = e^x + e^{2y}$, where $x + y = 3$.
13. Maximize $T = xe^y$, where $x + y = 2$.
14. Minimize $U = xe^{-y}$, where $x + y = 2$.
15. **Maximizing area.** A lifeguard needs to rope off a rectangular swimming area in front of Long Lake Beach, using 180 yd of rope and floats. What dimensions of the rectangle will maximize the area? What is the maximum area? (Note that the shoreline is one side of the rectangle.)

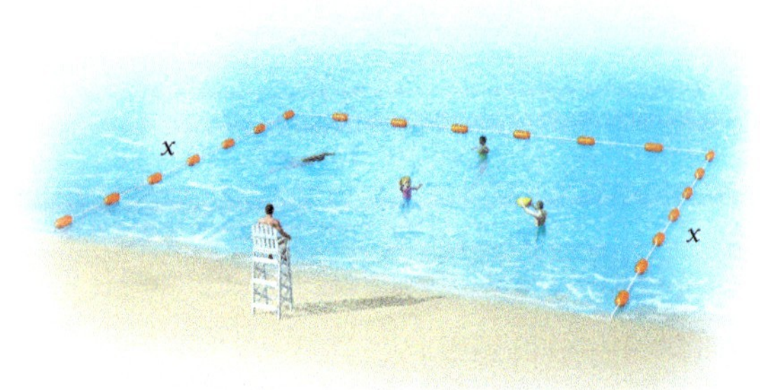

16. **Maximizing area.** A rancher wants to enclose two rectangular areas near a river, one for sheep and one for cattle. The rancher has 240 yd of fencing available. What is the largest total area that can be enclosed?

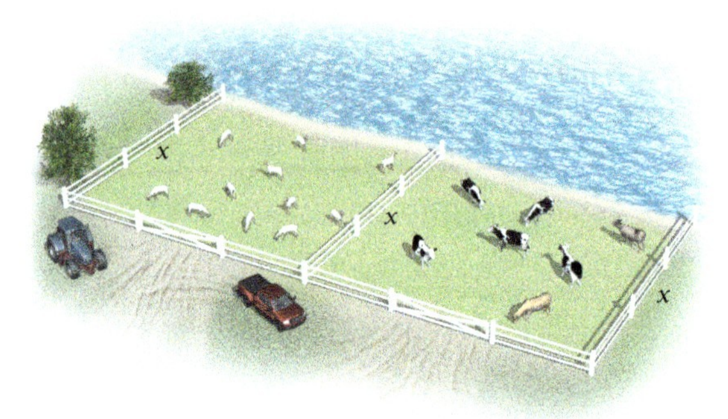

17. **Maximizing area.** Grayson Farms plans to enclose three parallel rectangular livestock pens within one large rectangular area using 600 m of fencing. One side of the enclosure is a pre-existing stone wall.
    a) If the three rectangular pens have their longer sides parallel to the stone wall, find the largest possible total area that can be enclosed.

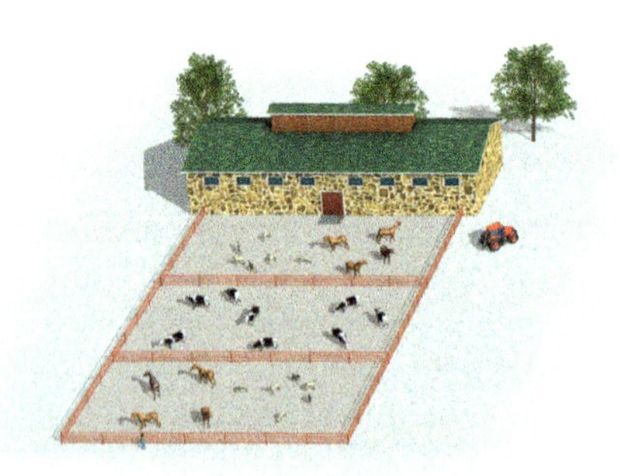

    b) If the three rectangular pens have their shorter sides perpendicular to the stone wall, find the largest possible total area that can be enclosed.

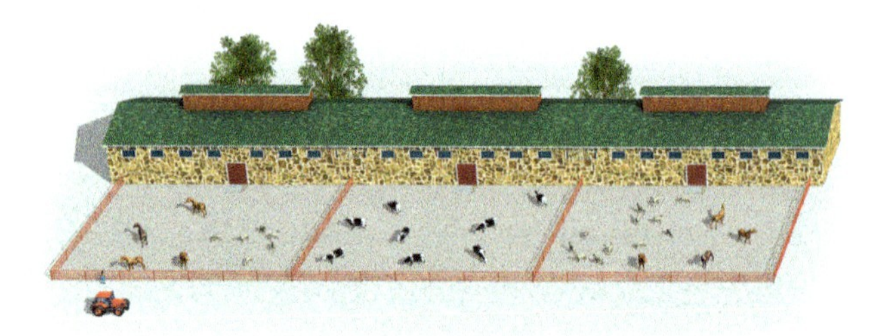

18. **Maximizing area.** Hentz Industries plans to enclose three parallel rectangular areas for sorting returned goods. The three areas are within one large rectangular area and 1200 yd of fencing is available. What is the largest total area that can be enclosed?

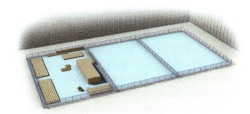

19. **Maximizing volume.** From a thin piece of cardboard 20 in. by 20 in., square corners are cut out so that the sides can be folded up to make a box. What dimensions will yield a box of maximum volume? What is the maximum volume?

20. **Maximizing volume.** From a 50-cm-by-50-cm sheet of aluminum, square corners are cut out so that the sides can be folded up to make a box. What dimensions will yield a box of maximum volume? What is the maximum volume?

21. **Minimizing surface area.** Mendoza Soup Company is constructing an open-top, square-based, rectangular metal tank that will have a volume of 32 ft^3. What dimensions will minimize surface area? What is the minimum surface area?

22. **Minimizing surface area.** Drum Tight Containers is designing an open-top, square-based, rectangular box that will have a volume of 62.5 in^3. What dimensions will minimize surface area? What is the minimum surface area?

23. **Minimizing surface area.** Open Air Waste Management is designing a rectangular construction dumpster that will be twice as long as it is wide and must hold 12 yd^3 of debris. Find the dimensions of the dumpster that will minimize its surface area.

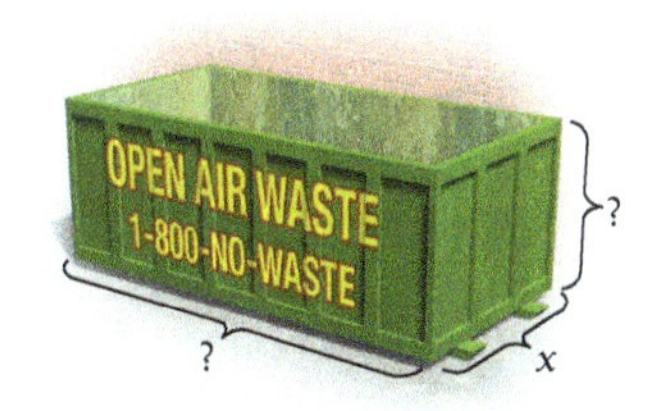

24. **Minimizing surface area.** Ever Green Gardening is designing a rectangular compost container that will be twice as tall as it is wide and must hold 18 ft^3 of composted food scraps. Find the dimensions of the compost container with minimal surface area (include the bottom and top).

APPLICATIONS

Business and Economics

Maximizing profit. *For Exercises 25–30, find the maximum profit and the number of units that must be produced and sold in order to achieve that profit. Assume that revenue, $R(x)$, and cost, $C(x)$, are in dollars and x is the number of units for Exercises 25–28.*

25. $R(x) = 50x - 0.5x^2, \quad C(x) = 4x + 10$

26. $R(x) = 50x - 0.5x^2, \quad C(x) = 10x + 3$

27. $R(x) = 2x, \quad C(x) = 0.01x^2 + 0.6x + 30$

28. $R(x) = 5x, \quad C(x) = 0.001x^2 + 1.2x + 60$

29. $R(x) = 9x - 2x^2, \quad C(x) = x^3 - 3x^2 + 4x + 1$; assume that $R(x)$ and $C(x)$ are in thousands of dollars, and x is in thousands of units.

30. $R(x) = 100x - x^2, C(x) = \frac{1}{3}x^3 - 6x^2 + 89x + 100$; assume that $R(x)$ and $C(x)$ are in thousands of dollars, and x is in thousands of units.

31. **Maximizing profit.** Riverside Appliances is marketing a new convection oven. It determines that in order to sell x ovens, the price per oven must be

$$p = 280 - 0.4x.$$

It also determines that the total cost of producing x ovens is given by

$$C(x) = 5000 + 0.6x^2.$$

a) Find the total revenue, $R(x)$.
b) Find the total profit, $P(x)$.
c) How many convection ovens must be produced and sold in order to maximize profit?
d) What is the maximum profit?
e) What price per oven will maximize profit?

32. **Maximizing profit.** Raggs, Ltd., a clothing firm, determines that in order to sell x suits, the price per suit must be

$$p = 150 - 0.5x.$$

It also determines that the total cost of producing x suits is given by

$$C(x) = 4000 + 0.25x^2.$$

a) Find the total revenue, $R(x)$.
b) Find the total profit, $P(x)$.
c) How many suits must be produced and sold in order to maximize profit?
d) What is the maximum profit?
e) What price per suit will maximize profit?

33. **Maximizing profit.** Gritz-Charlston is a 300-unit luxury hotel. All rooms are occupied when the hotel charges \$80 per day for a room. For every increase of x dollars in the daily room rate, there are x rooms vacant. Each occupied room costs \$22 per day to service and maintain. What should the hotel charge per day in order to maximize profit?

34. **Maximizing revenue.** Edwards University wants to determine what price to charge for tickets to football games. At \$18 per ticket, attendance averages 40,000 people per game. Every decrease of \$3 to the ticket price adds 10,000 people to the average attendance. Every person at a game spends an average of \$4.50 on concessions. What price per ticket will maximize revenue? How many people will attend at that price?

35. **Maximizing parking tickets.** Oak Glen currently employs 8 patrollers who each write an average of 24 parking tickets per day. For every additional patroller, the average number of parking tickets per day written by each patroller decreases by 4. How many additional patrollers should be working in order to maximize the number of parking tickets written per day?

36. **Maximizing yield.** Hood Apple Farm harvests an average of 30 bushels of apples per tree when 20 trees are planted on an acre of ground. If 1 more tree is planted per acre, the yield decreases by 1 bushel (bu) per tree as a result of crowding. How many trees should be planted on an acre in order to get the highest yield?

37. **Vanity license plates.** According to a pricing model, increasing the fee for vanity license plates by \$1 decreases the percentage of a state's population that will request them by 0.04%. (*Source*: E. D. Craft, "The demand for vanity (plates): Elasticities, net revenue maximization, and deadweight loss," *Contemporary Economic Policy*, Vol. 20, 133–144 (2002).)

   a) Recently, the fee for vanity license plates in Maryland was \$25, and the percentage of the state's population that had vanity plates was 2.13%. Use this information to construct the demand function, $q(x)$, for the percentage of Maryland's population that will request vanity license plates for a fee of x dollars.

   b) Find the fee, x, that will maximize revenue from vanity plates.

38. **Nitrogen prices.** During 2001, nitrogen prices fell by 41%. Over the same year, nitrogen demand went up by 12%. (*Source*: *Chemical Week*.)

   a) Assuming a linear change in demand, find the demand function, $q(x)$, by finding the equation of the line that passes through the points (1, 1) and (0.59, 1.12). Here x is the price as a fraction of the January 2001 price, and $q(x)$ is the demand as a fraction of the demand in January.

   b) As a percentage of the January 2001 price, what price of nitrogen will maximize revenue?

39. **Maximizing revenue.** When the Marchant Discount Theater charges \$5 for admission, there is an average attendance of 180 people. For every \$0.10 increase in admission, there is a loss of 1 customer from the average number. What admission should be charged in order to maximize revenue?

40. **Minimizing costs.** A rectangular box with a volume of 320 ft^3 is to be constructed with a square base and top. The cost per square foot for the bottom is 15¢, for the top is 10¢, and for the sides is 2.5¢. What dimensions will minimize the cost?

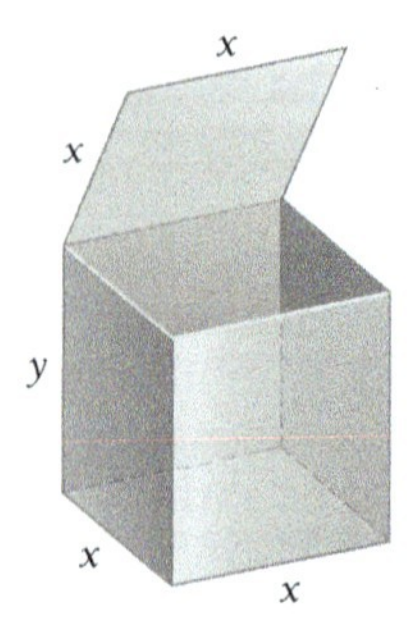

41. **Minimizing cost.** A rectangular parking area measuring 5000 ft^2 is to be enclosed on three sides using chain-link fencing that costs \$9.50 per foot. The fourth side will be a wooden fence that costs \$13 per foot. What dimensions will minimize the total cost to enclose this area, and what is the minimum cost (rounded to the nearest dollar)?

42. **Minimizing cost.** A rectangular garden with area 1200 yd^2 is to be enclosed on two parallel sides by stone wall that costs \$35 per yd and the other two sides by wooden fencing that costs \$28 per yd. What dimensions will minimize the total cost of enclosing this garden, and what is the minimum cost (rounded to the nearest dollar)?

43. **Maximizing area.** Bradley Publishing decides that each page in a new book must have an area of 73.125 in^2, a 0.75-in. margin at the top and at the bottom of each page, and a 0.5-in. margin on each side. What should the outside dimensions of each page be so that the printed area is a maximum?

44. **Minimizing inventory costs.** Big Break Billiards sells 100 pool tables per year. It costs \$20 to store one pool table for a year. To reorder, there is a fixed cost of \$40 per shipment plus \$16 for each pool table. How many times per year should the store order pool tables, and in what lot size, in order to minimize inventory costs?

45. **Minimizing inventory costs.** The Bowling Pro sells 200 bowling balls per year. It costs \$4 to store one bowling ball for a year. To reorder, there is a fixed cost of \$1, plus \$0.50 for each bowling ball. How many times per year should the shop order bowling balls, and in what lot size, in order to minimize inventory costs?

46. **Minimizing inventory costs.** A retail outlet for Boxowitz Calculators sells 720 calculators per year. It costs \$2 to store one calculator for a year. To reorder, there is a fixed cost of \$5, plus \$2.50 for each calculator. How many times per year should the store order calculators, and in what lot size, in order to minimize inventory costs?

47. **Minimizing inventory costs.** Bon Temps Surf and Scuba Shop sells 360 surfboards per year. It costs \$8 to store one surfboard for a year. Each reorder costs \$10, plus an additional \$5 for each surfboard ordered. How many times per year should the store order surfboards, and in what lot size, in order to minimize inventory costs?

48. **Minimizing inventory costs.** Repeat Exercise 46 using the same data, but assume yearly sales of 256 calculators with the fixed cost of each reorder set at \$4.

49. **Minimizing inventory costs.** Repeat Exercise 47 using the same data, but change the reorder costs from an additional \$5 per surfboard to \$6 per surfboard.

50. **Minimizing surface area.** A closed-top cylindrical can is to have a volume of 250 in^3. What dimensions (radius and height) will minimize the surface area?

51. **Minimizing surface area.** An open-top cylindrical cup is to have a volume of 400 cm^3. What dimensions (radius and height) will minimize the surface area?

52. **Minimizing cost.** Assume that the costs of the materials for making the can described in Exercise 50 are \$0.005/in^2 for the circular base and top and \$0.003/in^2 for the side. What dimensions will minimize the cost of materials?

53. Minimizing cost. Assume that the costs of the materials for making the cup described in Exercise 51 are $\$0.008/\text{cm}^2$ for the base and $\$0.0015/\text{cm}^2$ for the side. What dimensions will minimize the cost of materials?

54. Maximizing volume. The postal service places a limit of 84 in. on the combined length and girth of (distance around) a package to be sent parcel post. What dimensions of a rectangular box with square cross-section will contain the largest volume that can be mailed? (*Hint*: There are two different girths.)

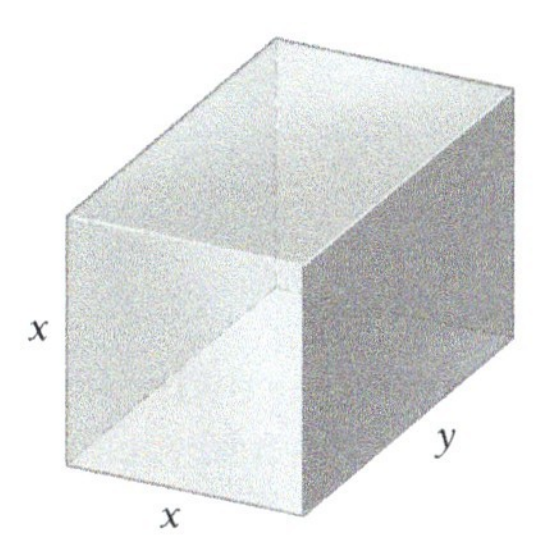

55. Minimizing cost. A rectangular play area of 48 yd^2 is to be fenced off in Jenny's yard. The next-door neighbor agrees to pay half the cost of the fence on the side of the play area that lies along the property line. What dimensions will minimize Jenny's cost for the fence?

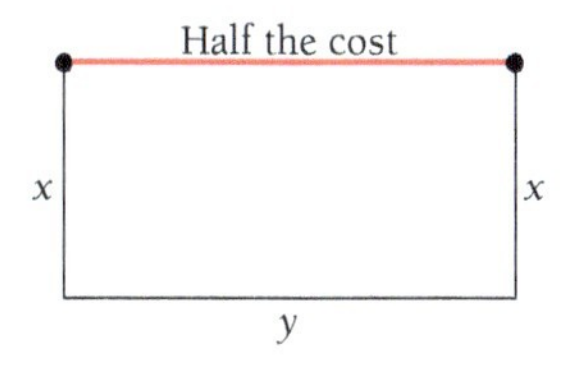

56. Maximizing light. A Norman window is a rectangle with a semicircle on top. Suppose that the perimeter of a particular Norman window is to be 24 ft. What should its dimensions be in order to allow the maximum amount of light to enter through the window?

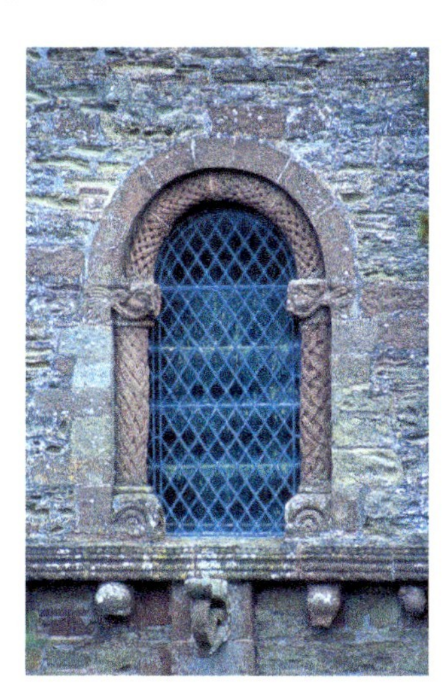

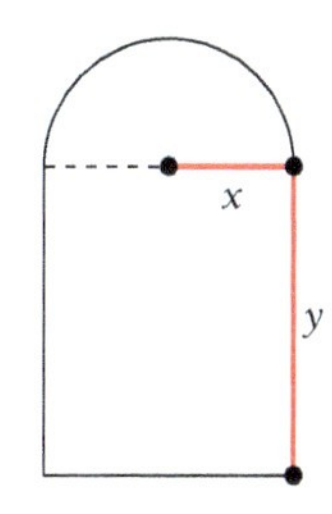

57. Maximizing light. Repeat Exercise 56, but assume that the semicircle is to be stained glass, which transmits only half as much light as clear glass does.

58. Minimizing cost. A grain silo in the shape of a circular cylinder topped with a hemisphere is to have a volume of 12,000 yd^3. The cost of materials is \$80 per square yard for the sides (the cylinder) and \$90 per square yard for the hemispherical top. Assume that the base is a pre-existing concrete pad.

a) What dimensions (radius and height) minimize the cost of materials? (*Hint*: The surface area of a hemisphere is $A = 2\pi r^2$.)
b) What is the minimum cost of materials for the silo?

59. Minimizing cost. A grain silo in the shape of a circular cylinder topped with a hemisphere is to have a volume of 10,000 yd^3. The cost of materials is \$90 per square yard for both the sides and the hemispherical top. Assume that the base is a pre-existing concrete pad.

a) What dimensions (radius and height) minimize the cost of materials? (*Hint*: The surface area of a hemisphere is $A = 2\pi r^2$.)
b) What is the minimum cost of materials for the silo?
c) Describe the shape of this silo.

60. Minimizing distance and cost. Relative to the center of a town, a power line runs on a straight line from a point 10 miles north of the town to a point 5 miles east of the town. A spur line is to be built from this main line to the center of town. The cost to build a spur line is \$45,000 per mile. (*Hint*: Let the town be at the origin, and minimize the distance between the origin and the line $y = 10 - 2x$.)

a) At what point along the power line should the spur line be built in order to minimize the cost of the spur?
b) What is the minimum cost?

61. Concentration. A sugar solution is administered into the bloodstream of a patient. The concentration of sugar, $C(t)$, in the bloodstream, in micrograms per deciliter (μg/dL), t minutes after the solution is administered is given by $C(t) = 40te^{-0.025t}$. What is the peak concentration of the sugar solution in the bloodstream, and when does this peak occur?

62. Concentration. A drug is administered into the bloodstream of a patient. The concentration of the drug, $C(t)$, in the bloodstream, in nanograms per milliliter (ng/mL), t minutes after being administered is given by $C(t) = 110te^{-0.006t}$. What is the peak concentration of the drug in the bloodstream, and when does this peak occur?

63. Minimizing distance and cost. A new farm is being developed. Relative to its location, a water main runs on a straight line from a point 8 miles north of the site to a point 6 miles west of the site. The cost to connect the farm to the water main via a secondary main is \$15,000 per mile.

a) Find the point along the water main at which the secondary main should begin to minimize the cost of the secondary main.
b) What is the minimum cost?

64. A 24-in. piece of wire is cut in two pieces. One piece is used to form a circle and the other to form a square. How should the wire be cut so that the sum of the areas is a minimum? A maximum?

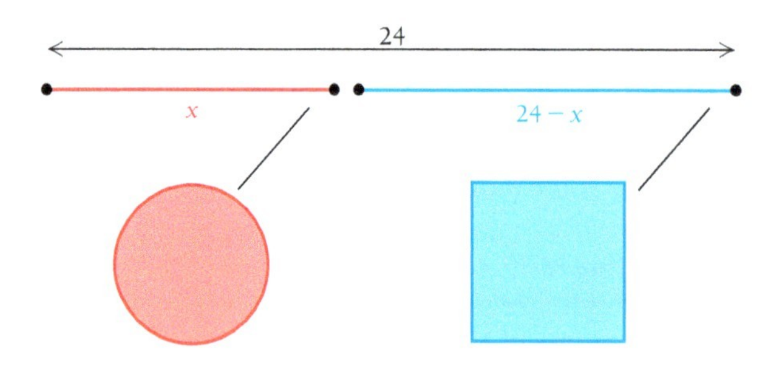

65. Business: minimizing costs. A power line is to be constructed from a power station at point A to an island at point C, which is 1 mi directly out in the water from a point B on the shore. Point B is 4 mi downshore from the power station at A. It costs \$5000 per mile to lay the power line under water and \$3000 per mile to lay the line under ground. At what point S downshore from A should the line come to the shore in order to minimize cost? Note that S could very well be B or A. (*Hint*: The length of CS is $\sqrt{1 + x^2}$.)

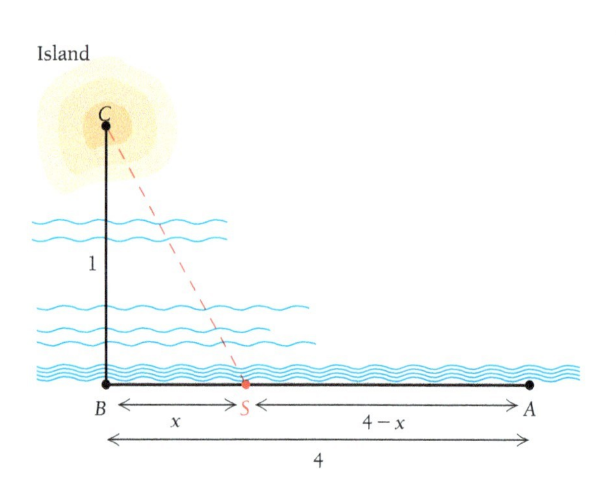

66. Life science: flights of homing pigeons. It is known that homing pigeons tend to avoid flying over water in the daytime, perhaps because downdrafts of air over water make flying difficult. Suppose a homing pigeon is released on an island at point C, which is 3 mi directly out in the water from a point B on shore. Point B is 8 mi downshore from the pigeon's home loft at point A. Assume that a pigeon flying over water uses energy at a rate 1.28 times the rate over land. Toward what point S downshore from A should the pigeon fly in order to minimize the total energy required to get to the home loft at A? Assume that

Total energy =
(Energy rate over water) • (Distance over water)
+ (Energy rate over land) • (Distance over land).

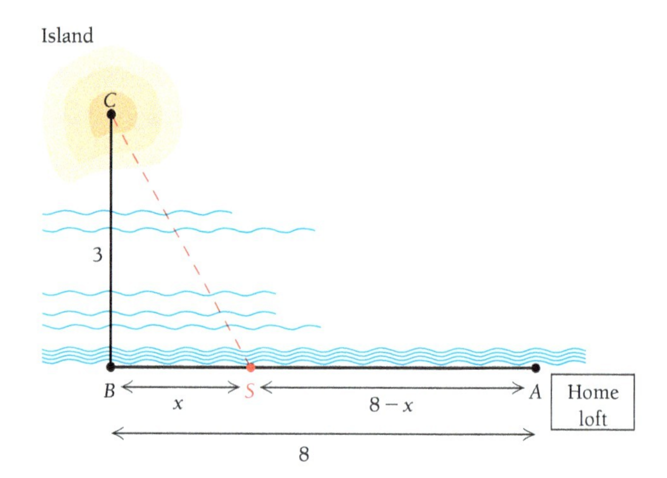

SYNTHESIS

67. A rectangular field is being divided into two parallel rectangular areas, as shown in the figure below. If the total fencing available is k units, show that, in order to maximize the area enclosed, the length of each of the three parallel fences will be $k/6$ units.

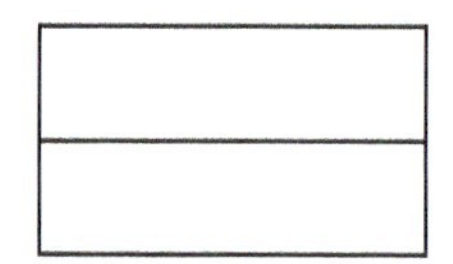

68. Business: minimizing distance. A road is being built between two cities C_1 and C_2, which are on opposite sides of a river of uniform width r. C_1 is a units from the river, and C_2 is b units from the river, with $a \leq b$. A bridge will span the river. Where should the bridge be located in order to minimize the total distance between the cities? Give a general solution using the constants a, b, p, and r as shown in the figure.

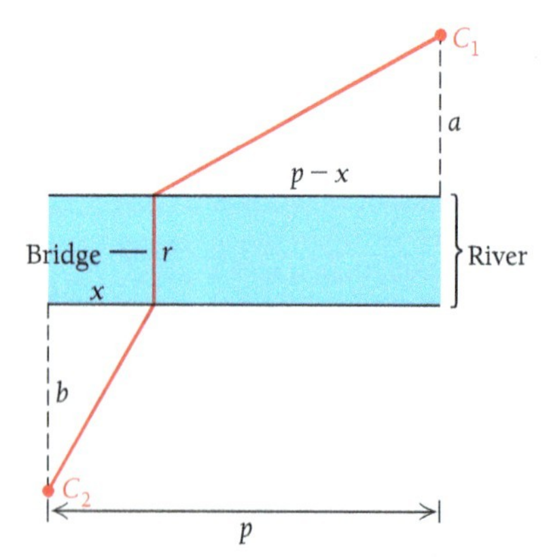

69. Business: minimizing cost. The total cost, in dollars, of producing x units of a certain product is given by

$$C(x) = 8x + 20 + \frac{x^3}{100}.$$

a) Find the average cost, $\overline{C}(x) = C(x)/x$.
b) Find $C'(x)$ and $\overline{C}'(x)$.
c) Find the minimum of $\overline{C}(x)$ and the value x_0 at which it occurs. Find $C'(x_0)$.
d) Compare $\overline{C}(x_0)$ and $C'(x_0)$.

70. Business: minimizing cost. Consider $\overline{C}(x) = C(x)/x$.

a) Express $\overline{C}'(x)$ in terms of $C'(x)$ and $C(x)$.

b) Show that if $\overline{C}(x)$ has a minimum, then it will occur at that value of x_0 for which

$$C'(x_0) = \overline{C}(x_0) = \frac{C(x_0)}{x_0}.$$

This result shows that if average cost can be minimized, such a minimum will occur when marginal cost equals average cost.

71. Business: minimizing inventory costs—a general solution. A store sells Q units of a product per year. It costs a dollars to store one unit for a year. To reorder, there is a fixed cost of b dollars, plus c dollars for each unit. How many times per year should the store reorder, and in what lot size, in order to minimize inventory costs?

72. Business: minimizing inventory costs. Use the general solution found in Exercise 71 to find how many times per year a store should reorder, and in what lot size, when $Q = 2500$, $a = \$10$, $b = \$20$, and $c = \$9$.

73. Prove that when the sum of two numbers is n, their maximum product is $\frac{n^2}{4}$.

74. Prove that the largest possible area of a rectangle where the perimeter is n is $\frac{n^2}{16}$.

Technology Connection

In Exercises 75–78, use a spreadsheet to maximize Q. Assume that all variables are positive, and state all answers to two decimal places.

75. $Q = xy$, where $2x + 3y = 100$

76. $Q = x^2y$, where $x^2 + y^2 = 16$

77. $Q = xy^3$, where $x^2 + 2y^2 = 20$

78. $Q = x^2y^2$, where $x^2 + y^2 = 50$

79. Explain why a table might be a better way to estimate the maximum of Q in Exercises 77 and 78.

Answers to Quick Checks

1. With 100 ft of fencing, the dimensions are 50 ft by 50 ft (2500 ft^2 area); in general, n feet of fencing gives $n/2$ ft by $n/2$ ft ($n^2/4$ ft^2 area). **2.** The dimensions are approximately 1.667 in. by 6.667 in. by 6.667 in.; the volume is 74.074 in^3. **3.** $r \approx 5.3$ cm, $h \approx 2.83$ cm, $C \approx \$0.212$/can **4.** The maximum concentration, 1839.4 ng/mL, occurs after about 100.53 min.
5. **(a)** $R(x) = 1750x - 2x^2$; **(b)** $P(x) = -2x^2 + 1735x - 2250$; **(c)** $x = 434$ units; **(d)** maximum profit = \$374,028; **(e)** price per unit = \$882.00 **6.** \$23.50 **7.** $x \approx 63$; the store should place 8 orders for 63 TVs and 39 orders for 64 TVs.

3.6 Marginals, Differentials, and Linearization

- Find marginal cost, revenue, and profit.
- Find Δy and dy.
- Use differentials for approximations.
- Find the linearization of a function at $x = a$.

In this section, we consider ways of using calculus to make approximations. Suppose, for example, that a company is considering an increase in production. Usually the company wants approximations of the resulting changes in *cost*, *revenue*, and *profit*.

Marginal Cost, Revenue, and Profit

Suppose that an animal rescue organization is considering increasing its monthly production of public service announcements (PSAs) from 12 to 13. To estimate the resulting increase in cost, it would be reasonable to find the rate at which cost is increasing when 12 PSAs are produced and add that to the cost of producing 12 PSAs. That is,

$$C(13) \approx C(12) + C'(12).$$

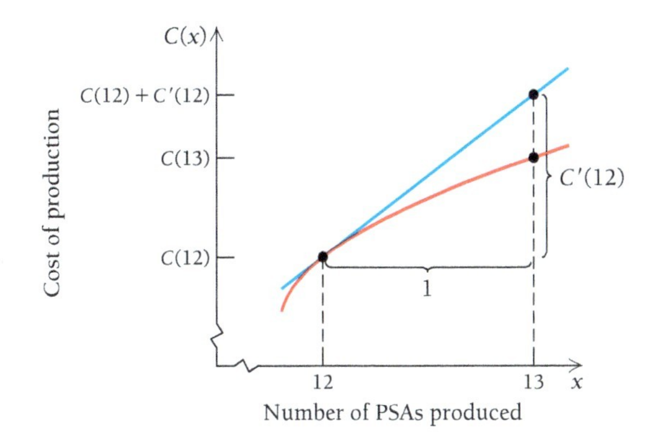

The number $C'(12)$ is called the *marginal cost at 12*. Remember that $C'(12)$ is the slope of the tangent line at the point $(12, C(12))$. If, for example, this slope is $\frac{3}{4}$, we can regard it as a vertical change of $\frac{3}{4}$ with a horizontal change of 1. This can be seen in the graph. It is possible that the organization has never produced 13 PSAs in a month, so the actual cost, $C(13)$, is unknown. But information would be known about the cost of producing 12 PSAs and the per-unit cost of producing the 12th PSA, making it reasonable to use $C(12) + C'(12)$ as an estimate for $C(13)$. Note in the figure that $C'(12)$ is slightly more than the difference between $C(13)$ and $C(12)$, or $C(13) - C(12)$. For other curves, $C'(12)$ may be slightly less than $C(13) - C(12)$.

Generalizing, we have the following.

DEFINITIONS

Let $C(x)$, $R(x)$, and $P(x)$ represent, respectively, the total cost, total revenue, and total profit from the production and sale of x items.

The **marginal cost** at x, given by $C'(x)$, is the approximate cost of the $(x + 1)$st item:

$$C'(x) \approx C(x + 1) - C(x), \text{ or } C(x + 1) \approx C(x) + C'(x).$$

The **marginal revenue** at x, given by $R'(x)$, is the approximate revenue from the $(x + 1)$st item:

$$R'(x) \approx R(x + 1) - R(x), \text{ or } R(x + 1) \approx R(x) + R'(x).$$

The **marginal profit** at x, given by $P'(x)$, is the approximate profit from the $(x + 1)$st item:

$$P'(x) \approx P(x + 1) - P(x), \text{ or } P(x + 1) \approx P(x) + P'(x).$$

The student can confirm that $P'(x) = R'(x) - C'(x)$.

EXAMPLE 1 **Business: Marginal Cost, Revenue, and Profit.** Given

$$C(x) = 62x^2 + 27{,}500 \text{ and } R(x) = x^3 - 12x^2 + 40x + 10,$$

find each of the following.

a) Total profit, $P(x)$

b) Total cost, revenue, and profit from the production and sale of 50 units of the product

c) The marginal cost, marginal revenue, and marginal profit when 50 units are produced and sold

Solution

a) Total profit $= P(x) = R(x) - C(x)$

$$= x^3 - 12x^2 + 40x + 10 - (62x^2 + 27{,}500)$$

$$= x^3 - 74x^2 + 40x - 27{,}490$$

b) We have

$$C(50) = 62 \cdot 50^2 + 27{,}500 = \$182{,}500$$ The total cost of producing the first 50 units

$$R(50) = 50^3 - 12 \cdot 50^2 + 40 \cdot 50 + 10 = \$97{,}010$$ The total revenue from the sale of the first 50 units

$$P(50) = R(50) - C(50)$$

$$= \$97{,}010 - \$182{,}500$$ We could also use $P(x)$ from part (a).

$$= -\$85{,}490$$ There is a *loss* of \$85,490 when 50 units are produced and sold.

c) We have

$$C'(x) = 124x,$$

$$C'(50) = 124 \cdot 50 = \$6200$$ Once 50 units have been made, the approximate cost of the 51st unit (marginal cost) is \$6200.

$$R'(x) = 3x^2 - 24x + 40,$$

$$R'(50) = 3 \cdot 50^2 - 24 \cdot 50 + 40 = \$6340$$ Once 50 units have been sold, the approximate revenue from the 51st unit (marginal revenue) is \$6340.

$$P'(x) = 3x^2 - 148x + 40,$$

$$P'(50) = 3 \cdot 50^2 - 148 \cdot 50 + 40 = \$140$$ Once 50 units have been produced and sold, the approximate profit from the sale of the 51st unit (marginal profit) is \$140. 1 ✓

Quick Check 1 ✓

Given

$$C(x) = 10x + 3$$

and

$$R(x) = 50x - 0.5x^2,$$

find each of the following.

a) $P(x)$

b) Total cost, revenue, and profit from the production and sale of 40 units

c) The marginal cost, marginal revenue, and marginal profit when 40 units are produced and sold

Technology Connection

To check the accuracy of $R'(50)$ as an estimate of $R(51) - R(50)$, let $y_1 = x^3 - 12x^2 + 40x + 10$, $y_2 = y_1(x + 1) - y_1(x)$, and $y_3 = \text{nDeriv}(y_1, x, x)$. By using TABLE with Indpnt: Ask, we can display a table in which y_2 (the difference between $y_1(x + 1)$ and $y_1(x)$) can be compared with $y_1'(x)$.

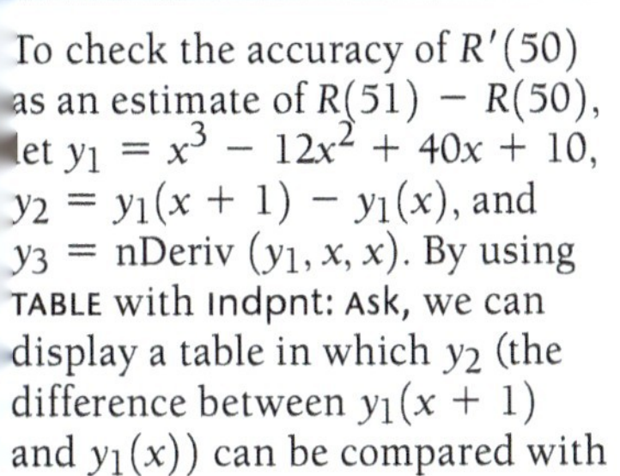

X	Y2	Y3
40	3989	3880
48	5933	5800
50	6479	6340

X =

EXERCISE

1. Create a table to check the accuracy of $P'(50)$ as an estimate of $P(51) - P(50)$.

Often, in business, formulas for $C(x)$, $R(x)$, and $P(x)$ are not known, but information may exist about the cost, revenue, and profit trends at a particular value $x = a$. For example, $C(a)$ and $C'(a)$ may be known, allowing for a reasonable prediction about $C(a + 1)$. In a similar manner, predictions can be made for $R(a + 1)$ and $P(a + 1)$. In Example 1, formulas *do* exist, so it is possible to see how accurate our predictions were. We check $C(51) - C(50)$ and leave the checks of $R(51) - R(50)$ and $P(51) - P(50)$ to the student (see the Technology Connection in the margin):

$$C(51) - C(50) = 62 \cdot 51^2 + 27{,}500 - (62 \cdot 50^2 + 27{,}500)$$
$$= 6262,$$

whereas

$$C'(50) = 6200.$$

In this case, $C'(50)$ provides an approximation of $C(51) - C(50)$ that is within 1% of the actual value.

Note that marginal cost is different from *average* cost:

$$\text{Average cost per unit for 50 units} = \frac{C(50)}{50} \quad \begin{matrix}\leftarrow \text{Total cost of 50 units} \\ \leftarrow \text{The number of units, 50}\end{matrix}$$
$$= \frac{182{,}500}{50} = \$3650 \text{ per unit,}$$

whereas

$$\text{Marginal cost when 50 units are produced} = \$6200$$
$$\approx \text{cost of the 51st unit.}$$

EXAMPLE 2 Donaldson's Milliners produces hats. It costs $C(x)$, in thousands of dollars, to produce x thousand hats, where

$$C(x) = 40 - 18e^{-0.08x}.$$

Find the marginal cost when 10,000 hats are produced, and estimate the cost of producing 11,000 hats.

Solution Here, $x = 10$ represents 10,000 hats. We have

$$C(10) = 40 - 18e^{-0.08(10)} \approx 31.912, \quad \text{or about } \$31{,}912.$$

The derivative is

$$C'(x) = -18e^{-0.08x}(-0.08) \qquad \text{Using the Chain Rule}$$
$$= 1.44e^{-0.08x} \qquad \text{Simplifying}$$

Evaluated at $x = 10$, this gives us the marginal cost when 10,000 hats are produced:

$$C'(10) = 1.44e^{-0.08(10)} \approx 0.647, \quad \text{or about } \$647 \text{ per 1000 hats.}$$

This marginal cost is the approximate additional cost to produce another 1000 hats, when 10,000 hats have already been produced. Thus, the estimated cost to produce 11,000 hats is

$$C(11) = C(10) + C'(10)$$
$$= \$31{,}912 + \$647$$
$$= \$32{,}559.$$

This marginal cost was found in terms of a group of a thousand units. A manufacturer producing in high volume may not find it useful to consider the marginal cost of one extra unit and will instead consider the marginal cost of a more typical group. 2 ✓

Quick Check 2 ✓

Barclay's Shoes determines that the cost to produce x hundred pairs of shoes is given by

$$C(x) = 35 - 9e^{-0.2x},$$

where $C(x)$ is in thousands of dollars. Find the marginal cost when 650 pairs of shoes are produced and sold, and estimate the cost to produce 750 pairs of shoes.

Differentials and Delta Notation

Just as marginal cost $C'(x_0)$ is used to estimate $C(x_0 + 1)$, the value of $f'(x_0)$ can be used to estimate values of $f(x)$ for x-values near x_0. To do so, we need to develop some notation.

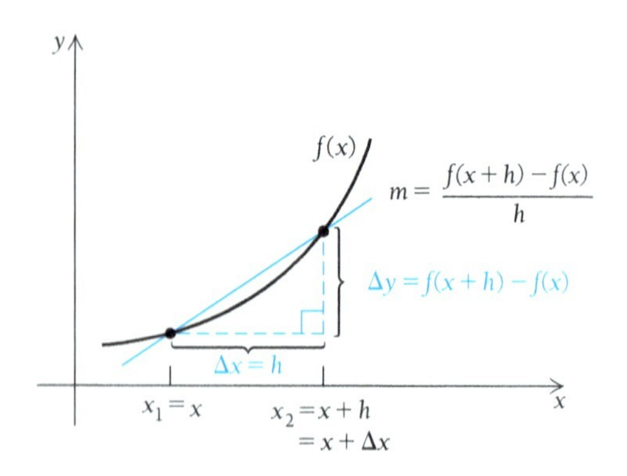

Recall that the difference quotient,

$$\frac{f(x+h)-f(x)}{h},$$

represents the slope of a secant line, as shown in the graph. The number h is regarded as the *change* in x. Another notation for such a change is Δx (read "delta x"), called **delta notation**. Thus,

$$\Delta x = (x+h) - x = h.$$

If subscripts are used for the first and second values of x, we have

$$\Delta x = x_2 - x_1, \quad \text{or} \quad x_2 = x_1 + \Delta x.$$

Note that the value of Δx can be positive or negative. For example,

if $x_1 = 4$ and $\Delta x = 0.7$, then $x_2 = 4.7$,

and if $x_1 = 4$ and $\Delta x = -0.7$, then $x_2 = 3.3$.

We generally omit the subscripts and use x and $x + \Delta x$. Now suppose we have a function given by $y = f(x)$. A change in x from x to $x + \Delta x$ yields a change in y from $f(x)$ to $f(x + \Delta x)$. The change in y is given by

$$\Delta y = f(x+\Delta x) - f(x).$$

EXAMPLE 3 Find Δy in each case.

a) $y = x^2$, with $x = 4$ and $\Delta x = 0.1$

b) $y = x^3$, with $x = 2$ and $\Delta x = -0.1$

Solution

a) We have

$$\begin{aligned}\Delta y &= (4+0.1)^2 - 4^2\\ &= (4.1)^2 - 4^2\\ &= 16.81 - 16\\ &= 0.81.\end{aligned}$$

b) We have

$$\begin{aligned}\Delta y &= [2+(-0.1)]^3 - 2^3\\ &= (1.9)^3 - 2^3\\ &= 6.859 - 8\\ &= -1.141.\end{aligned}$$

3 ✓

Quick Check 3 ✓

For $y = 2x^4 + x$, with $x = 2$ and $\Delta x = -0.05$, find Δy.

Let's now use calculus to predict function values. With delta notation, the difference quotient

$$\frac{f(x+h)-f(x)}{h}$$

becomes

$$\frac{f(x+\Delta x)-f(x)}{\Delta x} = \frac{\Delta y}{\Delta x}.$$

We can then express the derivative as

$$\frac{dy}{dx} = \lim_{\Delta x \to 0} \frac{\Delta y}{\Delta x}.$$

For values of Δx close to 0, we have the approximation

$$\frac{dy}{dx} \approx \frac{\Delta y}{\Delta x}, \quad \text{or} \quad f'(x) \approx \frac{\Delta y}{\Delta x}.$$

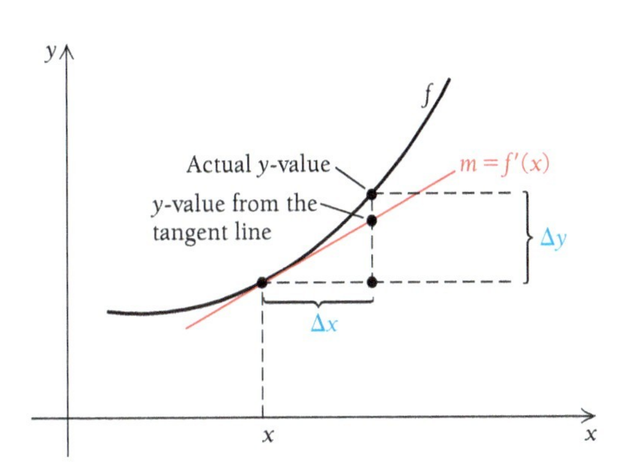

Multiplying both sides by Δx, we have

$$\Delta y \approx f'(x)\,\Delta x.$$

We can see in the graph at the left that, for small values of Δx, the y-values on the tangent line can be used to estimate y-values on the curve.

> For f, a continuous, differentiable function, and small Δx,
>
> $$f'(x) \approx \frac{\Delta y}{\Delta x} \quad \text{and} \quad \Delta y \approx f'(x) \cdot \Delta x.$$

Up to now, we have treated dy/dx as one expression. We now define dy and dx as separate expressions, called **differentials**.

> **DEFINITION**
>
> For $y = f(x)$, we define
>
> dx, called the **differential of x**, by $dx = \Delta x$
>
> and dy, called the **differential of y**, by $dy = f'(x)\,dx$.

We can illustrate dx and dy as shown at the right. Note that $dx = \Delta x$, but, in general, $dy \neq \Delta y$, though $dy \approx \Delta y$ for small values of dx.

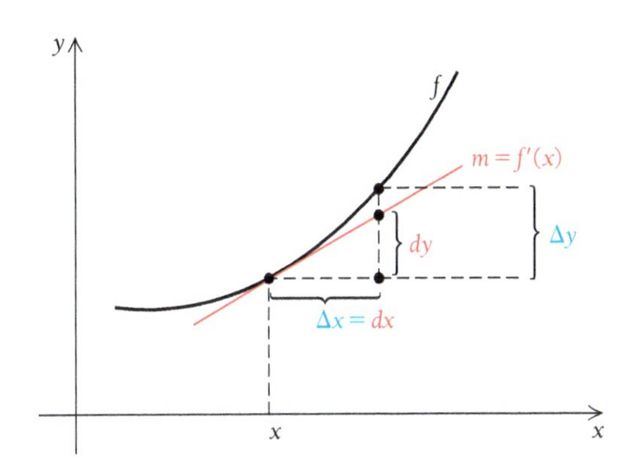

EXAMPLE 4 Consider the function given by $y = f(x) = \sqrt{x}$.

a) Find dy when $x = 9$ and $dx = 1$.

b) Use the result of part (a) to estimate $\sqrt{10}$.

c) Find the difference between the approximation found in part (b) and the actual value of $\sqrt{10}$.

Solution

a) We find dy/dx, then dy:

$$\frac{dy}{dx} = \frac{1}{2\sqrt{x}} \qquad \text{Differentiating } y = x^{1/2} \text{ with respect to } x$$

$$dy = \frac{1}{2\sqrt{x}}\,dx.$$

To find dy when $x = 9$ and $dx = 1$, we substitute:

$$dy = \frac{1}{2\sqrt{9}}(1) = \frac{1}{6} = 0.166666\ldots.$$

Quick Check 4 ✓

For $y = \sqrt{x}$, find dy when $x = 100$ and $dx = -2$. Estimate the value of $\sqrt{98}$, and compare the estimated value with the actual value of $\sqrt{98}$ found using a calculator.

b) Since $dy \approx \sqrt{10} - \sqrt{9}$, we have

$$\begin{aligned} \sqrt{10} &\approx \sqrt{9} + dy && \text{Adding } \sqrt{9} \text{ to both sides} \\ &\approx 3 + 0.166666\ldots && \text{Using } dy \text{ from part (a)} \\ &\approx 3.166666\ldots. \end{aligned}$$

c) Using a calculator, we obtain $\sqrt{10} = 3.16227766\ldots$. The estimated value, $\sqrt{10} \approx 3.166666\ldots$, differs from this by only about 0.004. **4 ✓**

We see that the approximation dy and the actual change Δy are reasonably close. It is often easier to calculate the approximation since that involves fewer steps, but the trade-off is some loss in accuracy. As long as dx is small, this loss in accuracy is often acceptable, as the following example illustrates.

EXAMPLE 5 **Business: Cost and Tolerance.** In preparation for laying new tile, Michelle measures the floor of a banquet hall and finds it to be square, measuring 100 ft by 100 ft. Suppose these measurements are accurate to ± 6 in. (the tolerance).

a) Use a differential to estimate the difference in area (dA) due to the tolerance.

b) Compare the result from part (a) with the actual difference in area (ΔA).

c) If each tile covers 1 ft^2 and a box of 12 tiles costs \$24, how many extra boxes of tiles should Michelle buy for covering the floor? What is the extra cost?

Solution

a) The floor is a square, with a presumed measurement of 100 ft per side and a tolerance of ± 6 in. $= \pm 0.5$ ft. The area A in square feet (ft^2) for a square of side length x ft is

$$A(x) = x^2.$$

The derivative is $dA/dx = 2x$, and solving for dA gives the differential of A:

$$dA = 2x\,dx.$$

To find dA, we substitute $x = 100$ and $dx = \pm 0.5$:

$$dA = 2(100)(\pm 0.5) = \pm 100.$$

The value of dA is the approximate difference in area due to the inexactness in measuring. Therefore, if Michelle's measurements are off by half a foot, the total area can differ by approximately ± 100 ft^2. A small "error" in measurement can lead to a significant difference in the resulting area.

b) To calculate the actual difference in area, ΔA, we set $x_1 = 100$ ft, and let x_2 represent the length plus or minus the tolerance.

If the true length is at the low end, we have $x_2 = 99.5$ ft. The floor's area is then $99.5^2 = 9900.25$ ft^2. The actual difference in area is then

$$\begin{aligned} \Delta A &= A(x_2) - A(x_1) \\ &= A(99.5) - A(100) \\ &= 99.5^2 - 100^2 \\ &= 9900.25 - 10{,}000 \\ &= -99.75 \text{ ft}^2. \end{aligned}$$

If the true length is at the high end, we have $x_2 = 100.5$ ft. The floor's area is then $100.5^2 = 10{,}100.25$ ft^2. The actual difference in area is

$$\begin{aligned} \Delta A &= A(x_2) - A(x_1) \\ &= A(100.5) - A(100) \\ &= 100.5^2 - 100^2 \\ &= 10{,}100.25 - 10{,}000 \\ &= 100.25 \text{ ft}^2. \end{aligned}$$

Quick Check 5 ✓

The four walls of a room measure 10 ft by 10 ft each, with a tolerance of ± 0.25 ft.

a) Calculate the approximate difference in area, dA, for the four walls.

b) Workers will texture the four walls using "knockdown" spray. Each bottle of knockdown spray costs \$9 and covers 12 ft^2. How many extra bottles should the workers buy to allow for overage in wall area? What will the extra cost be?

We see that ΔA, the actual difference in area, can range from $-99.75\ \text{ft}^2$ to $100.25\ \text{ft}^2$. Both values compare well with the approximate value of $dA = \pm 100\ \text{ft}^2$.

c) The tiles (each measuring 1 ft^2) come 12 to a box. Thus, if the room were exactly 100 ft by 100 ft (an area of 10,000 ft^2), Michelle would need $10{,}000/12 = 833.33\ldots$, or 834 boxes to cover the floor. To take into account the possibility that the room is larger by 100 ft^2, she needs a total of $10{,}100/12 = 841.67\ldots$, or 842 boxes of tiles. Therefore, she should buy $842 - 834$, or 8 extra boxes of tiles, for an extra cost of $(8)(24) = \$192$. **5 ✓**

Historically, differentials were quite valuable when used to make approximations in lengthy calculations. With the advent of computers and calculators, such use has diminished. The use of marginals remains important in the study of business and economics.

Linearization

Let $y = f(x)$ be differentiable at $x = a$. We can find the equation of the tangent line to f in a process called *linearization*. At the point $(a, f(a))$, the slope of the tangent line is $m = f'(a)$. Using the point–slope formula for the equation of a line, we have

$$y - y_1 = m(x - x_1) \qquad \text{The point–slope formula}$$
$$y - f(a) = f'(a)(x - a) \qquad \text{Substituting}$$
$$y = f(a) + f'(a)(x - a). \qquad \text{Adding } f(a) \text{ to both sides}$$

This leads to a general definition.

DEFINITION

Let $y = f(x)$ be differentiable at $x = a$. The **linearization of f at $x = a$** is given by

$$y = f(a) + f'(a)(x - a).$$

This is the equation of the tangent line to f at $x = a$.

The notation $L(x) = f(a) + f'(a)(x - a)$ is sometimes used to represent the linearization of f at $x = a$. For values of x close to a, the tangent line to f at $x = a$ closely approximates the graph of f, as shown in the figure below.

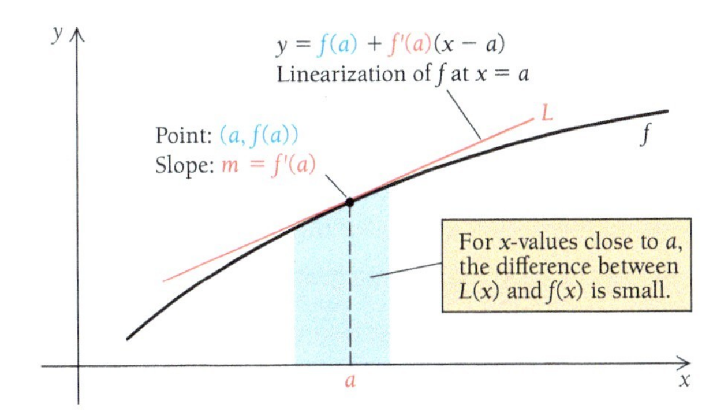

EXAMPLE 6 Find the linearization of $f(x) = \sqrt[3]{x}$ at $a = 8$, and use it to approximate $\sqrt[3]{9}$.

Solution We find $f(8)$:

$$f(8) = \sqrt[3]{8} = 2.$$

We then find $f'(x)$:

$$f'(x) = \frac{1}{3}x^{-2/3} = \frac{1}{3\sqrt[3]{x^2}}.$$

The slope of the tangent line to f at $a = 8$ is

$$f'(8) = \frac{1}{3\sqrt[3]{8^2}} = \frac{1}{3\sqrt[3]{64}} = \frac{1}{3 \cdot 4} = \frac{1}{12}.$$

We now find the linearization of f at $a = 8$; that is, we find the equation of the tangent line:

$$y = f(a) + f'(a)(x - a)$$

$$= 2 + \tfrac{1}{12}(x - 8) \quad \text{Substituting}$$

$$= 2 + \tfrac{1}{12}x - \tfrac{2}{3} \quad \text{Multiplying to clear parentheses}$$

$$= \tfrac{1}{12}x + \tfrac{4}{3}. \quad \text{Simplifying}$$

The graphs of $f(x) = \sqrt[3]{x}$ and the line $L(x) = \frac{1}{12}x + \frac{4}{3}$ are shown below. Note that the line is tangent to the graph of f at (8, 2) and closely approximates the graph "near" $a = 8$.

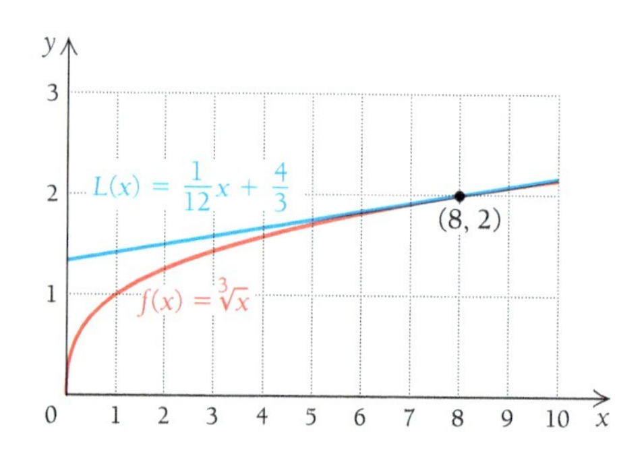

To approximate $\sqrt[3]{9}$, we substitute $x = 9$ into the linearization equation:

$$L(9) = \tfrac{1}{12}(9) + \tfrac{4}{3}$$

$$= \tfrac{3}{4} + \tfrac{4}{3}$$

$$= \tfrac{25}{12}, \quad \text{or } 2\tfrac{1}{12}.$$

Thus, $\sqrt[3]{9} \approx 2\frac{1}{12} = 2.08333\ldots$. Using a calculator, we find that the actual value of $\sqrt[3]{9}$ is $2.080083823\ldots$. The approximated value is only about 0.003 more than the actual value. **6 ✓**

Quick Check 6 ✓

Find the linearization of $f(x) = \sqrt{x}$ at $a = 9$, and use it to approximate $\sqrt{10}$.

Using differentials to approximate values (as in Examples 4 and 5) and using linearization to approximate values (as in Example 6) are similar processes, and in most cases, either method works well.

Section Summary

- If $C(x)$ represents the cost of producing x items, then *marginal cost* $C'(x)$ is its derivative, and $C'(x) \approx C(x + 1) - C(x)$. Thus, the cost to produce the $(x + 1)$st item can be approximated by $C(x + 1) \approx C(x) + C'(x)$.
- If $R(x)$ represents the revenue from selling x items, then *marginal revenue* $R'(x)$ is its derivative, and $R'(x) \approx R(x + 1) - R(x)$. Thus, the revenue from the $(x + 1)$st item can be approximated by $R(x + 1) \approx R(x) + R'(x)$.

- If $P(x)$ represents profit from selling x items, then *marginal profit* $P'(x)$ is its derivative, and $P'(x) \approx P(x+1) - P(x)$. Thus, the profit from the $(x+1)$st item can be approximated by $P(x+1) \approx P(x) + P'(x)$.
- In *delta notation*, $\Delta x = (x+h) - x = h$, and $\Delta y = f(x+h) - f(x)$. For small values of Δx, we have $\frac{\Delta y}{\Delta x} \approx f'(x)$, which is equivalent to $\Delta y \approx f'(x)\,\Delta x$.
- The *differential* of x is $dx = \Delta x$. Since $\frac{dy}{dx} = f'(x)$, we have $dy = f'(x)\,dx$. In general, $dy \approx \Delta y$, and the approximation is often very close for sufficiently small dx.
- Let $y = f(x)$ be differentiable at $x = a$. The *linearization of f at* $x = a$ is given by $y = L(x) = f(a) + f'(a)(x - a)$.

3.6 Exercise Set

In Exercises 1–12, find **(a)** Δy *for the given x and* Δx *values,* **(b)** $dy = f'(x)\,dx$*, and* **(c)** dy *for the given x and* $dx\ (= \Delta x)$ *values.*

1. $f(x) = x^3, x = 2, \Delta x = 0.01$

2. $f(x) = x^2, x = 5, \Delta x = 0.03$

3. $f(x) = x + x^2, x = 3, \Delta x = 0.04$

4. $f(x) = x - x^2, x = 3, \Delta x = 0.02$

5. $f(x) = \frac{1}{x}, x = 1, \Delta x = 0.2$

6. $f(x) = \frac{1}{x^2}, x = 1, \Delta x = 0.5$

7. $f(x) = 3x - 1, x = 4, \Delta x = -2$

8. $f(x) = 2x - 3, x = 8, \Delta x = 0.5$

9. $f(x) = e^x, x = 3, \Delta x = 0.1$

10. $f(x) = e^{-x}, x = 1, \Delta x = -0.2$

11. $f(x) = \ln x, x = 2, \Delta x = -0.03$

12. $f(x) = 2\ln x, x = 4, \Delta x = -0.05$

Use $\Delta y \approx f'(x)\,\Delta x$ *to find a decimal approximation of each radical expression. In each case, select a convenient y-value before calculating* $f'(x)$ *and* Δx*. Round to three decimal places.*

13. $\sqrt{26}$ **14.** $\sqrt{8}$ **15.** $\sqrt{102}$

16. $\sqrt{103}$ **17.** $\sqrt[3]{1005}$ **18.** $\sqrt[3]{28}$

19. Let $f(x) = x^2$.
  a) Find the linearization $L(x)$ of f at $a = 3$.
  b) Use the linearization to approximate 3.1^2.
  c) Find 3.1^2 using a calculator.
  d) What is the difference between the approximation and the actual value of 3.1^2?

20. Let $g(x) = x^3$.
  a) Find the linearization $L(x)$ of g at $a = 4$.
  b) Use the linearization to approximate 3.9^3.
  c) Find 3.9^3 using a calculator.
  d) What is difference between the approximation and the actual value of 3.9^3?

21. Let $h(x) = \sqrt{x}$.
  a) Find the linearization $L(x)$ of h at $a = 16$.
  b) Use the linearization to approximate $\sqrt{17}$.
  c) Find $\sqrt{17}$ using a calculator.
  d) What is the difference between the approximation and the actual value of $\sqrt{17}$?

22. Let $k(x) = 1/\sqrt{x}$.
  a) Find the linearization $L(x)$ of k at $a = 4$.
  b) Use the linearization to approximate $1/\sqrt{3}$.
  c) Find $1/\sqrt{3}$. using a calculator.
  d) What is the difference between the approximation and the actual value of $1/\sqrt{3}$?

23. Let $f(x) = e^x$.
  a) Find the linearization $L(x)$ of f at $a = 2$.
  b) Use the linearization to approximate $e^{2.1}$.
  c) Find $e^{2.1}$ using a calculator.
  d) What is the difference between the approximation and the actual value of $e^{2.1}$?

24. Let $f(x) = \ln x$.
  a) Find the linearization $L(x)$ of f at $a = e$.
  b) Use the linearization to approximate $\ln 2.72$.
  c) Find $\ln 2.72$ using a calculator.
  d) What is the difference between the approximation and the actual value of $\ln 2.72$?

APPLICATIONS

Business and Economics

25. Marginal revenue, cost, and profit. Let $R(x)$, $C(x)$, and $P(x)$ be, respectively, the revenue, cost, and profit, in dollars, from the production and sale of x items. If

$$R(x) = 50x - 0.5x^2 \quad \text{and} \quad C(x) = 4x + 10,$$

find each of the following.
  a) $P(x)$
  b) $R(20)$, $C(20)$, and $P(20)$
  c) $R'(x)$, $C'(x)$, and $P'(x)$
  d) $R'(20)$, $C'(20)$, and $P'(20)$
  e) Explain what each quantity in parts (b) and (d) represents.

26. Marginal revenue, cost, and profit. Let $R(x)$, $C(x)$, and $P(x)$ be, respectively, the revenue, cost, and profit, in dollars, from the production and sale of x items. If

$$R(x) = 5x \quad \text{and} \quad C(x) = 0.001x^2 + 1.2x + 60,$$

find each of the following.

a) $P(x)$
b) $R(100)$, $C(100)$, and $P(100)$
c) $R'(x)$, $C'(x)$, and $P'(x)$
d) $R'(100)$, $C'(100)$, and $P'(100)$
e) Explain what each quantity in parts (b) and (d) represents.

27. Marginal cost. Suppose the daily cost, in hundreds of dollars, of producing x security systems is

$$C(x) = 0.002x^3 + 0.1x^2 + 42x + 300,$$

and currently 40 security systems are produced daily.

a) What is the current daily cost?
b) What is the marginal cost when $x = 40$?
c) Use the result from part (b) to estimate the daily cost of increasing production to 42 security systems daily.
d) What would be the actual additional daily cost of increasing production to 42 security systems daily?

28. Marginal cost. Suppose the monthly cost, in dollars, of producing x daypacks is

$$C(x) = 0.001x^3 + 0.07x^2 + 19x + 700,$$

and currently 25 daypacks are produced monthly.

a) What is the current monthly cost?
b) What is the marginal cost when $x = 25$?
c) Use marginal cost to estimate the difference in cost between producing 25 and 27 daypacks per month.
d) Use the answer from part (c) to predict $C(27)$.

29. Marginal revenue. Pierce Manufacturing determines that the daily revenue, in dollars, from the sale of x lawn chairs is

$$R(x) = 0.005x^3 + 0.01x^2 + 0.5x.$$

Currently, Pierce sells 70 lawn chairs daily.

a) What is the current daily revenue?
b) What is the marginal revenue when 70 lawn chairs are sold daily?
c) How much would revenue increase if 73 lawn chairs were sold each day?
d) Use the answer from part (b) to estimate $R(71)$, $R(72)$, and $R(73)$.

30. Marginal profit. For Sunshine Motors, the weekly profit, in dollars, from selling x cars is

$$P(x) = -0.006x^3 - 0.2x^2 + 900x - 1200,$$

and currently 60 cars are sold weekly.

a) What is the current weekly profit?
b) What is the marginal profit when $x = 60$?
c) Use marginal profit to estimate the weekly profit if sales increase to 61 cars weekly.

31. Marginal revenue. Solano Carriers finds that its weekly revenue, in dollars, from the sale of x carry-on suitcases is

$$R(x) = 0.007x^3 - 0.5x^2 + 150x.$$

Currently Solano is selling 26 carry-on suitcases weekly.

a) What is the current weekly revenue?
b) How much would revenue increase if sales increased from 26 to 28 suitcases?
c) What is the marginal revenue when 26 suitcases are sold?
d) Use the answers from parts (a) and (c) to estimate the revenue resulting from selling 27 suitcases per week.

32. Marginal profit. Crawford Computing finds that its weekly profit, in dollars, from the production and sale of x laptop computers is

$$P(x) = -0.004x^3 - 0.3x^2 + 600x - 800.$$

Currently Crawford builds and sells 9 laptops weekly.

a) What is the current weekly profit?
b) How much profit would be lost if production and sales dropped to 8 laptops weekly?
c) What is the marginal profit when $x = 9$?
d) Use the answers from parts (a) and (c) to estimate the profit resulting from the production and sale of 10 laptops weekly.

33. Sales. Let $N(x)$ be the number of computers sold annually when the price is x dollars per computer. Explain in words what occurs if $N(1000) = 500{,}000$ and $N'(1000) = -100$.

34. Sales. Use the answer from Exercise 33 to estimate the number of computers sold if the price is raised to \$1025.

For Exercises 35–40, assume that $C(x)$ and $R(x)$ are in dollars and x is the number of units produced and sold.

35. For the total-cost function

$$C(x) = 0.01x^2 + 1.6x + 100,$$

find ΔC and $C'(x)$ when $x = 80$ and $\Delta x = 1$.

36. For the total-cost function

$$C(x) = 0.01x^2 + 0.6x + 30,$$

find ΔC and $C'(x)$ when $x = 70$ and $\Delta x = 1$.

37. For the total-revenue function

$$R(x) = 200 \ln x,$$

find ΔR and $R'(x)$ when $x = 70$ and $\Delta x = 1$.

38. For the total-revenue function

$$R(x) = 3000 \ln x,$$

find ΔR and $R'(x)$ when $x = 80$ and $\Delta x = 1$.

39. a) Using $C(x)$ from Exercise 35 and $R(x)$ from Exercise 38, find the total profit, $P(x)$.
b) Find ΔP and $P'(x)$ when $x = 80$ and $\Delta x = 1$.

40. a) Using $C(x)$ from Exercise 36 and $R(x)$ from Exercise 37, find the total profit, $P(x)$.
b) Find ΔP and $P'(x)$ when $x = 70$ and $\Delta x = 1$.

41. Marginal supply. The supply S, of a new rollerball pen is given by

$$S = 0.007p^3 - 0.5p^2 + 150p,$$

where p is the price in dollars.

a) Find the rate of change of quantity with respect to price, dS/dp.
b) How many units will producers want to supply when the price is \$25 per unit?
c) Find the rate of change at $p = 25$, and interpret this result.
d) Would you expect dS/dp to be positive or negative? Why?

42. Average cost. The average cost for Turtlehead, Inc., to produce x units of its thermal outerwear is given by

$$\overline{C}(x) = \frac{13x + 100}{x}.$$

Use $\overline{C}'(x)$ to estimate the change in average cost as production goes from 100 units to 101 units.

43. Marginal cost. Braden Foundry determines that the cost to produce x hundred tons of steel is given by

$$C(x) = 2.5x^2 + 5.65x + 8.75,$$

where $C(x)$ is in thousands of dollars.

a) Find the cost of producing 1500 tons of steel.
b) Find the marginal cost when 1500 tons of steel is produced.
c) Use the results from parts (a) and (b) to estimate the cost of producing 1600 tons of steel.

44. Marginal profit. Tuttle Automotive manufactures seat covers. The company has determined that the cost of producing x thousand seat covers is given by

$$C(x) = 0.0025x^3 + 0.3x^2 - 3.4x + 15,$$

where $C(x)$ is in thousands of dollars.

a) Find the cost of producing 6000 seat covers.
b) Find the marginal cost when 6000 seat covers are produced.
c) Use the results from parts (a) and (b) to estimate the cost to produce 7000 seat covers.

45. Marginal productivity. An employee's monthly productivity, $M(t)$, in number of units produced, is found to be a function of the number of years of employment, t. For a certain product, the productivity function is given by

$$M(t) = -2t^2 + 100t + 180.$$

a) Find the productivity of an employee after 5 yr, 10 yr, 25 yr, and 45 yr of employment.
b) Find the marginal productivity.
c) Find the marginal productivity at $t = 5$, $t = 10$, $t = 25$, $t = 45$; and interpret the results.

46. Supply. A supply function for a certain product is given by

$$S(p) = 0.08p^3 + 2p^2 + 10p + 11,$$

where $S(p)$ is the number of items produced when the price is p dollars. Use $S'(p)$ to estimate how many more units a producer will supply when the price changes from \$18.00 per unit to \$18.20 per unit.

47. Gross domestic product. The U.S. gross domestic product, in billions of current dollars, may be modeled by the function

$$P(x) = 1.025e^{0.0247x},$$

where x is the number of years since 1990. (*Source*: U.S. Bureau for Economic Analysis.) Use $P'(x)$ to estimate the increase in the gross domestic product from 2019 to 2020.

48. Advertising. Norris Inc. finds that it sells $N(x)$ thousand units of a product after spending x thousands of dollars on advertising, where

$$N(x) = 2500 - 1500e^{-0.05x}.$$

Use $N'(x)$ to estimate how many more units Norris will sell by increasing its advertising expenditure from \$100,000 to \$101,000.

Marginal tax rate. *Businesses and individuals are frequently concerned about their marginal tax rate, or the rate at which the next dollar earned is taxed. In progressive taxation, the 80,001st dollar earned is taxed at a higher rate than the 25,001st dollar earned and at a lower rate than the 140,001st dollar earned. Use the following graph, showing the marginal tax rate for 2018 for single filers, to answer Exercises 49–52.*

Single Filer's Income Bracket	Rate
0–\$9524	10%
\$9525–\$38,699	12%
\$38,700–\$82,499	22%
\$82,500–\$157,499	25%
\$157,500–\$199,999	32%
\$200,000–\$499,999	35%
\$500,000+	37%

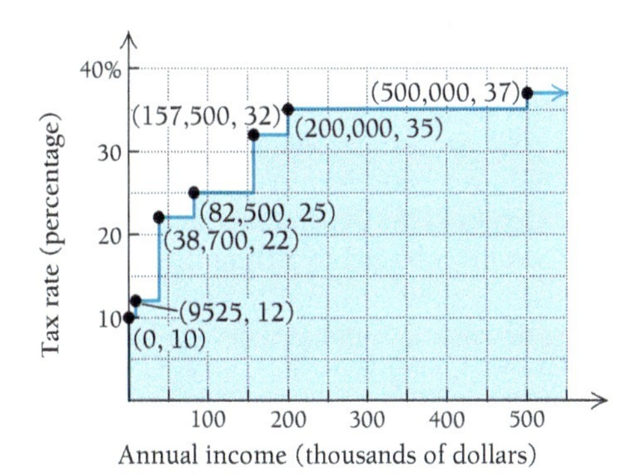

(*Source*: irs.gov, 2018.)

49. Was the taxation in 2018 progressive? Why or why not?

50. Marcy and Tyrone work for the same marketing agency. Because she is not yet a partner, Marcy's year-end income is approximately \$95,000; Tyrone's year-end income is approximately \$190,000. Suppose one of them is to receive another \$5000 in income for the year. Which one would keep more of that \$5000 after taxes? Why?

51. Elaine earns \$85,000 per year and is considering a second job that would earn her another \$10,000 annually. At what rate will her tax liability (the amount she must pay in taxes) change if she takes the extra job? Express your answer in tax dollars paid per dollar earned.

52. Gary earns \$50,000 per year and is considering extra work that would earn him an extra \$3000 annually. At what rate will his tax liability grow if he takes the extra work?

53. Tolerance. Each side of a cube-shaped shed is 15 ft long, with a measurement tolerance of ± 2 in. Find dA, the approximate difference in the exposed surface area (the four sides and the roof) due to the tolerance.

54. **Expansion due to heat.** A storage silo in the shape of a cylinder has a radius equal to its height. The height and radius are each measured to be 50 ft with a tolerance of ± 6 in. Find dV, the approximate change in volume when expansion due to heat occurs.

Business and Economics

55. **Cost and tolerance.** A firm contracts to paint the exterior of a large water tank in the shape of a half-dome (a hemisphere). The radius of the tank is measured to be 100 ft with a tolerance of ± 6 in. (± 0.5 ft). (The formula for the surface area of a hemisphere is $A = 2\pi r^2$; use 3.14 as an approximation for π.) Each can of paint costs \$30 and covers 300 ft^2.
   a) Calculate dA, the approximate difference in the surface area due to the tolerance.
   b) Assuming the painters cannot bring partial cans of paint to the job, how many extra cans should they bring to cover the extra area they may encounter?
   c) How much extra should the painters plan to spend on paint to account for the possible extra area?

56. **Strategic oil supply.** The U.S. Strategic Petroleum Reserve (SPR) stores petroleum in large spherical caverns built into salt deposits along the Gulf of Mexico. (*Source*: U.S. Department of Energy.) These caverns can be enlarged by filling the void with water, which dissolves the surrounding salt, and then pumping brine out. Suppose a cavern has a radius of 400 ft, which engineers want to enlarge by 2 ft. Use a differential to estimate how much volume will be added to form the enlarged cavern. (The formula for the volume of a sphere is $V = \frac{4}{3}\pi r^3$; use 3.14 as an approximation for π.)

Life and Physical Sciences

57. **Body surface area.** Certain chemotherapy dosages depend on a patient's surface area. According to the Gehan and George model,

$$S = 0.02235h^{0.42246}w^{0.51456},$$

where h is the patient's height in centimeters, w is his or her weight in kilograms, and S is the approximation to his or her surface area in square meters. (*Source*: www.halls.md.) Joanne is 160 cm tall and weighs 60 kg. Use a differential to estimate how much her surface area changes after her weight decreases by 1 kg.

58. **Medical dosage.** The function

$$N(t) = \frac{0.8t + 1000}{5t + 4}$$

gives the bodily concentration $N(t)$, in parts per million, of a certain medication after t hours. Use differentials to determine whether the concentration changes more from 1.0 hr to 1.1 hr or from 2.8 hr to 2.9 hr.

SYNTHESIS

59. Let $f(x) = \sqrt{x}$.
   a) Find $L(x)$, the linearization of f at $a = 36$.
   b) Using a spreadsheet or a calculator's TABLE feature, find b such that $L(x)$ and $f(x)$ differ by at most 0.05 over the interval $[36, b]$. Express b to the nearest tenth.

60. Let $f(x) = x^5$.
   a) Find $L(x)$, the linearization of f at $a = 2$.
   b) Using a spreadsheet or a calculator's TABLE feature, find b such that $L(x)$ and $f(x)$ differ by at most 0.1 over the interval $[2, b]$. Express b to the nearest hundredth.

61. **Approximating square roots.** The ancient Greek mathematicians used the formula $\sqrt{x^2 + b} \approx x + \frac{b}{2x}$ to approximate square roots. For example,
$\sqrt{38} = \sqrt{6^2 + 2} \approx 6 + \frac{2}{12}$.
   a) Derive this formula, using the linearization of $f(x) = \sqrt{x}$ at (a^2, a).
   b) Use the formula to approximate $\sqrt{5}, \sqrt{18}, \sqrt{24}$, and $\sqrt{104}$. Write the answers as mixed fractions.
   c) What observations can you make about the accuracy of this formula in terms of b and x^2?

62. **Approximating cube roots.** A formula similar to that in Exercise 61 is $\sqrt[3]{x^3 + b} \approx x + \frac{b}{3x^2}$, which is used to approximate cube roots.
   a) Derive this formula, using the linearization of $f(x) = \sqrt[3]{x}$ at (a^3, a).
   b) Use this formula to approximate $\sqrt[3]{7}, \sqrt[3]{10}, \sqrt[3]{29}$, and $\sqrt[3]{66}$. Write the answers as mixed fractions.
   c) What observations can you make about the accuracy of this formula in terms of b and x^3?

63. Why might estimating using differentials be easier than simply calculating a desired value?

64. Let $L(x)$ be the linearization of $f(x) = x^3$ at $x = a$. Explain why $L(x)$ always overestimates $f(x)$ for $a < 0$ and underestimates $f(x)$ for $a > 0$.

Answers to Quick Checks

1. (a) $P(x) = -0.5x^2 + 40x - 3$; **(b)** $C(40) = 403$, $R(40) = 1200$, $P(40) = 797$; **(c)** $C'(40) = 10$, $R'(40) = 10$, $P'(40) = 0$ **2.** Marginal cost: \$491; estimated cost to produce 750 pairs of shoes: \$33,038 **3.** $\Delta y = -3.1319875$ **4.** $dy = -0.1$; $\sqrt{98} \approx 9.9$. The actual value of $\sqrt{98}$ is 9.899494936 . . . , so the approximation is very close. **5. (a)** ± 20 ft^2; **(b)** \$18 (for 2 extra bottles) **6.** $y = \frac{1}{6}x + \frac{3}{2}$; at $x = 10$, $y = \frac{1}{6}(10) + \frac{3}{2} = \frac{19}{6} = 3\frac{1}{6} = 3.16666\ldots$

3.7

- Find the elasticity of a demand function.
- Find the maximum of a total-revenue function.
- Characterize demand in terms of elasticity.

Elasticity of Demand

A demand function, $q = D(x)$, relates the quantity q of units purchased to the price x, in dollars per unit, and it is usually a decreasing function. Retailers and manufacturers often need to know how a small increase in price will affect demand and total revenue.

A small increase in price may result in a relatively small drop in demand, but higher revenue. In such a case, a price increase may be wise. However, if a small price increase results in a significant drop in demand and lower total revenue, then the price increase may not be wise. In fact, the retailer may want to lower the price. To measure the sensitivity of demand to a small increase in price, economists calculate the *elasticity of demand*.

Suppose Klix Video Games has found that the demand for one of its popular video games is given by

$$q = D(x) = 120 - 20x,$$

where q is the number of games rented per day at x dollars per rental. Klix Video Games wants to determine what effect a small increase in the price per rental will have on demand and on revenue.

If the price per rental is currently \$2, the demand is

$$\begin{aligned} q &= D(2) \\ &= 120 - 20(2) \\ &= 80 \text{ rentals per day.} \end{aligned}$$

Thus, total revenue per day is $2 \cdot 80 = \$160$ per day. If the price is raised by 10%, to \$2.20 per rental, the demand will be

$$\begin{aligned} q &= D(2.2) \\ &= 120 - 20(2.2) \\ &= 76 \text{ rentals per day,} \end{aligned}$$

and total revenue will be $2.20 \cdot 76 = \$167.20$ per day. Note that a 10% increase in the price resulted in a 5% decrease in demand, but an increase in total revenue. In this case, raising the price per rental to \$2.20 may be wise.

Suppose the price per rental is \$5. The demand is then

$$q = D(5) = 120 - 20(5) = 20 \text{ rentals per day.}$$

Total revenue per day will be $5 \cdot 20 = \$100$ per day. If the price is raised by 10%, to \$5.50, the demand will be

$$q = D(5.5) = 120 - 20(5.5) = 10 \text{ rentals per day,}$$

and total revenue will be $5.50 \cdot 10 = \$55.00$ per day. Here, a 10% increase in price results in a 50% decrease in demand, and a drop in total revenue. In this case, raising the price would not be wise. Klix may want to lower the price per rental instead.

Let's develop a general formula for elasticity of demand. We begin with the demand function, $q = D(x)$. For any change, Δx, in the price per unit, the percent change (expressed as a decimal) in price is

$$\frac{\Delta x}{x}.$$

A change in price produces a change, Δq, in the quantity demanded, and the percent change in this quantity is

$$\frac{\Delta q}{q}.$$

The ratio of percent change in quantity sold to percent change in price is

$$\frac{\Delta q/q}{\Delta x/x},$$

which can be expressed as

$$\frac{x}{q} \cdot \frac{\Delta q}{\Delta x}.$$

Since, for differentiable functions,

$$\lim_{\Delta x \to 0} \frac{\Delta q}{\Delta x} = \frac{dq}{dx},$$

we have

$$\lim_{\Delta x \to 0} \frac{x}{q} \cdot \frac{\Delta q}{\Delta x} = \frac{x}{q} \cdot \frac{dq}{dx} = \frac{x}{q} \cdot D'(x) = \frac{x}{D(x)} \cdot D'(x).$$

This result is the basis of the following definition.

DEFINITION

The **elasticity of demand** E is given as a function of price x by

$$E(x) = -\frac{x \cdot D'(x)}{D(x)}.$$

Note that the price, x, and the demand, $D(x)$, are both nonnegative. Since $D(x)$ is normally decreasing, $D'(x)$ is usually negative. Inserting a negative sign in the definition makes $E(x)$ a positive quantity.

There are three possible cases:

- When $E(x) < 1$, the demand is *inelastic*. A small rise in price will result in an increase in total revenue.
- When $E(x) > 1$, the demand is *elastic*. A small rise in price will result in a decrease in total revenue.
- When $E(x) = 1$, total revenue is maximized. This case is called *unit elasticity*.

In the video game example above, demand is inelastic at $2 per rental, but elastic at $5 per rental.

This suggests the following theorem.

THEOREM 11

Total revenue is increasing at those x-values for which $E(x) < 1$.
Total revenue is decreasing at those x-values for which $E(x) > 1$.
Total revenue is maximized at the value(s) of x for which $E(x) = 1$.

Proof: We know that

$$R(x) = x \cdot D(x),$$

so

$$R'(x) = x \cdot D'(x) + D(x) \cdot 1 \qquad \text{Using the Product Rule}$$

$$= D(x)\left[\frac{x \cdot D'(x)}{D(x)} + 1\right] \qquad \text{Factoring; check this by multiplying.}$$

$$= D(x)[-E(x) + 1]$$

$$= D(x)[1 - E(x)].$$

Since we can assume that $D(x) > 0$, it follows that $R'(x)$ is positive for $E(x) < 1$, is negative for $E(x) > 1$, and is 0 when $E(x) = 1$. Thus, total revenue is increasing for $E(x) < 1$, is decreasing for $E(x) > 1$, and is maximized when $E(x) = 1$. ■

EXAMPLE 1 **Economics: Elasticity of Demand for Video Game Rentals.** The demand for video game rentals at Klix Video Games is given by

$$q = D(x) = 120 - 20x,$$

where q is the number of video games rented per day at x dollars per rental.

a) Find the elasticity of demand as a function of x.

b) Find the elasticity at $x = 2$ and at $x = 5$. Interpret the meaning of these values of the elasticity.

c) Find the value of x for which $E(x) = 1$. What is the significance of this price?

Solution

a) To find the elasticity, we first find the derivative, $D'(x)$:

$$D'(x) = -20.$$

Then we substitute -20 for $D'(x)$ and $120 - 20x$ for $D(x)$ in the expression for elasticity:

$$E(x) = -\frac{x \cdot D'(x)}{D(x)} = -\frac{x \cdot (-20)}{120 - 20x} = \frac{20x}{120 - 20x} = \frac{x}{6 - x}.$$

b) $E(2) = \dfrac{2}{6 - 2} = \dfrac{1}{2}$

At $x = 2$, the elasticity is $\frac{1}{2}$, which is less than 1. Thus, the ratio of percent change in quantity to percent change in price is less than 1. A small percentage increase in price will cause an even smaller percentage decrease in the quantity demanded. At $x = 2$, demand is inelastic, and raising the price of each rental by a small amount will increase total revenue.

$$E(5) = \frac{5}{6 - 5} = 5$$

At $x = 5$, the elasticity is 5, which is greater than 1. Thus, the ratio of percent change in quantity to percent change in price is greater than 1. A small percentage increase in price will cause a larger percentage decrease in the quantity demanded. At $x = 5$, demand is elastic, and raising the price of each rental by a small amount will decrease total revenue.

c) We set $E(x) = 1$ and solve for x:

$$\frac{x}{6 - x} = 1$$

$$x = 6 - x \quad \text{We multiply both sides by } 6 - x, \text{ assuming that } x \neq 6.$$

$$2x = 6$$

$$x = 3.$$

This is the price that results in unit elasticity: At \$3 per rental, Klix Video Games will maximize its total revenue. The demand is $q = D(3) = 120 - 20(3) = 60$ rentals per day, and the revenue is $3 \cdot 60 = \$180$ per day. **1 ✓**

Quick Check 1 ✓

Economics: Elasticity of Demand. The demand for organic chewing gum is given by

$$q = D(x) = 30 - 5x.$$

a) Find the quantity demanded when the price is \$2 per pack, \$3 per pack, and \$5 per pack.

b) Find the elasticity of demand as a function of x.

c) Find the elasticity at $x = 2$, $x = 3$, and $x = 5$. Interpret the meaning of these values.

d) Find the value of x for which $E(x) = 1$. Interpret the meaning of this price.

In a typical economy, goods with inelastic demands tend to be items people purchase regularly, such as food, clothing, and fuel. These goods tend to be purchased in set amounts, regardless of small fluctuations in price. Goods with elastic demands tend to be larger items purchased occasionally, such as a vehicle or furniture. Purchases of such items can be delayed until the price drops.

Elasticity and Revenue: A Summary

For a particular value of the price x:

1. Demand is *inelastic* if $E(x) < 1$. A small increase in price creates an increase in revenue. If demand is inelastic, then revenue is increasing.
2. Demand has *unit elasticity* if $E(x) = 1$. The demand has unit elasticity when revenue is at a maximum.
3. Demand is *elastic* if $E(x) > 1$. A small increase in price creates a decrease in revenue. If demand is elastic, then revenue is decreasing.

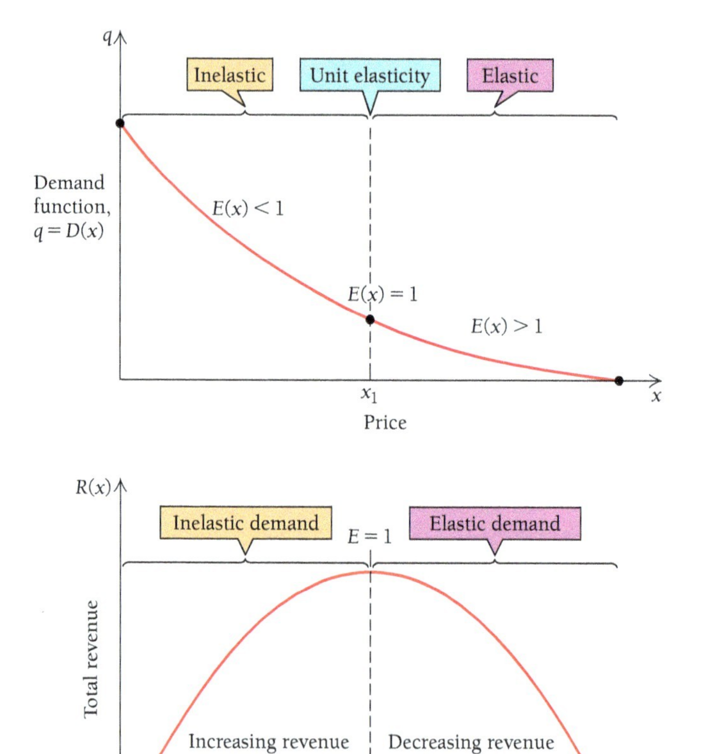

EXAMPLE 2 **Business: Elasticity of Demand.** Wayne's Honey Farm sells honey-based moisturizing cream for \$12 per jar. At this price, it sells 14,500 jars per month. To see if the price is too high or too low, Wayne's Honey Farm raises the price to \$18 per jar. At this price, it sells 10,750 jars per month.

a) Find a linear demand function, $q = D(x)$, that models this situation.

b) Find the elasticity of demand, $E(x)$.

c) Find $E(12)$ and $E(18)$, and interpret the meaning of each result.

d) Find the price at which demand has unit elasticity, and interpret its meaning.

Solution

a) If $q = D(x)$ is the line that includes the ordered pairs (12, 14,500) and (18, 10,750), then the equation of this line is

$$y = -625x + 22{,}000.$$ Using techniques developed in Section R.4

Thus, the demand function is given by $q = D(x) = -625x + 22{,}000$.

b) With $D(x) = -625x + 22{,}000$ and $D'(x) = -625$, the elasticity of demand is

$$E(x) = -\frac{x \cdot D'(x)}{D(x)}$$

$$= -\frac{x(-625)}{-625x + 22{,}000} \qquad \text{Substituting}$$

$$= \frac{625x}{22{,}000 - 625x}$$

$$= \frac{5x}{176 - 5x}. \qquad \text{Simplifying}$$

c) We have

$$E(12) = \frac{5(12)}{176 - 5(12)} = 0.517\ldots < 1,$$

$$\text{and} \quad E(18) = \frac{5(18)}{176 - 5(18)} = 1.046\ldots > 1.$$

At \$12 per jar, the demand is inelastic, and a small increase in price causes total monthly revenue to increase. At \$18 per jar, demand is elastic, and a small increase in price causes a drop in total monthly revenue.

d) We set $E(x) = 1$, and solve for x:

$$\frac{5x}{176 - 5x} = 1$$

$$5x = 176 - 5x \qquad \text{Multiplying both sides by } 176 - 5x$$

$$10x = 176$$

$$x = 17.6.$$

At \$17.60 per jar, demand has unit elasticity. This is the price at which Wayne's Honey Farm should sell its moisturizing cream to maximize total monthly revenue. Total revenue, $R(x) = x \cdot D(x)$, is then

$$R(17.6) = 17.6 \cdot D(17.6)$$

$$= 17.6(22{,}000 - 625(17.6))$$

$$= \$193{,}600.$$

Comparing this value to the total revenue at \$12 per jar,

$$R(12) = 12(22{,}000 - 625(12)) = \$174{,}000,$$

and the total revenue at \$18 per jar,

$$R(18) = 18(22{,}000 - 625(18)) = \$193{,}500,$$

serves as a check that at \$17.60 per jar, revenue is maximized.

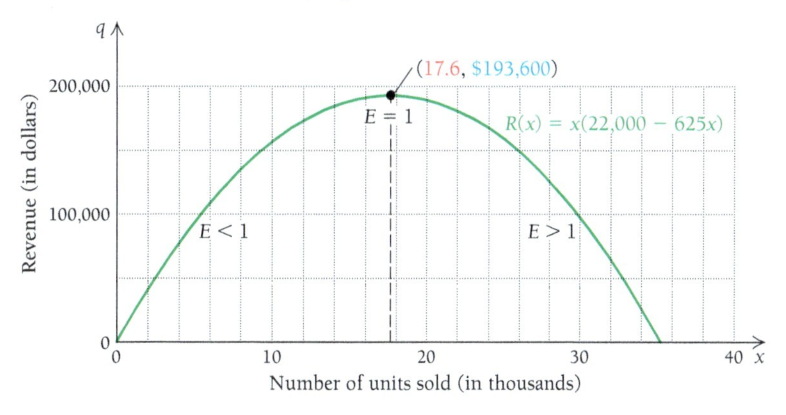

Quick Check 2 ✓

Raggs, Ltd., sells women's coats. At a price of \$60 per coat, Raggs sells 7500 coats, and at \$81, Raggs sells 5750 coats.

a) Find a linear demand function, $q = D(x)$, that models this situation.

b) Find the elasticity of demand, $E(x)$.

c) Find $E(60)$ and $E(81)$, and interpret the meaning of each result.

d) Find the price at which demand has unit elasticity, and interpret its meaning. Also find the revenue at that price.

Based on this linear demand function, Wayne's Honey Farm discovers that \$12 per jar is too low a price to maximize revenue. By raising the price to about \$17.60 per jar, it can expect to maximize its monthly revenue. **2 ✓**

Exponential Demand Functions

Linear demand functions, such as $q = D(x) = 22{,}000 - 625x$ (see Example 2) have limitations. For example, at a price of \$36 per jar, using this linear demand function, Wayne's Honey Farm would expect to sell $D(36) = 22{,}000 - 625(36) = -500$ jars per month. Although a high price per jar would reduce demand, it is impossible to sell a negative quantity of jars.

Exponential functions of the form $y = P_0e^{-kx}$, where $k > 0$, can be used to model demand. These are decreasing functions that allow for any price $x > 0$ to be considered.

EXAMPLE 3 Use the same data points, (12, 14,500) and (18, 10,750), given in Example 2.

a) Using regression, find an exponential demand function of the form $q = D(x) = P_0e^{-kx}$.

b) Find the elasticity of demand, $E(x)$.

c) Find the price x at which Wayne's Honey Farm should sell its jars of moisturizing cream for demand to have unit elasticity. Also, give the resulting total monthly revenue.

Solution

a) Using regression, we have

$$q = D(x) = 26{,}380.746e^{-0.04987x}.$$

b) The elasticity of demand is

$$\begin{aligned} E(x) &= -\frac{x \cdot D'(x)}{D(x)} \\ &= -\frac{x \cdot 26{,}380.746(-0.04987)e^{-0.04987x}}{26{,}380.746e^{-0.04987x}} \quad \text{Substituting} \\ &= 0.04987x. \end{aligned}$$

c) We set $E(x) = 1$, and solve for x:

$$\begin{aligned} 0.04987x &= 1 \\ x &= \frac{1}{0.04987} \\ &\approx 20.05. \end{aligned}$$

With this exponential demand function, at a price of \$20.05 per jar, Wayne's Honey Farm can expect total monthly revenue of

$$\begin{aligned} R(20.05) &= 20.05 \cdot 26{,}380.746e^{-0.04987(20.05)} \\ &\approx \$194{,}600. \quad \text{Rounding to the nearest hundred} \end{aligned}$$

Quick Check 3 ✓

Use the data points from Quick Check 2.

a) Using regression, find an exponential demand function of the form $q = D(x) = P_0 e^{-kx}$.

b) Find the elasticity of demand, $E(x)$.

c) Find the price x at which Raggs, Ltd., should sell its women's coats for demand to have unit elasticity. Give the resulting total revenue.

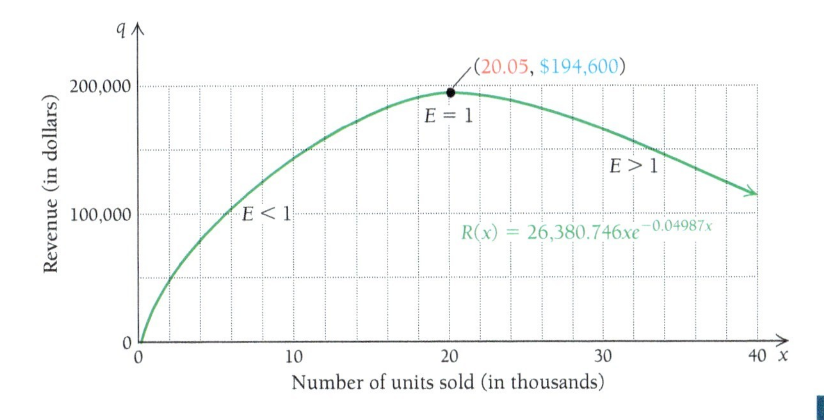

3 ✓

Two data points do not provide a lot of information, but both models suggest that a price in the \$17–\$20 range maximizes total monthly revenue for Wayne's Honey Farm. It might consider selling jars at different prices to gather more data points, from which to create more accurate regression functions to model the data.

Section Summary

- For a demand function $q = D(x)$, where x is in dollars, the **elasticity of demand** is
$$E(x) = -\frac{x \cdot D'(x)}{D(x)}.$$
- Demand is **inelastic** when $E(x) < 1$. If demand is inelastic, then with a small increase in price, revenue increases.
- Demand is **elastic** when $E(x) > 1$. If demand is elastic, then with a small increase in price, revenue decreases.
- Demand has **unit elasticity** when $E(x) = 1$. If demand has unit elasticity at price x, then revenue is maximized.

3.7 Exercise Set

For the demand function given in each of Exercises 1–12, find the following.

a) *The elasticity*

b) *The elasticity at the given price, stating whether the demand is elastic or inelastic*

c) *The value(s) of x for which total revenue is a maximum (assume that x is in dollars)*

1. $q = D(x) = 400 - x; \quad x = 125$

2. $q = D(x) = 500 - x; \quad x = 38$

3. $q = D(x) = 200 - 4x; \quad x = 46$

4. $q = D(x) = 500 - 2x; \quad x = 57$

5. $q = D(x) = \frac{400}{x}; \quad x = 50$

6. $q = D(x) = \frac{3000}{x}; \quad x = 60$

7. $q = D(x) = \sqrt{600 - x}; \quad x = 100$

8. $q = D(x) = \sqrt{300 - x}; \quad x = 250$

9. $q = D(x) = \frac{100}{(x + 3)^2}; \quad x = 1$

10. $q = D(x) = \frac{500}{(2x + 12)^2}; \quad x = 8$

11. $q = D(x) = 100e^{-0.25x}; \quad x = 10$

12. $q = D(x) = 200e^{-0.05x}; \quad x = 80$

APPLICATIONS

Business and Economics

13. Demand for chocolate drops. Good Time Chocolates determines that the demand function for its chocolate drops is

$$q = D(x) = 967 - 25x,$$

where q is the quantity of chocolate drops sold when the price is x cents per drop.

a) Find the elasticity.
b) At what price is elasticity of demand equal to 1?
c) At what prices is demand elastic?
d) At what prices is demand inelastic?
e) At what price is the revenue a maximum?
f) At a price of 20¢ per drop, will a small increase in price cause total revenue to increase or decrease?

14. Demand for oil. Suppose you have been hired as an economic consultant concerning the world demand for oil. The demand function is

$$q = D(x) = 35{,}000 + 150x - 4x^2, \quad \text{for } 0 \le x \le 180,$$

where q is measured in millions of barrels of oil per day at a price of x dollars per barrel.

a) Find the elasticity.
b) Find the elasticity at a price of \$45 per barrel, stating whether demand is elastic or inelastic at that price.
c) Find the elasticity at a price of \$60 per barrel, stating whether demand is elastic or inelastic at that price.
d) Find the elasticity at a price of \$75 per barrel, stating whether demand is elastic or inelastic at that price.
e) At what price is revenue a maximum?
f) What quantity of oil will be sold at the price that maximizes revenue? Compare the current world price to your answer.
g) In August 2017, a barrel of crude oil was selling for about \$48. (*Source*: West Texas Intermediate, NYSE.) At this price, will a small increase in price cause total revenue to increase or decrease?

15. Demand for computer apps. High Wire Graphx determines the following demand function for a new app:

$$q = D(x) = 50e^{-0.12x},$$

where q is the number of apps sold per day when the price is x dollars per app.

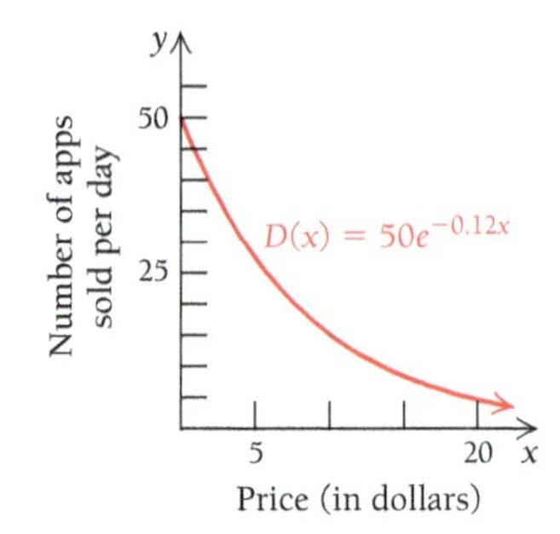

a) Find the elasticity.
b) Find the elasticity when $x = 3$.
c) At $x = 3$, will a small increase in price cause total revenue to increase or decrease?

16. Demand for tomato plants. Sunshine Gardens determines the following demand function during early summer for tomato plants:

$$q = D(x) = \frac{2x + 300}{10x + 11},$$

where q is the number of plants sold per day at x dollars per plant.

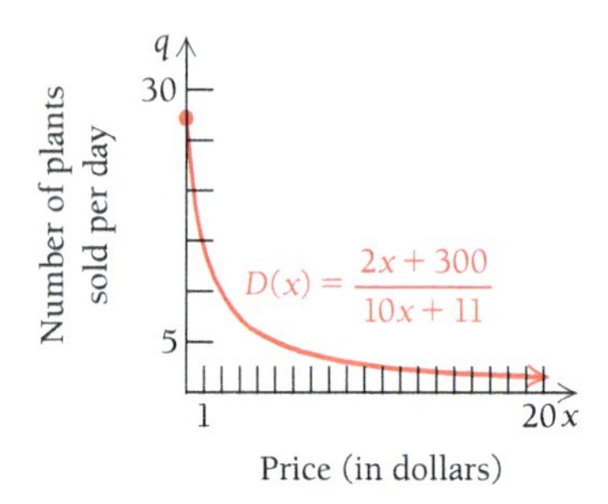

a) Find the elasticity.
b) Find the elasticity when $x = 3$.
c) At \$3 per plant, will a small increase in price cause total revenue to increase or decrease?

17. Demand for planters. Peacock Pottery sells large planters. At \$45 per unit, it sells 1200 units per month, and at \$55 per unit, it sells 1050 units per month.

a) Find a linear demand function, $q = D(x)$, that models this situation.
b) Find the elasticity of demand, $E(x)$.
c) Find $E(45)$ and $E(55)$, and interpret the meaning of each result.
d) Find the price x at which Peacock Pottery should sell its planters for demand to have unit elasticity, and give the resulting total revenue.

18. Demand for a new book. Drake Publishing releases a new autobiography. At \$19 per book, it sells 4500 books per month, and at \$24 per book, it sells 3200 books per month.

a) Find a linear demand function, $q = D(x)$, that models this situation.
b) Find the elasticity of demand, $E(x)$.
c) Find $E(19)$ and $E(24)$, and interpret the meaning of each result.
d) Find the price x at which Drake Publishing should sell its new autobiography for demand to have unit elasticity, and give the resulting total revenue.

19. Demand for planters. Use the data points given in Exercise 17.

a) Using regression, find an exponential demand function of the form $q = D(x) = P_0e^{-kx}$.
b) Find the elasticity of demand, $E(x)$.
c) Find the price x at which Peacock Pottery should sell its planters for demand to have unit elasticity, and give the resulting total revenue.

20. **Demand for a new book.** Use the data points given in Exercise 18.

a) Using regression, find an exponential demand function of the form $q = D(x) = P_0e^{-kx}$.

b) Find the elasticity of demand, $E(x)$.

c) Find the price x at which Drake Publishing should sell its new autobiography for demand to have unit elasticity, and give the resulting total revenue.

SYNTHESIS

21. **Business.** Tipton Industries determines that the demand function for its sunglass cases is

$$q = D(x) = 180 - 10x,$$

where q is the quantity of sunglass cases sold at x dollars per case.

a) Find the elasticity of demand.

b) Find the elasticity when $x = 8$.

c) At what price is revenue a maximum?

d) If the price is \$8 and Tipton Industries raises the price by 20%, will revenue increase or decrease? Does this contradict the answers to parts (b) and (c)? Why or why not?

22. **Economics: constant elasticity curve.**

a) Find the elasticity of the demand function

$$q = D(x) = \frac{k}{x^n},$$

where k is a positive constant and n is an integer greater than 0.

b) Is the value of the elasticity dependent on the price per unit?

c) For what value of n does total revenue have a maximum?

23. **Economics: exponential demand curve.**

a) Find the elasticity of the demand function

$$q = D(x) = Ae^{-kx},$$

where A and k are positive constants.

b) Is the value of the elasticity dependent on the price per unit?

c) At what x-value (expressed in terms of k) is the total revenue maximized?

24. Explain in your own words the concept of elasticity and its usefulness to economists. Do research or speak with an economist to determine when and how this concept was first developed.

25. Explain how the elasticity of demand for a product can be affected by the availability of substitutes for the product.

26. Show that for a demand function of the form $D(x) = b - ax$, unit elasticity occurs when $x = \dfrac{b}{2a}$.

Technology Connection 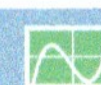

27. In order to raise funds to maintain a section of a popular hiking trail, a college's environmental organization is selling t-shirts. To determine an optimal price, the organization asks 100 students the *maximum* price they would be willing to pay for a shirt, with the results given in the table below:

Price, x	Number of Students, y
\$ 8	5
\$10	12
\$12	17
\$14	21
\$16	18
\$18	11
\$20	10
\$22	6

Assume that each student is willing to pay any price up to his or her stated maximum price. For example, all 100 students are willing to pay \$8, but at a price of \$10, the demand drops to 95 students willing to pay that amount. The demand, $q(x)$, is the total number of students who are willing to pay up to and including x dollars for a t-shirt.

a) Using the data in the above table, create a table showing the demand, $q(x)$, at price x.

b) Using regression, find linear, cubic, and logistic demand functions that model the data from part (a).

c) Find the elasticity of demand for each model from part (b).

d) Using the linear model, find the price that results in unit elasticity and the total revenue if the t-shirts are sold at this price.

e) Using the cubic model, find the price that results in unit elasticity and the total revenue if the t-shirts are sold at this price.

f) Using the logistic model, find the price that results in unit elasticity and the total revenue if the t-shirts are sold at this price.

g) Based on the results from parts (d)–(f), how might the environmental organization decide on the price per shirt?

Answers to Quick Check

1. (a) 20, 15, 5; (b) $E(x) = \dfrac{x}{6 - x}$; (c) 0.5, 1, 5 (see Example 1 for the interpretations); (d) \$3

2. (a) $D(x) = 12{,}500 - \frac{250}{3}x$; (b) $E(x) = \dfrac{x}{150 - x}$; (c) $E(60) = \frac{2}{3} < 1$, inelastic; $E(81) = \frac{27}{23} > 1$, elastic; (d) at a price of \$75, revenue is maximized, at \$468,750.

3. (a) $D(x) = 16{,}023.476e^{-0.0127x}$; (b) $E(x) = 0.0127x$; (c) \$78.74, \$464,150

3.8 Implicit Differentiation and Logarithmic Differentiation

- Differentiate implicitly.
- Use logarithmic differentiation to find the derivatives of certain functions.

We often write a function with the output variable (such as y) isolated on one side of the equation. For example, when we write $y = x^3$, we are expressing y as an *explicit* function of x. With an equation like $y^3 + x^2y^5 - x^4 = -11$, it may be difficult to isolate the output variable. In such a case, we have an *implicit* relationship between the variables x and y and can find the derivative of y with respect to x using *implicit differentiation*.

Implicit Differentiation

A method known as **implicit differentiation** allows us to find dy/dx without first solving for y. To do so, we differentiate both sides of the given equation, treating y as a function of x.

For example, we know from our earlier work that the derivative of $y = \sqrt[3]{x}$ is

$$y' = \tfrac{1}{3}x^{-2/3}. \quad (1)$$

However, if we solve $y = \sqrt[3]{x}$ for x, we have $y^3 = x$. To find dy/dx without first solving for y, we differentiate both sides of this equation with respect to x, using the Chain Rule:

$$\frac{d}{dx}(y^3) = \frac{d}{dx}(x).$$

The derivative on the left side is found using the Extended Power Rule:

$$3y^2\frac{dy}{dx} = 1. \qquad \text{Remembering that the derivative of } y \text{ with respect to } x \text{ is written } dy/dx$$

Finally, we solve for dy/dx by dividing both sides by $3y^2$:

$$\frac{dy}{dx} = \frac{1}{3y^2}, \quad \text{or} \quad \frac{1}{3}y^{-2}.$$

We can show that this indeed gives us the same answer as equation (1) by replacing y with $x^{1/3}$:

$$\frac{dy}{dx} = \frac{1}{3}y^{-2} = \frac{1}{3}(x^{1/3})^{-2} = \frac{1}{3}x^{-2/3}.$$

Equations like

$$y^3 + x^2y^5 - x^4 = -11$$

determine y as a function of x, but are difficult to solve for y. We can nevertheless find a formula for the derivative of y *without* solving for y. To do so usually involves using the Extended Power Rule in the form

$$\frac{d}{dx}y^n = ny^{n-1}\cdot\frac{dy}{dx}.$$

EXAMPLE 1 For $y^3 + x^2y^5 - x^4 = -11$:

a) Find dy/dx using implicit differentiation.

b) Find the slope of the tangent line to the curve at the point (2, 1).

Solution

a) We differentiate the term x^2y^5 using the Product Rule. Because y is a function of x, it is critical that dy/dx is included any time a term involving y is differentiated. When an expression involving just x is differentiated, there is no factor dy/dx.

$$\frac{d}{dx}(y^3 + x^2y^5 - x^4) = \frac{d}{dx}(-11) \quad \text{Differentiating both sides with respect to } x$$

$$\frac{d}{dx}y^3 + \frac{d}{dx}x^2y^5 - \frac{d}{dx}x^4 = 0$$

$$3y^2 \cdot \frac{dy}{dx} + x^2 \cdot 5y^4 \cdot \frac{dy}{dx} + y^5 \cdot 2x - 4x^3 = 0. \quad \text{Using the Extended Power Rule and the Product Rule}$$

We next isolate all terms with dy/dx as a factor on one side:

$$3y^2 \cdot \frac{dy}{dx} + 5x^2y^4 \cdot \frac{dy}{dx} = 4x^3 - 2xy^5 \quad \text{Adding } 4x^3 - 2xy^5 \text{ to both sides}$$

$$(3y^2 + 5x^2y^4)\frac{dy}{dx} = 4x^3 - 2xy^5 \quad \text{Factoring } dy/dx$$

$$\frac{dy}{dx} = \frac{4x^3 - 2xy^5}{3y^2 + 5x^2y^4}. \quad \text{Solving for } dy/dx \text{ and leaving the answer in terms of } x \text{ and } y$$

b) To find the slope of the tangent line to the curve at (2, 1), we replace x with 2 and y with 1:

$$\frac{dy}{dx} = \frac{4 \cdot 2^3 - 2 \cdot 2 \cdot 1^5}{3 \cdot 1^2 + 5 \cdot 2^2 \cdot 1^4} = \frac{28}{23}.$$

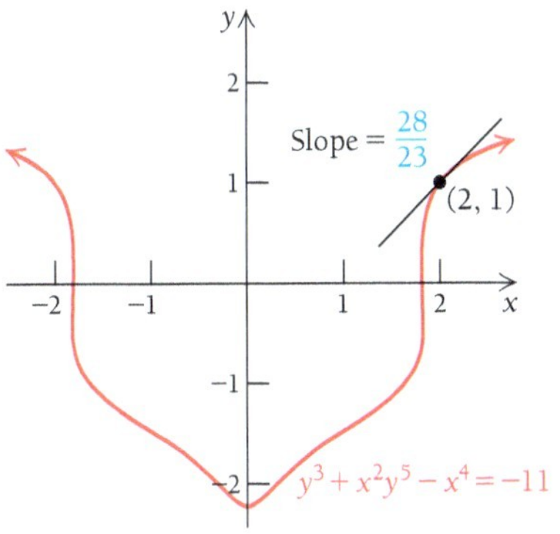

1 ✓

Quick Check 1 ✓

For $y^2x + 2x^3y^3 = y + 1$, find dy/dx using implicit differentiation.

It is common for the expression for dy/dx to contain *both* variables x and y. When this occurs, we calculate a slope by evaluating the derivative at both the x-value and the y-value of the point of tangency, as we did in part (b) of Example 1. The steps in Example 1 are typical of those used when differentiating implicitly.

The demand function for a product (see Section R.5) is often given implicitly.

EXAMPLE 2 Differentiate $x = \sqrt{200 - p^3}$ implicitly to find dp/dx.

Solution

$$\frac{d}{dx}(x) = \frac{d}{dx}\left(\sqrt{200 - p^3}\right)$$

$$1 = \frac{1}{2}(200 - p^3)^{-1/2} \cdot (-3p^2) \cdot \frac{dp}{dx} \quad \text{Using the Extended Power Rule twice}$$

$$1 = \frac{-3p^2}{2\sqrt{200 - p^3}} \cdot \frac{dp}{dx}$$

$$\frac{2\sqrt{200 - p^3}}{-3p^2} = \frac{dp}{dx}$$

2 ✓

Quick Check 2 ✓

Differentiate

$$y = 2\sqrt{1 + p^2}$$

implicitly to find $\frac{dp}{dy}$.

Logarithmic Differentiation

When differentiating functions such as $y = (x^4 + 3x - 1)^3 \cdot \sqrt{1 - 3x^5}$, we can use some combination of the Product, Quotient, and Chain Rules, but this approach can be complicated. An alternative to finding the derivative in such cases is a process called **logarithmic differentiation**, which relies on implicit differentiation and the properties of logarithms. Given a function of the form $y = f(x)$, we find the natural logarithm of both sides:

$$\ln(y) = \ln(f(x)).$$

Differentiating implicitly with respect to x, and using the Chain Rule, we have

$$\frac{d}{dx}(\ln(y)) = \frac{d}{dx}(\ln(f(x))) \quad \text{Implicitly differentiating both sides with respect to } x$$

$$\frac{1}{y} \cdot \frac{dy}{dx} = \frac{d}{dx}(\ln(f(x))). \quad \text{Using the Chain Rule}$$

The properties of logarithms can then be used to simplify $\ln(f(x))$ before differentiating. Finally, both sides of the equation are multiplied by $y = f(x)$ to isolate dy/dx:

$$\frac{dy}{dx} = y \cdot \frac{d}{dx}(\ln(f(x))), \quad \text{or} \quad \frac{dy}{dx} = f(x) \cdot \frac{d}{dx}(\ln(f(x))).$$

This approach is illustrated in the following example.

EXAMPLE 3 Given $y = (x^4 + 3x - 1)^3 \cdot \sqrt{1 - 3x^5}$, find dy/dx.

Solution We find the natural logarithm of both sides:

$$\ln(y) = \ln\left((x^4 + 3x - 1)^3 \cdot \sqrt{1 - 3x^5}\right)$$

$$= \ln(x^4 + 3x - 1)^3 + \ln(1 - 3x^5)^{1/2}. \quad \text{Using the property } \ln(MN) = \ln M + \ln N$$

Using the property $\ln a^k = k \ln a$, we simplify further:

$$\ln y = 3 \ln(x^4 + 3x - 1) + \tfrac{1}{2}\ln(1 - 3x^5).$$

Next, we implicitly differentiate both sides with respect to x. We use the Chain Rule $\frac{d}{dx}(\ln f(x)) = \frac{f'(x)}{f(x)}$, where $\frac{d}{dx}(\ln y) = \frac{1}{y} \cdot \frac{dy}{dx}$:

$$\frac{d}{dx}(\ln y) = \frac{d}{dx}\left(3\ln(x^4 + 3x - 1) + \frac{1}{2}\ln(1 - 3x^5)\right)$$

$$\frac{1}{y} \cdot \frac{dy}{dx} = 3 \cdot \frac{4x^3 + 3}{x^4 + 3x - 1} + \frac{1}{2} \cdot \left(\frac{-15x^4}{1 - 3x^5}\right)$$

$$\frac{1}{y} \cdot \frac{dy}{dx} = \frac{12x^3 + 9}{x^4 + 3x - 1} - \frac{15x^4}{2(1 - 3x^5)}. \quad \text{Simplifying}$$

Now, we multiply both sides by y to isolate dy/dx:

$$\frac{dy}{dx} = y\left(\frac{12x^3 + 9}{x^4 + 3x - 1} - \frac{15x^4}{2(1 - 3x^5)}\right).$$

Since $y = (x^4 + 3x - 1)^3 \cdot \sqrt{1 - 3x^5}$, we have

$$\frac{dy}{dx} = (x^4 + 3x - 1)^3 \cdot \sqrt{1 - 3x^5}\left(\frac{12x^3 + 9}{x^4 + 3x - 1} - \frac{15x^4}{2(1 - 3x^5)}\right).$$

3 ✓

Quick Check 3 ✓

Given $y = \frac{(2x + 4)^3}{(x^2 + x + 1)^7}$, find $\frac{dy}{dx}$.

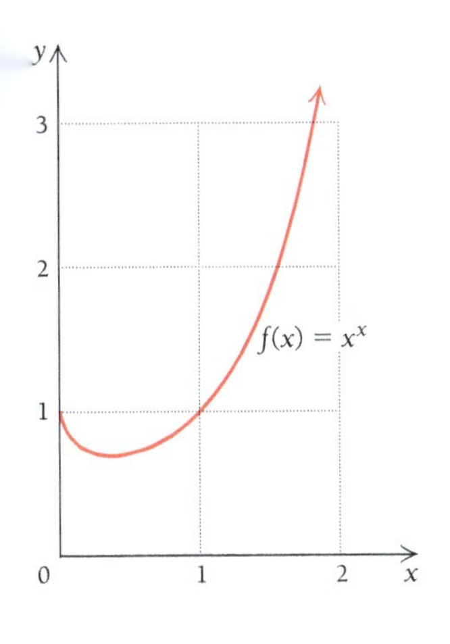
f(x) = x^x

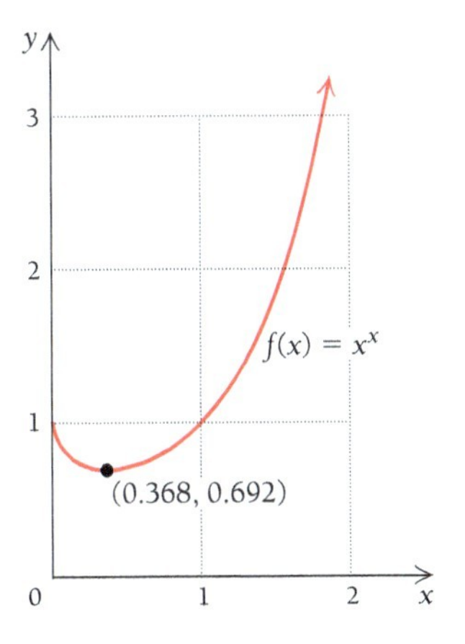
f(x) = x^x
(0.368, 0.692)

Quick Check 4 ✓

Find the absolute maximum value of $y = g(x) = x^{-x}$ over the interval $(0, \infty)$.

EXAMPLE 4 Find the absolute minimum value of $y = f(x) = x^x$ over $(0, \infty)$.

Solution The function x^x is neither a polynomial nor an exponential. Its graph, shown at the left, is defined only for positive x and has no x-intercepts.

To differentiate, we first find the natural logarithm of both sides:

$$\ln y = \ln x^x$$
$$= x \ln x \qquad \text{Using a property of logarithms}$$

Next, we implicitly differentiate both sides with respect to x, and solve for dy/dx:

$$\frac{d}{dx}(\ln y) = \frac{d}{dx}(x \ln x)$$
$$\frac{1}{y} \cdot \frac{dy}{dx} = x\left(\frac{1}{x}\right) + (1) \ln x \qquad \text{Using the Product Rule}$$
$$\frac{1}{y} \cdot \frac{dy}{dx} = 1 + \ln x \qquad \text{Simplifying}$$
$$\frac{dy}{dx} = y(1 + \ln x) \qquad \text{Multiplying both sides by } y$$
$$\frac{dy}{dx} = x^x(1 + \ln x) \qquad \text{Substituting } y = x^x$$

We now set the derivative equal to 0, and solve for any critical values. Using the Principle of Zero Products, we can ignore the factor x^x since it never equals 0. We have

$$x^x(1 + \ln x) = 0$$
$$1 + \ln x = 0 \qquad \text{The factor } 1 + \ln x \text{ can equal 0, but } x^x \text{ cannot.}$$
$$\ln x = -1$$
$$x = e^{-1} \approx 0.368.$$

Using the First-Derivative Test, we see that the graph of f is decreasing over the interval $(0, e^{-1})$ and increasing over (e^{-1}, ∞). Thus, the point $(e^{-1}, f(e^{-1}))$ is a relative minimum. Furthermore, this is the only critical point in the interval $(0, \infty)$, and by Maximum–Minimum Principle 2, it must be an absolute minimum.

Using a calculator, we find that $f(e^{-1}) = (e^{-1})^{e^{-1}} \approx 0.692$. This is the absolute minimum value of $y = f(x) = x^x$ over the interval $(0, \infty)$. 4 ✓

Application: Point of Diminishing Returns

In Example 5, we will show that the logistic function $f(t) = \dfrac{L}{1 + Ce^{-rt}}$ (see Section 2.4) has a point of inflection at $\left(\dfrac{\ln C}{r}, \dfrac{L}{2}\right)$. At this point, the rate of change of $f'(t)$ is maximized. Beyond this point, the output $f(t)$ continues to increase, but at a slower rate than before. The point $\left(\dfrac{\ln C}{r}, \dfrac{L}{2}\right)$ is called the **point of diminishing returns**.

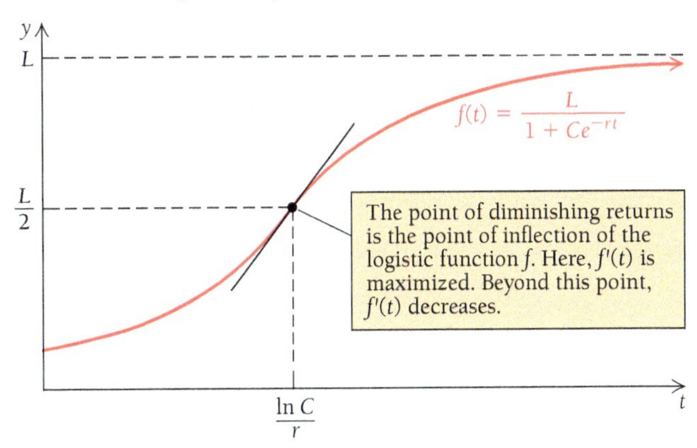
y
L
L/2
f(t) = L/(1 + Ce^{-rt})
The point of diminishing returns is the point of inflection of the logistic function f. Here, f′(t) is maximized. Beyond this point, f′(t) decreases.
ln C/r
t

EXAMPLE 5 **Business: Point of Diminishing Returns.** Use logarithmic differentiation to show that the point of inflection of $f(t) = \frac{L}{1 + Ce^{-rt}}$ occurs at $\left(\frac{\ln C}{r}, \frac{L}{2}\right)$.

Solution Using the Quotient Rule, we first find $f'(t)$:

$$f'(t) = \frac{(1 + Ce^{-rt})(0) - L(-Cre^{-rt})}{(1 + Ce^{-rt})^2} = \frac{LCre^{-rt}}{(1 + Ce^{-rt})^2}.$$

To find the second derivative, $f''(x)$, we use logarithmic differentiation to simplify the process. Finding the natural logarithm of both sides, we have

$$\ln(f'(t)) = \ln\left(\frac{LCre^{-rt}}{(1 + Ce^{-rt})^2}\right).$$

We use the properties of natural logarithms to simplify the right side:

$$\begin{aligned} \ln(f'(t)) &= \ln(LCr) + \ln(e^{-rt}) - \ln(1 + Ce^{-rt})^2 \\ &= \ln(LCr) - rt - 2\ln(1 + Ce^{-rt}). \end{aligned}$$ Using the properties of natural logarithms

We now differentiate implicitly:

$$\frac{d}{dt}(\ln(f'(t))) = \frac{d}{dt}(\ln(LCr) - rt - 2\ln(1 + Ce^{-rt}))$$

$$\frac{1}{f'(t)} \cdot \frac{d}{dt}[f'(t)] = 0 - r - 2\left(\frac{-Cre^{-rt}}{1 + Ce^{-rt}}\right)$$ Noting that $\ln(LCr)$ is a constant

$$\frac{1}{f'(t)} \cdot \frac{d}{dt}[f'(t)] = -r + \frac{2Cre^{-rt}}{1 + Ce^{-rt}}$$ Simplifying

$$\frac{d}{dt}[f'(t)] = f'(t)\left(-r + \frac{2Cre^{-rt}}{1 + Ce^{-rt}}\right)$$ Multiplying both sides by $f'(t)$

$$f''(t) = \frac{LCre^{-rt}}{(1 + Ce^{-rt})^2}\left(-r + \frac{2Cre^{-rt}}{1 + Ce^{-rt}}\right).$$ Substituting

To find the point of inflection, we solve $f''(t) = 0$. The first factor, $\frac{LCre^{-rt}}{(1 + Ce^{-rt})^2}$, is never 0, so it can be ignored. Using the second factor, we have

$$-r + \frac{2Cre^{-rt}}{1 + Ce^{-rt}} = 0$$

$$\frac{2Cre^{-rt}}{1 + Ce^{-rt}} = r$$

$$2Cre^{-rt} = r(1 + Ce^{-rt})$$ Multiplying both sides by $1 + Ce^{-rt}$ to clear fractions

$$2Cre^{-rt} = r + Cre^{-rt}$$

$$Cre^{-rt} = r$$ Adding $-Cre^{-rt}$ to both sides

$$Ce^{-rt} = 1$$ Dividing both sides by r; $r \neq 0$

$$e^{-rt} = \frac{1}{C}$$

$$-rt = \ln\left(\frac{1}{C}\right)$$ Finding the natural logarithm of both sides

$$-rt = -\ln C$$ Using the fact that $\ln\left(\frac{1}{C}\right) = \ln C^{-1} = -\ln C$

$$t = \frac{\ln C}{r}.$$

Quick Check 5 ✓

Suppose that sales of a popular book t weeks after it is published are given by $f(t) = \frac{2{,}000{,}000}{1 + 49e^{-0.04t}}$. When is the rate of sales maximized?

Evaluating $f(t)$ at $t = \frac{\ln C}{r}$, we have

$$f\left(\frac{\ln C}{r}\right) = \frac{L}{1 + Ce^{-r(\ln(C)/r)}} = \frac{L}{1 + Ce^{-\ln C}}.$$

The expression $e^{-\ln C}$ is equivalent to $e^{\ln C^{-1}} = C^{-1}$:

$$\frac{L}{1 + Ce^{-\ln C}} = \frac{L}{1 + C(C^{-1})} = \frac{L}{1 + 1} = \frac{L}{2}.$$

Thus, the point of inflection occurs at $\left(\frac{\ln C}{r}, \frac{L}{2}\right)$. **5 ✓**

Section Summary

- If variables x and y are related to one another by an equation but neither variable is isolated on one side of the equation, we say that x and y have an implicit relationship. To find dy/dx without solving such an equation for y, we use *implicit differentiation*.
- Whenever we implicitly differentiate y with respect to x, the factor dy/dx will appear as a result of the Chain Rule.
- To determine the slope of a tangent line at a point on the graph of an implicit relationship, we may need to evaluate the derivative by inserting both the x-value and the y-value of the point of tangency.
- *Logarithmic differentiation* can be used to differentiate certain functions. To do this with a function $y = f(x)$, the natural logarithm is taken on both sides: $\ln y = \ln f(x)$. This function can then be differentiated implicitly to find dy/dx.
- A logistic function of the form $f(t) = \frac{L}{1 + Ce^{-rt}}$ has its point of inflection at $\left(\frac{\ln C}{r}, \frac{L}{2}\right)$, where its rate of change is maximized. This is called the *point of diminishing returns*.

3.8 Exercise Set

Differentiate implicitly to find dy/dx.

1. $x^2 + 2xy = 3y^2$
2. $2xy + 3 = 0$
3. $x^2 - y^2 = 16$
4. $x^2 + y^2 = 25$
5. $y^3 = x^5$
6. $y^5 = x^3$
7. $x^2y^3 + x^3y^4 = 11$
8. $x^3y^2 + x^5y^3 = -19$
9. $e^y + y^2 = 3x$
10. $e^{-y} - y^3 = x^2$
11. $\ln(x^2 + y) = 2x + 1$
12. $3 - x^2 = \ln(x + y^3)$
13. $e^{2y} + x = \ln y$
14. $e^{3y} + 4x^3 = 2 \ln y$

Differentiate implicitly to find dy/dx. Then find the slope of the curve at the given point.

15. $3x^3 - y^2 = 8;\ (2, 4)$
16. $x^3 + 2y^3 = 6;\ (2, -1)$
17. $2x^3 + 4y^2 = -12;\ (-2, -1)$
18. $2x^2 - 3y^3 = 5;\ (-2, 1)$
19. $x^2 + y^2 = 1;\ \left(\frac{1}{2}, \frac{\sqrt{3}}{2}\right)$
20. $x^2 - y^2 = 1;\ (\sqrt{3}, \sqrt{2})$
21. $2x^3y^2 = -18;\ (-1, 3)$
22. $3x^2y^4 = 12;\ (2, -1)$
23. $x^4 - x^2y^3 = 12;\ (-2, 1)$
24. $x^3 - x^2y^2 = -9;\ (3, -2)$
25. $xy + y^2 - 2x = 0;\ (1, -2)$
26. $xy - x + 2y = 3;\ \left(-5, \frac{2}{3}\right)$
27. $4x^3 - y^4 - 3y + 5x + 1 = 0;\ (1, -2)$
28. $x^2y - 2x^3 - y^3 + 1 = 0;\ (2, -3)$

For each demand equation in Exercises 29–36, differentiate implicitly to find dp/dx.

29. $p^2 + p + 2x = 40$
30. $p^3 + p - 3x = 50$
31. $xp^3 = 24$
32. $x^3p^2 = 108$
33. $\frac{x^2p + xp + 1}{2x + p} = 1$ (*Hint*: Clear the fraction first.)

34. $\frac{xp}{x+p} = 2$ (*Hint*: Clear the fraction first.)

35. $(p+4)(x+3) = 48$

36. $1000 - 300p + 25p^2 = x$

Use logarithmic differentiation to find y'.

37. $y = (x^2+4)^{10}(2x-5)^8$

38. $y = (x^3-1)^9(5-2x^7)^{14}$

39. $y = (x+7)^3(2x-5)^6(x^3-2x+1)^7$

40. $y = (2x+1)^5(3x-2)^9(x^5-4x+9)^{11}$

41. $y = \frac{(2x-3)^5}{(3x+5)^4}$

42. $y = \frac{(3x+8)^{13}}{(9x-1)^6}$

43. $y = \frac{\sqrt{5-3x}(x^2+1)^2}{x^2+2x+5}$

44. $y = \frac{(x^4+3)^7\sqrt{1-7x}}{x^3+5x+7}$

45. $y = x^5e^{x^2+6x+7}$

46. $y = 4x^3e^{x^3+4x^2+8x-3}$

47. $y = \frac{\sqrt{x^2+5x+9}}{e^{x^4+2x^2+2}}$

48. $y = \frac{e^{8x^7+5x^4+2}}{\sqrt{4x^3-5x+7}}$

49. $y = \frac{xe^{\sqrt{x^2+1}}}{2x^3+5x}$

50. $y = \frac{x^2\sqrt{x^4+5}}{e^{x-x^4}}$

51. Find the absolute minimum of $y = x^{\sqrt{x}}$ over the interval $(0, \infty)$.

52. Find the absolute minimum of $y = (2x)^x$ over the interval $(0, \infty)$.

APPLICATIONS

Business and Economics

53. **Sales.** The new pop song "You're My Math Boo" is released on iSongz. The number of times the song has been downloaded t weeks after its initial release is given by

$$f(t) = \frac{3{,}500{,}000}{1 + 500e^{-0.65t}}.$$

a) After how many weeks is the rate of change of the number of downloads maximized?
b) What is the rate of change of the number of downloads at the time found in part (a)?
c) How many times has the song been downloaded at the time found in part (a)?

54. **Sales.** Sales of the self-help book *I Can Differentiate* t weeks after it is published are given by

$$f(t) = \frac{750{,}000}{1 + 355e^{-0.07t}}.$$

a) After how many weeks is the rate of change of sales maximized?
b) What is the rate of change of sales at the time found in part (a)?
c) How many times has the book been purchased at the time found in part (a)?

55. **Worker productivity.** Having more employees work on a task does not always result in increased efficiency and production. DynaCom Inc. discovers that its yearly production of cell-phone batteries by x employees is given by

$$P(x) = \frac{500{,}000}{1 + 435e^{-0.075x}}.$$

a) What number of employees will maximize the rate of production?
b) If DynaCom Inc. hires 20 more employees than the number found in part (a), then production will increase. Using calculus, explain why efficiency will decrease, even though production will increase.

56. **Worker productivity.** ShipMasters finds that the number of orders it can fill per day when x people are employed at its shipping center is given by

$$N(x) = \frac{20{,}000}{1 + 67e^{-0.3x}}.$$

a) What number of employees will maximize the rate of order fulfillment?
b) A new manager suggests that doubling the number of employees will double the order fulfillments. Explain why this will not occur. What would the number of orders filled and the rate of order fulfillment be if there were twice the number of employees found in part (a)?

General Interest

57. **Spread of a disease.** A dorm at Rubidoux College houses 1200 students. One day, 20 of the students become ill with the flu, which spreads quickly. Assume that the total number of students who have been infected after t days is given by

$$N(t) = \frac{1200}{1 + 13e^{-0.85t}}.$$

a) After how many days is the flu spreading the fastest?
b) Approximately how many students per day are catching the flu on the day found in part (a)?
c) How many students have been infected on the day found in part (a)?

58. **Spread of a rumor.** A new rumor spreads within a company with 500 employees. The number of employees who have heard the rumor after t hours is given by

$$N(t) = \frac{500}{1 + 25e^{-0.7t}}.$$

a) After how many hours is the rumor spreading most quickly?
b) Approximately how many employees per hour are first hearing the rumor at the time found in part (a)?
c) How many employees have heard the rumor at the time found in part (a)?

SYNTHESIS

59. **Business: revenue.** Revenue, in dollars, from sales of a popular new puzzle t weeks after its release is modeled by a logistic function of the form $R(t) = \dfrac{L}{1 + Ce^{-rt}}$. Initial revenue (at $t = 0$) was \$25,000, and revenue was increasing the fastest after 15 weeks, when total revenue was \$14,000,000.
    a) Find the logistic function that models the revenue after t weeks.
    b) How fast was revenue increasing at $t = 15$ weeks?

60. **Business: effect of advertising.** An advertising agency discovers that as it continues to air a television ad for a certain product, sales of that product increase. However, if it airs the ad too often, the rate of change of sales is not as high as before. Sales of the product when the ad is aired x times are given by $S(x) = \dfrac{L}{1 + Ce^{-rx}}$. When no ads were aired ($x = 0$), only 500 units were sold. When 45 ads were aired, sales were increasing the fastest. The upper limit of sales is expected to be about 15,000,000 units.
    a) Find the logistic function that models sales when the ad is aired x times.
    b) How fast were sales increasing when the ad was aired 45 times?

In Exercises 61–64, use logarithmic differentiation to find d^2y/dx^2.

61. $y = xe^{3x-2}$
62. $y = x^2(x^3 + 2)^3$
63. $y = x^x$ (*Hint*: See Example 4.)
64. $y = (2x)^x$

65. Given a logistic function of the form $f(t) = \dfrac{L}{1 + Ce^{-rt}}$, with inflection point $\left(\dfrac{\ln C}{r}, \dfrac{L}{2}\right)$, explain why doubling the time t does not result in double the output.

66. Let $y = (x^4 + 5)^3(3x^2 + 1)^7$.
    a) Find $y' = f'(x)$ using the Product and Chain Rules.
    b) Find $y' = f'(x)$ using logarithmic differentiation, and show that the result is the same as in part (a).
    c) Explain the advantages of each method for differentiating the given function.

Differentiate implicitly to find d^2y/dx^2.

67. $xy + x - 2y = 4$
68. $y^2 - xy + x^2 = 5$
69. $x^2 - y^2 = 5$
70. $x^3 - y^3 = 8$
71. Explain the usefulness of implicit differentiation.
72. Look up the word "implicit" in a dictionary. Explain how that definition can be related to the concept of a function that is defined "implicitly."

Technology Connection 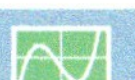

Graph each of the following equations. Equations must be solved for y before they can be entered into most calculators.

73. $x^2 + y^2 = 4$
    Note: You will probably need to sketch the graph in two parts: $y = \sqrt{4 - x^2}$ and $y = -\sqrt{4 - x^2}$. Then graph the tangent line to the graph at the point $(-1, \sqrt{3})$.
74. $x^4 = y^2 + x^6$
    Then graph the tangent line to the graph at the point $(-0.8, 0.384)$.

Answers to Quick Checks

1. $\dfrac{dy}{dx} = \dfrac{y^2 + 6x^2y^3}{1 - 2xy - 6x^3y^2}$
2. $\dfrac{dp}{dy} = \dfrac{\sqrt{1 + p^2}}{2p}$
3. $\dfrac{dy}{dx} = \dfrac{(2x + 4)^3}{(x^2 + x + 1)^7}\left(\dfrac{3}{x + 2} - \dfrac{14x + 7}{x^2 + x + 1}\right)$
4. At approximately (0.368, 1.445)
5. At $t \approx 97.3$ weeks

3.9 Related Rates*

- Solve related-rate problems.
- Solve applied problems involving related rates.

Any equation that contains two or more rates, expressed as derivatives, is called a *related-rates equation*. For example, the equation

$$2x\frac{dy}{dt} + 3y = \frac{dx}{dt}$$

is a related-rates equation, since it contains two rates, dx/dt and dy/dt. To solve a related-rates equation, we use implicit differentiation.

Suppose y is a function of x,

$$y = f(x),$$

and x is, itself, a function of time, t. Since y depends on x and x depends on t, it follows that y is also a function of t. Differentiating and using the Chain Rule gives the following:

$$\frac{dy}{dt} = \frac{dy}{dx} \cdot \frac{dx}{dt}.$$

* This section can be omitted without loss of continuity.

Thus, the rate of change of y with respect to t is *related* to the rate of change of x with respect to t.

EXAMPLE 1 Given $y = 3\sqrt{x}$, find dy/dt when $x = 9$ and $dx/dt = -4$.

Solution We differentiate implicitly with respect to t on both sides of the equation:

$$\frac{d}{dt}(y) = \frac{d}{dt}(3\sqrt{x})$$

$$= \frac{d}{dt}(3x^{1/2})$$

$$= \frac{3}{2}x^{-1/2} \cdot \frac{dx}{dt} \qquad \text{Using the Chain Rule}$$

$$= \frac{3}{2\sqrt{x}} \cdot \frac{dx}{dt}. \qquad \text{Simplifying}$$

Thus, we have a related-rates equation:

$$\frac{dy}{dt} = \frac{3}{2\sqrt{x}} \cdot \frac{dx}{dt}.$$

Substituting $x = 9$ and $dx/dt = -4$, we have

$$\frac{dy}{dt} = 3 \cdot \frac{1}{2\sqrt{9}} \cdot (-4)$$

$$= -\frac{12}{2 \cdot 3}$$

$$= -2.$$

Quick Check 1✓

Given $y = 4x^3$, find dx/dt when $x = 2$ and $dy/dt = 5$.

1✓

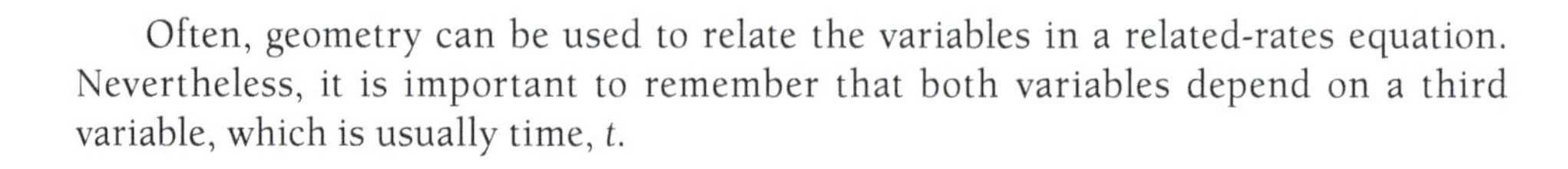

Often, geometry can be used to relate the variables in a related-rates equation. Nevertheless, it is important to remember that both variables depend on a third variable, which is usually time, t.

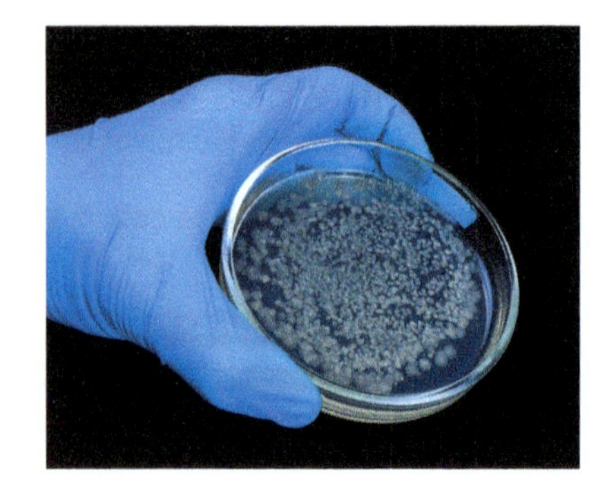

EXAMPLE 2 A colony of bacteria in a petri dish forms a circle whose radius is increasing by 0.7 mm per minute. Find the rate of change in the colony's area at the moment when its radius is 12 mm.

Solution We have two variables: A represents the area of the colony, and r represents the radius of the colony. The area A of a circle of radius r is given by

$$A = \pi r^2.$$

However, both A and r are functions of time t (in minutes). Thus, the above equation can be written in terms of t:

$$A(t) = \pi(r(t))^2.$$

Differentiating both sides implicitly with respect to t, we have

$$\frac{d}{dt}(A(t)) = \frac{d}{dt}(\pi(r(t))^2)$$

$$\frac{d}{dt}A(t) = 2\pi r(t) \cdot \frac{d}{dt}r(t) \qquad \text{Using the Chain Rule}$$

$$\frac{dA}{dt} = 2\pi r\frac{dr}{dt} \qquad \text{Simplifying; this is a related-rates equation.}$$

Quick Check 2 ✓

A restaurant supplier services the restaurants in a circular area whose radius is increasing at the rate of 2 mi per year at the moment when $r = 5$ mi. At that moment, how fast is the area of service changing?

To find how fast the area is changing (represented by dA/dt) when $dr/dt = 0.7$ mm per minute and $r = 12$ mm, we substitute

$$\frac{dA}{dt} = 2\pi(12)(0.7) \qquad \text{Substituting}$$

$$\approx 52.78. \qquad \text{Using a calculator}$$

The area of the colony is growing by about 52.78 mm^2 per minute at the moment its radius is 12 mm. **2 ✓**

EXAMPLE 3 **Business: Rates of Change of Revenue, Cost, and Profit.** For Luce Landscaping, the total revenue and the total cost, in dollars, for yard maintenance of x homes are given by

$$R(x) = 1000x - x^2 \quad \text{and} \quad C(x) = 3000 + 20x.$$

Suppose that Luce is adding 10 homes per day at the moment when the 400th customer is signed. At that moment, what is the rate of change of **(a)** total revenue, **(b)** total cost, and **(c)** total profit?

Solution

a) We regard $R(x) = 1000x - x^2$ as $R = 1000x - x^2$. Implicitly differentiating with respect to time t, we have

$$\frac{dR}{dt} = 1000 \cdot \frac{dx}{dt} - 2x \cdot \frac{dx}{dt} \qquad \text{Differentiating both sides with respect to time}$$

$$= 1000 \cdot 10 - 2(400)10 \qquad \text{Substituting 10 for } dx/dt \text{ and 400 for } x$$

$$= \$2000 \text{ per day.}$$

b) We regard $C(x) = 3000 + 20x$ as $C = 3000 + 20x$. Implicitly differentiating with respect to time t, we have

$$\frac{dC}{dt} = 20 \cdot \frac{dx}{dt} \qquad \text{Differentiating both sides with respect to time}$$

$$= 20(10)$$

$$= \$200 \text{ per day.}$$

c) Since $P(x) = R(x) - C(x)$, we have

$$\frac{dP}{dt} = \frac{dR}{dt} - \frac{dC}{dt}$$

$$= \$2000 \text{ per day} - \$200 \text{ per day}$$

$$= \$1800 \text{ per day.}$$

Related-rate equations can involve more than two variables. As with the two-variable equations, each variable is typically treated as a function of time t.

EXAMPLE 4 **Business: Revenue.** Suppose that in a highly volatile market, 10,000 shares of a stock have been sold at $45 per share and that the number of shares sold is increasing by 150 shares per day, while total revenue is decreasing by $18,250 per day. What is the rate at which the price of a share is changing?

Solution Here, total revenue, R, is equal to price p, in dollars, times quantity sold, q. We differentiate implicitly:

$$\frac{d}{dt}(R) = \frac{d}{dt}(pq) \qquad \text{Differentiating implicitly with respect to } t$$

$$\frac{dR}{dt} = p \cdot \frac{dq}{dt} + q \cdot \frac{dp}{dt}. \qquad \text{Using the Product Rule}$$

We make the following substitutions: $dR/dt = -18{,}250$ (since R is decreasing), $dq/dt = 150$, $p = 45$, and $q = 10{,}000$:

$$-18{,}250 = (45)(150) + (10{,}000)\frac{dp}{dt} \quad \text{Substituting}$$

$$-18{,}250 = 6750 + 10{,}000\frac{dp}{dt}$$

$$-25{,}000 = 10{,}000\frac{dp}{dt}$$

$$-2.5 = \frac{dp}{dt}. \quad \text{Solving for } \frac{dp}{dt}$$

Thus, the price of a share is *decreasing* at the rate of $2.50 per day. 3 ✓

Quick Check 3 ✓

Suppose that 5000 units of ProDuct have been sold at $20 per unit, with the price increasing by $1.75 per day and total revenue increasing by $10,750 per day. Find the rate at which the number of units sold is changing.

Section Summary

- If two or more variables are related to one another by an equation, then we may implicitly differentiate with respect to time t. The result is a *related rate*.
- Geometric formulas are often used to help solve related-rate problems.

3.9 Exercise Set

Find the indicated rate.

1. Given $y = x^3$, find dy/dt when $x = 2$ and $dx/dt = -4$.

2. Given $y = x^4$, find dy/dt when $x = 3$ and $dx/dt = 1.5$.

3. Given $y = 2x^2 + x$, find dy/dt when $x = -3$ and $dx/dt = 2$.

4. Given $y = -3x^2 + 2x$, find dy/dt when $x = -2$ and $dx/dt = 6$.

5. Given $y = 2x^3$, find dx/dt when $x = 1$ and $dy/dt = 10$.

6. Given $y = 4x^2$, find dx/dt when $x = 5$ and $dy/dt = -3$.

7. Given $y = x - x^4$, find dx/dt when $x = 2$ and $dy/dt = -5$.

8. Given $y = 5x - x^2$, find dx/dt when $x = -2$ and $dy/dt = 2.5$.

9. Given $y = e^{2x+1}$, find dy/dt when $x = 4$ and $dx/dt = 0.5$.

10. Given $y = e^{1-3x}$, find dy/dt when $x = 2$ and $dx/dt = -\frac{1}{3}$.

11. Given $y = \ln x$, find dy/dt when $x = -9$ and $dx/dt = 0.25$.

12. Given $y = \ln x$, find dx/dt when $x = 4$ and $dy/dt = 3$.

13. Given $y = \sqrt{x}$, find dx/dt when $y = 4$ and $dy/dt = 1.75$.

14. Given $y = \frac{1}{x^2}$, find dx/dt when $y = 16$ and $dy/dt = -0.8$.

15. Given $y = pq$, find dp/dt when $p = 30$, $q = 250$, $dq/dt = -200$, and $dy/dt = -5250$.

16. Given $y = pq$, find dq/dt when $p = 150$, $q = 75$, $dp/dt = 60$, and $dy/dt = 7500$.

17. Given $y = p^2q$, find dq/dt when $p = 15$, $q = 40$, $dp/dt = 55$, and $dy/dt = 54{,}750$.

18. Given $y = pq^3$, find dp/dt when $p = 80$, $q = 135$, $dq/dt = -5$, and $dy/dt = 7{,}654{,}500$.

19. Given $a^2 = b^2 + c^2$, where $a \geq 0$, $b \geq 0$, and $c \geq 0$, find da/dt when $a = 13$, $b = 12$, $db/dt = 0.25$, and $dc/dt = 2$.

20. Given $a^2 = b^2 + c^2$, where $a \geq 0$, $b \geq 0$, and $c \geq 0$, find dc/dt when $b = 7$, $c = 24$, $db/dt = 3$, and $da/dt = 0.84$.

Use geometry and implicit differentiation to find the unknown rate.

21. A circle is shrinking, losing 15 cm^2 of area per minute. Find the rate at which the radius is changing at the moment when the radius is 7 cm.

22. A circle is growing, its radius increasing by 3 mm per second. Find the rate at which the area is changing at the moment when the radius is 25 mm.

23. A spherical balloon is decreasing in size, losing 60 cm^3 of air per minute. Find the rate at which the radius is changing at the moment when the radius is 25 cm.

24. A spherical balloon is expanding, gaining 125 cm^3 of air per minute. Find the rate at which the radius is changing at the moment when the radius is 60 cm.

25. A spherical balloon is expanding, its radius increasing by 0.5 cm per minute. Find the rate at which its surface area is changing at the moment when the radius is 40 cm. (*Hint*: The surface area of a sphere is given by $A = 4\pi r^2$.)

26. A spherical balloon is shrinking, its radius changing by -5 cm per minute. Find the rate at which its surface area is changing at the moment when the radius is 22 cm.

27. A large ice cube is melting, each side shrinking by 0.8 cm per minute. Find the rate at which the volume is changing at the moment when the length of an edge is 20 cm. Assume that the cube maintains its shape.

28. A large ice cube is melting, each side shrinking by 2 in. per minute. Find the rate at which the volume is changing at the moment when the length of an edge is 15 in. Assume that the cube maintains its shape.

29. A large ice cube is melting, each side shrinking by 3 cm per minute. Find the rate at which the surface area is changing at the moment when the length of an edge is 40 cm. Assume that the cube maintains its shape.

30. An ice cube in a freezer is growing due to accretion, each edge increasing by 0.2 cm per minute. Find the rate at which the surface area is changing at the moment when the length of one side is 8 cm. Assume that the cube maintains its shape.

31. Nonnegative variable quantities G and H are related by

$$G^2 + H^2 = 25.$$

What is the rate of change dH/dt when $dG/dt = 3$ and $G = 0$? $G = 1$? $G = 3$?

32. Variable quantities A and B are related by

$$A^3 + B^3 = 9.$$

What is the rate of change dA/dt at the moment when $A = 2$ and $dB/dt = 3$?

APPLICATIONS

Business and Economics

Rates of change of total revenue, cost, and profit. *In Exercises 33–36, find the rates of change of total revenue, cost, and profit with respect to time. Assume that $R(x)$ and $C(x)$ are in dollars.*

33. $R(x) = 50x - 0.5x^2$,

$C(x) = 10x + 3$,

when $x = 10$ and $dx/dt = 5$ units per day

34. $R(x) = 50x - 0.5x^2$,

$C(x) = 4x + 10$,

when $x = 30$ and $dx/dt = 20$ units per day

35. $R(x) = 280x - 0.4x^2$,

$C(x) = 5000 + 0.6x^2$,

when $x = 200$ and $dx/dt = 300$ units per day

36. $R(x) = 2x$,

$C(x) = 0.01x^2 + 0.6x + 30$,

when $x = 20$ and $dx/dt = 8$ units per day

37. Change of sales. Suppose that the price p, in dollars, and number of sales, x, of a mechanical pencil are related by

$$5p + 4x + 2px = 60.$$

If p and x are both functions of time, measured in days, find the rate at which x is changing when

$$x = 3,\ p = 5, \text{ and } dp/dt = 1.5.$$

38. Change of revenue. For x and p as described in Exercise 37, find the rate at which total revenue is changing when

$$x = 3,\ p = 5, \text{ and } dp/dt = 1.5.$$

39. Change in revenue. A precious metal is selling at \$150 per ounce, and its price is increasing by \$2.50 per hour. If 300 ounces have been sold and revenue is growing by \$4500 per hour at this moment, find the rate at which the quantity (in ounces) being sold is changing.

40. Change in revenue. A barrel of heating oil is selling for \$200, and its price is increasing by \$1.75 per day. Find the rate at which the number of barrels being sold is changing when 4000 barrels have been sold and revenue is increasing by \$5000 per day.

Life and Physical Sciences

41. Rate of change of the Arctic ice cap. In a trend that scientists attribute, at least in part, to global warming, the floating cap of sea ice on the Arctic Ocean has been shrinking since 1980. The ice cap always shrinks in summer and grows in winter. Average minimum size of the ice cap, in square miles, can be approximated by

$$A = \pi r^2.$$

In 2017, the radius of the ice cap was approximately 1005 mi and was shrinking at a rate of approximately 5 mi/yr. (*Source*: Based on data from nsidc.org.) How fast was the area changing at that time?

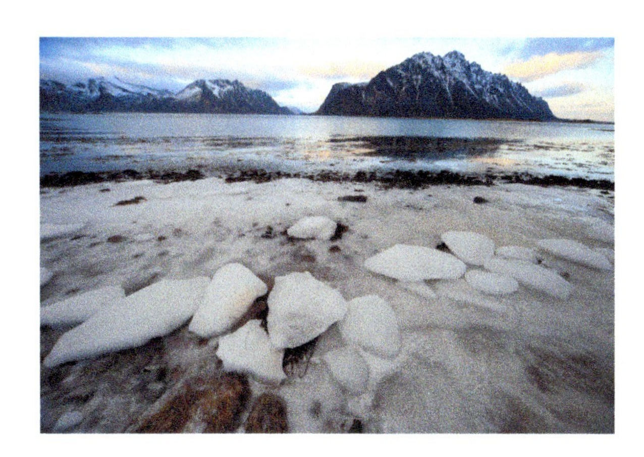

42. Rate of change of a healing wound. The area of a healing wound is given by

$$A = \pi r^2.$$

The radius is decreasing at the rate of 1 millimeter per day (-1 mm/day) at the moment when $r = 25$ mm. How fast is the area decreasing at that moment?

43. Body surface area. Certain chemotherapy dosages depend on a patient's surface area. According to the Mosteller model,

$$S = \frac{\sqrt{hw}}{60},$$

where h is the patient's height in centimeters, w is the patient's weight in kilograms, and S is the approximation of the patient's surface area in square meters. (*Source*: www.halls.md.) Assume that Kim's height is a constant 165 cm, but she is losing weight. If she loses 2 kg per month, how fast is her surface area decreasing at the instant she weighs 70 kg?

Poiseuille's Law. *The flow of blood in a blood vessel is faster toward the center of the vessel and slower toward the outside. The speed of the blood, V, in millimeters per second* (mm/sec), *is given by*

$$V = \frac{p}{4Lv}(R^2 - r^2),$$

where R is the radius of the blood vessel, r is the distance of the blood from the center of the vessel, and p, L, and v are physical constants related to blood pressure, length of the blood vessel, and viscosity of the blood, respectively. Assume that dV/dt is measured in millimeters per second squared (mm/sec^2). *Use this formula for Exercises 44 and 45.*

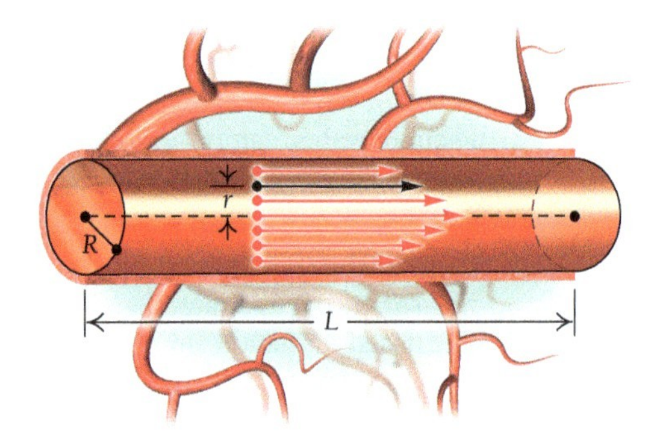

44. Assume that r is a constant as well as p, L, and v.

a) Find the rate of change dV/dt in terms of R and dR/dt when $L = 80$ mm, $p = 500$, and $v = 0.003$.

b) A person goes out into the cold to shovel snow. Cold air has the effect of contracting blood vessels far from the heart. Suppose a blood vessel contracts at a rate of

$$\frac{dR}{dt} = -0.0002 \text{ mm/sec}$$

at a place where the radius of the vessel is $R = 0.075$ mm. Find the rate of change, dV/dt, at that location.

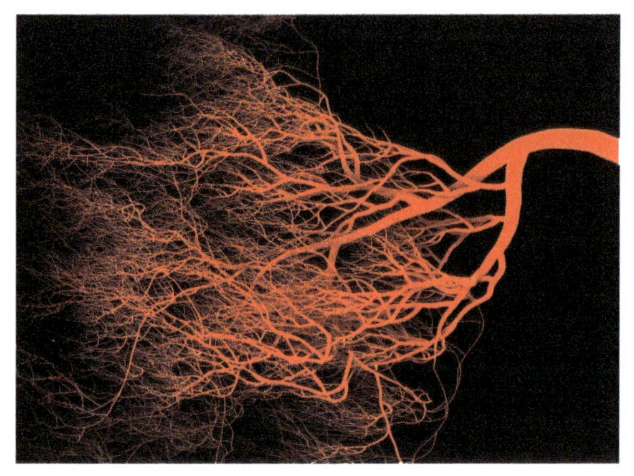

The flow of blood in a blood vessel can be modeled by Poiseuille's Law.

45. Assume that r is a constant as well as p, L, and v.

a) Find the rate of change dV/dt in terms of R and dR/dt when $L = 70$ mm, $p = 400$, and $v = 0.003$.

b) When shoveling snow in cold air, a person with a history of heart trouble can develop angina (chest pains) due to contracting blood vessels. To counteract this, he or she may take a nitroglycerin tablet, which dilates the blood vessels. Suppose, after a nitroglycerin tablet is taken, a blood vessel dilates at a rate of

$$\frac{dR}{dt} = 0.00015 \text{ mm/sec}$$

at a place where the radius of the vessel is $R = 0.1$ mm. Find the rate of change, dV/dt.

46. View to the horizon. The view to the horizon, V, is the distance to the horizon when one has a clear view over level land or water. From a height h, in feet, V, in miles, is given by $V = 1.22\sqrt{h}$.

a) A pirate on a ship in the middle of the ocean stands in the rigging 60 ft above the water. How far from him, in miles, is the horizon he sees from this height?

b) How fast is his view to the horizon changing if he is climbing at the rate of 2 ft per second, at the moment when he is 65 ft above the water?

c) How fast is the area he can view changing at the instant in part (b)?

General Interest

47. Two cars start from the same point at the same time. One travels north at 25 mph, and the other travels east at 60 mph. How fast is the distance between them increasing at the end of 1 hr? (*Hint*: $D^2 = x^2 + y^2$. To find D after 1 hr, solve $D^2 = 25^2 + 60^2$.)

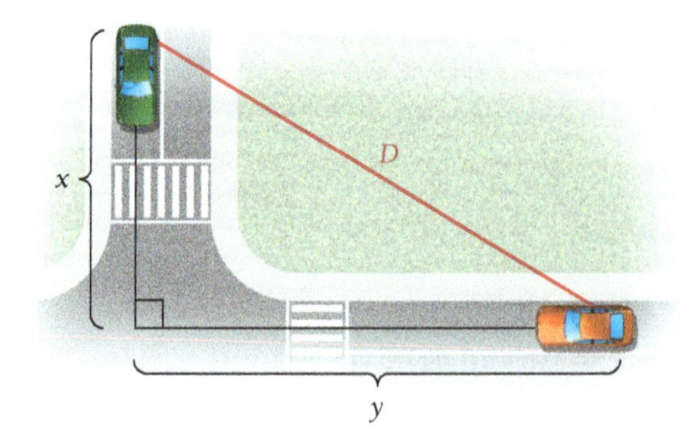

48. A ladder 26 ft long leans against a vertical wall. If the lower end is being moved away from the wall at the rate of 5 ft/sec, how fast is the height of the top changing (this will be a negative rate) when the lower end is 10 ft from the wall?

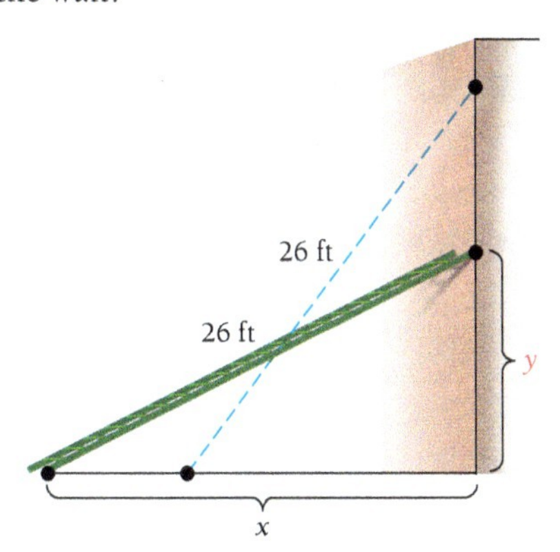

49. An inner city revitalization zone is a rectangle that is twice as long as it is wide. A diagonal through the region is growing at a rate of 90 m per year at a time when the region is 440 m wide. How fast is the area changing at that point in time?

50. The volume of a cantaloupe is approximated by

$$V = \tfrac{4}{3}\pi r^3.$$

The radius is growing at the rate of 0.7 cm/week at a time when the radius is 7.5 cm. How fast is the volume changing at that moment?

51. A pyramid with a square base of side length x and a height h is being built. The length of each side is increasing by 2 m per week, and the height is increasing by 1.5 m per week. Find the rate at which the volume of the pyramid is changing when each side is 100 m long and the height is 90 m. (*Hint*: The volume of such a pyramid is given by $V = \frac{1}{3}x^2h$.)

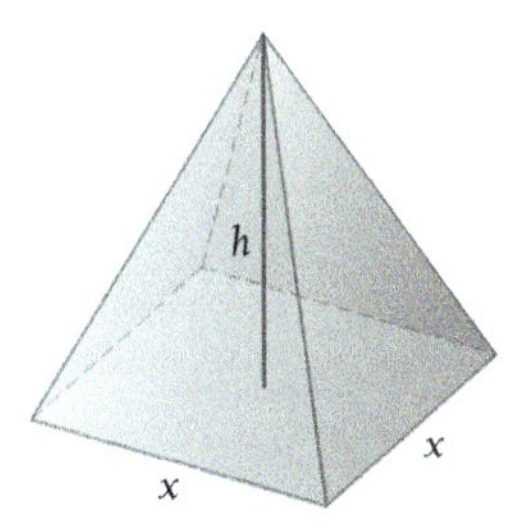

52. A doughnut-shaped object, called a *torus* (shown below), is increasing in size such that its major radius R is changing by 3 cm per hour and its minor radius r is changing by 0.2 cm per hour. Find the rate at which the volume is changing at the moment when the major radius is 100 cm and the minor radius is 15 cm. (*Hint*: The volume of a torus is given by $V = 2\pi^2 r^2 R$.)

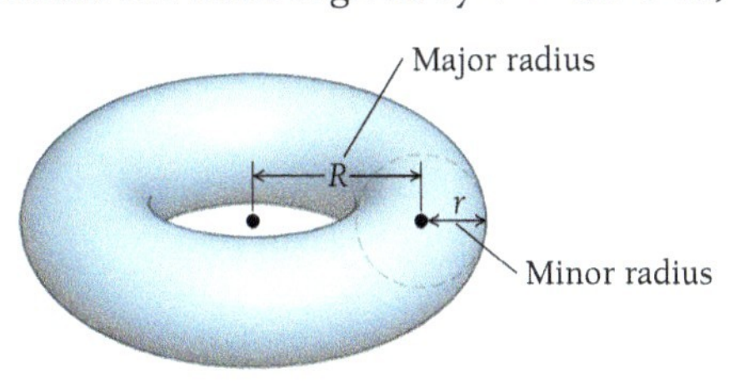

SYNTHESIS

53. A spherical soap bubble is growing in volume at a rate of 25 mm^3 per minute. Find the rate at which its surface area is increasing when the radius is 10 mm.

54. A large ice cube is melting, losing 200 cm^3 of volume per minute. Find the rate at which its surface area is changing when the length of a side is 30 cm.

55. **Volume of an octahedron.** The volume of an octahedron (an eight-sided solid with triangular faces and sides of the same length) is given by

$$V = \frac{\sqrt{2}}{3}x^3,$$ where x is the length of each edge. Find the rate at which the length of an edge is changing if the volume of an octahedron is increasing by 25 in^3 per minute, at the moment when the volume is 200 in^3.

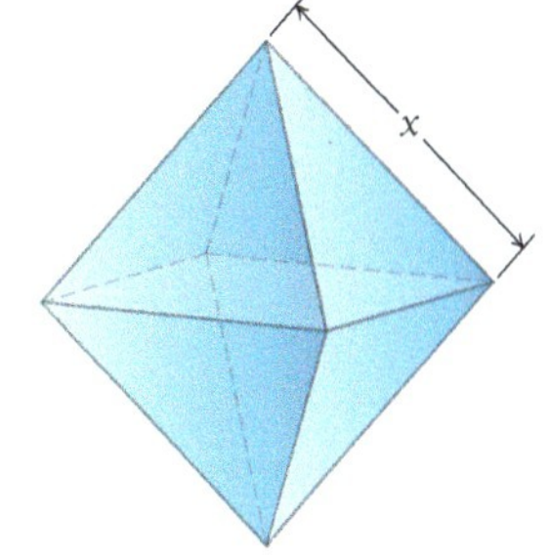

56. **Surface area of an octahedron.** The surface area of an octahedron with edge length x is given by $A = 2\sqrt{3}x^2$. Find the rate at which the surface area is changing at the moment when the volume of the octahedron is 200 in^3 and is increasing by 25 in^3 per minute.

57. A circular puddle is increasing in size, its radius growing at a rate of 0.5 cm per minute.

a) Find the rate at which the circumference is changing at the moment when the radius is 10 cm.

b) Find the rate at which the circumference is changing at the moment when the radius is 20 cm.

c) Find the rate at which the circumference is changing at the moment when the radius is 30 cm.

d) Based on your results for parts (a)–(c), explain why the rate of change of the circumference is not affected by the radius at any given time.

58. A square is increasing in size, its side length growing at a rate of 0.2 mm per minute.

a) Find the rate at which the perimeter is changing at the moment when each side length is 20 cm.

b) Find the rate at which the perimeter is changing at the moment when each side length is 200 cm.

c) Find the rate at which the perimeter is changing at the moment when each side length is 2000 cm.

d) Based on your results for parts (a)–(c), explain why the rate of change of the perimeter is not affected by the side length at any given time.

59. Let $y = pqr$. Find the rate at which y is changing when $p = 2, q = 3, r = 5, dp/dt = 0.1, dq/dt = -0.2$, and $dr/dt = 0.3$.

60. Let $y = pqr$. Find the rate at which p is changing when $y = 40, q = 5, r = 2, dy/dt = 0.6, dq/dt = 0.03$, and $dr/dt = -0.04$.

Answers to Quick Checks

1. $\frac{5}{48}$ **2.** 63 mi^2 per yr **3.** 100 units per day

Chapter 3 Summary

KEY TERMS AND CONCEPTS

EXAMPLES

SECTION 3.1

A function is **increasing** over an open interval I if, for all x in I, $f'(x) > 0$.

A function is **decreasing** over an open interval I if, for all x in I, $f'(x) < 0$.

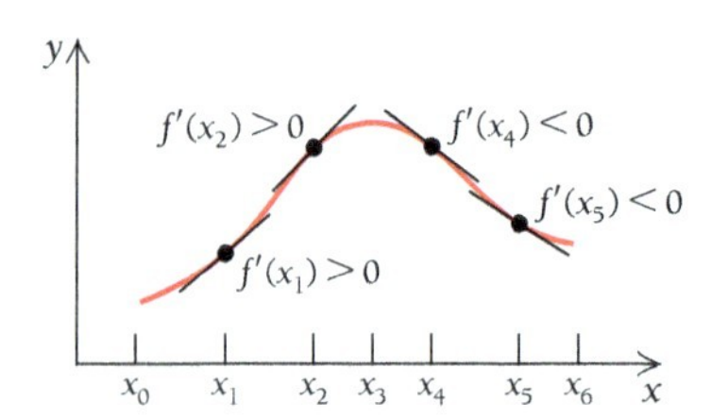

f is increasing over the interval (x_0, x_3) and decreasing over (x_3, x_6).

If f is a continuous function, then a **critical value** is any number c in the domain of f for which $f'(c) = 0$ or $f'(c)$ does not exist.

In both cases, the ordered pair $(c, f(c))$ is called a **critical point**.

If $f'(c)$ does not exist, then the graph of f may have a corner or a vertical tangent at $(c, f(c))$.

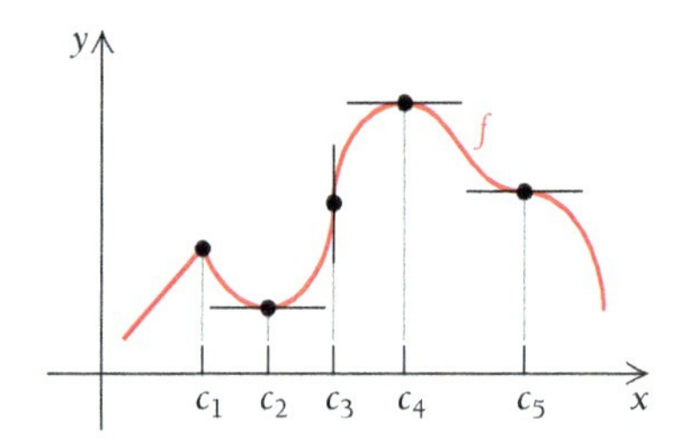

The values c_1, c_2, c_3, c_4, and c_5 are critical values of f.

- $f'(c_1)$ does not exist (corner).
- $f'(c_2) = 0$.
- $f'(c_3)$ does not exist (vertical tangent).
- $f'(c_4) = 0$.
- $f'(c_5) = 0$.

If f is a continuous function, then any **relative extremum (maximum** or **minimum)** occurs at a critical value.

The converse is not true: a critical value may not correspond to an extremum.

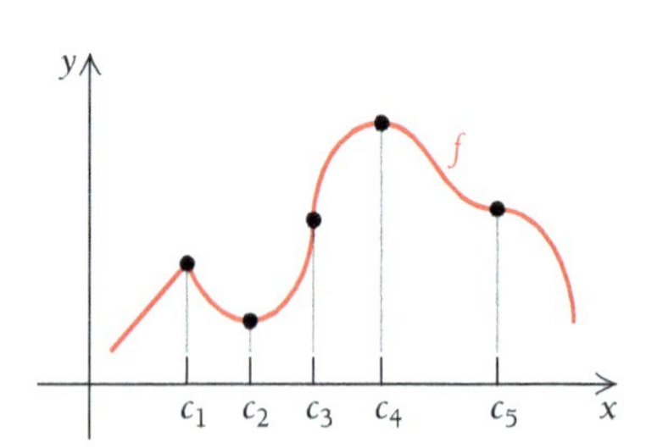

- The critical point $(c_1, f(c_1))$ is a relative maximum.
- The critical point $(c_2, f(c_2))$ is a relative minimum.
- The critical point $(c_3, f(c_3))$ is neither a relative maximum nor a relative minimum.
- The critical point $(c_4, f(c_4))$ is a relative maximum.
- The critical point $(c_5, f(c_5))$ is neither a relative maximum nor a relative minimum.

KEY TERMS AND CONCEPTS	EXAMPLES

SECTION 3.1 (continued)

The **First-Derivative Test** is used to classify a critical value as a relative maximum, a relative minimum, or neither.

Find the relative extrema of the function given by

$$f(x) = \frac{1}{3}x^3 - \frac{1}{2}x^2 - 20x + 7.$$

Critical values occur where $f'(x) = 0$ or $f'(x)$ does not exist. The derivative $f'(x) = x^2 - x - 20$ exists for all real numbers, so the only critical values occur when $f'(x) = 0$. Setting $x^2 - x - 20 = 0$ and solving gives $x = -4$ and $x = 5$ as the critical values.

To apply the First-Derivative Test, check the sign of $f'(x)$ to the left and right of each critical value, using test values:

Test Value	$x = -5$	$x = 0$	$x = 6$
Sign of $f'(x)$	$f'(-5) > 0$	$f'(0) < 0$	$f'(6) > 0$
Result	f increasing on $(-\infty, -4)$	f decreasing on $(-4, 5)$	f increasing on $(5, \infty)$

Therefore, there is a relative maximum at $x = -4$: $f(-4) = 57\frac{2}{3}$. There is a relative minimum at $x = 5$: $f(5) = -63\frac{5}{6}$.

SECTION 3.2

The **second derivative**, $f''(x)$, can be used to determine the **concavity** of a graph.

If $f''(x) > 0$ for all x in an open interval I, then the graph of f is **concave up** over I.

If $f''(x) < 0$ for all x in an open interval I, then the graph of f is **concave down** over I.

A **point of inflection** occurs at $(x_0, f(x_0))$ if $f''(x_0) = 0$ and there is a change in concavity on either side of x_0.

The function given by

$$f(x) = \frac{1}{3}x^3 - \frac{1}{2}x^2 - 20x + 7$$

has the second derivative $f''(x) = 2x - 1$. Setting the second derivative equal to 0 gives $x_0 = \frac{1}{2}$. Test values are used to check the concavity on either side of $x_0 = \frac{1}{2}$:

Test Value	$x = 0$	$x = 1$
Sign of $f''(x)$	$f''(0) < 0$	$f''(1) > 0$
Result	f is concave down on $\left(-\infty, \frac{1}{2}\right)$	f is concave up on $\left(\frac{1}{2}, \infty\right)$

Therefore, the graph of f is concave down over the interval $\left(-\infty, \frac{1}{2}\right)$ and concave up over the interval $\left(\frac{1}{2}, \infty\right)$. Since there is a change in concavity on either side of $x_0 = \frac{1}{2}$, it follows that the point $\left(\frac{1}{2}, -3\frac{1}{12}\right)$ is a point of inflection, where $f\left(\frac{1}{2}\right) = -3\frac{1}{12}$.

The **Second-Derivative Test** can also be used to classify relative extrema:

If $f'(c) = 0$ and $f''(c) > 0$, then $f(c)$ is a relative minimum.

If $f'(c) = 0$ and $f''(c) < 0$, then $f(c)$ is a relative maximum.

If $f'(c) = 0$ and $f''(c) = 0$, then the First-Derivative Test must be used to classify $f(c)$.

For the function

$$f(x) = \frac{1}{3}x^3 - \frac{1}{2}x^2 - 20x + 7,$$

evaluating the second derivative, $f''(x) = 2x - 1$, at the critical values yields the following conclusions:

- At $x = -4$, the evaluation gives $f''(-4) < 0$. Since $f'(-4) = 0$ and the graph is concave down, it follows that there is a relative maximum at $x = -4$.
- At $x = 5$, the evaluation gives $f''(5) > 0$. Since $f'(5) = 0$ and the graph is concave up, it follows that there is a relative minimum at $x = 5$.

KEY TERMS AND CONCEPTS	EXAMPLES
SECTION 3.3	
A line $x = a$ is a **vertical asymptote** if $$\lim_{x \to a^-} f(x) = \infty,$$ $$\lim_{x \to a^-} f(x) = -\infty,$$ $$\lim_{x \to a^+} f(x) = \infty,$$ or $$\lim_{x \to a^+} f(x) = -\infty.$$	Consider the function given by $$f(x) = \frac{x^2 - 1}{x^2 + x - 6}.$$ Factoring gives $$f(x) = \frac{(x + 1)(x - 1)}{(x + 3)(x - 2)}.$$ This expression is simplified. Therefore, $x = -3$ and $x = 2$ are vertical asymptotes since $$\lim_{x \to -3^-} f(x) = \infty \quad \text{and} \quad \lim_{x \to -3^+} f(x) = -\infty$$ and $$\lim_{x \to 2^-} f(x) = -\infty \quad \text{and} \quad \lim_{x \to 2^+} f(x) = \infty.$$
An asymptote is usually represented as a dashed line; it is not part of the graph itself. A line $y = b$ is a **horizontal asymptote** if $$\lim_{x \to -\infty} f(x) = b$$ or $$\lim_{x \to \infty} f(x) = b.$$	For the function given by $$f(x) = \frac{x^2 - 1}{x^2 + x - 6},$$ the limits evaluated at infinity are $$\lim_{x \to -\infty} f(x) = 1 \quad \text{and} \quad \lim_{x \to \infty} f(x) = 1.$$ Thus, the line $y = 1$ is a horizontal asymptote. 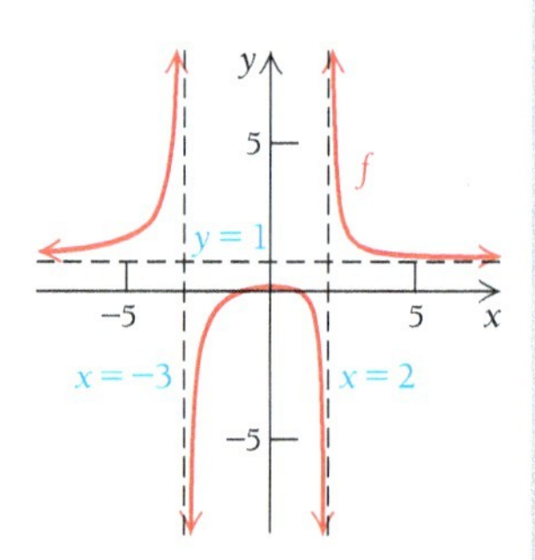
For a rational function of the form $f(x) = P(x)/Q(x)$, a **slant asymptote** occurs if the degree of the numerator is 1 greater than the degree of the denominator.	Let $f(x) = \frac{x^2 + 1}{x + 3}$. Division yields $$f(x) = x - 3 + \frac{10}{x + 3}.$$ As $x \to \infty$ or $x \to -\infty$, the remainder $\frac{10}{x + 3} \to 0$. Therefore, the slant asymptote is $y = x - 3$. 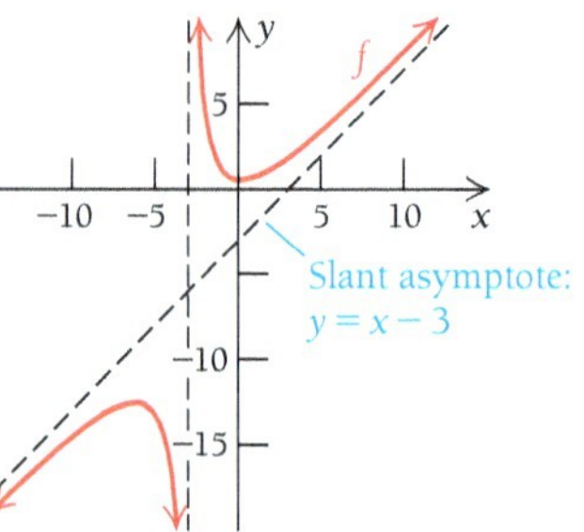
Asymptotes, extrema, x- and y-intercepts, points of inflection, concavity, and intervals over which the function is increasing or decreasing are all used in the strategy for accurate graph sketching.	Consider the function given by $$f(x) = \tfrac{1}{3}x^3 - \tfrac{1}{2}x^2 - 20x + 7.$$ • f has a relative maximum point at $(-4, 57\tfrac{2}{3})$ and a relative minimum point at $(5, -63\tfrac{5}{6})$. • f has a point of inflection at $(\tfrac{1}{2}, -3\tfrac{1}{12})$. • f is increasing over the intervals $(-\infty, -4)$ and $(5, \infty)$, decreasing over the interval $(-4, 5)$, concave down over the interval $(-\infty, \tfrac{1}{2})$, and concave up over the interval $(\tfrac{1}{2}, \infty)$. • f has a y-intercept at $(0, 7)$. 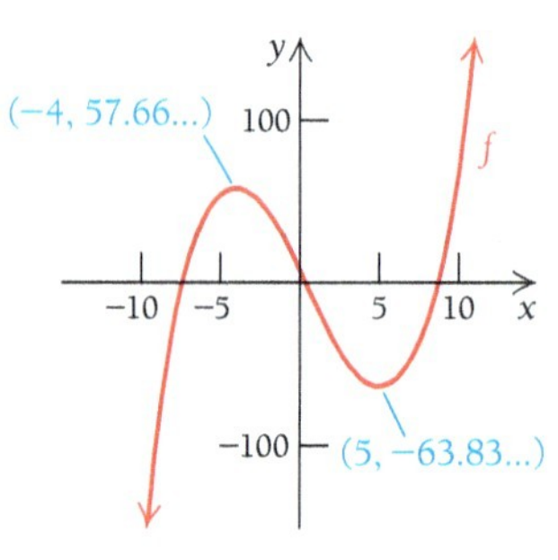

KEY TERMS AND CONCEPTS

EXAMPLES

SECTION 3.3 (continued)

Consider the function given by

$$f(x) = \frac{x^2 - 1}{x^2 + x - 6}.$$

- f has vertical asymptotes $x = -3$ and $x = 2$.
- f has a horizontal asymptote given by $y = 1$.
- f has a y-intercept at $(0, \frac{1}{6})$.
- f has x-intercepts at $(-1, 0)$ and $(1, 0)$.
- f has a relative maximum at $(0.101, 0.168)$ and a relative minimum at $(9.899, 0.952)$.
- f is concave up on $(-\infty, -3)$ and $(2, 14.929)$, and concave down on $(-3, 2)$ and $(14.929, \infty)$.

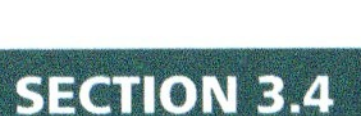

SECTION 3.4

If f is continuous over $[a, b]$, then the **Extreme-Value Theorem** tells us that f will have both an absolute maximum value and an absolute minimum value over this interval. One or both absolute extrema may occur at an endpoint of this interval.

Maximum–Minimum Principle 1 can be used to determine these absolute extrema: we find all critical values $c_1, c_2, c_3, \ldots, c_n$, in $[a, b]$, then evaluate $f(a), f(c_1), f(c_2), f(c_3), \ldots, f(c_n), f(b)$.

The largest of these is the **absolute maximum**, and the smallest is the **absolute minimum**.

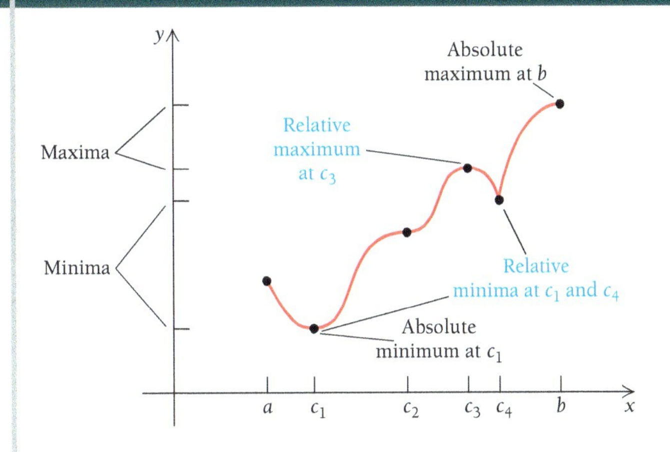

If f is differentiable for all x in an interval I, and there is exactly one critical value c in I such that $f'(c) = 0$, then, according to **Maximum–Minimum Principle 2**, $f(c)$ is an absolute extremum over I.

Let $f(x) = x + \frac{2}{x}$, for $x > 0$. The derivative is $f'(x) = 1 - \frac{2}{x^2}$. Solving for the critical value yields

$$1 - \frac{2}{x^2} = 0$$

$$x^2 = 2$$

$$x = \pm\sqrt{2}.$$

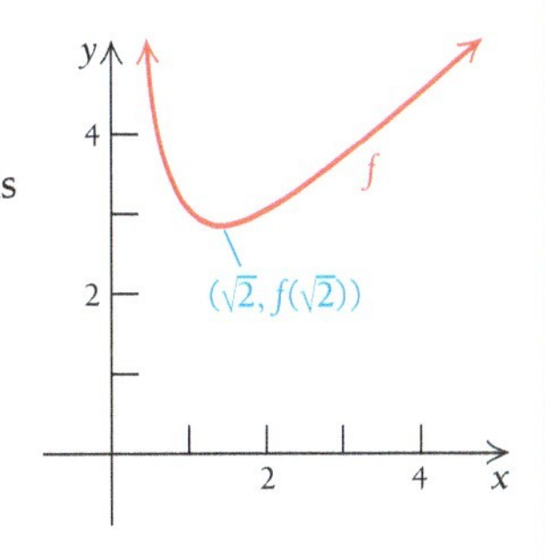

The only critical value over the interval where $x > 0$ is $x = \sqrt{2}$. The second derivative is $f''(x) = \frac{4}{x^3}$. It follows that $f''(\sqrt{2}) = \frac{4}{(\sqrt{2})^3} > 0$. Therefore, $(\sqrt{2}, f(\sqrt{2}))$ is an absolute minimum.

KEY TERMS AND CONCEPTS	EXAMPLES

SECTION 3.5

Many real-world applications involve maximum–minimum problems. In many such optimization problems, we seek to find the absolute maximum or absolute minimum point on the graph of a function f, called the **objective function**, where the independent variable may be subject to a **constraint**.

Maximize the quantity $Q = xy$ such that $3x + y = 30$.

Solving the constraint equation $3x + y = 30$ for y gives $y = 30 - 3x$. Substituting this expression for y in the equation $Q = xy$ gives

$$Q = x(30 - 3x) \quad \text{Substituting}$$
$$Q(x) = 30x - 3x^2. \quad \text{Simplifying}$$

The objective function is $Q(x) = 30x - 3x^2$. Differentiating gives $Q'(x) = 30 - 6x$. Since $Q'(x)$ is defined for all real numbers x, the only critical value occurs where $Q'(x) = 0$. Solving $30 - 6x = 0$ gives $x = 5$. The Second-Derivative Test is used to classify the critical point. Since $Q''(x) = -6 < 0$, by Maximum–Minimum Principle 2, the critical point $(5, 75)$ is the absolute maximum point, where $Q(5) = 75$.

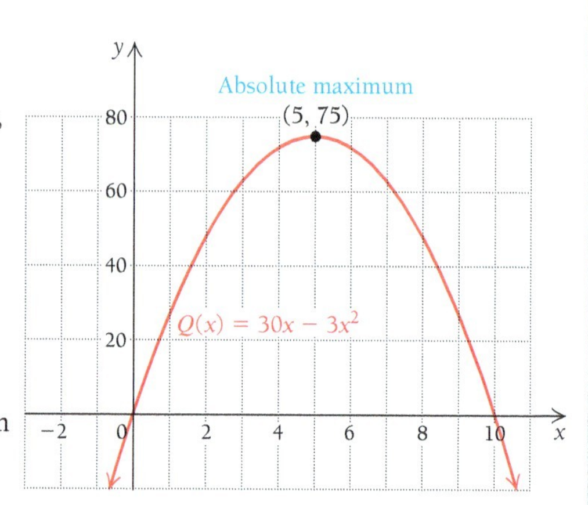

SECTION 3.6

Marginal cost, marginal revenue, and **marginal profit** are estimates of the cost, revenue, and profit for the $(x + 1)$st item produced:

- $C'(x) \approx C(x + 1) - C(x)$, so $C(x + 1) \approx C(x) + C'(x)$.
- $R'(x) \approx R(x + 1) - R(x)$, so $R(x + 1) \approx R(x) + R'(x)$.
- $P'(x) \approx P(x + 1) - P(x)$, so $P(x + 1) \approx P(x) + P'(x)$.

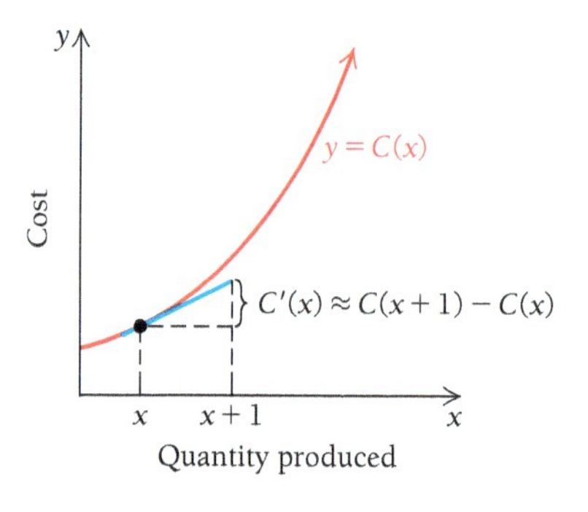

Delta notation represents the change in a variable:

$$\Delta x = x_2 - x_1$$

and

$$\Delta y = f(x_2) - f(x_1).$$

If $x_2 = x_1 + h$, then $\Delta x = h$.

If Δx is small, then the derivative can be used to approximate Δy:

$$\Delta y \approx f'(x) \cdot \Delta x.$$

For $f(x) = x^2$, let $x_1 = 2$ and $x_2 = 2.1$. Then, $\Delta x = 2.1 - 2 = 0.1$. Since $f(x_1) = f(2) = 4$ and $f(x_2) = f(2.1) = 4.41$,

$$\Delta y = f(x_2) - f(x_1) = 4.41 - 4 = 0.41.$$

Since $\Delta x = 0.1$ is small, Δy is approximated by

$$\Delta y \approx f'(x)\,\Delta x.$$

The derivative is $f'(x) = 2x$. Therefore,

$$\Delta y \approx f'(2) \cdot (0.1) = 2(2) \cdot (0.1) = 0.4.$$

This approximation, 0.4, is very close to the actual difference, 0.41.

KEY TERMS AND CONCEPTS | EXAMPLES

SECTION 3.6 (*continued*)

Differentials allow us to approximate changes in the output variable y given a change in the input variable x:

$$dx = \Delta x$$

and

$$dy = f'(x)\,dx.$$

If Δx is small, then $dy \approx \Delta y$.

In practice, it is often simpler to calculate dy, and it provides a close approximation for Δy.

For $y = \sqrt[3]{x}$, find dy when $x = 27$ and $dx = 2$.

Note that $\frac{dy}{dx} = \frac{1}{3\sqrt[3]{x^2}}$. Thus, $dy = \frac{1}{3\sqrt[3]{x^2}}\,dx$. Evaluating gives

$$dy = \frac{1}{3\sqrt[3]{(27)^2}}(2) = \frac{2}{27}.$$

This result can be used to approximate the value of $\sqrt[3]{29}$, using the fact that $\sqrt[3]{29} \approx \sqrt[3]{27} + dy$:

$$\sqrt[3]{29} \approx \sqrt[3]{27} + dy = 3 + \frac{2}{27} \approx 3.074.$$

Thus, the approximation $\sqrt[3]{29} \approx 3.074$ is very close to the actual value, $\sqrt[3]{29} = 3.07231\ldots$, found with a calculator.

If f is differentiable at $x = a$, then the **linearization** of f at $x = a$ is given by

$$y = L(x) = f(a) + f'(a)(x - a).$$

This is the equation of the tangent line to f at $x = a$.

Let $f(x) = x^3$. Find the linearization of f at $x = 2$.

The point of tangency is $f(2) = 8$, and differentiating, $f'(x) = 3x^2$, so $f'(2) = 3(2)^2 = 12$. Thus, the linearization of f at $x = 2$ is

$$y = L(x) = 8 + 12(x - 2)$$
$$L(x) = 12x - 16. \quad \text{Simplifying}$$

The linearization can be used to estimate points on f near $x = 2$. For example, $L(2.1) = 12(2.1) - 16 = 9.2$. This estimate compares well to the actual value of $f(2.1) = (2.1)^3 = 9.261$, found using a calculator.

SECTION 3.7

The **elasticity of demand** E is a function of x, the price:

$$E(x) = -\frac{x \cdot D'(x)}{D(x)}.$$

When $E(x) > 1$, total revenue is decreasing;

when $E(x) < 1$, total revenue is increasing;

and

when $E(x) = 1$, total revenue is maximized.

Business. The Leslie Davis Band finds that demand for its CD at performances is given by

$$q = D(x) = 50 - 2x,$$

where x is the price, in dollars, of each CD sold and q is the number of CDs sold at a performance. Find the elasticity when the price is \$10 per CD, and interpret the result. Then, find the price at which revenue is maximized.

Elasticity at x is given by

$$E(x) = -\frac{x \cdot D'(x)}{D(x)}$$
$$= -\frac{x(-2)}{50 - 2x}$$
$$= -\frac{-2x}{50 - 2x} = \frac{x}{25 - x}.$$

Thus, $E(10) = \frac{10}{25 - 10} = \frac{2}{3}$.

Since $E(10)$ is less than 1, the demand for the CD is *inelastic*, and a modest increase in price will increase revenue.

KEY TERMS AND CONCEPTS	EXAMPLES
SECTION 3.7 (*continued*)	
	Revenue is maximized when $E(x) = 1$: $$\frac{x}{25 - x} = 1$$ $$x = 25 - x$$ $$2x = 25$$ $$x = 12.5.$$ At a price of \$12.50 per CD, revenue will be maximized.
SECTION 3.8	
If an equation has variables x and y and y is not isolated on one side of the equation, the derivative dy/dx can be found without solving for y using **implicit differentiation**.	Find $\frac{dy}{dx}$ if $y^5 = x^3 + 7$. Differentiate both sides with respect to x, and then solve for $\frac{dy}{dx}$. $$\frac{d}{dx}y^5 = \frac{d}{dx}x^3 + \frac{d}{dx}7$$ $$5y^4\frac{dy}{dx} = 3x^2$$ $$\frac{dy}{dx} = \frac{3x^2}{5y^4}.$$
To differentiate complicated functions, we use **logarithmic differentiation**. Given a function $y = f(x)$, we find the natural logarithm of both sides: $$\ln y = \ln f(x).$$ The properties of logarithms are used to simplify $\ln f(x)$. The equation $\ln y = \ln f(x)$ is then differentiated implicitly with respect to x.	To find the derivative of $y = \frac{x^2e^{3x-1}}{(x^2 + 4x + 1)^7}$, find the natural logarithm of both sides: $$\ln(y) = \ln\left(\frac{x^2e^{3x-1}}{(x^2 + 4x + 1)^7}\right).$$ The right side is then simplified using the properties of logarithms: $$\ln y = \ln x^2 + \ln e^{3x-1} - \ln(x^2 + 4x + 1)^7$$ $$= 2\ln x + 3x - 1 - 7\ln(x^2 + 4x + 1).$$ Now, differentiate implicitly with respect to x: $$\frac{d}{dx}(\ln y) = \frac{d}{dx}(2\ln x + 3x - 1 - 7\ln(x^2 + 4x + 1))$$ $$\frac{1}{y}\cdot\frac{dy}{dx} = \frac{2}{x} + 3 - 7\left(\frac{2x + 4}{x^2 + 4x + 1}\right)$$ $$\frac{dy}{dx} = y\left(\frac{2}{x} + 3 - 7\left(\frac{2x + 4}{x^2 + 4x + 1}\right)\right)$$ $$= \frac{x^2e^{3x-1}}{(x^2 + 4x + 1)^7}\left(\frac{2}{x} + 3 - \frac{14x + 28}{x^2 + 4x + 1}\right).$$

KEY TERMS AND CONCEPTS	EXAMPLES
SECTION 3.8 (*continued*)	
The point of inflection of the logistic function $f(t) = \frac{L}{1 + Ce^{-rt}}$ is $\left(\frac{\ln C}{r}, \frac{L}{2}\right)$ and is called the **point of diminishing returns**. It is where the rate of change of f is maximized.	**Business.** The Leslie Davis Band releases its new single on iSongz, and the number of downloads t days after the song is released is given by $$N(t) = \frac{30{,}000}{1 + 49e^{-0.048t}}.$$ The point of inflection is $\left(\frac{\ln 49}{0.048}, \frac{30{,}000}{2}\right) \approx (81.1, 15{,}000)$. On the 81st day, the total number of downloads of the song is 15,000, and the rate of downloads is at its maximum: $N'(81.1) \approx 360$ downloads per day. After this day, total downloads will continue to increase, but the rate of downloads per day will decrease, eventually to 0 once the market has been saturated.
SECTION 3.9	
A **related rate** occurs when the rate of change of one variable (with respect to time) can be calculated in terms of the rate of change (with respect to time) of another variable of which it is a function.	A large cube of ice is melting, losing 30 cm^3 of its volume, V, per minute. When the length of a side is 20 cm, how fast is that length decreasing? Since $V = x^3$ and both V and x are changing with time, differentiate each variable with respect to time: $$\frac{dV}{dt} = 3x^2\frac{dx}{dt}.$$ Evaluating at $x = 20$ and $\frac{dV}{dt} = -30$ gives $$-30 = 3(20)^2\frac{dx}{dt}$$ or $$\frac{dx}{dt} = -\frac{30}{3(20)^2} = -0.025 \text{ cm/min}.$$
A related-rates equation may contain more than two variables. As for the two-variable case, all variables are differentiated with respect to time, t.	Revenue is found by multiplying price p by the quantity sold q: $R = pq$. Suppose that 15,000 units of a product have been sold at \$45 each, and that price is increasing by \$1.50 per day and revenue is changing by \$18,450 per day. Find the rate at which the quantity sold is changing. Differentiate $R = pq$ with respect to t: $$\frac{dR}{dt} = p\frac{dq}{dt} + q\frac{dp}{dt}.$$ Using the Product Rule. Substitute and solve for dq/dt: $$18{,}450 = 45\frac{dq}{dt} + 15{,}000(1.50)$$ $$18{,}450 = 45\frac{dq}{dt} + 22{,}500$$ $$-4050 = 45\frac{dq}{dt}$$ $$\frac{dq}{dt} = -\frac{4050}{45} = -90 \text{ units per day.}$$

Chapter 3 Review Exercises

These review exercises are for test preparation. They can also be used as a practice test. Answers are at the back of the book. The red bracketed section references tell you what part(s) of the chapter to restudy if your answer is incorrect.

CONCEPT REINFORCEMENT

Match each description in column A with the most appropriate graph in column B. [3.1–3.4]

Column A

1. A function with a relative maximum but no absolute extrema

2. A function with both a vertical asymptote and a horizontal asymptote

3. A function that is concave up and decreasing

4. A function that is concave up and increasing

5. A function with three critical values

6. A function with one critical value and a second derivative that is always positive

7. A function with a first derivative that is always positive

Column B

a)

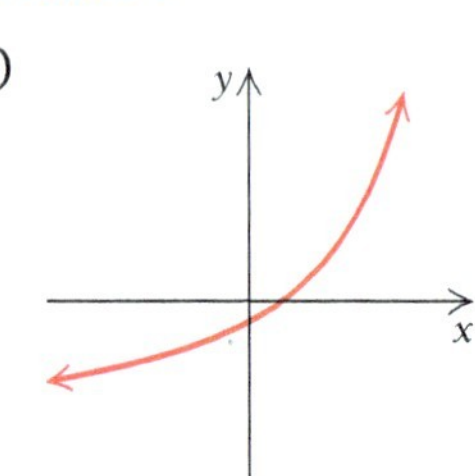

b)

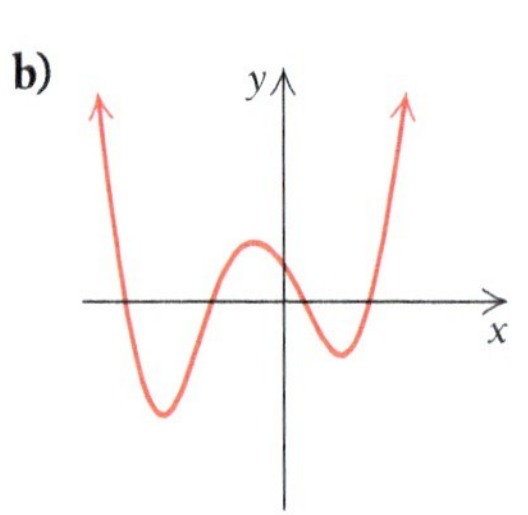

c)

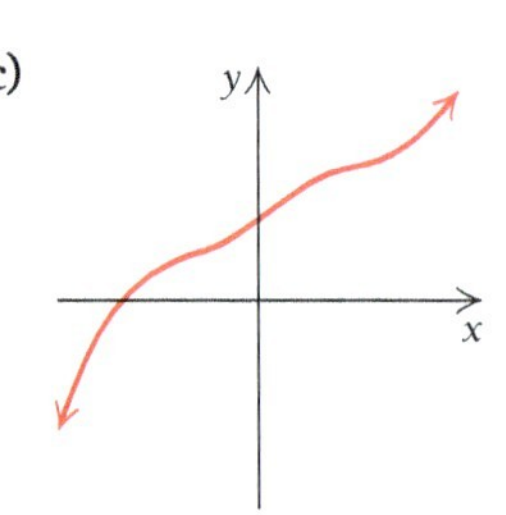

d)

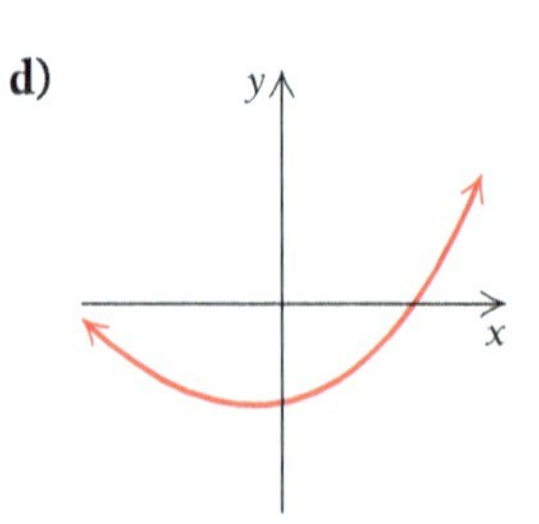

e)

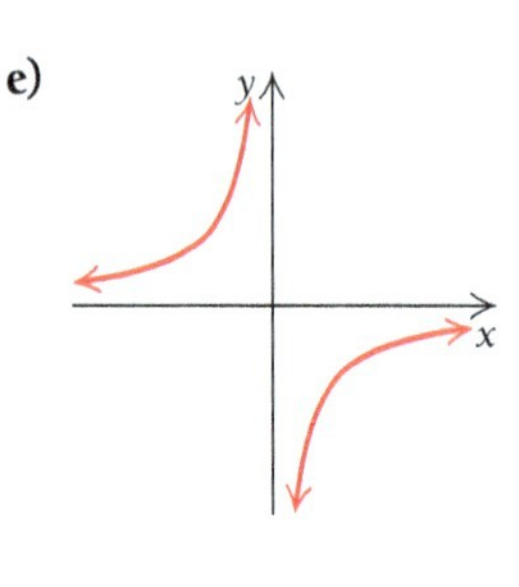

f)

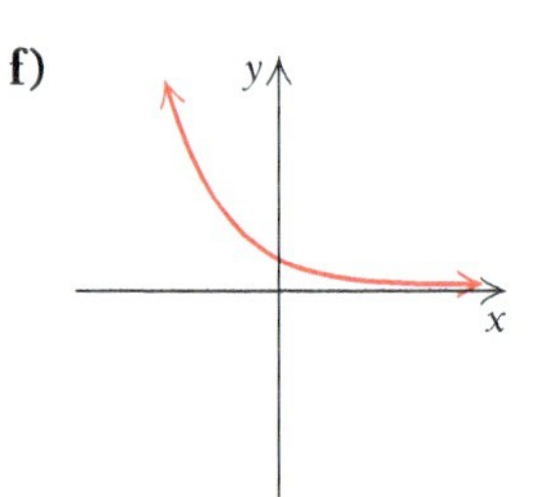

g)

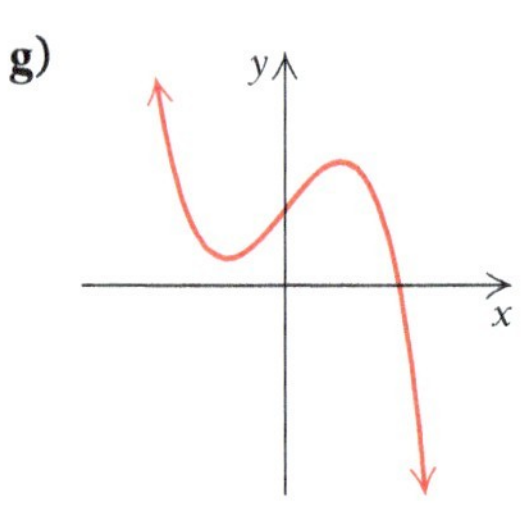

In Exercises 8–17, classify each statement as either true or false.

8. Every continuous function has at least one critical value. [3.1]

9. If a continuous function $y = f(x)$ has extrema, they will always occur where $f'(x) = 0$. [3.1]

10. If $f'(c) = 0$ and $f''(c) > 0$, then $f(c)$ is a relative minimum. [3.2]

11. If $f'(c) = 0$ and $f''(c) = 0$, then $f(c)$ cannot be a relative minimum. [3.2]

12. If the graph of $f(x) = P(x)/Q(x)$ has a horizontal asymptote, then the degree of the polynomial $P(x)$ is less than or equal to that of the polynomial $Q(x)$. [3.3]

13. Absolute extrema of a continuous function f always occur at the endpoints of a closed interval. [3.4]

14. In general, if f is a continuous function, then $\Delta x = dx$ and $\Delta y \geq dy$. [3.6]

15. If the elasticity of demand at a certain price x is 1, then revenue is maximized at this price. [3.7]

16. For a logistic function of the form $f(t) = \dfrac{L}{1 + Ce^{-rt}}$, where f is the total number of units sold after t days, the maximum number of units sold occurs at the point of inflection. [3.8]

17. In a related-rate problem, the variables are commonly differentiated implicitly with respect to time, t. [3.9]

REVIEW EXERCISES

For each function given, find any extrema, along with the x-value at which each one occurs. Then sketch a graph of the function. [3.1]

18. $f(x) = 4 - 3x - x^2$

19. $f(x) = \dfrac{-8x}{x^2 + 1}$

20. $f(x) = xe^{-6x}$

21. $f(x) = x^3 + x^2 - x + 3$

22. $f(x) = 3x^{2/3}$

23. $f(x) = e^{5x} - e^{2x}$

24. $f(x) = x^3 - 3x + 2$

Sketch the graph of each function. List any minimum or maximum values, where they occur, and any points of inflection. State where the function is increasing or decreasing and where it is concave up or concave down. [3.2]

25. $f(x) = \frac{1}{3}x^3 + 3x^2 + 9x + 2$

26. $f(x) = x^2 - 10x + 8$

27. $f(x) = e^{2x} - e^{4x}$

28. $f(x) = \ln(x^2 + 10x + 26)$

29. $f(x) = 3x^4 + 2x^3 - 3x^2 + 1$ (Round to three decimal places where appropriate.)

30. $f(x) = \frac{1}{5}x^5 + \frac{3}{4}x^4 - \frac{4}{3}x^3 + 8$ (Round to three decimal places where appropriate.)

Sketch the graph of each function. Indicate where each function is increasing or decreasing, the coordinates at which any relative extrema occur, where any asymptotes occur, where the graph is concave up or concave down, and where any intercepts occur. [3.3]

31. $f(x) = \dfrac{2x + 5}{x + 1}$

32. $f(x) = \dfrac{x}{x - 2}$

33. $f(x) = \dfrac{5}{x^2 - 16}$

34. $f(x) = -\dfrac{x + 1}{x^2 - x - 2}$

35. $f(x) = \dfrac{1000}{1 + 24e^{-0.05x}}$

36. $f(x) = \dfrac{x^2 + 3}{x}$

For each function, find any absolute extrema over the indicated interval. Indicate the x-value at which each extremum occurs. Where no interval is specified, use the real line. [3.4]

37. $f(x) = x^4 - 2x^2 + 3;\ [0, 3]$

38. $f(x) = e^{-3x} + 8x;\ [-1, 2]$

39. $f(x) = x + \dfrac{50}{x};\ (0, \infty)$

40. $f(x) = x^4 - 2x^2 + 1$

41. Maximize $Q = xy$, where $3x + 4y = 24$. [3.5]

42. Find the minimum value of $Q = x^2 - 2y^2$, where $x - 2y = 1$. [3.5]

43. Business: maximizing profit. If $R(x) = 52x - 0.5x^2$ and $C(x) = 22x - 1$, find the maximum profit and the number of units that must be produced and sold in order to yield this maximum profit. Assume that $R(x)$ and $C(x)$ are in dollars. [3.5]

44. Business: minimizing cost. A rectangular steel storage container with a square base and a cover is to have a volume of $2500\ \text{ft}^3$. If the cost of material is $\$2/\text{ft}^2$ for the bottom, $\$3/\text{ft}^2$ for the top, and $\$1/\text{ft}^2$ for the sides, what should the dimensions of the container be in order to minimize the cost of material? What is the cost? [3.5]

45. Business: minimizing inventory cost. Venice Cyclery sells 360 hybrid bicycles per year. It costs \$8 to store one bicycle for a year. To reorder, there is a fixed cost of \$10, plus \$2 for each bicycle. How many times per year should the shop order bicycles, and in what lot size, in order to minimize inventory costs? [3.5]

46. Business: marginal revenue. Crane Foods determines that its daily revenue, $R(x)$, in dollars, from the sale of x frozen dinners is given by

$$R(x) = 4x^{3/4}.$$ [3.6]

a) What is Crane's daily revenue when 81 frozen dinners are sold?

b) What is Crane's marginal revenue when 81 frozen dinners are sold?

c) Use the answers from parts (a) and (b) to estimate $R(82)$.

For Exercises 47–49, $y = f(x) = 2x^3 + x$. [3.6]

47. Find Δy and dy, given that $x = 1$ and $\Delta x = -0.05$.

48. a) Find dy.
b) Find dy when $x = -2$ and $dx = 0.01$.

49. a) Find the linearization of f at $x = 3$.
b) Use the linearization from part (a) to approximate $f(2.9)$; then compare the approximation to the actual value of $f(2.9)$ found using a calculator.

50. Approximate $\sqrt{83}$ using $\Delta y \approx f'(x)\,\Delta x$. [3.6]

51. Physical science: waste storage. The Waste Isolation Pilot Plant (WIPP) in New Mexico consists of large rooms carved into a salt deposit and is used for long-term storage of radioactive waste. (*Source*: www.wipp.energy.gov.) A new storage room in the shape of a cube with an edge length of 200 ft is to be carved into the salt. Use a differential to estimate the potential difference in the volume of this room if the edge measurements have a tolerance of ± 2 ft. [3.6]

52. Economics: elasticity of demand. Schneider's Bakery sells cakes. At a price of \$20 per cake, it sells 300 cakes per week. At a price of \$50, it sells 150 cakes per week. [3.7]

a) Find a linear demand function $D(x)$ that models this situation.

b) Find the elasticity of demand.

c) Find $E(20)$ and $E(50)$, and explain what these numbers represent.

d) Using the linear demand function from part (a), find the price x that results in unit elasticity, and explain what this number represents. Also, determine the weekly revenue at this price.

e) Find an exponential demand function of the form $y = P_0e^{-kx}$.

f) Using the demand function from part (e), find the price x that results in unit elasticity, and explain what this number represents. Also, determine the weekly revenue at this price.

53. Differentiate the following implicitly to find dy/dx. Then find the slope of the curve at the given point.

$$2x^3 + 2y^3 = -9xy; \quad (-1, -2) \quad [3.8]$$

54. Use logarithmic differentiation to differentiate $y = (x^2 + 1)^8\sqrt{x^4 + 2x - 7}$. [3.8]

55. Life science. A scientist studies the population P of deer on an island, and determines that it is best modeled by $P(t) = \dfrac{550}{1 + 27e^{-0.033t}}$, where t is in months since observations began. [3.8]

a) After how many months is the population increasing the fastest?

b) What is the rate of change in the population at the time found in part (a)?

c) Why might the scientist have chosen the logistic function to model the population?

56. Given $y = x^2 + 5x$, find dy/dt when $x = 3$ and $dx/dt = -0.5$. [3.9]

57. Business. Ardosh Delivery Services slowly expands its delivery area, which is circular with a radius of 15 mi. How fast is the delivery area increasing if the radius is increasing by 3 miles per year? [3.9]

58. A ladder 25 ft long leans against a vertical wall. If the bottom moves away from the wall at the rate of 6 ft/sec, how fast is the height of the top changing when the lower end is 7 ft from the wall? [3.8]

59. Business: total revenue, cost, and profit. Find the rates of change, with respect to time, of total revenue, cost, and profit for

$$R(x) = 120x - 0.5x^2 \quad \text{and} \quad C(x) = 15x + 6,$$

when $x = 100$ and $dx/dt = 30$ units per day. Assume that $R(x)$ and $C(x)$ are in dollars. [3.8]

SYNTHESIS

60. Find the absolute maximum and minimum values of the piecewise-defined function given by

$$f(x) = \begin{cases} 2 - x^2, & \text{for } -2 \leq x \leq 1, \\ 3x - 2, & \text{for } \ 1 < x < 2, \\ (x - 4)^2, & \text{for } \ 2 \leq x \leq 6. \end{cases} \quad [3.4]$$

61. Differentiate implicitly to find dy/dx:

$$(x - y)^4 + (x + y)^4 = x^6 + y^6. \quad [3.8]$$

62. Find any relative maxima and minima of

$$y = x^4 - 8x^3 - 270x^2. \quad [3.1, 3.2]$$

63. Determine a rational function f whose graph has a vertical asymptote at $x = -2$ and a horizontal asymptote at $y = 3$ and includes the point (1, 2). [3.3]

64. A spherical balloon is being inflated, and its surface area is increasing by 140 cm^2 per minute. Find the rate at which its volume is changing when the radius is 9 cm. [3.9]

Technology Connection

Use a calculator to estimate the relative extrema of each function. [3.1, 3.2]

65. $f(x) = 3.8x^5 - 18.6x^3$

66. $f(x) = xe^{x^2+3x+1}$

67. $f(x) = x^2e^{3x} - 2xe^x$

68. Life and physical sciences: incidence of breast cancer. The following table provides data relating the incidence of breast cancer per 100,000 women of various ages.

a) Use REGRESSION to fit linear, quadratic, cubic, and quartic functions to the data.

Age	Incidence per 100,000
0	0
27	10
32	25
37	60
42	125
47	187
52	224
57	270
62	340
67	408
72	437
77	475
82	460
87	420

(*Source:* National Cancer Institute.)

b) Which function best fits the data?

c) Determine a reasonable domain of the function on the basis of the function and the problem situation.

d) Determine the maximum value of the function over the domain. At what age is the incidence of breast cancer the greatest? [3.1, 3.2]

Chapter 3 Test

Find all relative minimum or maximum values as well as the x-values at which they occur. State where each function is increasing or decreasing. Then sketch a graph of the function.

1. $f(x) = x^2 - 4x - 5$
2. $f(x) = 2xe^{-4x}$
3. $f(x) = (x - 2)^{2/3} - 4$
4. $f(x) = \dfrac{16}{x^2 + 4}$

Sketch a graph of each function. List any extrema, and indicate any asymptotes or points of inflection.

5. $f(x) = x^3 + x^2 - x + 1$
6. $f(x) = 2x^4 - 4x^2 + 1$
7. $f(x) = (x - 2)^3 + 3$
8. $f(x) = x\sqrt{9 - x^2}$
9. $f(x) = 5xe^{-8x}$
10. $f(x) = \dfrac{-8}{x^2 - 4}$
11. $f(x) = \dfrac{x^2 - 1}{x}$
12. $f(x) = \ln(x^2 - 2x + 3)$

Find the absolute maximum and minimum points, if they exist, of each function over the indicated interval. Where no interval is specified, use the real line.

13. $f(x) = x(6 - x)$
14. $f(x) = x^3 + x^2 - x + 1; \left[-2, \frac{1}{2}\right]$
15. $f(x) = -x^2 + 8.6x + 10$
16. $f(x) = e^{-2x} + 3x; [-2, 1]$
17. $f(x) = -2x + 5$
18. $f(x) = 3x^2 - x - 1$
19. $f(x) = x^2 + \dfrac{128}{x}; (0, \infty)$
20. Maximize $Q = xy^2$, where $x + 2y = 50$.
21. Minimize $Q = x^2 + y^2$, where $x - y = 10$.
22. **Business: maximum profit.** Find the maximum profit and the number of units, x, of a leather briefcase that must be produced and sold in order to yield that maximum profit. Assume that $R(x)$ and $C(x)$ are the revenue and cost, in dollars, when x units are produced:

$$R(x) = x^2 + 110x + 60,$$
$$C(x) = 1.1x^2 + 10x + 80.$$

23. **Business: maximizing area.** Comstock Pyrotechnics plans to build a rectangular storage yard with an area of 2000 ft^2 adjacent to an existing building. The side opposite the wall of the building will be a brick wall and cost \$75 per foot to build, while the two other parallel sides will be chain-link fences costing \$30 per foot to build.
    a) Find the dimensions that minimize the cost of building the storage yard.
    b) What is the lowest cost?

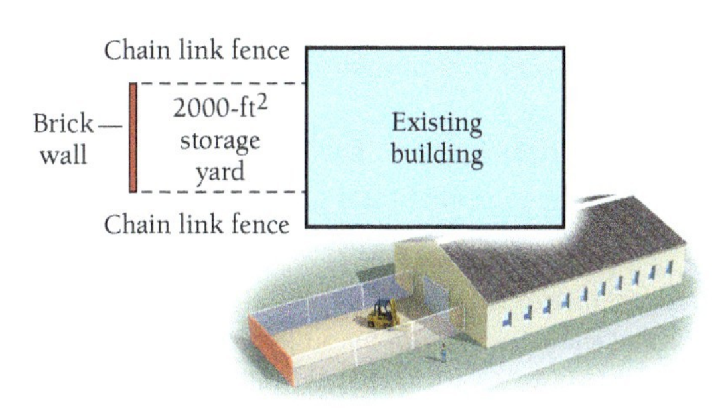

24. **Business: minimizing inventory costs.** Ironside Sports sells 1225 tennis rackets per year. It costs \$2 to store one tennis racket for a year. To reorder, there is a fixed cost of \$1, plus \$0.50 for each tennis racket. How many times per year should Ironside order tennis rackets, and in what lot size, in order to minimize inventory costs?
25. For $y = f(x) = x^2 - 3$, $x = 5$, and $\Delta x = 0.1$, find Δy and $f'(x)\,\Delta x$.
26. Approximate $\sqrt{50}$ using $\Delta y \approx f'(x)\,\Delta x$.
27. For $y = \sqrt{x^2 + 3}$:
    a) Find dy.
    b) Find dy when $x = 2$ and $dx = 0.01$.
28. Let $f(x) = \sqrt{x}$.
    a) Find $L(x)$, the linearization of f at $x = 16$.
    b) Use the linearization from part (a) to estimate $f(15)$. Compare your estimate to the actual value of $f(15)$.
29. **Economics: elasticity of demand.** Consider the demand function given by

$$q = D(x) = \frac{600}{(x + 4)^2}.$$

   a) Find the elasticity.
   b) Find the elasticity at $x = 1$, stating whether demand is elastic or inelastic.
   c) Find the elasticity at $x = 12$, stating whether demand is elastic or inelastic.
   d) At a price of \$12, will a small increase in price cause total revenue to increase or decrease?
   e) Find the price at which total revenue is a maximum.

30. Differentiate the following implicitly to find dy/dx. Then find the slope of the curve at $(1, 2)$:

$$x^3 + y^3 = 9.$$

31. Use logarithmic differentiation to differentiate

$$y = \frac{\sqrt{x^3 + 5x}}{e^{x^2+7x+1}}.$$

32. Business: point of diminishing returns. The total gross revenue of the movie *It Came from the Math Department* is given by $R(t) = \dfrac{45{,}000{,}000}{1 + 4999e^{-0.4t}}$, where t is the number of weeks since the movie's release.

a) Find the point of diminishing returns.

b) Find the rate at which total gross revenue is increasing at the time found in part (a).

c) What is the expected total gross revenue of this movie?

33. Business: rate of change. A stock sells for \$80 per share, and its price is increasing by \$2 per day. One day, 2500 shares of this stock were sold. Find the rate at which shares are being purchased if the total revenue on this day was growing by \$14,600 per day.

SYNTHESIS

34. Find the absolute maximum and minimum values of the following function, if they exist, over $[0, \infty)$:

$$f(x) = \frac{x^2}{1 + x^3}.$$

35. Business: minimizing average cost. The total cost in dollars of producing x units of a visor is given by

$$C(x) = 100x + 100\sqrt{x} + \frac{\sqrt{x^3}}{100}.$$

How many units should be produced to minimize average cost?

Technology Connection 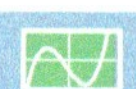

36. Estimate any extrema of the function given by

$$f(x) = 5x^3 - 30x^2 + 45x + 5\sqrt{x}.$$

37. Estimate any extrema of the function given by

$$f(x) = x^2 + x + e^{-0.1x};\ [-2, 1].$$

38. Maximize $Q = x^2y^2$, where $x^2 + y = 20$ and x and y are positive.

39. Business: advertising. The business of manufacturing and selling bowling balls is one of frequent changes. Companies introduce new models to the market about every 3 to 4 months. Typically, a new model is created because of advances in technology such as new surface stock or a new way to place weight blocks in a ball. To decide how to best use advertising dollars, companies track sales in relation to amount spent on advertising. Suppose a company has the following data from past sales.

Amount Spent on Advertising (in thousands)	Number of Bowling Balls Sold, N
\$ 0	8
50	13,115
100	19,780
150	22,612
200	20,083
250	12,430
300	4

a) Use REGRESSION to fit linear, quadratic, cubic, and quartic functions to the data.

b) Determine the domain of the function in part (a) that best fits the data and the problem situation. How did you arrive at your answer?

c) Using the cubic or quadratic model, determine the maximum value of the function over the domain. How much should the company spend on advertising a new model in order to maximize the number of bowling balls sold?

EXTENDED TECHNOLOGY APPLICATION 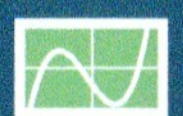

Maximum Sustainable Harvest

In certain situations, biologists are able to determine what is called a **reproduction curve**. This is a function

$$y = f(P)$$

such that if P is the population at a given point in time, then $f(P)$ is the population a year later. Such a curve is shown below.

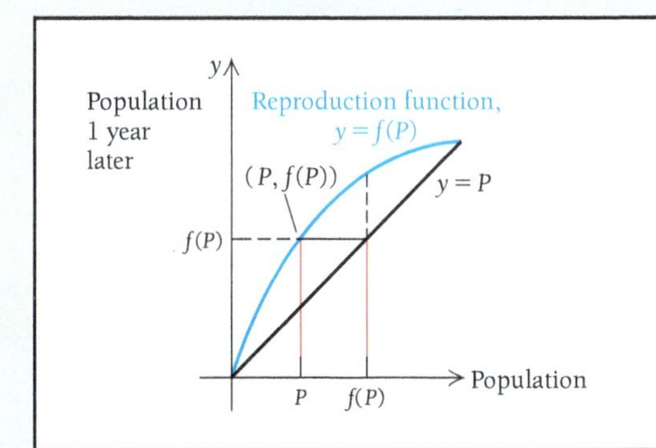

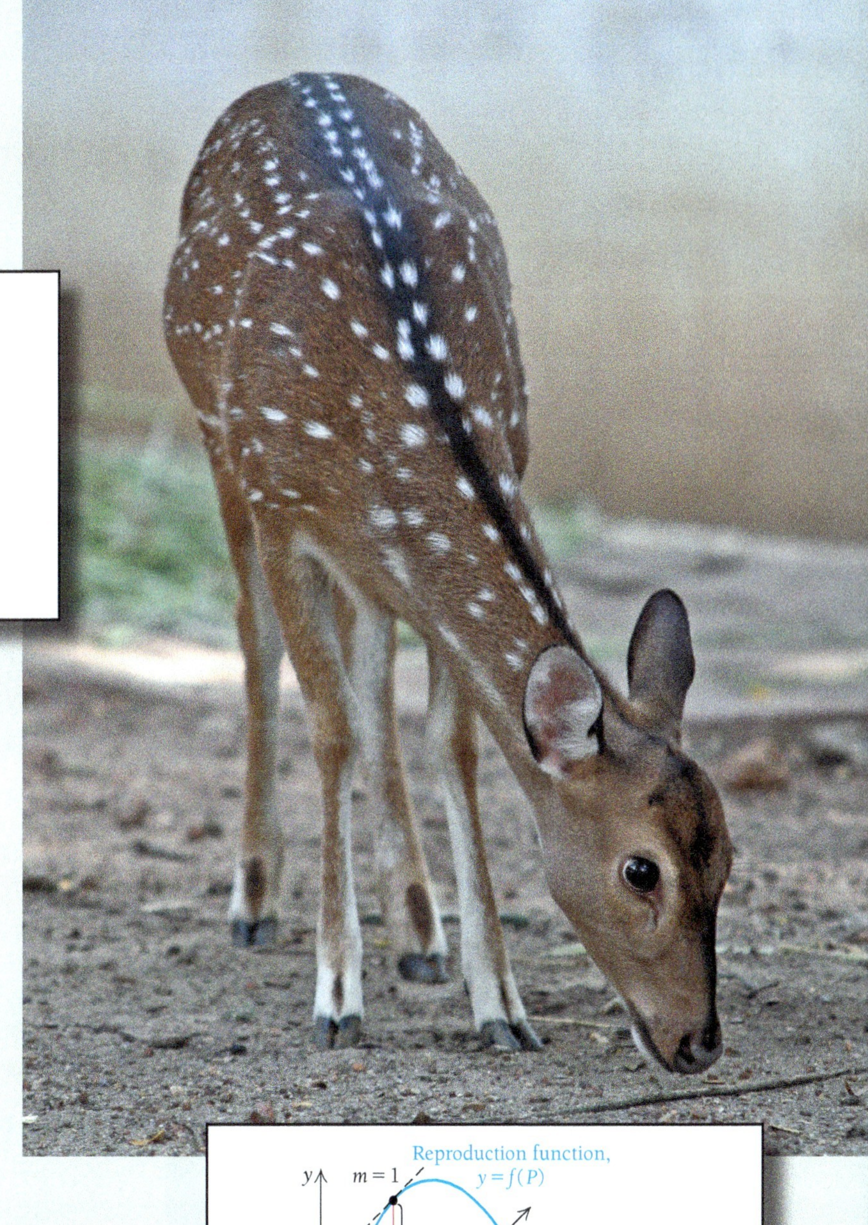

The line $y = P$ is significant because if it coincides with the curve $y = f(P)$, then we know that the population stays the same from year to year. Here the graph of f lies mostly above the line, indicating that the population is increasing.

Too many deer in a forest can deplete the food supply and cause the population to decrease. In such cases, hunters are often allowed to "harvest" some of the deer. Then with a greater food supply, the remaining deer population may prosper and increase.

We know that a population P will grow to a population $f(P)$ in a year. If the population were increasing, then hunters could "harvest" the amount

$$f(P) - P$$

each year without shrinking the initial population P. If the population were remaining the same or decreasing, then such a harvest would deplete the population.

Suppose we want to know the value of P_0 that will allow the harvest to be the largest. If we could determine that P_0, we could let the population grow until it reached that level and then begin harvesting year after year the amount $f(P_0) - P_0$.

Let the harvest function H be given by

$$H(P) = f(P) - P.$$

Then $H'(P) = f'(P) - 1.$

Now, if we assume that $H'(P)$ exists for all values of P and that there is only one critical value, it follows that the *maximum sustainable harvest* occurs at that value P_0 such that

$$H'(P_0) = f'(P_0) - 1 = 0$$

and $H''(P_0) = f''(P_0) < 0.$

Or, equivalently, we have the following.

THEOREM

The **maximum sustainable harvest** occurs at P_0 such that

$$f'(P_0) = 1 \quad \text{and} \quad f''(P_0) < 0,$$

and is given by

$$H(P_0) = f(P_0) - P_0.$$

Exercises

For Exercises 1–3, do the following.

a) *Graph the reproduction curve, the line $y = P$, and the harvest function using the same viewing window.*

b) *Find the population at which the maximum sustainable harvest occurs. Use both a graphical solution and a calculus solution.*

c) *Find the maximum sustainable harvest.*

1. $f(P) = P(10 - P)$, where P is measured in thousands.

2. $f(P) = -0.025P^2 + 4P$, where P is measured in thousands. This is the reproduction curve in the Hudson Bay area for the snowshoe hare.

3. $f(P) = -0.01P^2 + 2P$, where P is measured in thousands. This is the reproduction curve in the Hudson Bay area for the lynx.

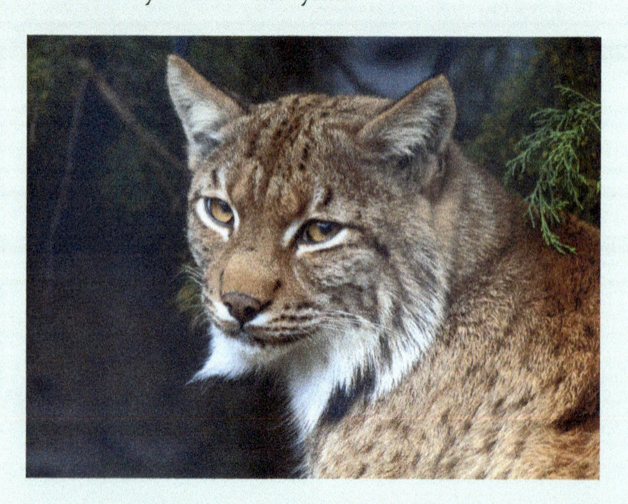

For Exercises 4 and 5, do the following.

a) *Graph the reproduction curve, the line $y = P$, and the harvest function using the same viewing window.*

b) *Graphically determine the population at which the maximum sustainable harvest occurs.*

c) *Find the maximum sustainable harvest.*

4. $f(P) = 40\sqrt{P}$, where P is measured in thousands. Assume that this is the reproduction curve for the brown trout population in a large lake.

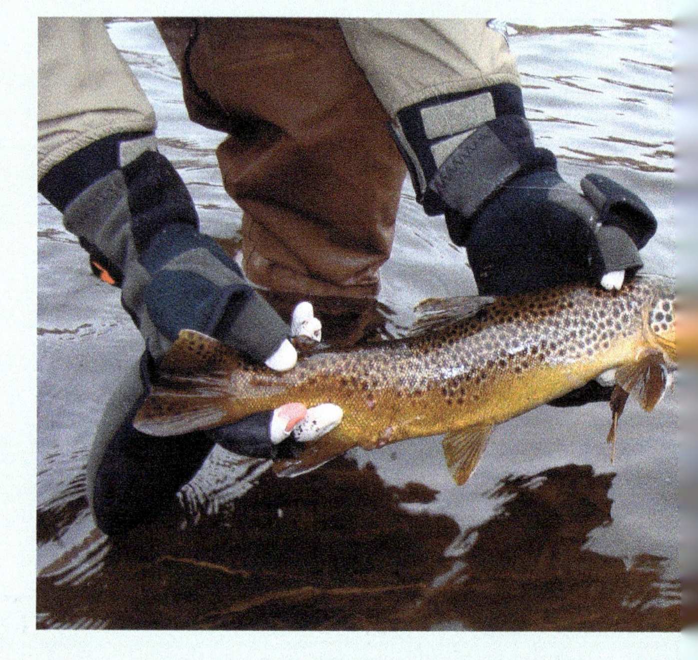

5. $f(P) = 0.237P\sqrt{2000 - P^2}$, where P is measured in thousands.

6. The table below lists data regarding the reproduction of a certain animal.

a) Use REGRESSION to fit a cubic polynomial to these data.

b) Graph the reproduction curve, the line $y = P$, and the harvest function using the same viewing window.

c) Graphically determine the population at which the maximum sustainable harvest occurs.

Population, P (in thousands)	Population, $f(P)$, 1 Year Later
10	9.7
20	23.1
30	37.4
40	46.2
50	42.6

Another common model used to determine the maximum sustainable harvest is the logistic function, $P(t) = \frac{L}{1 + Ce^{-rt}}$, where $r = Lk$. Recall that this function solves the differential equation

$$\frac{dP}{dt} = kP(L - P).$$ See Exercise 50, Section 2.4.

An equivalent form of this differential equation is

$$\frac{dP}{dt} = kP\left(1 - \frac{P}{L}\right).$$

It can be shown through substitution that $P(t) = \frac{L}{1 + Ce^{-Lkt}}$ solves this form of the differential equation.

When the population P is small, the ratio P/L is very small, so $\left(1 - \frac{P}{L}\right) \approx 1$. In this case, the population grows according to the model

$$\frac{dP}{dt} = kP \cdot 1, \quad \text{or} \quad \frac{dP}{dt} = kP,$$

which is the unconstrained model for growth. The external factors that may inhibit a population's growth, such as physical space, availability of food, or number of predators, do not yet have a strong effect on suppressing the population. Harvesting individuals at this point would not be wise, as it would remove mating couples from an already small population.

As the population grows, it nears its carrying capacity, so the ratio P/L approaches 1. The factor $\left(1 - \frac{P}{L}\right)$ approaches 0, and the differential equation becomes $dP/dt = kP \cdot 0$, meaning that the rate of change of growth is slowing and approaching 0. Harvesting individuals at this point may be wise, but is there a better time at which to harvest rather than waiting for the population to reach carrying capacity? We see that harvesting too early removes mating couples from the population, whereas waiting until P is close to L may be too late; other factors may then affect the population adversely.

Under these conditions, the maximum sustainable harvest should occur at the point where the population is increasing the fastest, so that once the excess individuals are harvested, the population can quickly replenish. This point occurs at the point of inflection, $\left(\frac{\ln C}{r}, \frac{L}{2}\right)$, or at half the carrying capacity. The harvest rate, h, will match the growth rate at this point, so $h = P'\left(\frac{\ln C}{r}\right)$.

Exercises

7. Show that under this assumption, the maximum sustainable harvest rate is $h = \frac{Lr}{4}$.

8. A scientist studying feral pigs on an island determines that the population is modeled by $P(t) = \frac{1250}{1 + 45e^{-0.081t}}$, where t is measured in months.

a) When does the population experience its fastest rate of growth?

b) What is the rate of growth at the time found in part (a)?

c) What is the recommended harvest rate that will maintain sustainability of the feral pig population?

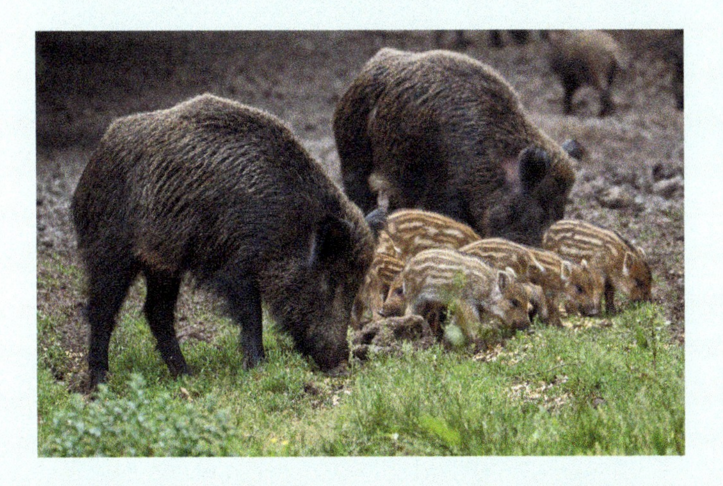

9. In reality, the maximum sustainable harvest often occurs when the population is about at 30% of carrying capacity, rather than at 50%. Why might it be unwise to harvest at the 50% figure?

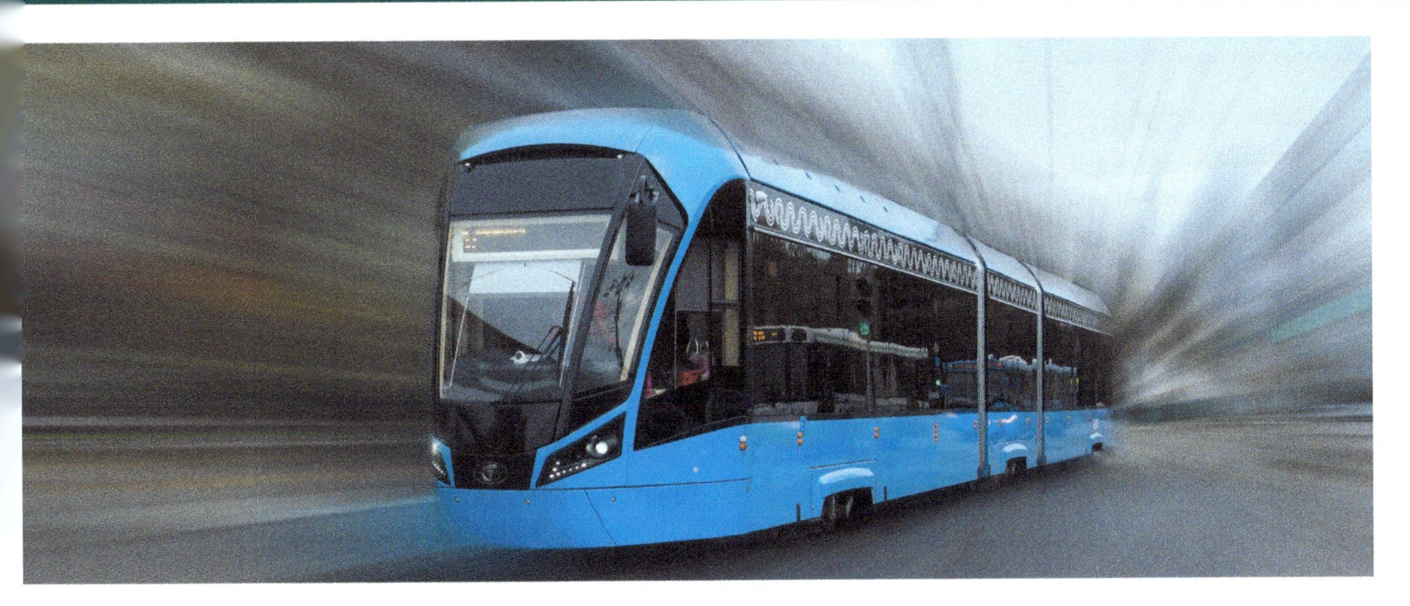

4 Integration

What You'll Learn

Why It's Important

When a vehicle moves, it accumulates distance traveled. Is it possible to determine the distance a vehicle has traveled if we know its velocity function? Similarly, for every unit of product sold, a company accumulates profit. Can we determine a company's total profit if we know its marginal-profit function? We can, using a process called *integration*, which is one of the two main branches of calculus, the other being differentiation. In this chapter, we explore some of the many practical applications of integration in science, business, and statistics.

Where It's Used

Fossil Fuel Displacement: Since 2013, the rate of change in the amount of fossil fuel displaced (not needed) globally because of electric vehicles can be approximated by

$$D'(t) = 1696t^3 - 14{,}091t^2 + 30{,}420t - 7808,$$

where $D'(t)$ is in thousands of barrels of fossil fuel displaced per year and t is the number of years since 2013. In 2016, approximately 24,638 thousand barrels of fossil fuel were displaced worldwide. Find a function $D(t)$ that models the amount of fossil fuel displaced t years since 2013, and estimate the amount of fossil fuel that will be displaced in 2020.

(This problem appears as Example 7 in Section 4.1.)

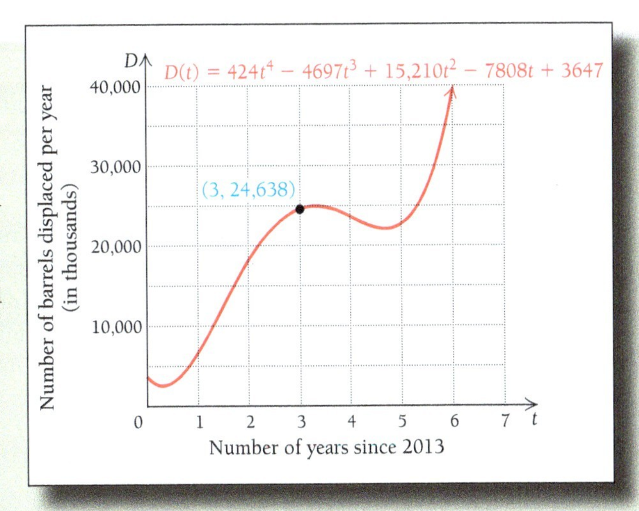

4.1

- Find an antiderivative of a function.
- Evaluate indefinite integrals using basic rules of antidifferentiation.
- Use initial conditions to determine an antiderivative.

Antidifferentiation

In this chapter, we explore *integration*, which is one of the two principal branches of calculus (*differential calculus*, which we have studied in Chapters 1–3, being the other). With *integral calculus*, we are able to determine accumulation of a quantity based on a given rate function, for example:

- Given a function $y = v(t)$, the velocity of an object at time t, we can determine an object's *distance traveled* over an interval of time.
- Given a function $y = P'(x)$, the marginal profit of a business after x units have been sold, we can determine the business's *total profit* after x units have been sold.
- Given a function $y = f(t)$, the rate of change of a population after t years, we can determine the *total population growth* after t years.

Finding Antiderivatives

One aspect of integral calculus is **antidifferentiation**, which is the process of differentiation performed in reverse. Given a function f, we find another function F such that

$$\frac{d}{dx}F(x) = f(x).$$

The function F is an **antiderivative** of f. For example, if $f(x) = 2x$, then $F(x) = x^2$ is an antiderivative of f since

$$\frac{d}{dx}(x^2) = 2x.$$

Note that functions like $F(x) = x^2 + 5$ and $F(x) = x^2 - 17$ are also antiderivatives of $f(x) = 2x$ since

$$\frac{d}{dx}(x^2 + 5) = 2x + 0 = 2x; \quad \text{and} \quad \frac{d}{dx}(x^2 - 17) = 2x + 0 = 2x.$$

Thus, an antiderivative of $f(x) = 2x$ is any function that can be written in the form $F(x) = x^2 + C$, where C is any constant. This leads us to the following theorem.

THEOREM 1

The **antiderivative** of $f(x)$ is the set of functions $F(x) + C$ such that

$$\frac{d}{dx}[F(x) + C] = f(x).$$

The constant C is called the **constant of integration**.

If F is an antiderivative of f, we write

$$\int f(x)\, dx = F(x) + C.$$

This equation is read as "the antiderivative of $f(x)$, with respect to x, is $F(x) + C$" or as "the integral of $f(x)$, with respect to x, is $F(x) + C$." The expression on the left side is called an **indefinite integral**. The symbol $\int$ is the *integral sign*, and $f(x)$ is the *integrand*. The symbol dx can be regarded as indicating that x is the variable of integration, similar to d/dx indicating that the expression that follows it is to be differentiated with respect to x.

EXAMPLE 1 Determine these indefinite integrals. That is, find the antiderivative of each integrand:

a) $\int 8\, dx$; **b)** $\int 3x^2\, dx$; **c)** $\int e^x\, dx$; **d)** $\displaystyle\int \frac{1}{x}\, dx,\ x \neq 0$.

Solution We have seen these integrands before as derivatives of other functions.

a) $\int 8\,dx = 8x + C$ **Check:** $\frac{d}{dx}(8x + C) = 8$

b) $\int 3x^2\,dx = x^3 + C$ **Check:** $\frac{d}{dx}(x^3 + C) = 3x^2$

c) $\int e^x\,dx = e^x + C$ **Check:** $\frac{d}{dx}(e^x + C) = e^x$

d) $\int \frac{1}{x}\,dx = \ln|x| + C$ **Check:** $\frac{d}{dx}(\ln|x| + C) = \frac{1}{x}$

Every antiderivative can be checked by differentiation.

The results of Example 1 suggest some rules for antiderivatives, which are summarized in Theorem 2.

THEOREM 2 Rules for Antiderivatives

A1. Constant Rule:

$$\int k\,dx = kx + C.$$

A2. Power Rule (where $n \neq -1$):

$$\int x^n\,dx = \frac{1}{n+1}x^{n+1} + C.$$

A3. Natural Logarithm Rule:

$$\int \frac{1}{x}\,dx = \ln|x| + C, \text{ and for } x > 0, \int \frac{1}{x}\,dx = \ln x + C.$$

A4. Exponential Rule (base e):

$$\int e^{ax}\,dx = \frac{1}{a}e^{ax} + C, \qquad a \neq 0.$$

The Power Rule for Antiderivatives can be viewed as a two-step process:

$$\int x^n\,dx = \frac{1}{n+1}x^{n+1} + C$$

1. Increase the exponent by 1.
2. Divide the term by the new power.

EXAMPLE 2 Find the following indefinite integrals:

a) $\int x^7\,dx$; **b)** $\int \sqrt{x}\,dx$; **c)** $\int \frac{1}{x^3}\,dx$.

Check each answer by differentiation.

Solution

a) $$\int x^7\,dx = \frac{x^{7+1}}{7+1} + C = \frac{1}{8}x^8 + C$$

Check: $$\frac{d}{dx}\left(\frac{1}{8}x^8 + C\right) = \frac{1}{8}(8x^7) = x^7$$

b) Recall that $\sqrt{x} = x^{1/2}$. Therefore,

$$\int \sqrt{x}\,dx = \int x^{1/2}\,dx = \frac{x^{(1/2)+1}}{\left(\frac{1}{2}\right)+1} + C = \frac{x^{3/2}}{\frac{3}{2}} + C$$

$$= \frac{2}{3}x^{3/2} + C, \quad \text{or } \frac{2}{3}x\sqrt{x} + C.$$

Check: $\frac{d}{dx}\left(\frac{2}{3}x^{3/2} + C\right) = \frac{2}{3}\left(\frac{3}{2}x^{1/2}\right) = x^{1/2} = \sqrt{x}$

c) Recall that $\frac{1}{x^3} = x^{-3}$. Therefore,

$$\int \frac{1}{x^3}\,dx = \int x^{-3}\,dx = \frac{x^{-3+1}}{-3+1} + C = -\frac{1}{2}x^{-2} + C$$

$$= -\frac{1}{2x^2} + C.$$

Check: $\frac{d}{dx}\left(-\frac{1}{2}x^{-2} + C\right) = -\frac{1}{2}(-2x^{-3}) = x^{-3} = \frac{1}{x^3}$ **1 ✓**

Quick Check 1 ✓

Find these indefinite integrals:

a) $\int x^{10}\,dx$;

b) $\int \sqrt[6]{x}\,dx$;

c) $\int \frac{1}{x^4}\,dx$.

The Power Rule for Antiderivatives is valid for all real numbers n, except for $n = -1$. As we saw in Example 1(d), for $n = -1$, we have $x^{-1} = \frac{1}{x}$, which is the derivative of the natural logarithm function, $y = \ln|x|$. Therefore,

$$\int \frac{1}{x}\,dx = \ln|x| + C, \text{ and for } x > 0, \int \frac{1}{x}\,dx = \ln x + C.$$

In Example 3, we explore the case of $f(x) = e^{ax}$.

EXAMPLE 3 Find $\int e^{4x}\,dx$.

Solution By Rule A4 of Theorem 2, we have

$$\int e^{4x}\,dx = \frac{1}{4}e^{4x} + C.$$

Check: $\frac{d}{dx}\left(\frac{1}{4}e^{4x} + C\right) = \frac{1}{4}(4e^{4x}) = e^{4x}$ **2 ✓**

Quick Check 2 ✓

Find each antiderivative:

a) $\int e^{-3x}\,dx$;

b) $\int e^{(1/2)x}\,dx$.

Two useful properties of antiderivatives are presented in Theorem 3.

THEOREM 3 Properties of Antiderivatives

P1. A constant multiplier can be factored to the front of the indefinite integral:

$$\int [c \cdot f(x)]\,dx = c \cdot \int f(x)\,dx.$$

P2. The antiderivative of a sum or difference is the sum or difference of the antiderivatives:

$$\int [f(x) \pm g(x)]\,dx = \int f(x)\,dx \pm \int g(x)\,dx.$$

EXAMPLE 4 Find each antiderivative. Assume $x > 0$.

a) $\int (3x^5 + 7x^2 + 8)\,dx$; **b)** $\int \frac{4 + 3x + 2x^4}{x}\,dx$.

Solution

a) We find the antiderivative of each term separately:

$$\int (3x^5 + 7x^2 + 8)\,dx = \int 3x^5\,dx + \int 7x^2\,dx + \int 8\,dx$$ Using Property P2 of Theorem 3

$$= 3\left(\tfrac{1}{6}x^6\right) + 7\left(\tfrac{1}{3}x^3\right) + 8x + C$$ Using Property P1 and Rules A1 and A2

$$= \tfrac{1}{2}x^6 + \tfrac{7}{3}x^3 + 8x + C.$$ Simplifying coefficients and writing just one constant of integration

b) We use x as a common denominator and then simplify each ratio as much as possible:

$$\frac{4 + 3x + 2x^4}{x} = \frac{4}{x} + \frac{3x}{x} + \frac{2x^4}{x} = \frac{4}{x} + 3 + 2x^3.$$

Therefore,

$$\int \frac{4 + 3x + 2x^4}{x}\,dx = \int \left(\frac{4}{x} + 3 + 2x^3\right) dx$$

$$= 4 \ln x + 3x + \tfrac{1}{2}x^4 + C.$$ Using Properties P1 and P2 and Rules A1, A2, and A3

3 ✓

Quick Check 3 ✓

Find each integral:

a) $\int (2x^4 + 3x^3 - 7x^2)\,dx$;

b) $\int \frac{x^2 - 7x + 2}{x^2}\,dx$, $x > 0$.

Initial Conditions

When a point that is a solution of an antiderivative is given, it is possible to solve for C. The given point is called an **initial condition**.

EXAMPLE 5 Find $\int (2x + 3)\,dx$ given that $F(1) = -2$.

Solution If we specify that $F'(x) = 2x + 3$, then we have

$$F(x) = \int (2x + 3)\,dx = x^2 + 3x + C.$$

Since $F(1) = -2$, we can substitute and solve for C:

$$-2 = (1)^2 + 3(1) + C.$$

Simplifying, we have $-2 = 4 + C$, or $C = -6$. Therefore, the specific antiderivative that satisfies the initial condition is

$$F(x) = x^2 + 3x - 6.$$

4 ✓

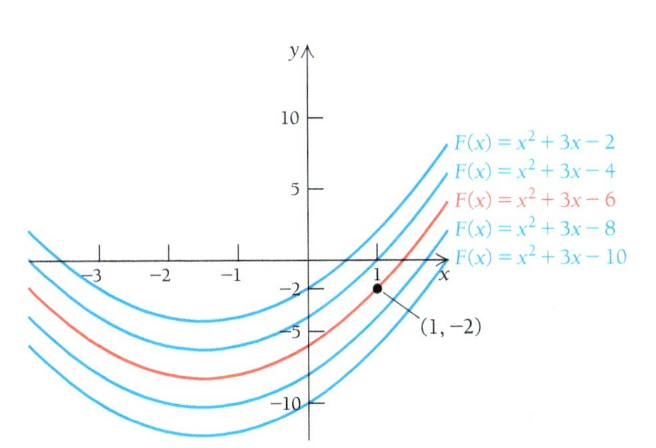

A visualization of Example 5

Quick Check 4 ✓

Find an antiderivative of $g(x) = e^{2x}$ such that the point $(0, 3)$ is a solution of the antiderivative.

The antiderivative of a function has many applications. For example, in Section 1.8, we saw that the derivative of a distance function is velocity. Therefore, if we are given a velocity function, its antiderivative is a function that describes the moving object's distance from a starting point. If the distance traveled after some time t is known (an initial condition), then we can find distances traveled over other intervals of time.

EXAMPLE 6 **Physical Science: Height of a Thrown Object.** A rock thrown upward with the initial velocity 50 ft/sec from 10 ft above the ground has a velocity modeled by $v(t) = -32t + 50$, where t is the number of seconds after the rock is released and $v(t)$ is in feet per second.

a) Determine a distance function h as a function of t (in this case, "distance" is the height of the rock).

b) Find the height and the velocity of the rock after 3 sec.

Solution

a) Since distance (height) is the antiderivative of velocity, we have

$$h(t) = \int(-32t + 50)\,dt = -16t^2 + 50t + C.$$

The initial height, 10 ft, gives us the ordered pair (0, 10) as an initial condition. We substitute 0 for t and 10 for $h(t)$, and solve for C:

$$10 = -16(0)^2 + 50(0) + C$$
$$10 = C.$$

Therefore, the distance function is given by $h(t) = -16t^2 + 50t + 10$.

b) To find the height of the rock after 3 sec, we substitute 3 for t in the distance function:

$$h(3) = -16(3)^2 + 50(3) + 10 = 16 \text{ ft}.$$

The velocity after 3 sec is

$$v(3) = -32(3) + 50 = -46 \text{ ft/sec}.$$

After 3 sec, the rock is 16 ft above the ground, but the negative velocity indicates that it is moving downward. 5 ✓

Quick Check 5 ✓

An arrow shot directly upward from the ground has a velocity modeled by $v(t) = -32t + 125$, where t is the number of seconds after the arrow is released and $v(t)$ is in feet per second. Find the arrow's height and velocity after 5 sec.

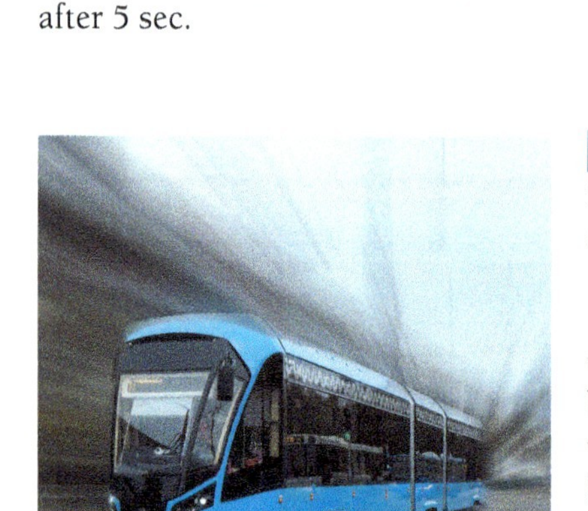

EXAMPLE 7 **Life Science: Fossil Fuel Displacement.** Since 2013, the rate of change in the amount of fossil fuel displaced (not needed) globally because of electric vehicles can be approximated by

$$D'(t) = 1696t^3 - 14{,}091t^2 + 30{,}420t - 7808,$$

where $D'(t)$ is in thousands of barrels of fossil fuel displaced per year and t is the number of years since 2013. In 2016, approximately 24,638 thousand barrels of fossil fuel were displaced globally. (*Source*: Based on data from *Bloomberg New Energy Finance*, May 2018.)

a) Find a function $D(t)$ that models the amount of fossil fuel displaced t years since 2013.

b) Estimate the amount of fossil fuel that will be displaced in 2020.

Solution

a) To find $D(t)$, we find an antiderivative for the rate-of-change model:

$$D(t) = \int(1696t^3 - 14{,}091t^2 + 30{,}420t - 7808)\,dt$$

$$= 1696\left(\frac{1}{4}t^4\right) - 14{,}091\left(\frac{1}{3}t^3\right) + 30{,}420\left(\frac{1}{2}t^2\right) - 7808t + C \quad \text{Using Properties P1 and P2}$$

$$= 424t^4 - 4697t^3 + 15{,}210t^2 - 7808t + C. \quad \text{Simplifying}$$

To find C, we use the initial condition (3, 24,638), where $t = 3$ represents the number of years since 2013:

$$24{,}638 = 424(3)^4 - 4697(3)^3 + 15{,}210(3)^2 - 7808(3) + C \quad \text{Substituting}$$
$$24{,}638 = 20{,}991 + C$$
$$3647 = C.$$

Therefore, the amount of displaced fossil fuel each year, in thousands of barrels, t years since 2013 is given by

$$D(t) = 424t^4 - 4697t^3 + 15{,}210t^2 - 7808t + 3647.$$

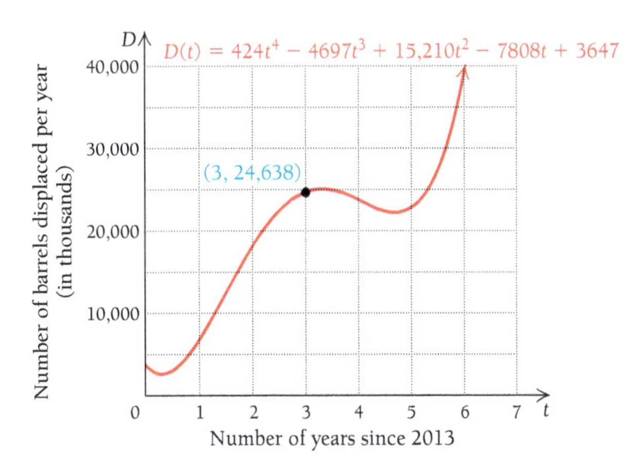

Quick Check 6 ✓

Waltonville's rate of population change is modeled by $P'(t) = 34t + 16$, where t is the number of years since 2000 and $P'(t)$ is in people per year.

a) Find the population model for Waltonville if it is known that in 2010, the population was 2500.

b) Estimate the town's population in 2028.

b) To estimate the number of barrels of fossil fuel displaced in 2020, we substitute 7 for t in the model:

$$D(7) = 424(7)^4 - 4697(7)^3 + 15{,}210(7)^2 - 7808(7) + 3647$$
$$= 101{,}234. \quad \text{Using a calculator}$$

Using this model, the amount of fossil fuel displaced worldwide in 2020 will be about 101,234 thousand, or about 101 million, barrels. **6 ✓**

Section Summary

- An *antiderivative* of a function f is a function F such that
$$\frac{d}{dx}F(x) = f(x).$$
- An antiderivative is denoted by an *indefinite integral* using the integral sign, $\int$. If F is an antiderivative of f, we write
$$\int f(x)\,dx = F(x) + C,$$
where the constant C is called the *constant of integration*. We check that an antiderivative is correct by differentiating it.
- The *Constant Rule for Antiderivatives* is
$$\int k\,dx = kx + C.$$
- The *Power Rule for Antiderivatives* is
$$\int x^n\,dx = \frac{1}{n+1}x^{n+1} + C, \quad \text{for } n \neq -1.$$
- The *Natural Logarithm Rule for Antiderivatives* is
$$\int \frac{1}{x}\,dx = \ln|x| + C,$$
or, for $x > 0$,
$$\int \frac{1}{x}\,dx = \ln x + C.$$
- The *Exponential Rule* (base e) *for Antiderivatives* is
$$\int e^{ax}\,dx = \frac{1}{a}e^{ax} + C, \quad \text{for } a \neq 0.$$
- An *initial condition* is an ordered pair that is a solution of a particular antiderivative of an integrand.

4.1 Exercise Set

Find each integral.

1. $\int 2\,dx$

2. $\int 4\,dx$

3. $\int x^6\,dx$

4. $\int x^7\,dx$

5. $\int x^{1/4}\,dx$

6. $\int x^{1/3}\,dx$

7. $\int (x^2 + x - 1)\,dx$

8. $\int (x^2 - x + 2)\,dx$

9. $\int (2t^2 + 5t - 3)\,dt$

10. $\int (3t^2 - 4t + 7)\,dt$

11. $\int \frac{1}{x^3}\,dx$

12. $\int \frac{1}{x^5}\,dx$

13. $\int \sqrt[6]{x}\,dx$

14. $\int \sqrt[7]{x}\,dx$

15. $\int \sqrt{x^5}\,dx$

16. $\int \sqrt[3]{x^2}\,dx$

17. $\int \frac{dx}{x^4}$

18. $\int \frac{dx}{x^2}$

19. $\int \frac{10}{x}\,dx$

20. $\int \frac{2}{x}\,dx$

21. $\int \left(\frac{3}{x} + \frac{5}{x^2}\right)dx$

22. $\int \left(\frac{4}{x^3} + \frac{7}{x}\right)dx$

23. $\int \frac{-7}{\sqrt[3]{x^2}}\,dx$

24. $\int \frac{5}{\sqrt[4]{x^3}}\,dx$

25. $\int e^{3x}\,dx$

26. $\int e^{5x}\,dx$

27. $\int 2e^{2x}\,dx$

28. $\int 4e^{4x}\,dx$

29. $\int 6e^{x/2}\,dx$

30. $\int 15e^{x/3}\,dx$

31. $\int 100e^{0.02x}\,dx$

32. $\int 2500e^{-0.075x}\,dx$

33. $\int e^{3x}(e^x - e^{4x})\,dx$ (*Hint:* Multiply first.)

34. $\int e^{-2x}(e^{3x} + e^{2x})\,dx$

35. $\int (x^3 + 4\sqrt{x} + e^{-6x})\,dx$

36. $\int \left(2x^4 + \frac{1}{x^2} - e^{-9x}\right)dx$

37. $\int \frac{4x^2 - 8x + 3}{x}\,dx$

38. $\int \frac{2x^2 - x + 5}{x}\,dx$

39. $\int \frac{3x^2 + 2x + 5}{x^2}\,dx$

40. $\int \frac{5x^2 + 7x - 11}{x^2}\,dx$

41. $\int (3x + 2)^2\,dx$ (*Hint:* Expand first.)

42. $\int (x + 4)^2\,dx$

43. $\int \frac{1 + \sqrt{x}}{\sqrt{x}}\,dx$

44. $\int \frac{2 + \sqrt[3]{x}}{\sqrt[3]{x}}\,dx$

45. $\int (3 + 2\sqrt{x})^2\,dx$

46. $\int (\sqrt{x} + 6)^2\,dx$

Find f such that:

47. $f'(x) = x - 3, \quad f(2) = 9$

48. $f'(x) = x - 5, \quad f(1) = 6$

49. $f'(x) = x^2 - 4, \quad f(0) = 7$

50. $f'(x) = x^2 + 1, \quad f(0) = 8$

51. $f'(x) = 8x^2 + 4x - 2, \quad f(0) = 6$

52. $f'(x) = 6x^2 - 4x + 2, \quad f(1) = 9$

53. $f'(x) = 5e^{2x}, \quad f(0) = \frac{1}{2}$

54. $f'(x) = 3e^{4x}, \quad f(0) = \frac{7}{4}$

55. $f'(x) = \frac{4}{\sqrt{x}}, \quad f(1) = -5$

56. $f'(x) = \frac{2}{\sqrt[3]{x}}, \quad f(1) = 1$

APPLICATIONS

Business and Economics

Credit market debt. *Since 2013, the annual rate of change in the national consumer revolving credit market debt can be modeled by the function*

$$D'(t) = 12.922t + 11.474,$$

where $D'(t)$ is in billions of dollars per year and t is the number of years since January 2013. (Source: Based on data from federalreserve.gov/releases/g19/current.) Use the preceding information for Exercises 57 and 58.

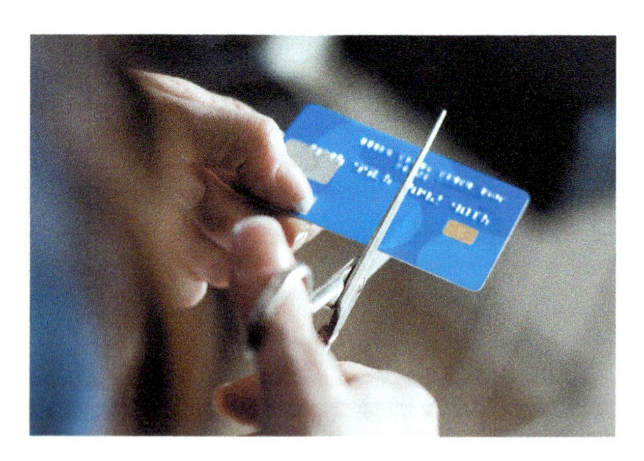

57. Find the credit market debt, $D(t)$, since 2013, given that $D(0) = 848.8$.

58. Estimate the credit market debt in 2020. (*Hint:* See Exercise 57.)

59. **Business: electric vehicle sales.** The rate of change in worldwide sales of electric vehicles t years since 2013 is given by

$$S'(t) = 96.2885e^{0.427t},$$

where $S'(t)$ is in thousands of vehicles sold per year. In 2016, approximately 774,000 electric vehicles were sold worldwide. (*Source:* Based on data from www.ev-volumes.com.)

a) Find a function $S(t)$ that models the yearly worldwide sales of electric vehicles t years since 2013.

b) Estimate the yearly worldwide sales in 2020.

60. Total cost from marginal cost. Solid Rock Industries determines that the marginal cost, $C'(x)$, of producing the xth climbing harness is given by

$$C'(x) = x^3 - x.$$

Find the total-cost function, C, assuming that $C(x)$ is in dollars and that fixed costs are \$6500.

61. Total profit from marginal profit. Eloy Chutes determines that the marginal profit, $P'(x)$, in hundreds of dollars per unit, from selling the xth parachute is given by

$$P'(x) = 0.02x - 1.45.$$

a) Find the total-profit function, P, assuming that $P(0) = 0$.

b) How many parachutes does Eloy Chutes need to sell to break even?

62. Total revenue from marginal revenue. Taylor Ceramics determines that the marginal revenue, $R'(x)$, in dollars per unit, from selling the xth vase is given by

$$R'(x) = 1.68x^2 + x + 2.5.$$

Find the total-revenue function, R, assuming that $R(0) = 0$.

63. Supply from marginal supply. Keans Corporation finds that the rate at which it supplies plates changes with respect to price and is given by the marginal-supply function

$$S'(x) = 0.24x^2 + 4x + 10,$$

where x is the price per plate, in dollars. Find the supply function if it is known that Keans sells 121 plates when the price is \$5 per plate.

64. Demand from marginal demand. Lessard & Company finds that the rate at which the quantity of flameless candles that consumers demand changes with respect to price is given by the marginal-demand function

$$D'(x) = -\frac{4000}{x^2},$$

where x is the price per candle, in dollars. Find the demand function if 1003 candles are demanded by consumers when the price is \$4 per candle.

65. Efficiency of a machine operator. The rate at which a machine operator's efficiency, E (expressed as a percentage), changes with respect to time t is given by

$$\frac{dE}{dt} = 40 - 10t,$$

where t is the number of hours the operator has worked.

a) Find $E(t)$, given that the operator's efficiency after working 3 hr is 56%; that is, $E(3) = 56$.

b) Use the answer to part (a) to find the operator's efficiency after 4 hr; after 7 hr.

66. Efficiency of a machine operator. The rate at which a machine operator's efficiency, E (expressed as a percentage), changes with respect to time t is given by

$$\frac{dE}{dt} = 30 - 10t,$$

where t is the number of hours the operator has worked.

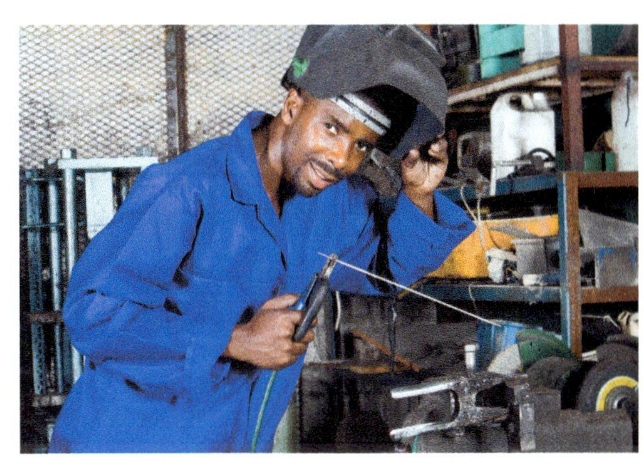

A machine operator's efficiency changes with respect to time.

a) Find $E(t)$, given that the operator's efficiency after working 2 hr is 72%; that is, $E(2) = 72$.

b) Use the answer to part (a) to find the operator's efficiency after 3 hr; after 5 hr.

Social and Life Sciences

67. Memory. In a memory experiment, the rate at which students memorize Spanish vocabulary is estimated by

$$M'(t) = 0.15\sqrt{t} + \frac{0.005}{\sqrt{t}},$$

where $M(t)$ is the number of words memorized in t minutes.

a) Find $M(t)$ if it is known that $M(0) = 0$.

b) How many words are memorized in 1 hr?

68. Heart rate. The rate of change in Trisha's pulse (in beats per minute per minute) t minutes after she stops exercising is given by

$$R'(t) = -46.964e^{-0.796t}.$$

a) Find $R(t)$ if Trisha's pulse is 78 beats per minute 2 min after she has stopped exercising.

b) Find Trisha's pulse rate 4 min after she has stopped exercising.

c) Find the rate of change in Trisha's pulse after 4 min.

d) How can $R(t)$ and $R'(t)$ be used to find Trisha's resting pulse rate?

Physical Sciences

69. Physics: height of an object. A football player punts a football, which leaves his foot 3 ft above the ground and with an initial upward velocity of 70 ft/sec. The vertical velocity of the football t seconds after it is punted is given by

$$v(t) = -32t + 70,$$

where $v(t)$ is in feet per second.

a) Find the function h that gives the height (in feet) of the football after t seconds.
b) What are the height and the velocity of the football after 1.5 sec?
c) After how many seconds does the ball reach its highest point, and how high is the ball at this point?
d) The punt returner catches the football 5 ft above the ground. What is the vertical velocity of the ball at the moment it is being caught?

70. Physics: height of a thrown baseball. A baseball is thrown directly upward with an initial velocity of 75 ft/sec from an initial height of 30 ft. The velocity of the baseball t seconds after being released is given by

$$v(t) = -32t + 75,$$

where $v(t)$ is in feet per second.

a) Find the function h that gives the height (in feet) of the baseball after t seconds.
b) What are the height and the velocity of the baseball 2 sec after it is released?
c) After how many seconds does the ball reach its highest point? (*Hint*: The ball "stops" for an instant before starting its downward fall.)
d) How high is the ball at its highest point?
e) After how many seconds will the ball hit the ground?
f) What is the ball's velocity at the moment it hits the ground?

General Interest

71. Population growth. The rates of change in population for two cities are as follows:

Alphaville: $P'(t) = 45$,

Betaburgh: $Q'(t) = 105e^{0.03t}$,

where t is the number of years since 2010, and both $P'(x)$ and $Q'(x)$ are measured in people per year. In 2010, Alphaville had a population of 5000, and Betaburgh had a population of 3500.

a) Determine a population model for each city.
b) What are the populations of Alphaville and Betaburgh, to the nearest hundred, in 2020?
c) Graph each city's population model, and estimate the year in which the two cities have the same population.

72. Comparing rates of change. Jim is offered a job that will pay him \$50 on the first day, \$100 on the second day, \$150 on the third day, and so on; thus, the rate of change of his pay t days after starting the job is given by $J'(t) = 50$. Larry is offered the same job, but the rate of change of his pay is given by $L'(t) = e^{0.1t}$. Both $J'(t)$ and $L'(t)$ are measured in dollars per day.

a) Determine the total pay model for Jim and for Larry.
b) After 30 days, what are Jim's total pay and Larry's total pay?
c) On what day does Larry's daily pay first exceed Jim's daily pay?
d) In general, how does exponential growth compare to linear growth? Explain.

SYNTHESIS

Exponential and logarithmic base-*a* functions. *Two common antiderivative forms involving a^x and $\log_a x$, (see Section 2.6), are*

$$\int a^x\,dx = \frac{1}{\ln a}a^x + C \quad \text{and} \quad \int \frac{1}{x \ln a}\,dx = \log_a x + C$$

where $x \neq 0$ and $a \neq 1$, $a > 0$. In Exercises 73–80, use these forms to solve each indefinite integral.

73. $\int 3^x\,dx$

74. $\int 5^x\,dx$

75. $\int 1.25^x\,dx$

76. $\int 3.025^x\,dx$

77. $\int 1.48(1.00325)^x\,dx$

78. $\int 2.667(1.0425)^x\,dx$

79. $\int \frac{2}{x \ln 3}\,dx$

80. $\int \frac{5}{x \ln 4}\,dx$

Solve each integral. Solutions can be found using rules developed in this section, but some algebra may be required. State any restrictions on the variable of integration.

81. $\int (5t + 4)^2 t^4\,dt$

82. $\int (x - 1)^2 x^3\,dx$

83. $\int \frac{(t + 3)^2}{\sqrt{t}}\,dt$

84. $\int \frac{x^4 - 6x^2 - 7}{x^3}\,dx$

85. $\int (t + 1)^3\,dt$

86. $\int be^{ax}\,dx$

87. $\int (3x - 5)(2x + 1)^2\,dx$

88. $\int \sqrt[3]{64x^4}\,dx$

89. $\int \frac{x^2 - 1}{x + 1}\,dx$

90. $\int \frac{t^3 + 8}{t + 2}\,dt$

91. $\int \frac{2^x + 3^x}{4^x}\,dx$

92. $\int \frac{1 + 5^x}{3^x}\,dx$

93. On a test, a student makes this statement: "The function given by $f(x) = x^2$ has a unique antiderivative." Is this a true statement? Why or why not?

94. Since $\frac{d}{dx}(4) = 0$, then is it true that $\int 0\,dx = 4$? Why or why not?

Answers to Quick Checks

1. (a) $\frac{1}{11}x^{11} + C$; **(b)** $\frac{6}{7}\sqrt[6]{x^7} + C$; **(c)** $-\frac{1}{3x^3} + C$

2. (a) $-\frac{1}{3}e^{-3x} + C$; **(b)** $2e^{(1/2)x} + C$

3. (a) $\frac{2}{5}x^5 + \frac{3}{4}x^4 - \frac{7}{3}x^3 + C$;

(b) $x - 7\ln x - \frac{2}{x} + C$ **4.** $G(x) = \frac{1}{2}e^{2x} + \frac{5}{2}$

5. 225 ft, −35 ft/sec **6. (a)** $P(t) = 17t^2 + 16t + 640$; **(b)** $P(28) = 14{,}416$ people

4.2 Antiderivatives as Areas

- Find the area under a graph and use it to solve real-world problems.
- Use rectangles to approximate the area under a graph.

Integral calculus studies the *accumulation* of units as the input variable increases. For example, suppose a jogger maintains a constant velocity of 5 mi/hr. As she runs, she "accumulates" distance. After 1 hr, she has run 5 mi. Between the first hour and the second hour, she has run another 5 mi, so that for the first 2 hr, she has accumulated a distance of 10 mi.

We can view accumulations graphically, as shown in the following example.

EXAMPLE 1 Emma drives her motor scooter at 15 mi/hr for an extended period of time.

a) How far has she traveled after 1 hr?

b) How far has she traveled between the first hour and the second hour?

c) How far has she traveled cumulatively over the first 2 hr?

d) What function $f(t)$ gives Emma's total distance traveled after t hours?

Solution Emma's velocity after t hours is given by $v(t) = 15$, where $v(t)$ is in miles per hour. We graph v, noting that its graph is a horizontal line.

a) On the graph, we shade a rectangular area between $t = 0$ and $t = 1$. This area represents $(1\,\text{hr})\left(15\,\frac{\text{mi}}{\text{hr}}\right) = 15\,\text{mi}$. Thus, Emma has traveled 15 mi after 1 hr.

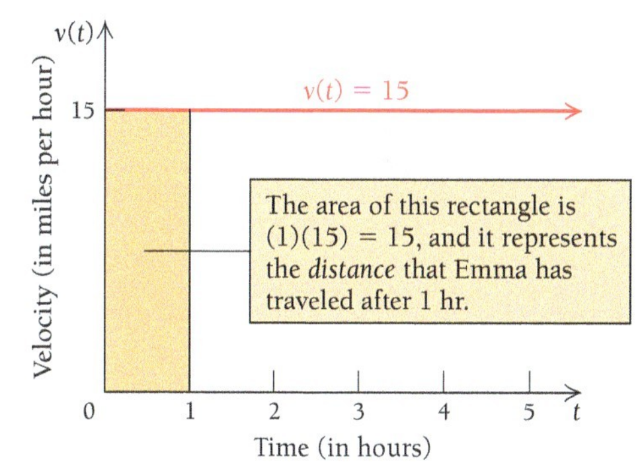

v(t)
15
v(t) = 15
The area of this rectangle is (1)(15) = 15, and it represents the *distance* that Emma has traveled after 1 hr.
Velocity (in miles per hour)
0
1
2
3
4
5
t
Time (in hours)

b) On the graph, we shade a rectangular area between $t = 1$ and $t = 2$. This rectangle has width 1 and height 15. Thus, in this 1-hr period, Emma has traveled another 15 mi.

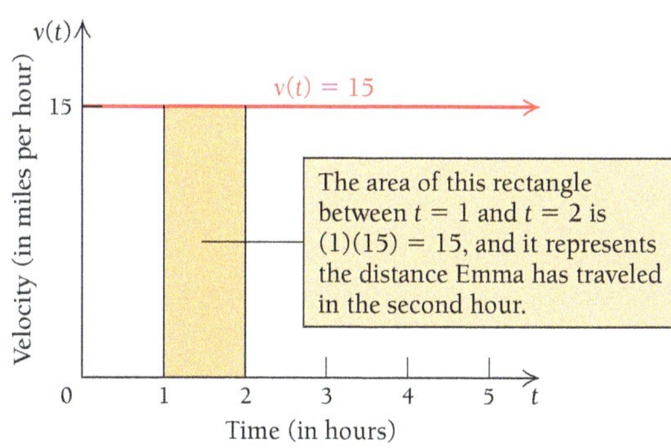

v(t)
15
v(t) = 15
The area of this rectangle between t = 1 and t = 2 is (1)(15) = 15, and it represents the distance Emma has traveled in the second hour.
Velocity (in miles per hour)
0
1
2
3
4
5
t
Time (in hours)

c) Emma has accumulated a total of $15 + 15 = 30$ mi traveled over the first 2 hr. Graphically, her total distance traveled after 2 hr is the area of the rectangle between $t = 0$ and $t = 2$, with width 2 and height 15.

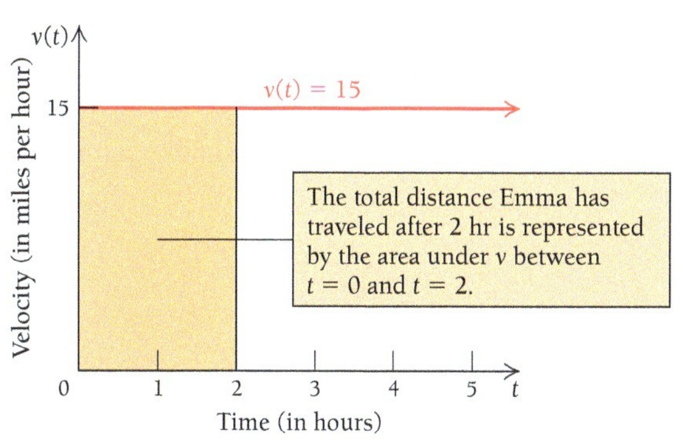

v(t)
15
v(t) = 15
The total distance Emma has traveled after 2 hr is represented by the area under v between t = 0 and t = 2.
Velocity (in miles per hour)
0
1
2
3
4
5
t
Time (in hours)

Quick Check 1 ✓

Green Leaf Skateboards determines that its cost of production is \$40 per skateboard. Find:

a) the cost to produce 10 skateboards;

b) the cost to produce 10 more skateboards;

c) the cumulative cost to produce 20 skateboards; and

d) a function $C(x)$ that gives the *total* cost to produce x skateboards.

d) We set up an input-output table for v, including a third column showing distance traveled in each hour and a fourth column showing total *accumulated* (or *cumulative*) distance traveled:

Time t (in hours)	Velocity, $v(t)$ (in miles per hour)	Distance Traveled in Each Hour	Accumulated Distance Traveled
1	15	15	15
2	15	15	30
3	15	15	45
4	15	15	60

The accumulated distances traveled suggest that $f(t) = 15t$ gives Emma's *total* distance traveled, in miles, after t hours. Note that $f(t) = 15t$ is an antiderivative of $v(t) = 15$. 1 ✓

Geometry and Areas

Example 1 suggests that the antiderivative plays a role in determining area under a graph. For linear functions, we can use geometry to find the area under the graph of a function. Two formulas, where b = base and h = height, are useful:

Area of a rectangle: $A = bh$

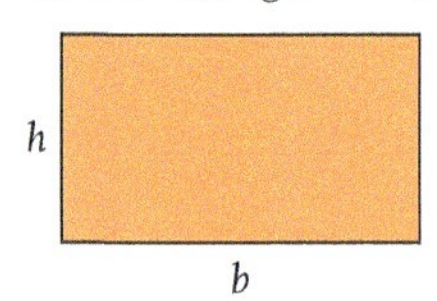

Area of a triangle: $A = \frac{1}{2}bh$

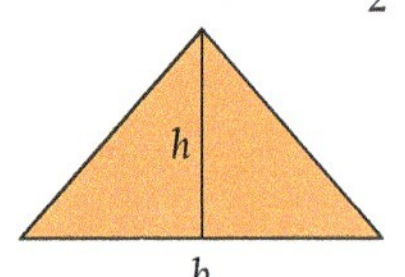

EXAMPLE 2 **Physical Science: Distance as Area.** A toy drone flies in a straight line, and its velocity t seconds after takeoff is given by $v(t) = 2t$, where $v(t)$ is in meters per second.

a) Find the distance the drone has flown after 1 sec.

b) Find the distance the drone has flown between $t = 1$ sec and $t = 2$ sec.

c) Find the cumulative distance the drone has flown over the first 2 sec.

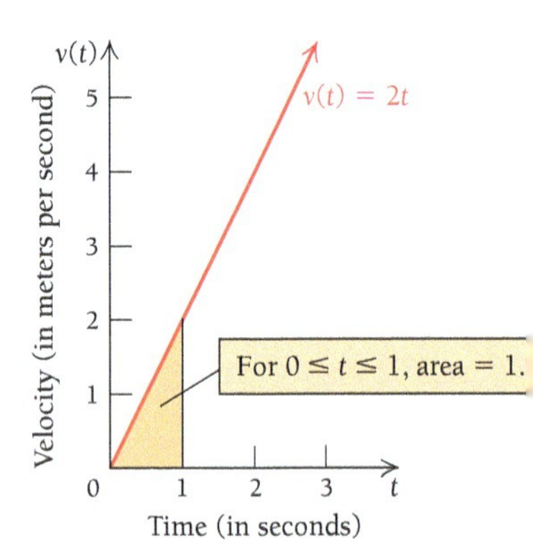

Solution We graph $v(t) = 2t$, noting that it is a linear function. Thus, we can use geometry to find the areas under its graph.

a) To find the distance flown after 1 sec, we form a triangular area under v from $t = 0$ to $t = 1$. The area is given by $A = \frac{1}{2}bh$. Here, $b = 1$ and $h = 2$, so after 1 sec, the drone has flown

$$A = \frac{1}{2}(1\text{ sec})\left(2\,\frac{\text{m}}{\text{sec}}\right) = 1\text{ m}.$$

b) To find the distance traveled between $t = 1$ sec and $t = 2$ sec, we form a trapezoidal area under v over $[1, 2]$. This can be regarded as a rectangle and a triangle, as shown in the figure. The rectangle has area $(1)(2) = 2$, and the triangle has area $\frac{1}{2}(1)(2) = 1$. Thus, the drone has flown a distance of $2 + 1 = 3$ m between $t = 1$ sec and $t = 2$ sec.

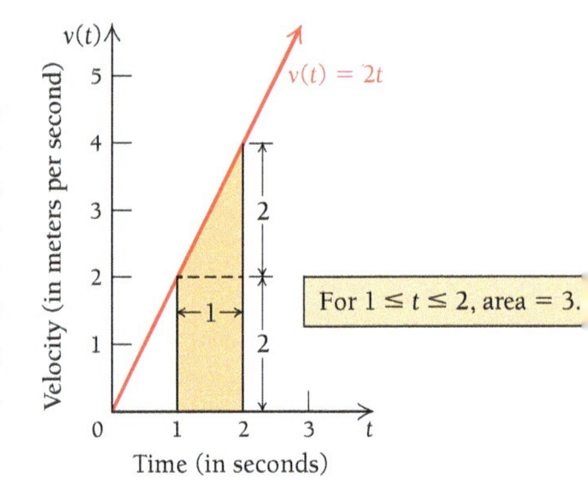

Quick Check 2 ✓

The velocity of a model helicopter is given by $v(t) = 3t$, where t is in seconds and $v(t)$ is in feet per second. Find:

a) the distance the helicopter has flown after 4 sec;

b) the distance the helicopter has flown between $t = 4$ sec and $t = 6$ sec; and

c) the cumulative distance the helicopter has flown over the first 6 sec.

c) The cumulative distance flown after 2 sec is 1 m [from part (a)] plus 3 m [from part (b)], or a total of 4 m. We can also view the cumulative distance as the area of the entire triangle over [0, 2], or $\frac{1}{2}(2)(4) = 4$ m.

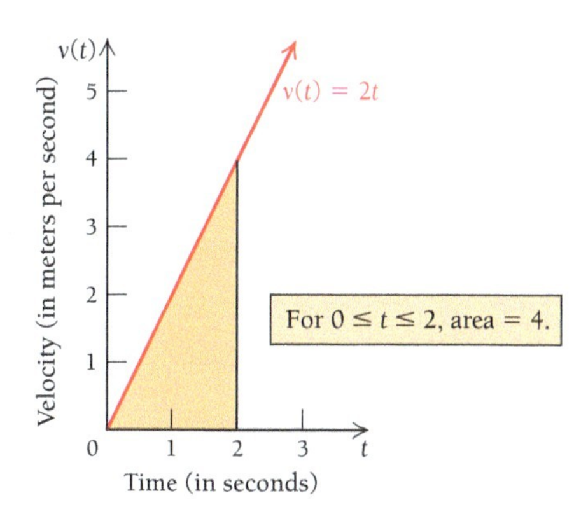

2 ✓

Examples 1 and 2 in this section suggest a pattern:

- The graph of $f(x) = k$, where k is a constant, is a horizontal line of height k. The region under this graph over the interval $[0, x]$ is a rectangle, and its area is $A = kx$ (height times base).

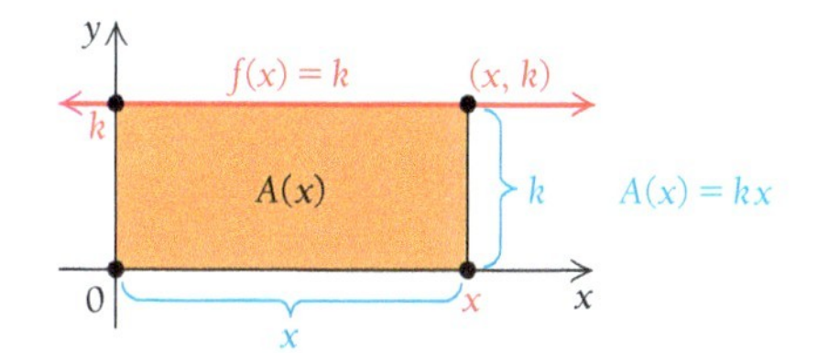

- The graph of $f(x) = mx$ is a line with slope m, passing through the origin. The region under this graph over the interval $[0, x]$ is a triangle, and its area is $A = \frac{1}{2}(x)(mx) = \frac{1}{2}mx^2$.

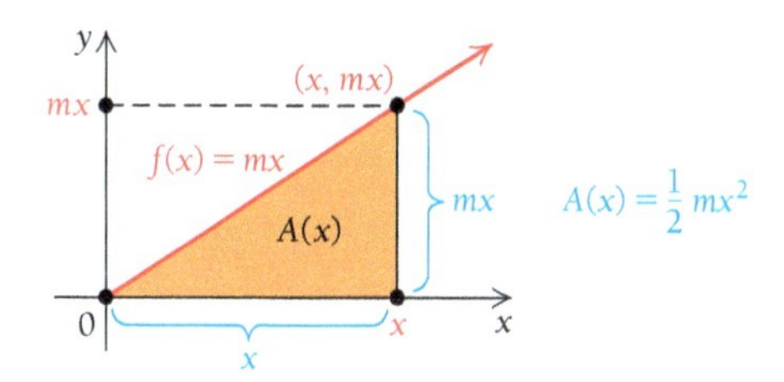

In Example 2, note that the antiderivative of $v(t) = 2t$ is $V(t) = t^2$, and that $V(2) = 2^2 = 4$ is the area under v over [0, 2]. For both Example 1 and Example 2, the area function is an antiderivative of the graphed function. In Section 4.3, we show that this can be generalized. But how do we find areas under curved graphs for which area formulas and antiderivatives are not known? We investigate these questions using geometry, in a procedure called *Riemann summation* (pronounced "Ree-mahn") in honor of the German mathematician G. F. Bernhard Riemann (1826–1866).

EXAMPLE 3 **Business: Total Cost.** Green Leaf Skateboards has the following marginal-cost function for producing skateboards: For up to 50 skateboards, the cost is \$40 per skateboard. For quantities from 51 through 125 skateboards, the cost drops to \$30 per skateboard. After 125 skateboards, it drops to \$25 per skateboard. If x represents the number of skateboards produced, we have

$$C'(x) = \begin{cases} 40, & \text{for } 0 \le x \le 50, \\ 30, & \text{for } 50 < x \le 125, \\ 25, & \text{for } 125 < x, \end{cases}$$

where $C'(x)$ is the cost per skateboard, in dollars. Find the total cost of producing 150 skateboards.

Solution We calculate the areas of the rectangles formed under the graph of C' over the intervals [0, 50], [50, 125], and [125, 150].

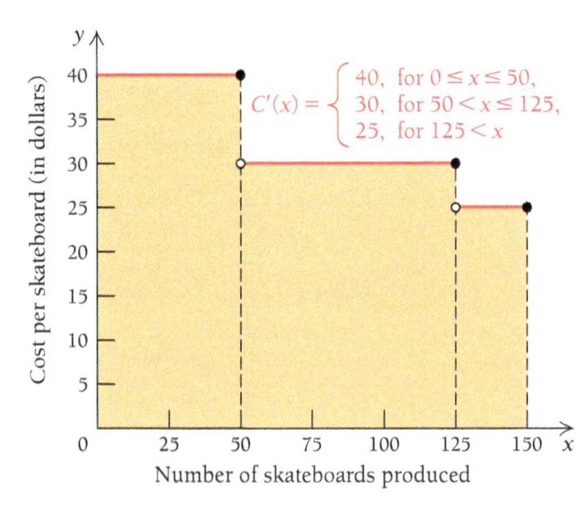

The total cost of producing 150 skateboards is the sum of these three areas:

$$\text{Total cost} = (40)(50) + (30)(75) + (25)(25) = \$4875.$$

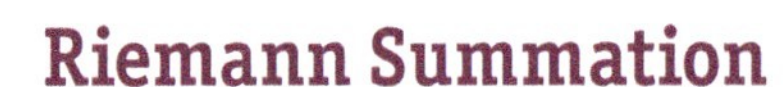

Riemann Summation

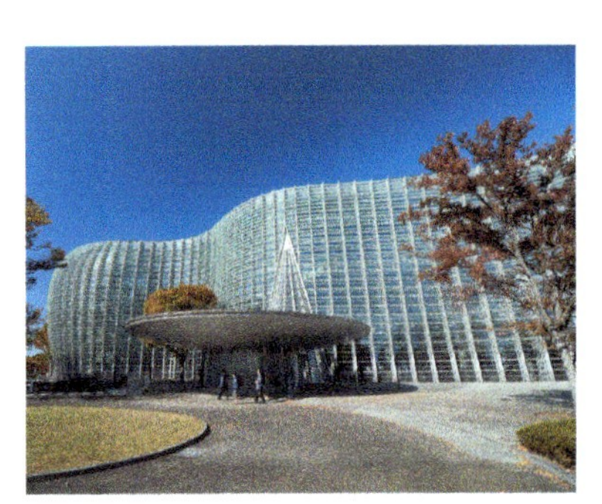

The area under a curve can be approximated by a sum of rectangular areas.

In **Riemann summation**, rectangles can be used to approximate the area under the graph of a continuous function.

In the following figure, $[a, b]$ is divided into four subintervals, each having width $\Delta x = (b - a)/4$.

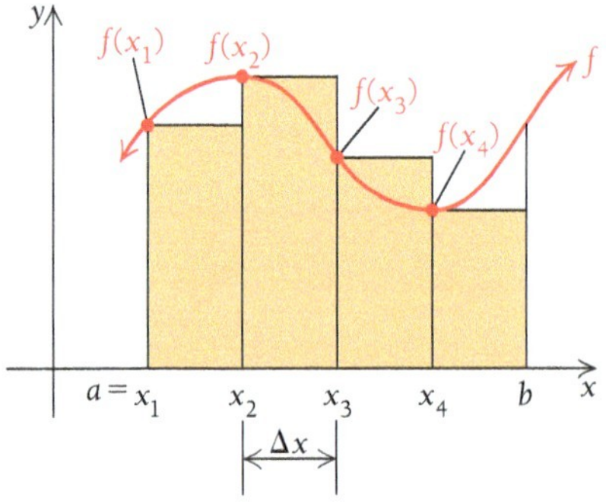

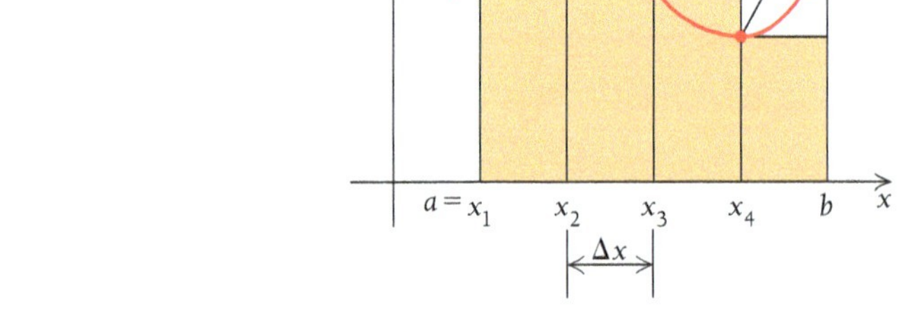

The heights of the rectangles shown are $f(x_1)$, $f(x_2)$, $f(x_3)$, and $f(x_4)$, and the area of the region under the curve is approximately the sum of the areas of the four rectangles:

$$f(x_1)\,\Delta x + f(x_2)\,\Delta x + f(x_3)\,\Delta x + f(x_4)\,\Delta x. \qquad \text{This is a Riemann sum.}$$

We can denote this sum with **summation**, or **sigma**, **notation**, which uses the Greek capital letter sigma, Σ:

$$\sum_{i=1}^{4} f(x_i)\,\Delta x.$$

This is read "the sum of the product $f(x_i)\,\Delta x$ from $i = 1$ to $i = 4$." To recover the original expression, we substitute the numbers 1 through 4 successively for i in $f(x_i)\,\Delta x$ and write plus signs between the results.

Before we continue, let's consider some examples involving summation notation.

Quick Check 3 ✓

Express $\sum_{i=1}^{6} (i^2 + i)$ without using summation notation.

EXAMPLE 4 Express $\sum_{i=1}^{5} h(x_i)\Delta x$ without using summation notation.

Solution We have

$$\sum_{i=1}^{5} h(x_i)\Delta x = h(x_1)\Delta x + h(x_2)\Delta x + h(x_3)\Delta x + h(x_4)\Delta x + h(x_5)\Delta x.$$ **3 ✓**

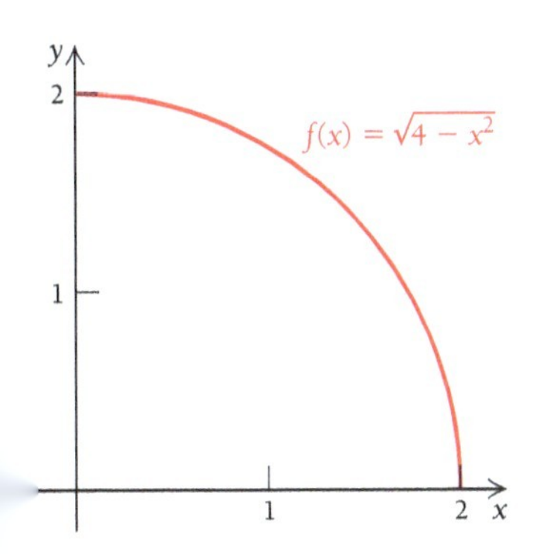

EXAMPLE 5 Consider the graph of $f(x) = \sqrt{4 - x^2}$ over the interval $[0, 2]$. This is a quarter-circle of radius 2. Use a Riemann sum to approximate the area under the graph using 4 equally sized subintervals and then 8 equally sized subintervals. Then use geometry to find the area under f over $[0, 2]$, and compare this value to your approximations.

Solution Dividing $[0, 2]$ into 4 subintervals of equal width, we have

$$\Delta x = \frac{2-0}{4} = \frac{1}{2}. \qquad \text{This is the width of each rectangle.}$$

We then let x_i range from $x_1 = 0$ to $x_4 = \frac{3}{2}$ in increments of $\frac{1}{2}$. The area under the graph of f is then approximately

$$\begin{aligned}\sum_{i=1}^{4} f(x_i)\,\Delta x &= f(0)\cdot\frac{1}{2} + f\left(\frac{1}{2}\right)\cdot\frac{1}{2} + f(1)\cdot\frac{1}{2} + f\left(\frac{3}{2}\right)\cdot\frac{1}{2}\\ &= \frac{1}{2}\left(f(0) + f\left(\frac{1}{2}\right) + f(1) + f\left(\frac{3}{2}\right)\right) && \text{Factoring}\\ &\approx \frac{1}{2}(2 + 1.93649 + 1.73205 + 1.32288) && \text{Using a calculator}\\ &= \frac{1}{2}(6.99142)\\ &= 3.49571.\end{aligned}$$

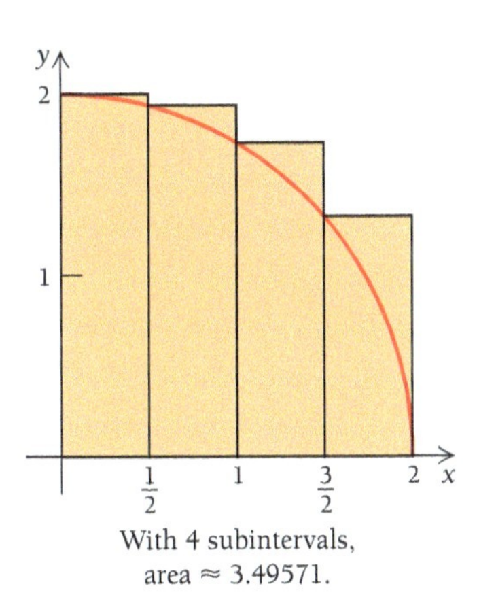

With 4 subintervals, area ≈ 3.49571.

Thus, the area under f over $[0, 2]$ is approximately 3.49571 square units. Note that this approximation is greater than the actual area of the quarter-circle.

Dividing $[0, 2]$ into 8 subintervals of equal width, we have $\Delta x = \frac{2-0}{8} = \frac{1}{4}$, with x_i ranging from $x_1 = 0$ to $x_8 = \frac{7}{4}$ in increments of $\frac{1}{4}$. This gives another approximation of the area under the graph:

$$\begin{aligned}\sum_{i=1}^{8} f(x_i)\,\Delta x &= f(0)\cdot\frac{1}{4} + f\left(\frac{1}{4}\right)\cdot\frac{1}{4} + f\left(\frac{1}{2}\right)\cdot\frac{1}{4} + f\left(\frac{3}{4}\right)\cdot\frac{1}{4} + f(1)\cdot\frac{1}{4}\\ &\quad + f\left(\frac{5}{4}\right)\cdot\frac{1}{4} + f\left(\frac{3}{2}\right)\cdot\frac{1}{4} + f\left(\frac{7}{4}\right)\cdot\frac{1}{4}\\ &= \frac{1}{4}\left(f(0) + f\left(\frac{1}{4}\right) + f\left(\frac{1}{2}\right) + f\left(\frac{3}{4}\right) + f(1) + f\left(\frac{5}{4}\right)\right.\\ &\quad \left. + f\left(\frac{3}{2}\right) + f\left(\frac{7}{4}\right)\right)\\ &\approx \frac{1}{4}(2 + 1.98431 + 1.93649 + 1.85405 + 1.73205 + 1.56125\\ &\quad + 1.32288 + 0.96825)\\ &= 3.33982.\end{aligned}$$

Using 8 subintervals, we have refined the estimate of the area under f over $[0, 2]$ to 3.33982 square units. This approximation is still greater than the actual area of the quarter-circle, but the difference is less than when we used 4 subintervals.

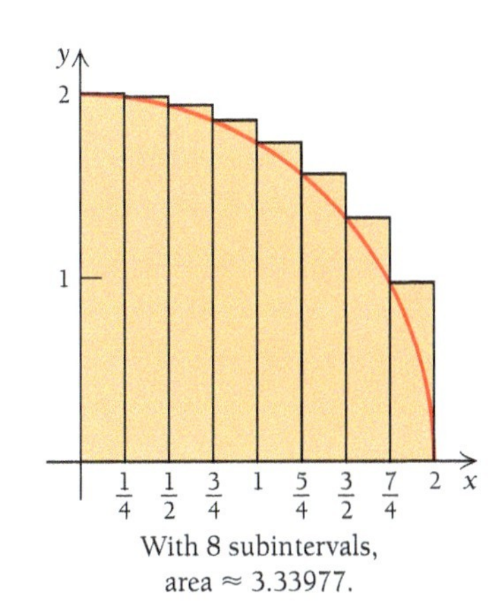

With 8 subintervals, area ≈ 3.33977.

Quick Check 4 ✓

Consider the graph of $g(x) = \sqrt{x}$ over the interval [0, 9]. Use Riemann sums to approximate the area under the graph of g using **(a)** 3 equally sized subintervals and **(b)** 9 equally sized subintervals.

The graph of $f(x) = \sqrt{4 - x^2}$ over [0, 2] is a quarter-circle of radius 2. Using geometry, the area of a circle of radius 2 is $A = \pi(2)^2 = 4\pi$. Dividing by 4, the area under the graph of $f(x) = \sqrt{4 - x^2}$ over [0, 2] is $4\pi/4 = \pi \approx 3.1415926$. The approximations are close, but the better approximation was found using more subintervals of smaller width. 4 ✓

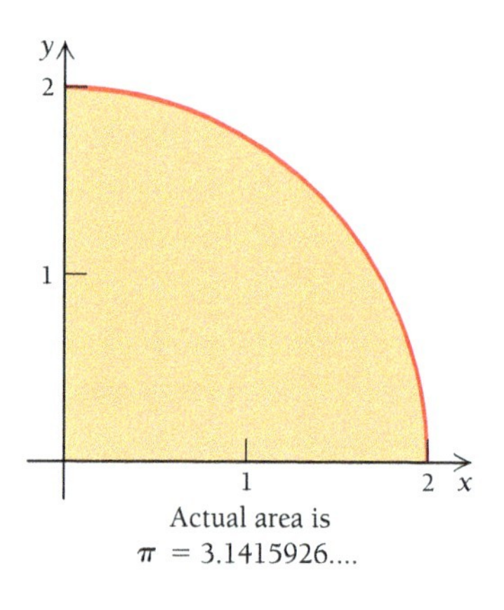

Actual area is $\pi = 3.1415926....$

EXAMPLE 6 Use 5 subintervals to approximate the area under the graph of $f(x) = 0.1x^3 - 2.3x^2 + 12x + 25$ over the interval [1, 16].

Solution We divide [1, 16] into 5 subintervals of size $\Delta x = (16 - 1)/5 = 3$, with x_i ranging from $x_1 = 1$ to $x_5 = 13$ in increments of 3, as shown below.

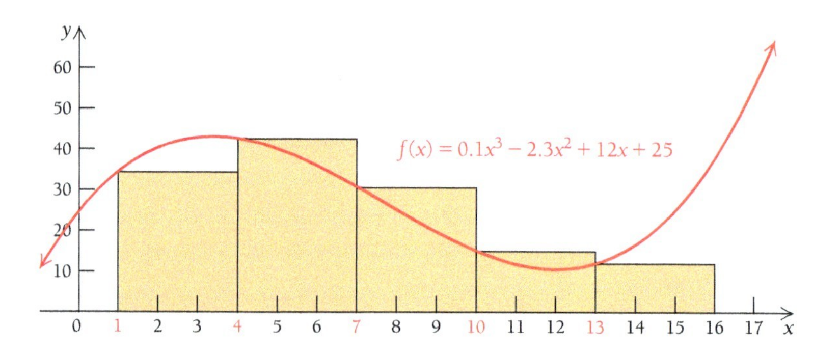

The area under the curve from 1 to 16 is approximately

$$\begin{aligned}\sum_{i=1}^{5} f(x_i)\,\Delta x &= f(1)\cdot 3 + f(4)\cdot 3 + f(7)\cdot 3 + f(10)\cdot 3 + f(13)\cdot 3 \\ &= 3(34.8 + 42.6 + 30.6 + 15 + 12) \\ &= 405.\end{aligned}$$

5 ✓

Quick Check 5 ✓

Use 6 subintervals to approximate the area under the graph of the function in Example 6 over the interval [0, 12].

Definite Integrals

The key concept being developed in this section is that the more subintervals we use, the more accurate the approximation of area becomes. As the number of subdivisions n increases, the width of each rectangle, Δx, decreases. If n approaches infinity, then Δx approaches 0, and the Riemann sum approaches the exact area under the graph. The *exact* area under the graph of a continuous function $y = f(x)$ over an interval $[a, b]$ is given by a *definite integral*.

DEFINITION

Let $y = f(x)$ be continuous and nonnegative over an interval $[a, b]$. A **definite integral** is the limit as $n \to \infty$ (equivalently, $\Delta x \to 0$) of the Riemann sum of the areas of rectangles under the graph of $y = f(x)$ over $[a, b]$.

$$\text{Exact area} = \lim_{\Delta x \to 0} \sum_{i=1}^{n} f(x_i)\cdot \Delta x = \int_a^b f(x)\,dx.$$

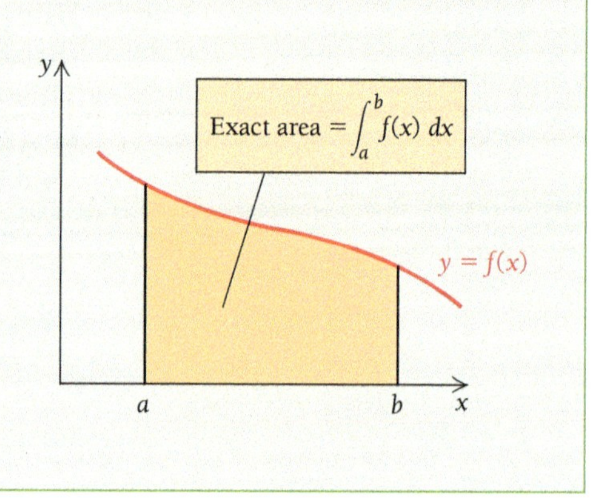

Notice that the summation symbol becomes an integral sign (the elongated "s" is Leibniz notation representing "sum") and Δx becomes dx. The interval endpoints a and b are placed at the bottom and top, respectively, of the integral sign.

For $f(x) \geq 0$ over $[a, b]$, *the definite integral represents area.* The definite integral is also defined for $f(x) < 0$. We will discuss its interpretation in Section 4.3.

We can use geometry to determine the value of some definite integrals, as the following example suggests.

EXAMPLE 7 Find the value of $\int_0^2 (3x + 2)\, dx$.

Solution We sketch the graph over the interval [0, 2] and note that the region is a trapezoid. Thus, we can use geometry to determine this area.

Using the method of Example 2(b), we find that the area is 10. Therefore,

$$\int_0^2 (3x + 2)\, dx = 2 \cdot 2 + \frac{1}{2} \cdot 2 \cdot 6$$
$$= 10.$$

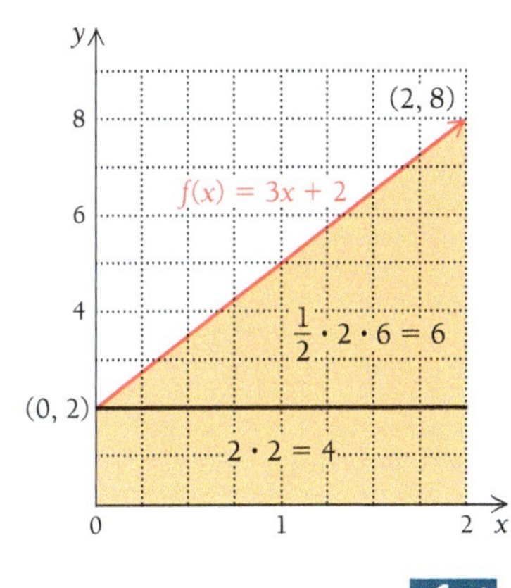

6 ✓

Quick Check 6 ✓

Use geometry to determine the values of these definite integrals:

a) $\int_0^3 (x + 1)\, dx$;

b) $\int_4^7 (15 - 2x)\, dx$.

Section Summary

- The area under a curve can often be interpreted as an accumulation of smaller units of area.
- Geometry can be used to find areas of regions formed by graphs of linear functions.
- *Riemann summation* uses rectangles to approximate the area under the graph of a function. The more rectangles, the better the approximation.
- The *definite integral*, $\int_a^b f(x)\, dx$, represents the exact area under the graph of a continuous function $y = f(x)$, where $f(x) \geq 0$, over the interval $[a, b]$.

4.2 Exercise Set

In Exercises 1–14, use geometry to evaluate each definite integral.

1. $\int_0^2 2\, dx$

2. $\int_0^5 6\, dx$

3. $\int_2^6 3\, dx$

4. $\int_{-1}^4 4\, dx$

5. $\int_0^3 x\, dx$

6. $\int_0^5 4x\, dx$

7. $\int_0^{10} \frac{1}{2}x\, dx$

8. $\int_0^5 (2x + 5)\, dx$

9. $\int_1^5 3x\, dx$

10. $\int_2^7 \frac{1}{4}x\, dx$

11. $\int_0^6 (2x + 3)\, dx$

12. $\int_0^{10} (4x + 1)\, dx$

13. $\int_0^3 \sqrt{9 - x^2}\, dx$

14. $\int_{-4}^4 \sqrt{16 - x^2}\, dx$

15. Lillian hikes at a constant pace; her velocity is given by $v(t) = 3$, where t is in hours and $v(t)$ is in miles per hour.

a) How far did she hike in the first 1 hr?

b) How far did she hike between $t = 1$ hr and $t = 2$ hr?

c) What is the cumulative distance she has hiked after 2 hr?

16. Paul rides his bicycle at a constant speed; his velocity is given by $v(t) = 12$, where t is in hours and $v(t)$ is in miles per hour.

a) How far did he ride in the first 2 hr?

b) How far did he ride between $t = 2$ hr and $t = 4$ hr?

c) What is the cumulative distance he has ridden after 4 hr?

17. Physical science: falling object. The velocity of a falling object on Earth can be approximated by $v(t) = 9.8t$, where t is in seconds and $v(t)$ is in meters per second.

a) How far has an object fallen 1 sec after being dropped on Earth?

b) How far does the object fall between $t = 1$ sec and $t = 2$ sec?

c) What is the cumulative distance the object has fallen after 2 sec?

18. Physical science: falling object. The velocity of a falling object on the moon is given by $v(t) = 1.62t$, where t is in seconds and $v(t)$ is in meters per second.

a) How far has an object fallen 3 sec after being dropped on the moon?

b) How far does the object fall between $t = 3$ sec and $t = 5$ sec?

c) What is the cumulative distance the object has fallen after 5 sec?

19. a) Approximate the area under the following graph of $f(x) = \frac{1}{x^2}$ over the interval [1, 7] by computing the area of each rectangle to four decimal places and then adding.

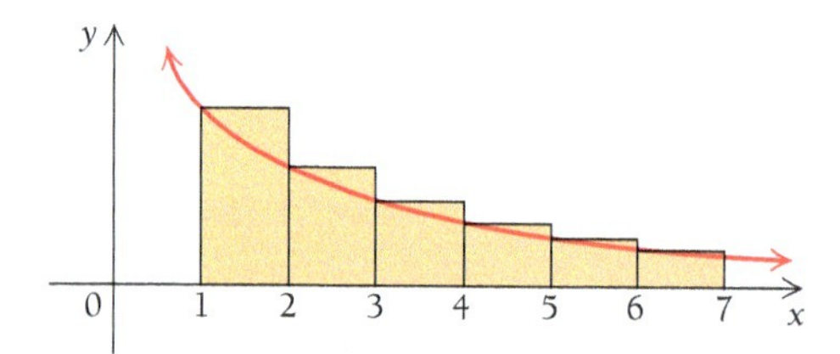

b) Approximate the area under the graph of $f(x) = \frac{1}{x^2}$ over the interval [1, 7] by computing the area of each rectangle to four decimal places and then adding. Compare your answer to that for part (a).

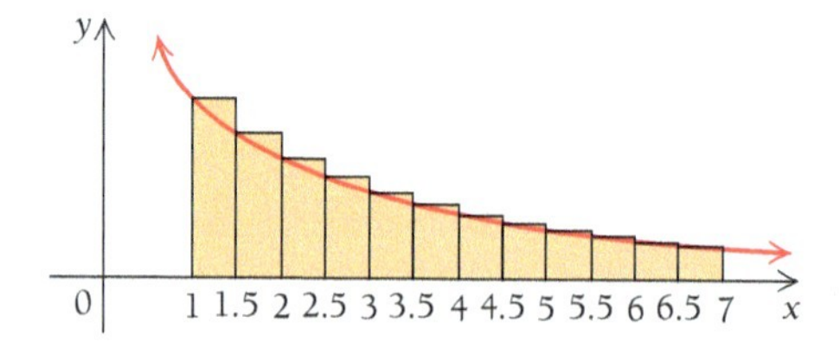

20. a) Approximate the area under the graph of $f(x) = x^2 + 1$ over the interval [0, 5] by computing the area of each rectangle and then adding.

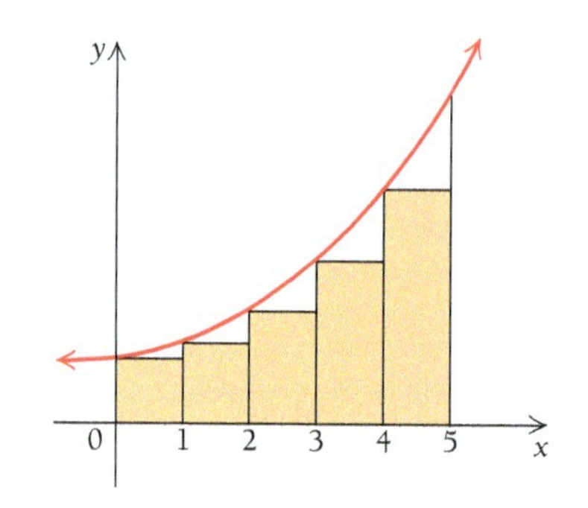

b) Approximate the area under the graph of $f(x) = x^2 + 1$ over the interval [0, 5] by computing the area of each rectangle and then adding. Compare your answer to that for part (a).

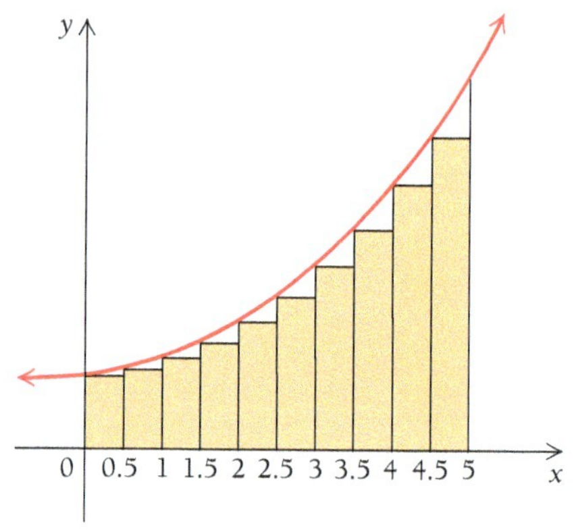

21. Approximate the area under the graph of

$$f(x) = 0.01x^4 - 1.44x^2 + 60$$

over the interval [2, 10] using 4 subintervals.

22. Approximate the area under the graph of

$$g(x) = -0.02x^4 + 0.28x^3 - 0.3x^2 + 20$$

over the interval [3, 12] using 4 subintervals.

23. Approximate the area under the graph of

$$F(x) = 0.2x^3 + 2x^2 - 0.2x - 2$$

over the interval $[-8, -3]$ using 5 subintervals.

24. Approximate the area under the graph of

$$G(x) = 0.1x^3 + 1.2x^2 - 0.4x - 4.8$$

over the interval $[-10, -4]$ using 6 subintervals.

25. Approximate the area under the graph of $H(x) = 50e^{0.04x}$ over the interval [0, 18] using 6 subintervals.

26. Approximate the area under the graph of $K(x) = \ln x$ over the interval [1, 11] using 5 subintervals.

APPLICATIONS

Business and Economics

In Exercises 27–44, calculate total cost (disregarding any fixed costs) or total profit.

27. Total profit from marginal profit. A concert promoter sells x tickets and has a marginal-profit function given by

$$P'(x) = 2x - 150,$$

where $P'(x)$ is in dollars per ticket. This means that the rate of change of total profit with respect to the number of tickets sold, x, is $P'(x)$. Find the total profit from the sale of the 75th ticket through the 300th ticket.

28. Total profit from marginal profit. Poyse Inc. has a marginal-profit function given by

$$P'(x) = -2x + 80,$$

where $P'(x)$ is in dollars per unit. This means that the rate of change of total profit with respect to the number of units produced, x, is $P'(x)$. Find the total profit from the production and sale of the first 40 units.

29. **Total cost from marginal cost.** Sylvie's Old World Cheeses has found that its marginal cost, in dollars per kilogram, is

$$C'(x) = -0.003x + 4.25, \quad \text{for } x \le 500,$$

where x is the number of kilograms of cheese produced. Find the total cost of producing 400 kg of cheese.

30. **Total cost from marginal cost.** Redline Roasting has found that its marginal cost, in dollars per pound, is

$$C'(x) = -0.012x + 6.50, \quad \text{for } x \le 300,$$

where x is the number of pounds of coffee roasted. Find the total cost of roasting 200 lb of coffee.

31. **Total cost from marginal cost.** Cleo's Custom Fabrics has found that its marginal cost, in dollars per yard, is

$$C'(x) = -0.007x + 12, \quad \text{for } x \le 350,$$

where x is the number of yards of fabric produced. Find the total cost of producing 200 yd of this fabric.

32. **Total cost from marginal cost.** Photos from Nature has found that its marginal cost, in cents per card, is

$$C'(x) = -0.04x + 85, \quad \text{for } x \le 1000,$$

where x is the number of cards produced. Find the total cost of producing 650 cards.

33. **Total cost from marginal cost.** Raggs, Ltd., determines that its marginal cost, in dollars per dress, is given by

$$C'(x) = -\frac{2}{25}x + 50, \quad \text{for } x \le 450.$$

Find the total cost of producing the first 200 dresses.

34. **Total cost from marginal cost.** Using the information and answer from Exercise 33, find the cost of producing the 201st dress through the 400th dress.

35. **Total cost from marginal cost.** Beuerlein Industries has found that its marginal cost, in dollars per yard, is

$$C'(x) = -0.015x + 15.50,$$

where x is the number of yards of audio cable produced. Find the total cost of producing 200 yards of audio cable.

36. **Total cost from marginal cost.** Stevens Bakery has found that its marginal cost, in dollars per wedding cake, is

$$C'(x) = -0.12x + 40,$$

where x is the number of wedding cakes produced. Find the total cost of producing 50 wedding cakes.

37. **Total profit from marginal profit.** Holcomb Hill Fitness has found that its marginal profit, $P'(x)$, in cents, is given by

$$P'(x) = -0.0006x^3 + 0.28x^2 + 55.6x, \quad \text{for } x \le 500,$$

where x is the number of members currently enrolled at the health club.

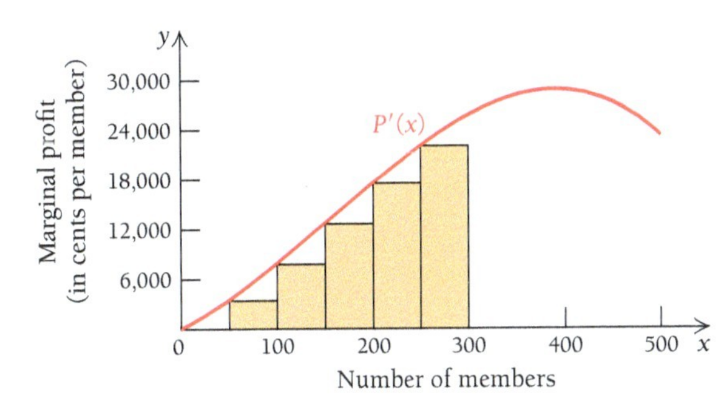

Approximate the total profit when 300 members are enrolled by computing

$$\sum_{i=1}^{6} P'(x_i)\,\Delta x, \quad \text{with} \quad \Delta x = 50.$$

38. **Total cost from marginal cost.** Raggs, Ltd., has found that its marginal cost, in dollars, for the xth jacket produced is given by

$$C'(x) = 0.0003x^2 - 0.2x + 50.$$

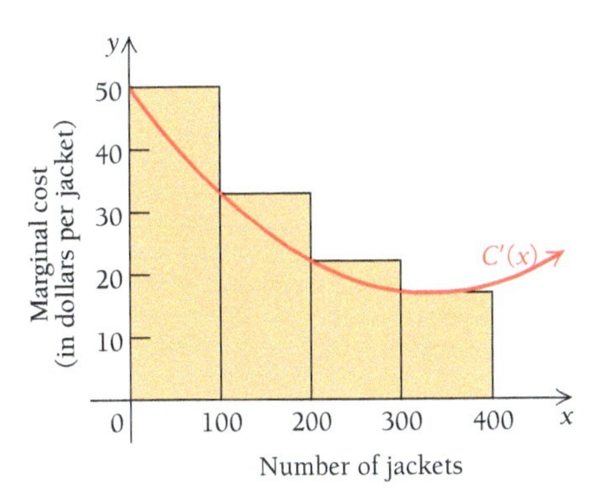

Approximate the total cost of producing 400 jackets by computing

$$\sum_{i=1}^{4} C'(x_i)\,\Delta x, \quad \text{with } \Delta x = 100.$$

39. **Total cost from marginal cost.** Ship Shape Woodworkers has found that the marginal cost of producing x feet of custom molding is given by

$$C'(x) = -0.00002x^2 - 0.04x + 45, \quad \text{for } x \le 800,$$

where $C'(x)$ is in cents. Approximate the total cost of manufacturing 800 ft of molding, using 5 subintervals over $[0, 800]$ and the left endpoint of each subinterval.

40. **Total cost from marginal cost.** Soulful Scents has found that the marginal cost of producing x ounces of a new fragrance is given by

$$C'(x) = 0.0005x^2 - 0.1x + 30, \quad \text{for } x \le 125,$$

where $C'(x)$ is in dollars. Use 5 subintervals over $[0, 100]$ and the left endpoint of each subinterval to approximate the total cost of producing 100 oz of the fragrance.

41. **Total cost from marginal cost.** Shelly's Roadside Fruit has found that the marginal cost of producing x pints of fresh-squeezed orange juice is given by

$$C'(x) = 0.000008x^2 - 0.004x + 2, \quad \text{for } x \le 350,$$

where $C'(x)$ is in dollars. Approximate the total cost of producing 270 pt of juice, using 3 subintervals over $[0, 270]$ and the left endpoint of each subinterval.

42. **Total cost from marginal cost.** Mangianello Paving, Inc., has found that the marginal cost, in dollars, of paving a road surface with asphalt is given by

$$C'(x) = \frac{1}{6}x^2 - 20x + 1800, \quad \text{for } x \le 80,$$

where x is measured in hundreds of feet. Use 4 subintervals over $[0, 40]$ and the left endpoint of each subinterval to approximate the total cost of paving 4000 ft of road surface.

43. **Total cost from marginal cost.** Henson Hatmakers finds that the marginal cost of manufacturing x baseball caps is given by

$$C'(x) = \begin{cases} 6.50, & 0 \le x \le 20 \\ 5.50, & 20 < x \le 35 \\ 3.75, & x > 35, \end{cases}$$

where $C'(x)$ is in dollars per cap. The price breaks are not retroactive; that is, if 25 caps are manufactured, the first 20 are produced at \$6.50 per cap, and the next 5 at \$5.50 per cap. Find the total cost of manufacturing 60 caps.

44. **Total cost from marginal cost.** Steve's Airport Shuttle charges customers a fixed rate per mile, with certain price breaks that are not retroactive. The marginal cost of transporting a passenger x miles is given by

$$C'(x) = \begin{cases} 0.80, & 0 \le x \le 100 \\ 0.60, & 100 < x \le 150 \\ 0.45, & x > 150, \end{cases}$$

where $C'(x)$ is in dollars per mile. Find the total cost of transporting a passenger 200 mi.

SYNTHESIS

Use geometry to evaluate each definite integral.

45. $\int_{-4}^{6} |x|\,dx$

46. $\int_{-3}^{7} |x|\,dx$

47. $\int_{0}^{10} |x - 4|\,dx$

48. $\int_{-2}^{12} |x - 5|\,dx$

49. Use the following graph of $y = f(x)$ to evaluate each definite integral.

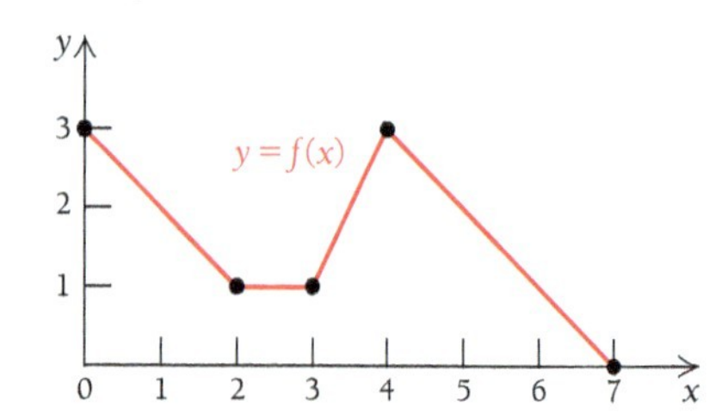

a) $\int_{0}^{2} f(x)\,dx$

b) $\int_{2}^{3} f(x)\,dx$

c) $\int_{3}^{4} f(x)\,dx$

d) $\int_{4}^{7} f(x)\,dx$

e) Use the results from parts (a)–(d) to evaluate $\int_{0}^{7} f(x)\,dx$.

50. Use geometry and the following graph of $f(x) = \frac{1}{2}x$ to evaluate each definite integral.

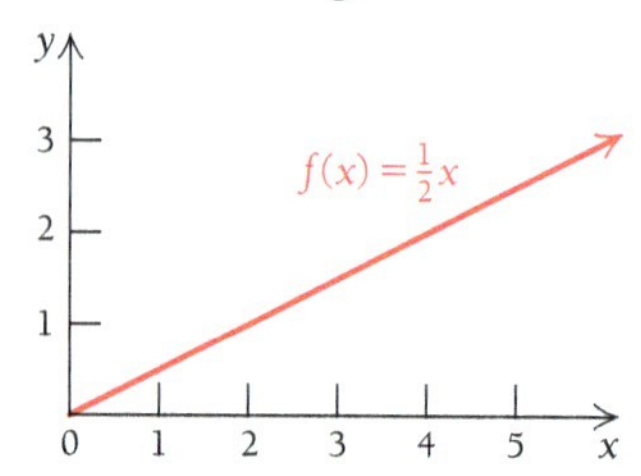

a) $\int_{0}^{1} f(x)\,dx$

b) $\int_{1}^{3} f(x)\,dx$

c) Find c such that $\int_{0}^{c} f(x)\,dx = 4$.

d) Find c such that $\int_{0}^{c} f(x)\,dx = 3$.

51. When using Riemann summation to approximate the area under the graph of a function, is it necessary to construct rectangles that have their upper-left corners touching the graph? Would the method work if their upper-right corners touched the graph instead? Why or why not?

52. When using Riemann summation to approximate the area under the graph of a function, is it necessary to divide the interval $[a, b]$ into subintervals of equal width? Why or why not?

Technology Connection 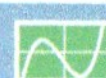

It can be shown that the exact area under the graph of $y = b - x^2$ over the interval $[0, \sqrt{b}]$ is given by $A = \frac{2}{3}b\sqrt{b}$. Use this formula in Exercises 53 and 54.

53. Let $\int_{0}^{3} (9 - x^2)\,dx$. Approximate the area using 6 subintervals; then use the formula to find the exact area.

54. Let $\int_{0}^{5} (25 - x^2)\,dx$. Approximate the area using 10 subintervals; then use the formula to find the exact area.

Answers to Quick Checks

1. **(a)** \$400; **(b)** \$400; **(c)** \$800; **(d)** $C(x) = 40x$
2. **(a)** 24 ft; **(b)** 30 ft; **(c)** 54 ft **3.** 112
4. **(a)** 12.545 square units; **(b)** 16.306 square units
5. 368 **6.** **(a)** 7.5; **(b)** 12

4.3 Area and Definite Integrals

- Find the area under the graph of a nonnegative function over a given closed interval.
- Evaluate a definite integral.
- Solve applied problems involving definite integrals.

In Sections 4.1 and 4.2, we considered examples in which we showed a relationship between the area under the graph of a function f and the function's antiderivative, F. In this section, we show that this relationship is true for any continuous function over a closed interval. This result is known as the *Fundamental Theorem of Calculus*.

The Fundamental Theorem of Calculus

The area under the graph of a nonnegative continuous function f over an interval $[a, b]$ is determined by an area function A, which is an antiderivative of f; that is, $\frac{d}{dx}A(x) = f(x)$. We have established this fact for cases in which f is a constant or linear function by using formulas for areas of a rectangle and a triangle. When the graph of f is a curve, we can approximate the area under the graph using a Riemann sum, which suggests a general method for calculating the area under the graph of *any* nonnegative continuous function f.

In Section 4.2, we found that the area under the graph of $f(x) = k$ is given by $A(x) = kx$ and the area under the graph of $f(x) = mx$ is given by $A(x) = \frac{1}{2}mx^2$. In both cases, the derivative of the area function, $A(x)$, is $f(x)$. Is this always the case?

To answer this, we let $A(x)$ represent the area under a nonnegative continuous function f over the interval $[0, x]$. To find $A'(x)$, we use the definition of derivative:

$$A'(x) = \lim_{h \to 0} \frac{A(x + h) - A(x)}{h}.$$

Since the area under f over $[0, x + h]$ is $A(x + h)$, it follows that the area under f between x and $x + h$ is $A(x + h) - A(x)$.

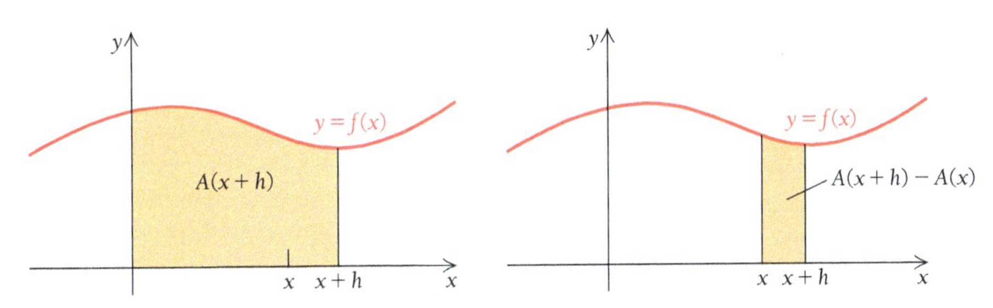

The area represented by $A(x + h) - A(x)$ can be approximated by a rectangle with width h and height $f(x)$. That is, for small values of h,

$$A(x + h) - A(x) \approx h \cdot f(x).$$

Thus, $$\frac{A(x + h) - A(x)}{h} \approx f(x).$$ Dividing both sides by h

As h approaches 0, the approximation becomes more exact. Taking the limit of both sides, we have

$$\lim_{h \to 0} \frac{A(x + h) - A(x)}{h} = \lim_{h \to 0} f(x).$$

Since $\lim_{h \to 0} f(x) = f(x)$, we see that $A'(x) = f(x)$. We have proved the following:

THEOREM 4

Let f be a nonnegative continuous function over $[0, b]$, and let $A(x)$ be the area between the graph of f and the x-axis over $[0, x]$, with $0 < x < b$. Then $A(x)$ is a differentiable function of x and $A'(x) = f(x)$.

y = f(x)

A(a)

A(b) − A(a)

Theorem 4 answers the question posed earlier: The derivative of the area function is always the function under which the area is being calculated. We now adapt Theorem 4 for cases in which f is defined over *any* interval $[a, b]$. Referring to the graph on the left, we see that the area over $[a, b]$ is the same as the area over $[0, b]$ minus the area over $[0, a]$, or $A(b) - A(a)$.

In Section 4.1, we found that a function's antiderivatives can differ only by a constant. Thus, if F is another antiderivative of f, then $A(x) = F(x) + C$, for some constant C, and

$$\text{Area} = A(b) - A(a) = F(b) + C - (F(a) + C) = F(b) - F(a).$$

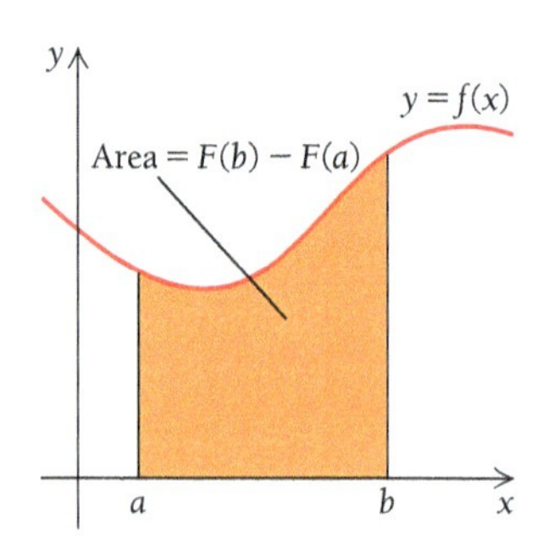

This result tells us that as long as an area is computed by substituting an interval's endpoints into an antiderivative and then subtracting, *any* antiderivative—and any choice of C—can be used. It generally simplifies computations to choose 0 as the value of C.

EXAMPLE 1 Find the area under the graph of $f(x) = \frac{1}{5}x^2 + 3$ over $[2, 5]$.

Solution Although making a drawing is not required, doing so helps us visualize the problem. The interval is $[2, 5]$, so we have $a = 2$ and $b = 5$.

Note that every antiderivative of $f(x) = \frac{1}{5}x^2 + 3$ is of the form

$$F(x) = \tfrac{1}{15}x^3 + 3x + C.$$

Check: $$\frac{d}{dx}\left[\frac{1}{15}x^3 + 3x + C\right] = \frac{1}{5}x^2 + 3 = f(x)$$

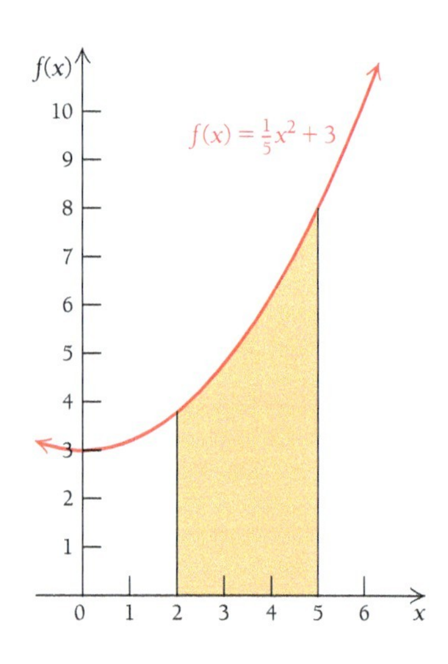

For simplicity, we set $C = 0$, so that $F(x) = \frac{1}{15}x^3 + 3x$ and

$$\begin{aligned}
\text{Area over } [2, 5] &= F(5) - F(2) \\
&= \tfrac{1}{15}(5)^3 + 3(5) - \left[\tfrac{1}{15}(2)^3 + 3(2)\right] && \text{Evaluating the antiderivative at the endpoints} \\
&= \left(\tfrac{125}{15} + 15\right) - \left(\tfrac{8}{15} + 6\right) && \text{Subtracting; this is } F(b) - F(a). \\
&= 16\tfrac{4}{5}.
\end{aligned}$$

EXAMPLE 2 Find the area under the graph of $y = x^2 + 1$ over $[-1, 2]$.

Solution In this case, $f(x) = x^2 + 1$, with $a = -1$ and $b = 2$.

First, we find any antiderivative F of f. We choose the simplest one:

$$F(x) = \frac{x^3}{3} + x. \qquad \text{Choosing } C = 0 \text{ as the constant term}$$

Then we substitute the endpoints, 2 and -1, and find the difference $F(2) - F(-1)$:

$$\begin{aligned}
F(2) - F(-1) &= \left[\frac{2^3}{3} + 2\right] - \left[\frac{(-1)^3}{3} + (-1)\right] \\
&= \frac{8}{3} + 2 - \left[\frac{-1}{3} - 1\right] \\
&= \frac{8}{3} + 2 + \frac{1}{3} + 1 \\
&= 6.
\end{aligned}$$

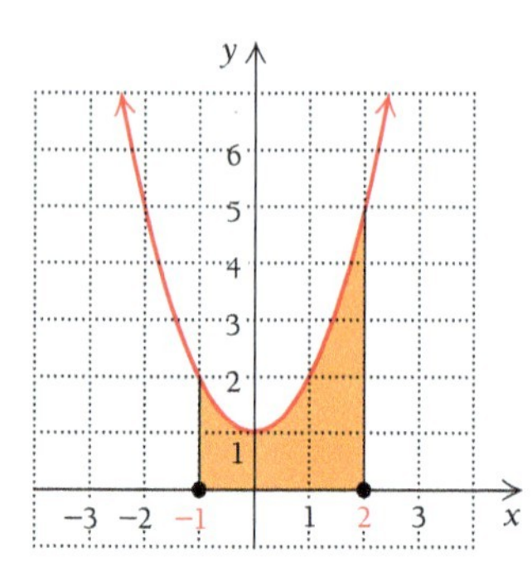

As a partial check, we can count the squares and parts of squares shaded on the graph above.

Quick Check 1 ✓

Refer to the function and graph in Example 2.

a) Calculate the area over $[0, 3]$.

b) Calculate the area over $[-2, 2]$.

c) Can you suggest a shortcut for part (b)?

Number of kilowatts generated per day

Number of days since solar array began operating

EXAMPLE 3 Let $y = x^3$ represent the number of kilowatts (kW) generated by a new community-owned solar array each day, x days after going operational. Find the area under the graph of $y = x^3$ over $[0, 5]$, and explain what this area represents.

Solution In this case, $f(x) = x^3$, $a = 0$, and $b = 5$.

We find any antiderivative F of f. We choose the simplest one:

$$F(x) = \frac{x^4}{4}.$$

We then substitute 5 and 0, and find the difference $F(5) - F(0)$:

$$F(5) - F(0) = \frac{5^4}{4} - \frac{0^4}{4} = \frac{625}{4} = 156\tfrac{1}{4}.$$

The area represents the total number of kilowatts generated during the first 5 days. To see this, note that the unit of the area is the product of the units on the two axes: $(\text{kW}/\text{day})(\text{days}) = \text{kW}$.

The difference $F(b) - F(a)$ is the same for all antiderivatives F of a function f whether the function f is nonnegative or not. It is called the *definite integral* of f from a to b.

DEFINITION

Let f be any continuous function over $[a, b]$ and F be any antiderivative of f. Then the **definite integral** of f from a to b is

$$\int_a^b f(x)\,dx = F(b) - F(a).$$

Evaluating definite integrals is called *integration*. The numbers a and b are the **limits of integration.** Note that this use of the word *limit* indicates an endpoint of an interval, not a value that is being approached, as presented in Chapter 1.

It is often convenient to use an intermediate notation:

$$\int_a^b f(x)\,dx = [F(x)]_a^b = F(b) - F(a),$$

where $F(x)$ is an antiderivative of $f(x)$.

EXAMPLE 4 Evaluate each of the following:

a) $\int_{-1}^{4} (x^2 - x)\,dx$; **b)** $\int_0^2 e^x\,dx$; **c)** $\int_2^5 \frac{1}{x}\,dx$; **d)** $\int_{-4}^{-1} \frac{1}{x}\,dx$.

Solution

a)
$$\int_{-1}^{4} (x^2 - x)\,dx = \left[\frac{x^3}{3} - \frac{x^2}{2}\right]_{-1}^{4} = \left(\frac{4^3}{3} - \frac{4^2}{2}\right) - \left(\frac{(-1)^3}{3} - \frac{(-1)^2}{2}\right)$$
$$= \left(\frac{64}{3} - \frac{16}{2}\right) - \left(\frac{-1}{3} - \frac{1}{2}\right)$$
$$= \frac{64}{3} - 8 + \frac{1}{3} + \frac{1}{2} = 14\tfrac{1}{6}$$

b)
$$\int_0^2 e^x\,dx = [e^x]_0^2 = e^2 - e^0 = e^2 - 1 \approx 6.389$$ Using a calculator

c) $\displaystyle\int_2^5 \frac{1}{x}\,dx = \left[\ln x\right]_2^5$ Using the absolute value of x is unnecessary here since $x > 0$ on $[2, 5]$.

$= \ln 5 - \ln 2$

≈ 0.916 Using a calculator

Quick Check 2 ✓

Evaluate each of the following:

a) $\displaystyle\int_2^4 (2x^3 - 3x)\,dx$;

b) $\displaystyle\int_0^{\ln 4} 2e^x\,dx$.

d) $\displaystyle\int_{-4}^{-1} \frac{1}{x}\,dx = \left[\ln|x|\right]_{-4}^{-1}$

$= \ln|-1| - \ln|-4|$ Here, using the absolute value is necessary.

$= \ln 1 - \ln 4$

$= 0 - \ln 4$

≈ -1.386 Using a calculator **2 ✓**

The fact that we can express the integral of a function either as a limit of a sum or in terms of an antiderivative is so important that it has a name: the *Fundamental Theorem of Integral Calculus.*

The Fundamental Theorem of Integral Calculus

If a continuous function f has an antiderivative F over $[a, b]$, where n is the number of subdivisions of $[a, b]$, then

$$\lim_{n\to\infty}\sum_{i=1}^{n} f(x_i)\,\Delta x = \int_a^b f(x)\,dx = F(b) - F(a).$$

It is helpful to envision taking the limit as stretching the summation sign, Σ, into something resembling an S (the integral sign) and redefining Δx as dx. Because Δx is used in the limit, dx appears in the integral notation to indicate that integration is being carried out *with respect to* x. Later we will see that more than one variable can be used.

More on Area

When we evaluate the definite integral of a nonnegative function f over $[a, b]$, we get the area under the graph of f over that interval.

EXAMPLE 5 Find the area under the graph of $y = 1/x^2$ over $[1, 10]$.

Solution

$$\int_1^{10} \frac{dx}{x^2} = \int_1^{10} x^{-2}\,dx$$

$$= \left[\frac{x^{-2+1}}{-2+1}\right]_1^{10}$$

$$= \left[\frac{x^{-1}}{-1}\right]_1^{10} = \left[-\frac{1}{x}\right]_1^{10}$$

$$= \left(-\frac{1}{10}\right) - \left(-\frac{1}{1}\right)$$

$$= 1 - \tfrac{1}{10} = 0.9$$

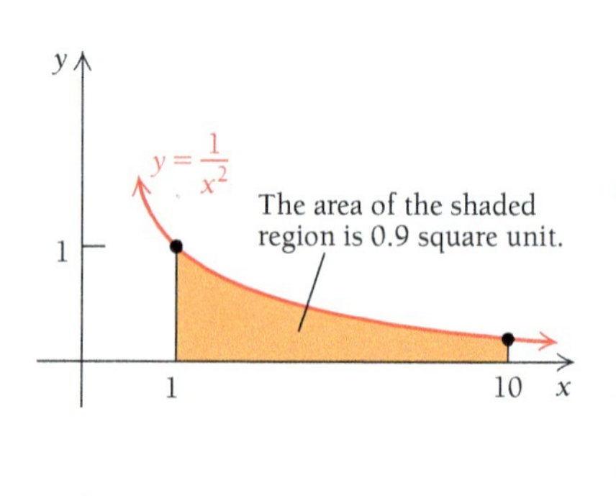

EXAMPLE 6 Suppose that y is profit, in dollars, per mile traveled and x is number of miles traveled, in thousands, and $y = 1/x$. Find the area under $y = 1/x$ over the interval $[1, 4]$, and explain what this area represents.

Solution

$$\int_1^4 \frac{dx}{x} = \left[\ln x\right]_1^4 = \ln 4 - \ln 1$$

$$= \ln 4 - 0 \approx 1.3863$$

Considering the units, (dollars/mile) • thousands of miles = thousands of dollars, we see that the area represents a profit of \$1386.30 when the miles traveled increase from 1000 to 4000.

Now let's compare two similar definite integrals:

$$\int_0^2 x^2\,dx = \left[\frac{x^3}{3}\right]_0^2 = \frac{2^3}{3} - \frac{0^3}{3} = \frac{8}{3} \qquad \int_0^2 -x^2\,dx = \left[-\frac{x^3}{3}\right]_0^2 = -\frac{2^3}{3} + \frac{0^3}{3} = -\frac{8}{3}$$

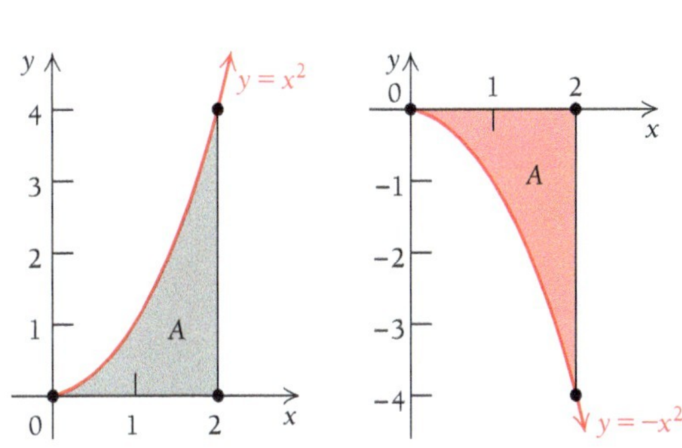

The graphs of $y = x^2$ and $y = -x^2$ are reflections of each other across the x-axis. Thus, the shaded areas are the same, $\frac{8}{3}$. The integral involving $y = -x^2$ gives $-\frac{8}{3}$. This shows that for negative-valued functions, the definite integral gives us the opposite of the area between the curve and the x-axis.

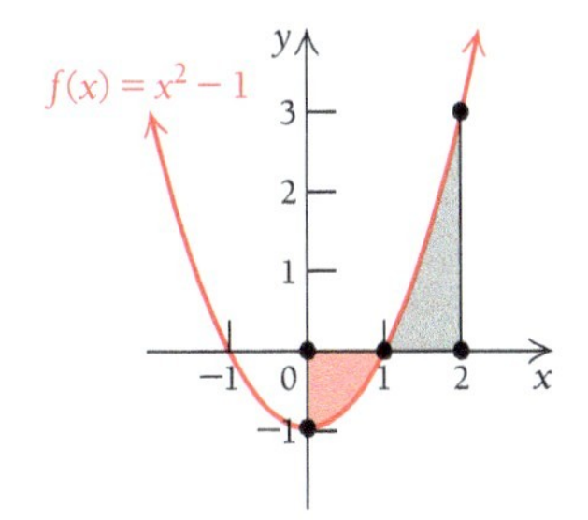

Next, let's consider $f(x) = x^2 - 1$ over $[0, 2]$. Here $f(x)$ has both positive and negative values. We can find $\int_0^2 f(x)\,dx$ in two ways.

First, let's use the fact that for any a, b, and c, if $a < c < b$, then

$$\int_a^b f(x)\,dx = \int_a^c f(x)\,dx + \int_c^b f(x)\,dx.$$

The area from a to c plus the area from c to b is the area from a to b.

(We will consider this property of integrals again in Section 4.4.) Because 1 is the x-intercept in $[0, 2]$, we first integrate from 0 to 1 and then from 1 to 2:

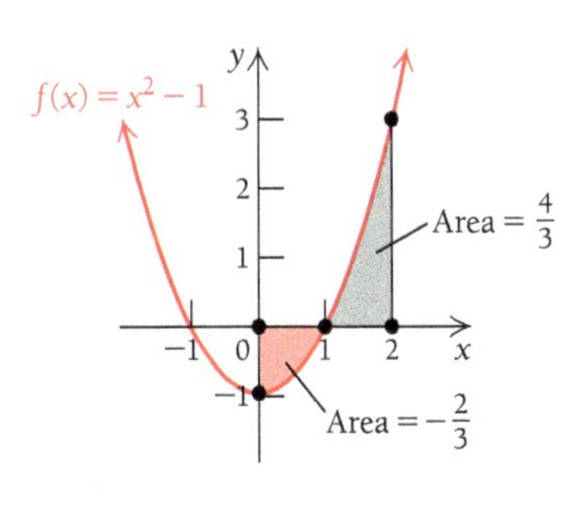

$$\int_0^2 (x^2 - 1)\,dx = \int_0^1 (x^2 - 1)\,dx + \int_1^2 (x^2 - 1)\,dx$$

$$= \left[\frac{x^3}{3} - x\right]_0^1 + \left[\frac{x^3}{3} - x\right]_1^2$$

$$= \left[\left(\frac{1^3}{3} - 1\right) - \left(\frac{0^3}{3} - 0\right)\right] + \left[\left(\frac{2^3}{3} - 2\right) - \left(\frac{1^3}{3} - 1\right)\right]$$

$$= \left[\frac{1}{3} - 1\right] + \left[\frac{8}{3} - 2 - \frac{1}{3} + 1\right]$$

$$= -\frac{2}{3} + \frac{4}{3} = \frac{2}{3}.$$

Note that $\frac{1}{3} - \frac{1}{3} = 0$ and $-1 + 1 = 0$.

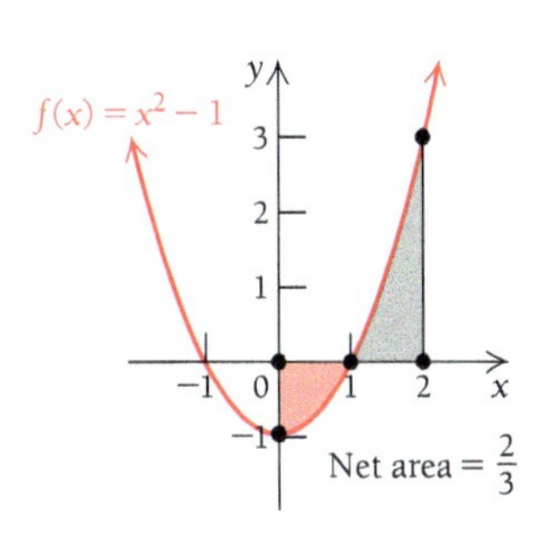

This shows that the area above the x-axis exceeds the area below the x-axis by $\frac{2}{3}$ unit.

Now let's evaluate the original integral in another, more direct, way:

$$\int_0^2 (x^2 - 1)\,dx = \left[\frac{x^3}{3} - x\right]_0^2 = \left(\frac{2^3}{3} - 2\right) - \left(\frac{0^3}{3} - 0\right)$$

$$= \left(\frac{8}{3} - 2\right) - 0 = \frac{2}{3}.$$

The definite integral of a continuous function over an interval is the area above the x-axis minus the area below the x-axis.

Quick Check 3 ✓

a) By examining the graph of $f(x) = x^4 - x^2$ shown below, predict the sign of $\int_0^2 f(x)\,dx$.

b) Evaluate this integral.

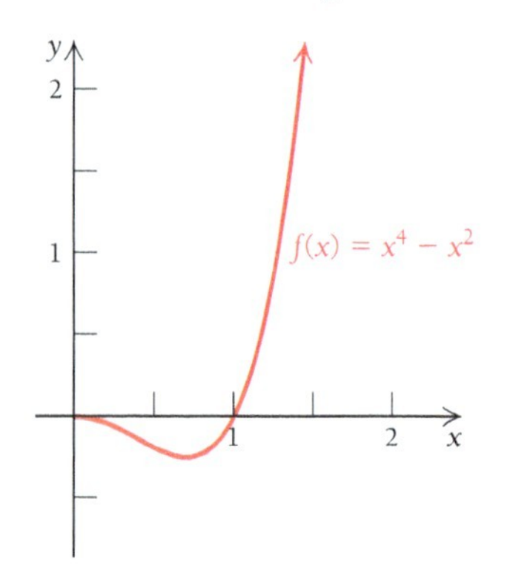

EXAMPLE 7 Consider $\int_{-1}^{2}(-x^3 + 3x - 1)\,dx$. Predict the sign of the result by examining the graph, shown to the right, and then evaluate the integral.

Solution From the graph, it appears that there is more area below the x-axis than above. Thus, we expect that

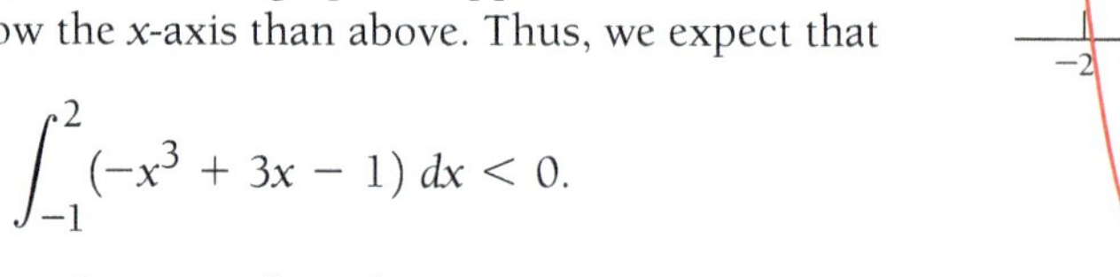

$$\int_{-1}^{2} (-x^3 + 3x - 1)\,dx < 0.$$

Evaluating the integral, we have

$$\int_{-1}^{2} (-x^3 + 3x - 1)\,dx = \left[-\frac{x^4}{4} + \frac{3}{2}x^2 - x\right]_{-1}^{2}$$

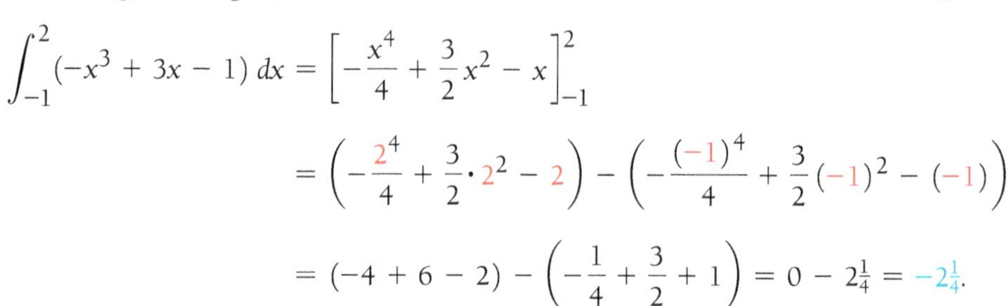

$$= \left(-\frac{2^4}{4} + \frac{3}{2}\cdot 2^2 - 2\right) - \left(-\frac{(-1)^4}{4} + \frac{3}{2}(-1)^2 - (-1)\right)$$

$$= (-4 + 6 - 2) - \left(-\frac{1}{4} + \frac{3}{2} + 1\right) = 0 - 2\tfrac{1}{4} = -2\tfrac{1}{4}.$$

As a partial check, we note that the result is negative, as expected. **3 ✓**

Applications Involving Definite Integrals

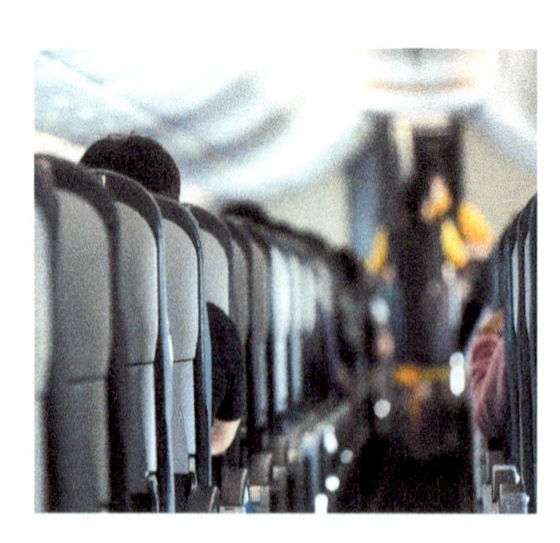

EXAMPLE 8 **Business: Total Profit from Marginal Profit.** Northeast Airlines determines that the marginal profit, in hundreds of dollars per seat, from the sale of x seats on a jet traveling from Atlanta to Kansas City is given by

$$P'(x) = \sqrt{x} - 6.$$

Find the total profit when 60 seats are sold.

Solution We integrate to find $P(60)$:

$$P(60) = \int_0^{60} P'(x)\,dx$$

$$= \int_0^{60} (\sqrt{x} - 6)\,dx$$

$$= \left[\frac{2}{3}x^{3/2} - 6x\right]_0^{60}$$

$$\approx -50.1613. \quad \text{Using a calculator}$$

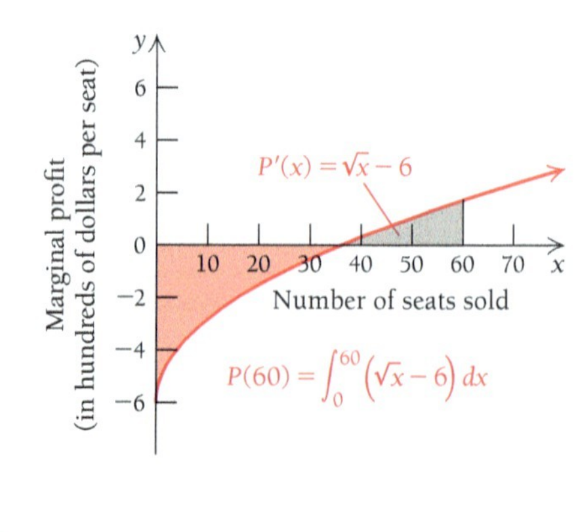

When 60 seats are sold, Northeast's profit is −\$5016.13. That is, the airline will lose \$5016.13 on the flight. **4 ✓**

Quick Check 4 ✓

Business. Referring to Example 8, find the total profit of Northeast Airlines when 140 seats are sold.

Technology Connection 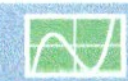

Approximating Definite Integrals

There are two methods for evaluating definite integrals with a calculator. Let's consider the function from Example 7: $f(x) = -x^3 + 3x - 1$.

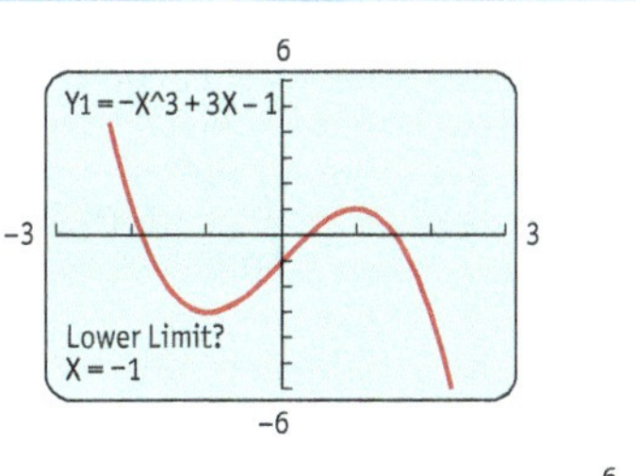

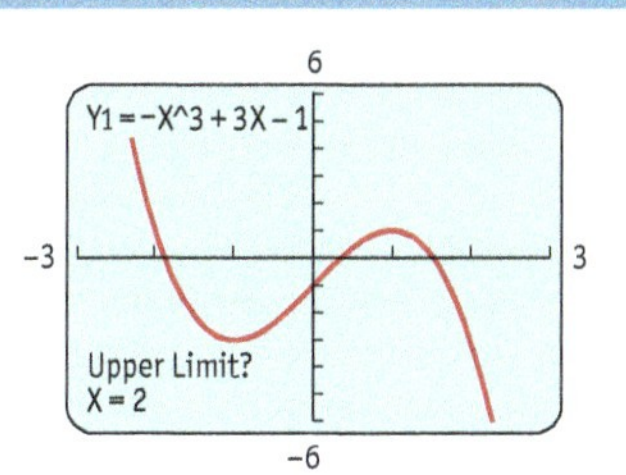

Method 1: fnInt

First, we select fnInt from the MATH menu. Next, we enter the function, the variable, and the endpoints of the interval over which we are integrating. The calculator returns the same value for the integral as we found in Example 7.

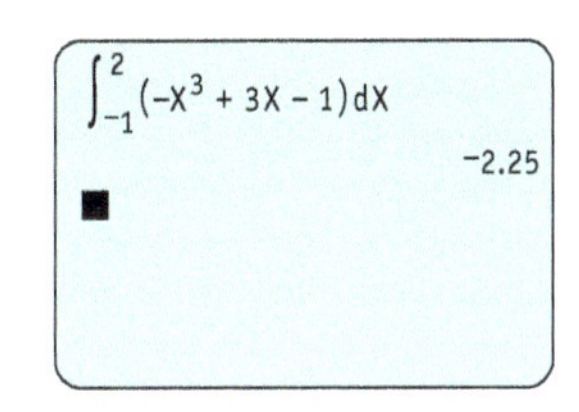

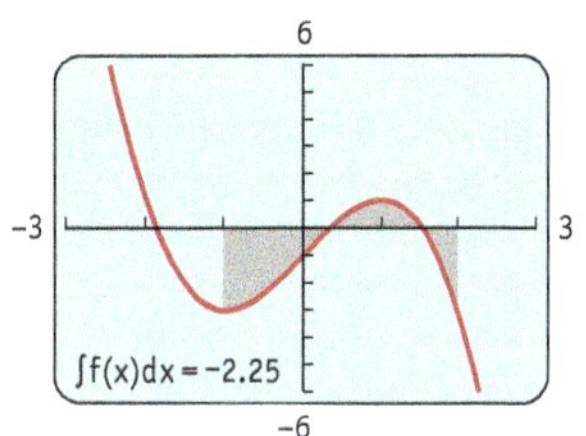

Method 2: ∫f(x)dx

We first graph $y_1 = -x^3 + 3x - 1$. Then we select ∫f(x)dx from the CALC menu and enter the lower and upper limits of integration. The calculator shades the area and returns the value found in Example 7.

EXERCISES

Evaluate each definite integral.

1. $\displaystyle\int_{-1}^{2} (x^2 - 1)\, dx$

2. $\displaystyle\int_{-2}^{3} (x^3 - 3x + 1)\, dx$

3. $\displaystyle\int_{1}^{6} \frac{\ln x}{x^2}\, dx$

4. $\displaystyle\int_{-8}^{2} \frac{4}{(1 + e^x)^2}\, dx$

5. $\displaystyle\int_{-10}^{10} (0.002x^4 - 0.3x^2 + 4x - 7)\, dx$

If the location of an object relative to a starting point is $s(t)$ at time t, then

$$s'(t) = v(t) = \text{the } \textbf{velocity} \text{ at time } t,$$
$$s''(t) = v'(t) = a(t) = \text{the } \textbf{acceleration} \text{ at time } t.$$

Thus, if we are given information about the acceleration of an object, we may be able to use integration to determine information about the object's velocity and location.

EXAMPLE 9 **Physical Science: Braking Distance.** Juanita is driving her car at 40 mi/hr (58.67 ft/sec) when she applies the brakes, and the car comes to a stop after 7 sec. Her acceleration during the time she slows to a stop is given by $a(t) = -2.394t$, where $0 \le t \le 7$.

a) Find Juanita's velocity function, $v(t)$, over $[0, 7]$.

b) How far did the car travel while Juanita was braking?

Solution

a) To find velocity, we integrate $a(t)$:

$$\begin{aligned} v(t) &= \int -2.394t\, dt \\ &= -2.394\left(\tfrac{1}{2}t^2\right) + C \\ &= -1.197t^2 + C. \qquad \text{Simplifying} \end{aligned}$$

When Juanita applied the brakes ($t = 0$), her velocity was 58.67 ft/sec. We use this initial condition to solve for C:

$$58.67 = -1.197(0)^2 + C$$
$$C = 58.67.$$

Thus, Juanita's velocity function is $v(t) = -1.197t^2 + 58.67$.

b) The distance the car traveled is given by the definite integral of $v(t)$ over the interval $0 \le t \le 7$, the time during which Juanita was braking:

$$\int_0^7 (-1.197t^2 + 58.67)\,dt = \left[-\frac{1.197}{3}t^3 + 58.67t\right]_0^7$$
$$= -\frac{1.197}{3}(7)^3 + 58.67(7) - 0$$
$$= 273.83 \text{ ft.}$$

In the graph of v, the shaded area represents the distance the car traveled during the 7 sec.

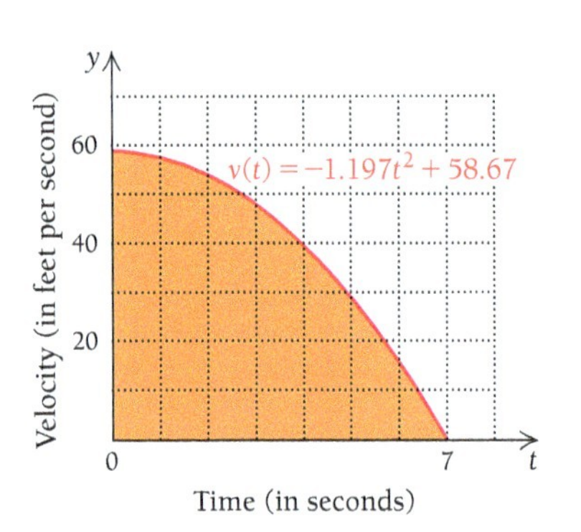

Quick Check 5 ✓

Suppose that the driver in Example 9 braked to a stop in 7 sec but did so "linearly," according to the velocity function $v(t) = 58.67 - 8.38t$. Find the braking distance in feet.

5 ✓

Section Summary

- The area between the x-axis and the graph of the nonnegative continuous function $y = f(x)$ over $[a, b]$ is found by evaluating the *definite integral*

$$\int_a^b f(x)\,dx = F(b) - F(a),$$

where F is an antiderivative of f.

- If a function has areas both below and above the x-axis, the definite integral gives the net total area, or the difference between the sum of the areas above the x-axis and the sum of the areas below the x-axis.
  - If there is more area above the x-axis than below, then the definite integral is positive.
  - If there is more area below the x-axis than above, then the definite integral is negative.
  - If the areas above and below the x-axis are the same, then the definite integral is 0.

4.3 Exercise Set

Find the area under the given curve over the indicated interval.

1. $y = 5$; $[1, 3]$

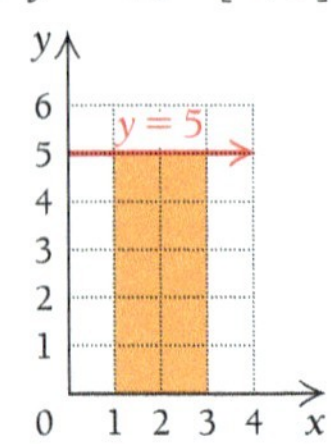

2. $y = 4$; $[1, 3]$

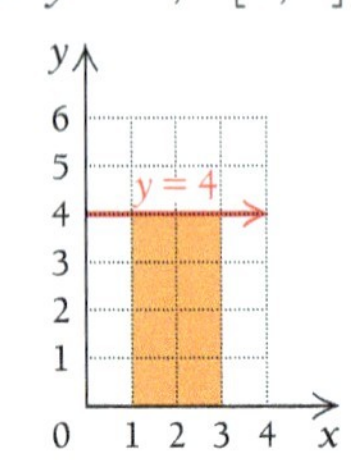

3. $y = 5x$; $[1, 2]$

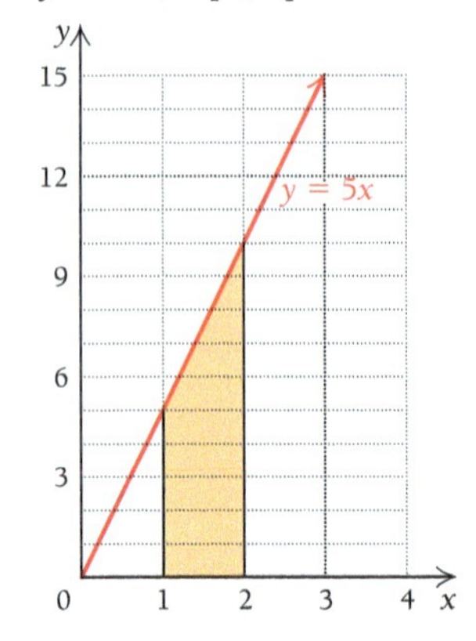

4. $y = 2x$; $[1, 3]$

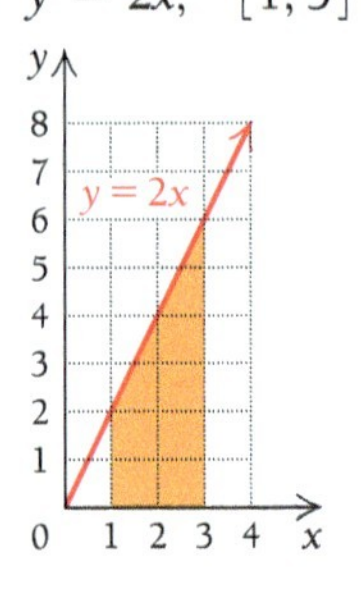

5. $y = x^2$; $[0, 3]$

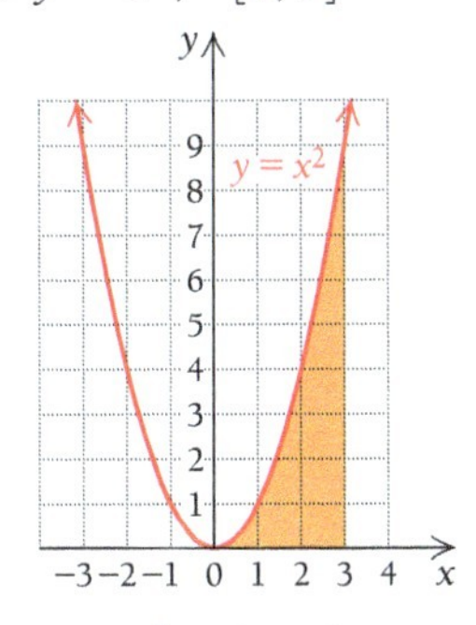

6. $y = x^2$; $[0, 5]$

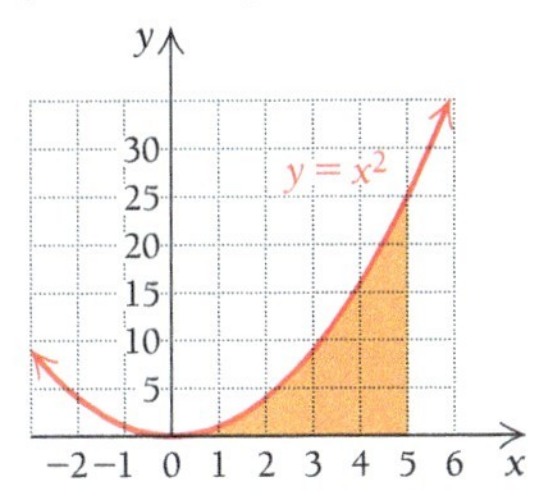

7. $y = x^3$; $[0, 2]$

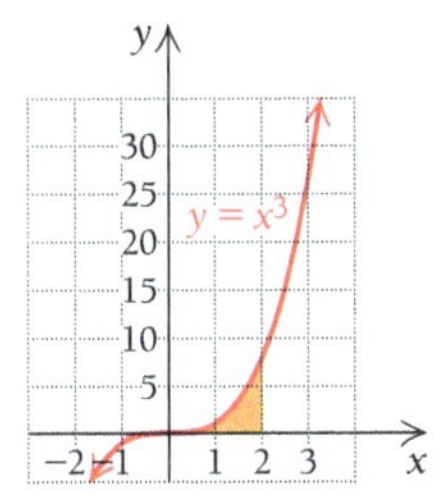

8. $y = x^3$; $[0, 1]$

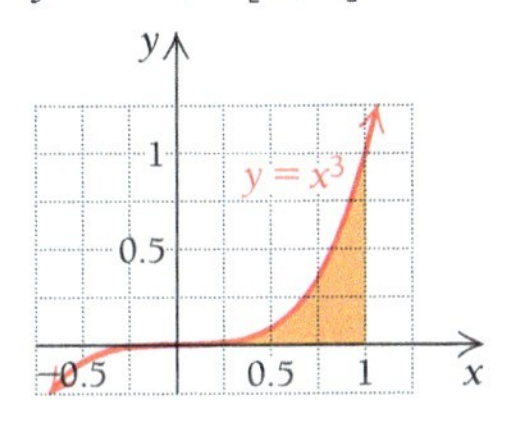

9. $y = 1 - x^2$; $[-1, 1]$

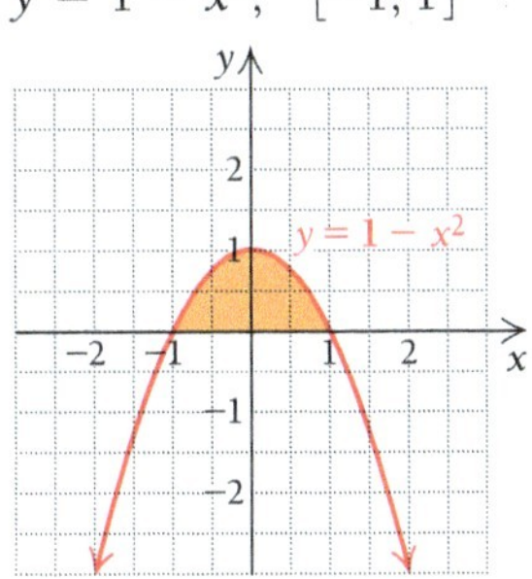

10. $y = 4 - x^2$; $[-2, 2]$

11. $y = e^x$; $[2, 4]$

12. $y = e^x$; $[0, 3]$

13. $y = \frac{2}{x}$; $[1, 4]$

14. $y = \frac{3}{x}$; $[-6, -1]$

In each of Exercises 15–24, explain what the shaded area represents.

15.

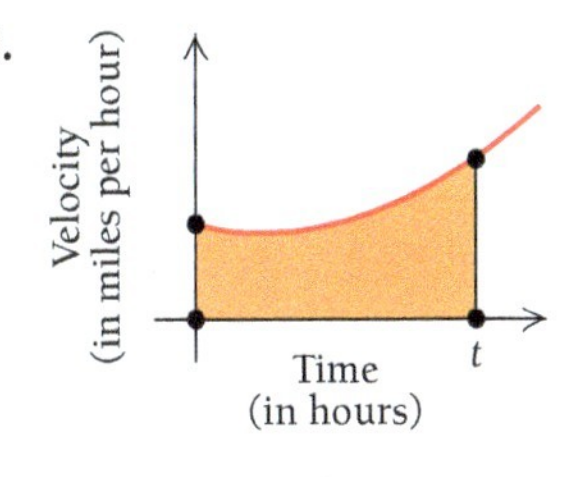

16.

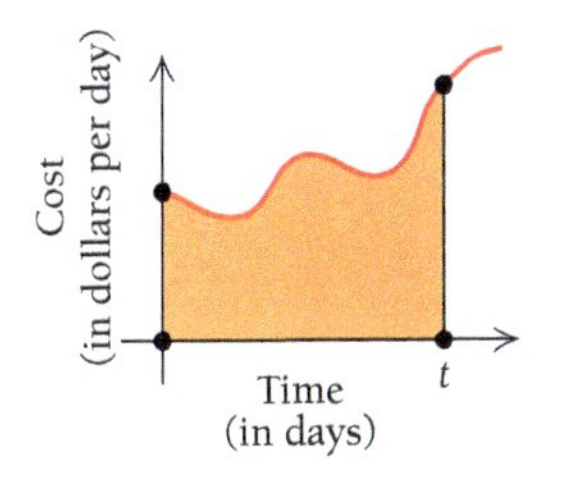

17.

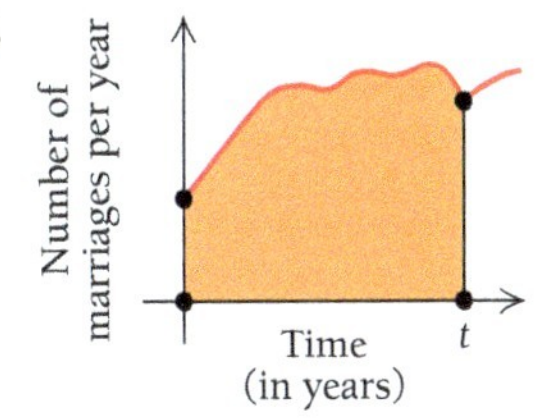

18.

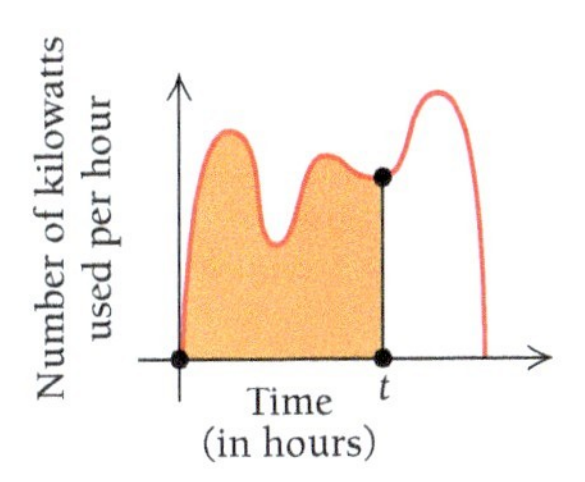

19.

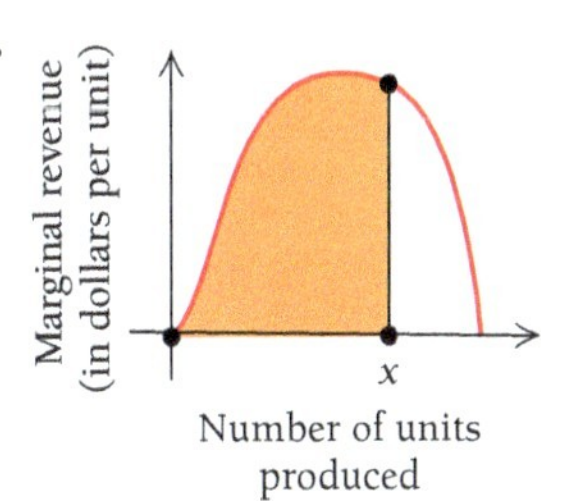

20.

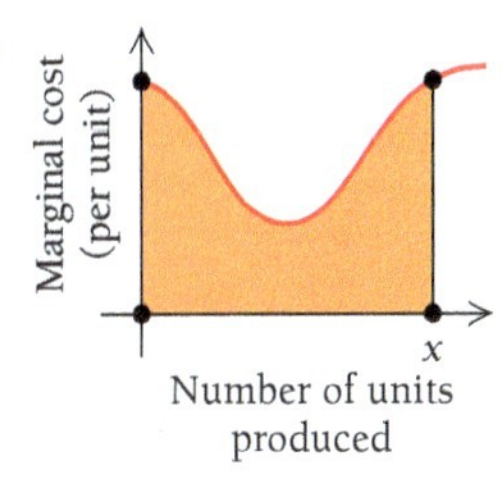

21.

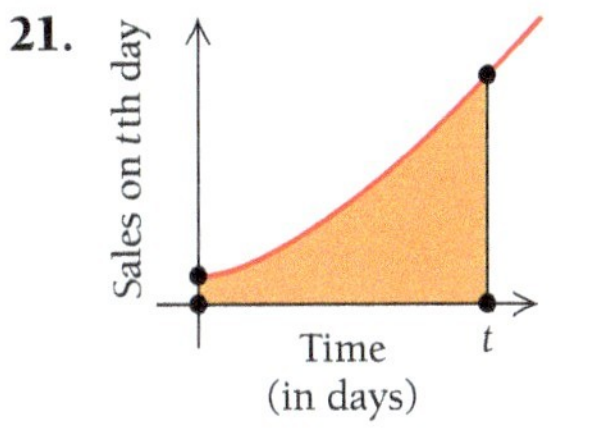

22.

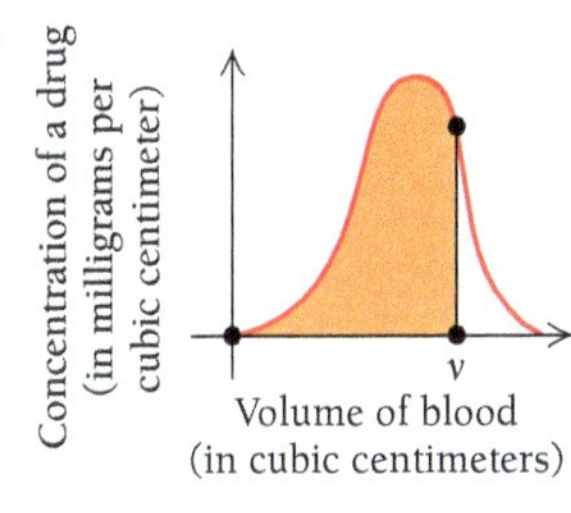

23.

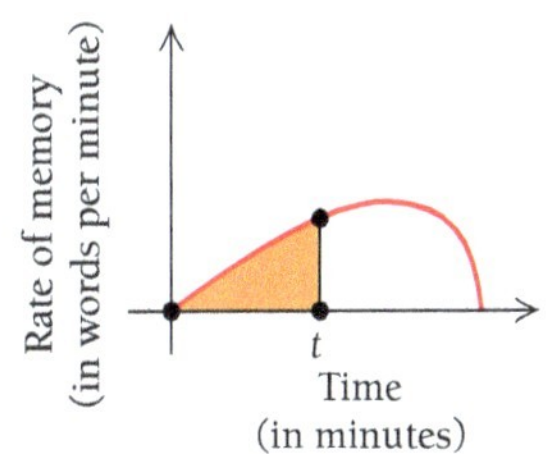

24.

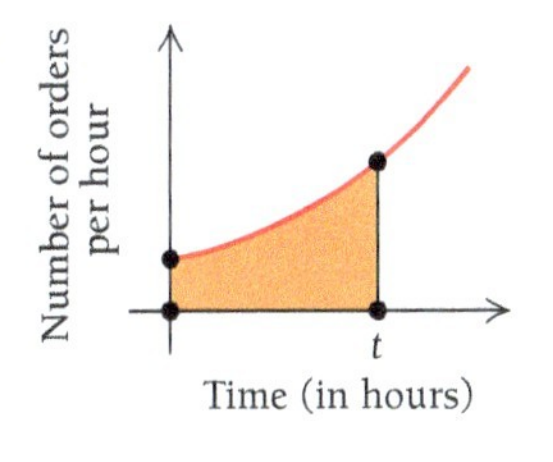

Find the area under the graph of each function over the given interval.

25. $y = x^3$; $[1, 3]$

26. $y = x^4$; $[0, 1]$

27. $y = x^2 + x + 1$; $[2, 3]$

28. $y = 2 - x - x^2$; $[-2, 1]$

29. $y = 5 - x^2$; $[-1, 2]$

30. $y = e^{2x}$; $[-2, 3]$

31. $y = e^{3x}$; $[-1, 5]$

32. $y = 2x + \frac{1}{x^2}$; $[1, 4]$

In Exercises 33 and 34, determine visually whether $\int_a^b f(x)\,dx$ is positive, negative, or zero, and express $\int_a^b f(x)\,dx$ in terms of area A.

33. a)

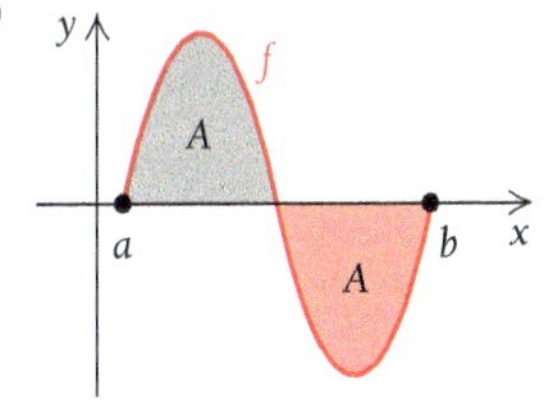

b)

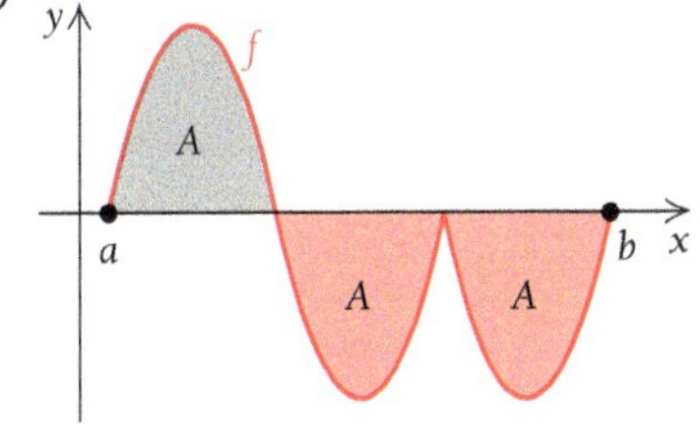

34. **a)**

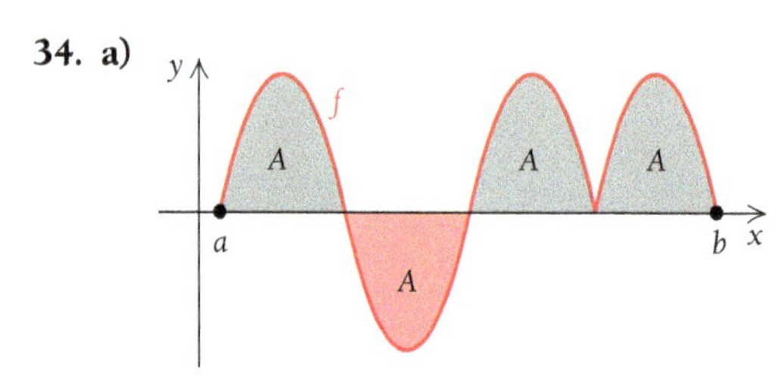

b)

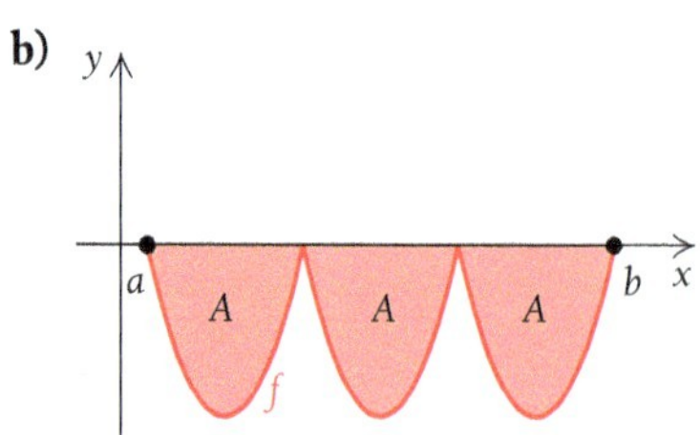

Evaluate each integral. Then state whether the result indicates that there is more area above or below the x-axis or that the areas above and below the axis are equal.

35. $\int_0^{1.5} (x - x^2)\, dx$

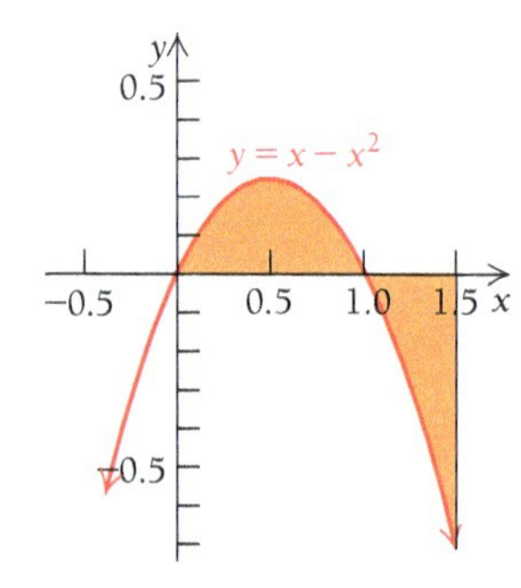

36. $\int_0^2 (x^2 - x)\, dx$

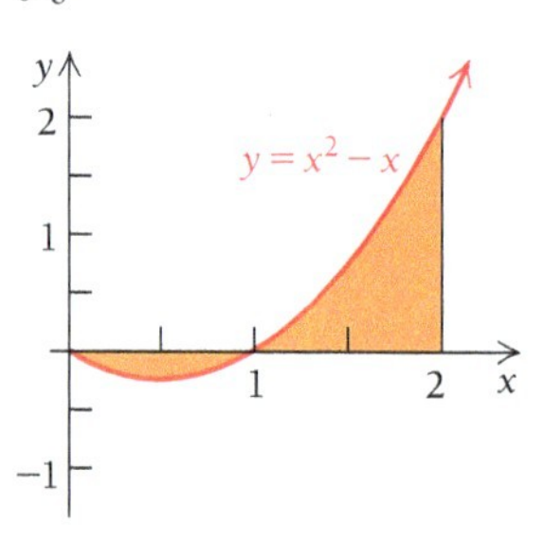

37. $\int_{-1}^{1} (x^3 - 3x)\, dx$

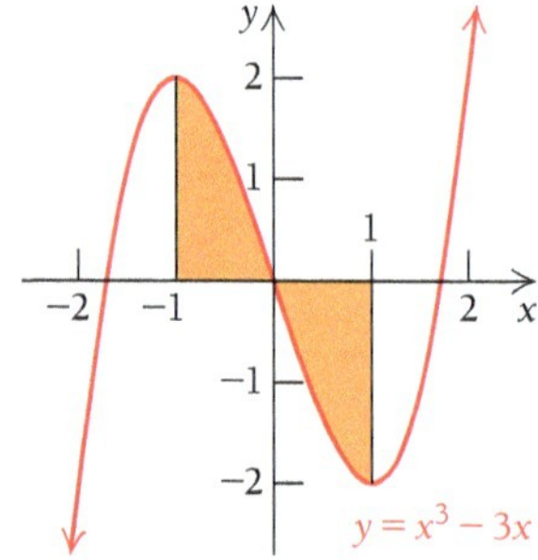

38. $\int_0^b -2e^{3x}\, dx$

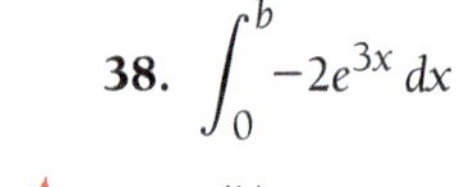

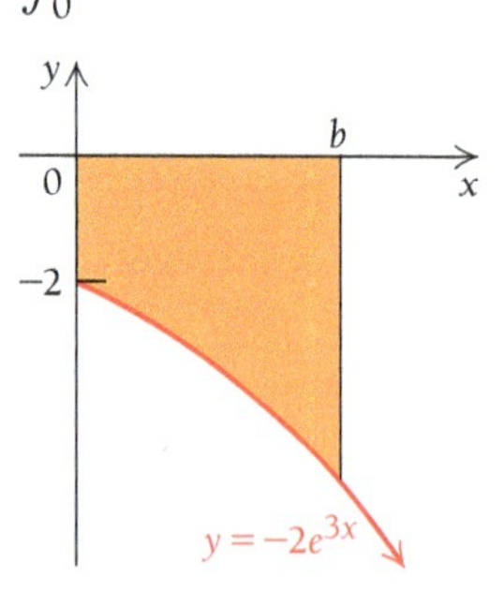

Evaluate.

39. $\int_1^3 (3t^2 + 7)\, dt$

40. $\int_1^2 (4t^3 - 1)\, dt$

41. $\int_1^4 (\sqrt{x} - 1)\, dx$

42. $\int_1^8 (\sqrt[3]{x} - 2)\, dx$

43. $\int_{-2}^{5} (2x^2 - 3x + 7)\, dx$

44. $\int_{-2}^{3} (-x^2 + 4x - 5)\, dx$

45. $\int_{-5}^{2} e^t\, dt$

46. $\int_{-2}^{3} e^{-t}\, dt$

47. $\int_a^b \frac{1}{2}x^2\, dx$

48. $\int_a^b \frac{1}{5}x^3\, dx$

49. $\int_a^b e^{2t}\, dt$

50. $\int_a^b -e^t\, dt$

51. $\int_0^{\ln 4} e^{3x}\, dx$

52. $\int_0^{\ln 6} e^{2x}\, dx$

53. $\int_{\ln 3}^{\ln 7} 4e^{-x}\, dx$

54. $\int_{\ln 8}^{\ln 15} 3e^{-2x}\, dx$

55. $\int_1^e \left(x + \frac{1}{x}\right) dx$

56. $\int_{-5}^{-e} \left(x - \frac{1}{x}\right) dx$

57. $\int_0^2 \sqrt{2x}\, dx$ (*Hint*: Simplify first.)

58. $\int_0^{27} \sqrt{3x}\, dx$

APPLICATIONS

Business and Economics

59. Business: total profit. Pure Water Enterprises finds that the marginal profit, in dollars per foot, from drilling a well that is x feet deep is given by

$$P'(x) = \sqrt[5]{x}.$$

Find the total profit when a well 250 ft deep is drilled.

60. Business: total revenue. Sally's Sweets finds that the marginal revenue, in dollars per pound, from the sale of x pounds of maple-coated pecans is given by

$$R'(x) = 2x^{1/6}.$$

Find the total revenue when 300 lb of maple-coated pecans are produced.

61. Business: increasing total cost. Kitchens-to-Please Contracting determines that the marginal cost, in dollars per square foot, of installing x square feet of kitchen countertop is given by

$$C'(x) = 4x^{1/3}.$$

a) Find the cost of installing 50 ft^2 of countertop.
b) Find the cost of installing an extra 14 ft^2 of countertop after 50 ft^2 have already been installed.

62. Business: increasing total profit. Laso Industries finds that the marginal profit, in dollars per board, from the sale of x digital control boards is given by

$$P'(x) = 2.6x^{0.1}.$$

a) Find the cost of producing 1200 digital control boards.
b) A customer orders 1200 digital control boards and later increases the order to 1500. Find the extra profit resulting from the increase in order size.

63. Accumulated sales. Melanie's Crafts estimates that its sales are growing continuously at a rate given by

$$S'(t) = 20e^t,$$

where $S'(t)$ is in dollars per day, on day t.

a) Find the accumulated sales for the first 5 days.
b) Find the accumulated sales from the beginning of the 2nd day through the 5th day.

64. **Accumulated sales.** Raggs, Ltd., estimates that its sales are growing continuously at a rate given by

$$S'(t) = 10e^t,$$

where $S'(t)$ is in dollars per day, on day t.

a) Find the accumulated sales for the first 5 days.
b) Find the accumulated sales from the beginning of the 2nd day through the 5th day.

Credit market debt. *Since 2013, the annual rate of change in the national consumer revolving credit market debt can be modeled by the function*

$$D'(t) = 12.922t + 11.474,$$

where $D'(t)$ is in billions of dollars per year and t is the number of years since January 2013. (Source: Based on data from federalreserve.gov/releases/g19/current.) Use the preceding information for Exercises 65 and 66.

65. By how much did the credit market debt increase between 2013 and 2017?

66. By how much did the credit market debt increase between 2016 and 2019?

Industrial learning curve. *A company is producing a new product, and the time required to produce each unit decreases as workers gain experience. It is determined that*

$$T(x) = 2 + 0.3\left(\frac{1}{x}\right),$$

where $T(x)$ is the time, in hours, required to produce the xth unit. Use this information for Exercises 67 and 68.

67. Find the total time required for a worker to produce units 1 through 10; units 20 through 30.

68. Find the total time required for a worker to produce units 1 through 20; units 20 through 40.

Social Sciences

Memorizing. *The rate of memorizing information initially increases. Eventually, however, a maximum rate is reached, after which the rate begins to decrease.*

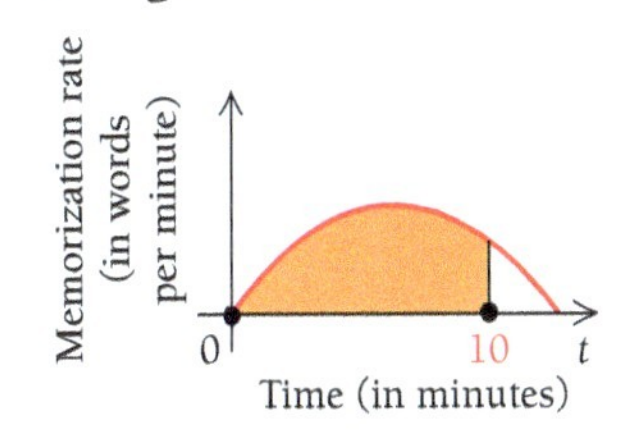

69. Suppose an experiment finds that the memorization rate is given by

$$M'(t) = -0.009t^2 + 0.2t,$$

where $M'(t)$ is the rate, in words per minute. How many words are memorized in the first 10 min (from $t = 0$ to $t = 10$)?

70. Suppose another experiment finds that the memorization rate is given by

$$M'(t) = -0.003t^2 + 0.2t,$$

where $M'(t)$ is the rate, in words per minute. How many words are memorized in the first 10 min (from $t = 0$ to $t = 10$)?

71. See Exercise 69. How many words are memorized during minutes 10–15?

72. See Exercise 70. How many words are memorized during minutes 10–17?

Life and Physical Sciences

In Exercises 73–78, $s(t)$, $v(t)$, and $a(t)$ represent, respectively, an object's position (in meters), velocity (in meters per second), and acceleration (in meters per second per second).

Find $s(t)$.

73. $v(t) = 3t^2$, $s(0) = 4$ 74. $v(t) = 2t$, $s(0) = 10$

Find $v(t)$.

75. $a(t) = 4t$, $v(0) = 20$ 76. $a(t) = 6t$, $v(0) = 30$

Find $s(t)$.

77. $a(t) = -2t + 6$, with $v(0) = 6$ and $s(0) = 10$

78. $a(t) = -6t + 7$, with $v(0) = 10$ and $s(0) = 20$

79. **Physics.** A particle is released as part of an experiment. Its speed t seconds after release is given by $v(t) = -0.5t^2 + 10t$, where $v(t)$ is in meters per second.

a) How far does the particle travel during the first 5 sec?
b) How far does it travel during the second 5 sec?

80. **Physics.** A particle is released during an experiment. Its speed t minutes after release is given by $v(t) = -0.3t^2 + 9t$, where $v(t)$ is in kilometers per minute.

a) How far does the particle travel during the first 10 min?
b) How far does it travel during the second 10 min?

81. **Distance and speed.** A motorcyclist being monitored by radar accelerates at a constant rate from 0 mph ($v(0) = 0$) to 60 mph in 15 sec. How far has she traveled after 15 sec? (*Hint*: Convert seconds to hours.)

82. **Distance and speed.** A car under surveillance accelerates at a constant rate from 0 mph to 60 mph in 30 sec. How far has it traveled after 30 sec?

83. **Distance and speed.** A bicycle racer decelerates at a constant rate from 30 km/hr to a complete stop in 45 sec.

a) How fast is the bicyclist traveling after 20 sec?
b) How far has the bicyclist traveled after 45 sec?

84. **Distance and speed.** A cheetah decelerates at a constant rate from 50 km/hr to a complete stop in 20 sec.

a) How fast is the cheetah moving after 10 sec?
b) How far has the cheetah traveled after 20 sec?

85. **Braking distance.** A motorist slows from 30 mi/hr (44 ft/sec) to a stop in 5 sec; his acceleration is given by $a(t) = -3.52t$, where $a(t)$ is in ft/sec^2 and t is in seconds, with $0 \le t \le 5$.

a) Find his velocity function, $v(t)$, over $[0, 5]$.
b) How far did the car travel while he was slowing to a stop?

86. **Stopping distance.** A skateboarder slows from 18 mi/hr (26.41 ft/sec) to a stop in 3 sec; her acceleration is given by $a(t) = -5.868t$, where $a(t)$ is in ft/sec^2 and t is in seconds, with $0 \le t \le 3$.

a) Find her velocity function, $v(t)$.
b) How far did she travel while she was slowing to a stop?

87. **Top-fuel dragster.** A top-fuel dragster's acceleration is given by $a(t) = 183.4$, where t is in seconds and $a(t)$ is in ft/sec^2. (*Source*: Based on data from www.nhra.com.)

a) Assuming that the dragster starts from a stationary position, find its velocity function, $v(t)$.
b) How fast is the dragster moving after 0.8 sec?
c) How far has the dragster traveled after 0.8 sec?
d) Restate the answer to part (b) in miles per hour.

88. **Top-fuel dragster.** A top-fuel dragster slows (with the help of chutes) from a top speed of 330 mi/hr (484 ft/sec) to a complete stop in a period of 10 sec. Assume that the dragster slows at a constant rate during this time.

a) Find the dragster's velocity function, $v(t)$.
b) How far does the dragster travel during the time it takes to come to a complete stop?

SYNTHESIS

89. **Total pollution.** A factory is polluting a lake in such a way that the rate of pollutants entering the lake after t months is

$$N'(t) = 280t^{3/2},$$

where $N(t)$ is the total number of pounds of pollutants in the lake after t months.

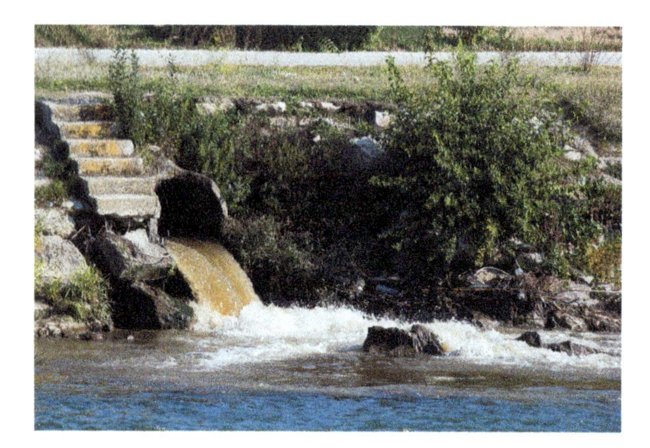

a) How many pounds of pollutants enter the lake over the first 16 months?
b) An environmental board ordered the factory to begin cleanup procedures after 50,000 lb of pollutants had already entered the lake. When was the order issued?

90. **Accumulated sales.** Bluetape, Inc., estimates that its sales are growing continuously at a rate given by

$$S'(t) = 0.5e^t,$$

where $S'(t)$ is in dollars per day, on day t. On what day will accumulated sales first exceed $10,000?

Evaluate.

91. $\displaystyle\int_2^3 \frac{x^2 - 1}{x - 1}\,dx$

92. $\displaystyle\int_0^1 (x + 2)^3\,dx$

93. $\displaystyle\int_4^{16} (x - 1)\sqrt{x}\,dx$

94. $\displaystyle\int_1^8 \frac{\sqrt[3]{x^2} - 1}{\sqrt[3]{x}}\,dx$

95. $\displaystyle\int_2^5 (t + \sqrt{3})(t - \sqrt{3})\,dt$

96. $\displaystyle\int_1^3 \left(x - \frac{1}{x}\right)^2 dx$

97. $\displaystyle\int_1^3 \frac{t^5 - t}{t^3}\,dt$

98. $\displaystyle\int_4^9 \frac{t + 1}{\sqrt{t}}\,dt$

Integrals as functions. *Certain functions may be defined by an integral of the form* $f(t) = \int_a^t g(u)\,du$, *where* a *is a constant,* u *is a "dummy" variable, and* t *is the independent variable. Defining functions in this manner is not uncommon. For example, the definition of the natural logarithm function is*

$$\ln t = \int_1^t \frac{1}{u}\,du.$$

99. Let $f(t) = \displaystyle\int_0^t 2u\,du$.

a) Find $f(0)$, $f(1)$, $f(2)$, and $f(3)$.
b) Find $f'(t)$.
c) Find $f'(t)$ if $f(t) = \displaystyle\int_1^t 2u\,du$.
d) Explain why the answers to parts (b) and (c) are the same.

100. Let $f(t) = \displaystyle\int_0^t 3u^2\,du$.

a) Find $f(0)$, $f(1)$, $f(2)$, and $f(3)$.
b) Find $f'(t)$.
c) Find $f'(t)$ if $f(t) = \displaystyle\int_2^t 3u^2\,du$.
d) Explain why the answers to parts (b) and (c) are the same.

101. Let $f(t) = \displaystyle\int_0^t e^{2u}\,du$.

a) Find $f'(t)$.
b) Find $f'(t)$ if $f(t) = \displaystyle\int_t^0 e^{2u}\,du$.

102. Let $f(t) = \displaystyle\int_0^t \sqrt{1 + 2u}\,du$.

a) Find $f'(t)$.
b) Find $f'(t)$ if $f(t) = \displaystyle\int_t^{-3} \sqrt{1 + 2u}\,du$.

103. Find $f'(t)$ if $f(t) = \displaystyle\int_0^{2t} (u + 1)^3\,du$.

104. Find $f'(t)$ if $f(t) = \displaystyle\int_0^{3t} \frac{1}{5x + 2}\,dx$.

Explain the error that has been made in each of Exercises 105 and 106.

105.
$$\int_1^2 (x^2 - x)\,dx = \left[\frac{1}{3}x^3 - \frac{1}{2}x^2\right]_1^2$$
$$= \left(\frac{1}{3}\cdot 2^3 - \frac{1}{2}\cdot 1^2\right)$$
$$= \frac{13}{6}$$

106. $\int_1^2 (\ln x - e^x)\,dx = \left[\frac{1}{x} - e^x\right]_1^2$

$= \left(\frac{1}{2} - e^2\right) - (1 - e^1)$

$= e - e^2 - \frac{1}{2}$

107. Prove that $\int_a^b f(x)\,dx = -\int_b^a f(x)\,dx.$

Technology Connection

Evaluate.

108. $\int_{-8}^{1.4} (x^4 + 4x^3 - 36x^2 - 160x + 300)\,dx$

109. $\int_{-2}^{2} \sqrt{4 - x^2}\,dx$

110. $\int_0^8 x(x-5)^4\,dx$

111. $\int_2^4 \frac{x^2 - 4}{x^2 - 3}\,dx$

Answers to Quick Checks

1. (a) 12; **(b)** $9\frac{1}{3}$, or $\frac{28}{3}$; **(c)** integrate from 0 to 2, then double the result
2. (a) 102; **(b)** 6 **3. (a)** Positive; **(b)** $\frac{56}{15}$
4. Approximately $26,433.49
5. Approximately 205.38 ft

4.4 Properties of Definite Integrals: Additive Property, Average Value, and Moving Average

- Use properties of definite integrals to find the area between curves.
- Solve applied problems involving definite integrals.
- Determine the average value of a function.
- Find the moving average of a function.

The Additive Property of Definite Integrals

The definite integral

$$\int_a^b f(x)\,dx$$

can be regarded as the area under the graph of f over the interval $[a, b]$. Thus, for c such that $a < c < b$, the above integral can be expressed as a sum of two definite integrals. This **additive property of definite integrals** is stated in the following theorem.

THEOREM 5

For $a < c < b$,

$$\int_a^b f(x)\,dx = \int_a^c f(x)\,dx + \int_c^b f(x)\,dx.$$

For any number c between a and b, the integral from a to b is the integral from a to c plus the integral from c to b.

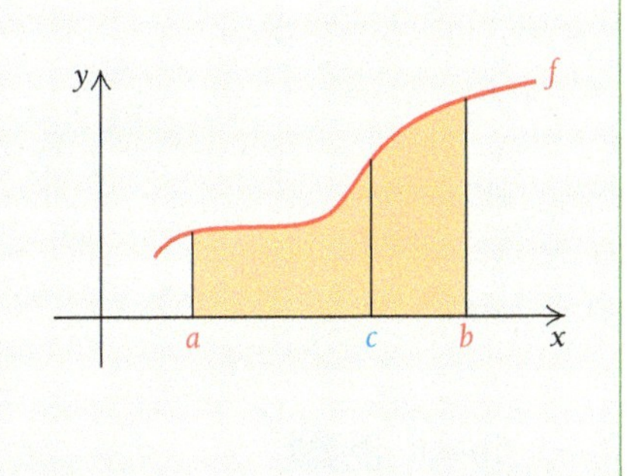

Theorem 5 can be used to integrate continuous piecewise-defined functions.

EXAMPLE 1 Find the area under the graph of f from -4 to 5, where

$$f(x) = \begin{cases} 9, & \text{for } x < 3, \\ x^2, & \text{for } x \geq 3. \end{cases}$$

Solution We express the definite integral of f over $[-4, 5]$ as the sum of two definite integrals, one over $[-4, 3]$ and the other over $[3, 5]$:

$$\int_{-4}^{5} f(x)\,dx = \int_{-4}^{3} f(x)\,dx + \int_{3}^{5} f(x)\,dx$$

$$= \int_{-4}^{3} 9\,dx + \int_{3}^{5} x^2\,dx$$

$$= 9\big[x\big]_{-4}^{3} + \left[\frac{x^3}{3}\right]_3^5$$

$$= 9(3 - (-4)) + \left(\frac{5^3}{3} - \frac{3^3}{3}\right)$$

$$= 95\tfrac{2}{3}.$$

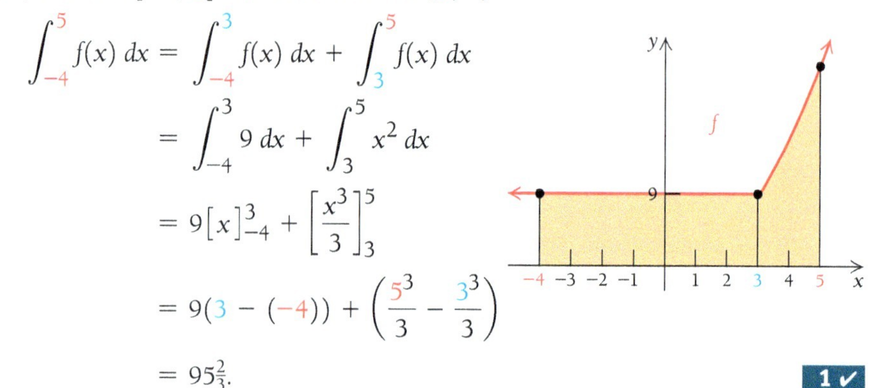

Quick Check 1 ✓

Find the area under the graph of g from -3 to 6, where

$$g(x) = \begin{cases} x^2, & \text{for } x \le 2, \\ 6 - x, & \text{for } x > 2. \end{cases}$$

1 ✓

EXAMPLE 2 Evaluate $\int_0^3 |1 - x^2|\,dx.$

Solution The graph of $f(x) = |1 - x^2|$ is the graph of $y = 1 - x^2$, where any portion of the graph below the x-axis (that is, where $y < 0$) is reflected above the x-axis.

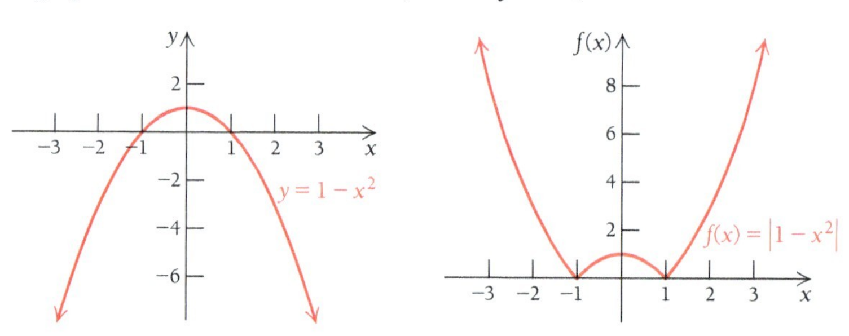

We see that y is negative for $x < -1$ or $x > 1$. Therefore, the function is defined piecewise, as follows. Note that $-(1 - x^2) = x^2 - 1$.

$$f(x) = |1 - x^2| = \begin{cases} x^2 - 1, & \text{for } x < -1 \text{ or } x > 1, \\ 1 - x^2, & \text{for } -1 \le x \le 1. \end{cases}$$

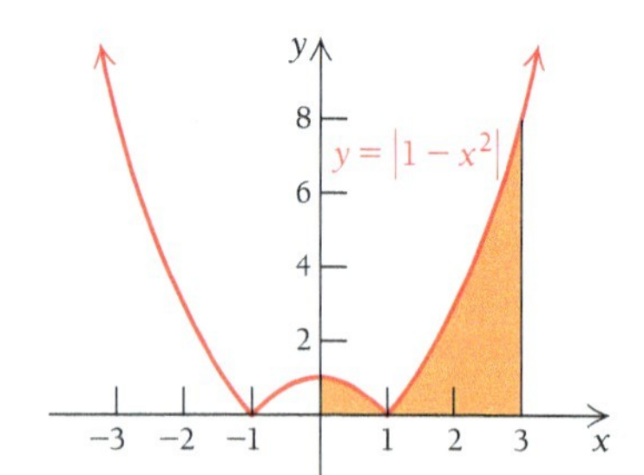

The definite integral of $f(x) = |1 - x^2|$ over $[0, 3]$ is the sum of two definite integrals, of $y = 1 - x^2$ over $[0, 1]$ and of $y = x^2 - 1$ over $[1, 3]$:

$$\int_0^3 |1 - x^2|\,dx = \int_0^1 (1 - x^2)\,dx + \int_1^3 (x^2 - 1)\,dx$$

$$= \left[x - \frac{1}{3}x^3\right]_0^1 + \left[\frac{1}{3}x^3 - x\right]_1^3$$

$$= \left[\left(1 - \frac{1}{3}\cdot 1^3\right) - \left(0 - \frac{1}{3}\cdot 0^3\right)\right] + \left[\left(\frac{1}{3}\cdot 3^3 - 3\right) - \left(\frac{1}{3}\cdot 1^3 - 1\right)\right]$$

$$= \frac{22}{3}.$$

Quick Check 2 ✓

Evaluate $\int_0^7 |2x^2 - 8|\,dx$.

2 ✓

The Area of a Region Bounded by Two Graphs

Suppose we want to find the area of region A, which is bounded by the graphs of f and g, as shown at the top of the next page. Note that over $[a, b]$, we have $f(x) \ge g(x)$, so we say that region A is *bounded above* by f and *bounded below* by g. The area of A is the area of A_2, which is the area below f over $[a, b]$, minus the area of A_1, which is the area below g over $[a, b]$:

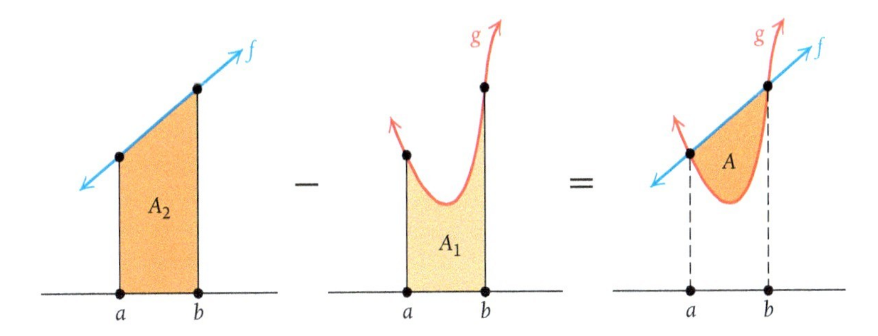

Thus,

$$A = \underbrace{\int_a^b f(x)\,dx}_{A_2} - \underbrace{\int_a^b g(x)\,dx}_{A_1},$$

or
$$A = \int_a^b [f(x) - g(x)]\,dx.$$

Generalizing, we have the following theorem.

THEOREM 6

Let f and g be continuous functions with $f(x) \geq g(x)$ over $[a, b]$. Then the area of the region between the two curves, from $x = a$ to $x = b$, is

$$\int_a^b [f(x) - g(x)]\,dx.$$

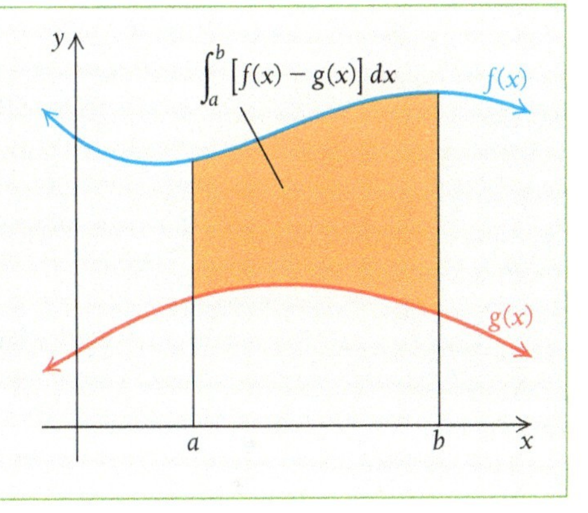

Sometimes, we need to find where f and g intersect, as illustrated in the following example.

EXAMPLE 3 Find the area of the region bounded by the graphs of $f(x) = 2x + 1$ and $g(x) = x^2 + 1$.

Solution Graphing both functions shows that f and g enclose region A, which is bounded above by f and below by g. To determine the bounds of integration, we set $f(x)$ equal to $g(x)$ and solve.

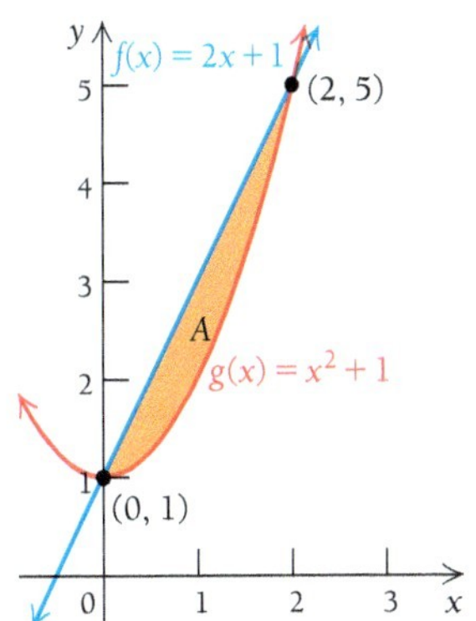

$$\begin{aligned} f(x) &= g(x) \\ 2x + 1 &= x^2 + 1 \\ 0 &= x^2 - 2x \\ 0 &= x(x - 2) \\ x = 0 \quad &or \quad x = 2. \end{aligned}$$

We now compute the area as follows:

$$\int_0^2 [\underbrace{(2x + 1)}_{f(x),\text{ above } A} - \underbrace{(x^2 + 1)}_{g(x),\text{ below } A}]\,dx = \int_0^2 (2x - x^2)\,dx$$

$$= \left[x^2 - \frac{x^3}{3}\right]_0^2$$

$$= \left(2^2 - \frac{2^3}{3}\right) - \left(0^2 - \frac{0^3}{3}\right)$$

$$= 4 - \frac{8}{3} = \frac{4}{3}.$$

3 ✓

Quick Check 3 ✓

Find the area of the region bounded by the graphs of $y = \sqrt{x}$ and $y = \frac{1}{3}x$.

EXAMPLE 4 **Life Science: Emission Control.** A college student develops an engine that is believed to meet all state standards for emission control. The new engine's rate of emission is given by

$$E(t) = 2t^2,$$

where $E(t)$ is the emissions, in billions of particulates per year, at time t, in years. Suppose the emission rate of a conventional engine is given by

$$C(t) = 9 + t^2.$$

The graphs of both curves are shown at the right.

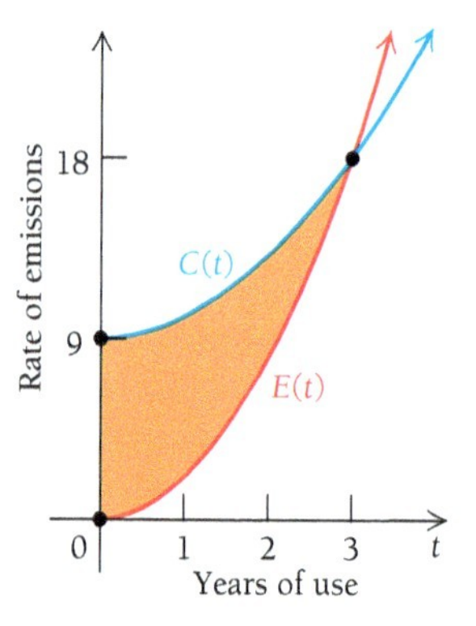

a) At what point in time will the emission rates be the same?

b) What reduction in emissions results with the student's engine up to the time found in part (a)?

Solution

a) The rate of emission will be the same when $E(t) = C(t)$, or

$$2t^2 = 9 + t^2$$
$$t^2 - 9 = 0$$
$$(t - 3)(t + 3) = 0$$
$$t = 3 \quad or \quad t = -3.$$

Since negative time values have no meaning here, the emission rates will be the same when $t = 3$ yr.

b) The reduction in emissions is represented by the area of the shaded region in the figure above. It is the area between $C(t) = 9 + t^2$ and $E(t) = 2t^2$, from $t = 0$ to $t = 3$, and is computed as follows:

$$\int_0^3 [(9 + t^2) - 2t^2]\,dt = \int_0^3 (9 - t^2)\,dt$$

$$= \left[9t - \frac{t^3}{3}\right]_0^3$$

$$= \left(9 \cdot 3 - \frac{3^3}{3}\right) - \left(9 \cdot 0 - \frac{0^3}{3}\right)$$

$$= 27 - 9 = 18.$$

Over 3 yr, the student's engine reduces emissions by 18 billion particulates. 4 ✓

Quick Check 4 ✓

Two rockets are fired upward simultaneously. The first rocket's velocity is given by $v_1(t) = 4t$; the second rocket's velocity is given by $v_2(t) = \frac{1}{10}t^2$. In both cases, t is in seconds and velocity is in feet per second.

a) After how many seconds will the velocities of the two rockets be the same?

b) How far ahead (in feet) of the second rocket is the first rocket after the number of seconds found in part (a)?

Average Value of a Continuous Function

Another important use of the area under a curve is in finding the average value of a continuous function over a closed interval.

Suppose that

$$T = f(t)$$

is the temperature at time t recorded at a weather station on a certain day. The station uses a 24-hr clock, so the domain of the temperature function is $[0, 24]$. The function is continuous, as shown in the following graph.

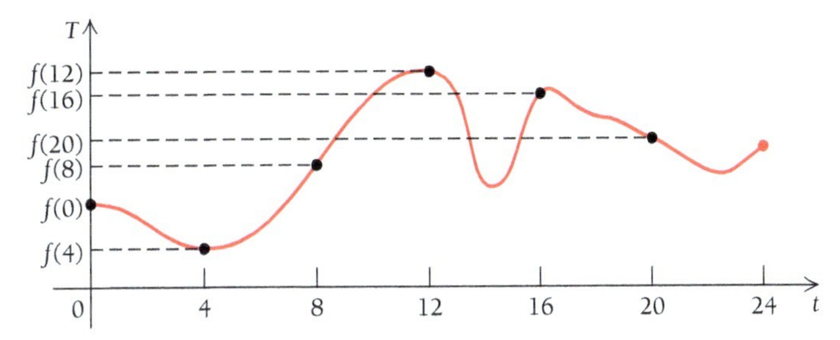

To find the average temperature for the day, we might take six temperature readings at 4-hr intervals, starting at midnight:

$$T_0 = f(0), \quad T_1 = f(4), \quad T_2 = f(8), \quad T_3 = f(12), \quad T_4 = f(16), \quad T_5 = f(20).$$

The average reading would then be the sum of these six readings divided by 6:

$$T_{av} = \frac{T_0 + T_1 + T_2 + T_3 + T_4 + T_5}{6}.$$

This computation of the average temperature has limitations. For example, suppose it is a hot summer day, and at 2:00 in the afternoon (hour 14 on the 24-hr clock), a short thunderstorm cools the air for an hour between our readings. This temporary dip would not show up in the average computed above.

What can we do? We could take 48 readings at half-hour intervals. This should give us a better result. In fact, the shorter the time between readings, the better the result should be. It seems reasonable that we might define the **average value** of T over $[0, 24]$ to be the limit, as n approaches ∞, of the average of n values:

$$\text{Average value of } T \text{ over } [0, 24] = \lim_{n \to \infty} \left(\frac{1}{n} \sum_{i=1}^{n} T_i \right) = \lim_{n \to \infty} \left(\frac{1}{n} \sum_{i=1}^{n} f(t_i) \right).$$

Note that this is not too far from our definition of an integral. All we need is to get Δt, which is $(24 - 0)/n$, or $24/n$, into the summation. We accomplish this by multiplying by 1, writing 1 as $\frac{1}{\Delta t} \cdot \Delta t$:

$$\text{Average value of } T \text{ over } [0, 24] = \lim_{n \to \infty} \left(\frac{1}{\Delta t} \cdot \frac{1}{n} \sum_{i=1}^{n} f(t_i)\, \Delta t \right) \qquad \text{Note that } \Delta t = \frac{24}{n}.$$

$$= \lim_{n \to \infty} \left(\frac{n}{24} \cdot \frac{1}{n} \sum_{i=1}^{n} f(t_i)\, \Delta t \right) \qquad \Delta t = \frac{24}{n}, \text{ so } \frac{1}{\Delta t} = \frac{n}{24}$$

$$= \frac{1}{24} \lim_{n \to \infty} \sum_{i=1}^{n} f(t_i)\, \Delta t \qquad \text{Using a limit property}$$

$$= \frac{1}{24} \int_0^{24} f(t)\, dt.$$

DEFINITION

For f, a continuous function over $[a, b]$, the **average value**, y_{av}, is given by

$$y_{av} = \frac{1}{b - a} \int_a^b f(x)\, dx.$$

We can look at average value another way. If we multiply both sides of

$$y_{av} = \frac{1}{b-a}\int_a^b f(x)\,dx$$

by $b - a$, we get

$$(b-a)y_{av} = \int_a^b f(x)\,dx.$$

The expression on the left is the area of a rectangle of length $b - a$ and height y_{av}. That area is the same as the area under the graph of f over $[a, b]$, as shown in the figure at the left. Note that the units of y_{av} will be the same as the units of f.

EXAMPLE 5 Find the average value of $f(x) = x^2$ over $[0, 2]$.

Solution The average value is

$$\frac{1}{2-0}\int_0^2 x^2\,dx = \frac{1}{2}\left[\frac{x^3}{3}\right]_0^2$$

$$= \frac{1}{2}\left(\frac{2^3}{3} - \frac{0^3}{3}\right)$$

$$= \frac{1}{2}\cdot\frac{8}{3} = \frac{4}{3}, \quad \text{or } 1\frac{1}{3}.$$

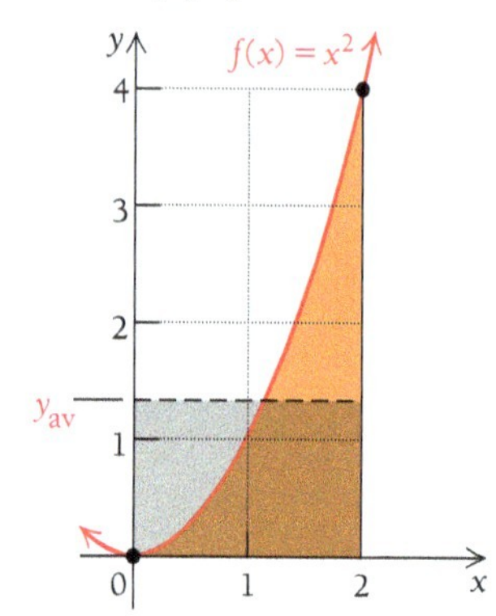

EXAMPLE 6 Rico is standing in a very long line, waiting to enter an arena to attend a concert. His speed, in feet per minute, t minutes after getting in line, is given by

$$v(t) = -\frac{1}{200}t^3 + \frac{3}{20}t^2 - \frac{3}{8}t + 60, \quad t \le 30.$$

From 5 min after getting in line to 25 min after doing so, what is Rico's average speed? How far does he move over that time interval?

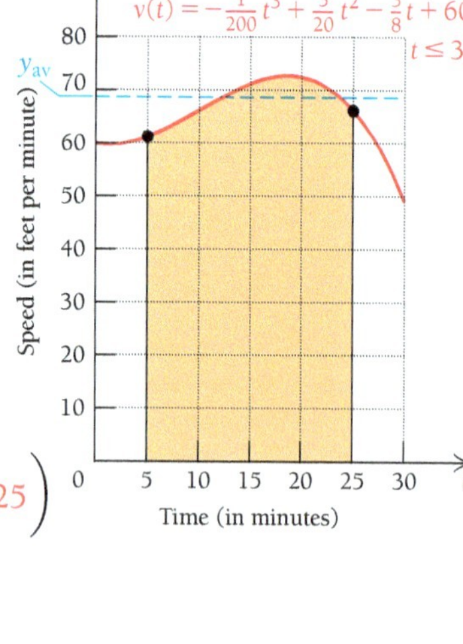

Solution Rico's average speed is

$$\frac{1}{25-5}\int_5^{25}\left(-\frac{1}{200}t^3 + \frac{3}{20}t^2 - \frac{3}{8}t + 60\right)dt$$

$$= \frac{1}{20}\left[-\frac{1}{800}t^4 + \frac{1}{20}t^3 - \frac{3}{16}t^2 + 60t\right]_5^{25}$$

$$= \frac{1}{20}\left[\left(-\frac{1}{800}\cdot 25^4 + \frac{1}{20}\cdot 25^3 - \frac{3}{16}\cdot 25^2 + 60\cdot 25\right) - \left(-\frac{1}{800}\cdot 5^4 + \frac{1}{20}\cdot 5^3 - \frac{3}{16}\cdot 5^2 + 60\cdot 5\right)\right]$$

$$= \frac{1}{20}\left(\frac{53{,}625}{32} - \frac{9625}{32}\right) = 68\tfrac{3}{4}\text{ ft/min.}$$

To find how far Rico moves over the time interval $[5, 25]$, we multiply by $25 - 5 = 20$. Thus, the distance he moves over $[5, 25]$ is

$$20\cdot 68\tfrac{3}{4} = 1375\text{ ft.}$$

5 ✓

Quick Check 5 ✓

The temperature, $T(x)$, in degrees Fahrenheit, in Minneapolis on a winter's day can be modeled by

$T(x) =$

$-0.012x^3 + 0.38x^2 - 1.99x - 10.1,$

where x is the number of hours from midnight $(0 \le x \le 24)$. Find the average temperature in Minneapolis during this 24-hour period.

Moving Average*

In business, data can fluctuate, which makes forecasting difficult. Averaging data over a fixed interval of time and allowing that interval of time to move yields a *moving*

*This section can be skipped without loss of continuity.

average, which often improves the quality of the forecasts. For example, the red curve in the graph below shows the number of workers in the United States aged 85 or older, for each month since 2005.

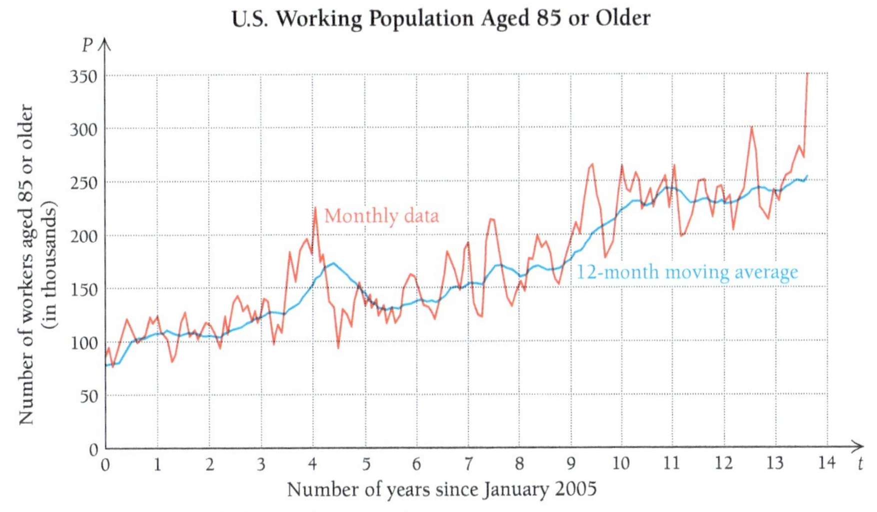

(*Sources*: U.S. Department of Labor; *Washington Post*.)

The number of workers aged 85 or older varies significantly from month to month, as you can see from the red curve. However, graphing the 12-month moving average of the data gives the blue curve, which shows the general trend of the monthly data but with the spikes and dips smoothed out.

DEFINITION

Let f be a continuous function over $[a, b]$. The **moving average function** of f is given by

$$f_{\text{av}}(x) = \frac{1}{L}\int_x^{x+L} f(t)\,dt,$$

where L is a constant representing a fixed interval of time.

For a given input x, the moving average function finds the average value of f over $[x, x + L]$. It "smooths" the behavior of f, and allows us to view general trends that are less affected by sudden rises or dips in the data. Because x is a bound of the definite integral, we use a different variable, t, in the integrand of the moving average function.

EXAMPLE 7 **Business: Moving Average.** The weekly revenue, $R(x)$, in thousands of dollars, of Trux Rentals x weeks since the start of the year is given by

$$R(x) = 0.05x^4 - 1.2x^3 + 9.6x^2 - 28.6x + 38.3,$$

where $0 \le x \le 10$. Find the moving average over 3-week intervals.

Solution We have $L = 3$. To find the moving average for the first 3 weeks, we set $x = 0$:

$$\begin{aligned} R_{\text{av}}(0) &= \frac{1}{3}\int_0^{0+3} R(t)\,dt \quad \text{Substituting} \\ &= \frac{1}{3}\int_0^{3} (0.05t^4 - 1.2t^3 + 9.6t^2 - 28.6t + 38.3)\,dt \\ &= \frac{1}{3}\left[0.01t^5 - 0.3t^4 + 3.2t^3 - 14.3t^2 + 38.3t\right]_0^3 \\ &\approx \frac{1}{3}(50.73) = 16.91. \end{aligned}$$

Thus, over the first 3 weeks of the year, Trux Rentals had an average revenue of \$16,910 per week.

The moving average over the second 3 weeks—that is, between $x = 1$ and $x = 4$—is

$$R_{av}(1) = \frac{1}{3}\int_{1}^{1+3} R(t)\,dt \qquad \text{Substituting}$$

$$= \frac{1}{3}\int_{1}^{4} (0.05t^4 - 1.2t^3 + 9.6t^2 - 28.6t + 38.3)\,dt$$

$$= \frac{1}{3}\left[0.01t^5 - 0.3t^4 + 3.2t^3 - 14.3t^2 + 38.3t\right]_1^4$$

$$\approx \frac{1}{3}(35.73) = 11.91.$$

Trux Rentals had an average weekly revenue of \$11,910 over these 3 weeks.

In a similar way, we find the average revenue over successive 3-week periods:

Between weeks 2 and 5: $R_{av}(2) = \frac{1}{3}\int_{2}^{5} R(t)\,dt \approx 12.41$, or \$12,410 per week;

Between weeks 3 and 6: $R_{av}(3) = \frac{1}{3}\int_{3}^{6} R(t)\,dt \approx 14.81$, or \$14,810 per week;

Between weeks 4 and 7: $R_{av}(4) = \frac{1}{3}\int_{4}^{7} R(t)\,dt \approx 16.71$, or \$16,710 per week;

Between weeks 5 and 8: $R_{av}(5) = \frac{1}{3}\int_{5}^{8} R(t)\,dt \approx 16.91$, or \$16,910 per week;

Between weeks 6 and 9: $R_{av}(6) = \frac{1}{3}\int_{6}^{9} R(t)\,dt \approx 15.41$, or \$15,410 per week;

Between weeks 7 and 10: $R_{av}(7) = \frac{1}{3}\int_{7}^{10} R(t)\,dt \approx 13.41$, or \$13,410 per week.

The graph below displays R, along with a graph of the moving average, R_{av}, over these seven 3-week periods of time. The graph of the moving average retains the general shape of the graph of R but reduces the fluctuations, making the general trend easier to see.

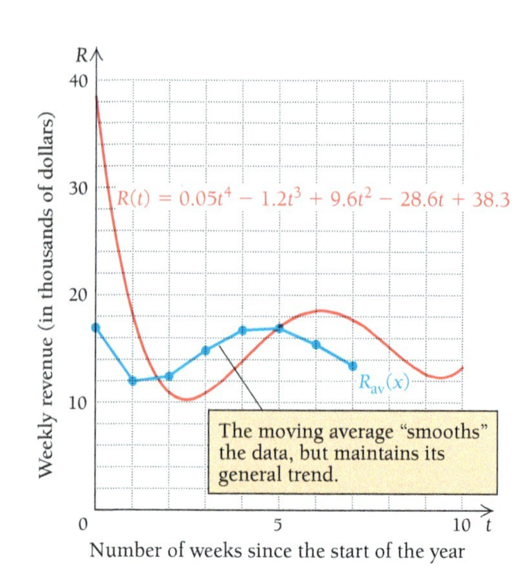

Quick Check 6 ✓

Using the function R in Example 7, find the moving averages over 4-week intervals, for $x = 0, 2, 4,$ and 6.

6 ✓

Section Summary

- The *additive property of definite integrals* states that a definite integral can be expressed as the sum of two (or more) other definite integrals. If f is continuous over $[a, b]$ and we choose c such that $a < c < b$, then

$$\int_a^b f(x)\,dx = \int_a^c f(x)\,dx + \int_c^b f(x)\,dx.$$

- The area of a region bounded by the graphs of two functions, f and g, with $f(x) \geq g(x)$ over $[a, b]$, is

$$A = \int_a^b [f(x) - g(x)]\,dx.$$

- The *average value* of a continuous function f over $[a, b]$ is

$$y_{av} = \frac{1}{b-a}\int_a^b f(x)\,dx.$$

- Let f be a continuous function over $[a, b]$. The *moving average function* of f is given by

$$f_{av}(x) = \frac{1}{L}\int_x^{x+L} f(t)\,dt,$$

where L is a constant representing a fixed interval of time.

4.4 Exercise Set

Find the area under the graph of f over $[1, 5]$.

1. $f(x) = \begin{cases} x + 5, & \text{for } x \leq 4, \\ 11 - \frac{1}{2}x, & \text{for } x > 4 \end{cases}$

2. $f(x) = \begin{cases} 2x + 1, & \text{for } x \leq 3, \\ 10 - x, & \text{for } x > 3 \end{cases}$

Find the area under the graph of g over $[-2, 3]$.

3. $g(x) = \begin{cases} -x^2 + 5, & \text{for } x \leq 0, \\ x + 5, & \text{for } x > 0 \end{cases}$

4. $g(x) = \begin{cases} x^2 + 4, & \text{for } x \leq 0, \\ 4 - x, & \text{for } x > 0 \end{cases}$

Find the area under the graph of f over $[-6, 4]$.

5. $f(x) = \begin{cases} -x - 1, & \text{for } x < -1, \\ -x^2 + 4x + 5, & \text{for } x \geq -1 \end{cases}$

6. $f(x) = \begin{cases} -x^2 - 6x + 8, & \text{for } x < 1, \\ 2x - 1, & \text{for } x \geq 1 \end{cases}$

Find the area represented by each definite integral.

7. $\int_{-3}^{4} |x^3|\,dx$

8. $\int_0^2 |x^3 - 1|\,dx$

9. $\int_0^4 |x - 3|\,dx$

10. $\int_{-1}^{1} |3x - 2|\,dx$

Find the area of the shaded region.

11. $f(x) = 2x + x^2 - x^3$, $g(x) = 0$

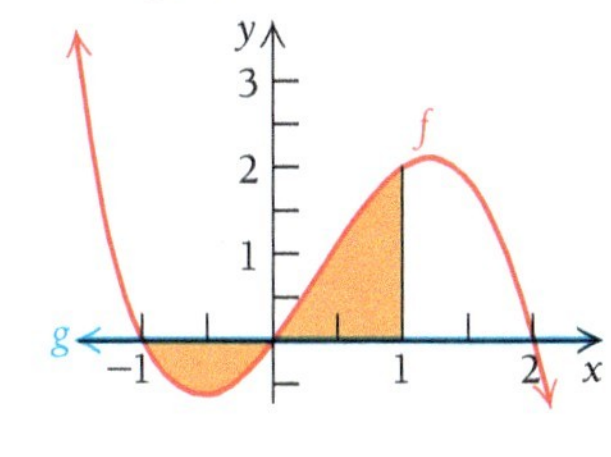

12. $f(x) = x^3 + 3x^2 - 9x - 12$, $g(x) = 4x + 3$

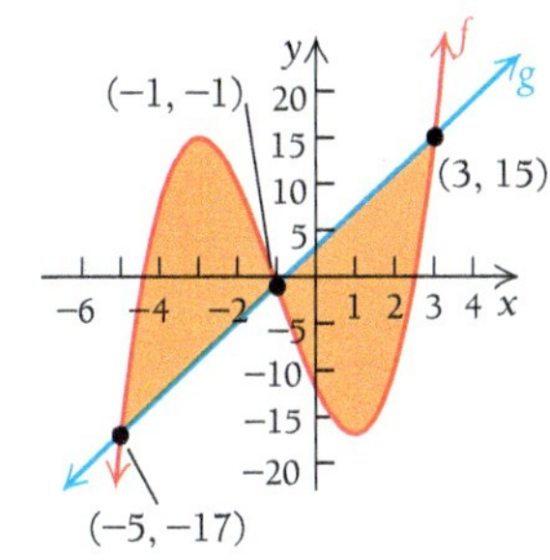

13. $f(x) = 4x - x^2$, $g(x) = x^2 - 6x + 8$

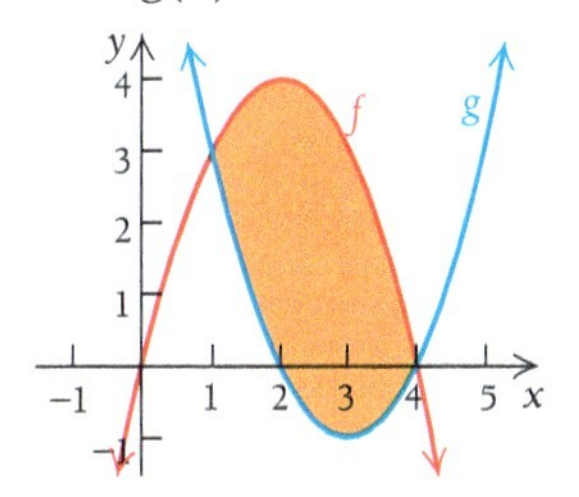

14. $f(x) = x^4 - 8x^3 + 18x^2$, $g(x) = x + 28$

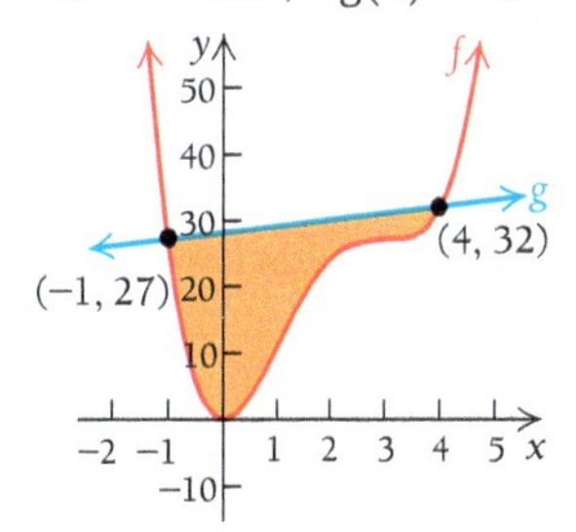

Find the area of the region bounded by the graphs of the given equations.

15. $y = x, y = x^4$

16. $y = x, y = x^3, x = 0, x = 1$

17. $y = x + 2, y = x^2$

18. $y = x^2 - 2x, y = x$

19. $y = 6x - x^2, y = x$

20. $y = x^2 - 6x, y = -x$

21. $y = x^2, y = \sqrt{x}$

22. $y = 2x - x^2, y = -x$

23. $y = x, y = \sqrt[4]{x}$

24. $y = 3, y = x, x = 0$

25. $y = 5, y = \sqrt{x}, x = 0$

26. $y = x^2, y = x^3$

27. $y = x^2 + 1, y = x^2, x = 1, x = 3$

28. $y = 4 - x^2, y = 4 - 4x$

29. $y = x^2 + 3, y = x^2, x = 1, x = 2$

30. $f(x) = x^2 - x - 5$, $g(x) = x + 10$

31. $f(x) = x^2 - 7x + 20$, $g(x) = 2x + 6$

32. $y = 2x^2 - 6x + 5, y = x^2 + 6x - 15$

33. $y = 2x^2 - x - 3, y = x^2 + x$

Find the average function value over the given interval.

34. $y = 4 - x^2;\ [-2, 2]$

35. $y = 2x^3;\ [-1, 1]$

36. $y = e^x;\ [0, 1]$

37. $y = e^{-x};\ [0, 1]$

38. $y = x^2 - x + 1;\ [0, 2]$

39. $f(x) = x^2 + x - 2;\ [0, 4]$

40. $f(x) = mx + 1;\ [0, 2]$

41. $f(x) = \frac{1}{x};\ [1, 3]$

42. $g(x) = \frac{1}{x};\ [4, 8]$

43. $y = \frac{3}{x^2};\ [1, 5]$

44. $y = \frac{2}{x^3};\ [-3, -1]$

APPLICATIONS

Business and Economics

45. Total and average daily profit. Great Green, Inc., determines that its marginal revenue per day is given by

$$R'(t) = 75e^t - 2t, \quad R(0) = 0,$$

where $R(t)$ is the total accumulated revenue, in dollars, on day t. The company's marginal cost per day is given by

$$C'(t) = 75 - 3t, \quad C(0) = 0,$$

where $C(t)$ is the total accumulated cost, in dollars, on day t.

a) Find the total profit from $t = 0$ to $t = 10$. *Note*:

$$P(T) = R(T) - C(T) = \int_0^T [R'(t) - C'(t)]\,dt.$$

b) Find the average daily profit for the first 10 days.

46. Total and average daily profit. Shylls, Inc., determines that its marginal revenue per day is given by

$$R'(t) = 100e^t, \quad R(0) = 0,$$

where $R(t)$ is the total accumulated revenue, in dollars, on day t. The company's marginal cost per day is given by

$$C'(t) = 100 - 0.2t, \quad C(0) = 0,$$

where $C(t)$ is the total accumulated cost, in dollars, on day t.

a) Find the total profit from $t = 0$ to $t = 10$ (the first 10 days).

b) Find the average daily profit for the first 10 days (from $t = 0$ to $t = 10$).

47. Accumulated sales. Music Manager, Ltd., estimates that monthly revenue, $R(t)$, in thousands of dollars, attributable to its Web site, t months after the site was launched, is given by

$$R(t) = 0.5e^t.$$

Find the average monthly revenue attributable to the site for its first 4 months of operation.

48. Accumulated sales. ProArt, Inc., estimates that its weekly online sales, $S(t)$, in hundreds of dollars, t weeks after online sales began, is given by

$$S(t) = 9e^t.$$

Find the average weekly sales for the first 5 weeks after online sales began.

49. Refer to Exercise 47. Find the average monthly revenue from Music Manager's Web site for months 3 through 5 ($t = 2$ to $t = 5$).

50. Refer to Exercise 48. Find ProArt's average weekly online sales for weeks 2 through 5 ($t = 1$ to $t = 5$).

Social Sciences

51. Memorizing. In a memory experiment, Alan is able to memorize words at the rate (in words per minute) given by

$$m'(t) = 2t - 0.09t^2.$$

In the same memory experiment, Bonnie is able to memorize words at the rate given by

$$M'(t) = 2t - 0.06t^2.$$

a) Who has memorized more words after 10 min? How many more words?

b) Over the first 10 min of the experiment, on average, how many words per minute did Alan memorize?

c) Over the first 10 min of the experiment, on average, how many words per minute did Bonnie memorize?

52. Vocabulary test. While studying for a German vocabulary test, Celia is able to memorize words at a rate, in words per hour, given by

$$s(t) = t^2, \quad 0 \le t \le 5.$$

Dan is also studying for the German vocabulary test, and he can memorize words at a rate given by

$$S(t) = 10t, \quad 0 \le t \le 5,$$

where $S(t)$ is the rate, in words per hour, at which he is memorizing after t hours.

a) For $0 < t < 5$, who will memorize more words?

b) Find the average value of $s(t)$ over $[0, 3]$, and explain what it represents.

c) Find the average value of $S(t)$ over $[2, 5]$, and explain what it represents.

d) Assuming that both students have the same study habits and are equally likely to study for any number of hours, t, in $[0, 5]$, on average, what is the difference in the number of words memorized?

53. Results of practice. A keyboarder's speed over a 5-min interval is given by

$$W(t) = -6t^2 + 12t + 90, \quad t \text{ in } [0, 5],$$

where $W(t)$ is the speed, in words per minute, at time t.

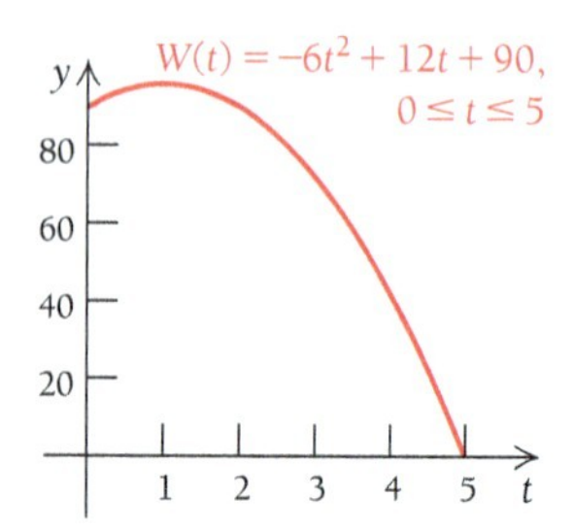

a) Find the speed at the beginning of the interval.

b) Find the maximum speed and when it occurs.

c) Find the average speed over the 5-min interval.

54. Average population. The population of the United States can be approximated by

$$P(t) = 310.65e^{0.00722t},$$

where $P(t)$ is in millions and t is the number of years since 2010. (*Source:* Population Division, U.S. Census Bureau.) Find the average value of the population from 2012 to 2019.

Life and Physical Sciences

55. Average drug dose. The concentration, $C(t)$, of phenylbutazone, in micrograms per milliliter (μg/mL), in the plasma of a calf injected with this anti-inflammatory agent is approximately

$$C(t) = 42.03e^{-0.01050t},$$

where t is the number of hours after the injection and $0 \leq t \leq 120$. (*Source:* A. K. Arifah and P. Lees, "Pharmacodynamics and Pharmacokinetics of Phenylbutazone in Calves," *Journal of Veterinary Pharmacology and Therapeutics*, Vol. 25, 299–309 (2002).)

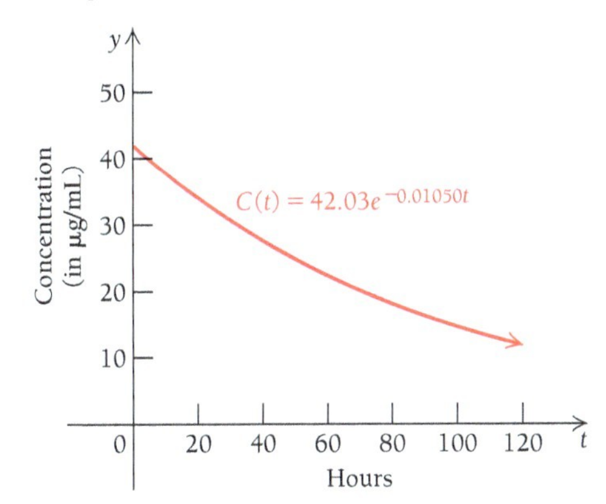

a) Given that this model is accurate for $0 \leq t \leq 120$, what is the initial dosage?
b) What is the average amount of phenylbutazone in the calf's body for the time between 10 and 120 hours?

56. New York temperature. For any date, the average temperature in New York City can be approximated by

$$T(x) = 43.5 - 18.4x + 8.57x^2 - 0.996x^3 + 0.0338x^4,$$

where T represents the temperature in degrees Fahrenheit x months from mid-December. That is, $x = 1$ represents the middle of January, $x = 2$ represents the middle of February, and so on. (*Source:* Based on data from www.worldclimate.com.) Compute the average temperature in New York over the whole year to the nearest degree.

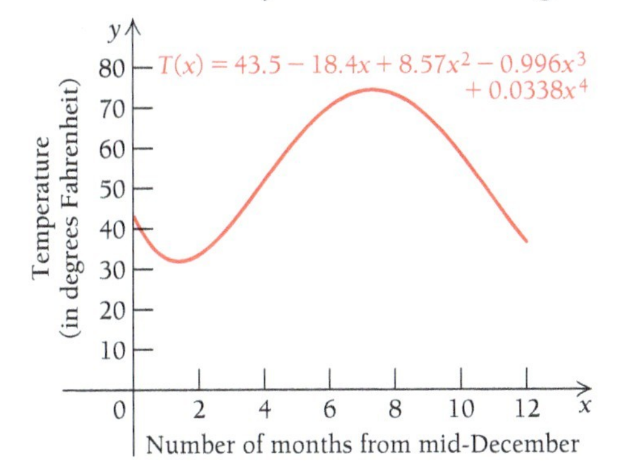

57. Outside temperature. Suppose the temperature in degrees Celsius over a 10-hr period is given by

$$f(t) = -t^2 + 5t + 40, \quad 0 \leq t \leq 10.$$

a) Find the average temperature.
b) Find the minimum temperature.
c) Find the maximum temperature.

58. Engine emissions. The emissions of an engine are given by

$$E(t) = 2t^2,$$

where $E(t)$ is the engine's rate of emission, in billions of particulates per year, after t years. Find the average emissions from $t = 1$ to $t = 5$.

59. Engine emissions. Suppose emissions from an older engine are given by $f(x) = x$, and those from a redesigned engine are given by $g(x) = \frac{1}{2}x^2$, where x is in years and both $f(x)$ and $g(x)$ are in billions of particulates emitted per year. Assume $x > 0$.

a) When will the emissions rate be the same for both engines?
b) Which engine has emitted more particulates in the time found in part (a), and how much more?

60. Engine emissions. Suppose emissions from an older engine are given by $f(x) = \frac{1}{3}x$, and those from a redesigned engine are given by $g(x) = \frac{1}{10}x^2$, where x is in years and both $f(x)$ and $g(x)$ are in billions of particulates emitted per year. Assume $x > 0$.

a) Find the time when the emissions rate is the same for both engines.
b) Which engine has emitted more particulates in the time found in part (a), and how much more?

61. Areas as distance. The velocity of Beth's remote-control car is given by $v_1(t) = \frac{1}{2}t$, and the velocity of James's remote-control car is given by $v_2(t) = \frac{1}{15}t^2$, where t is in seconds and the velocities are in feet per second. Assume that both cars start on a race course at the same time.

a) Which car is ahead after 5 sec, and by how much?
b) When are the cars traveling at the same velocity?
c) Which car is ahead at the time found in part (b), and by how much?

62. Areas as distance. The velocity of Phil's remote-control drone is given by $v_1(t) = \frac{1}{4}t^2$, and the velocity of Allison's remote-control drone is given by $v_2(t) = \sqrt{t}$, where t is in seconds and the velocities are in feet per second. Assume that both drones start at the same time.

a) Which drone is ahead after 2 sec, and by how much?
b) When are the drones traveling at the same velocity?
c) Which drone is ahead at the time found in part (b), and by how much?

In Exercises 63 and 64, find the moving averages of the given function, for the given values of x and interval length L.

63. $f(x) = x^3 - x^2 - 4x + 6; \quad x = 0, 1, 2, 3, 4, 5$ and $L = 2$

64. $g(x) = x^4 - x^3 + 5x - 1; \quad x = 0, 2, 4, 6$ and $L = 4$

65. **Moving averages.** The monthly profit, $P(x)$, in thousands of dollars, t months after January 1, for Ferguson's Family Fun Center, is given by

$$P(x) = -0.04x^4 + 1.04x^3 - 8.53x^2 + 26.46x + 10.5.$$

a) Find the 2-month moving averages for $x = 0, 1, 2, 3, 4,$ and 5.
b) Graph P, for $0 \leq x \leq 8$, and the moving averages, on the same graph.
c) Do the moving averages follow the same general trend as the graph of P? Why or why not?

66. **Moving averages.** The weekly revenue, $R(x)$, in thousands of dollars, t weeks after January 1, for Yeager Neckwear, is given by

$$R(x) = -0.003x^3 - 0.79x^2 + 8.33x + 72.9.$$

a) Find the 3-month moving averages for $x = 0, 2, 4,$ and 6.
b) Graph R, for $0 \leq x \leq 9$, and the moving averages, on the same graph.
c) Do the moving averages follow the same general trend as the graph of P? Why or why not?

SYNTHESIS

Find the area of the region bounded by the given graphs.

67. $y = e^x, y = e^{-x}, x = -2$

68. $y = x + 6, y = -2x, y = x^3$

69. Find the area bounded by $y = 3x^5 - 20x^3$, the x-axis, and the first coordinates of the relative maximum and minimum values of the function.

70. Find the area bounded by $y = x^3 - 3x + 2$, the x-axis, and the first coordinates of the relative maximum and minimum values of the function.

71. **Life science: Poiseuille's Law.** The flow of blood in a blood vessel is faster toward the center of the vessel and slower toward the outside. The speed of the blood is given by

$$V = \frac{p}{4Lv}(R^2 - r^2),$$

where R is the radius of the blood vessel, r is the distance of the blood from the center of the vessel, and p, v, and L are physical constants related to the pressure and viscosity of the blood and the length of the blood vessel. If R is constant, we can regard V as a function of r:

$$V(r) = \frac{p}{4Lv}(R^2 - r^2).$$

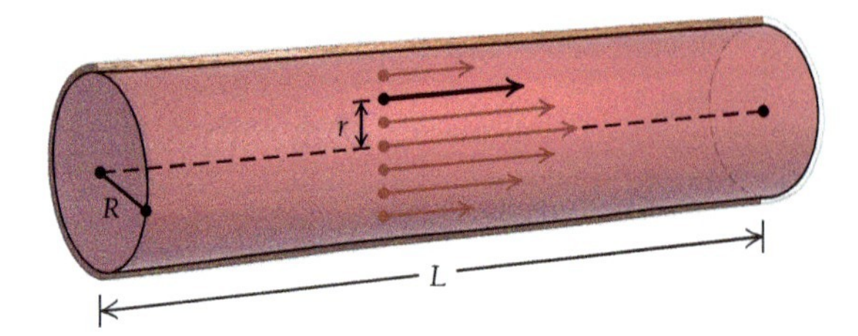

The total blood flow, Q, is given by

$$Q = \int_0^R 2\pi \cdot V(r) \cdot r \cdot dr.$$

Find Q.

72. Solve for K, given that

$$\int_1^2 [(3x^2 + 5x) - (3x + K)]\, dx = 6.$$

73. **Engine emissions.** As in Exercise 59, two engines have rates of emissions given by $f(x) = x$ and $g(x) = \frac{1}{2}x^2$, where x is in years and both $f(x)$ and $g(x)$ are in billions of particulates emitted per year. When will both engines have emitted the same total number of particulates?

74. **Engine emissions.** As in Exercise 60, two engines have rates of emissions given by $f(x) = \frac{1}{3}x$ and $g(x) = \frac{1}{10}x^2$, where x is in years and both $f(x)$ and $g(x)$ are in billions of particulates emitted per year. When will both engines have emitted the same total number of particulates?

75. **Areas as distance.** As in Exercise 61, the velocity of Beth's remote-control car is given by $v_1(t) = \frac{1}{2}t$, and the velocity of James's remote-control car is given by $v_2(t) = \frac{1}{15}t^2$, where t is in seconds and the velocities are in feet per second.

a) Find the time at which the two cars are side by side.
b) How far have the cars traveled at the time found in part (a)?

76. **Areas as distance.** As in Exercise 62, the velocity of Phil's remote-control drone is given by $v_1(t) = \frac{1}{4}t^2$, and the velocity of Allison's remote-control drone is given by $v_2(t) = \sqrt{t}$, where t is in seconds and the velocities are in feet per second.

a) Find the time at which the two drones are side by side.
b) How far have the drones traveled at the time found in part (a)?

Technology Connection

Find the area of the region enclosed by the given graphs.

77. $y = x\sqrt{4 - x^2}, y = \frac{-4x}{x^2 + 1}, x = 0, x = 2$

78. $y = 2x^2 + x - 4, y = 1 - x + 8x^2 - 4x^4$

79. $y = \sqrt{1 - x^2}, y = 1 - x^2, x = -1, x = 1$

80. Consider the following functions:

$$f(x) = 3.8x^5 - 18.6x^3, \quad g(x) = 19x^4 - 55.8x^2.$$

a) Graph f and g in the window $[-3, 3, -80, 80]$, with Yscl = 10.
b) Estimate the first coordinates a, b, and c of the three points of intersection of f and g.
c) Find the area between the curves over $[a, b]$.
d) Find the area between the curves over $[b, c]$.

81. For the moving averages found in Exercise 65, use REGRESSION to find a curve that best fits those points; then use the curve to estimate the 2-month average monthly profit for Ferguson's Family Fun Center for $x = 6$.

82. For the moving averages found in Exercise 66, use REGRESSION to find a curve that best fits those points; then use the curve to estimate the 3-month average monthly profit for Yeager Neckwear for $x = 8$.

Answers to Quick Checks

1. $\frac{59}{3}$ **2.** 194 **3.** $\frac{9}{2}$, or $4\frac{1}{2}$ **4.** **(a)** 40 sec; **(b)** $1066\frac{2}{3}$ ft **5.** Approximately -2.5°F
6. $R_{av}(0) = 15.66$, or \$15,660/week over weeks 0 through 4; $R_{av}(2) = 13.66$, or \$13,660/week over weeks 2 through 6; $R_{av}(4) = 16.46$, or \$16,460/week over weeks 4 through 8; $R_{av}(6) = 14.46$, or \$14,460/week over weeks 6 through 10

4.5 Integration Techniques: Substitution

- Evaluate integrals using substitution.
- Solve applied problems involving integration by substitution.

The following formulas provide a basis for an integration technique called **substitution**, a process that is, as we will see, the reverse of differentiation using the Chain Rule.

A. $\displaystyle\int u^r\,du = \frac{u^{r+1}}{r+1} + C$, assuming $r \neq -1$

B. $\displaystyle\int e^u\,du = e^u + C$

C. $\displaystyle\int \frac{1}{u}\,du = \ln|u| + C$; and $\displaystyle\int \frac{1}{u}\,du = \ln u + C, \quad u > 0$

In the above formulas, the variable u represents some function of x and du is the derivative of u with respect to x. Recall that we solve $\int x^7\,dx$ using the Power Rule for Antiderivatives:

$$\int x^7\,dx = \frac{x^{7+1}}{7+1} + C = \frac{x^8}{8} + C, \quad \text{or} \quad \frac{1}{8}x^8 + C.$$

But, what about an integral like $\int (3x-4)^7\,dx$? Suppose we thought the antiderivative was

$$\frac{(3x-4)^8}{8} + C.$$

If we check by differentiating, we get

$$8 \cdot \frac{1}{8} \cdot (3x-4)^7 \cdot 3 \cdot dx. \qquad \text{Using the Extended Power Rule}$$

This simplifies to

$$3(3x-4)^7, \quad \textit{not } (3x-4)^7.$$

To correct our antiderivative, let's make this substitution:

$$u = 3x - 4.$$

Then $du/dx = 3$, and recalling our work with differentials (Section 3.6), we have

$$du = 3 \cdot dx, \quad \text{and} \quad \frac{du}{3} = dx.$$

With *substitution*, our original integral, $\int (3x-4)^7\,dx$, takes the form

$$\int (3x-4)^7\,dx = \int u^7 \cdot \frac{du}{3} \qquad \text{Substituting } u \text{ for } 3x-4 \text{ and } \frac{du}{3} \text{ for } dx$$

$$= \frac{1}{3}\cdot \int u^7\,du \qquad \text{Factoring out the constant } \frac{1}{3}$$

$$= \frac{1}{3}\cdot \frac{u^8}{8} + C \qquad \text{Using formula A}$$

$$= \frac{1}{3\cdot 8}\cdot (3x-4)^8 + C = \frac{1}{24}(3x-4)^8 + C.$$

We leave it to the student to check that this is indeed the antiderivative. Note how this procedure reverses the Chain Rule.

Throughout this section, it is important to recall that

$$\frac{dy}{dx} = f'(x) \qquad \text{and} \qquad dy = f'(x)\,dx.$$

EXAMPLE 1 Find dy for each function:

a) $y = f(x) = x^3$;
b) $y = f(x) = x^{2/3}$;
c) $y = g(x) = \ln x$;
d) $y = f(x) = e^{x^2}$

Solution

a) We have

$$\frac{dy}{dx} = f'(x) = 3x^2,$$

so $\quad dy = f'(x)\,dx = 3x^2\,dx.$

b) We have

$$\frac{dy}{dx} = f'(x) = \tfrac{2}{3}x^{-1/3},$$

so $\quad dy = f'(x)\,dx = \tfrac{2}{3}x^{-1/3}\,dx.$

c) We have

$$\frac{dy}{dx} = g'(x) = \frac{1}{x},$$

so $\quad dy = g'(x)\,dx = \dfrac{1}{x}\,dx, \quad \text{or} \quad \dfrac{dx}{x}.$

d) Using the Chain Rule, we have

$$\frac{dy}{dx} = f'(x) = e^{x^2}\cdot 2x,$$

so $\quad dy = f'(x)\,dx = 2xe^{x^2}\,dx.$ **1 ✓**

Quick Check 1 ✓

Find each differential.

a) For $y = \sqrt{x}$, find dy.

b) For $u = x^2 - 3x$, find du.

c) For $y = \dfrac{1}{x^3}$, find dy.

d) For $u = 4x - 3$, find du.

So far, the dx in

$$\int f(x)\,dx$$

has played no role in integration other than to indicate the variable of integration. Now it becomes convenient to make use of dx. Consider the integral

$$\int 2xe^{x^2}\,dx.$$

If we note that $2xe^{x^2} = e^{x^2} \cdot 2x$, we see in Example 1(d) that $f(x) = e^{x^2}$ is an antiderivative of $f'(x) = 2xe^{x^2}$. How might we find such an antiderivative directly? Suppose we let $u = x^2$. Since

$$\frac{du}{dx} = 2x, \quad \text{we have} \quad du = 2x\,dx.$$

We substitute u for x^2 and du for $2x\,dx$:

$$\int 2xe^{x^2}\,dx = \int e^{x^2}\,2x\,dx = \int e^u\,du.$$

Since

$$\int e^u\,du = e^u + C,$$

it follows that

$$\int 2xe^{x^2}\,dx = \int e^u\,du = e^u + C$$

$$= e^{x^2} + C. \qquad \text{Replacing } u \text{ with } x^2$$

In effect, we have applied the Chain Rule in reverse. The procedure is referred to as *substitution*, or *change of variable*. We can check the result by differentiating. While many integrals cannot be solved using substitution, any integral that fits formula A, B, or C on page 429 can be solved with this procedure.

When using substitution, we choose what u represents so that we obtain an equivalent integral in which the "original" variables (using x and dx) no longer appear and which is more easily solved.

EXAMPLE 2 Evaluate: $\int 3x^2(x^3 + 1)^{10}\,dx$.

Solution Note that $3x^2$ is the derivative of $x^3 + 1$. Thus,

$$\int 3x^2(x^3+1)^{10}\,dx = \int (x^3+1)^{10}\,3x^2\,dx \qquad \text{Our choice of substitution } \boxed{u = x^3 + 1,\ du = 3x^2\,dx}$$

$$= \int u^{10}\,du$$

$$= \frac{u^{11}}{11} + C$$

$$= \tfrac{1}{11}(x^3+1)^{11} + C. \qquad \text{Reversing the substitution}$$

To check, we differentiate:

$$\frac{d}{dx}\left[\tfrac{1}{11}(x^3+1)^{11} + C\right] = \tfrac{11}{11}(x^3+1)^{10} \cdot 3x^2 + 0$$

$$= (x^3+1)^{10} \cdot 3x^2 = 3x^2(x^3+1)^{10}.$$

2 ✓

Quick Check 2 ✓
Evaluate: $\int 4x(2x^2 + 3)^3\,dx$.

EXAMPLE 3 Evaluate: $\displaystyle\int \frac{2x\,dx}{1 + x^2}$.

Solution Note that $2x$ is the derivative of $1 + x^2$. We have

$$\int \frac{2x\,dx}{1+x^2} = \int \frac{du}{u} \qquad \text{Our choice of substitution } \boxed{u = 1 + x^2,\ du = 2x\,dx}$$

$$= \ln u + C \qquad \text{Remember: } \int \frac{du}{u} = \int \frac{1}{u} \cdot du.$$

$$= \ln(1 + x^2) + C \qquad \text{Using absolute value is not necessary here since } 1 + x^2 > 0 \text{ for all } x.$$

3 ✓

Quick Check 3 ✓
Evaluate: $\displaystyle\int \frac{e^x}{1 + e^x}\,dx$.

EXAMPLE 4 Evaluate: $\int \frac{2x\,dx}{(1 + x^2)^5}$.

Solution As in Example 3, note that $\frac{d}{dx}(1 + x^2) = 2x$:

$$\int \frac{2x\,dx}{(1 + x^2)^5} = \int \frac{du}{u^5}$$

Our choice of substitution: $u = 1 + x^2$, $du = 2x\,dx$

$$= \int u^{-5}\,du$$

$$= \frac{u^{-4}}{-4} + C$$

$$= -\frac{1}{4u^4} + C$$

$$= -\frac{1}{4(1 + x^2)^4} + C.$$

Don't forget to reverse the substitution.

Quick Check 4 ✓

Evaluate: $\int \frac{6x^2}{\sqrt{3 + 2x^3}}\,dx$.

4 ✓

EXAMPLE 5 Evaluate: $\int \frac{\ln(3x)\,dx}{x}$, $x > 0$.

Solution Note that $\frac{d}{dx}\ln(3x) = \frac{1}{3x} \cdot 3 = \frac{1}{x}$. Thus,

$$\int \frac{\ln(3x)\,dx}{x} = \int u\,du$$

Our choice of substitution: $u = \ln(3x)$, $du = \frac{1}{x}\,dx$

$$= \frac{u^2}{2} + C$$

$$= \frac{(\ln(3x))^2}{2} + C. \quad \text{Substituting}$$

Quick Check 5 ✓

Evaluate:

$$\int \frac{(\ln x)^2}{x}\,dx, \quad x > 0.$$

5 ✓

EXAMPLE 6 Evaluate: $\int xe^{x^2}\,dx$.

Solution We let $u = x^2$, so $du = 2x\,dx$. Since the integrand contains $x\,dx$, we need a "new" factor of 2.

$$\int xe^{x^2}\,dx = \int e^{x^2}\,x\,dx \quad \text{Grouping } x \text{ and } dx$$

$$= \int e^u\left(\frac{du}{2}\right)$$

Our choice of substitution: $u = x^2$, $du = 2x\,dx$, so that $x\,dx = du/2$

$$= \frac{1}{2}\int e^u\,du$$

$$= \tfrac{1}{2}e^u + C = \tfrac{1}{2}e^{x^2} + C$$

Quick Check 6 ✓

Evaluate: $\int x^2 e^{4x^3}\,dx$.

6 ✓

EXAMPLE 7 Evaluate: $\int \frac{dx}{6x + 1}$, $x \neq -\frac{1}{6}$.

Solution

$$\int \frac{dx}{6x + 1} = \int \frac{du}{6u}$$

Our choice of substitution: $u = 6x + 1$, $du = 6\,dx$, so that $dx = du/6$

$$= \frac{1}{6}\int \frac{du}{u}$$

$$= \frac{1}{6}\ln|u| + C \quad \text{Finding the antiderivative with respect to } u$$

$$= \tfrac{1}{6}\ln|6x + 1| + C \quad \text{Substituting}$$

EXAMPLE 8 Evaluate: $\int_0^1 5x\sqrt{x^2+3}\,dx$. Round to the nearest thousandth.

Solution We first find the antiderivative. We move the factor 5 in front of the integral and group x and dx:

$$\int 5x\sqrt{x^2+3}\,dx = 5\int \sqrt{x^2+3}\,x\,dx$$

$$= 5\int \sqrt{x^2+3}\,x\,dx$$

$$= 5\int \sqrt{u}\,\frac{du}{2}$$ Our choice of substitution $u = x^2+3$, $du = 2x\,dx$

$$= \frac{5}{2}\int u^{1/2}\,du$$ Simplifying

$$= \frac{5}{2}\cdot\frac{2}{3}u^{3/2} + C$$ Finding the antiderivative with respect to u

$$= \frac{5}{3}(x^2+3)^{3/2} + C.$$ Reversing the substitution before evaluating the bounds

Using 0 for C, we evaluate the antiderivative:

$$\int_0^1 5x\sqrt{x^2+3}\,dx = \left[\frac{5}{3}(x^2+3)^{3/2}\right]_0^1$$

$$= \frac{5}{3}(1^2+3)^{3/2} - \frac{5}{3}(0^2+3)^{3/2}$$

$$= \frac{5}{3}\left[4^{3/2} - 3^{3/2}\right]$$ Simplifying

$$\approx 4.673.$$ Using a calculator

7 ✓

Quick Check 7 ✓
Evaluate:

$$\int_0^2 7x(x^2+3)^4\,dx.$$

In some cases, after a substitution is made, a further simplification can allow us to complete an integration.

EXAMPLE 9 Evaluate: $\int \frac{x}{x+2}\,dx$. Assume $x > -2$.

Solution We substitute $u = x+2$ and $du = dx$. Note that $u > 0$ and $x = u - 2$. The substitutions are made:

$$\int \frac{x}{x+2}\,dx = \int \frac{u-2}{u}\,du$$ Our choice of substitution $u = x+2$, $du = dx$, $x = u-2$

$$= \int\left(1 - \frac{2}{u}\right)du$$ $\frac{u-2}{u} = \frac{u}{u} - \frac{2}{u} = 1 - \frac{2}{u}$

$$= u - 2\ln u + C_1$$

$$= x + 2 - 2\ln(x+2) + C_1$$ Reversing the substitution

$$= x - 2\ln(x+2) + C$$ Collecting constant terms: $C = C_1 + 2$

8 ✓

Quick Check 8 ✓

Evaluate $\int \frac{x}{(x-1)^3}\,dx$ by letting $u = x - 1$. Assume that $x > 1$.

Section Summary

- Integration by substitution anticipates the application of the Chain Rule, when an antiderivative is differentiated.
- Substitutions must be reversed after the integration has been performed so that the original variables appear in the solution.
- All antiderivatives should be checked using differentiation.

4.5 Exercise Set

Evaluate. (Be sure to check by differentiating!)

1. $\int (x^2 - 7)^6\, 2x\, dx$

2. $\int (8 + x^3)^5\, 3x^2\, dx$

3. $\int (x^2 - 6)^7 x\, dx$

4. $\int (x^3 + 1)^4 x^2\, dx$

5. $\int (2t^5 - 3)t^4\, dt$

6. $\int (3t^4 + 2)t^3\, dt$

7. $\int \frac{2}{1 + 2x}\, dx,\ x \neq -\frac{1}{2}$

8. $\int \frac{5}{5x + 7}\, dx,\ x \neq -\frac{7}{5}$

9. $\int \frac{(\ln x)^7}{x}\, dx,\ x > 0$

10. $\int \frac{(\ln x)^3}{x}\, dx,\ x > 0$

11. $\int e^{3x}\, dx$

12. $\int e^{7x}\, dx$

13. $\int e^{x/2}\, dx$

14. $\int e^{x/3}\, dx$

15. $\int x^4 e^{x^5}\, dx$

16. $\int x^3 e^{x^4}\, dx$

17. $\int t^2 e^{-t^3}\, dt$

18. $\int t e^{-t^2}\, dt$

19. $\int \frac{1}{5 + 2x}\, dx,\ x \neq -\frac{5}{2}$

20. $\int \frac{1}{2 + 8x}\, dx,\ x \neq -\frac{1}{4}$

21. $\int \frac{dx}{1 + 7x},\ x \neq -\frac{1}{7}$

22. $\int \frac{dx}{12 + 3x},\ x \neq -4$

23. $\int \frac{dx}{1 - x},\ x \neq 1$

24. $\int \frac{dx}{4 - x},\ x \neq 4$

25. $\int t^2(t^3 - 1)^7\, dt$

26. $\int t(t^2 - 1)^5\, dt$

27. $\int (x^4 + x^3 + x^2)^7(4x^3 + 3x^2 + 2x)\, dx$

28. $\int (x^3 - x^2 - x)^9(3x^2 - 2x - 1)\, dx$

29. $\int \frac{e^t\, dt}{3 + e^t}$

30. $\int \frac{e^x\, dx}{4 + e^x}$

31. $\int \frac{\ln x^2}{x}\, dx,\ x > 0$
(*Hint:* Use the properties of logarithms.)

32. $\int \frac{(\ln x)^2}{x}\, dx,\ x > 0$

33. $\int \frac{dx}{x \ln x^2},\ x > 1$

34. $\int \frac{dx}{x \ln x},\ x > 1$

35. $\int x\sqrt{ax^2 + b}\, dx$

36. $\int \sqrt{ax + b}\, dx$

37. $\int be^{ax}\, dx$

38. $\int P_0 e^{kt}\, dt$

39. $\int \frac{x^3\, dx}{(2 - x^4)^7}$

40. $\int \frac{3x^2\, dx}{(1 + x^3)^5}$

41. $\int 5x\sqrt[4]{1 - x^2}\, dx$

42. $\int 12x\sqrt[5]{1 + 6x^2}\, dx$

43. $\int \frac{3e^{2x}}{e^{2x} + 5}\, dx$

44. $\int \frac{4e^{-x}}{3 + e^{-x}}\, dx$

Evaluate.

45. $\int_0^1 3x^2 e^{x^3}\, dx$

46. $\int_0^1 2xe^{x^2}\, dx$

47. $\int_1^2 x(x^2 - 1)^7\, dx$

48. $\int_0^1 x(x^2 + 1)^5\, dx$

49. $\int_0^2 e^{4x}\, dx$

50. $\int_0^4 \frac{dt}{1 + t}$

51. $\int_1^3 \frac{2x + 3}{x^2 + 3x}\, dx$

52. $\int_1^4 \frac{2x + 1}{x^2 + x - 1}\, dx$

53. $\int_0^b 2e^{-2x}\, dx$

54. $\int_0^b e^{-x}\, dx$

55. $\int_0^b ke^{-kx}\, dx$

56. $\int_0^b me^{-mx}\, dx$

57. $\int_0^3 (x - 5)^2\, dx$

58. $\int_0^4 (x - 6)^2\, dx$

59. $\int_{-1}^0 \frac{x^3\, dx}{(2 - x^4)^7}$

60. $\int_0^2 \frac{3x^2\, dx}{(1 + x^3)^5}$

61. $\int_0^1 12x\sqrt[5]{1 - x^2}\, dx$

62. $\int_0^{\sqrt{7}} 7x\sqrt[3]{1 + x^2}\, dx$

63. $\int_0^{\ln 2} \frac{e^x}{e^x + 1} dx$

64. $\int_0^{\ln 4} \frac{e^{3x}}{2 + e^{3x}} dx$

65. $\int_1^3 (x + 1)e^{x^2+2x} dx$

66. $\int_1^4 \frac{e^{\sqrt{x}}}{\sqrt{x}} dx$

Evaluate. Use the technique of Example 9.

67. $\int \frac{x}{x - 5} dx$

68. $\int \frac{3x}{2x + 1} dx$

69. $\int \frac{x}{1 - 4x} dx$

70. $\int \frac{x + 3}{x - 2} dx$ (*Hint*: $u = x - 2$.)

71. $\int \frac{2x + 3}{3x - 2} dx$

72. $\int x^2(x + 1)^{10} dx$

73. $\int x^3(x + 2)^7 dx$

74. $\int x^2\sqrt{x - 2}\, dx$

APPLICATIONS

Business and Economics

75. Demand from marginal demand. Masterson Insoles, Inc., has the marginal-demand function

$$D'(x) = \frac{-2000x}{\sqrt{25 - x^2}},$$

where $D(x)$ is the number of units sold at x dollars per unit. Find the demand function given that $D = 13{,}000$ when $x = \$3$ per unit.

76. Profit from marginal profit. A firm has the marginal-profit function

$$\frac{dP}{dx} = \frac{9000 - 3000x}{(x^2 - 6x + 10)^2},$$

where $P(x)$ is the profit earned at x dollars per unit. Find the total-profit function given that $P = \$1500$ at $x = \$3$.

77. Cost from marginal cost. Bellyacher's Home Ice Cream, Inc., determines that its marginal cost, in dollars per unit, is given by

$$\frac{dC}{dx} = 25.765xe^{0.0035x^2},$$

where x is the number of home ice-cream makers produced. Find the total cost to produce 10 units.

78. Profit from marginal profit. Silinder Electronics determines that its marginal profit, in hundreds of dollars per speaker, is given by

$$\frac{dP}{dx} = 0.35x\sqrt{0.25x^2 + 1.75},$$

where x is the number of panorama stereo speakers produced and sold. Find the total profit when 8 speakers are sold.

Social Sciences

79. Marriage rate. The marriage rate in Nevada is approximated by

$$M(t) = 38.045e^{-0.045t},$$

where $M(t)$ is the number of marriages per 1000 people, per year, t years after 2010. (*Source*: Based on data from www.cdc.gov.)

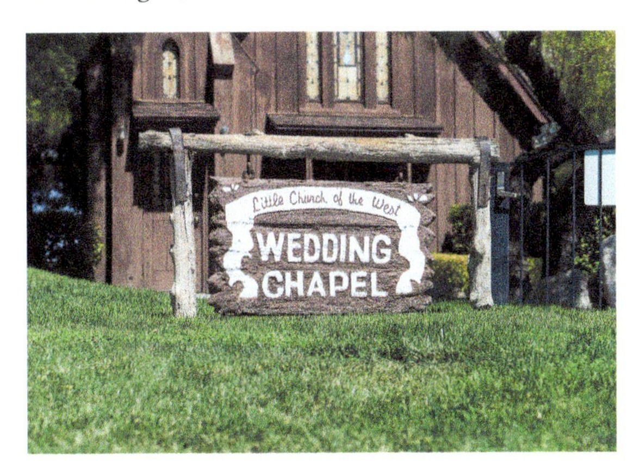

a) Find the total number of marriages per 1000 people in Nevada from 2010 to 2015.
b) Estimate the total number of marriages per 1000 people in Nevada between 2015 and 2020.

80. Divorce rate. The divorce rate in Texas is approximated by

$$D(t) = 33.3e^{-0.5t},$$

where $D(t)$ is the number of divorces per 1000 people per year, t years after 2010. (*Source*: Based on data from www.cdc.gov.)

a) Find the total number of divorces per 1000 people in Texas from 2010 to 2015.
b) Estimate the total number of divorces in Texas between 2015 and 2020.

SYNTHESIS

In Exercises 81–84, solve each integral, using the graph of $f(x) = y = x\sqrt{16 - x^2}$, shown below, as a hint.

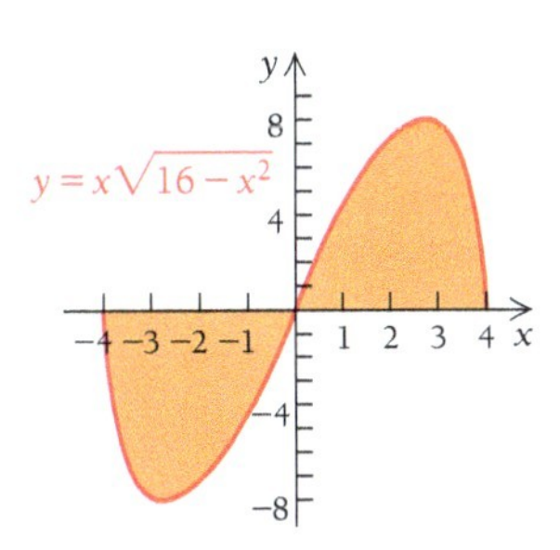

81. $\int_{-4}^{0} f(x)\, dx$

82. $\int_0^4 f(x)\, dx$

83. $\int_{-4}^{4} f(x)\, dx$

84. $\int_{-4}^{4} |f(x)|\, dx$

Evaluate.

85. $\int 5x\sqrt{1-4x^2}\,dx$

86. $\int \frac{dx}{ax+b}$

87. $\int \frac{x^2}{e^{x^3}}\,dx$

88. $\int \frac{e^{\sqrt{t}}}{\sqrt{t}}\,dt$

89. $\int \frac{x-3}{(x^2-6x)^{1/3}}\,dx$

90. $\int \frac{e^{1/t}}{t^2}\,dt$

91. $\int \frac{t^3\ln(t^4+8)}{t^4+8}\,dt$

92. $\int \frac{t^2+2t}{(t+1)^2}\,dt$ (*Hint*: $u = t + 1$.)

93. $\int \frac{x^2+6x}{(x+3)^2}\,dx$

94. $\int \frac{x+3}{x+1}\,dx$ $\left(\textit{Hint}: \frac{x+3}{x+1} = 1 + \frac{2}{x+1}.\right)$

95. $\int \frac{t-5}{t-4}\,dt$

96. $\int \frac{dx}{e^x+1}$ $\left(\textit{Hint}: \frac{1}{e^x+1} = \frac{e^{-x}}{1+e^{-x}}.\right)$

97. $\int \frac{e^x - e^{-x}}{e^x + e^{-x}}\,dx$

98. $\int \frac{e^{-mx}}{1-ae^{-mx}}\,dx$

99. Is the following a true statement? Why or why not?

$$\int [2f(x)]\,dx = [f(x)]^2 + C$$

100. Prove that $\int a^x\,dx = \frac{a^x}{\ln a} + C$.

[*Hint*: Rewrite $a^x = (e^{\ln a})^x = e^{x\ln a}$ and use a substitution.]

101. Total change in population. The rate of change of the population of Oronti Falls is given by

$$P'(t) = 437.52 \cdot (3)^{t/8},$$

where t is the number of years since 2010 and $P'(t)$ is the change in population in number of people per year.

a) Find the population of Oronti Falls in 2012, assuming a population of 3186 in 2010.

b) Estimate the total change in the population of Oronti Falls between 2012 and 2020.

102. Total change in population. The rate of change in the population of Red Bluff Lake is given by

$$P'(t) = 1104.382 \cdot (2)^{t/7},$$

where t is the number of years since 2010 and $P'(t)$ is the change in population in number of people per year.

a) Find the population of Red Bluff Lake in 2013, assuming a population of 11,153 in 2010.

b) Estimate the total change in the population of Red Bluff Lake between 2013 and 2020.

Answers to Quick Checks

1. a) $dy = \frac{1}{2\sqrt{x}}\,dx$; **b)** $du = (2x-3)\,dx$; **c)** $dy = -\frac{3}{x^4}\,dx$; **d)** $du = 4\,dx$ **2.** $\frac{1}{4}(2x^2+3)^4 + C$ **3.** $\ln(1+e^x) + C$ **4.** $2\sqrt{3+2x^3} + C$ **5.** $\frac{1}{3}(\ln x)^3 + C$ **6.** $\frac{1}{12}e^{4x^3} + C$ **7.** 11,594.8 **8.** $-\frac{1}{x-1} - \frac{1}{2(x-1)^2} + C$

4.6 Integration Techniques: Integration by Parts

- Evaluate integrals using the formula for integration by parts.
- Solve applied problems involving integration by parts.

The Product Rule leads to a useful technique for solving certain integrals. Called *integration by parts*, this technique is often used in situations where the integrand is a product of two (or more) factors and where techniques like substitution do not work.

Integration by Parts

Let $y = u(x)$ and $y = v(x)$ be two functions. Applying the Product Rule, we have

$$\frac{d}{dx}(u(x)\cdot v(x)) = u(x)\cdot\frac{d}{dx}v(x) + v(x)\cdot\frac{d}{dx}u(x).$$

Integrating both sides with respect to x, we have

$$\int\left[\frac{d}{dx}(u(x)\cdot v(x))\right]dx = \int\left[u(x)\cdot\frac{d}{dx}v(x)\right]dx + \int\left[v(x)\cdot\frac{d}{dx}u(x)\right]dx.$$

Note that $\int \left[\frac{d}{dx}(u(x) \cdot v(x))\right] dx = u(x) \cdot v(x)$. We simplify by writing u for $u(x)$, v for $v(x)$, du for $\frac{d}{dx}u(x)\, dx$ and dv for $\frac{d}{dx}v(x)\, dx$:

$$uv = \int u\, dv + \int v\, du.$$

Solving for $\int u\, dv$, we obtain the following theorem.

THEOREM 7 The Integration-by-Parts Formula

$$\int u\, dv = uv - \int v\, du$$

EXAMPLE 1 Evaluate: $\int xe^x\, dx$.

Solution We let

$$u = x \quad \text{and} \quad dv = e^x\, dx.$$

In this case, differentiating u gives

$$du = dx,$$

and integrating dv gives

$$v = e^x. \quad \text{We select } C = 0 \text{ to obtain the simplest antiderivative.}$$

The Integration-by-Parts Formula then gives us

$$\int \overset{u}{(x)}\overset{dv}{(e^x\, dx)} = \overset{u}{(x)}\overset{v}{(e^x)} - \int \overset{v}{(e^x)}\overset{du}{(dx)} \quad \text{The integral on the right is easily solved.}$$
$$= xe^x - e^x + C.$$

Quick Check 1 ✓
Evaluate: $\int 3xe^{2x}\, dx$.

To check, we differentiate the result. This check is left to the student. **1 ✓**

Note that integration by parts, like substitution, can be a trial-and-error process. In the preceding example, if we had reversed the roles of x and e^x, we would have obtained

$$u = e^x, \qquad dv = x\, dx,$$

$$du = e^x\, dx, \qquad v = \frac{x^2}{2},$$

and $$\int \overset{u}{(e^x)}\overset{dv}{(x\, dx)} = \overset{u}{(e^x)}\overset{v}{\left(\frac{x^2}{2}\right)} - \int \overset{v}{\left(\frac{x^2}{2}\right)}\overset{du}{(e^x\, dx)}.$$

Now the integrand on the right is *more* difficult to integrate than the one with which we began. We usually have a choice as to how to apply the Integration-by-Parts Formula. It may be that only one (or none) of the possibilities will work.

EXAMPLE 2 Evaluate: $\int x \ln x\, dx$, $x > 0$

Solution We let

$$u = \ln x \quad \text{and} \quad dv = x\, dx.$$

Then $$du = \frac{1}{x}dx \quad \text{and} \quad v = \frac{x^2}{2}.$$

Using the Integration-by-Parts Formula, we have

$$\int \underset{u}{x} \underset{dv}{\ln x\, dx} = \underset{u}{\ln x} \cdot \underset{v}{\frac{x^2}{2}} - \int \underset{v}{\frac{x^2}{2}} \underset{du}{\left(\frac{1}{x} dx\right)}$$

$$= \frac{x^2}{2} \ln x - \frac{1}{2} \int x\, dx$$

$$= \frac{x^2}{2} \ln x - \frac{x^2}{4} + C.$$

Check: $\frac{d}{dx}\left[\frac{x^2}{2} \ln x - \frac{x^2}{4} + C\right] = \frac{x^2}{2} \cdot \frac{1}{x} + \ln x \cdot x - \frac{x}{2}$ Using the Product Rule

$$= \frac{x}{2} + x \ln x - \frac{x}{2}$$

$= x \ln x$ This is the original integrand, so our answer checks. **2 ✓**

Quick Check 2 ✓

Evaluate: $\int 5x \ln(3x)\, dx$.

EXAMPLE 3 Evaluate: $\int x\sqrt{5x + 1}\, dx$.

Solution We let

$u = x$ and $dv = (5x + 1)^{1/2}\, dx$.

Then $du = dx$, and to find v, we use substitution:

$$v = \int (5x + 1)^{1/2}\, dx = \frac{1}{5} \int w^{1/2}\, dw$$

Substitution: $w = 5x + 1,\ dw = 5\, dx$

$$v = \frac{1}{5} \cdot \frac{w^{3/2}}{\frac{3}{2}} = \frac{2}{15} w^{3/2} = \frac{2}{15}(5x + 1)^{3/2}.$$

Using the Integration-by-Parts Formula gives us

$$\int \underset{u}{x}\underset{dv}{(\sqrt{5x + 1}\, dx)} = \underset{u}{x} \cdot \underset{v}{\tfrac{2}{15}(5x + 1)^{3/2}} - \int \underset{v}{\tfrac{2}{15}(5x + 1)^{3/2}}\, \underset{du}{dx}$$

$$= \tfrac{2}{15}x(5x + 1)^{3/2} - \tfrac{2}{15} \cdot \tfrac{2}{25}(5x + 1)^{5/2} + C$$

Using substitution to evaluate the integral on the right.

$$= \tfrac{2}{15}x(5x + 1)^{3/2} - \tfrac{4}{375}(5x + 1)^{5/2} + C.$$

This integral may also be evaluated using a substitution similar to that shown in Example 9 of Section 4.5. (See Exercise 41 at the end of this section.) **3 ✓**

Quick Check 3 ✓

Evaluate: $\int 2x\sqrt{3x - 2}\, dx$.

EXAMPLE 4 Evaluate: $\int \ln x\, dx$. Assume $x > 0$.

Solution Since we can differentiate $\ln x$, we let $u = \ln x$, so that $dv = dx$. Thus,

$du = \frac{1}{x} dx$ and $v = x$.

Using the Integration-by-Parts Formula gives

$$\int \underset{u}{(\ln x)}\underset{dv}{(dx)} = \underset{u}{(\ln x)}\underset{v}{x} - \int \underset{v}{x}\underset{du}{\left(\frac{1}{x} dx\right)}$$

$$= x \ln x - \int dx$$

$$= x \ln x - x + C.$$

Tips on Using Integration by Parts

1. **a)** Use integration by parts when other techniques are not effective and an integral can be written in the form

$$\int f(x)\, g(x)\, dx.$$

   b) Write the integral in the form

$$\int u\, dv$$

   by choosing one factor to be $u = f(x)$, where $f(x)$ can be differentiated, and the remaining factor to be $dv = g(x)\, dx$, where $\int g(x)\, dx$ can be solved.

2. Find du by differentiating and v by integrating.
3. If the resulting integral, $\int v\, du$, is more difficult to solve than the original, try another choice for u and dv.
4. Check your result by differentiating.

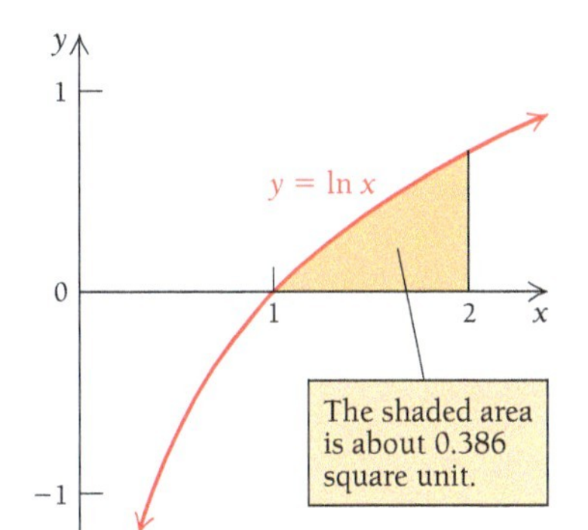

EXAMPLE 5 Evaluate: $\int_1^2 \ln x\, dx$.

Solution First, we find the antiderivative (see Example 4). Next, we evaluate the definite integral:

$$\int_1^2 \ln x\, dx = [x \ln x - x]_1^2 \quad \text{Using the result from Example 4}$$
$$= (2 \ln 2 - 2) - (1 \cdot \ln 1 - 1)$$
$$= 2 \ln 2 - 2 + 1$$
$$= 2 \ln 2 - 1 \approx 0.386.$$

4 ✓

Quick Check 4 ✓

Evaluate: $\int_1^4 x \ln x\, dx$.

EXAMPLE 6 **Life Science: Population Decay.** The rate of change in a population of bacteria t hours after an antibiotic treatment begins is estimated by

$$P'(t) = te^{-0.04t},$$

where $P'(t)$ is the rate of change of the population, in thousands of bacteria per hour. Assume that when the treatment begins, the population consists of 1,500,000 bacteria.

a) Find the population of bacteria after 24 hr of treatment.

b) What is the total change in the population of bacteria from 24 hr to 36 hr after the treatment begins?

Solution To find $P(t)$, which gives the population of bacteria (in thousands), after t hours, we integrate $P'(t)$ using integration by parts. Here, we let $u = t$, so that $dv = e^{-0.04t}\, dt$. Thus, $du = dt$ and $v = -\frac{1}{0.04}e^{-0.04t}$:

$$P(t) = \int te^{-0.04t}\, dt = t\left(-\frac{1}{0.04}e^{-0.04t}\right) - \int \left(-\frac{1}{0.04}e^{-0.04t}\right) dt$$
$$= -25te^{-0.04t} + 25\int e^{-0.04t}\, dt$$
$$= -25te^{-0.04t} + 25\left(-\frac{1}{0.04}e^{-0.04t}\right) + C$$
$$= -25te^{-0.04t} - 625e^{-0.04t} + C.$$

To find C, we note that $P(0) = 1500$ (where 1,500,000 is 1500 thousand):

$$1500 = -25(0)e^{-0.04(0)} - 625e^{-0.04(0)} + C \quad \text{Substituting}$$
$$1500 = -625 + C$$
$$C = 2125.$$

Thus, the population of bacteria t hours after the treatment begins is given by

$$P(t) = -25te^{-0.04t} - 625e^{-0.04t} + 2125.$$

a) The population of bacteria 24 hr after the treatment begins is found by substituting $t = 24$:

$$P(24) = -25(24)e^{-0.04(24)} - 625e^{-0.04(24)} + 2125$$
$$\approx 1655.956. \quad \text{Using a calculator}$$

There are about 1,655,956 bacteria present 24 hr after the treatment begins.

b) The total change in the population of bacteria between 24 hr and 36 hr is given by

$$\int_{24}^{36} P'(t)\,dt = P(36) - P(24).$$

Using $P(t)$ from above, we have

$$P(36) - P(24) = 1763.685 - 1655.956$$
$$\approx 107.729, \text{ or about } 107{,}729 \text{ bacteria.}$$

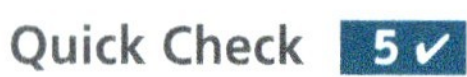

Quick Check 5 ✓

The rate of change of a population of bacteria t hours after an antibiotic treatment begins is estimated by $P'(t) = te^{-0.03125t}$, where $P'(t)$ is the rate of change of the population, in thousands of bacteria per hour. When the treatment begins, the population consists of 600,000 bacteria. What is the total change in the population of bacteria from 48 hr to 72 hr after the treatment begins?

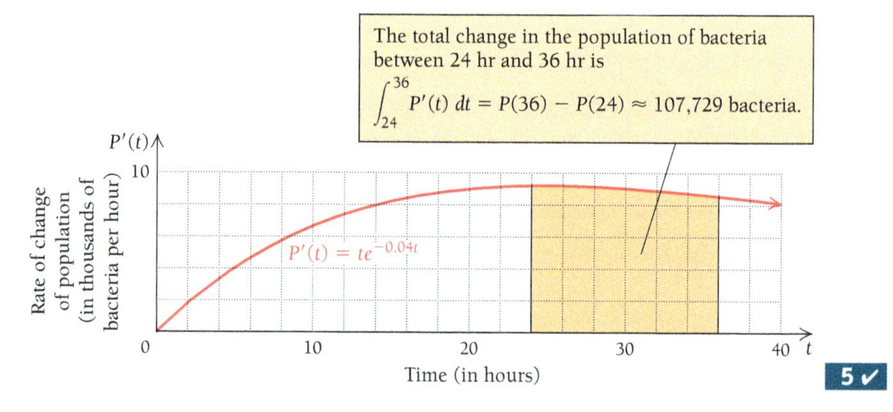

5 ✓

Repeated Integration by Parts

In some cases, we may need to apply the Integration-by-Parts Formula more than once.

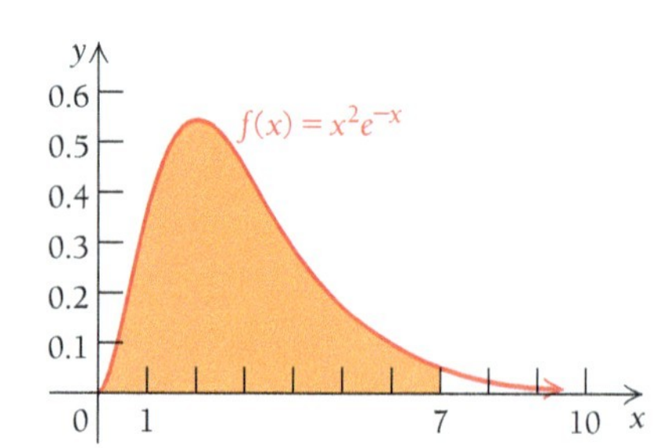

EXAMPLE 7 Evaluate $\int_0^7 x^2e^{-x}\,dx$ to find the shaded area in the graph at the left.

Solution We first let

$$u = x^2 \quad \text{and} \quad dv = e^{-x}\,dx.$$

Then $\quad du = 2x\,dx \quad \text{and} \quad v = -e^{-x}.$

Using the Integration-by-Parts Formula, we have

$$\int \overset{u}{x^2}(\overset{dv}{e^{-x}\,dx}) = \overset{u}{x^2}(\overset{v}{-e^{-x}}) - \int \overset{v}{-e^{-x}}(\overset{du}{2x\,dx})$$
$$= -x^2e^{-x} + \int 2xe^{-x}\,dx. \quad (1)$$

Technology Connection 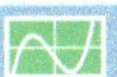

Exploratory

Use a calculator to evaluate

$$\int_0^7 x^2 e^{-x}\, dx.$$

To evaluate the integral on the right, we use integration by parts again:

$$u = 2x \quad \text{and} \quad dv = e^{-x}\, dx.$$

$$\text{so} \quad du = 2\, dx \quad \text{and} \quad v = -e^{-x}.$$

Using the Integration-by-Parts Formula once again, we get

$$\int \overset{u}{2x}(\overset{dv}{e^{-x}\, dx}) = \overset{u}{2x}(\overset{v}{-e^{-x}}) - \int \overset{v}{-e^{-x}}(\overset{du}{2\, dx})$$

$$= -2xe^{-x} - 2e^{-x} + C. \qquad (2)$$

When we substitute from equation (2) into (1), the original integral becomes

$$\int x^2e^{-x}\, dx = -x^2e^{-x} - 2xe^{-x} - 2e^{-x} + C \qquad \text{Substituting}$$

$$= -e^{-x}(x^2 + 2x + 2) + C. \qquad \text{Factoring simplifies the next step.}$$

We now evaluate the definite integral:

$$\int_0^7 x^2e^{-x}dx = \left[-e^{-x}(x^2 + 2x + 2)\right]_0^7 \qquad \text{We again let } C = 0.$$

$$= \left[-e^{-7}(7^2 + 2(7) + 2)\right] - \left[-e^{-0}(0^2 + 2(0) + 2)\right]$$

$$= -65e^{-7} + 2 \approx 1.94. \qquad 6 ✓$$

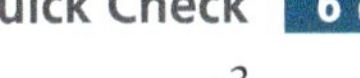

Quick Check 6 ✓

Evaluate: $\displaystyle\int_0^3 \frac{x}{\sqrt{x+1}}\, dx.$

Tabular Integration by Parts

In situations similar to Example 7, we have an integral,

$$\int f(x)\, g(x)\, dx,$$

for which $f(x)$ is a polynomial that can be easily differentiated repeatedly, leading to a higher-order derivative that is 0. The function $g(x)$ can also be easily integrated repeatedly. In such situations, we can use integration by parts more than once to evaluate the integral. This approach is made easier if we use a table and is thus called *tabular integration by parts.*

EXAMPLE 8 Evaluate: $\int x^2e^{-x}dx$ (from Example 7) using tabular integration by parts.

Solution We create a table with two columns: one for $f(x) = x^2$, which will be repeatedly differentiated until we reach a derivative of 0, and the other for $g(x) = e^{-x}$, which will be repeatedly integrated each time we differentiate $f(x)$.

$f(x)$ and Its Derivatives	$g(x)$ and Its Antiderivatives
x^2	e^{-x}
$2x$	$-e^{-x}$
2	e^{-x}
0	$-e^{-x}$

We then draw an arrow from the first entry in the first column to the second entry in the second column, and so on. We multiply along each arrow, alternating signs and starting with a positive sign, as shown in the table below:

f and Its Derivatives		g and Its Antiderivatives
x^2	$(+)$	e^{-x}
$2x$	$(-)$	$-e^{-x}$
2	$(+)$	e^{-x}
0		$-e^{-x}$

Thus, we have

$$\int x^2e^{-x}\,dx = +(x^2)(-e^{-x}) - (2x)(e^{-x}) + (2)(-e^{-x}) + C$$ Note the alternating signs.

$$= -x^2e^{-x} - 2xe^{-x} - 2e^{-x} + C$$ Simplifying

$$= -e^{-x}(x^2 + 2x + 2) + C$$ Factoring; compare this expression with that obtained in Example 7.

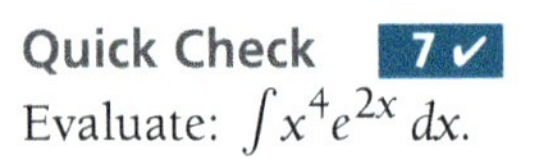
Quick Check 7 ✓

Evaluate: $\int x^4e^{2x}\,dx$.

7 ✓

Section Summary

- The *Integration-by-Parts Formula*, which makes use of the Product Rule, is
$$\int u\,dv = uv - \int v\,du.$$
- The choices for u and dv should be such that $\int v\,du$ is simpler than the original integral. If this does not occur, other choices should be tried.
- Tabular integration can be used when repeated integration by parts is necessary.

4.6 Exercise Set

Evaluate. (Assume $u > 0$ in $\ln u$.) Check by differentiating.

1. $\int 3xe^{4x}\,dx$
2. $\int 4xe^{3x}\,dx$
3. $\int xe^{5x}\,dx$
4. $\int 2xe^{4x}\,dx$
5. $\int xe^{-2x}\,dx$
6. $\int xe^{-x}\,dx$
7. $\int x^2\ln x\,dx$
8. $\int x^3\ln x\,dx$
9. $\int x\ln\sqrt{x}\,dx$
10. $\int x^2\ln x^3\,dx$
11. $\int \ln(x + 5)\,dx$
12. $\int \ln(x + 4)\,dx$
13. $\int (x + 2)\ln x\,dx$
14. $\int (x + 1)\ln x\,dx$
15. $\int (x - 1)\ln x\,dx$
16. $\int (x - 2)\ln x\,dx$
17. $\int x\sqrt{x + 2}\,dx$
18. $\int x\sqrt{x + 5}\,dx$
19. $\int x^3\ln(2x)\,dx$
20. $\int x^2\ln(5x)\,dx$
21. $\int x^2e^x\,dx$
22. $\int 10x\ln(2x)\,dx$
23. $\int x^2e^{2x}\,dx$
24. $\int x^5e^{-3x}\,dx$
25. $\int x^3e^{-2x}\,dx$
26. $\int x^5e^{4x}\,dx$
27. $\int (x^4 + 4)e^{3x}\,dx$
28. $\int (x^3 - x + 1)e^{-x}\,dx$

Evaluate using integration by parts.

29. $\int_1^2 x^2\ln x\,dx$
30. $\int_1^2 x^3\ln x\,dx$

31. $\int_1^3 \ln(2x)\,dx$

32. $\int_1^6 \ln(5x)\,dx$

33. $\int_0^1 xe^x\,dx$

34. $\int_0^1 (x^3 + 2x^2 + 3)e^{-2x}\,dx$

35. $\int_0^8 x\sqrt{x+1}\,dx$

36. $\int_0^{\ln 3} x^2e^{2x}\,dx$

37. **Cost from marginal cost.** Larry's Lawn Chairs determines that its marginal-cost function is given by

$$C'(x) = 4x\sqrt{x+3},$$

where x is the number of lawn chairs sold and $C'(x)$ is the marginal cost in dollars per chair. Find the total cost given that $C(13) = \$1126.40$.

38. **Profit from marginal profit.** Nevin Patio Contractors determines that its marginal-profit function is given by

$$P'(x) = 1000x^2e^{-0.2x},$$

where x is the number of patios built and $P'(x)$ is the marginal profit, in dollars per patio. Find the total profit given that $P(0) = -\$2000$.

Life and Physical Sciences

39. **Drug dosage.** Suppose an oral dose of a drug is taken. Over time, the drug is assimilated in the body and excreted in the urine. The total amount of the drug that passes through the body in T hours is given by

$$\int_0^T E(t)\,dt,$$

where $E(t)$ is the rate of excretion of the drug, in milligrams per hour. A typical rate-of-excretion function is

$$E(t) = te^{-kt},$$

where $k > 0$ and t is the time, in hours.

a) Find a formula for

$$\int_0^T E(t)\,dt.$$

b) Find

$$\int_0^{10} E(t)\,dt, \quad \text{when } k = 0.2 \text{ mg/hr}.$$

40. **Electrical energy use.** The rate at which electrical energy is used by the Ortiz family, in kilowatt-hours (kW-h) per hour, is given by

$$K(t) = 10te^{-t},$$

where t is time, in hours.

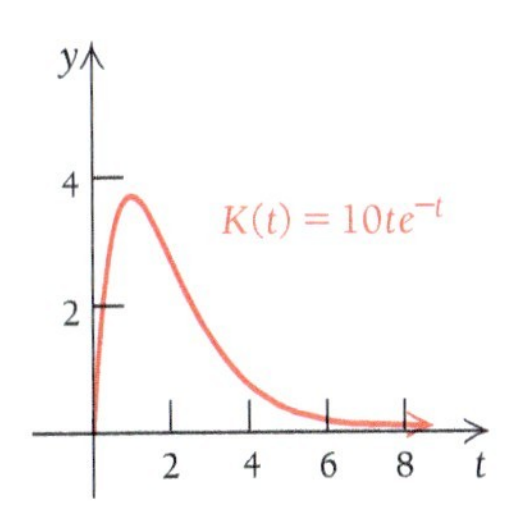

a) How many kilowatt-hours does the family use in the first T hours of a day ($t = 0$ to $t = T$)?

b) How many kilowatt-hours does the family use in the first 4 hours of the day?

SYNTHESIS

In Exercises 41 and 42, evaluate the given indefinite integral using substitution. Refer to Example 9 in Section 4.5 to review the technique.

41. Evaluate $\int x\sqrt{5x+1}\,dx$ by letting $u = 5x + 1$ and $du = 5\,dx$ (so that $dx = \frac{1}{5}\,du$) and observing that $x = \frac{u-1}{5}$. Compare your answer to that found in Example 3 of this section. Are they the same? (*Hint:* Simplify both forms of the answer into a common third form.)

42. Consider $\int \frac{x}{\sqrt{x-3}}\,dx$.

a) Evaluate this integral using integration by parts.

b) Evaluate this integral using the substitution $u = x - 3$ and observing that $x = u + 3$.

c) Show algebraically that the answers from parts (a) and (b) are equivalent.

In Exercises 43 and 44, both substitution and integration by parts are used to determine the indefinite integral.

43. Evaluate $\int e^{\sqrt{x}}\,dx$ by letting $u = \sqrt{x}$. Note that $x = u^2$, so $dx = 2u\,du$. Make the substitutions and solve the new integral using integration by parts.

44. Evaluate $\int \frac{1}{1+\sqrt{x}}\,dx$ by letting $u = \sqrt{x}$ and following the procedure used in Exercise 43.

45. Differentiate to confirm that

$$\int axe^{bx}\,dx = e^{bx}\left(\frac{abx - a}{b^2}\right) + C.$$

46. Differentiate to confirm that

$$\int x^n \ln x\,dx = \frac{x^{n+1}}{n+1}\left(\ln x - \frac{1}{n+1}\right) + C, \text{ where } n \text{ is}$$

any real number such that $n \neq -1$ and $x > 0$.

47. Differentiate to confirm that for any positive integer n,

$$\int x^ne^x\,dx = x^ne^x - n\int x^{n-1}e^x\,dx.$$

48. Differentiate to confirm that for any positive integer n,

$$\int (\ln x)^n\,dx = x(\ln x)^n - n\int (\ln x)^{n-1}\,dx.$$

49. Differentiate to confirm that

$$\int \ln(ax+b)\,dx = \frac{ax+b}{a}\ln(ax+b) - x + C,$$

where $x > -\frac{b}{a}$.

Evaluate.

50. $\int \ln(5x+7)\,dx$ (*Hint:* Use the result from Exercise 49.)

51. $\int \ln(3x - 8)\, dx$

52. $\int_2^6 \ln(3x + 1)\, dx$

53. $\int_0^5 \ln(6x + 7)\, dx$

54. $\int \sqrt{x} \ln x\, dx$

55. $\int \frac{te^t}{(t + 1)^2}\, dt$

56. $\int \frac{\ln x}{\sqrt{x}}\, dx$

57. $\int x^2(\ln x)^2\, dx$

58. $\int x \cdot 3^x\, dx$

59. $\int 2x \cdot 5^x\, dx$

60. $\int 3x \cdot 2^{1-x}\, dx$

61. $\int 4x \cdot 6^{2+3x}$

62. Is the following a true statement?

$$\int f(x)g(x)\, dx = \int f(x)\, dx \cdot \int g(x)\, dx.$$

Why or why not?

63. Compare the methods of integration by substitution and integration by parts. For an integral for which the method of solution is not clear, which method would you try first, and why?

64. Evaluate $\int_0^b x^2 e^{-x}\, dx$, where $b > 0$ is the critical value corresponding to the local maximum of the integrand.

Recurring integrals. *Occasionally, integration by parts yields an integral of the form $\int u\, dv$ that is identical to the original integral. In some cases, we can then solve for $\int u\, dv$ algebraically. For example, to find $\int 2^x e^x\, dx$, we let $u = 2^x$ and $dv = e^x\, dx$, so $du = (\ln 2)2^x\, dx$ and $v = e^x$. Using integration by parts, we have*

$$\int 2^x e^x\, dx = 2^x e^x - \ln 2 \int 2^x e^x\, dx.$$

Note that $\int 2^x e^x\, dx$ appears twice. Adding $\ln 2 \int 2^x e^x\, dx$ to both sides, we have

$$\int 2^x e^x\, dx + \ln 2 \int 2^x e^x\, dx = 2^x e^x$$

$$(1 + \ln 2) \int 2^x e^x\, dx = 2^x e^x$$

$$\int 2^x e^x\, dx = \frac{2^x e^x}{1 + \ln 2} + C.$$

Use this method to evaluate the integrals in Exercises 65–68.

65. $\int 3^x e^x\, dx$

66. $\int 5^x e^{2x}\, dx$

67. $\int 10^x e^{3x}\, dx$

68. $\int x \ln x\, dx$ (*Hint:* Let $u = x \ln x$ and $dv = dx$. Assume $x > 0$.)

Technology Connection 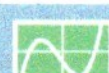

Use a graphing calculator to evaluate each integral.

69. $\int_1^{10} x^5 \ln x\, dx$

70. $\int_1^4 x^7 e^{2x}\, dx$

Answers to Quick Checks

1. $\frac{3}{2}e^{2x}(x - \frac{1}{2}) + C$ **2.** $\frac{5}{2}x^2(\ln(3x) - \frac{1}{2}) + C$
3. $\frac{4}{9}x(3x - 2)^{3/2} - \frac{8}{135}(3x - 2)^{5/2} + C$
4. $8 \ln 4 - \frac{15}{4} \approx 7.34$ **5.** About 220,445 bacteria
6. $\frac{8}{3}$ **7.** $e^{2x}(\frac{1}{2}x^4 - x^3 + \frac{3}{2}x^2 - \frac{3}{2}x + \frac{3}{4}) + C$

4.7 Numerical Integration

- Solve problems using numerical integration methods such as Riemann sums, the Midpoint Rule, the Trapezoidal Rule, and Simpson's Rule.

In many situations, it may be difficult or impossible to evaluate a definite integral using an antiderivative. To address this difficulty, we develop ways to approximate the value of a definite integral using geometry—a process called **numerical integration**. Two common situations can require the use of numerical integration:

- When finding an antiderivative is difficult or impossible. An example of this situation occurs in trying to evaluate $\int_a^b e^{-x^2}\, dx$, an integral used in statistics. There is no way to antidifferentiate $f(x) = e^{-x^2}$.
- When the data may not be easily modeled by a continuous function.

Let's consider a situation where the data consist of individual points. We will discover that it is not necessary to find a continuous function that models the data.

Riemann Sums

The most common geometric method for approximating area is to use rectangles, as we did in Section 4.2. We subdivide $[a, b]$ into n subintervals, $[a, x_1]$, $[x_1, x_2]$, $[x_2, x_3]$, and so on, through $[x_{n-1}, b]$, where a is x_0 and b is x_n. If we require the subintervals to be equal in size, then each subinterval has width $\Delta x = \dfrac{b-a}{n}$. To illustrate, the graph to the right shows the rate of exertion, measured in calories expended per hour, after t 30-second intervals of exercise by a certain individual.

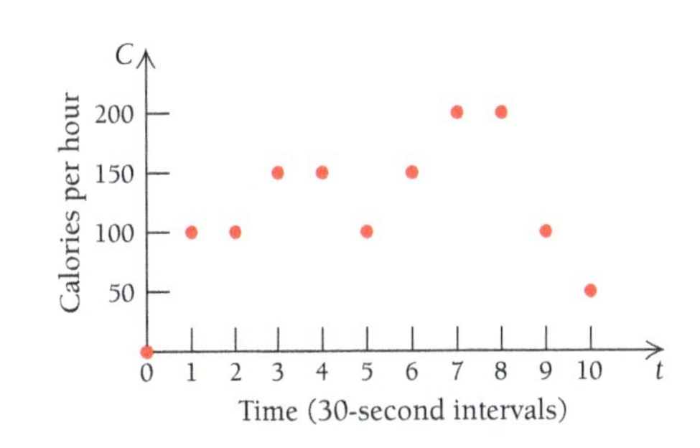

The total number of calories expended is approximated by the area under a graph of the data. Over each subinterval, a rectangle is drawn. One approach uses each data point as the top-left corner of such a rectangle. The resulting Riemann sum is consistent with our work in Section 4.2.

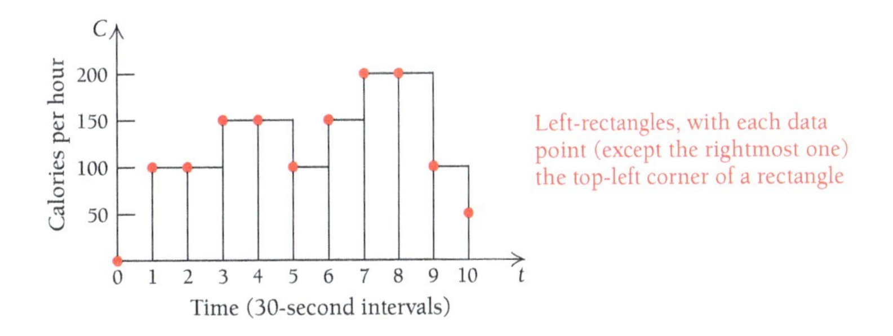

Since C is measured in calories per hour, we view each 30-sec interval as $\frac{1}{120}$ of an hour. Thus, each rectangle has a width of $\frac{1}{120}$ and a height corresponding to the data point at the top-left corner. The sum of these **left-rectangles** is denoted as L_n, where n is the number of subintervals. We use a table to calculate the area of each rectangle, rounded to three decimal places. Note that the rightmost data point is not used.

Subinterval	Width	Height (x = left endpoint)	Area
$[0, 1]$	$\frac{1}{120}$ hr	$C(0) = 0$ cal/hr	$\frac{1}{120} \cdot 0 = 0$ cal
$[1, 2]$	$\frac{1}{120}$ hr	$C(1) = 100$ cal/hr	$\frac{1}{120} \cdot 100 \approx 0.833$ cal
$[2, 3]$	$\frac{1}{120}$ hr	$C(2) = 100$ cal/hr	$\frac{1}{120} \cdot 100 \approx 0.833$ cal
$[3, 4]$	$\frac{1}{120}$ hr	$C(3) = 150$ cal/hr	$\frac{1}{120} \cdot 150 = 1.250$ cal
$[4, 5]$	$\frac{1}{120}$ hr	$C(4) = 150$ cal/hr	$\frac{1}{120} \cdot 150 = 1.250$ cal
$[5, 6]$	$\frac{1}{120}$ hr	$C(5) = 100$ cal/hr	$\frac{1}{120} \cdot 100 \approx 0.833$ cal
$[6, 7]$	$\frac{1}{120}$ hr	$C(6) = 150$ cal/hr	$\frac{1}{120} \cdot 150 = 1.250$ cal
$[7, 8]$	$\frac{1}{120}$ hr	$C(7) = 200$ cal/hr	$\frac{1}{120} \cdot 200 \approx 1.667$ cal
$[8, 9]$	$\frac{1}{120}$ hr	$C(8) = 200$ cal/hr	$\frac{1}{120} \cdot 200 \approx 1.667$ cal
$[9, 10]$	$\frac{1}{120}$ hr	$C(9) = 100$ cal/hr	$\frac{1}{120} \cdot 100 \approx 0.833$ cal

The sum of the values in the last column is the total area of the 10 rectangles. This sum, L_{10}, approximates the total calories expended during 5 minutes of exercising. We have $L_{10} = 0 + 0.833 + 0.833 + 1.250 + 1.250 + 0.833 + 1.250 + 1.667 + 1.667 + 0.833 \approx 10.416$ cal.

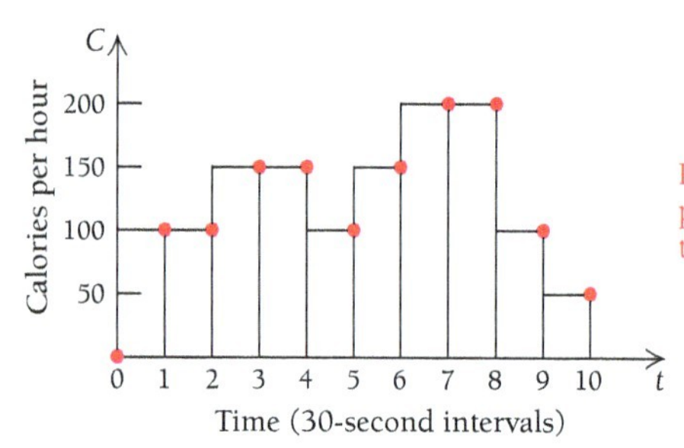

Right-rectangles, with each data point (except the leftmost one) the top-right corner of a rectangle

We can also draw the rectangles so that each data point is the top-right corner of a rectangle. The sum of these **right-rectangles** is denoted as R_n, where n is the number of subintervals. The leftmost data point is not used.

We again use a table to find the area of each rectangle, rounded to three decimal places, and add the areas in the last column to approximate the total number of calories expended.

Subinterval	Width	Height (x = right endpoint)	Area
$[0, 1]$	$\frac{1}{120}$ hr	$C(1) = 100$ cal/hr	$\frac{1}{120} \cdot 100 \approx 0.833$ cal
$[1, 2]$	$\frac{1}{120}$ hr	$C(2) = 100$ cal/hr	$\frac{1}{120} \cdot 100 \approx 0.833$ cal
$[2, 3]$	$\frac{1}{120}$ hr	$C(3) = 150$ cal/hr	$\frac{1}{120} \cdot 150 = 1.250$ cal
$[3, 4]$	$\frac{1}{120}$ hr	$C(4) = 150$ cal/hr	$\frac{1}{120} \cdot 150 = 1.250$ cal
$[4, 5]$	$\frac{1}{120}$ hr	$C(5) = 100$ cal/hr	$\frac{1}{120} \cdot 100 \approx 0.833$ cal
$[5, 6]$	$\frac{1}{120}$ hr	$C(6) = 150$ cal/hr	$\frac{1}{120} \cdot 150 = 1.250$ cal
$[6, 7]$	$\frac{1}{120}$ hr	$C(7) = 200$ cal/hr	$\frac{1}{120} \cdot 200 \approx 1.667$ cal
$[7, 8]$	$\frac{1}{120}$ hr	$C(8) = 200$ cal/hr	$\frac{1}{120} \cdot 200 \approx 1.667$ cal
$[8, 9]$	$\frac{1}{120}$ hr	$C(9) = 100$ cal/hr	$\frac{1}{120} \cdot 100 \approx 0.833$ cal
$[9, 10]$	$\frac{1}{120}$ hr	$C(10) = 50$ cal/hr	$\frac{1}{120} \cdot 50 \approx 0.417$ cal

We have

$$\begin{aligned} R_{10} &= 0.833 + 0.833 + 1.250 + 1.250 + 0.833 + 1.250 + 1.667 \\ &\quad + 1.667 + 0.833 + 0.417 \\ &\approx 10.833 \text{ calories.} \end{aligned}$$

Averaging L_{10} and R_{10}, we can conclude that the total number of calories expended is about

$$\frac{L_{10} + R_{10}}{2} = \frac{10.416 + 10.833}{2} = 10.625 \text{ calories.}$$

The method of Riemann sums is summarized below.

DEFINITION Riemann Sums

Let $[a, b]$ be subdivided into n equal subintervals, $[a, x_1], [x_1, x_2], [x_2, x_3], \dots, [x_{n-1}, b]$, each with width $\Delta x = \frac{b - a}{n}$. Assume that f is defined for $a, x_1, x_2, \dots, x_{n-1}, b$. The approximate value of $\int_a^b f(x)\,dx$ is given by L_n, where

$$L_n = \frac{b - a}{n} \cdot (f(a) + f(x_1) + f(x_2) + \cdots + f(x_{n-2}) + f(x_{n-1})).$$

The approximate value of $\int_a^b f(x)\,dx$ is also given by R_n, where

$$R_n = \frac{b - a}{n} \cdot (f(x_1) + f(x_2) + \cdots + f(x_{n-2}) + f(x_{n-1}) + f(b)).$$

In the following example, we use Riemann sums to approximate a total distance given velocity data for 1-minute intervals.

EXAMPLE 1 **Approximating Total Distance.** Ken rides his bicycle for 10 min. The table below shows Ken's speed, $v(t)$, in miles per hour, for each 1-min interval of time. Find L_{10} to approximate the total distance Ken travels during the 10 min.

t (min)	0	1	2	3	4	5	6	7	8	9	10
$v(t)$, mi/hr	10	12	18	20	20	8	6	15	18	20	16

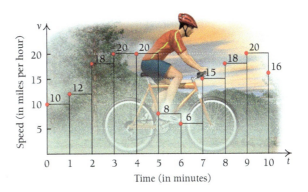

Solution For consistency of units, note that each 1-min interval is equivalent to $\frac{1}{60}$ of an hour. Since we are using left-rectangles, the rightmost data point will not be used. The following table summarizes the calculations:

Subinterval	Width	Height (x = left endpoint)	Area
$[0, 1]$	$\frac{1}{60}$ hr	$v(0) = 10$ mi/hr	$\frac{1}{60} \cdot 10 \approx 0.167$ mi
$[1, 2]$	$\frac{1}{60}$ hr	$v(1) = 12$ mi/hr	$\frac{1}{60} \cdot 12 = 0.2$ mi
$[2, 3]$	$\frac{1}{60}$ hr	$v(2) = 18$ mi/hr	$\frac{1}{60} \cdot 18 = 0.3$ mi
$[3, 4]$	$\frac{1}{60}$ hr	$v(3) = 20$ mi/hr	$\frac{1}{60} \cdot 20 \approx 0.333$ mi
$[4, 5]$	$\frac{1}{60}$ hr	$v(4) = 20$ mi/hr	$\frac{1}{60} \cdot 20 \approx 0.333$ mi
$[5, 6]$	$\frac{1}{60}$ hr	$v(5) = 8$ mi/hr	$\frac{1}{60} \cdot 8 \approx 0.133$ mi
$[6, 7]$	$\frac{1}{60}$ hr	$v(6) = 6$ mi/hr	$\frac{1}{60} \cdot 6 = 0.1$ mi
$[7, 8]$	$\frac{1}{60}$ hr	$v(7) = 15$ mi/hr	$\frac{1}{60} \cdot 15 = 0.25$ mi
$[8, 9]$	$\frac{1}{60}$ hr	$v(8) = 18$ mi/hr	$\frac{1}{60} \cdot 18 = 0.3$ mi
$[9, 10]$	$\frac{1}{60}$ hr	$v(9) = 20$ mi/hr	$\frac{1}{60} \cdot 20 \approx 0.333$ mi

Quick Check 1 ✓

Use the table in Example 1 to find R_{10}, an approximation of Ken's total distance traveled, and then find the average of L_{10} and R_{10}.

Thus, Ken travels approximately

$$L_{10} = 0.167 + 0.2 + 0.3 + 0.333 + 0.333 + 0.133 + 0.1 + 0.25 + 0.3 + 0.333$$
$$= 2.449 \text{ mi.}$$

1 ✓

Many continuous functions have antiderivatives that are not easily found. For example, it is not possible to find the antiderivative of $f(x) = \sqrt{1 + x^3}$ using the procedures developed thus far. The following example approximates such a definite integral using Riemann sums.

EXAMPLE 2 Approximate $\int_0^3 \sqrt{1 + x^3}\, dx$, using L_6, R_6, and their average.

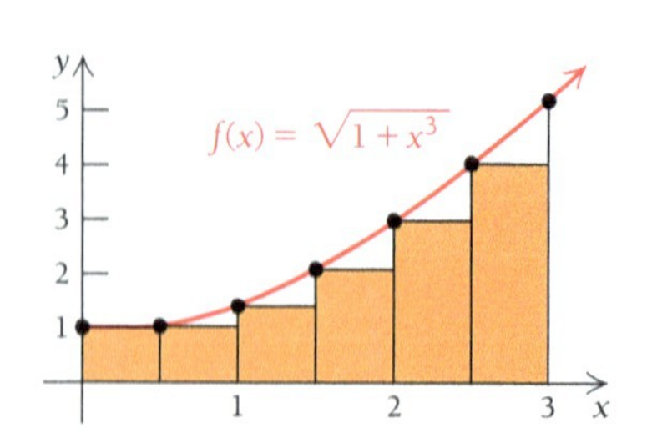

Solution To approximate this definite integral using L_6, we subdivide [0, 3] into six equal subintervals of width 0.5. We then graph $f(x) = \sqrt{1 + x^3}$ over [0, 3] and draw six left-rectangles. We evaluate $y = f(x)$ at the left endpoint of each subinterval, rounding each area to three decimal places. The following table lists the areas of the rectangles, which we will add together.

Subinterval	Width	Height (x = left endpoint)	Area
[0, 0.5]	0.5	$f(0) = 1$	$0.5 \cdot 1 = 0.500$
[0.5, 1]	0.5	$f(0.5) \approx 1.061$	$0.5 \cdot 1.061 \approx 0.531$
[1, 1.5]	0.5	$f(1) \approx 1.414$	$0.5 \cdot 1.414 \approx 0.707$
[1.5, 2]	0.5	$f(1.5) \approx 2.092$	$0.5 \cdot 2.092 \approx 1.046$
[2, 2.5]	0.5	$f(2) = 3$	$0.5 \cdot 3 = 1.500$
[2.5, 3]	0.5	$f(2.5) \approx 4.077$	$0.5 \cdot 4.077 \approx 2.039$

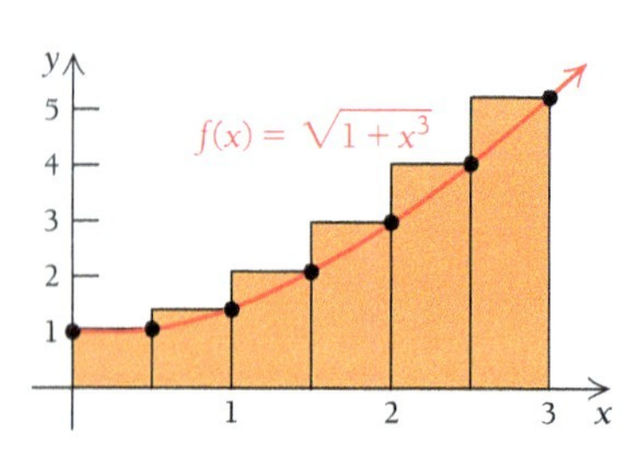

Thus, we have

$$L_6 = 0.500 + 0.531 + 0.707 + 1.046 + 1.500 + 2.039 = 6.323.$$

To find R_6, the height of each rectangle is found by evaluating $y = f(x)$ at the right endpoint of each subinterval.

Subinterval	Width	Height (x = right endpoint)	Area
[0, 0.5]	0.5	$f(0.5) \approx 1.061$	$0.5 \cdot 1.061 \approx 0.531$
[0.5, 1]	0.5	$f(1) \approx 1.414$	$0.5 \cdot 1.414 \approx 0.707$
[1, 1.5]	0.5	$f(1.5) \approx 2.092$	$0.5 \cdot 2.092 \approx 1.046$
[1.5, 2]	0.5	$f(2) = 3$	$0.5 \cdot 3 = 1.500$
[2, 2.5]	0.5	$f(2.5) \approx 4.077$	$0.5 \cdot 4.077 \approx 2.039$
[2.5, 3]	0.5	$f(3) \approx 5.292$	$0.5 \cdot 5.292 \approx 2.646$

We have $R_6 = 0.531 + 0.707 + 1.046 + 1.500 + 2.039 + 2.646 = 8.469$. Averaging the two sums gives us a third approximation of the definite integral:

$$\int_0^3 \sqrt{1 + x^3}\, dx \approx \frac{6.323 + 8.469}{2} = 7.396.$$

A calculator or calculus software shows that to three decimal places, the value of $\int_0^3 \sqrt{1 + x^3}\, dx$ is 7.341. Thus, using six rectangles, we have found a value that is within 0.055 square unit of the true area. **2 ✓**

Quick Check 2 ✓
Approximate

$$\int_0^2 \ln(x + 1)\, dx$$

by finding L_4, R_4, and their average.

Midpoint Rule

Instead of using the left or right endpoint of each subinterval to evaluate $y = f(x)$, we can evaluate the function at the *midpoint* of each subinterval. This is the basis of the **Midpoint Rule**, which gives an approximation M_n that is the sum of the areas of n rectangles whose heights are measured at the midpoints of the subintervals. The midpoint of each subinterval is the average of its left and right endpoints.

> **DEFINITION Midpoint Rule**
>
> Let $[a, b]$ be subdivided into n equal subintervals with width $\Delta x = \dfrac{b-a}{n}$, and assume that f is defined for $\dfrac{a+x_1}{2}, \dfrac{x_1+x_2}{2}, \ldots, \dfrac{x_{n-1}+b}{2}$. The approximate value of $\int_a^b f(x)\,dx$ is given by M_n, where
>
> $$M_n = \frac{b-a}{n} \cdot \left(f\left(\frac{a+x_1}{2}\right) + f\left(\frac{x_1+x_2}{2}\right) + f\left(\frac{x_2+x_3}{2}\right) + \cdots + f\left(\frac{x_{n-2}+x_{n-1}}{2}\right) + f\left(\frac{x_{n-1}+b}{2}\right)\right).$$

Let's find an approximation of $\int_0^3 \sqrt{1+x^3}\,dx$ (from Example 2) using the Midpoint Rule.

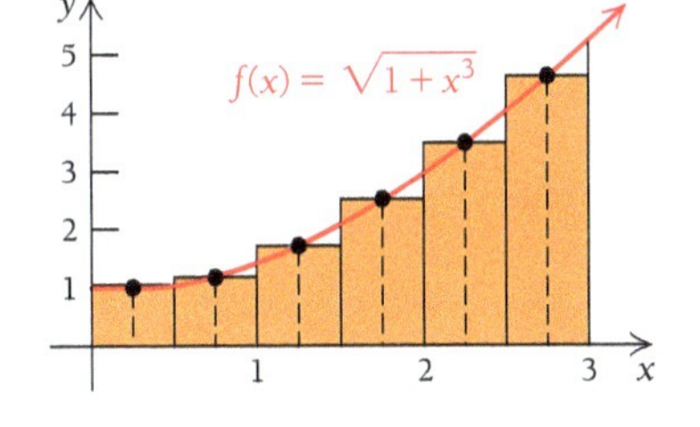

EXAMPLE 3 Use the Midpoint Rule to find M_6, an approximation of $\int_0^3 \sqrt{1+x^3}\,dx$.

Solution We subdivide [0, 3] into six subintervals, each with width 0.5, and then find the midpoint of each subinterval using the average of the endpoints.

A table is used to find the area of each rectangle. To find the height of each rectangle, we evaluate $y = f(x)$ at the midpoint of each subinterval. Heights and areas are rounded to three decimal places.

Subinterval	Midpoint	Width	Height (x = midpoint)	Area
[0, 0.5]	0.25	0.5	$f(0.25) \approx 1.008$	$0.5 \cdot 1.008 \approx 0.504$
[0.5, 1]	0.75	0.5	$f(0.75) \approx 1.192$	$0.5 \cdot 1.192 \approx 0.596$
[1, 1.5]	1.25	0.5	$f(1.25) \approx 1.718$	$0.5 \cdot 1.718 \approx 0.859$
[1.5, 2]	1.75	0.5	$f(1.75) \approx 2.522$	$0.5 \cdot 2.522 \approx 1.261$
[2, 2.5]	2.25	0.5	$f(2.25) \approx 3.520$	$0.5 \cdot 3.520 \approx 1.760$
[2.5, 3]	2.75	0.5	$f(2.75) \approx 4.669$	$0.5 \cdot 4.669 \approx 2.335$

Quick Check 3 ✓
Use the Midpoint Rule to find M_8, an approximation of $\int_0^2 \ln(x+1)\,dx$.

Since $M_6 = 0.504 + 0.596 + 0.859 + 1.261 + 1.760 + 2.335 = 7.315$, we conclude that $\int_0^3 \sqrt{1+x^3}\,dx \approx 7.315$. This compares well with the values found in Example 2. **3 ✓**

The Trapezoidal Rule

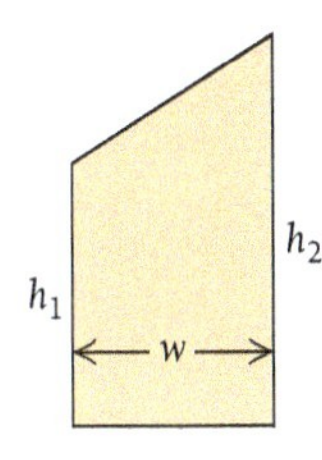

We may also use trapezoids to approximate the area under a curve. Recall that a *trapezoid* is a four-sided polygon of which two sides are parallel. If the parallel sides have lengths h_1 and h_2 and are w units apart, then the area of the trapezoid is $A = \left(\dfrac{h_1+h_2}{2}\right) \cdot w$, where $\dfrac{h_1+h_2}{2}$ is the average of the lengths h_1 and h_2.

Suppose we want to approximate the value of $\int_a^b f(x)\,dx$ using trapezoids, with $y = f(x)$ as shown below. Trapezoids are drawn over each subinterval with their parallel sides extending to the curve f. Assume that each trapezoid has width Δx.

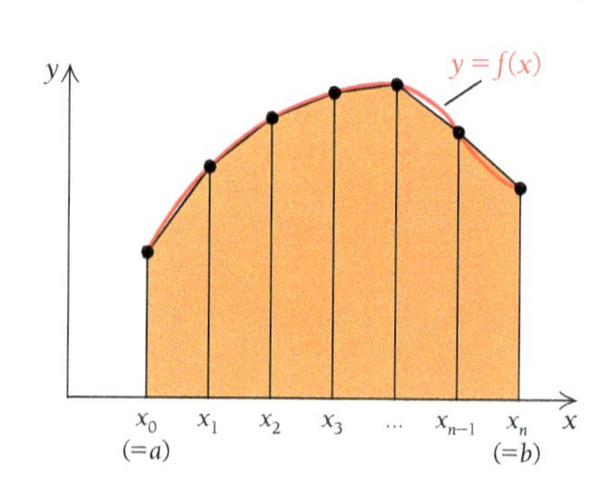

The first trapezoid has a width Δx and heights $f(x_0)$ and $f(x_1)$. Thus, the area of the first trapezoid is $\dfrac{f(x_0) + f(x_1)}{2} \cdot \Delta x$, the area of the second trapezoid is $\dfrac{f(x_1) + f(x_2)}{2} \cdot \Delta x$, and so on. Adding areas, we have

$$\int_a^b f(x)\,dx \approx \frac{f(x_0) + f(x_1)}{2} \cdot \Delta x + \frac{f(x_1) + f(x_2)}{2} \cdot \Delta x + \cdots + \frac{f(x_{n-1}) + f(x_n)}{2} \cdot \Delta x.$$

We now factor out Δx and express each fraction as a sum:

$$\int_a^b f(x)\,dx \approx \Delta x \cdot \left(\frac{f(x_0)}{2} + \frac{f(x_1)}{2} + \frac{f(x_1)}{2} + \frac{f(x_2)}{2} + \frac{f(x_2)}{2} + \cdots + \frac{f(x_{n-1})}{2} + \frac{f(x_{n-1})}{2} + \frac{f(x_n)}{2}\right).$$

Note that $\dfrac{f(x_1)}{2} + \dfrac{f(x_1)}{2} = f(x_1)$, $\dfrac{f(x_2)}{2} + \dfrac{f(x_2)}{2} = f(x_2)$, and so on. Only $\dfrac{f(x_0)}{2}$ and $\dfrac{f(x_n)}{2}$ cannot be combined. Thus, we have

$$\int_a^b f(x)\,dx \approx \Delta x \cdot \left(\frac{f(x_0)}{2} + f(x_1) + f(x_2) + \cdots + f(x_{n-1}) + \frac{f(x_n)}{2}\right).$$

This result leads to the **Trapezoidal Rule**.

DEFINITION Trapezoidal Rule

Let $[a, b]$ be subdivided into n equal subintervals with width $\Delta x = \dfrac{b - a}{n}$, and assume that f is defined for $a, x_1, x_2, \ldots, x_{n-1}, b$. The approximate value of $\int_a^b f(x)\,dx$ is given by T_n, where

$$T_n = \frac{b - a}{n} \cdot \left(\frac{f(a)}{2} + f(x_1) + f(x_2) + \cdots + f(x_{n-1}) + \frac{f(b)}{2}\right).$$

EXAMPLE 4 Use the Trapezoidal Rule to find T_4, an approximation of $\int_1^3 \sqrt[3]{x + x^6}\,dx$.

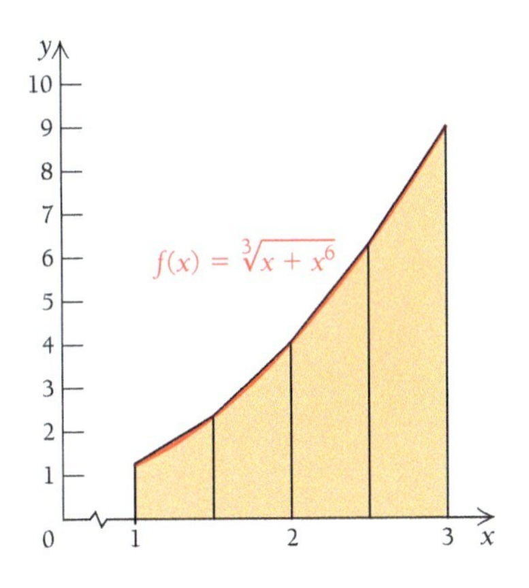

Solution The interval [1, 3] is subdivided into four equal subintervals, [1, 1.5], [1.5, 2], [2, 2.5], and [2.5, 3], each having width $\Delta x = \frac{3 - 1}{4} = \frac{1}{2}$. Using a calculator, we have

$$f(1) = 1.260,\ f(1.5) = 2.345,\ f(2) = 4.041,\ f(2.5) = 6.271,\ f(3) = 9.012.$$

Therefore,

$$T_4 = \frac{1}{2} \cdot \left(\frac{f(1)}{2} + f(1.5) + f(2) + f(2.5) + \frac{f(3)}{2}\right)$$

$$\approx \frac{1}{2} \cdot \left(\frac{1.260}{2} + 2.345 + 4.041 + 6.271 + \frac{9.012}{2}\right)$$

$$= 8.897.$$

Thus, $\int_1^3 \sqrt[3]{x + x6}\, dx \approx T_4 = 8.897.$ **4 ✓**

Quick Check 4 ✓
Use the Trapezoidal Rule to find T_6, an approximation of $\int_0^3 \sqrt{1 + x^5}\, dx$.

Simpson's Rule

When working with Riemann sums, the Midpoint Rule, and the Trapezoidal Rule, we use line segments to approximate the curve of the graph of $y = f(x)$. We can also approximate the curve using parabolas. This is the basis of *Simpson's Rule*, which gives an approximation denoted by S_n, where n is the number of subdivisions of the interval of integration. We will find that with Simpson's Rule, n must be even.

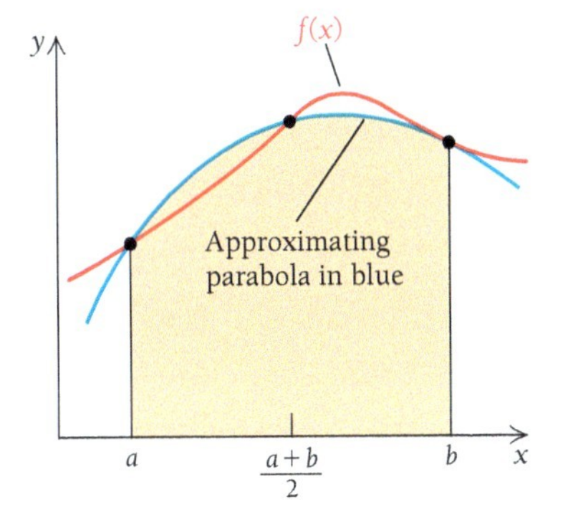

Consider $\int_a^b f(x)\, dx$ with $[a, b]$ subdivided into two subintervals, $\left[a, \frac{a + b}{2}\right]$ and $\left[\frac{a + b}{2}, b\right]$, where $\frac{a + b}{2}$ is the midpoint of $[a, b]$. This provides three points: $(a, f(a))$, $\left(\frac{a + b}{2}, f\left(\frac{a + b}{2}\right)\right)$, and $(b, f(b))$. We can find a parabola that passes through these three points. The area under this parabola is determined by integration and, after simplification, is used to approximate $\int_a^b f(x)\, dx$:

$$\int_a^b f(x)\, dx \approx \frac{b - a}{3n} \cdot \left(f(a) + 4f\left(\frac{a + b}{2}\right) + f(b)\right).$$

The proof of this formula is outlined in Exercise 57.

We now extend this rule to include more subdivisions. If n is even, then $n/2$ is a whole number and represents the number of parabolas. Again, $[a, b]$ is subdivided by $x_0, x_1, x_2, x_3, \ldots, x_{n-1}, x_n$, where $x_0 = a$ and $x_n = b$. A parabola is fitted to the first, second, and third points; another parabola is fitted to the third, fourth, and fifth points, and so on. This leads us to Simpson's Rule.

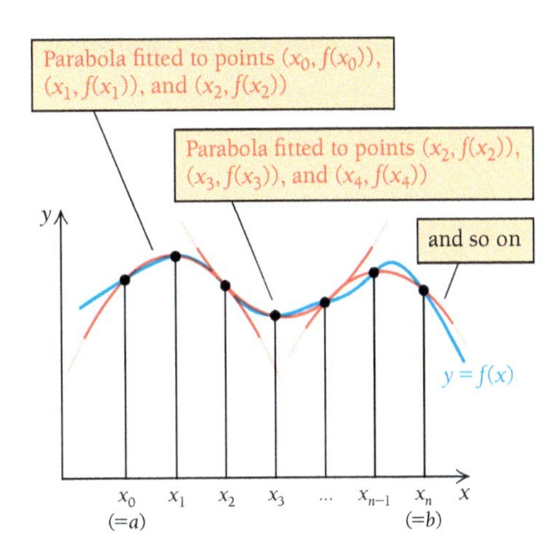

DEFINITION Simpson's Rule

Let $[a, b]$ be subdivided into an even number n of equal subintervals with width $\Delta x = \frac{b-a}{n}$, and assume that f is defined for $a, x_1, x_2, \ldots, x_{n-1}, b$. The approximate value of $\int_a^b f(x)\,dx$ is given by S_n, where

$$S_n = \frac{b-a}{3n} \cdot (f(a) + 4f(x_1) + 2f(x_2) + 4f(x_3) + \cdots + 2f(x_{n-2}) + 4f(x_{n-1}) + f(b)).$$

EXAMPLE 5 Use Simpson's Rule to find S_2 and S_4, approximations of $\int_0^2 \sqrt{9-x^2}\,dx$.

Solution For S_2, we subdivide $[0, 2]$ into two equal subintervals, $[0, 1]$ and $[1, 2]$. Note that $x_0 = 0$, $x_1 = 1$, and $x_2 = 2$. Thus, we have

$$S_2 = \frac{2-0}{3 \cdot 2} \cdot (f(0) + 4f(1) + f(2)) \quad \text{Substituting}$$

$$\approx \tfrac{1}{3}(3 + 4 \cdot 2.828 + 2.236) \quad \text{Calculating } f(0), f(1), \text{ and } f(2)$$

$$= 5.516 \text{ (rounded)}.$$

For S_4, we subdivide $[0, 2]$ into four equal subintervals, $[0, 0.5]$, $[0.5, 1]$, $[1, 1.5]$, and $[1.5, 2]$. We have $x_0 = 0$, $x_1 = 0.5$, $x_2 = 1$, $x_3 = 1.5$, and $x_4 = 2$. Thus,

$$S_4 = \frac{2-0}{3 \cdot 4} \cdot (f(0) + 4f(0.5) + 2f(1) + 4f(1.5) + f(2))$$

$$\approx \tfrac{1}{6} \cdot (3 + 4 \cdot 2.958 + 2 \cdot 2.828 + 4 \cdot 2.598 + 2.236)$$

$$= 5.519 \text{ (rounded)}.$$

Calculus software shows that, to four decimal places, the value of $\int_0^2 \sqrt{9-x^2}\,dx$ is 5.5198. Thus, both S_2 and S_4 are very accurate approximations of $\int_0^2 \sqrt{9-x^2}\,dx$. 5 ✓

Quick Check 5 ✓
Use Simpson's Rule to find S_2 and S_4, approximations of $\int_{-1}^1 e^{-x^2}\,dx$.

Section Summary

- The process of numerically approximating the value of $\int_a^b f(x)\,dx$ using geometry is called *numerical integration*. To do this, we subdivide $[a, b]$ into n subintervals, $[a, x_1], [x_1, x_2], \ldots, [x_{n-1}, b]$, regarding a as x_0 and b as x_n, and assume that f is defined for $a, x_1, x_2, \ldots, x_{n-1}, b$. If the subintervals are equal in size, then each subinterval has a width of $\Delta x = \frac{b-a}{n}$. We may then use any of the following techniques.
  - *Riemann sums using rectangles*: Rectangles are drawn over the subintervals. With *left-rectangles*, the height of each rectangle is evaluated at the left endpoint of the subinterval. The sum of the areas of all rectangles is denoted as L_n.

$$L_n = \frac{b-a}{n} \cdot (f(a) + f(x_1) + f(x_2) + \cdots + f(x_{n-2}) + f(x_{n-1})).$$

With *right-rectangles*, the height of each rectangle is evaluated at the right endpoint of the subinterval. The sum of the areas of all rectangles is denoted as R_n.

$$R_n = \frac{b-a}{n} \cdot (f(x_1) + f(x_2) + \cdots + f(x_{n-2}) + f(x_{n-1}) + f(b)).$$

We can average L_n and R_n (or use a larger value of n) to obtain what is usually a better approximation of $\int_a^b f(x)\,dx$.

- *Midpoint Rule*: Using rectangles, the height of each rectangle is evaluated at the midpoint of the subinterval, assuming that f is defined for $\frac{a + x_1}{2}, \frac{x_1 + x_2}{2}, \ldots, \frac{x_{n-1} + b}{2}$. The sum of the areas of all rectangles is denoted as M_n.

$$M_n = \frac{b-a}{n} \cdot \left(f\left(\frac{a + x_1}{2}\right) + f\left(\frac{x_1 + x_2}{2}\right) + f\left(\frac{x_2 + x_3}{2}\right) + \cdots + f\left(\frac{x_{n-2} + x_{n-1}}{2}\right) + f\left(\frac{x_{n-1} + b}{2}\right)\right).$$

- *Trapezoidal Rule*: Trapezoids are drawn over each subinterval. The sum of the areas of all the trapezoids is denoted T_n, where

$$T_n = \frac{b-a}{n} \cdot \left(\frac{f(a)}{2} + f(x_1) + f(x_2) + \cdots + f(x_{n-1}) + \frac{f(b)}{2}\right).$$

- *Simpson's Rule*: The interval $[a, b]$ is divided into n subintervals, where n is even. The graph of f is then approximated by $n/2$ parabolas, and the area under f is approximated by S_n, where

$$S_n = \frac{b-a}{3n} \cdot \left(f(a) + 4f(x_1) + 2f(x_2) + 4f(x_3) + \cdots + 2f(x_{n-2}) + 4f(x_{n-1}) + f(b)\right).$$

4.7 Exercise Set

In Exercises 1–10, find L_n, R_n, and their average for each definite integral using the indicated value of n. Give all answers to three decimal places.

1. $\int_0^4 (x^2 + 1)\,dx,\ n = 4$
2. $\int_2^6 (x^3 - 1)\,dx,\ n = 4$
3. $\int_0^3 (2x^3 - x)\,dx,\ n = 6$
4. $\int_{-1}^2 (x^2 + 2x)\,dx,\ n = 6$
5. $\int_2^4 \frac{1}{x}\,dx,\ n = 8$
6. $\int_3^8 \frac{1}{x-2}\,dx,\ n = 5$
7. $\int_0^3 e^{2x}\,dx,\ n = 6$
8. $\int_{-2}^0 e^{-x}\,dx,\ n = 4$
9. $\int_1^5 x(x^2 + 1)^2\,dx,\ n = 8$
10. $\int_0^5 x^2(x^3 + 2)^2\,dx,\ n = 10$

11–20. Find M_n to three decimal places for each definite integral in Exercises 1–10, using the indicated value of n.

In Exercises 21–28, use the Trapezoidal Rule to find T_n using the indicated value of n. Give all answers to three decimal places.

21. $\int_0^2 \sqrt{x^2 + 1}\,dx,\ n = 4$
22. $\int_1^4 \sqrt{x^2 + 3}\,dx,\ n = 6$
23. $\int_0^4 \frac{1}{x^2 + 1}\,dx,\ n = 8$
24. $\int_3^4 \frac{1}{x^2 - 1}\,dx,\ n = 3$
25. $\int_0^5 e^{\sqrt{x}}\,dx,\ n = 5$
26. $\int_1^3 e^{-\sqrt{x}}\,dx,\ n = 6$
27. $\int_0^4 \frac{1}{x^3 + 1}\,dx,\ n = 4$
28. $\int_1^6 \frac{x}{x^2 + 1}\,dx,\ n = 5$

In Exercises 29–36, use Simpson's Rule to find S_n using the indicated value of n. Give all answers to three decimal places.

29. $\int_2^4 \sqrt{x^2 - 1}\,dx,\ n = 4$
30. $\int_5^8 \sqrt{x^2 - 4}\,dx,\ n = 6$
31. $\int_{-1}^1 e^{-x^3}\,dx,\ n = 6$
32. $\int_0^1 e^{x^2}\,dx,\ n = 4$
33. $\int_1^3 \ln(x^2 + 1)\,dx,\ n = 6$
34. $\int_2^3 (1 + \ln x)^2\,dx,\ n = 4$
35. $\int_1^5 \frac{1}{\sqrt{x^2 + 1}}\,dx,\ n = 4$
36. $\int_{-1}^3 \frac{x}{\sqrt{x^3 + 2}}\,dx,\ n = 4$

APPLICATIONS

General Interest

37. **Total distance.** Walt goes for a 12-min walk. His pedometer shows his speed, $v(t)$, in miles per hour, for 1-min intervals. Use L_{12}, R_{12}, and their average to approximate the distance Walt travels to three decimal places. (*Hint*: 1 min $= \frac{1}{60}$ hr.)

t (min)	0	1	2	3	4	5	6	7	8	9	10	11	12
$v(t)$ (mi/hr)	0	4	4	6	6	4	5	2	1	3	5	6	6

38. **Total distance.** Moira drives her car for 8 min. Her speed, $v(t)$, in miles per hour, for 1-min intervals, is shown below. Use L_8, R_8, and their average to approximate the distance Moira travels to three decimal places.

t (min)	0	1	2	3	4	5	6	7	8
$v(t)$ (mi/hr)	0	25	30	35	30	22	20	10	10

39. Surface area. The following diagram shows the distances across a pond, in feet, measured at 6-foot intervals. Use the Trapezoidal Rule to approximate the surface area of the pond to three decimal places.

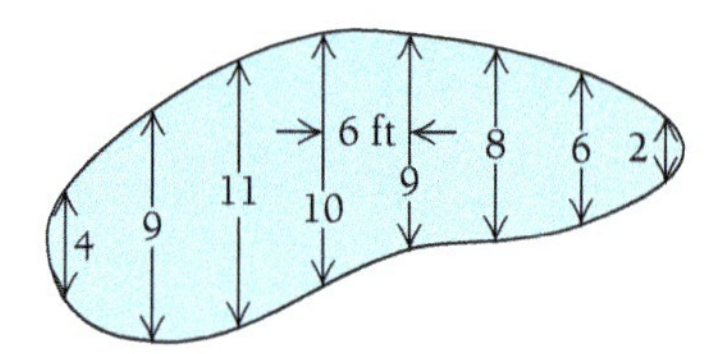

40. Cross-sectional area. A stream channel has the following profile, where the depths are in feet and measured at 2-ft intervals across the stream's width. Use the Trapezoidal Rule to approximate the cross-sectional area of the stream channel to two decimal places.

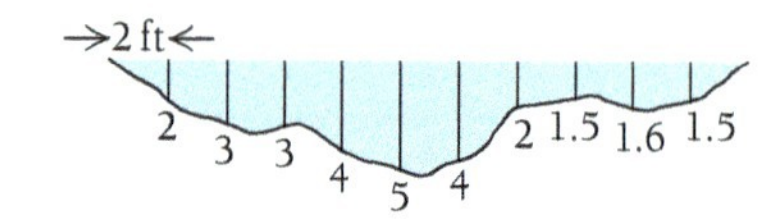

41. Area inside an ellipse. An ellipse is centered at the origin and has x-intercepts $(-5, 0)$ and $(5, 0)$ and y-intercepts $(0, -2)$ and $(0, 2)$. The portion of the ellipse in the first quadrant is given by $f(x) = \frac{2}{5}\sqrt{25 - x^2}$, for $0 \le x \le 5$.

a) Approximate the area of the portion of the ellipse that is in the first quadrant by finding T_{10} to three decimal places.

b) Estimate the total area enclosed within the ellipse.

42. Area inside an ellipse. An ellipse is centered at the origin and has x-intercepts $(-4, 0)$ and $(4, 0)$ and y-intercepts $(0, -3)$ and $(0, 3)$. The portion of the ellipse in the first quadrant is given by $f(x) = \frac{3}{4}\sqrt{16 - x^2}$, for $0 \le x \le 4$.

a) Approximate the area of the portion of the ellipse that is in the first quadrant by finding T_8 to three decimal places.

b) Estimate the total area enclosed within the ellipse.

For Exercises 43–46, the length of any differentiable curve $y = f(x)$ over $[a, b]$ is given by $\int_a^b \sqrt{1 + [f'(x)]^2}\, dx$.

43. Circumference of a circle. The portion of a unit circle that is in the first quadrant is given by $f(x) = \sqrt{1 - x^2}$, for $0 \le x \le 1$.

a) Approximate the length of this curve, $\int_a^b \sqrt{1 + [f'(x)]^2}\, dx$, by finding M_6.

b) Use a geometric formula to find the exact length of the curve.

44. Circumference of a circle. The portion of a circle of radius 2 that is in the first quadrant is given by $f(x) = \sqrt{4 - x^2}$, for $0 \le x \le 2$.

a) Approximate the length of this curve, $\int_a^b \sqrt{1 + [f'(x)]^2}\, dx$, by finding M_8 to three decimal places.

b) Use a geometric formula to find the exact length of the curve.

45. Length of a curve. Using $\int_a^b \sqrt{1 + [f'(x)]^2}\, dx$, approximate the length of the curve $f(x) = 4 - x^2$ over $[-2, 2]$ by finding S_8 to three decimal places.

46. Length of a curve. Using $\int_a^b \sqrt{1 + [f'(x)]^2}\, dx$, approximate the length of the curve $f(x) = e^x$ over $[-1, 2]$ by finding S_6 to three decimal places.

Business and Economics

47. Total cost. The shape of a wall in a museum is shown below, where heights (in feet) are given at 6-ft intervals. The wall is to be paneled, at a cost of \$3.50 per square foot. Find the approximate cost of paneling the wall.

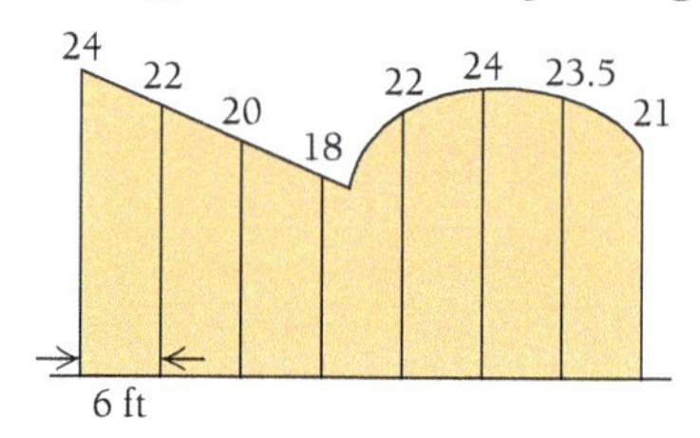

48. Total cost. The back of a storage shed is in the shape shown below, where the heights (in feet) are given at 3-ft intervals. The cost to install metal sheeting over this surface is \$6 per square foot. Approximately how much will it cost to cover the back of the shed with metal sheeting? Assume that the shed is symmetrical.

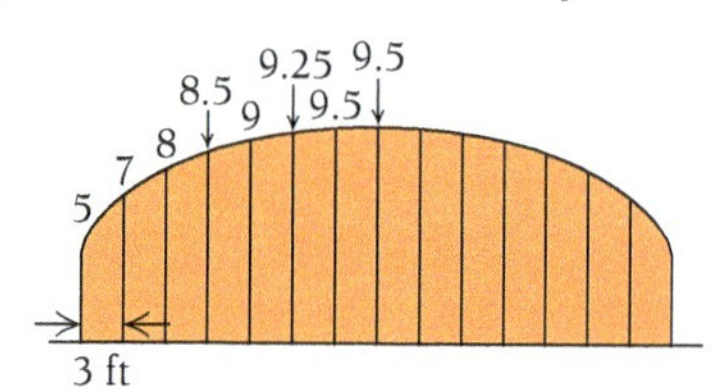

49. Total cost to maintain a green. The 17th green (called the "Island Green") at the Sawgrass TPC Golf Course in Ponte Vedra Beach, Florida, has the measurements shown below.

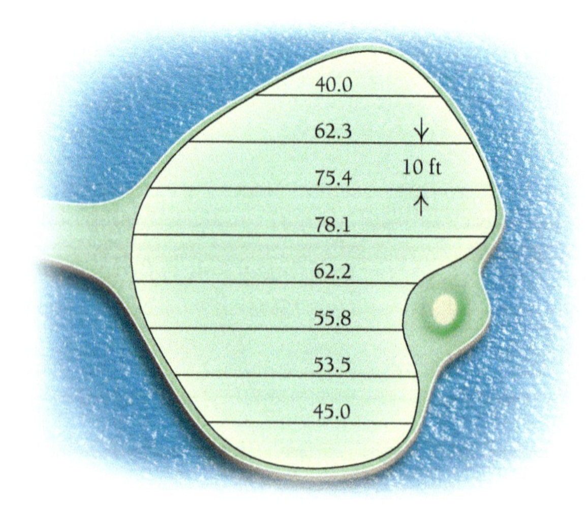

a) Use a numerical integration technique to approximate the area of the green.

b) If the cost to maintain the 17th green is \$6.00 per square foot per month, what is the approximate total monthly cost of maintaining the green?

50. Finding total area. Fair territory at Dodger Stadium in Los Angeles, California, is shown below, with distances, in feet, from the right-field foul line to the opposite side of the field given at 30-ft intervals. Estimate the total area of fair territory.

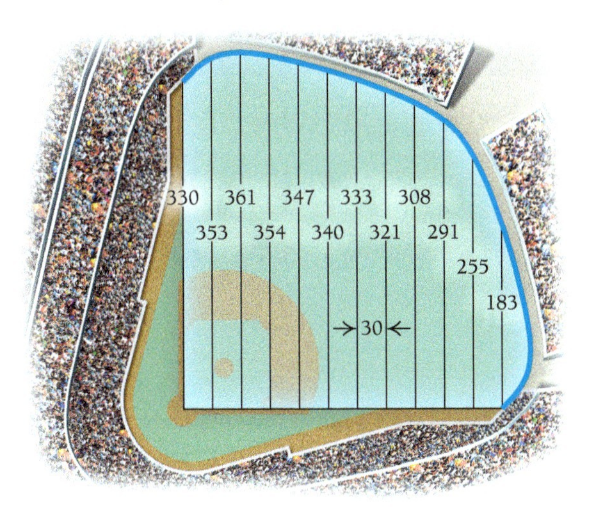

SYNTHESIS

51. Suppose $y = f(x)$ is differentiable, increasing, and concave up on $[a, b]$. Fill in each blank with $<$ or $>$.

a) L_n ____ $\int_a^b f(x)\,dx$ b) R_n ____ $\int_a^b f(x)\,dx$

c) T_n ____ $\int_a^b f(x)\,dx$

52. Suppose $y = f(x)$ is differentiable, decreasing, and concave up on $[a, b]$. Fill in each blank with $<$ or $>$.

a) L_n ____ $\int_a^b f(x)\,dx$ b) R_n ____ $\int_a^b f(x)\,dx$

c) T_n ____ $\int_a^b f(x)\,dx$

53. Suppose $y = f(x)$ is differentiable, increasing, and concave down on $[a, b]$. Fill in each blank with $<$ or $>$.

a) L_n ____ $\int_a^b f(x)\,dx$ b) R_n ____ $\int_a^b f(x)\,dx$

c) T_n ____ $\int_a^b f(x)\,dx$

54. Suppose $y = f(x)$ is differentiable, decreasing, and concave down on $[a, b]$. Fill in each blank with $<$ or $>$.

a) L_n ____ $\int_a^b f(x)\,dx$ b) R_n ____ $\int_a^b f(x)\,dx$

c) T_n ____ $\int_a^b f(x)\,dx$

55. Explain why the Trapezoidal Rule always gives an exact value for $\int_a^b (Cx + D)\,dx$.

56. Explain why Simpson's Rule always gives an exact value for $\int_a^b (Cx^2 + Dx + E)\,dx$.

57. The following is an outline of a proof of Simpson's Rule for the special case where $n = 2$ with f continuous over $[-1, 1]$. Here, $a = -1$, $b = 1$, and $\frac{a+b}{2} = 0$. We will show that

$$\int_{-1}^{1} f(x)\,dx \approx \frac{1}{3}\cdot\left(f(-1) + 4f(0) + f(1)\right).$$

a) Let $(-1, y_1)$, $(0, y_2)$, and $(1, y_3)$ be three points, where $y_1 = f(-1)$, $y_2 = f(0)$, and $y_3 = f(1)$, and let $y = Ax^2 + Bx + C$ be a parabola that passes through these three points. Find values for A, B, and C in terms of y_1, y_2, and y_3. (*Hint:* Evaluate $y = Ax^2 + Bx + C$ at each point. You should be able to solve for C immediately. Then substitute and find expressions for A and B.)

b) Evaluate $\int_{-1}^{1}(Ax^2 + Bx + C)\,dx$. Your answer will be in terms of y_1, y_2, and y_3. Write each term over a single common denominator.

58. Assume that f is continuous over the interval $[-1, 3]$. Using a method similar to that in Exercise 57, we can show that $\int_1^3 f(x)\,dx \approx \frac{1}{3}\cdot\left(f(1) + 4f(2) + f(3)\right)$. Use the fact that $\int_{-1}^{1} f(x)\,dx \approx \frac{1}{3}\cdot\left(f(-1) + 4f(0) + f(1)\right)$ (from Exercise 57) to show that

$$\int_{-1}^{3} f(x)\,dx \approx \frac{1}{3}\cdot\left(f(-1) + 4f(0) + 2f(1) + 4f(2) + f(3)\right),$$

where $n = 4$.

59. Does the Midpoint Rule always give a better approximation than that found using left- or right-rectangles? Why or why not?

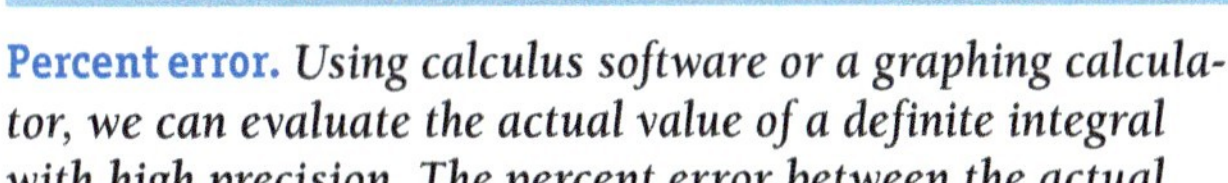

Percent error. *Using calculus software or a graphing calculator, we can evaluate the actual value of a definite integral with high precision. The percent error between the actual value and an approximation is given by*

$$\text{Percent error} = \frac{\text{approximation} - \text{actual value}}{\text{actual value}} \times 100.$$

60–75. Using calculus software or a graphing calculator, find (a) the actual value of each definite integral in Exercises 21–36 to three decimal places and (b) the percent error between the approximation and the actual value of each integral.

Answers to Quick Checks

1. $R_{10} = 2.549$; average $= 2.50$ mi
2. $L_4 = 1.007$, $R_4 = 1.557$; average $= 1.282$
3. $M_8 = 1.268$ **4.** $T_6 = 14.674$
5. $S_2 = 1.579$, $S_4 = 1.494$

Chapter 4 Summary

KEY TERMS AND CONCEPTS	EXAMPLES
SECTION 4.1	
A function F is an **antiderivative** of a function f if $$\frac{d}{dx}F(x) = f(x).$$ Antiderivatives of a function f all differ by a constant C, called the **constant of integration.**	• $F(x) = x^2$ is an antiderivative of $f(x) = 2x$ because $\frac{d}{dx}(x^2) = 2x$. • $G(x) = \ln x$ is an antiderivative of $g(x) = \frac{1}{x}$ because $\frac{d}{dx}(\ln x) = \frac{1}{x}$. Antiderivatives of $f(x) = 2x$ have the form $x^2 + C$. These antiderivatives can be expressed by $\int 2x\,dx = x^2 + C$.
An **indefinite integral** of a function f is written $$\int f(x)\,dx = F(x) + C,$$ where $f(x)$ is called the **integrand.**	In the indefinite integral $\int (x^{-4} + x + e^x)\,dx$, the integrand is $x^{-4} + x + e^x$. The antiderivative is the set of functions of the form $-\frac{1}{3x^3} + \frac{1}{2}x^2 + e^x + C$.
Rules for Antiderivatives:	
A1. $\int k\,dx = kx + C$	• $\int 9\,dx = 9x + C$ A1
A2. $\int x^n\,dx = \frac{x^{n+1}}{n+1} + C, \quad n \neq -1$	• $\int x^6\,dx = \frac{1}{7}x^7 + C$ A2
A3. $\int \frac{1}{x}\,dx = \ln\lvert x\rvert + C,$ or, for $x > 0$, $\int \frac{1}{x}\,dx = \ln x + C$	• $\int \frac{5}{x}\,dx = 5\ln\lvert x\rvert + C$ A3
A4. $\int e^{ax}\,dx = \frac{1}{a}e^{ax} + C$	• $\int e^{3x}\,dx = \frac{1}{3}e^{3x} + C$ A4
Properties of Indefinite Integrals:	
P1. $\int [c \cdot f(x)]\,dx = c\int f(x)\,dx$	• $\int (3x^4 + 4x - 5)\,dx = \frac{3}{5}x^5 + 2x^2 - 5x + C$ A1, A2, P1, P2
P2. $\int [f(x) \pm g(x)]\,dx = \int f(x)\,dx \pm \int g(x)\,dx.$	• $\int (x + 4)^2\,dx = \int (x^2 + 8x + 16)\,dx = \frac{1}{3}x^3 + 4x^2 + 16x + C$ A1, A2, P1, P2

KEY TERMS AND CONCEPTS	EXAMPLES

SECTION 4.1 (*continued*)

An **initial condition** is a point that is a solution of a particular antiderivative.

Find $\int (3x - 2)\,dx$, given that (1, 4) is a solution of the antiderivative.

Find the antiderivative: $\displaystyle\int (3x - 2)\,dx = \frac{3}{2}x^2 - 2x + C$, so

$F(x) = \frac{3}{2}x^2 - 2x + C$. Since (1, 4) is an initial condition, substitute 1 for x and 4 for $F(x)$ and solve for C:

$$4 = \frac{3}{2}(1)^2 - 2(1) + C \qquad \text{Substituting}$$
$$4 = \frac{3}{2} - 2 + C$$
$$4 = -\frac{1}{2} + C$$
$$C = \frac{9}{2}.$$

The particular antiderivative that meets the initial condition is

$F(x) = \frac{3}{2}x^2 - 2x + \frac{9}{2}.$

SECTION 4.2

The **area under the graph of a function** can be interpreted in a meaningful way. The units of the area are determined by multiplying the units of the input variable by the units of the output variable.

Physical Science. Suppose Josef's jogging speed, in miles per hour, is $v(t) = 6$, where t is in hours. In 3 hr, Josef runs $3\text{ hr} \cdot 6\,\frac{\text{mi}}{\text{hr}} = 18$ mi, which is the area under the graph representing his velocity function. Every hour, Josef travels 6 mi. His total distance traveled is modeled by $d(t) = 6t$. Note that $d(t)$ is the antiderivative of $v(t)$.

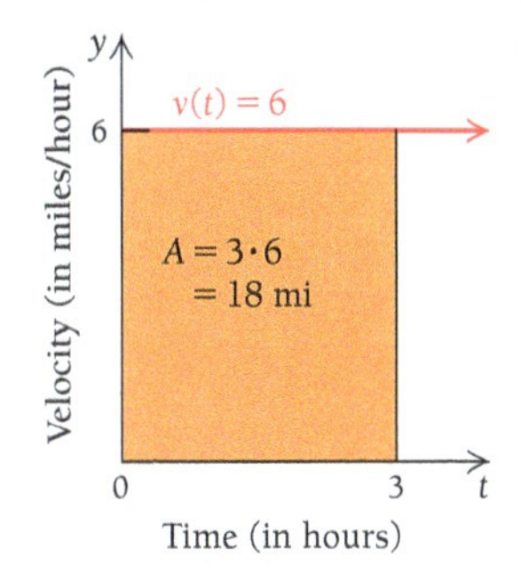

Common geometry formulas can sometimes be used to calculate area.

Business. McLean Furniture's marginal revenue is modeled by

$$R'(x) = 37x,$$

where x is the number of dining room sets sold and $R'(x)$ is in thousands of dollars per set. The total revenue from selling 100 sets is the area under the marginal revenue function.

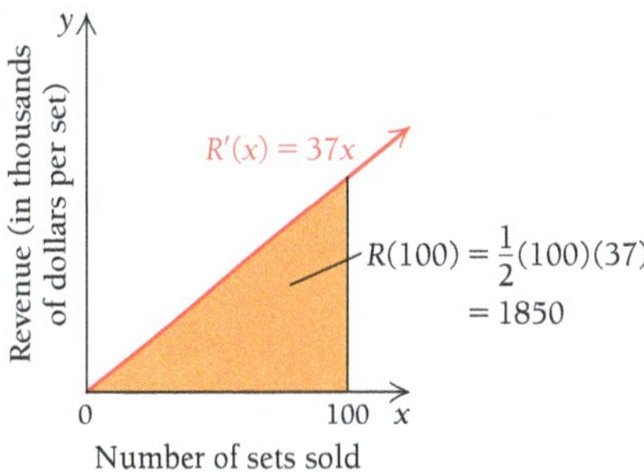

$$\text{Total revenue} = \frac{1}{2}(100 \text{ units})\left(37\,\frac{\text{thousands of dollars}}{\text{unit}}\right)$$
$$= 1850 \text{ thousand dollars, or } \$1{,}850{,}000.$$

KEY TERMS AND CONCEPTS | EXAMPLES

SECTION 4.2 (*continued*)

Riemann summation uses rectangles to approximate the area under a curve.

As the number of rectangles approaches infinity, we have a **definite integral**, which represents the exact area under the graph of a continuous and nonnegative function $f(x) \geq 0$ over an interval $[a, b]$:

$$\text{Exact area} = \int_a^b f(x)\,dx.$$

Approximate the area under the graph of $f(x) = -\frac{1}{3}x^2 + 3x$ over $[1, 7]$ using 3 equally sized subintervals.

Each subinterval will have width $\Delta x = \dfrac{7-1}{3} = 2$, with x_i ranging from $x_1 = 1$ to $x_3 = 5$ in increments of 2. The area under the curve over $[1, 7]$ is approximated as follows:

$$\sum_{i=1}^{3} f(x_i)\cdot\Delta x = f(1)\cdot 2 + f(3)\cdot 2 + f(5)\cdot 2$$

$$= \frac{8}{3}\cdot 2 + 6\cdot 2 + \frac{20}{3}\cdot 2$$

$$= 30.666\ldots.$$

Thus, the area under f is approximately 31 square units.

SECTION 4.3

The **Fundamental Theorem of Calculus** states that the exact area under a continuous function f over $[a, b]$ can be calculated directly using a definite integral:

$$\int_a^b f(x)\,dx = F(b) - F(a).$$

The function F is any antiderivative of f (we usually set the constant of integration equal to 0).

The exact area under the graph of $f(x) = -\frac{1}{3}x^2 + 3x$ over $[1, 7]$ is

$$\int_1^7 \left(-\frac{1}{3}x^2 + 3x\right)dx = \left[-\frac{1}{9}x^3 + \frac{3}{2}x^2\right]_1^7$$

$$= \left(-\frac{1}{9}(7)^3 + \frac{3}{2}(7)^2\right) - \left(-\frac{1}{9}(1)^3 + \frac{3}{2}(1)^2\right) = 34.$$

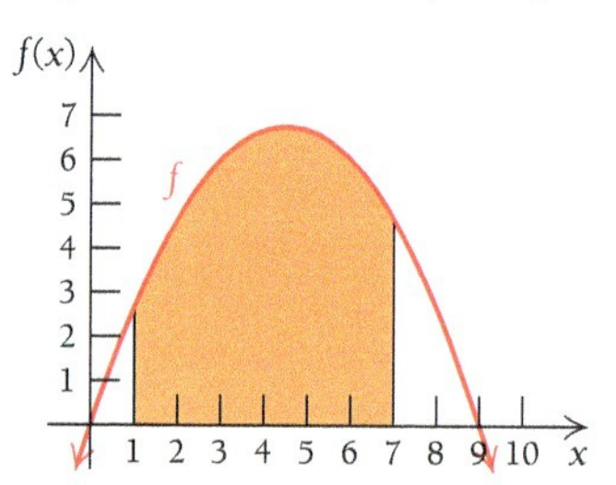

The Fundamental Theorem of Calculus is true for *all* continuous functions f over an interval $[a, b]$.

- If f is negative over $[a, b]$, then the definite integral is negative.
- If f has more area above the x-axis than below it over $[a, b]$, then the definite integral is positive.
- If f has more area below the x-axis than above it over $[a, b]$, then the definite integral is negative.
- If f has equal areas above and below the x-axis over $[a, b]$, then the definite integral is zero.

Evaluate the definite integral of $f(x) = x^2 - 1$ over $\left[-\frac{1}{2}, 1\right]$.

Since $f(x)$ is negative over $\left[-\frac{1}{2}, 1\right]$, the definite integral will be negative.

$$\int_{-1/2}^{1} (x^2 - 1)\,dx = \left[\frac{1}{3}x^3 - x\right]_{-1/2}^{1}$$

$$= \left(\frac{1}{3}(1)^3 - (1)\right) - \left(\frac{1}{3}\left(-\frac{1}{2}\right)^3 - \left(-\frac{1}{2}\right)\right) = -\frac{9}{8}.$$

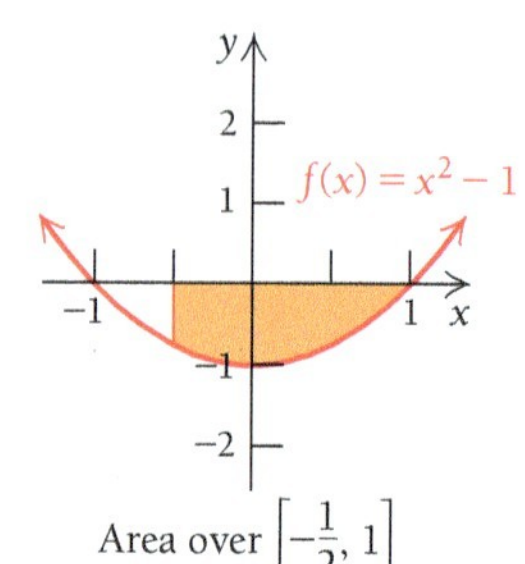

Area over $\left[-\frac{1}{2}, 1\right]$

KEY TERMS AND CONCEPTS	EXAMPLES

SECTION 4.3 (*continued*)

Evaluate the definite integral of $f(x) = x^2 - 1$ over $[0, 3]$.

Over $[0, 3]$, f has more area above the x-axis than below, so we expect a positive result.

$$\int_0^3 (x^2 - 1)\, dx = \left[\frac{1}{3}x^3 - x\right]_0^3 = (9 - 3) - (0) = 6$$

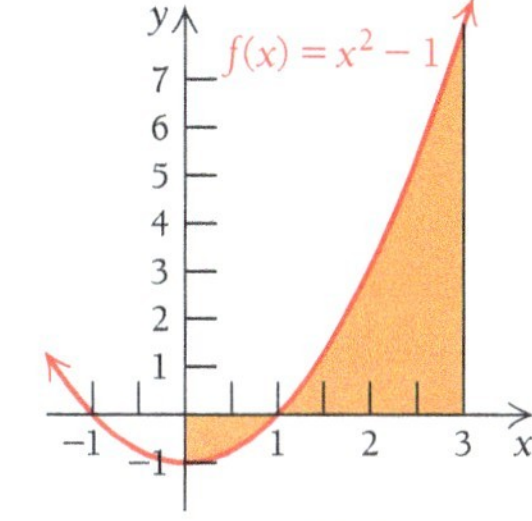

Area over $[0, 3]$

The function given by $g(x) = x - 2$ over $[0, 4]$ has equal areas below and above the x-axis. Therefore,

$$\int_0^4 (x - 2)\, dx = \left[\frac{1}{2}x^2 - 2x\right]_0^4 = 8 - 8 = 0.$$

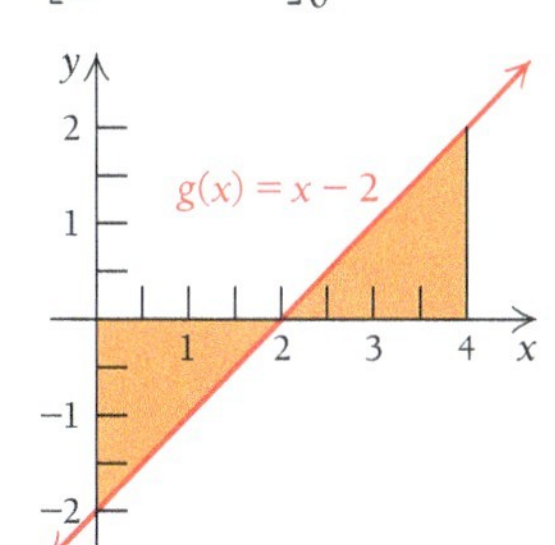

SECTION 4.4

There are many useful properties of definite integrals.

Additive property: For $a < c < b$, we have

$$\int_a^b f(x)\, dx = \int_a^c f(x)\, dx + \int_c^b f(x)\, dx.$$

The additive property is useful for piecewise-defined functions, including the absolute-value function. For example, if

$$f(x) = \begin{cases} -x + 1, & \text{for } x < 0, \\ \frac{1}{2}x + 1, & \text{for } x \geq 0, \end{cases}$$

then
$$\int_{-2}^3 f(x)\, dx = \int_{-2}^0 (-x + 1)\, dx + \int_0^3 \left(\frac{1}{2}x + 1\right) dx$$
$$= 4 + \frac{21}{4}$$
$$= \frac{37}{4}.$$

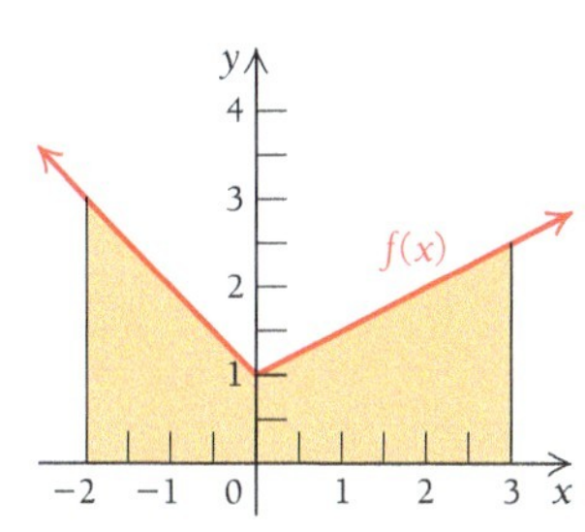

KEY TERMS AND CONCEPTS | **EXAMPLES**

SECTION 4.4 (*continued*)

Area of a region bounded by two curves: If $f(x) \geq g(x)$ over $[a, b]$, then the area between the graphs of f and g from $x = a$ to $x = b$ is

$$A = \int_a^b [f(x) - g(x)]\,dx.$$

Let $f(x) = x^2$ and $g(x) = x + 2$. Solving $f(x) = g(x)$, we find that the curves intersect at $x = -1$ and $x = 2$. Furthermore, we see that $g(x) \geq f(x)$ on $[-1, 2]$. Therefore, the area between these curves is

$$\begin{aligned} A &= \int_{-1}^{2} [g(x) - f(x)]\,dx \\ &= \int_{-1}^{2} (x + 2 - x^2)\,dx = \left[\frac{1}{2}x^2 + 2x - \frac{1}{3}x^3\right]_{-1}^{2} \\ &= \left(\frac{1}{2}(2)^2 + 2(2) - \frac{1}{3}(2)^3\right) - \left(\frac{1}{2}(-1)^2 + 2(-1) - \frac{1}{3}(-1)^3\right) \\ &= \frac{9}{2}. \end{aligned}$$

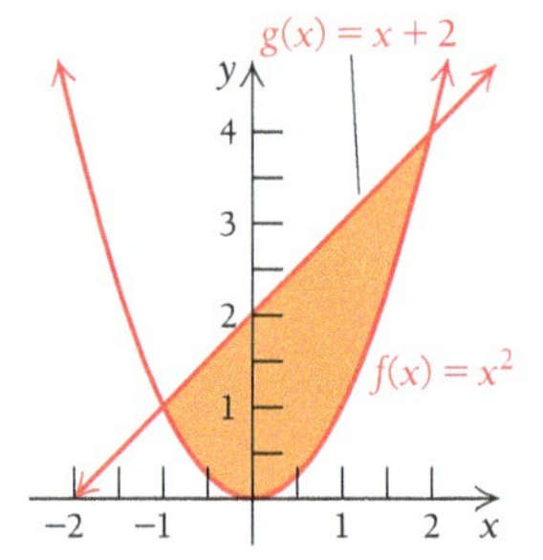

Average value: The average value of y, or $f(x)$, over $[a, b]$ is

$$y_{\text{av}} = \frac{1}{b - a}\int_a^b f(x)\,dx.$$

The average value of $y = x^3$ over $[1, 4]$ is

$$y_{\text{av}} = \frac{1}{3}\int_1^4 x^3\,dx = \left[\frac{1}{12}x^4\right]_1^4 = 21\frac{1}{4}.$$

SECTION 4.5

Integration by **substitution** is the reverse of applying the Chain Rule. We choose u, determine du, and rewrite the integrand in terms of u and du. *Results should be checked using differentiation!*

- Evaluate $\int 2x(x^2 + 1)^5\,dx$.

  Let $u = x^2 + 1$, so that $du = 2x\,dx$. Therefore, we have

  $$\int 2x(x^2 + 1)^5\,dx = \int u^5\,du = \frac{1}{6}u^6 + C = \frac{1}{6}(x^2 + 1)^6 + C.$$

- Evaluate $\displaystyle\int \frac{1}{3x - 2}\,dx$.

  Let $u = 3x - 2$, so that $du = 3\,dx$. Thus, $dx = du/3$.

  $$\begin{aligned} \int \frac{1}{3x - 2}\,dx &= \int \frac{1}{u}\frac{du}{3} = \frac{1}{3}\int \frac{1}{u}\,du \\ &= \frac{1}{3}\ln|u| + C = \frac{1}{3}\ln|3x - 2| + C. \end{aligned}$$

KEY TERMS AND CONCEPTS	EXAMPLES

SECTION 4.6

The **Integration-by-Parts Formula** is derived using the product rule for differentiation:

$$\int u\,dv = uv - \int v\,du.$$

Evaluate $\int x^3 \ln x\,dx$, where $x > 0$.

Let $u = \ln x$ and $dv = x^3\,dx$. Then $du = \frac{1}{x}\,dx$ and $v = \frac{1}{4}x^4$, and

$$\int u\,dv = uv - \int v\,du$$

$$\int x^3 \ln x\,dx = \frac{1}{4}x^4 \ln x - \int \left(\frac{1}{4}x^4\right)\left(\frac{1}{x}\,dx\right)$$

$$= \frac{1}{4}x^4 \ln x - \frac{1}{4}\int x^3\,dx$$

$$= \frac{1}{4}x^4 \ln x - \frac{1}{16}x^4 + C.$$

Tabular integration can be used when integration by parts has to be applied more than once to evaluate an integral.

Evaluate $\int x^3 e^{2x}\,dx$.

This will involve repeated integrations by parts. Since repeated differentiation of $f(x) = x^3$ eventually yields 0 and $g(x) = e^{2x}$ is easily integrable, we use tabular integration by parts:

$f(x)$ and Repeated Derivatives	Sign of Product	$g(x)$ and Repeated Integrals
x^3	$(+)$	e^{2x}
$3x^2$	$(-)$	$\frac{1}{2}e^{2x}$
$6x$	$(+)$	$\frac{1}{4}e^{2x}$
6	$(-)$	$\frac{1}{8}e^{2x}$
0		$\frac{1}{16}e^{2x}$

Multiply along the arrows, alternate signs, and simplify when possible. The antiderivative is

$$\int x^3 e^{2x}\,dx = \frac{1}{2}x^3e^{2x} - \frac{3}{4}x^2e^{2x} + \frac{6}{8}xe^{2x} - \frac{6}{16}e^{2x}$$

$$= e^{2x}\left(\frac{1}{2}x^3 - \frac{3}{4}x^2 + \frac{3}{4}x - \frac{3}{8}\right) + C.$$

SECTION 4.7

Numerical integration uses geometry to approximate a definite integral, $\int_a^b f(x)\,dx$. The interval $[a, b]$ is first subdivided into n equal subintervals, $[a, x_1], [x_1, x_2], \ldots, [x_{n-1}, b]$, each with width $\Delta x = \frac{b-a}{n}$.

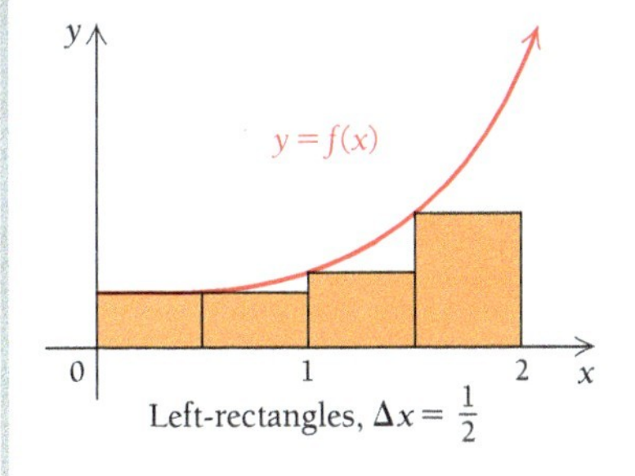

Left-rectangles, $\Delta x = \frac{1}{2}$

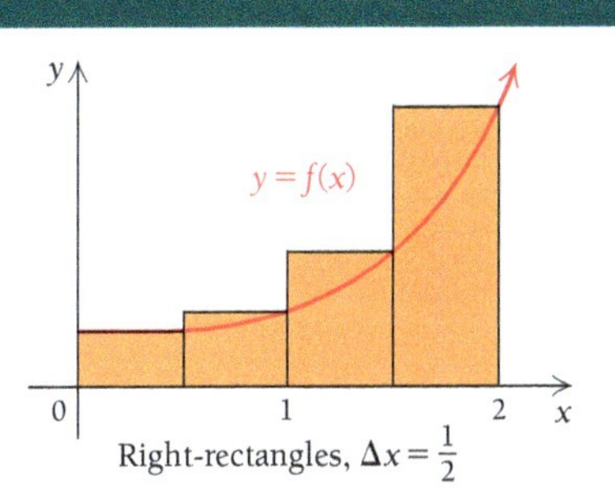

Right-rectangles, $\Delta x = \frac{1}{2}$

KEY TERMS AND CONCEPTS	EXAMPLES

SECTION 4.7 (*continued*)

Riemann sums use rectangles drawn above each subinterval to approximate the area. With **left-rectangles**, the height of each rectangle is the value of $f(x)$ at the left endpoint of that subinterval. The sum of the areas of all n rectangles is L_n, where

$$L_n = \frac{b-a}{n}\cdot(f(a) + f(x_1) + f(x_2) + \cdots + f(x_{n-2}) + f(x_{n-1})).$$

With **right-rectangles**, the height of each rectangle is the value of $f(x)$ at the right endpoint of that subinterval. The sum of the areas of all n rectangles is R_n, where

$$R_n = \frac{b-a}{n}\cdot(f(x_1) + f(x_2) + \cdots + f(x_{n-2}) + f(x_{n-1}) + f(b)).$$

The average of L_n and R_n usually provides a better approximation of $\int_a^b f(x)\,dx$.

Let $\int_0^2 \sqrt{1+x^4}\,dx$, with $n = 4$. Divide $[0, 2]$ into four subintervals, $[0, 0.5]$, $[0.5, 1]$, $[1, 1.5]$, and $[1.5, 2]$. Each subinterval has a width $\Delta x = \frac{2-0}{4} = \frac{1}{2}$. Therefore,

$$\begin{aligned} L_4 &= \Delta x\cdot(f(0) + f(0.5) + f(1) + f(1.5)) \\ &= \frac{1}{2}\cdot(1 + 1.031 + 1.414 + 2.462) \\ &= 2.954, \end{aligned}$$

and

$$\begin{aligned} R_4 &= \Delta x\cdot(f(0.5) + f(1) + f(1.5) + f(2)) \\ &= \frac{1}{2}\cdot(1.031 + 1.414 + 2.462 + 4.123) \\ &= 4.515. \end{aligned}$$

The average of L_4 and R_4, $\frac{2.954 + 4.515}{2} = 3.735$, is an approximate value of $\int_0^2 \sqrt{1+x^4}\,dx$.

Midpoint Rule: Using rectangles, the height of each rectangle is the value of $f(x)$ at the midpoint of that subinterval. The sum of the areas of all n rectangles is M_n, where

$$M_n = \frac{b-a}{n}\cdot\left(f\left(\frac{a+x_1}{2}\right) + f\left(\frac{x_1+x_2}{2}\right) + f\left(\frac{x_2+x_3}{2}\right) + \cdots + f\left(\frac{x_{n-2}+x_{n-1}}{2}\right) + f\left(\frac{x_{n-1}+b}{2}\right)\right).$$

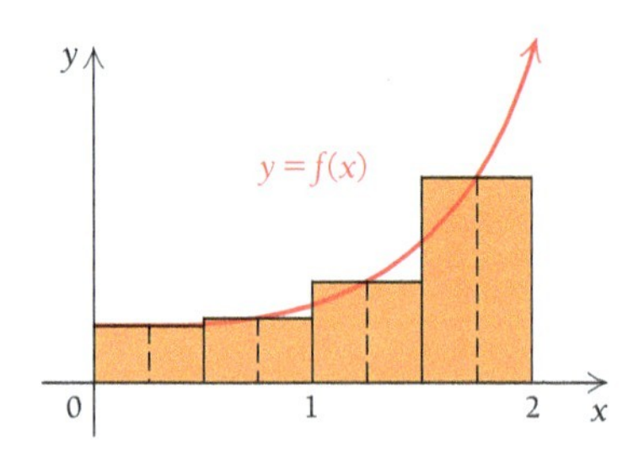

With $\int_0^2 \sqrt{1+x^4}\,dx$ and $n = 4$, we have

$$\begin{aligned} M_4 &= \tfrac{1}{2}\cdot(f(0.25) + f(0.75) + f(1.25) + f(1.75)) \\ &= \tfrac{1}{2}\cdot(1.002 + 1.147 + 1.855 + 3.222) \\ &= 3.613. \end{aligned}$$

Trapezoidal Rule: A trapezoid is drawn above each subinterval, and the definite integral is approximated by T_n, where

$$T_n = \frac{b-a}{n}\cdot\left(\frac{f(a)}{2} + f(x_1) + f(x_2) + \cdots + f(x_{n-1}) + \frac{f(b)}{2}\right).$$

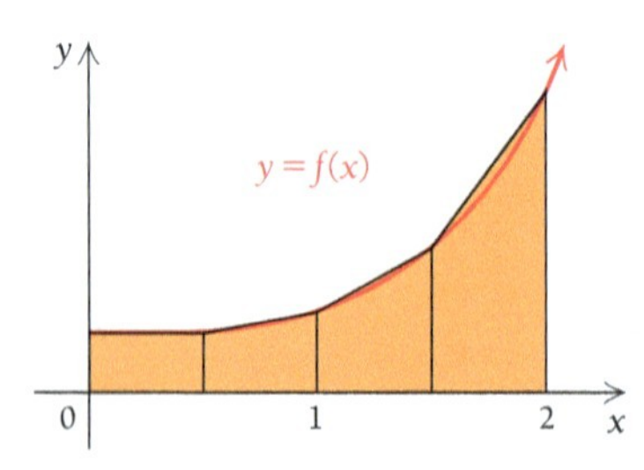

With $\int_0^2 \sqrt{1+x^4}\,dx$ and $n = 4$, we have

$$\begin{aligned} T_4 &= \frac{1}{2}\cdot\left(\frac{f(0)}{2} + f(0.5) + f(1) + f(1.5) + \frac{f(2)}{2}\right) \\ &= \frac{1}{2}\cdot\left(\frac{1}{2} + 1.031 + 1.414 + 2.462 + \frac{4.123}{2}\right) \\ &= 3.734. \end{aligned}$$

KEY TERMS AND CONCEPTS	EXAMPLES
SECTION 4.7 (continued)	
Simpson's Rule: The number of subintervals n is even, and $n/2$ parabolas are used to approximate the curve. The definite integral is approximated by S_n, where $S_n = \frac{b-a}{3n} \cdot (f(a) + 4f(x_1) + 2f(x_2) + 4f(x_3) + \cdots + 2f(x_{n-2}) + 4f(x_{n-1}) + f(b))$.	With $\int_0^2 \sqrt{1 + x^4}\, dx$ and $n = 4$, we have $S_4 = \frac{2-0}{3(4)} \cdot (f(0) + 4f(0.5) + 2f(1) + 4f(1.5) + f(2))$ $= \frac{1}{6} \cdot (1 + 4(1.031) + 2(1.414) + 4(2.462) + 4.123)$ $= 3.654$.

Chapter 4 Review Exercises

These review exercises are for test preparation. They can also be used as a practice test. Answers are at the back of the book. The red bracketed section references tell you what part(s) of the chapter to restudy if your answer is incorrect.

CONCEPT REINFORCEMENT

Classify each statement as either true or false.

1. Riemann sums are a way of approximating the area under a curve by using rectangles. [4.2]

2. If a and b are both negative, then $\int_a^b f(x)\, dx$ is negative. [4.3]

3. For any continuous function f defined over $[-1, 7]$, it follows that
$$\int_{-1}^{2} f(x)\, dx + \int_{2}^{7} f(x)\, dx = \int_{-1}^{7} f(x)\, dx. \quad [4.4]$$

4. Every integral can be evaluated using integration by parts. [4.6]

5. $\int x^2 e^x\, dx = \left(\frac{1}{3}x^3\right)e^x + C$ [4.1, 4.6]

For Exercises 6–11, match each integral in column A with the corresponding antiderivative in column B. [4.1, 4.5]

Column A	Column B
6. $\int \frac{1}{\sqrt{x}}\, dx$	a) $\ln x + C$
7. $\int (1 + 2x)^{-2}\, dx$	b) $-x^{-1} + C$
8. $\int \frac{1}{x}\, dx, \quad x > 0$	c) $-(1 + x^2)^{-1} + C$
9. $\int \frac{2x}{1 + x^2}\, dx$	d) $-\frac{1}{2}(1 + 2x)^{-1} + C$
10. $\int \frac{1}{x^2}\, dx$	e) $2x^{1/2} + C$
11. $\int \frac{2x}{(1 + x^2)^2}\, dx$	f) $\ln(1 + x^2) + C$

REVIEW EXERCISES

12. **Business: total cost.** The marginal cost, in dollars, of producing the xth car stereo is given by
$$C'(x) = 0.004x^2 - 2x + 500.$$

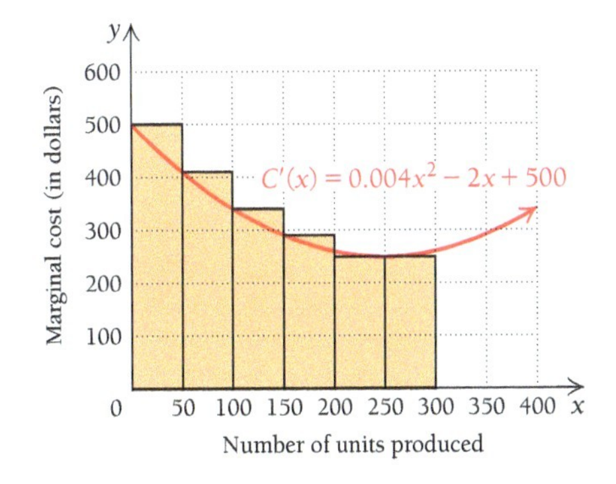

Approximate the total cost of producing 300 car stereos by computing the sum using left endpoints.
$$\sum_{i=1}^{6} C'(x_i)\, \Delta x, \quad \text{with } \Delta x = 50. \quad [4.2]$$

Find each antiderivative. [4.1]

13. $\int 20x^4\, dx$

14. $\int (3e^{4x} + 2)\, dx$

15. $\int \left(18t^2 + 6t + \frac{1}{2t}\right) dt \quad (\text{assume } t > 0)$

Find the area under each curve over the indicated interval. [4.3]

16. $y = 6 - x^2;\quad [-2, 1]$

17. $y = x^2 + 4x + 4;\quad [0, 3]$

In each case, give an interpretation of what the shaded region represents. [4.2, 4.3]

18.

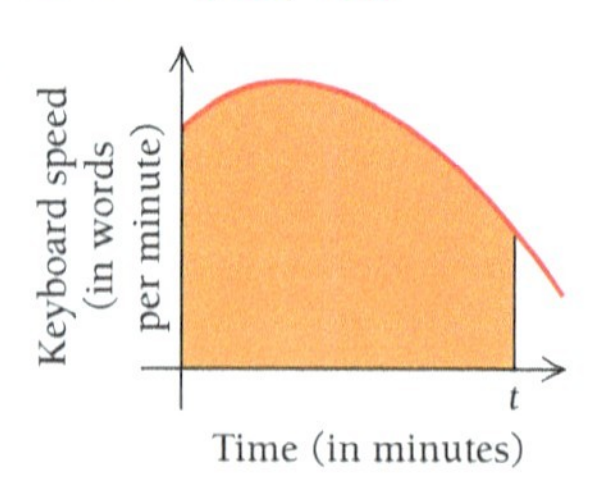

19.

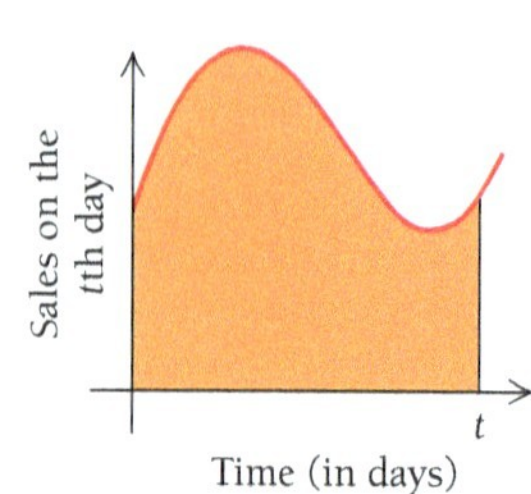

Evaluate. [4.3, 4.4]

20. $\int_2^4 g(x)\,dx$, for g as shown in the graph at right

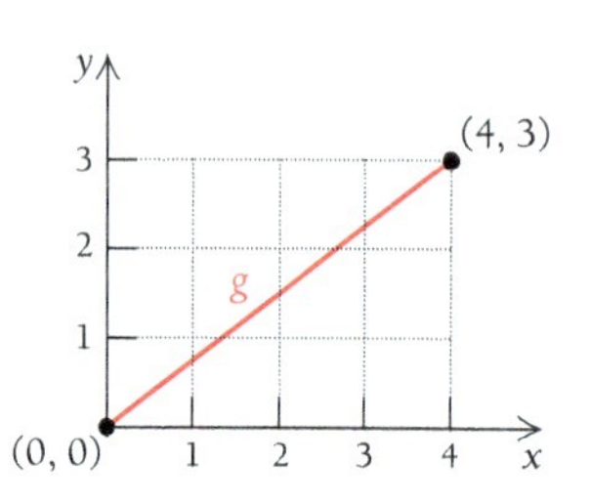

21. $\int_a^b x^5\,dx$

22. $\int_{-1}^{2} (x^3 - x^4)\,dx$

23. $\int_0^1 (e^{2x} + x)\,dx$

24. $\int_1^4 \frac{2}{x}\,dx$

25. $\int_{-2}^{4} f(x)\,dx$, where $f(x) = \begin{cases} x + 2, & \text{for } x \le 0, \\ 2 - \frac{1}{2}\sqrt{x}, & \text{for } x > 0 \end{cases}$

Decide whether $\int_a^b f(x)\,dx$ *is positive, negative, or zero.* [4.3]

26.

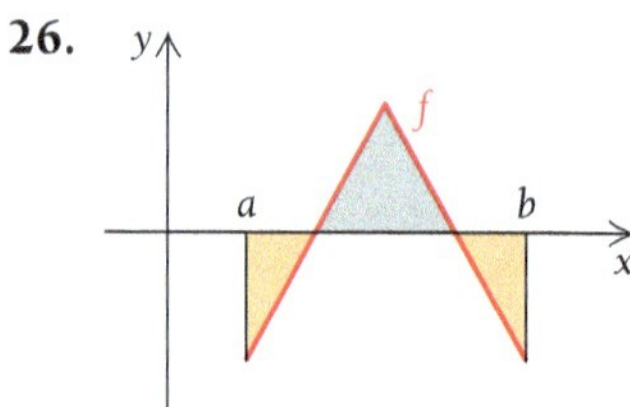

27.

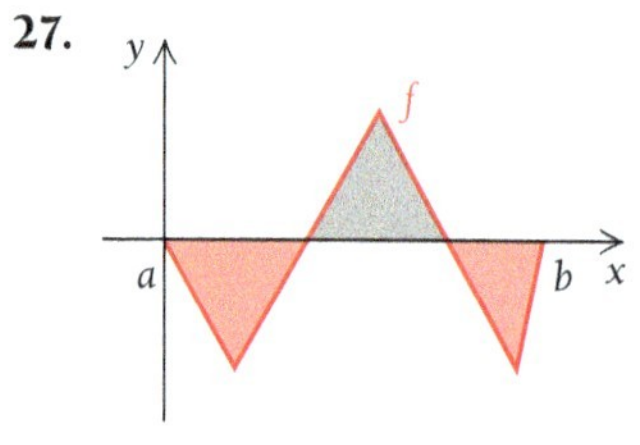

28.

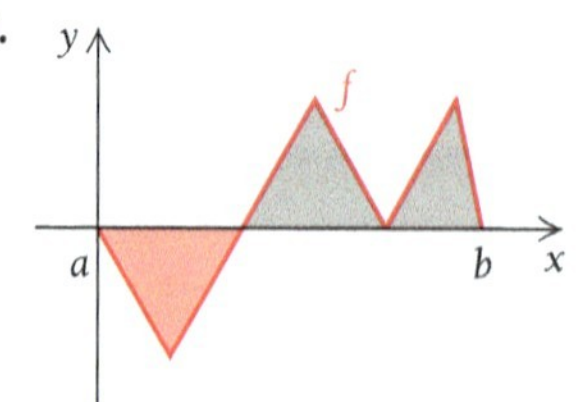

29. Find the area of the region bounded by

$$y = x^2 + 3x + 1 \text{ and } y = 6x - 1.\quad [4.4]$$

Evaluate, using substitution. [4.5]

30. $\int x^3 e^{x^4}\,dx$

31. $\int \frac{24t^5}{4t^6 + 3}\,dt$

32. $\int \frac{\ln(4x)}{2x}\,dx$

33. $\int \frac{e^{2x}}{e^{2x} + 2}\,dx$

Evaluate, using integration by parts. [4.6]

34. $\int 3xe^{4x}\,dx$

35. $\int \ln(4x + 9)\,dx$

36. $\int 5x^2 \ln x\,dx$

37. $\int x^4 e^{3x}\,dx$

38. Approximate the value of $\int_0^4 \sqrt{1 + e^x}\,dx$ by finding L_4, R_4, and their average. [4.7]

39. Approximate the value of $\int_1^5 \frac{1}{1 + x^3}\,dx$ by finding M_4. [4.7]

40. Approximate the value of $\int_{-1}^{2} \ln(1 + x^2)\,dx$ by finding T_6. [4.7]

41. Approximate the value of $\int_0^2 x\sqrt{1 + x^2}\,dx$ by finding S_4. [4.7]

42. A painter measures the height of an irregularly shaped wall that is 35 ft long. The height of the wall, measured every 5 ft along its base, is given in the following table. Find the approximate surface area of the wall. [4.7]

Distance along Base of Wall (in feet)	0	5	10	15	20	25	30	35
Height (in feet)	9.5	12.5	14	15.5	14	12.5	9.5	8.5

43. Business: total cost. Refer to Exercise 12. Calculate the total cost of producing 300 car stereos. [4.4]

44. Find the average value of $y = xe^{-x}$ over $[0, 2]$. [4.4]

45. A particle's velocity, $v(t)$, in miles per hour after t hours is given by $v(t) = 3t^2 + 2t$. Find the distance the particle travels during the first 4 hr (from $t = 0$ to $t = 4$). [4.3]

46. Business: total revenue. A company estimates that its revenue grows continuously at a rate given by $S'(t) = 3e^{3t}$, where t is the number of days since an innovation is introduced. Find the accumulated revenue for the first 4 days. [4.3]

Evaluate, using any method. [4.3–4.6]

47. $\int \frac{12t^2}{4t^3 + 7}\,dt$

48. $\int \frac{x\,dx}{\sqrt{4 + 5x}}$

49. $\int 5x^4 e^{x^5}\,dx$

50. $\int \frac{x}{x + 9}\,dx$

51. $\int t^7 (t^8 + 3)^{11}\,dt$

52. $\int \ln|7x|\,dx$

53. $\int x \ln|8x|\,dx$

SYNTHESIS

Find each antiderivative. [4.5, 4.6]

54. $\int \frac{t^4 \ln(t^5 + 3)}{t^5 + 3} dt$

55. $\int \frac{dx}{e^x + 2}$

56. $\int \frac{\ln \sqrt{x}}{x} dx$

57. $\int x^{91} \ln |x| dx$

58. $\int \ln \left| \frac{x - 3}{x - 4} \right| dx$

59. $\int \frac{dx}{x(\ln |x|)^4}$

60. $\int x \sqrt[3]{x + 3}\, dx$

61. $\int \frac{x^2}{2x + 1} dx$

Technology Connection

62. Use a graphing calculator to approximate the area between the following curves:

$$y = 2x^2 - 2x, \quad y = 12x^2 - 12x^3. \quad [4.4]$$

Chapter 4 Test

1. Approximate
$$\int_0^5 (25 - x^2)\, dx$$
by computing the area of each rectangle and adding.

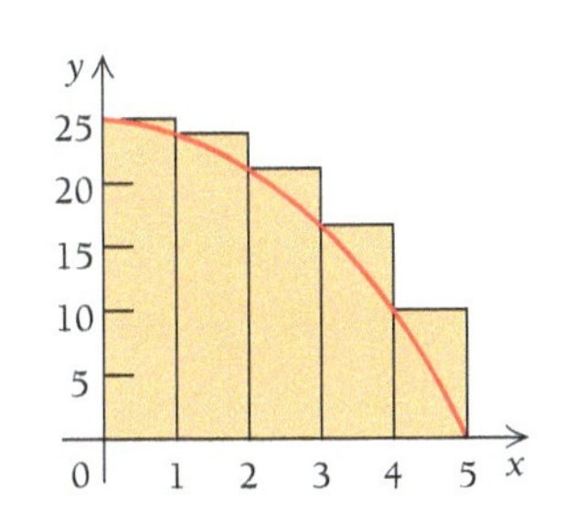

Evaluate.

2. $\int \sqrt{3x}\, dx$

3. $\int 300x^5\, dx$

4. $\int \left(e^{5x} + \frac{1}{x} + x^{3/8}\right) dx$ (assume $x > 0$)

Find the area under the graph of each equation over the indicated interval.

5. $y = x - x^2$; $[0, 1]$

6. $y = \frac{4}{x}$; $[1, 3]$

7. What does the area of the shaded region represent?

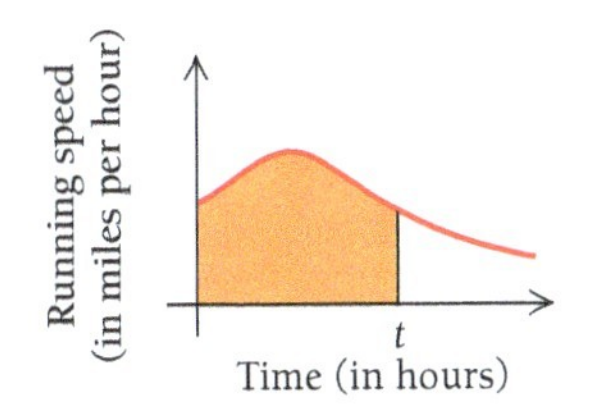

Evaluate.

8. $\int_{-1}^{2} (4x + 5x^2)\, dx$

9. $\int_0^1 e^{-2x}\, dx$

10. $\int_{e^3}^{e^5} \frac{dx}{x}$

11. $\int_0^5 g(x)\, dx$, where $g(x) = \begin{cases} x^2, & \text{for } x \leq 2, \\ 6 - x, & \text{for } x > 2 \end{cases}$

12. Find $\int_3^7 f(x)\, dx$, for f as shown in the graph.

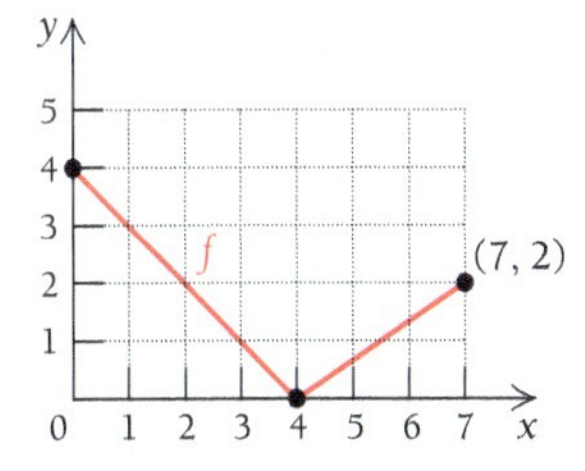

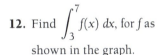

13. State whether $\int_a^b f(x)\, dx$ is positive, negative, or zero.

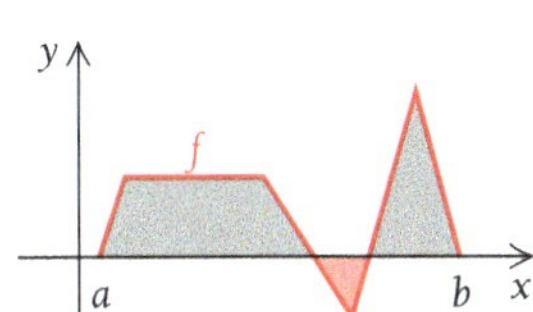

Find each antiderivative using substitution. Assume $u > 0$ if $\ln u$ appears.

14. $\int \frac{dx}{3x + 12}$

15. $\int e^{-0.5x}\, dx$

16. $\int t^3(t^4 + 3)^7\, dt$

Find each antiderivative using integration by parts.

17. $\int xe^{5x}\, dx$

18. $\int x^3 \ln x^4\, dx$

19. Estimate the value of $\int_2^5 \ln(x^2 - 1)\, dx$ by finding T_6.

20. Estimate the value of $\int_1^6 \frac{1}{\sqrt{7 - x}}\, dx$ by finding L_5, R_5, and their average.

21. **Total distance.** Eduardo runs for 10 min. His FitBit tracks his speed, $v(t)$, in miles per hour, over 1-min intervals. Use left- and right-rectangles and their average to approximate the total distance Eduardo runs. (*Hint:* 1 min $= \frac{1}{60}$ hr.)

1-min Intervals, t	1	2	3	4	5	6	7	8	9	10
Speed, $v(t)$, in mi/hr	9	10	10	8	8	7	6	6	5	3

22. Business: resodding a green. The following diagram shows the widths (in feet) of a golf green, measured at 5-ft intervals. If sod costs \$4.25 per square foot, find the approximate cost of resodding this green.

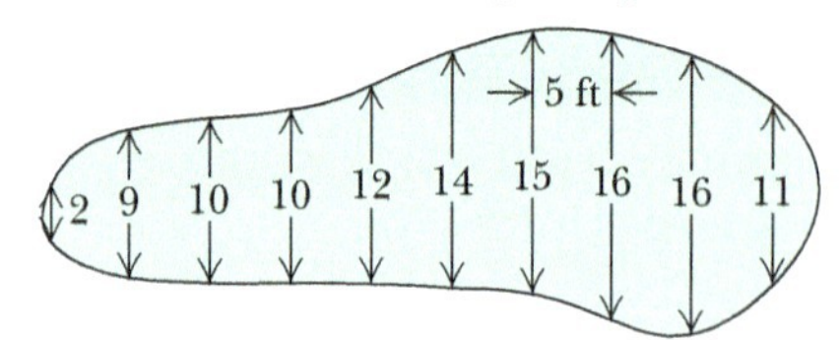

23. Find the average value of $y = 4t^3 + 2t$ over $[-1, 2]$.

24. Find the area of the region in the first quadrant bounded by $y = x$ and $y = x^6$.

25. Business: cost from marginal cost. An air conditioning company determines that the marginal cost, in dollars, for producing the xth air conditioner is given by

$$C'(x) = -0.2x + 500, \quad C(0) = 0.$$

Find the total cost of producing 250 air conditioners.

26. Social science: learning curve. A translator's speed over a 4-min interval is given by

$$W(t) = -6t^2 + 12t + 90, \quad t \text{ in } [0, 4],$$

where $W(t)$ is in words per minute, after t minutes. How many words are translated during the second minute (from $t = 1$ to $t = 2$)?

27. A drone has a velocity given by $v(t) = -0.4t^2 + 2t$, where $v(t)$ is in kilometers per hour and t is the number of hours since the drone took off. Find the total distance traveled during the first 4 hr.

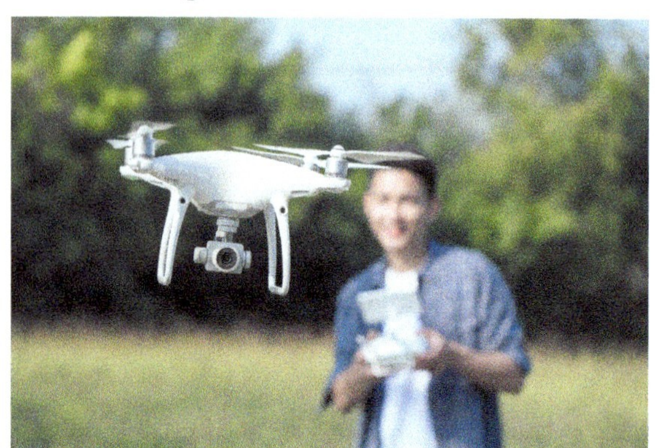

Evaluate each integral. Assume $u > 0$ if $\ln u$ appears.

28. $\int x^5 e^{x^6}\, dx$

29. $\int_4^9 \sqrt{x} \ln x\, dx$

30. $\int e^{3x}\sqrt{1 + e^{3x}}\, dx$

31. $\int_0^2 x^4 e^{-0.1x}\, dx$

32. $\int x \ln(13x)\, dx$

33. $\int \frac{x}{(x + 1)^2}\, dx$ (*Hint*: Let $u = x + 1$.)

34. $\int_{\ln 2}^{\ln 3} e^{2x}(e^{2x} + 1)^3\, dx$

35. $\int 12 \cdot 5^{x/4}\, dx$

36. Area as distance. Danah and Cameron start walking at the same time. Danah's velocity, t hours after starting, is given by $v_1(t) = \frac{1}{4}t$, where v_1 is in miles per hour. Cameron's velocity, t hours after starting, is given by $v_2(t) = \frac{1}{20}t^2$.

a) When Danah and Cameron are walking at the same velocity, who is ahead and by how far?

b) Find the time $T > 0$ at which Danah and Cameron are walking side by side and the distance both have walked at that time.

SYNTHESIS

37. The graphs of $f(x) = x^2$ and $g(x) = 2^x$ intersect three times at $x = a$, b, and c, where $a < b < c$.

a) Find a, b, and c.

b) Find the area enclosed by f and g over the interval $[a, b]$.

c) Find the area enclosed by f and g over the interval $[b, c]$.

d) Explain why $\int_a^c [g(x) - f(x)]\, dx$ is not equal to the sum of the areas found in parts (b) and (c).

38. Let $f(t) = \int_0^t 3x\, dx$.

a) Find $f(0)$, $f(1)$, $f(2)$, and $f(3)$.

b) Find $f'(t)$.

EXTENDED TECHNOLOGY APPLICATION 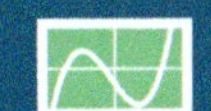

Business and Economics: Distribution of Wealth

Lorenz Functions and the Gini Coefficient

The distribution of wealth within a population is of great interest to many economists and sociologists. Let $y = f(x)$ represent the percentage of wealth owned by x percent of the population, with x and y expressed as decimals between 0 and 1. The assumptions are that 0% of the population owns 0% of the wealth and that 100% of the population owns 100% of the wealth. Given these requirements, the *Lorenz function* is defined to be any continuous, increasing, and concave upward function connecting the points (0, 0) and (1, 1). The function is named for economist Max Otto Lorenz (1880–1962), who developed these concepts as a graduate student in 1905–1906.

If the collective wealth of a society is equitably distributed among its population, we say that "x% of the population owns x% of the wealth," and this is modeled by the function $f(x) = x$, where $0 \leq x \leq 1$. This is called the *line of equality*.

In many societies, the distribution of wealth is not equitable. For example, the Lorenz function $f(x) = x^3$ represents a society in which a large percentage of the population owns a small percentage of the wealth. In this example, $f(0.7) = 0.7^3 = 0.343$, meaning that 70% of the population owns just 34.3% of the wealth, and the other 30% owns the remaining 65.7% of the wealth.

In the graphs below, we see the line of equality in the left-most graph, and increasingly inequitable distributions of wealth as we move to the right. Note that the area between the line of equality and the graph of the Lorenz function $f(x)$ is small if the distribution of wealth is close to equitable and is large when the distribution is very unequitable. The *Gini coefficient* (named for the Italian statistician and demographer Corrado Gini, 1884–1965) is a measure of the difference between the actual distribution of wealth in a society and the ideal distribution represented by the line of equality. It is the ratio of the area between the line of equality and the graph of the Lorenz function to the area below the line of equality and above the x-axis, as shown below:

$$\text{Gini coefficient} = \frac{A}{A + B}.$$

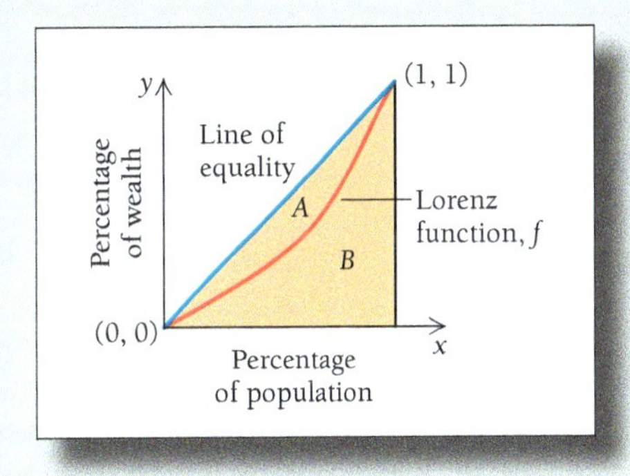

The area A is found by calculating the area between the graphs of $y = x$ and $y = f(x)$. We observe that $A + B$ is a triangle with area $\frac{1}{2}(1)(1) = \frac{1}{2}$. Thus,

$$\text{Gini coefficient} = \frac{A}{A + B} = \frac{\int_0^1 (x - f(x))\,dx}{\left(\frac{1}{2}\right)}$$

$$= 2\int_0^1 (x - f(x))\,dx.$$

For the most equitable distribution of wealth, the Gini coefficient is 0, since there will be no difference (area) between the graph of the Lorenz function and the line of equality; for the most inequitable distribution of wealth, the Gini coefficient is 1. Often, the Gini coefficient is multiplied by 100 to give the *Gini index*: a Gini coefficient of 0.34 gives a Gini index of 34.

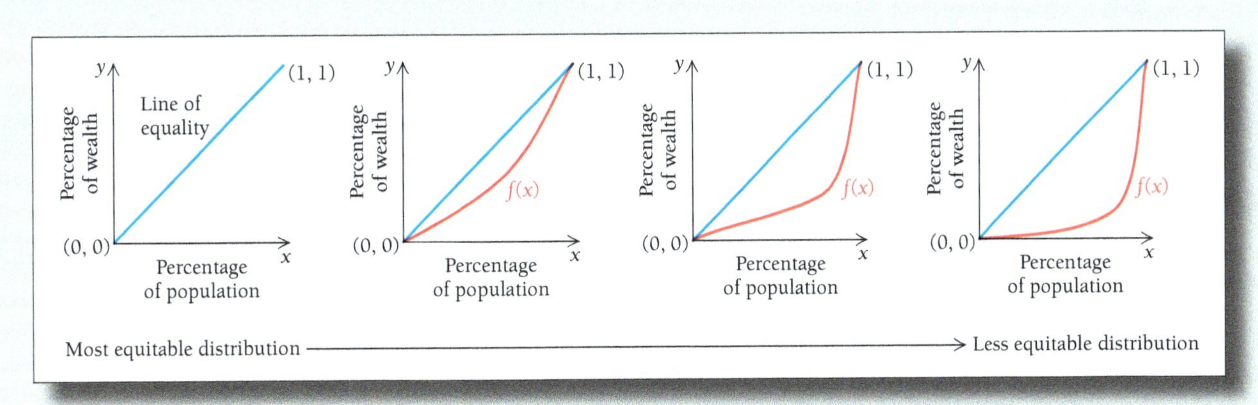

Exercises

1. Suppose the Lorenz function for a society is given by $f(x) = x^2, 0 \leq x \leq 1$.
   a) What percentage of the wealth is owned by 60% of the population?
   b) Calculate the Gini index.

2. Suppose the Lorenz function for a society is given by $f(x) = x^{3.5}, 0 \leq x \leq 1$.
   a) What percentage of the wealth is owned by 60% of the population?
   b) Calculate the Gini index.

Regression for Determining Lorenz Functions

If data exist on the distribution of wealth in a society, a Lorenz function can be determined using regression.

Exercises

3. The data in the table show the distribution of wealth, y, within a population, where x is the percentage (expressed as a decimal) of the population that owns that amount of the wealth.

x	0.1	0.2	0.3	0.4	0.5	0.6	0.7	0.8	0.9	1.0
y	0.0178	0.06	0.122	0.201	0.297	0.409	0.536	0.677	0.833	1.0

Use regression to determine a power function that best fits these data. [*Note:* Entering the point (0, 0) may cause an error message to appear.]
   a) Express the Lorenz function in the form $f(x) = x^n$. The coefficient should be 1, so you may have to do some rounding.
   b) Determine the Gini coefficient and the Gini index.
   c) What percentage of the wealth is owned by the lowest 74% of this population?

4. A fast-food chain has many hundreds of franchises nationwide. Ideally, all franchises would generate equal amounts of revenue, but in reality, some generate more than others. An internal audit reveals the following results: the lowest 30% of the franchises account for just 6% of the total revenue, the lowest 50% account for 20% of the total revenue, and the lowest 70% account for 43.5% of the total revenue. (Assume that 100% of the franchises account for 100% of the total revenue.)
   a) Use regression to determine a power function that models these data, and write the Lorenz function in the form $f(x) = x^n$. The coefficient should be 1, so you may have to do some rounding.
   b) Determine the Gini coefficient and the Gini index.
   c) What percentage of total revenue is generated by the lowest 45% of the franchises?
   d) What percentage of total revenue is generated by the top 10% of the franchises?

Gini Coefficient as a Function of n

Functions of the form $f(x) = x^n, 0 \le x \le 1$, where $n \ge 1$, meet the criteria for Lorenz functions. We can develop a function $G(n)$ that allows us to calculate the Gini coefficient directly, given a value of n.

$$\begin{aligned} G(n) &= 2\int_0^1 (x - x^n)\,dx \\ &= \left[2\left(\frac{1}{2}x^2 - \frac{1}{n+1}x^{n+1}\right)\right]_0^1 \\ &= 2\left(\frac{1}{2} - \frac{1}{n+1}\right) \\ &= 1 - \frac{2}{n+1} \\ &= \frac{n-1}{n+1}. \end{aligned}$$

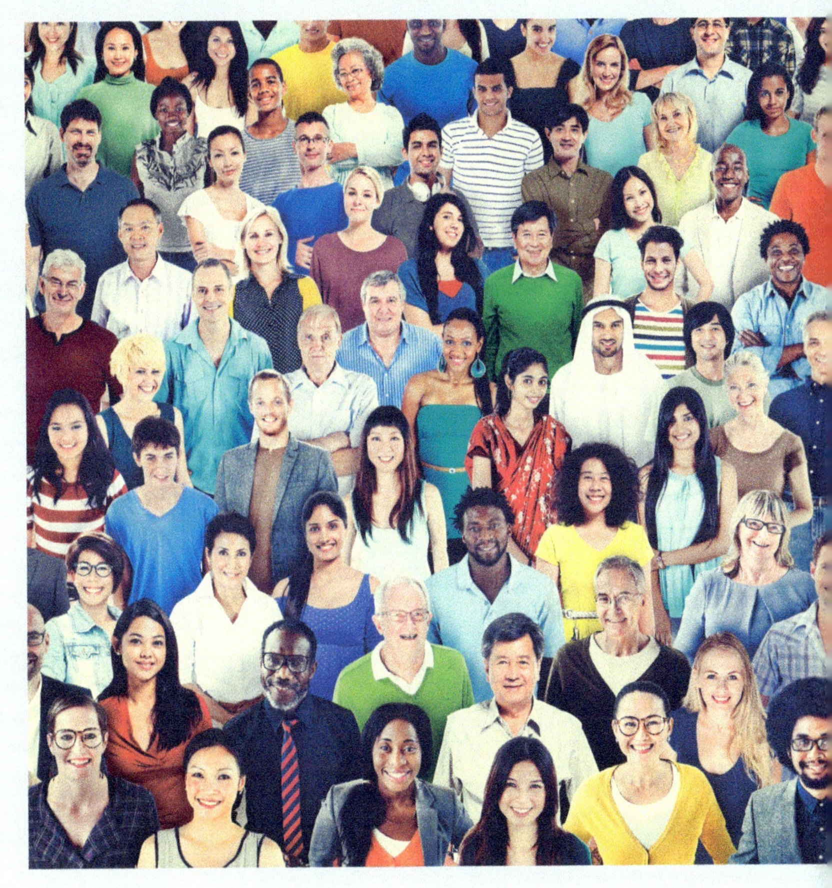

Exercises

5. Verify your results for Exercises 3 and 4 using $G(n) = \dfrac{n-1}{n+1}$.

6. The United States had a Gini index of 46.9, or as a decimal, 0.469, in 2013. (*Source*: www.census.gov.)

a) Solve for n, and write the Lorenz function in the form $f(x) = x^n$.

b) According to this model, what percentage of the wealth was owned by the least wealthy 55% of U.S. citizens in 2013?

7. Canada's Gini index is usually 30.0.

a) Determine the Lorenz function.

b) What percentage of wealth is owned by the least wealthy 55% of the citizens in Canada?

Sometimes, data may not fit "neatly" into the form $f(x) = x^n$, especially when a small percentage of the population holds most of the wealth. In these cases, an exponential function of the form $f(x) = a \cdot b^x, 0 \le x \le 1$ may work better than $f(x) = x^n$, as long as the value of a is extremely small.

8. In 2016, the distribution of net total worth within the United States was as given in the following table:

Percentage of Population	0.2	0.4	0.6	0.8	0.9	0.95	0.99	1.0
Percentage of Total Net Worth Held	0.002	0.005	0.029	0.082	0.193	0.314	0.585	1.0

(*Source*: Data prepared by Dr. E. N. Wolff, National Bureau of Economic Research, Nov. 2017.)

a) According to the table, what percentage of net worth was held by the top 1%?

b) Use regression to fit an exponential function $g(x) = a \cdot b^x$ to these data.

c) Determine the area between the line of equality and the graph of g over $[0, 1]$.

d) Determine the Gini coefficient and the Gini index.

e) Use the model from part (b) to find the percentage of total net worth held by the bottom 90% of the population, and compare your result to the value in the table. Why might the two values differ? What other regression models might be appropriate for this data?

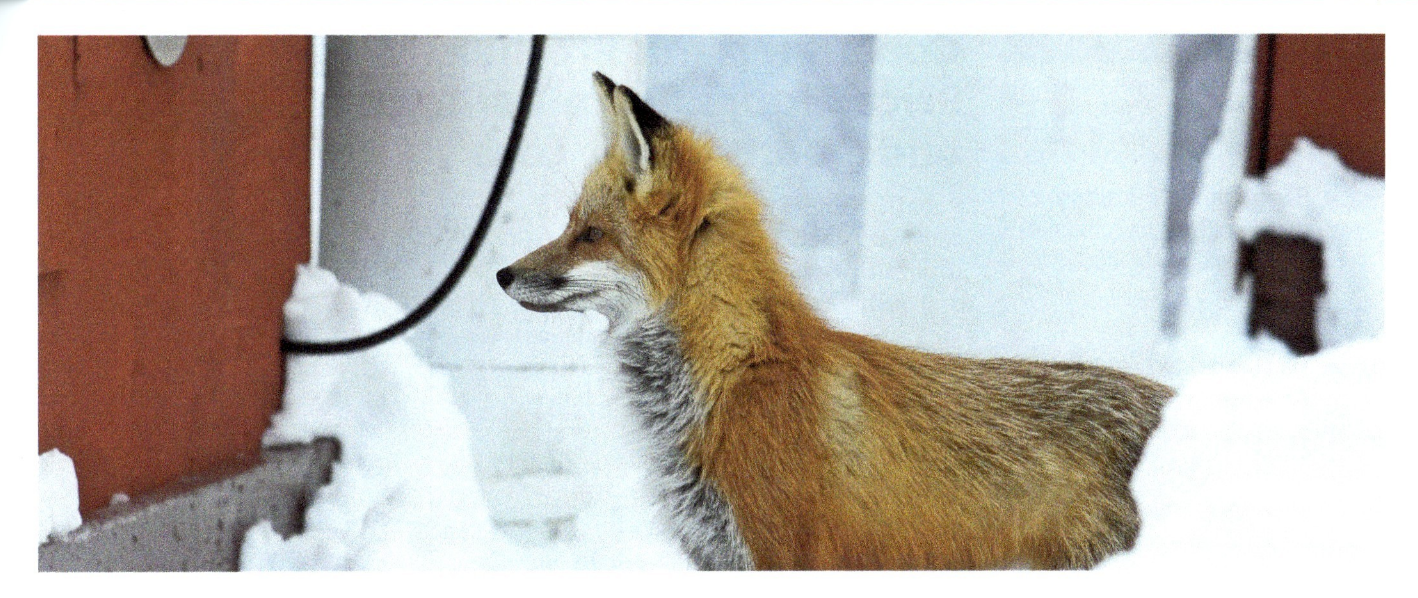

5 Applications of Integration

What You'll Learn

Why It's Important

In this chapter, we explore a variety of applications of integration in business and economics (consumer and producer surplus, deadweight loss, and income streams) and environmental science and finance (exponential growth and decay and expected value). We also consider how integration is used in constructing probability distributions, in finding the volumes of certain solids, and in solving differential equations.

Where It's Used

Price Ceiling: In a small isolated mountain town, demand for propane is given by $D(x) = 6.50 - 0.25x$, and supply is given by $S(x) = 2.10 + 0.15x$, where x is in gallons per month per customer and $D(x)$ and $S(x)$ are in dollars per gallon. Assume that a price ceiling of \$3 per gallon is imposed. Find the producer surplus, the consumer surplus, and the deadweight loss.

(This problem appears as Example 4 in Section 5.1.)

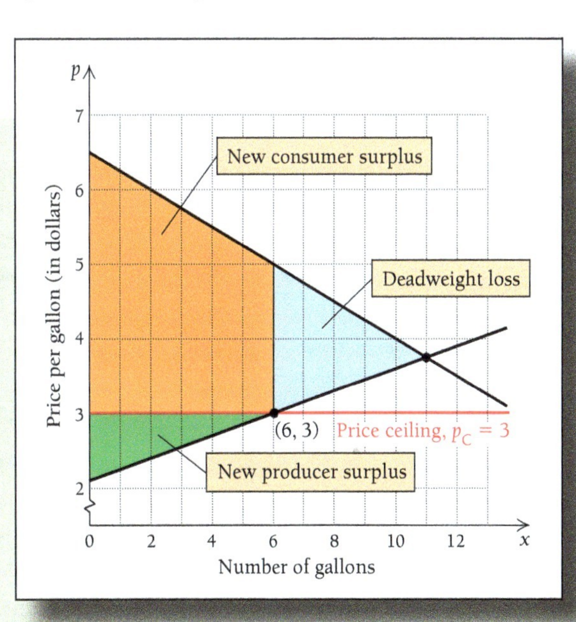

5.1 Consumer and Producer Surplus; Price Floors, Price Ceilings, and Deadweight Loss

- Given demand and supply functions, find the consumer surplus and the producer surplus at the equilibrium point.
- Find the deadweight loss for consumers and producers when a price ceiling or price floor is imposed.

Recall from Section R.5 that a consumer's **demand curve** is the graph of $p = D(x)$, which is the price per unit, p, that a consumer is willing to pay for x units of a product. It is usually a decreasing function since the consumer expects to pay less per unit for large quantities of the product. Also recall that a producer's **supply curve** is the graph of $p = S(x)$, which is the price per unit, p, that a producer is willing to accept for selling x units. It is usually an increasing function since a higher price per unit is an incentive for the producer to make more units available for sale. The *equilibrium point*, (x_E, p_E), is the intersection of these two curves.

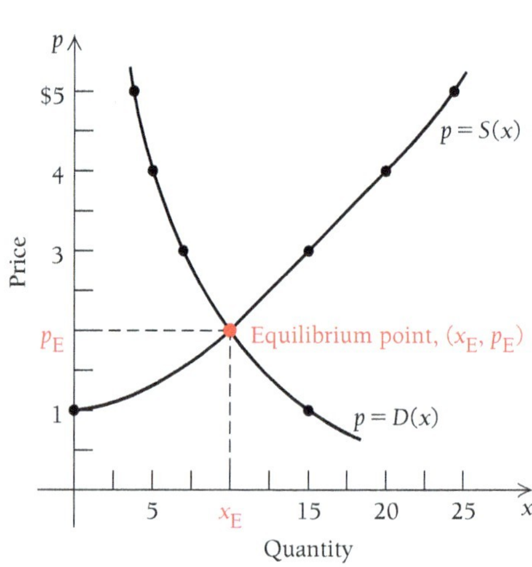

Consumer Surplus

Suppose that, at a price of \$10 per ticket, Louise will see no movies. At a price of \$8.75 per ticket, she will see one movie per month, and at \$7.50 per ticket, she will see two movies per month. As long as the number of movies, x, is small, Louise's demand function for movies can be modeled by $p = D(x) = 10 - 1.25x$.

At a ticket price of \$8.75, Louise sees one movie. Her total expenditure is (1)(\$8.75) = \$8.75, as shown by the blue rectangle in Fig. 1. However, the area under her demand curve over [0, 1] is \$9.38 (which the student can confirm). This is what going to one movie per month is worth to Louise. When she spends \$8.75, the difference in area, represented by the orange triangle, \$9.38 − \$8.75 = \$0.63, can be interpreted as the *consumer surplus*. It is the difference between what consumers are *willing* to pay, as determined by the area below their demand curve, and what they *actually* pay.

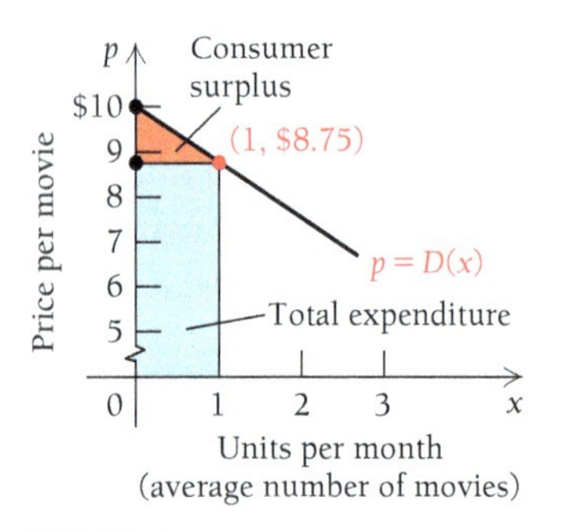

FIGURE 1

Now suppose that Louise goes to two movies per month at \$7.50 per ticket. Her total expenditure is (2)(\$7.50) = \$15.00, which is represented by the blue rectangle in Fig. 2. The area under Louise's demand curve over [0, 2] is \$17.50. Although Louise would be willing to spend \$17.50 to see two movies, she actually pays only \$15.00. Her consumer surplus is \$2.50.

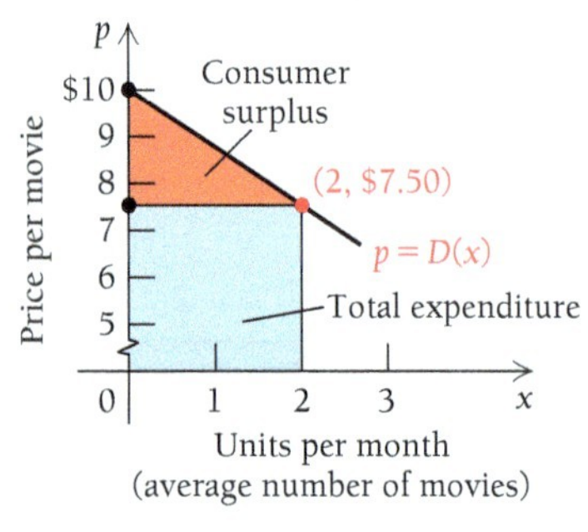

FIGURE 2

Generalizing, if the graph of a demand function is a curve, as shown below, and a consumer purchases Q items at P dollars per item, then the total expenditure is QP. The area under the curve over $[0, Q]$ is the total amount a consumer would be willing to pay for Q items:

$$\int_0^Q D(x)\,dx.$$

The *consumer surplus* is the difference between the area under the curve and the total expenditure, and it is given by

$$\int_0^Q D(x)\,dx - QP.$$

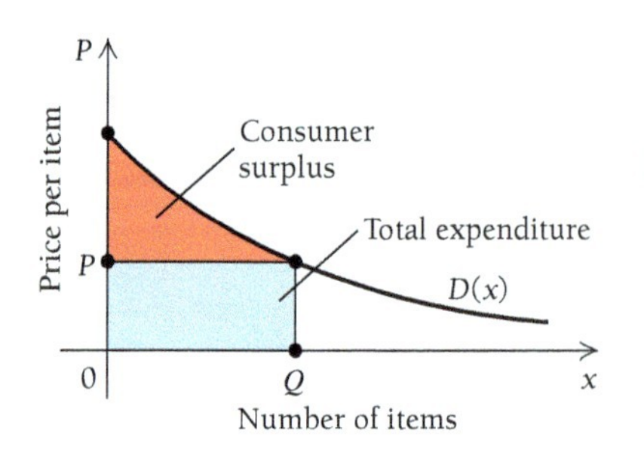

DEFINITION

Let $p = D(x)$ describe the demand function for a product. Then the **consumer surplus** for Q units of the product, at price P per unit, is

$$\int_0^Q D(x)\,dx - QP.$$

EXAMPLE 1 **Business: Consumer Surplus.** Arnold is shopping for high-quality sketchpads for his art class. His demand function is given by $p = D(x) = (x - 6)^2$. Find Arnold's consumer surplus if he purchases 2 sketchpads.

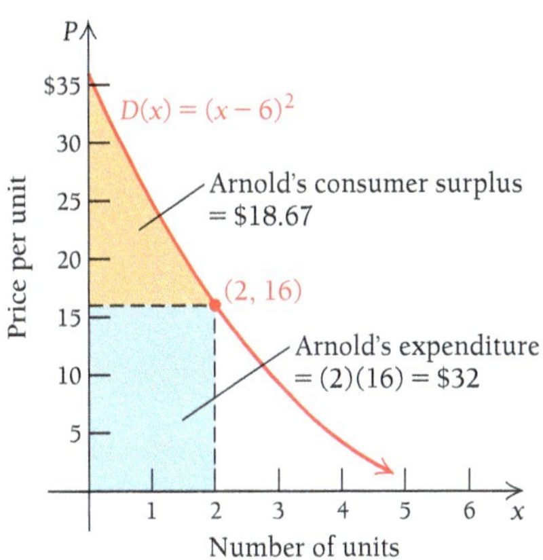

Solution At $x = 2$, Arnold pays

$$p = D(2) = (2 - 6)^2 = (-4)^2 = 16,$$

or \$16 per sketchpad.

If he purchases 2 sketchpads at \$16 per unit, Arnold's consumer surplus is

$$\begin{aligned}
\int_0^2 (x-6)^2\,dx - 2\cdot 16 &= \int_0^2 (x^2 - 12x + 36)\,dx - 32 \\
&= \left[\frac{x^3}{3} - 6x^2 + 36x\right]_0^2 - 32 \\
&= \left[\left(\frac{(2)^3}{3} - 6(2)^2 + 36(2)\right) - \left(\frac{(0)^3}{3} - 6(0)^2 + 36(0)\right)\right] - 32 \\
&= \left(\frac{8}{3} - 24 + 72\right) - 0 - 32 \\
&= \$18.67.
\end{aligned}$$

Quick Check 1 ✓

Find the consumer surplus for the demand function given by $D(x) = x^2 - 6x + 16$ when $x = 1$.

1 ✓

Producer Surplus

Let's now look at a supply curve for a movie theater, as shown in Figs. 3 and 4. Suppose the theater will not sell tickets to a movie for less than \$4 each, but will sell one ticket for \$5.75 or two tickets for \$7.50. For small numbers of movies, x, the theater's supply curve is modeled by $p = 4 + 1.75x$. The price \$5.75 is within what Louise is willing to pay for one movie, and the theater will take in (1)(\$5.75) = \$5.75 for selling her one ticket for one movie. The yellow area in Fig. 3 represents the minimum the theater wants to receive for one ticket for a movie, which is \$4.88. Since the theater's revenue is \$5.75 for selling one ticket, the difference, \$5.75 − \$4.88 = \$0.87, represents a bonus for the theater. Economists call this the *producer surplus.*

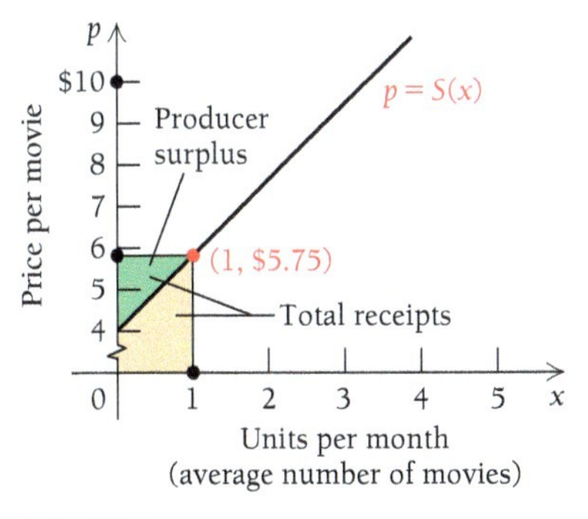

FIGURE 3

At a price of \$7.50, the theater will sell Louise two tickets and collect (2)(\$7.50), or \$15, in revenue. The yellow area in Fig. 4 represents what the theater needs to charge Louise (this may be close to its "cost") for two tickets, which is \$11.50. The area of the green triangle, \$15.00 − \$11.50 = \$3.50, is the producer surplus. It is part of the theater's profit.

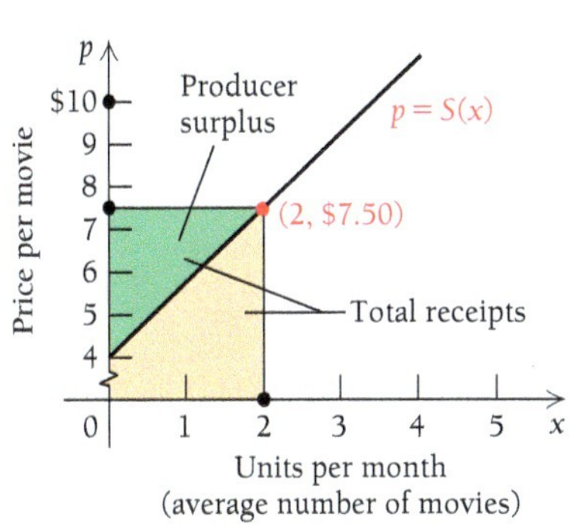

FIGURE 4

Generalizing, if the graph of a supply function is a curve, as shown at the right, and a producer sells Q items at P dollars per item, the total receipts are QP. The *producer surplus* is the total receipts minus the area under the curve:

$$QP - \int_0^Q S(x)\,dx.$$

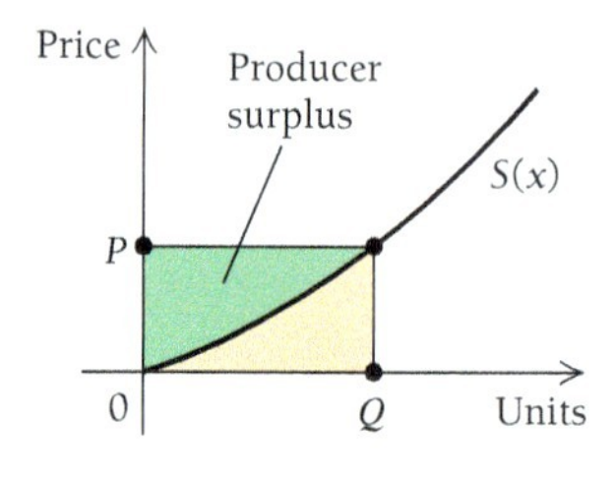

DEFINITION

Let $p = S(x)$ be a supply function for a product. Then the **producer surplus** for Q units of the product, at price P per unit, is

$$QP - \int_0^Q S(x)\,dx.$$

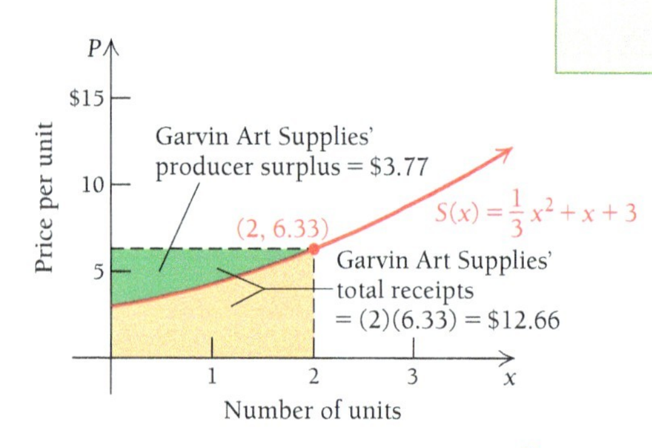

EXAMPLE 2 **Business: Producer Surplus.** Garvin Art Supplies sells artist's sketchpads, and its supply function for this product is given by $p = S(x) = \frac{1}{3}x^2 + x + 3$. Find the producer surplus when Garvin Art Supplies sells 2 sketchpads.

Solution At $x = 2$, Garvin receives $p = S(2) = \frac{1}{3}(2)^2 + (2) + 3 = 6.33$, or \$6.33 per sketchpad.

If Garvin sells 2 sketchpads at \$6.33 per unit, its producer surplus is

$$2 \cdot 6.33 - \int_0^2 \left(\frac{1}{3}x^2 + x + 3\right) dx = 12.66 - \left[\frac{x^3}{9} + \frac{x^2}{2} + 3x\right]_0^2$$

$$= 12.66 - \left[\left(\frac{(2)^3}{9} + \frac{(2)^2}{2} + 3(2)\right) - \left(\frac{(0)^3}{9} + \frac{(0)^2}{2} + 3(0)\right)\right]$$

$$= 12.66 - \left(\frac{8}{9} + 2 + 6 - 0\right)$$

$$= \$3.77.$$

2 ✓

Quick Check 2 ✓

Find the producer surplus for $S(x) = \frac{1}{3}x^2 + \frac{4}{3}x + 4$ when $x = 1$.

Equilibrium Point

The **equilibrium point**, (x_E, p_E), in Fig. 5 is the point at which the supply and demand curves intersect. It is the ideal point at which buyers and sellers come together and purchases and sales actually occur.

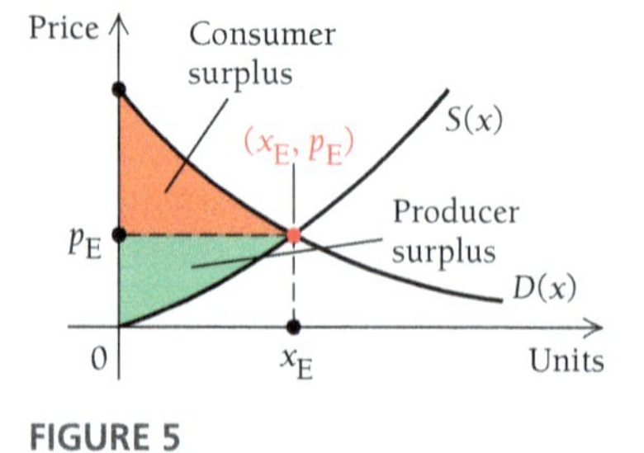

FIGURE 5

In the example involving Louise and the movie theater, suppose that the theater charges \$5.75 for one ticket, and Louise sees one movie. Since seeing one movie is worth \$9.38 to Louise, the difference, \$9.38 − \$5.75 = \$3.63, is her consumer surplus. To her, this is a good deal, since she paid less than she was willing to pay. However, the theater lost potential revenue by "undercharging" her.

As Fig. 6 shows, at \$7.50 per ticket, Louise's demand curve and the theater's supply curve intersect. This point is advantageous for both Louise and the theater, since she is willing to see two movies at \$7.50 per ticket, while the theater can increase its revenue by selling two tickets.

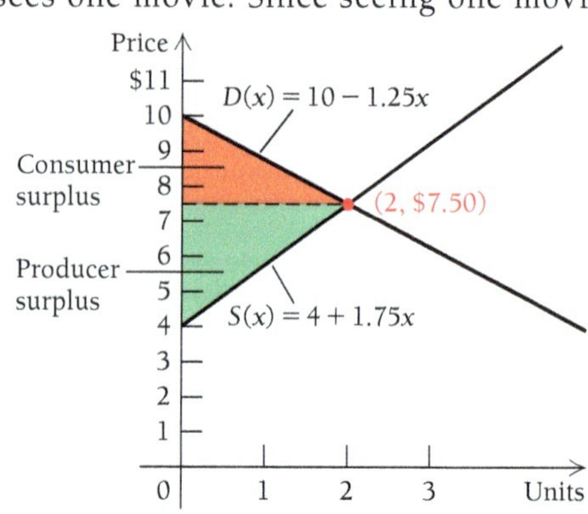

FIGURE 6

In other words, if the price per ticket is set too low, the theater will sell tickets but will lose revenue it could be receiving at a higher price, since Louise is willing to pay more according to her demand curve. On the other extreme, if the theater sets the price per ticket too high, it will sell fewer tickets and receive less revenue. The \$7.50 ticket price is the best "middle ground" for both producer and consumer in this case.

EXAMPLE 3 **Business: Equilibrium Point.** Given Arnold's demand function, $D(x) = (x - 6)^2$, and Garvin Art Supplies' supply function, $S(x) = \frac{1}{3}x^2 + x + 3$, find the equilibrium point, and explain what it represents. Assume $x \leq 5$.

Solution To find the equilibrium point, we set $D(x) = S(x)$ and solve:

$$
\begin{aligned}
(x-6)^2 &= \frac{1}{3}x^2 + x + 3 \\
3(x-6)^2 &= x^2 + 3x + 9 \qquad \text{Multiplying both sides by 3} \\
3(x^2 - 12x + 36) &= x^2 + 3x + 9 \\
3x^2 - 36x + 108 &= x^2 + 3x + 9 \\
2x^2 - 39x + 99 &= 0.
\end{aligned}
$$

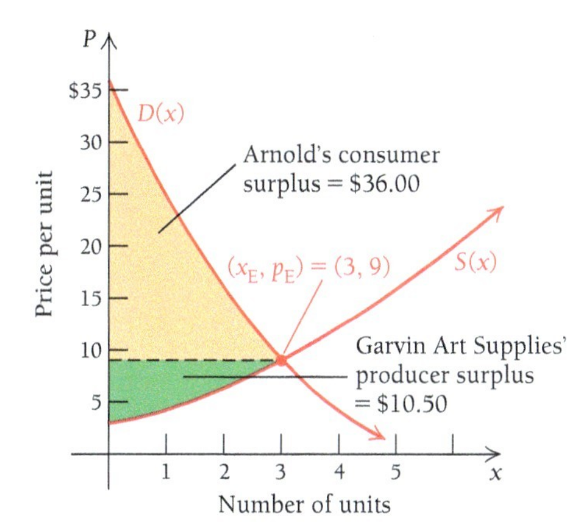

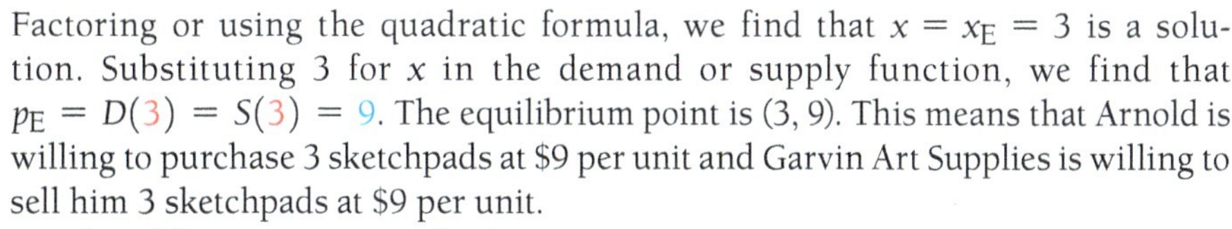

Factoring or using the quadratic formula, we find that $x = x_E = 3$ is a solution. Substituting 3 for x in the demand or supply function, we find that $p_E = D(3) = S(3) = 9$. The equilibrium point is (3, 9). This means that Arnold is willing to purchase 3 sketchpads at \$9 per unit and Garvin Art Supplies is willing to sell him 3 sketchpads at \$9 per unit.

Arnold's consumer surplus is

$$
\begin{aligned}
\int_0^3 (x-6)^2\,dx - 3\cdot 9 &= \int_0^3 (x^2 - 12x + 36)\,dx - 27 \\
&= \left[\frac{x^3}{3} - 6x^2 + 36x\right]_0^3 - 27 \\
&= \left[\left(\frac{(3)^3}{3} - 6(3)^2 + 36(3)\right) - \left(\frac{(0)^3}{3} - 6(0)^2 + 36(0)\right)\right] - 27 \\
&= (9 - 54 + 108) - 0 - 27 \\
&= \$36.00.
\end{aligned}
$$

Garvin Art Supplies' producer surplus is

$$
\begin{aligned}
3\cdot 9 - \int_0^3 \left(\frac{1}{3}x^2 + x + 3\right)dx &= 27 - \left[\frac{x^3}{9} + \frac{x^2}{2} + 3x\right]_0^3 \\
&= 27 - \left[\left(\frac{(3)^3}{9} + \frac{(3)^2}{2} + 3(3)\right) - \left(\frac{(0)^3}{9} + \frac{(0)^2}{2} + 3(0)\right)\right] \\
&= 27 - \left(3 + \frac{9}{2} + 9 - 0\right) \\
&= \$10.50.
\end{aligned}
$$

We saw in Example 1 that if Arnold buys 2 sketchpads at \$16 each, he spends \$32, but would have been willing to spend up to \$50.67 (the area under the demand function). The difference, \$18.67, is Arnold's consumer surplus. Similarly, we saw in Example 2 that if Garvin Art Supplies sells 2 sketchpads at \$6.33 per unit, it receives revenue of \$12.66, of which \$3.77 is the producer surplus, a contribution to its overall profit.

However, Arnold is willing to spend \$9 per unit for 3 sketchpads, and Garvin Art Supplies is willing to sell 3 sketchpads at \$9 per unit. At this point of equilibrium, Arnold spends more but also gains consumer surplus, while Garvin Art Supplies collects more revenue and gains more producer surplus. Both producer and consumer benefit from this transaction. **3 ✓**

Quick Check 3 ✓

Given $D(x) = x^2 - 6x + 16$ and $S(x) = \frac{1}{3}x^2 + \frac{4}{3}x + 4$, find each of the following. Assume that x is the number of units sold, $D(x)$ and $S(x)$ are in dollars per unit, and $x \leq 5$.

a) The equilibrium point

b) The consumer surplus at the equilibrium point

c) The producer surplus at the equilibrium point

Price Ceilings, Price Floors, and Deadweight Loss*

At the equilibrium point, p_E is the most advantageous price for both consumers and producers for purchasing or selling x_E units of a product. However, circumstances may require that a price ceiling be imposed (to protect consumers) or that a price floor be imposed (to protect producers). For example, a city may impose rent control (a price ceiling) to allow its residents to find affordable housing, or a country may impose a tariff (a price floor) to support one of its industries.

DEFINITIONS

A **price ceiling** is a price p_C such that $p_C < p_E$, and p_C is the maximum price for which the product may be sold.

A **price floor** is a price p_F such that $p_F > p_E$, and p_F is the minimum price for which the product may be sold.

The loss in surplus is called the **deadweight loss.**

The following table summarizes how a price ceiling or a price floor affects consumer surplus and producer surplus.

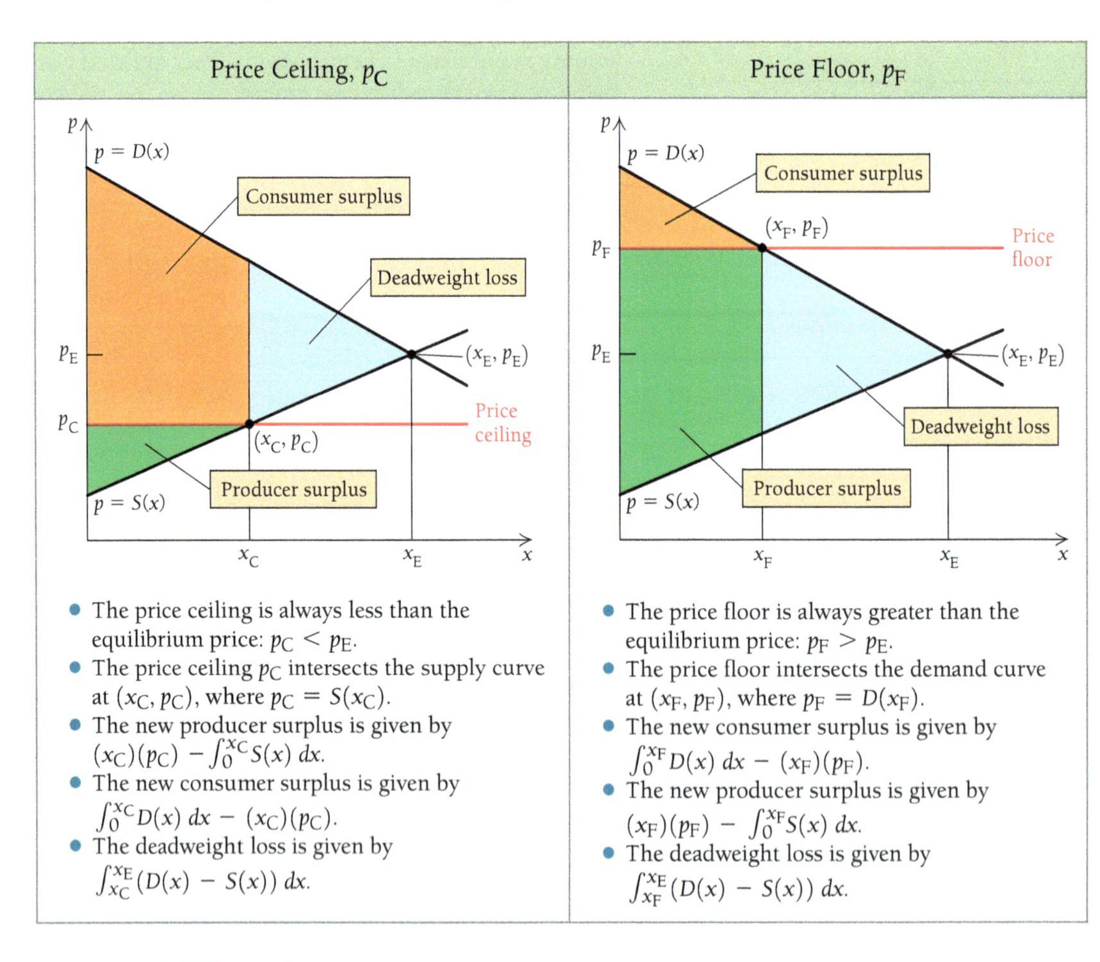

Price Ceiling, p_C	Price Floor, p_F
• The price ceiling is always less than the equilibrium price: $p_C < p_E$.	• The price floor is always greater than the equilibrium price: $p_F > p_E$.
• The price ceiling p_C intersects the supply curve at (x_C, p_C), where $p_C = S(x_C)$.	• The price floor intersects the demand curve at (x_F, p_F), where $p_F = D(x_F)$.
• The new producer surplus is given by $(x_C)(p_C) - \int_0^{x_C} S(x)\,dx$.	• The new consumer surplus is given by $\int_0^{x_F} D(x)\,dx - (x_F)(p_F)$.
• The new consumer surplus is given by $\int_0^{x_C} D(x)\,dx - (x_C)(p_C)$.	• The new producer surplus is given by $(x_F)(p_F) - \int_0^{x_F} S(x)\,dx$.
• The deadweight loss is given by $\int_{x_C}^{x_E} (D(x) - S(x))\,dx$.	• The deadweight loss is given by $\int_{x_F}^{x_E} (D(x) - S(x))\,dx$.

EXAMPLE 4 **Business: Price Ceiling.** In a small isolated mountain town, demand for propane is given by $D(x) = 6.50 - 0.25x$, and supply is given by $S(x) = 2.10 + 0.15x$, where x is in gallons per month per customer and $D(x)$ and $S(x)$ are dollars per gallon.

a) Find the equilibrium point, (x_E, p_E).

*This section can be omitted without loss of continuity.

b) Find the consumer surplus and the producer surplus at the equilibrium point.

c) Assume a price ceiling of \$3 per gallon of propane is imposed. Find the point (x_C, p_C).

d) Find the new producer surplus and the new consumer surplus at (x_C, p_C).

e) Find the deadweight loss.

Solution

a) To find the equilibrium point, (x_E, p_E), we set $D(x) = S(x)$ and solve:

$$6.50 - 0.25x = 2.10 + 0.15x$$
$$4.40 = 0.40x$$
$$x_E = \frac{4.40}{0.40} = 11.$$

Thus, $D(11) = 6.50 - 0.25(11) = 3.75$, and $S(11) = 2.10 + 0.15(11) = 3.75$. The point of equilibrium is $(x_E, p_E) = (11, 3.75)$. Consumers are willing to pay \$3.75 per gallon of propane to buy 11 gallons per month, and producers are willing to sell this amount of propane at this price.

b) The consumer surplus is

$$\int_0^{11} (6.50 - 0.25x)\,dx - (11)(3.75) = \left[6.50x - 0.125x^2\right]_0^{11} - 41.25$$
$$= \left[(6.50(11) - 0.125(11)^2) - 0\right] - 41.25$$
$$= 56.375 - 41.25 = \$15.125, \quad \text{or } \$15.13 \text{ (rounded)}.$$

The producer surplus is

$$(11)(3.75) - \int_0^{11} (2.10 + 0.15x)\,dx = 41.25 - \left[2.10x + 0.075x^2\right]_0^{11}$$
$$= 41.25 - \left[(2.10(11) + 0.075(11)^2) - 0\right]$$
$$= 41.25 - 32.175 = \$9.075, \quad \text{or } \$9.08 \text{ (rounded)}.$$

The consumer surplus and producer surplus are shown in the following graph.

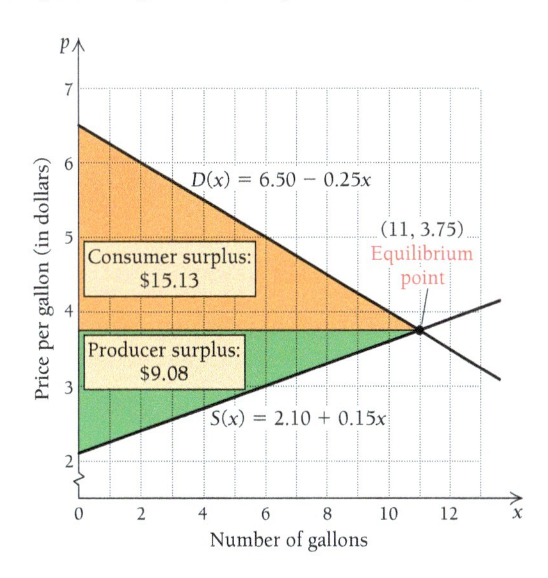

c) To find where the price ceiling $y = p_C = 3$ intersects the supply curve, we set $S(x) = 3$ and solve:

$$2.10 + 0.15x = 3$$
$$0.15x = 0.90$$
$$x_C = \frac{0.90}{0.15} = 6.$$

Thus, we have $(x_C, p_C) = (6, 3)$. Producers are willing to sell 6 gallons of propane (per month, per customer) at a price of \$3 per gallon. Consumers may purchase higher quantities, if producers make it available at that price.

d) With the price ceiling in effect, the new producer surplus is found over the interval [0, 6]:

$$(6)(3) - \int_0^6 (2.10 + 0.15x)\,dx = 18 - \left[2.10x + 0.075x^2\right]_0^6$$
$$= 18 - \left[(2.10(6) + 0.075(6)^2) - 0\right]$$
$$= 18 - 15.30$$
$$= \$2.70.$$

The new consumer surplus is the area between $D(x) = 6.50 - 0.25x$ and $p_C = 3$ over the interval [0, 6]. We have

$$\int_0^6 (6.50 - 0.25x)\,dx - (6)(3) = \left[6.50x - 0.125x^2\right]_0^6 - 18$$
$$= \left[6.50(6) - 0.125(6)^2\right] - 18$$
$$= \$16.50.$$

e) The deadweight loss is the area bounded above by $D(x)$ and below by $S(x)$ over the interval $[x_C, x_E]$, or [6, 11]:

$$\text{Deadweight loss} = \int_6^{11} \left[(6.50 - 0.25x) - (2.10 + 0.15x)\right] dx$$
$$= \int_6^{11} (4.40 - 0.40x)\,dx \qquad \text{Simplifying the integrand}$$
$$= \left[4.40x - 0.20x^2\right]_6^{11}$$
$$= \left[4.40(11) - 0.20(11)^2\right] - \left[4.40(6) - 0.20(6)^2\right]$$
$$= \$5.$$

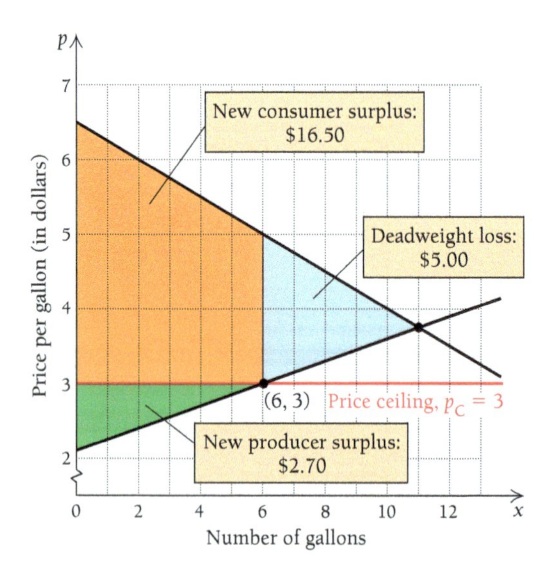

Note that with a price ceiling of \$3, consumers can purchase more than 6 gallons of propane per month. However, the producers may not be willing to supply more. 4 ✓

Quick Check 4 ✓

The demand for movie tickets in a certain town is given by $D(x) = 10 - 1.25x$, and the supply is given by $S(x) = 4 + 1.75x$, where x is the number of tickets. Suppose that the town council imposes a minimum price per ticket of \$8.75. Assume that $D(x)$ and $S(x)$ are the price, in dollars per ticket. Find:

a) the new consumer surplus;

b) the new producer surplus;

c) the deadweight loss.

Section Summary

- *A demand curve* is the graph of a function $p = D(x)$, which is the unit price p a consumer is willing to pay for x units. It is usually a decreasing function.
- *A supply curve* is the graph of a function $p = S(x)$, which is the unit price p a producer is willing to accept for x units. It is usually an increasing function.
- *Consumer surplus* for Q units at a price P per unit is

$$\int_0^Q D(x)\,dx - QP.$$

- *Producer surplus* for Q units at a price P per unit is

$$QP - \int_0^Q S(x)\,dx.$$

- The *equilibrium point*, (x_E, p_E), is the point at which the supply and demand curves intersect. The consumer surplus at the equilibrium point is

$$\int_0^{x_E} D(x)\,dx - x_E p_E.$$

The producer surplus at the equilibrium point is

$$x_E p_E - \int_0^{x_E} S(x)\,dx.$$

- A *price ceiling*, p_C, is the maximum price for which a product can be sold. It is always less than the equilibrium price, p_E. That is, $p_C < p_E$.
  - The price ceiling p_C intersects the supply curve at (x_C, p_C).
  - The new producer surplus is $(x_C)(p_C) - \int_0^{x_C} S(x)\,dx$.
  - The new consumer surplus is $\int_0^{x_C} D(x)\,dx - (x_C)(p_C)$.
  - The *deadweight loss* is $\int_{x_C}^{x_E} (D(x) - S(x))\,dx$.

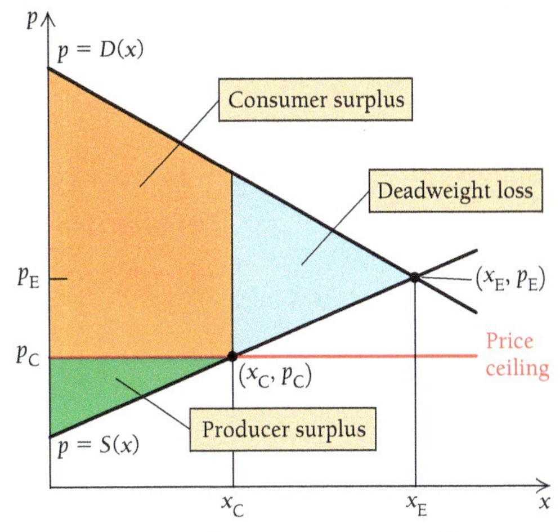

- A *price floor*, p_F, is the minimum price for which a product can be sold. It is always greater than the equilibrium price. That is, $p_F > p_E$.
  - The price floor intersects the demand curve at (x_F, p_F).
  - The new consumer surplus is $\int_0^{x_F} D(x)\,dx - (x_F)(p_F)$.
  - The new producer surplus is $(x_F)(p_F) - \int_0^{x_F} S(x)\,dx$.
  - The *deadweight loss* is $\int_{x_F}^{x_E} (D(x) - S(x))\,dx$.

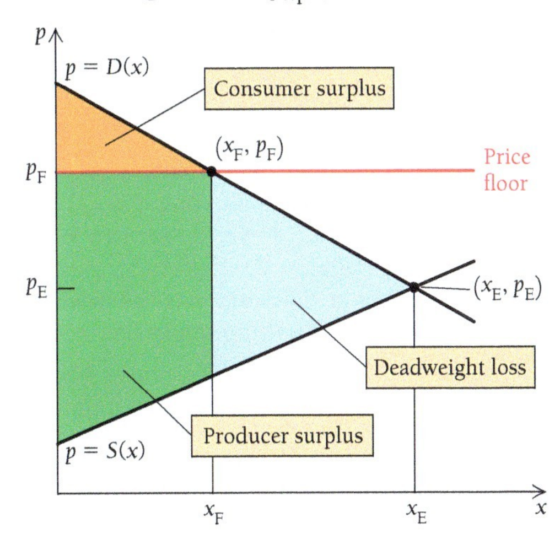

5.1 Exercise Set

In Exercises 1–14, $D(x)$ is the price, in dollars per unit, that consumers will pay for x units of an item, and $S(x)$ is the price, in dollars per unit, that producers will accept for x units. Find (a) the equilibrium point, (b) the consumer surplus at the equilibrium point, and (c) the producer surplus at the equilibrium point.

1. $D(x) = -\frac{5}{6}x + 9, \quad S(x) = \frac{1}{2}x + 1$
2. $D(x) = -3x + 7, \quad S(x) = 2x + 2$
3. $D(x) = (x - 3)^2, \quad S(x) = x^2 + 2x + 1$
4. $D(x) = (x - 4)^2, \quad S(x) = x^2 + 2x + 6$

5. $D(x) = (x - 6)^2, \quad S(x) = x^2$
6. $D(x) = (x - 8)^2, \quad S(x) = x^2$
7. $D(x) = 8800 - 30x, \quad S(x) = 7000 + 15x$
8. $D(x) = 1000 - 10x, \quad S(x) = 250 + 5x$
9. $D(x) = 5 - x, S(x) = \sqrt{x + 7}; \quad \text{for } 0 \le x \le 5$
10. $D(x) = 7 - x, S(x) = 2\sqrt{x + 1}; \quad \text{for } 0 \le x \le 7$
11. $D(x) = \dfrac{1800}{\sqrt{x + 1}}, \quad S(x) = 2\sqrt{x + 1}, \text{ for } x \ge 0$
12. $D(x) = \dfrac{100}{\sqrt{x}}, \quad S(x) = \sqrt{x}, \text{ for } x \ge 0$
13. $D(x) = (x - 4)^2, \quad S(x) = x^2 + 2x + 8$
14. $D(x) = 13 - x, \text{ for } 0 \le x \le 13; \quad S(x) = \sqrt{x + 17}, \text{ for } x \ge 0$

APPLICATIONS

Business and Economics

15. **Business: consumer and producer surplus.** Beth enjoys skydiving and is willing to pay p dollars per jump for x jumps, where $p = D(x) = 7.5x^2 - 60.5x + 254$.
    a) Find Beth's consumer surplus if she makes 2 jumps.
    b) Suppose the supply function for Aero Skydiving Center is given by $p = S(x) = 15x + 95$. Find the producer surplus if the center sells Beth 2 jumps.
    c) Find the equilibrium point and the consumer and producer surpluses at this point. Assume that Beth makes no more than 5 jumps.
    d) Explain what the equilibrium point represents to both Beth and Aero Skydiving Center.

16. **Business: consumer and producer surplus.** Chris is enjoying a day at the Splashorama Water Park. His demand function for sliding down El Monstro Water Slide is given by $p = D(x) = 0.425x^2 - 5.7x + 22.5$, where x is the number of slides and p is the price, in dollars per slide, that he is willing to pay.
    a) Find Chris's consumer surplus if he buys 3 slides.
    b) Suppose the supply function for Splashorama Water Park for the El Monstro Water Slide is given by $p = S(x) = 0.3x + 5.3$. Find the producer surplus if Chris is sold 3 slides.
    c) Find the equilibrium point and the consumer and producer surpluses at this point. Assume that Chris buys no more than 6 slides.
    d) Explain what the equilibrium point represents to both Chris and the Splashorama Water Park.

In Exercises 17–22, a price ceiling or price floor is given along with demand and supply functions, where D(x) is the price, in dollars per unit, that consumers will pay for x units, and S(x) is the price, in dollars per unit, at which producers will sell x units. Find (a) *the equilibrium point,* (b) *the point* (x_C, p_C) *or* (x_F, p_F), (c) *the new consumer surplus,* (d) *the new producer surplus, and* (e) *the deadweight loss.*

17. $D(x) = 50 - x, S(x) = 17 + 0.5x, p_C = \$24$
18. $D(x) = 75 - x, S(x) = 21 + 2x, p_C = \$50$
19. $D(x) = 100 - 1.25x, S(x) = 30 + 0.75x, p_F = \$80$
20. $D(x) = 125 - 2.25x, S(x) = 20 + 1.5x, p_F = \$90$
21. $D(x) = 30 + (x - 10)^2, S(x) = x^2, p_C = \$30$ (Assume $x \le 10$.)
22. $D(x) = 5 + (x - 12)^2, S(x) = 0.2x^2, p_F = \$40$ (Assume $x \le 12$.)

23. **Rent control.** Demand for apartments in Curtisville is $D(x) = 1500 - 5x$, and supply is $S(x) = 600 + 10x$, where x is the number of apartments, in hundreds, and $D(x)$ and $S(x)$ are the rent in dollars per month, per apartment.
    a) Find the equilibrium point.
    b) Find the consumer surplus and producer surplus at the equilibrium point.
    c) Suppose a maximum rent of \$1000 per month is imposed by the city council. Find the point (x_C, p_C).
    d) Find the new consumer surplus and new producer surplus.
    e) Find the deadweight loss.

24. **Rent control.** Demand for rental cabins in a beach town is $D(x) = 1000 - 2.5x$, and supply is $S(x) = 520 + 5x$, where x is the number of cabins, and $D(x)$ and $S(x)$ are the rent in dollars per month, per cabin.
    a) Find the equilibrium point.
    b) Find the consumer surplus and producer surplus at the equilibrium point.
    c) Suppose a maximum rent of \$800 per month is imposed by the town council. Find the point (x_C, p_C).
    d) Find the new consumer surplus and new producer surplus.
    e) Find the deadweight loss.

25. **Price floor.** Suppose the demand for bicycles in Ocean Shores is given by $D(x) = 275 - 1.25x$, and the supply is given by $S(x) = 135 + 0.5x$, where x is in thousands of bicycles and $D(x)$ and $S(x)$ are in dollars per bicycle.
    a) Find the equilibrium point.
    b) Find the consumer surplus and producer surplus at the equilibrium point.
    c) Suppose a minimum price of \$200 per bicycle is imposed. Find the point (x_F, p_F).
    d) Find the new consumer surplus and new producer surplus.
    e) Find the deadweight loss.
    f) Why might a price floor be imposed in this situation?

26. **Price floor.** Suppose the demand for milk is given by $D(x) = 5 - 0.06x$, and the supply is given by $S(x) = 1.5 + 0.03x$, where x is in gallons and $D(x)$ and $S(x)$ are in dollars per gallon.
    a) Find the equilibrium point.
    b) Find the consumer surplus and producer surplus at the equilibrium point.
    c) Suppose a minimum price of \$3.25 per gallon of milk is imposed. Find the point (x_F, p_F).
    d) Find the new consumer surplus and new producer surplus.
    e) Find the deadweight loss.
    f) Why might a price floor be imposed in this situation?

SYNTHESIS

For Exercises 27 and 28, follow the directions given for Exercises 1–14.

27. $D(x) = e^{-x+4.5}$, $S(x) = e^{x-5.5}$

28. $D(x) = \sqrt{56 - x}$, $S(x) = x$

29. Explain why both consumers and producers feel good when consumer and producer surpluses exist.

30. Explain why a price ceiling that is higher than the equilibrium price is unnecessary.

31. Explain why a price floor that is lower than the equilibrium price is unnecessary.

Technology Connection

For Exercises 32 and 33, graph each pair of demand and supply functions. Then:

a) *Find the equilibrium point using the* INTERSECT *feature or another feature that will allow you to find this point of intersection.*

b) *Graph* $y = D(x)$ and $S(x)$ *and identify the regions of both consumer and producer surpluses.*

c) *Find the consumer surplus.*

d) *Find the producer surplus.*

32. $D(x) = \dfrac{x + 8}{x + 1}$, $S(x) = \dfrac{x^2 + 4}{20}$

33. $D(x) = 15 - \frac{1}{3}x$, $S(x) = 2\sqrt[3]{x}$

34. Bungee jumping. Regina loves bungee jumping. The table shows the number of half-hours that Regina is willing to bungee jump at various prices.

a) Make a scatterplot of the data, and determine the type of function that you think fits best.

b) Fit that function to the data using REGRESSION.

c) If Regina goes bungee jumping for 6 half-hours per month, what is her consumer surplus?

d) At a price of $115.00 per half-hour, what is Regina's consumer surplus?

Time Spent (in half-hours per month)	Price (per half-hour)
8	$25.00
7	50.00
6	75.00
5	100.00
4	125.00
3	150.00
2	175.00
1	200.00

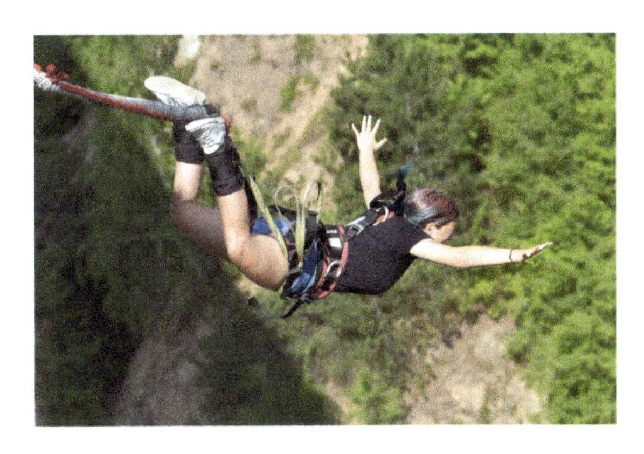

Answers to Quick Checks

1. $2.33 **2.** $0.89 **3. (a)** (2, 8); **(b)** $6.67; **(c)** $4.44 **4. (a)** $0.625; **(b)** $3.88; **(c)** $1.50

5.2 Integrating Growth and Decay Models

- Find the future value of an investment.
- Find the accumulated future value of a continuous income stream.
- Find the present value of an amount due in the future.
- Find the accumulated present value of an income stream.
- Calculate the total consumption of a natural resource.

We studied exponential growth and decay models using $P(t) = P_0e^{kt}$ and $P(t) = P_0e^{-kt}$ in Sections 2.4 and 2.5. In this section, we consider applications of the integrals of these functions. For convenience, we first derive formulas for evaluating these integrals. Recall that the interest rate k is expressed in decimal notation.

For the *growth* model, the formula is

$$\int_0^T P_0e^{kt}\,dt = \left[\frac{P_0}{k}\cdot e^{kt}\right]_0^T \qquad \text{Using the substitution } u = e^{kt}$$

$$= \frac{P_0}{k}(e^{kT} - e^{k\cdot 0}) \qquad \text{Evaluating the integral}$$

$$= \frac{P_0}{k}(e^{kT} - 1).$$

Similarly, for the *decay* model, the formula is $\int_0^T P_0e^{-kt}\,dt = \frac{P_0}{k}(1 - e^{-kT})$. Thus, we have the following integration formulas.

For exponential growth: $$\int_0^T P_0 e^{kt}\,dt = \frac{P_0}{k}\left(e^{kT} - 1\right) \qquad (1)$$

For exponential decay: $$\int_0^T P_0 e^{-kt}\,dt = \frac{P_0}{k}\left(1 - e^{-kT}\right) \qquad (2)$$

We now consider applications of these formulas to business and economics and environmental studies.

Future Value

Recall the basic model for the growth of an amount of money, presented in the following definition.

DEFINITION

If P_0 is invested for t years at interest rate k, compounded continuously (Section 2.4), then

$$P(t) = P_0 e^{kt}, \qquad (3)$$

where $P_0 = P(0)$. The value $P(t)$ is called the **future value** of P_0 dollars invested at interest rate k, compounded continuously, for t years.

EXAMPLE 1 **Business: Future Value of an Investment.** Find the future value of \$36,500 invested for 4 yr at an interest rate of 3%, compounded continuously.

Solution Using equation (3) with $P_0 = 36{,}500$, $k = 0.03$, and $t = 4$, we have

$$\begin{aligned} P(4) &= 36{,}500e^{0.03(4)} \\ &= 36{,}500e^{0.12} \\ &\approx 41{,}153.64. \quad \text{Using a calculator} \end{aligned}$$

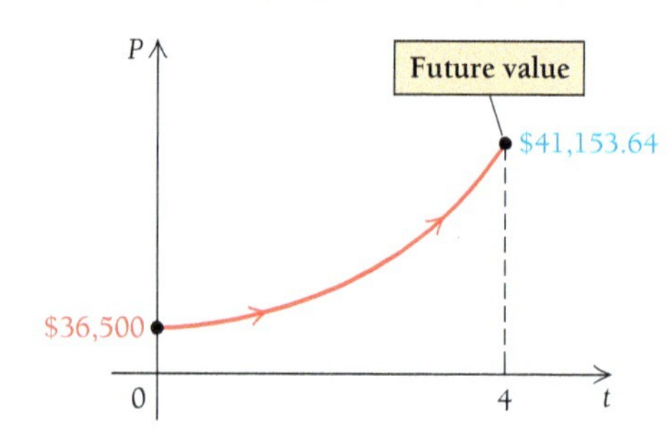

The future value of \$36,500 after 4 yr is about \$41,153.64.

1 ✓

Quick Check 1 ✓

Business: Future Value of an Investment. Find the future value of \$10,000 invested for 3 yr at an interest rate of 2.35%, compounded continuously.

Accumulated Future Value of a Continuous Income Stream

Let's consider a situation involving the accumulation of future values. The owner of a parking space near a convention center receives a yearly profit of \$36,500 at the end of each of 4 years; this is called an *income stream*. The owner invests the \$36,500 at 3% interest compounded continuously. When \$36,500 is received at the end of the first year, it is invested for $4 - 1$, or 3 yr. The future value is $36{,}500e^{0.03(4-1)}$, or \$39,937.36. The next \$36,500, received at the end of the second year, is invested for $4-2$, or 2 yr. The future value of this investment is $36{,}500e^{0.03(4-2)}$, or \$38,757.03. When \$36,500 is received at the end of the third year, it is invested for $4 - 3$, or 1 yr. Its future value is $36{,}500e^{0.03(4-3)}$, or \$37,611.59. When the last \$36,500 is received after the fourth year, it is invested for $4 - 4$, or 0 yr. This amount has no time to earn interest, so its future value is \$36,500. The *accumulated, or total, future value of the income stream* is the sum of the four future values:

$$\begin{aligned}
&\text{After 1st year, } t = 3: \quad \$36{,}500e^{0.03(3)} \longrightarrow \$39{,}937.36\\
&\text{After 2nd year, } t = 2: \quad \$36{,}500e^{0.03(2)} \longrightarrow \$38{,}757.03\\
&\text{After 3rd year, } t = 1: \quad \$36{,}500e^{0.03(1)} \longrightarrow \$37{,}611.59\\
&\text{After 4th year, } t = 0: \quad \$36{,}500e^{0.03(0)} \longrightarrow \$36{,}500.00\\
&\text{Total future value of the income stream} = \$152{,}805.98
\end{aligned}$$

Next, suppose the owner of the parking space receives the profit at a rate of \$36,500 per year but in 365 payments of \$100 per day. Each day, when the owner gets \$100, it is invested at 3%, compounded continuously, and due at the end of the fourth year. The *first* day's investment grows to

$$\frac{36{,}500}{365}e^{0.03(4-1/365)} = 100e^{0.03(4-1/365)} \approx \$112.74,$$

since it will be invested for 1 day, or 1/365 yr, less than the full 4 yr. The next investment, made on the *second* day, grows to

$$\frac{36{,}500}{365}e^{0.03(4-2/365)} = 100e^{0.03(4-2/365)} \approx \$112.73,$$

at the end of the fourth year, and so on, for every day in the 4-yr period. Assuming that all deposits are made into the same account, the total of the future values is

$$\underbrace{\overbrace{100e^{0.03(4-1/365)}}^{\text{First deposit}} + \overbrace{100e^{0.03(4-2/365)}}^{\text{Second deposit}} + \cdots + \overbrace{100e^{0.03(2/365)}}^{\text{Third-to-last deposit}} + \overbrace{100e^{0.03(1/365)}}^{\text{Second-to-last deposit}} + \overbrace{100}^{\text{Last deposit}}.}_{\substack{4 \text{ yr} \times 365 \text{ days} = 1460 \text{ daily deposits} \\ \text{(For simplicity, the leap day is ignored.)}}}$$

The above expression can be written as a summation, where i is in days:

$$\sum_{i=1}^{1460} 100e^{0.03(4-i/365)}.$$

Since t represents years, we have $t = \frac{i}{365}$, so the bounds are $\frac{1}{365}$ and $\frac{1460}{365}$ if t is used as the index. Furthermore, we can write 100 as $36{,}500 \cdot \frac{1}{365}$, so $\Delta t = \frac{1}{365}$.

Thus, the above summation is written

$$\begin{aligned}
\sum_{i=1}^{1460} 100e^{0.03(4-i/365)} &= 36{,}500\sum_{i=1}^{1460} e^{0.03(4-i/365)} \cdot \frac{1}{365} && \text{Rewriting 100 as } 36{,}500 \cdot \frac{1}{365}\\
&= 36{,}500 \sum_{t=1/365}^{1460/365} e^{0.03(4-t)} \cdot \Delta t && \text{Converting the index to } t \text{ using } \frac{1}{365} \text{ as } \Delta t\\
&= 36{,}500 \sum_{t=1/365}^{1460/365} e^{0.03(4-t)} \cdot \Delta t.
\end{aligned}$$

As the time between deposits, Δt, approaches 0, the lower bound approaches 0, and the sum can be regarded as a Riemann sum and approximated by a definite integral:

$$36{,}500 \sum_{t=1/365}^{1460/365} e^{0.03(4-t)} \cdot \Delta t \approx 36{,}500 \int_0^4 e^{0.03(4-t)}\,dt \qquad \text{Noting that } \frac{1460}{365} = 4$$

$$= 36{,}500 \int_0^4 e^{0.03(4)} e^{-0.03t}\,dt \qquad \text{Using a property of exponents: } e^{m+n} = e^m e^n$$

$$= e^{0.12} \int_0^4 36{,}500 e^{-0.03t}\,dt. \qquad \text{Using a property of integrals}$$

Instead of receiving an income stream at the rate of \$100 a day, suppose the owner receives the money *continuously* at a rate of \$36,500 *per year*. This means that over the course of 4 yr, profit is received at a constant rate of \$36,500 per year in what is called a *continuous income stream*, or *flow*. If at each instant the money is invested at 3%, compounded continuously, then the *accumulated future value of the continuous income stream* is approximated by the definite integral found above. Let's calculate it:

$$e^{0.12} \int_0^4 36{,}500\,e^{-0.03t}\,dt = -\frac{36{,}500\,e^{0.12}}{0.03}(e^{-0.12} - 1)$$

$$\approx \$155{,}121.17 \qquad \text{Using a calculator and rounding to the nearest dollar}$$

Economists call \$155,121.17 the **accumulated future value of a continuous income stream.**

DEFINITION Accumulated Future Value of a Continuous Income Stream

Let $R(t)$ represent the rate, per year, of a continuous income stream; let k be the interest rate, compounded continuously, at which the continuous income stream is invested; and let T be the number of years for which it is invested. Then the **accumulated future value of the continuous income stream** is given by

$$A = \int_0^T R(t)e^{k(T-t)}\,dt = e^{kT}\int_0^T R(t)e^{-kt}\,dt. \qquad (4)$$

If $R(t)$ is a constant, it can be factored out of the integral, and the formula becomes, after simplifying,

$$A = \frac{R(t)}{k}(e^{kT} - 1). \qquad (5)$$

If $R(t)$ is not a constant, then equation (5) does not apply and the integral in equation (4) must be evaluated using another integration technique.

EXAMPLE 2 **Business: Insurance Settlement.** A cardiac surgeon, Sarah Makahone, who earns \$450,000 per year, is involved in an automobile accident that prevents her from working. In a legal settlement with an insurance company, Sarah is granted a continuous income stream of \$225,000 per year for 20 yr. Sarah invests the money at 3.2%, compounded continuously, in the Halmos Global Equities Fund. Find the accumulated future value of the continuous income stream.

Solution Since this is an income stream flowing at a constant rate, we can use equation (5), with $R(t) = \$225{,}000$, $k = 0.032$, and $T = 20$. We have

$$A = \frac{225{,}000}{0.032}(e^{0.032(20)} - 1) \approx \$6{,}303{,}381. \qquad \text{Rounding to the nearest dollar}$$

2 ✓

Quick Check 2 ✓

Business: Insurance Settlement. Repeat Example 2 but assume that the insurance settlement is a continuous income stream of \$125,000 per year for 25 yr and the money is invested at 2.84%, compounded continuously.

Present Value

We saw in Example 1 that the future value of \$36,500 invested for 4 yr at a continuously compounded interest rate of 3% is \$41,153.64. We call \$36,500 the **present value** of \$41,153.64 invested for 4 yr at an interest rate of 3%, compounded continuously. It answers this question: "What do we have to invest now at a certain interest rate to attain a certain future value?"

In general, the present value P_0 of an amount P that results from an investment at interest rate k for t years is found by solving the growth equation for P_0:

$$P_0 e^{kt} = P$$

$$P_0 = \frac{P}{e^{kt}} = Pe^{-kt}.$$

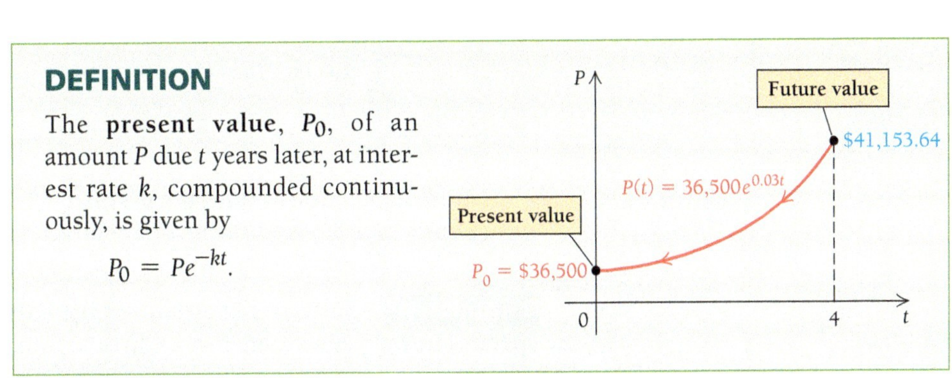

DEFINITION
The present value, P_0, of an amount P due t years later, at interest rate k, compounded continuously, is given by
$P_0 = Pe^{-kt}$.
P
Future value
\$41,153.64
$P(t) = 36{,}500e^{0.03t}$
Present value
P_0 = \$36,500
0
4
t

EXAMPLE 3 **Business: Finding the Present Value of a Trust.** In 10 years, Sam Bixby is going to receive \$250,000 under the terms of a trust established by his aunt. If the money in the trust fund is invested at 3.25% interest, compounded continuously, what is the present value of Sam's trust?

Solution Using the equation for present value, we have

$$P_0 = 250{,}000e^{-0.0325(10)} \approx \$180{,}631.84.$$

3 ✓

Quick Check 3 ✓

Business: Finding the Present Value of a Trust. Following the birth of a grandchild, Mira Bell wants to set up a trust fund that will be worth \$120,000 on the child's 18th birthday. Mira secures an interest rate of 3.6%, compounded continuously, for the time period. What amount should she deposit to achieve her goal?

Accumulated Present Value of a Continuous Income Stream

To find the **accumulated present value of a continuous income stream**, when $R(t)$ is constant, we can work backward from equation (5):

$$A = \frac{R(t)}{k}(e^{kT} - 1).$$

We are looking for the principal B, the amount of a one-time deposit, at the interest rate k, that will yield the same accumulated value as the income stream. We choose B such that $Be^{kT} = A$ in equation (5). Then we solve for B:

$$Be^{kT} = \frac{R(t)}{k}(e^{kT} - 1) \qquad \text{Substituting}$$

$$\frac{Be^{kT}}{e^{kT}} = \frac{R(t)}{k}\left(\frac{e^{kT} - 1}{e^{kT}}\right) \qquad \text{Dividing both sides by } e^{kT}$$

$$B = \frac{R(t)}{k}\left(\frac{e^{kT}}{e^{kT}} - \frac{1}{e^{kT}}\right)$$

$$B = \frac{R(t)}{k}(1 - e^{-kT}). \qquad \text{Simplifying}$$

DEFINITION Accumulated Present Value of a Continuous Income Stream

Let $R(t)$ represent the rate, per year, of a continuous income stream; let k be the interest rate, compounded continuously, at which the continuous income stream is invested; and let T be the number of years over which the income stream is received.

If $R(t)$ is a constant, then B, the **accumulated present value of the continuous income stream,** is given by

$$B = \frac{R(t)}{k}(1 - e^{-kT}). \tag{6}$$

If $R(t)$ is not a constant, the accumulated present value of the continuous income stream is given by

$$B = \int_0^T R(t)e^{-kt}\,dt. \tag{7}$$

Accumulated present value is a useful tool in business decision making when evaluating a purchase, an investment, or a contract. It allows for comparison of alternatives.

EXAMPLE 4 **Business: Determining the Value of a Franchise.** Silver Spoon, Inc., operates frozen yogurt franchises. Chris Nelson, yearning to be an entrepreneur, considers buying a franchise in his home town, Carmel, Indiana. As part of his decision to purchase, he wants to determine the accumulated present value of the income stream from the franchise over an 8-yr period. Silver Spoon tells Chris that he should expect a constant annual income stream given by

$$R_1(t) = \$275{,}000,$$

which Chris knows he can invest at an interest rate of 3.3%, compounded continuously.

However, Chris performs a linear regression on data from the annual reports of Silver Spoon, which indicates that there will be a nonconstant annual income stream of

$$R_2(t) = \$80{,}000t,$$

where t is the number of years the franchise is in operation.

a) Evaluate the accumulated future value of the income stream at rate $R_1(t)$. Then evaluate the accumulated present value of that income stream, and interpret the results.

b) Evaluate the accumulated future value of the income stream at rate $R_2(t)$. Then evaluate the accumulated present value of that income stream, and interpret the results.

Solution

a) Assuming a constant income stream of \$275,000 per year for 8 yr and using equation (5), we find that the accumulated *future* value is

$$\begin{aligned} A &= \frac{R_1(t)}{k}(e^{kT} - 1) \\ &= \frac{275{,}000}{0.033}(e^{0.033(8)} - 1) \approx \$2{,}517{,}734.97. \end{aligned}$$

This gives Chris a sense of the value of the franchise over the 8-yr period. The accumulated *present* value is found by using equation (6):

$$\begin{aligned} B &= \frac{R_1(t)}{k}(1 - e^{-kT}) \\ &= \frac{275{,}000}{0.033}\left(1 - e^{-0.033(8)}\right) \approx \$1{,}933{,}553.84. \end{aligned}$$

The first result tells us that if Chris were to buy the franchise now and invest the predicted income stream at 3.3%, compounded continuously, he would have \$2,517,734.97 in 8 yr. The second result tells us that \$2,517,734.97 is worth \$1,933,553.84 today.

b) With a nonconstant income stream, $R_2(t) = 80{,}000t$ per year, using equation (4), the accumulated *future* value is

$$e^{0.033(8)}\int_0^8 (80{,}000t)e^{-0.033t}\,dt = 80{,}000e^{0.264}\int_0^8 te^{-0.033t}\,dt$$

$$= 80{,}000e^{0.264}\left[-\frac{1}{0.033}te^{-0.033t} - \frac{1}{0.033^2}e^{-0.033t}\right]_0^8 \quad \text{Using integration by parts, with } u = t \text{ and } dv = e^{-0.033t}\,dt$$

$$= 80{,}000e^{0.264}\left[\left(-\frac{1}{0.033}(8)e^{-0.033(8)} - \frac{1}{0.033^2}e^{-0.033(8)}\right) - \left(-\frac{1}{0.033}(0)e^{-0.033(0)} - \frac{1}{0.033^2}e^{-0.033(0)}\right)\right]$$

$$= 80{,}000e^{0.264}\left[\left(-\frac{8}{0.033}e^{-0.264} - \frac{1}{0.033^2}e^{-0.264}\right) - \left(-\frac{1}{0.033^2}\right)\right] \approx \$2{,}800{,}969.43.$$

Quick Check 4 ✓

Business: Determining the Value of a Franchise. Repeat Example 4, but with the following income streams:

$$R_1(t) = \$265{,}000,$$

$$R_2(t) = 75{,}000t,$$

and an interest rate of 4%, compounded continuously.

This result tells us that if Chris were to buy the franchise now and invest the predicted income at an interest rate of 3.3%, compounded continuously, he would have \$2,800,969.43 in 8 yr.

Using equation (7), we find that the accumulated present value is

$$\int_0^8 (80{,}000t)e^{-0.033t}\,dt = 80{,}000\int_0^8 te^{-0.033t}\,dt \approx \$2{,}151{,}070.40.$$

This tells us that \$2,800,969.43 is worth about \$2,151,070.40 today.

These computations yield a higher accumulated present value than claimed by Silver Spoon, suggesting that Chris is dealing with a reputable company. 4 ✓

EXAMPLE 5 **Business: Creating a College Trust.** Emma and Jake Tuttle establish a college trust fund for their new grandchild, Erica, that will yield \$100,000 by her 18th birthday.

a) What lump sum do they need to deposit now, at 3.5% interest, compounded continuously, to yield \$100,000?

b) They discover that the required lump sum is more than they can afford at the time, so they decide to invest a constant stream of $R(t)$ dollars per year. Find $R(t)$ such that the accumulated future value of the continuous money stream is \$100,000, assuming that the interest rate is 3.5%, compounded continuously.

Solution

a) The lump sum is the *present value* of \$100,000, at 3.5% interest, compounded continuously, for 18 yr:

$$P_0 = Pe^{-kt} = 100{,}000e^{-0.035(18)} \approx \$53{,}259.18.$$

b) We want $R(t)$ such that

$$100{,}000 = \frac{R(t)}{0.035}(e^{0.035(18)} - 1) \quad \text{Using equation (5)}$$

$$0.035(100{,}000) = R(t)(e^{0.63} - 1)$$

$$\frac{3500}{(e^{0.63} - 1)} = R(t)$$

$$R(t) \approx \$3988.10.$$

Quick Check 5 ✓

Business: Creating a College Trust. Repeat Example 5 for a yield of \$50,000 and an interest rate of 4%.

A continuous money stream of \$3988.10 per year, invested at 3.5%, compounded continuously for 18 yr, will yield a *future value* of \$100,000. 5 ✓

EXAMPLE 6 **Business: Contract Buyout.** Gregory is playing basketball under a contract that pays him \$3,000,000 each year for 5 yr. After 2 yr, the team offers him a buyout of his contract. How much should the team offer him? Assume an annual percentage rate of 2.8%, compounded continuously.

Solution We view the \$3,000,000 as a continuous money stream. After 2 yr, the contract's accumulated future value, A_2, is

$$A_2 = \frac{3{,}000{,}000}{0.028}(e^{0.028(2)} - 1) \approx \$6{,}171{,}180.40.$$

If the contract were allowed to run the full 5 yr, the accumulated future value, A_5, would be

$$A_5 = \frac{3{,}000{,}000}{0.028}(e^{0.028(5)} - 1) \approx \$16{,}100{,}764.16.$$

The difference is

$$A_5 - A_2 = \$16{,}100{,}764.16 - \$6{,}171{,}180.40 = \$9{,}929{,}583.76.$$

Since the team is offering a lump sum payment to buy out the contract, Gregory should expect an amount that, if allowed to grow at 2.8%, compounded continuously for the remaining 3 yr, would yield \$9,929,583.76. That is, he should receive the present value of the difference, or

$$P_0 = \$9{,}929{,}583.76e^{-0.028(3)} \approx \$9{,}129{,}569.67.$$

6 ✓

Quick Check 6 ✓

Business: Contract Buyout. Repeat Example 6 for a \$4,000,000 contract and an interest rate of 3.2%.

Life and Physical Sciences: Consumption of Natural Resources

Another application of the integration of models of exponential growth uses

$$P(t) = P_0e^{kt}$$

as a model of the demand for natural resources. Suppose that P_0 represents the annual amount of a natural resource (such as natural gas or oil) used at time $t = 0$ and that the growth rate for the use of this resource is k. Then, assuming exponential growth in demand, the amount used annually t years in the future is $P(t)$, where

$$P(t) = P_0e^{kt}.$$

The total amount used during an interval $[0, T]$ is then given by

$$\int_0^T P(t)\,dt = \int_0^T P_0e^{kt}\,dt = \left[\frac{P_0}{k}e^{kt}\right]_0^T = \frac{P_0}{k}(e^{kT} - 1).$$

Consumption of a Natural Resource

Suppose $P(t)$ is the annual consumption of a natural resource in year t. If consumption of the resource is growing exponentially at growth rate k, then the total consumption of the resource after T years is given by

$$\int_0^T P_0e^{kt}\,dt = \frac{P_0}{k}(e^{kT} - 1), \quad \textbf{(8)}$$

where P_0 is the annual consumption at time $t = 0$.

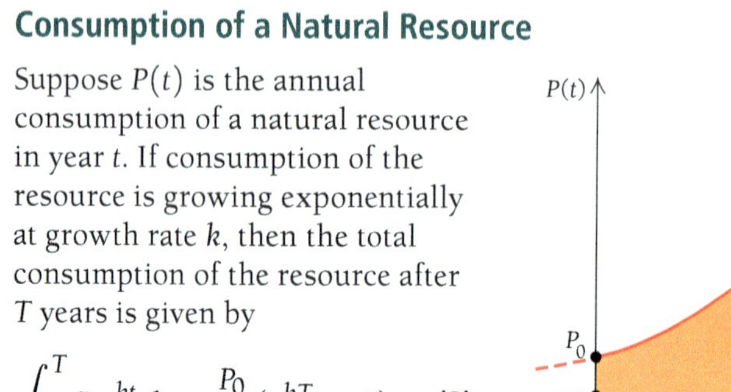

EXAMPLE 7 **Physical Science: Gold Mining.** In 2016 ($t = 0$), world production of gold was 3100 metric tons, and it was growing exponentially at the rate of 3.2% per year. (*Source*: minerals.usgs.gov.) If growth continues at this rate, how many tons of gold will be produced from 2016 to 2024?

Solution Using equation (8), we have

$$\int_0^8 3100e^{0.032t}\,dt = \frac{3100}{0.032}(e^{0.032(8)} - 1)$$
$$\approx 28{,}263.55.$$

From 2016 to 2024, approximately 28,264 metric tons of gold will be produced.

Quick Check 7 ✓

Physical Science: Silver.

a) In 2016, world production of silver was 27,200 metric tons, and it was growing at the rate of 7.6% per year. (*Source*: minerals.usgs.gov.) If growth continues at this rate, how many metric tons of silver will be produced from 2016 to 2024?

b) The world reserves of silver in 2016 were 570,000 metric tons. (*Source*: minerals.usgs .gov.) Assuming that the growth rate of 7.6% per year continues and that no new reserves are discovered, when will the world reserves of silver be depleted?

EXAMPLE 8 **Physical Science: Depletion of Gold Reserves.** The world reserves of gold in 2016 were estimated to be 56,000 metric tons. (*Source*: minerals.usgs.gov.) Assuming that the growth rate of 3.2% per year continues and that no new reserves are discovered, when will the world reserves of gold be depleted?

Solution Using equation (8), we want to find T such that

$$56{,}000 = \frac{3100}{0.032}(e^{0.032T} - 1).$$

We solve for T as follows:

$$56{,}000 = 96{,}875(e^{0.032T} - 1)$$
$$0.578 = e^{0.032T} - 1 \qquad \text{Dividing both sides by 96,875}$$
$$1.578 = e^{0.032T}$$
$$\ln 1.578 = \ln e^{0.032T} \qquad \text{Finding the natural logarithm of each side}$$
$$\ln 1.578 = 0.032T \qquad \text{Recall that } \ln e^k = k.$$
$$14.26 \approx T. \qquad \text{Dividing both sides by 0.032 and rounding}$$

Thus, assuming that world production of gold continues to increase at 3.2% per year and no new reserves are found, the world reserves of gold will be depleted 14.26 yr from 2016, or in 2030. 7 ✓

Section Summary

- If P_0 dollars is invested for t years at an interest rate k, compounded continuously, the *future value* is given by $P(t) = P_0e^{kt}$.
- If a continuous income stream $R(t)$, in dollars, is invested at an interest rate k, compounded continuously, for T years, then the *accumulated future value of the continuous income stream* is given by

$$A = e^{kT}\int_0^T R(t)e^{-kt}\,dt.$$

If $R(t)$ is constant, then

$$A = \frac{R(t)}{k}(e^{kT} - 1).$$

- To attain a future value P, the *present value*, P_0, that should be invested at an interest rate k, compounded continuously, for t years, is given by $P_0 = Pe^{-kt}$.
- If a continuous income stream $R(t)$, in dollars, is invested at an interest rate k, compounded continuously, for T years, the *accumulated present value of the continuous income stream* is given by

$$B = \int_0^T R(t)e^{-kt}\,dt$$

If $R(t)$ is constant, then

$$B = \frac{R(t)}{k}(1 - e^{-kT}).$$

5.2 Exercise Set

Find the future value P of each amount P_0 invested for time period t at interest rate k, compounded continuously. Round answers to the nearest dollar.

1. $P_0 = \$55{,}000, \quad t = 8 \text{ yr}, \quad k = 4\%$
2. $P_0 = \$100{,}000, \quad t = 6 \text{ yr}, \quad k = 3\%$
3. $P_0 = \$88{,}000, \quad t = 13 \text{ yr}, \quad k = 2.7\%$
4. $P_0 = \$140{,}000, \quad t = 9 \text{ yr}, \quad k = 3.8\%$

Find the present value P_0 of each amount P due t years in the future and invested at interest rate k, compounded continuously. Round answers to the nearest dollar.

5. $P = \$100{,}000, \quad t = 8 \text{ yr}, \quad k = 4\%$
6. $P = \$100{,}000, \quad t = 6 \text{ yr}, \quad k = 3\%$
7. $P = \$2{,}000{,}000, \quad t = 20 \text{ yr}, \quad k = 3.5\%$
8. $P = \$1{,}000{,}000, \quad t = 25 \text{ yr}, \quad k = 2.9\%$

Find the accumulated future value of each continuous income stream at rate $R(t)$, for the given time T and interest rate k, compounded continuously. Round answers to the nearest dollar.

9. $R(t) = \$125{,}000, \quad T = 20 \text{ yr}, \quad k = 3.1\%$
10. $R(t) = \$50{,}000, \quad T = 22 \text{ yr}, \quad k = 2.35\%$
11. $R(t) = \$50{,}000, \quad T = 22 \text{ yr}, \quad k = 2.75\%$
12. $R(t) = \$400{,}000, \quad T = 20 \text{ yr}, \quad k = 4\%$

Find the accumulated present value of each continuous income stream at rate $R(t)$, for the given time T and interest rate k, compounded continuously. Round answers to the nearest dollar.

13. $R(t) = \$425{,}000, \quad T = 15 \text{ yr}, \quad k = 3.5\%$
14. $R(t) = \$250{,}000, \quad T = 18 \text{ yr}, \quad k = 4\%$
15. $R(t) = \$520{,}000, \quad T = 25 \text{ yr}, \quad k = 2.05\%$
16. $R(t) = \$800{,}000, \quad T = 20 \text{ yr}, \quad k = 2.3\%$
17. $R(t) = \$6400t, \quad T = 20 \text{ yr}, \quad k = 3.33\%$
18. $R(t) = \$5200t, \quad T = 18 \text{ yr}, \quad k = 3.1\%$
19. $R(t) = \$t^2, \quad T = 40 \text{ yr}, \quad k = 4.25\%$
20. $R(t) = \$(2000t + 7), \quad T = 30 \text{ yr}, \quad k = 4.5\%$

APPLICATIONS

Business and Economics

21. **Present value of a trust.** In 16 yr, Claire Beasley is to receive \$180,000 under the terms of a trust established by her aunt. Assuming an interest rate of 4.2%, compounded continuously, what is the present value of Claire's trust?

22. **Present value of a trust.** In 18 yr, Maggie Oaks is to receive \$200,000 under the terms of a trust established by her grandparents. Assuming an interest rate of 3.8%, compounded continuously, what is the present value of Maggie's trust?

23. **Salary value.** At age 25, Del earns his CPA and accepts a position in an accounting firm. Del plans to retire at the age of 65, having received an annual salary of \$125,000. Assume an interest rate of 4%, compounded continuously.
    a) What is the accumulated present value of his position?
    b) What is the accumulated future value of his position?

24. **Salary value.** At age 35, Rochelle earns her MBA and accepts a position as vice president of a paving company. Assume that she will retire at age 65, having received an annual salary of \$95,000, and that the interest rate is 3.5%, compounded continuously.
    a) What is the accumulated present value of her position?
    b) What is the accumulated future value of her position?

25. **Future value of an inheritance.** Upon the death of his aunt, Burt receives an inheritance of \$80,000, which he invests for 20 yr at 3.9%, compounded continuously. What is the future value of the inheritance?

26. **Future value of an inheritance.** Upon the death of his uncle, David receives an inheritance of \$50,000, which he invests for 16 yr at 4.3%, compounded continuously. What is the future value of the inheritance?

27. **Decision making.** A group of entrepreneurs is considering the purchase of a mini-mart franchise. Franchise A predicts that it will bring in a constant revenue stream of \$1,200,000 per year for 8 yr. Franchise B predicts that it will bring in a constant revenue stream of \$950,000 per year for 12 yr. Based on a comparison of accumulated present values, which franchise is the better buy, assuming the interest rate is 3.7%, compounded continuously, and both franchises have the same purchase price?

28. **Decision making.** A group of entrepreneurs is considering the purchase of an online business. Firm A predicts that it will bring in a constant revenue stream of \$80,000 per year for 10 yr. Firm B predicts that it will bring in a constant revenue stream of \$95,000 per year for 8 yr. Based on a comparison of accumulated present values, which firm is the better buy, assuming the interest rate is 4.1%, compounded continuously, and both firms have the same purchase price?

29. **Capital outlay.** Chrome Solutions determines that the rate of revenue coming in from its new software is

$$R_1(t) = 8000 - 100t,$$

in dollars per year, for 8 yr, after which the software will be replaced. The company learns that an alternative program will yield revenue at a rate of

$$R_2(t) = 7600 - 85t, \quad \text{for 8 yr.}$$

    a) Find the accumulated present value of the income stream from each program at an interest rate of 5.8%, compounded continuously.
    b) Find the difference in the accumulated present values.

30. **Decision making.** Jonathan has job offers from two employers. Syntech Solutions offers a salary of $\$100{,}000t$ for 8 yr, and Digitalis, Inc., offers a salary of $\$83{,}000t$ for 9 yr, where t is in years.
    a) Based on the accumulated present values of the salaries, which employer has the better offer, assuming an interest rate of 4.2%, compounded continuously?
    b) What signing bonus should the employer with the lower offer give to equalize the offers?

31. **Trust fund.** Ted and Edith have a new grandchild, Kurt, and want to create a trust fund for him that will yield $1,000,000 on his 22nd birthday.
    a) What lump sum should they deposit now at 3.2%, compounded continuously, to achieve $1,000,000?
    b) The amount in part (a) is more than they can afford, so they decide to invest a constant amount, $R(t)$ dollars per year. Find $R(t)$ such that the accumulated future value of the continuous money stream is $1,000,000, assuming an interest rate of 3.2%, compounded continuously.

32. **Trust fund.** Bob and Ann have a new grandchild, Brenda, and want to create a trust fund for her that will yield $250,000 on her 24th birthday.
    a) What lump sum should they deposit now at 2.85%, compounded continuously, to achieve $250,000?
    b) The amount in part (a) is more than they can afford, so they decide to invest a constant amount, $R(t)$ dollars per year. Find $R(t)$ such that the accumulated future value of the continuous money stream is $250,000, assuming an interest rate of 2.85%, compounded continuously.

33. **Early sports retirement.** Tory signs a 10-yr contract to play for a soccer team at a salary of $5,000,000 per year. After 6 yr, his skills deteriorate, and the team offers to buy out the rest of his contract. What is the least amount Tory should accept for the buyout, to the nearest dollar, assuming an interest rate of 2.9%, compounded continuously?

34. **Early retirement.** Lauren signs a 10-yr contract as a loan officer for a bank, at a salary of $84,000 per year. After 7 yr, the bank offers her early retirement. What is the least amount the bank should offer Lauren, to the nearest dollar, assuming an interest rate of 2.7%, compounded continuously?

35. **Disability insurance settlement.** Dale was a furnace maintenance employee who earned a salary of $70,000 per year before she was injured on the job. Through a settlement with her employer's insurance company, she is granted a continuous income stream of $40,000 per year for 25 yr. Dale invests the money at 3%, compounded continuously.
    a) Find the accumulated future value of the continuous income stream. Round the answer to the nearest $10.
    b) Thinking that she might not live for 25 yr, Dale negotiates a flat sum payment from the insurance company, which is the accumulated present value of the continuous stream plus $100,000. What is that amount? Round the answer to the nearest $10.

36. **Disability insurance settlement.** A movie stuntman who receives an annual salary of $180,000 per year is injured and can no longer work. Through a settlement with an insurance company, he is granted a continuous income stream of $120,000 per year for 20 yr. The stuntman invests the money at 4%, compounded continuously.
    a) Find the accumulated future value of the continuous income stream. Round your answer to the nearest $10.
    b) Thinking that he might not live 20 yr, the stuntman negotiates a flat sum payment from the insurance company, which is the accumulated present value of the continuous income stream. What is that amount? Round your answer to the nearest $10.

37. **Lottery winnings and risk analysis.** Lucky Larry wins $1,000,000 in a state lottery. The standard way in which a state pays such lottery winnings is at a constant rate of $50,000 per year for 20 yr.
    a) If Lucky invests each payment from the state at 4.4%, compounded continuously, what is the accumulated future value of the income stream? Round your answer to the nearest $10.
    b) What is the accumulated present value of the income stream at 4.4%, compounded continuously? This amount represents what the state needs to invest at the start of its lottery payments, assuming the 4.4% interest rate holds.
    c) The risk for Lucky is that he doesn't know how long he will live or what the future interest rate will be; it might vary considerably over 20 yr. This is the *risk* he assumes in accepting payments of $50,000 a year over 20 yr. Lucky has studied business calculus so he is aware of the formulas for accumulated future value and present value. He calculates the accumulated present value of the income stream for interest rates of 3%, 4%, and 5%. What values does he obtain?
    d) Lucky thinks "a bird in the hand (present value) is worth two in the bush (future value)" and decides to negotiate with the state for immediate payment of his lottery winnings. He asks the state for $750,000. They offer $600,000. Discuss the pros and cons of each amount. Lucky finally accepts $675,000. Is this a good decision? Why or why not?

38. **Negotiating a sports contract.** Slick O'Houlihan is a professional baseball player who has just become a free agent. His attorney begins negotiations with an interested team by asking for a contract that provides Slick with an income stream given by $R_1(t) = 800{,}000 + 340{,}000t$, over 10 yr, where t is in years. (Round all answers to the nearest $100.)
    a) What is the accumulated future value of the offer, assuming an interest rate of 3.5%, compounded continuously?
    b) What is the accumulated present value of the offer, assuming an interest rate of 3.5%, compounded continuously?

c) The team counters by offering an income stream given by $R_2(t) = 600{,}000 + 210{,}000t$. What is the accumulated present value of this counteroffer?

d) Slick comes back with a demand for an income stream given by $R_3(t) = 750{,}000 + 360{,}000t$. What is the accumulated present value of this income stream?

e) Slick signs a contract for the income stream in part (d) but decides to live on $500,000 each year, investing the rest at 3.5%, compounded continuously. What is the accumulated future value of the remaining income, assuming an interest rate of 3.5%, compounded continuously?

39. Accumulated present value. The Wilkinsons want to have $500,000 in 10 yr for a down payment on a retirement home. Find the continuous money stream, $R(t)$ dollars per year, that they need to invest at 3.33%, compounded continuously, to generate $500,000.

40. Accumulated present value. Tania wants to have $40,000 in 5 yr to open her own restaurant. Find the continuous money stream, $R(t)$ dollars per year, that she needs to invest at 4.1%, compounded continuously, to generate $40,000.

Life and Physical Sciences

41. Demand for natural gas. In 2016 ($t = 0$), U.S. consumption of natural gas was approximately 27.5 trillion cubic feet and was growing exponentially at about 0.73% per year. (*Source:* U.S. Energy Information Administration.) If the demand continues to grow at this rate, how many cubic feet of natural gas will the United States use from 2020 to 2025?

42. Demand for aluminum ore (bauxite). In 2016 ($t = 0$), bauxite production was approximately 274 million metric tons, and the demand was growing exponentially at a rate of 11.8% per year. (*Source:* minerals.usgs.gov.) If the demand continues to grow at this rate, how many metric tons of bauxite will the world use from 2016 to 2030?

43. Depletion of natural gas. The 2016 U.S. reserves of natural gas were approximately 2355 trillion cubic feet. (*Source:* www.eia.com.) Assuming that the growth described in Exercise 41 continues and that no new reserves are found, when will the U.S. reserves of natural gas be depleted?

44. Depletion of aluminum ore (bauxite). In 2016, the world reserves of bauxite were about 28 billion metric tons. (*Source:* U.S. Geological Survey summaries, Jan. 2017.) Assuming that the growth described in Exercise 42 continues and that no new reserves are discovered, when will the world reserves of bauxite be depleted?

45. Demand for and depletion of oil. In 2016, annual world demand for crude oil was approximately 34.6 billion barrels, and it was projected to increase by 5.6% per year. (*Sources:* Based on information from www.iea.gov and www.cia.gov.)

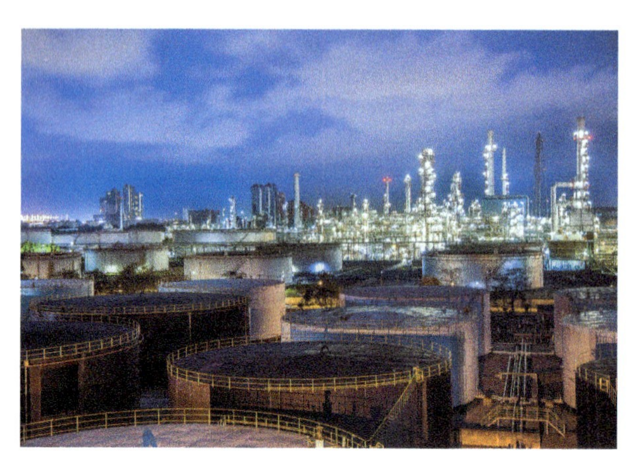

a) Assuming an exponential growth model, predict the demand in 2025.

b) World reserves of crude oil in 2016 were approximately 1492 billion barrels. Assuming that no new oil reserves are found, when will the reserves be depleted?

The model

$$\int_0^T Pe^{-kt}\,dt = \frac{P}{k}(1 - e^{-kT})$$

can be applied to calculate the buildup of a radioactive material that is being released into the atmosphere at a constant annual rate. Some of the material decays, but more continues to be released. The amount present at time T is given by the integral above, where P is the amount released per year and k is the half-life.

46. Radioactive buildup. Plutonium-239 has a decay rate of approximately 0.003% per year. Suppose plutonium-239 is released into the atmosphere for 20 yr at a constant rate of 1 lb per year. How much plutonium-239 will be present in the atmosphere after 20 yr?

47. Radioactive buildup. Cesium-137 has a decay rate of 2.3% per year. Suppose cesium-137 is released into the atmosphere for 20 yr at a rate of 1 lb per year. How much cesium-137 will be present in the atmosphere after 20 yr?

SYNTHESIS

Capitalized cost. *The capitalized cost, c, of an asset over its lifetime is the total of the initial cost and the present value of all maintenance expenses that will occur in the future. It is computed with the formula*

$$c = c_0 + \int_0^L m(t)e^{-kt}\,dt,$$

where c_0 is the initial cost of the asset, L is the lifetime (in years), k is the interest rate (compounded continuously), and m(t) is the annual cost of maintenance. In Exercises 48–51, find the capitalized cost under each set of assumptions.

48. $c_0 = \$500{,}000$, $k = 5\%$, $m(t) = \$20{,}000$, $L = 20$

49. $c_0 = \$400{,}000$, $k = 5.5\%$, $m(t) = \$10{,}000$, $L = 25$

50. $c_0 = \$600{,}000$, $k = 4\%$, $m(t) = \$40{,}000 + \$1000e^{0.01t}$, $L = 40$

51. $c_0 = \$300{,}000$, $k = 5\%$, $m(t) = \$30{,}000 + \$500t$, $L = 20$

52. How would you explain the concepts of present value and accumulated present value to a friend who has not studied this chapter?

53. Look up some data on rate of use and current world reserves of fresh water, iron, titanium, or phosphorus. Predict when the world reserves for that resource will be depleted.

Answers to Quick Checks

1. \$10,730.45 **2.** \$4,551,018 **3.** \$62,770.91 **4.** With R_1, accumulated future value is \$2,498,471, and accumulated present value is \$1,814,263. With R_2, accumulated future value is \$2,677,864, and accumulated present value is \$1,944,528. **5.** \$24,337.61, \$1896.75 **6.** \$12,198,227.08 **7. (a)** 299,470.00 metric tons; **(b)** 12.5 yr

5.3 Improper Integrals

- Show that an improper integral is convergent or divergent.
- Solve applied problems involving improper integrals.

Let's try to find the area under the graph of $y = 1/x^2$ over $[1, \infty)$. Note that this region is of infinite extent. To find the area of such a region, let's find the area over the interval from 1 to b, and then see what happens as b approaches ∞. The area under the graph over $[1, b]$ is

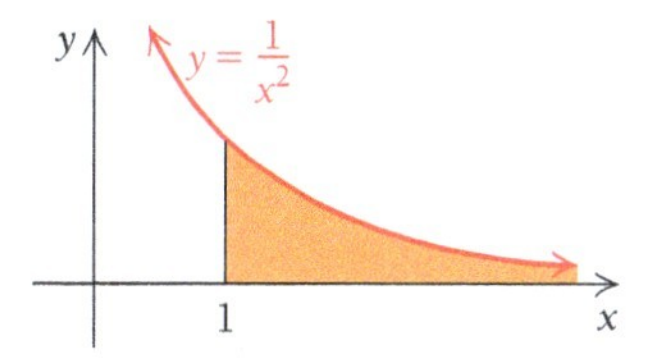

$$\int_1^b \frac{dx}{x^2} = \left[-\frac{1}{x}\right]_1^b$$
$$= \left(-\frac{1}{b}\right) - \left(-\frac{1}{1}\right)$$
$$= -\frac{1}{b} + 1$$
$$= 1 - \frac{1}{b}.$$

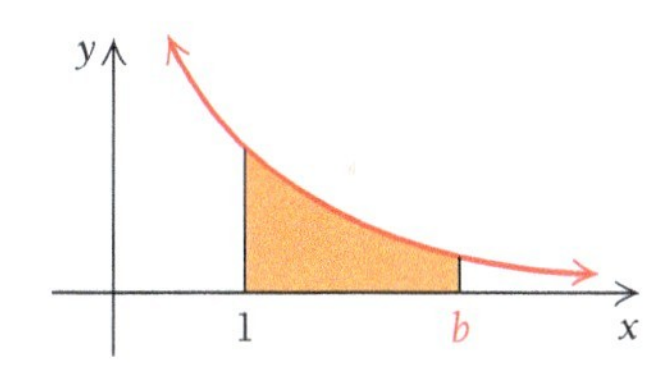

Then

$$\lim_{b\to\infty}\left(\int_1^b \frac{dx}{x^2}\right) = \lim_{b\to\infty}\left(1 - \frac{1}{b}\right) = 1.$$

We *define* the area from 1 to infinity to be this limit.

Similar areas may not be finite. Let's try to find the area under the graph of $y = \dfrac{1}{x}$ over $[1, \infty)$.

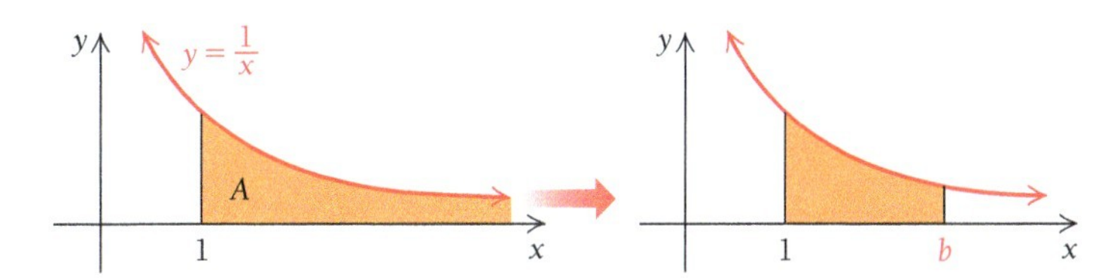

The area A, from 1 to infinity, is by definition the limit as b approaches ∞ of the area from 1 to b, so

$$A = \lim_{b\to\infty}\int_1^b \frac{dx}{x} = \lim_{b\to\infty}\left[\ln x\right]_1^b$$
$$= \lim_{b\to\infty}(\ln b - \ln 1)$$
$$= \lim_{b\to\infty}\ln b.$$

Technology Connection

Exploratory

1. Using a graphing calculator, find

$$\int_1^{10}\frac{dx}{x^3},$$
$$\int_1^{100}\frac{dx}{x^3}, \text{ and}$$
$$\int_1^{1000}\frac{dx}{x^3}.$$

2. Predict the value of

$$\int_1^{\infty}\frac{dx}{x^3}.$$

Technology Connection

Exploratory

1. Using a graphing calculator, find

$$\int_1^{10} \frac{dx}{x},$$

$$\int_1^{100} \frac{dx}{x},$$

$$\int_1^{1000} \frac{dx}{x},$$

and $\int_1^{10,000} \frac{dx}{x}$.

2. Based on the results from Exercise 1, predict the value of

$$\int_1^{\infty} \frac{dx}{x}.$$

In Section 2.1, we saw that the function $y = \ln x$ is always increasing. Therefore, the limit $\lim_{b \to \infty} \ln b$ approaches infinity. The area under $y = 1/x$ from 1 to infinity is infinite.

Note that the graphs of $y = 1/x^2$ and $y = 1/x$ have similar shapes over $[1, \infty)$, but the region under $y = 1/x^2$ has a finite area and the region under $y = 1/x$ does not.

An integral such as

$$\int_a^{\infty} f(x)\, dx,$$

with an upper limit of infinity, is an example of an **improper integral.** Its value is defined to be the following limit, if it exists.

DEFINITION

$$\int_a^{\infty} f(x)\, dx = \lim_{b \to \infty} \int_a^b f(x)\, dx$$

If the limit exists, then the improper integral **converges**, or is **convergent.** If the limit does not exist, then the improper integral **diverges**, or is **divergent.** Thus,

$$\int_1^{\infty} \frac{dx}{x^2} \text{ converges, and } \int_1^{\infty} \frac{dx}{x} \text{ diverges.}$$

In general, an improper integral of the form $\int_a^{\infty} \frac{1}{x^n}\, dx$, where $a > 0$, is convergent for $n > 1$ and is divergent for $n \le 1$. The proof is left as Exercise 59.

EXAMPLE 1 Determine whether each improper integral is convergent or divergent, and find its value if it is convergent.

a) $\int_1^{\infty} \frac{dx}{x^4}$ b) $\int_3^{\infty} \frac{dx}{\sqrt{x}}$ c) $\int_5^{\infty} \frac{x+1}{x^3}\, dx$

Solution

a) Since $4 > 1$, this improper integral is convergent. We have

$$\int_1^{\infty} \frac{dx}{x^4} = \lim_{b \to \infty} \int_1^b \frac{dx}{x^4}$$ Using the definition given above

$$= \lim_{b \to \infty} \left[-\frac{1}{3x^3}\right]_1^b$$ Note that $\int x^{-4}\, dx = -\frac{1}{3}x^{-3} + C$

$$= \lim_{b \to \infty} \left(-\frac{1}{3 \cdot b^3}\right) - \left(-\frac{1}{3 \cdot 1^3}\right)$$

$$= 0 - \left(-\frac{1}{3}\right)$$ Finding the limit as $b \to \infty$

$$= \frac{1}{3}.$$

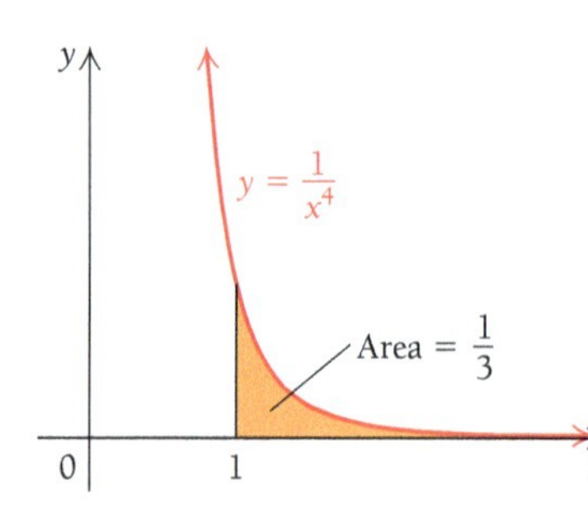

b) Since $\frac{1}{2} < 1$, the improper integral $\int_3^{\infty} \frac{dx}{\sqrt{x}}$ is divergent. The area represented by this integral is infinite.

c) We first simplify the integrand, then write the improper integral as a limit:

$$\int_5^{\infty} \frac{x+1}{x^3}\, dx = \int_5^{\infty} \left(\frac{x}{x^3} + \frac{1}{x^3}\right) dx = \int_5^{\infty} \left(\frac{1}{x^2} + \frac{1}{x^3}\right) dx,$$

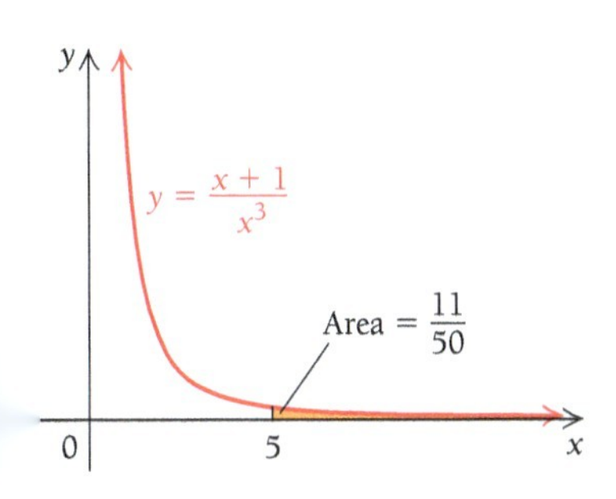

$$\text{and} \int_5^\infty \left(\frac{1}{x^2} + \frac{1}{x^3}\right) dx = \lim_{b\to\infty} \int_5^b \left(\frac{1}{x^2} + \frac{1}{x^3}\right) dx \quad \text{Using the definition given above}$$

$$= \lim_{b\to\infty}\left[-\frac{1}{x} - \frac{1}{2x^2}\right]_5^b$$

$$= \lim_{b\to\infty}\left(-\frac{1}{b} - \frac{1}{2b^2}\right) - \left(-\frac{1}{5} - \frac{1}{2(5)^2}\right)$$

$$= 0 + \frac{1}{5} + \frac{1}{50} \quad \text{Finding the limit as } b \to \infty$$

$$= \frac{11}{50}.$$

1 ✓

Quick Check 1 ✓

Determine whether each improper integral is convergent or divergent, and find its value if it is convergent.

a) $\int_2^\infty \frac{3}{x^5}\, dx$

b) $\int_7^\infty \frac{x+2}{x^2}\, dx$

EXAMPLE 2 Determine whether $\int_0^\infty 4e^{-2x}\, dx$ is convergent or divergent, and find its value if it is convergent.

Solution We have

$$\int_0^\infty 4e^{-2x}\, dx = \lim_{b\to\infty} \int_0^b 4e^{-2x}\, dx \quad \text{Using the definition given above}$$

$$= \lim_{b\to\infty}\left[\frac{4}{-2}e^{-2x}\right]_0^b$$

$$= \lim_{b\to\infty}\left[-2e^{-2x}\right]_0^b$$

$$= \lim_{b\to\infty}\left[-2e^{-2b} - (-2e^{-2\cdot 0})\right] \quad \text{Evaluating}$$

$$= \lim_{b\to\infty}\left(-2e^{-2b} + 2\right)$$

$$= \lim_{b\to\infty}\left(2 - \frac{2}{e^{2b}}\right).$$

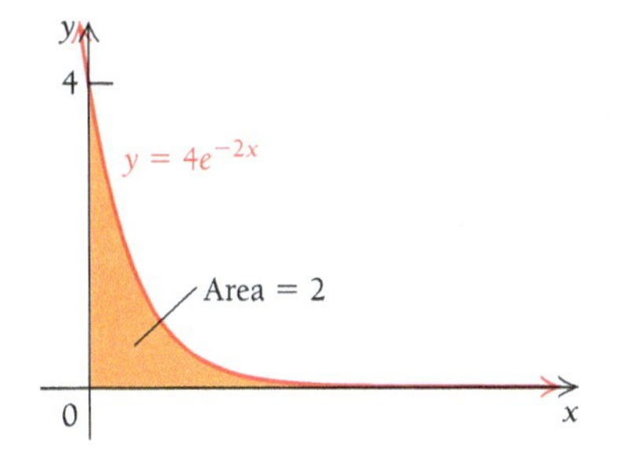

As b approaches ∞, we know that e^{2b} approaches ∞, so

$$\frac{2}{e^{2b}} \to 0 \quad \text{and} \quad \left(2 - \frac{2}{e^{2b}}\right) \to 2.$$

Thus, $$\int_0^\infty 4e^{-2x}\, dx = \lim_{b\to\infty}\left(2 - \frac{2}{e^{2b}}\right) = 2.$$

The integral is convergent.

2 ✓

Quick Check 2 ✓

Determine whether $\int_0^\infty 2e^{-5x}\, dx$ is convergent or divergent, and find its value if it is convergent.

Following are definitions of two other types of improper integrals.

DEFINITIONS

1. $$\int_{-\infty}^b f(x)\, dx = \lim_{a\to-\infty} \int_a^b f(x)\, dx$$

2. $$\int_{-\infty}^\infty f(x)\, dx = \int_{-\infty}^c f(x)\, dx + \int_c^\infty f(x)\, dx,$$

   where c can be any real number.

In order for $\int_{-\infty}^\infty f(x)\, dx$ to converge, both $\int_{-\infty}^c f(x)\, dx$ and $\int_c^\infty f(x)\, dx$ must converge.

Applications of Improper Integrals

In Section 5.2, we learned that the accumulated present value of a continuous money flow (income stream) of P dollars per year, at a constant rate, from now until T years in the future can be found using

$$\int_0^T Pe^{-kt}\,dt = \frac{P}{k}(1 - e^{-kT}),$$

where k is the interest rate and interest is compounded continuously. Suppose that the money flow is to continue perpetually (forever). Under this assumption, the accumulated present value of the money flow is

$$\begin{aligned}\int_0^\infty Pe^{-kt}\,dt &= \lim_{T\to\infty}\int_0^T Pe^{-kt}\,dt = \lim_{T\to\infty}\frac{P}{k}(1 - e^{-kT})\\ &= \lim_{T\to\infty}\frac{P}{k}\left(1 - \frac{1}{e^{kT}}\right)\\ &= \frac{P}{k}(1 - 0) \qquad \text{Taking the limit as } T\to\infty\\ &= \frac{P}{k}.\end{aligned}$$

THEOREM 1

The **accumulated present value** of a continuous money flow into an investment at the constant rate of P dollars per year perpetually is given by

$$\int_0^\infty Pe^{-kt}\,dt = \frac{P}{k},$$

where k is the annual interest rate, compounded continuously.

Quick Check 3 ✓

Find the accumulated present value of an investment for which there is a perpetual continuous money flow of \$10,000 per year. Assume that the interest rate is 3.5%, compounded continuously.

EXAMPLE 3 **Business: Accumulated Present Value.** Find the accumulated present value of an investment for which there is a perpetual continuous money flow of \$2000 per year. Assume that the interest rate is 5%, compounded continuously.

Solution Using Theorem 1, we see that the accumulated present value is $2000/0.05$, or \$40,000. **3 ✓**

Technology Connection 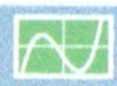

Exploratory

We can explore the situation of Example 3 with a calculator. To evaluate $\int_0^\infty 2000e^{-0.05x}\,dx$, we first consider

$$\int_0^t 2000e^{-0.05x}\,dx = \frac{2000}{0.05}(1 - e^{-0.05t}).$$

Then we examine what happens as t approaches infinity. Graph

$$f(x) = \frac{2000}{0.05}(1 - e^{-0.05x})$$

using the window [0, 10, 0, 50000], with Xscl = 1 and Yscl = 5000. On the same set of axes, graph $y = 40{,}000$. Then change the viewing window to [0, 50, 0, 50000], with Xscl = 10 and Yscl = 5000, and finally to [0, 100, 0, 50000]. What happens as x gets larger? What is the significance of 40,000?

When an amount P of radioactive material is being released into the atmosphere annually, the total amount that has been released up to time T is given by

$$\int_0^T Pe^{-kt}\,dt = \frac{P}{k}(1 - e^{-kT}).$$

As T approaches infinity (the radioactive material is released forever), the buildup of radioactive material approaches a limiting value P/k. It is no wonder that scientists and environmentalists are so concerned about radioactive waste. The radioactivity is "here to stay."

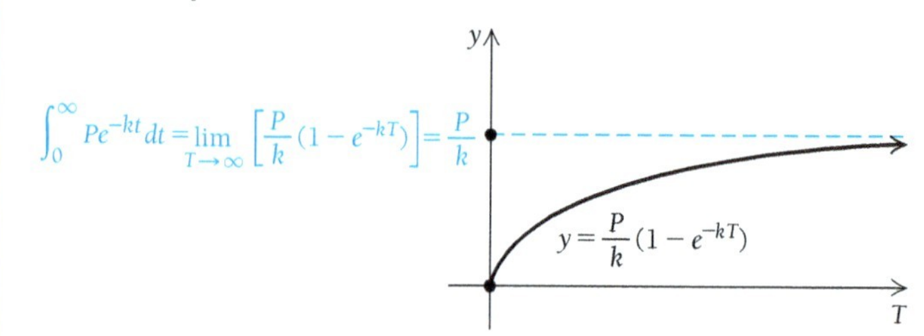

Section Summary

- An *improper integral* has infinity as one or both of its bounds and is evaluated using

$$\int_a^\infty f(x)\,dx = \lim_{b\to\infty}\int_a^b f(x)\,dx,$$

$$\int_{-\infty}^b f(x)\,dx = \lim_{a\to-\infty}\int_a^b f(x)\,dx,$$

and $$\int_{-\infty}^\infty f(x)\,dx = \int_{-\infty}^c f(x)\,dx + \int_c^\infty f(x)\,dx,$$

where c is any real number.

- The *accumulated present value* of a continuous money flow into an investment at the rate of P dollars per year perpetually is given by

$$\int_0^\infty Pe^{-kt}\,dt = \frac{P}{k},$$

where k is the annual interest rate, compounded continuously.

5.3 Exercise Set

Determine whether each improper integral is convergent or divergent, and find its value if it is convergent.

1. $\displaystyle\int_3^\infty \frac{dx}{x^2}$

2. $\displaystyle\int_5^\infty \frac{dx}{x^2}$

3. $\displaystyle\int_3^\infty \frac{dx}{x}$

4. $\displaystyle\int_4^\infty \frac{dx}{x}$

5. $\displaystyle\int_0^\infty 4e^{-4x}\,dx$

6. $\displaystyle\int_0^\infty 3e^{-3x}\,dx$

7. $\displaystyle\int_1^\infty \frac{dx}{x^3}$

8. $\displaystyle\int_1^\infty \frac{dx}{x^4}$

9. $\displaystyle\int_0^\infty \frac{4\,dx}{3+x}$

10. $\displaystyle\int_0^\infty \frac{dx}{2+x}$

11. $\displaystyle\int_2^\infty 4x^{-2}\,dx$

12. $\displaystyle\int_2^\infty 7x^{-2}\,dx$

13. $\displaystyle\int_0^\infty e^{2x}\,dx$

14. $\displaystyle\int_0^\infty e^{x}\,dx$

15. $\displaystyle\int_3^\infty x^2\,dx$

16. $\displaystyle\int_5^\infty x^4\,dx$

17. $\displaystyle\int_1^\infty \ln x\,dx$

18. $\displaystyle\int_0^\infty xe^{x}\,dx$

19. $\displaystyle\int_0^\infty Qe^{-kt}\,dt,\ k>0$

20. $\displaystyle\int_0^\infty me^{-mx}\,dx,\ m>0$

21. $\displaystyle\int_1^\infty \frac{dt}{t^{1.001}}$

22. $\displaystyle\int_1^\infty \frac{2t}{t^2+1}\,dt$

23. $\displaystyle\int_1^\infty \frac{3x^2}{(x^3+1)^2}\,dx$

24. $\displaystyle\int_{-\infty}^\infty t\,dt$

25. $\displaystyle\int_2^\infty \frac{x+3}{x^4}\,dx$

26. $\displaystyle\int_4^\infty \frac{2x-1}{x^3}\,dx$

27. $\displaystyle\int_1^\infty \frac{x+10}{x^2}\,dx$

28. $\displaystyle\int_6^\infty \frac{5x-2}{x^2}\,dx$

29. Find the area, if it is finite, of the region under the graph of $y = 1/x^2$ over $\left[\frac{1}{2}, \infty\right)$.

30. Find the area, if it is finite, of the region under the graph of $y = 1/x$ over $[2, \infty)$.

31. Find the area, if it is finite, of the region under the graph of $y = 2xe^{-x^2}$ over $[0, \infty)$.

32. Find the area, if it is finite, of the region under the graph of $y = 1/\sqrt{(3x-2)^3}$ over $[6, \infty)$.

APPLICATIONS

Business and Economics

33. **Total profit from marginal profit.** Myna's Fashions determines that its marginal profit, in dollars per shawl, from producing x shawls is given by

$$P'(x) = 200{,}000e^{-0.032x}.$$

Suppose it were possible for this firm to make infinitely many shawls. What would its total profit be?

34. **Total profit from marginal profit.** Find the total profit in Exercise 33 if

$$P'(x) = 200{,}000x^{-1.032}, \quad \text{where } x \ge 1.$$

35. **Total production.** A firm determines that it can produce $r(t)$ tires per year, where

$$r(t) = (2\times 10^6)e^{-0.42t},$$

and t is in years. Assuming that the firm endures forever (it never gets tired), how many tires can it make?

36. **Total cost from marginal cost.** Barton Novelties determines that its marginal cost, in dollars per keyholder, for producing x keyholders is given by

$$C'(x) = 3{,}600{,}000x^{-1.8}, \quad \text{where } x \ge 1.$$

Suppose it were possible for this company to make infinitely many keyholders. What would the total cost be?

37. **Accumulated present value.** Find the accumulated present value of an investment for which there is a perpetual continuous money flow of \$3500 per year at an interest rate of 3.1%, compounded continuously.

38. **Accumulated present value.** Find the accumulated present value of an investment for which there is a perpetual continuous money flow of \$3600 per year at an interest rate of 2.5%, compounded continuously.

39. **Accumulated present value.** Find the accumulated present value of an investment for which there is a perpetual continuous money flow of $\$2000e^{-0.01t}$ per year, assuming continuously compounded interest at a rate of 1.88%.

40. **Accumulated present value.** Find the accumulated present value of an investment for which there is a perpetual continuous money flow of \$5000 per year, assuming continuously compounded interest at a rate of 3.7%.

Capitalized cost. *The capitalized cost, c, of an asset for an unlimited lifetime is the total of the initial cost and the present value of all maintenance expenses that will occur in the future. It is computed with the formula*

$$c = c_0 + \int_0^{\infty} m(t)e^{-kt}\,dt,$$

where c_0 is the initial cost of the asset, k is the interest rate (compounded continuously), and $m(t)$ is the annual cost of maintenance. Find the capitalized cost under each set of assumptions.

41. $c_0 = \$700{,}000, \quad k = 3.07\%, \quad m(t) = \$30{,}000$

42. $c_0 = \$500{,}000, \quad k = 2.75\%, \quad m(t) = \$20{,}000$

Life and Physical Sciences

43. **Radioactive buildup.** Plutonium has a decay rate of 0.003% per year. Suppose a nuclear accident causes plutonium to be released into the atmosphere perpetually at the rate of 1 lb per year. What is the limiting value of the radioactive buildup?

44. **Radioactive buildup.** Cesium-137 has a decay rate of 2.3% per year. Suppose a nuclear accident causes cesium-137 to be released into the atmosphere perpetually at the rate of 1 lb per year. What is the limiting value of the radioactive buildup?

Radioactive implant treatments. *In the treatment of prostate cancer, radioactive implants are often used. The implants are left in the patient and never removed. The amount of energy that is transmitted to the body from the implant is measured in rem units and is given by*

$$E = \int_0^{a} P_0 e^{-kt}\,dt,$$

where k is the decay constant for the radioactive material, t is the number of years since the implant, a is the time (in years) until the rem measurement is made, and P_0 is the initial rate at which energy is transmitted. (Source: www.cancer.gov.) Use this information for Exercises 45 and 46.

45. Suppose the treatment uses iodine-125, which has a half-life of 60.1 days.
    a) Find the annual decay rate, k, of iodine-125.
    b) How much energy (measured in rems) is transmitted in the first month if the initial rate of transmission is 10 rems per year?
    c) What is the total amount of energy that the implant will transmit to the body?

46. Suppose the treatment uses palladium-103, which has a half-life of 16.99 days.
    a) Find the annual decay rate, k, of palladium-103.
    b) How much energy (measured in rems) is transmitted in the first month if the initial rate of transmission is 10 rems per year?
    c) What is the total amount of energy that the implant will transmit to the body?

SYNTHESIS

Determine whether each improper integral is convergent or divergent, and find its value if it is convergent.

47. $\displaystyle\int_3^{\infty} \frac{dx}{x^{2/3}}$

48. $\displaystyle\int_1^{\infty} \frac{dx}{\sqrt[4]{x}}$

49. $\displaystyle\int_0^{\infty} \frac{dx}{(x+1)^{3/2}}$

50. $\displaystyle\int_{-\infty}^{0} e^{2x}\,dx$

51. $\displaystyle\int_0^{\infty} xe^{-x}\,dx$

52. $\displaystyle\int_{-\infty}^{\infty} xe^{-x^2}\,dx$

Life science: drug dosage. *Suppose an oral dose of a drug is taken. Over time, the drug is assimilated in the body and excreted through the urine. The total amount of the drug that has passed through the body in T hours is given by*

$$\int_0^{T} E(t)\,dt,$$

where $E(t)$ is the rate of excretion of the drug. A typical rate-of-excretion function is $E(t) = te^{-kt}$, where $k > 0$ and t is the time, in hours. Use this information for Exercises 53 and 54.

53. Find $\int_0^{\infty} E(t)\,dt$, and interpret the answer. That is, what does the integral represent?

54. A physician prescribes a dosage of 100 mg. Find k.

Another form of improper integral occurs when a vertical asymptote appears at one of the bounds of integration. For example, to find the area under $f(x) = \dfrac{1}{\sqrt{x}}$ over $[0, 4]$, we note that f is not defined at $x = 0$ and that there is a vertical asymptote as x approaches 0 from the right. In such a case, we integrate over $[a, 4]$ and find the limit as a approaches 0 from the right. Use this technique for Exercises 55 and 56.

55. Find $\displaystyle\int_0^{4} \frac{1}{\sqrt{x}}\,dx.$

56. Find $\displaystyle\int_4^{5} \frac{3}{\sqrt[3]{x-5}}\,dx.$

57. Find n such that $\displaystyle\int_1^{\infty} \frac{1}{x^n}\,dx = \frac{2}{3}.$

58. Find a such that $\displaystyle\int_a^{\infty} \frac{1}{x^2}\,dx = \frac{3}{4}.$

59. Show that $\int_a^{\infty} \frac{1}{x^n}\,dx$, where $a > 0$, is convergent for $n > 1$ and is divergent for $n \le 1$.

60. Suppose you own a building that yields a continuous series of rental payments and you decide to sell the building. Explain how you would use the concept of the accumulated present value of a perpetual continuous money flow to determine a fair selling price.

61. Find and explain the error in the following calculation:

$$\int_{-1}^{2} \frac{1}{x^2}\,dx = \left[-\frac{1}{x}\right]_{-1}^{2} = \left(-\frac{1}{2}\right) - \left(-\frac{1}{(-1)}\right) = -\frac{3}{2}.$$

62. Explain why $\int_0^{\infty} \frac{dx}{\sqrt{x^2+1}}$ is divergent.

63. Suppose that $\int_1^{\infty} f(x)\,dx$ is convergent, where $f(x) > 0$ over $[1, \infty)$.

a) If $0 < g(x) \le f(x)$ over $[1, \infty)$, explain why $\int_1^{\infty} g(x)\,dx$ must also be convergent.

b) If $g(x) \ge f(x)$ over $[1, \infty)$, explain why $\int_1^{\infty} g(x)\,dx$ is not necessarily divergent.

64. Suppose that $\int_1^{\infty} f(x)\,dx$ is divergent, where $f(x) > 0$ over $[1, \infty)$.

a) If $0 < g(x) \le f(x)$ over $[1, \infty)$, explain why $\int_1^{\infty} g(x)\,dx$ is not necessarily convergent.

b) If $g(x) \ge f(x)$ over $[1, \infty)$, explain why $\int_1^{\infty} g(x)\,dx$ must also be divergent.

Technology Connection 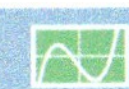

Approximate each integral.

65. $\int_1^{\infty} \frac{4}{1+x^2}\,dx$

66. $\int_1^{\infty} \frac{6}{5+e^x}\,dx$

67. $\int_{-\infty}^{\infty} \frac{1}{1+x^2}\,dx$

68. $\int_{-\infty}^{\infty} e^{-x^2}\,dx$

Answers to Quick Checks

1. (a) Convergent, $\frac{3}{64}$; **(b)** divergent
2. Convergent, $\frac{2}{5}$ **3.** \$285,714.29

5.4

- Verify certain properties of probability density functions.
- Solve applied problems involving probability density functions.

Probability

A number from 0 to 1 that represents the likelihood of an event occurring is referred to as the event's **probability**. A probability of 0 means that the event is certain *not* to occur, and a probability of 1 means that the event is certain to occur. In this section, we will see that integration is a useful tool for calculating some probabilities.

Experimental and Theoretical Probability

There are two types of probability, *experimental* and *theoretical*.

If we toss a coin a high number of times—say, 1000—and count the number of times we get heads, we can determine the probability of the coin landing heads up. If it lands heads up 503 times, we calculate the probability of it landing heads up to be

$$\frac{503}{1000}, \quad \text{or} \quad 0.503.$$

This is an **experimental** determination of probability. Such a determination is made through observation and study of data and is quite common and useful. For example, here are some probabilities that have been determined experimentally:

1. The lifetime probability (assuming a life span of 80 years) of being struck by lightning is about $\frac{1}{13{,}500}$. (*Source*: www.noaa.gov.)
2. According to one study, a person who is released from prison has a probability of 67.8% of returning to prison within 3 years. (*Source*: www.nij.gov.)
3. The probability that a basketball player will make a free throw is based on his or her past success rate (number of free throws made divided by total number of free throws attempted).

If we consider tossing a coin and reason that we are just as likely to get heads as tails, we would *calculate* the probability of it landing heads up to be $\frac{1}{2}$, or 0.5. This is a

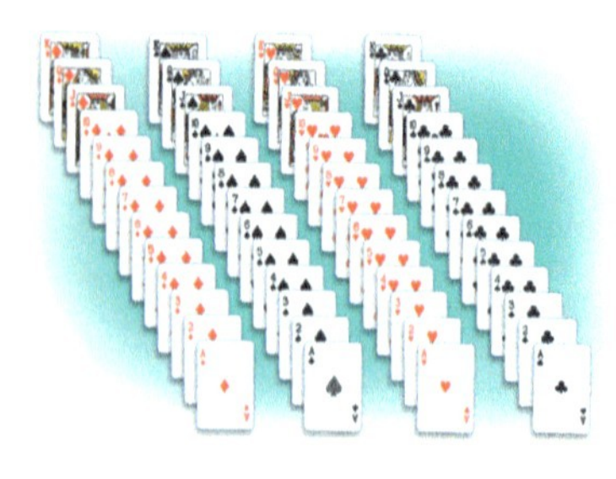

A desire to calculate odds in games of chance gave rise to the theory of probability.

theoretical determination of probability. Here, for example, are some probabilities that have been determined theoretically, using mathematics:

1. In any random group of 30 people, the probability that at least two of them have the same birthday (excluding year) is 0.706.
2. The probability of winning the Powerball lottery is $\frac{1}{175{,}223{,}510}$. (*Source:* powerball.com.)
3. The probability that two cards drawn from a standard deck of 52 cards (as shown at left) are both kings is $\frac{1}{221}$.

In summary, experimental probabilities are determined from observations and data. Theoretical probabilities are determined by mathematical reasoning. There are situations in which it is easier to determine one type of probability than the other. For example, it would be difficult to determine the theoretical probability of catching a cold.

In the discussion that follows, we consider primarily theoretical probabilities.

Quick Check 1 ✓

What is the probability of drawing each of the following from a well-shuffled deck of cards?

a) a three

b) a heart

c) the three of hearts

EXAMPLE 1 What is the probability of drawing an ace from a well-shuffled deck of cards?

Solution There are 52 possible cards that could be drawn, and each card has the same chance of being drawn. Since there are 4 aces, the probability of drawing an ace is $\frac{4}{52}$, or $\frac{1}{13}$, or about 7.7%. **1 ✓**

Quick Check 2 ✓

Assume that a jar has the same assortment of gumballs as in Example 2 and 1 gumball is randomly selected.

a) What is the probability that it is black or yellow?

b) What is the probability that it is not green?

EXAMPLE 2 A jar contains 7 black, 6 yellow, 4 green, and 3 red gumballs, all the same size and weight. The jar is shaken well, and 1 gumball is randomly selected.

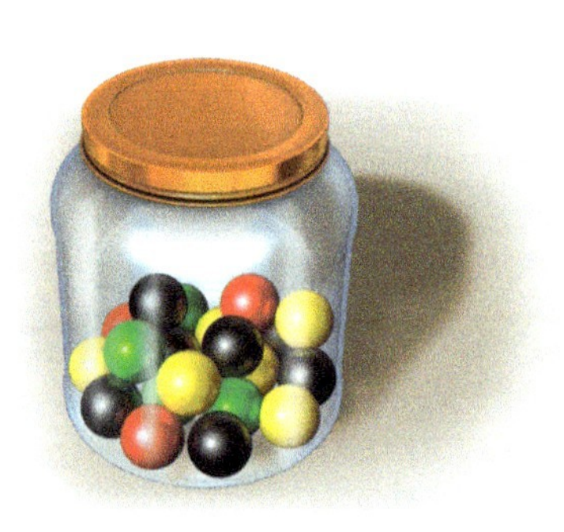

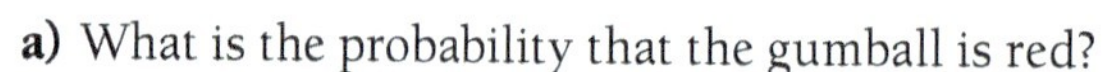

a) What is the probability that the gumball is red?

b) What is the probability that it is white?

Solution

a) There are 20 gumballs, of which 3 are red; so the probability of selecting a red one is $\frac{3}{20}$.

b) There are no white gumballs, so the probability of selecting a white one is $\frac{0}{20}$, or 0. **2 ✓**

Below is a table of probabilities for the situation in Example 2. Note that the sum of these probabilities is 1. We are certain that we will select a black, yellow, green, or red gumball, so the probability of that event is 1. We can arrange the data from the table into what is called a **relative frequency graph**, or **histogram**, which shows the proportion of times that each event occurs (the probability of each event). If we assign a width of 1 to each rectangle in this graph, then the sum of the areas of the rectangles is 1.

Color	Probability
Black (B)	$\frac{7}{20}$
Yellow (Y)	$\frac{6}{20}$
Green (G)	$\frac{4}{20}$
Red (R)	$\frac{3}{20}$

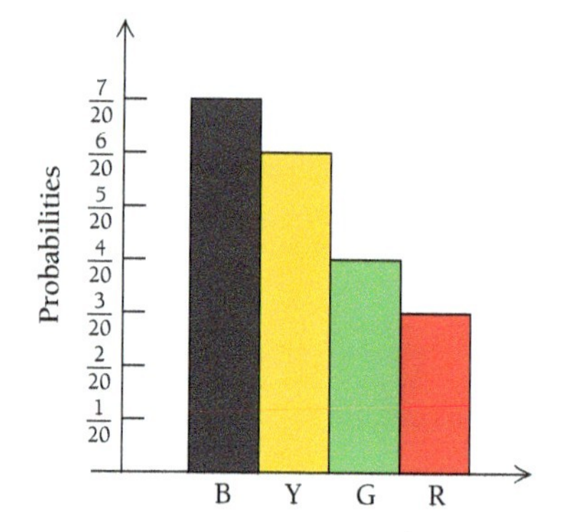

Continuous Random Variables

Suppose that we throw a dart at a number line in such a way that it always lands in the interval [3, 5]. Let x be the number where the dart lands. There is an infinite number of possibilities for x. Note that x can be observed (or measured) repeatedly and its possible values comprise an interval of real numbers. Such a variable is an example of a **continuous random variable**.

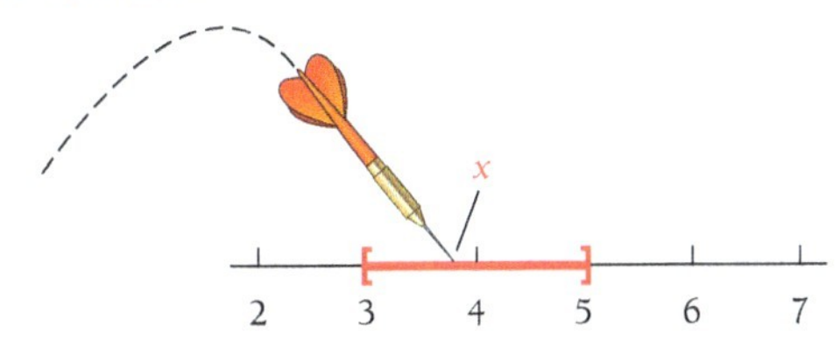

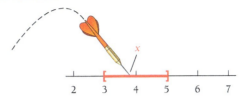

Suppose we throw the dart a large number of times and it lands 70% of the time in the subinterval [3.6, 4.8]. We can then conclude that the experimental probability of the dart landing in [3.6, 4.8] is 0.7.

Let's consider some other examples of continuous random variables.

- If x is the temperature at any point on Earth, with −128.6°F the lowest temperature ever recorded (at Vostok Station, Antarctica, in 1983) and 134°F the highest ever recorded (at Death Valley, California, in 1913), then x is a continuous random variable distributed over $[-128.6, 134]$. (*Source*: www.ncdc.noaa.gov.)

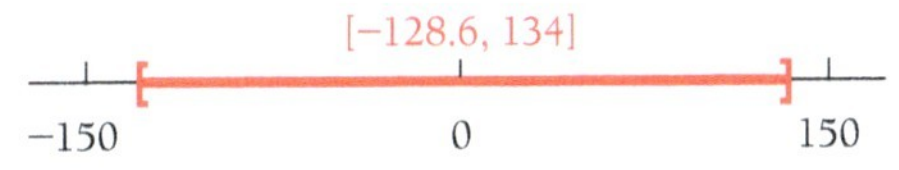

- If x is the volume, in milliliters, of fruit juice in a bottle, and any bottle with at least 498 mL and at most 505 mL of juice will pass quality control, then x is a continuous random variable distributed over [498, 505].

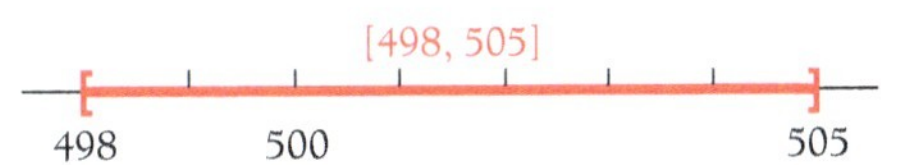

- If buses traveling from Philadelphia to Baltimore require at least 2 hr and at most 5 hr for the trip and x is the number of hours a bus takes to make the trip, then x is a continuous random variable distributed over [2, 5].

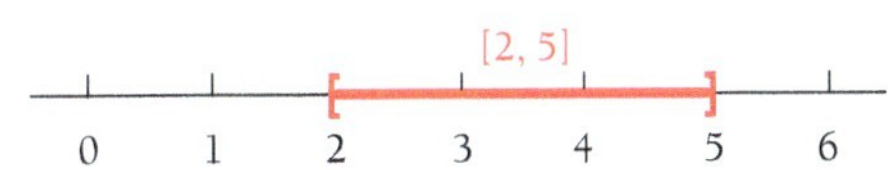

Probability Density Functions

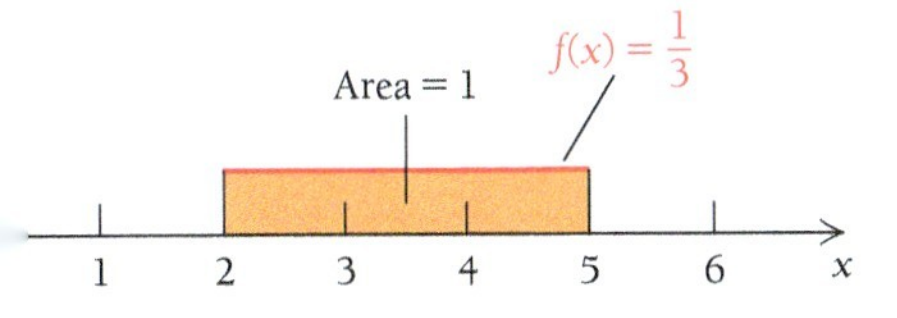

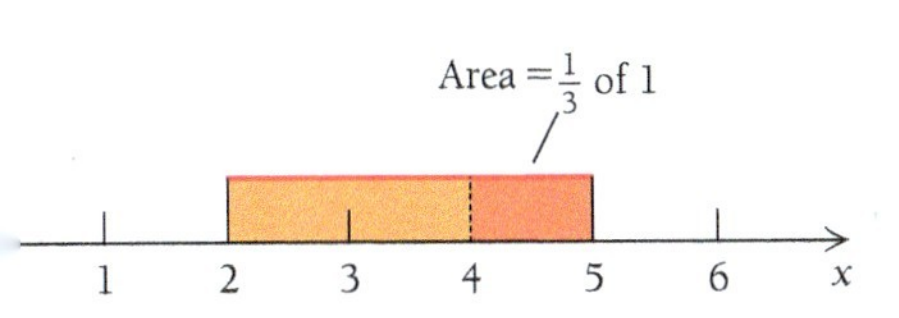

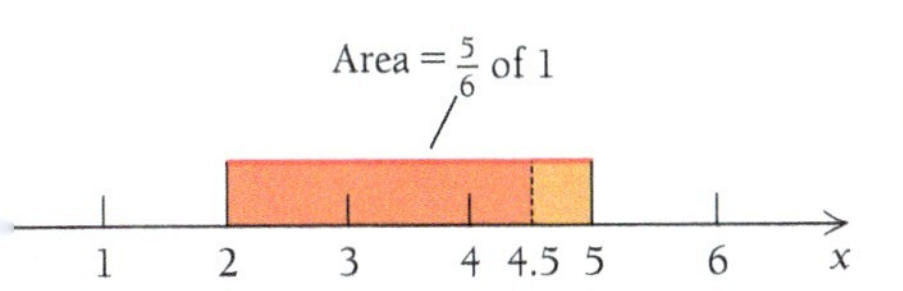

There may be a nonnegative function $y = f(x)$ defined over an interval $[a, b]$ such that the area under any subinterval gives the probability of x occurring in that subinterval. For example, suppose we let $f(x) = \frac{1}{3}$ over the interval [2, 5], describing the trip times for buses between Philadelphia and Baltimore. This indicates that all trip times from 2 hr to 5 hr are equally likely to occur. The area under the graph is $3 \cdot \frac{1}{3}$, or 1.

Using this graph, the probability that a trip takes 4 hr to 5 hr is the area that lies over the subinterval [4, 5]. That is,

$$P([4, 5]) = \tfrac{1}{3} = 33\tfrac{1}{3}\%.$$

The probability that a trip takes between 2 hr and 4.5 hr is $\frac{5}{6}$, or $83\frac{1}{3}\%$. This is the area of the rectangle over [2, 4.5].

Note that when $f(x) = \frac{1}{3}$, any interval between the numbers 2 and 5 of width 1 has probability $\frac{1}{3}$. This does not happen for all functions.

Suppose instead that

$$f(x) = \tfrac{3}{117}x^2, \quad \text{over } [2, 5].$$

Technology Connection 

Exploratory

Graph the function

$$f(x) = \tfrac{3}{117}x^2$$

using [0, 5, 0, 1] as the viewing window. Then successively evaluate each of the following integrals, shading the appropriate area if possible:

$$\int_2^3 \tfrac{3}{117}x^2\,dx,$$

$$\int_3^4 \tfrac{3}{117}x^2\,dx,$$

and $\int_4^5 \tfrac{3}{117}x^2\,dx.$

Add your results, and explain what the sum represents.

The area under the graph of f from 4 to 5 is given by the definite integral over [4, 5] and yields the probability that a trip takes 4 hr to 5 hr.

We have

$$P([4,5]) = \int_4^5 f(x)\,dx$$

$$= \int_4^5 \frac{3}{117}x^2\,dx$$

$$= \frac{1}{117}\Big[x^3\Big]_4^5$$

$$= \frac{1}{117}(5^3 - 4^3)$$

$$= \frac{61}{117} \approx 0.52.$$

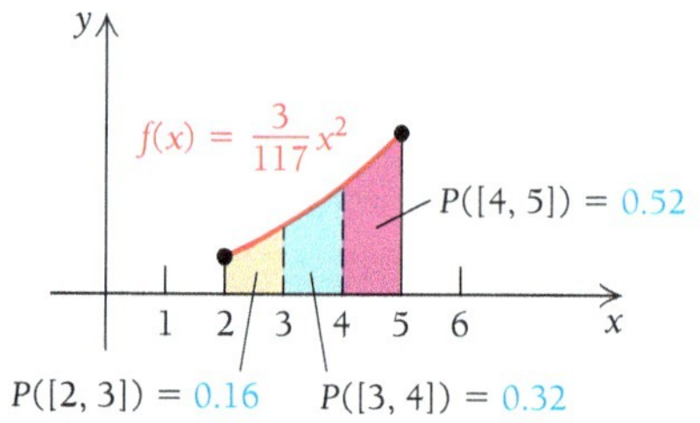

Thus, according to this model, there is a probability of 0.52 that a bus trip takes 4 hr to 5 hr. The function f is called a *probability density function*. Its integral over any subinterval gives the probability that x "lands" in that subinterval.

Similar calculations for the bus trip example are shown in the following table.

Trip Time	Probability That a Trip Time Occurs During the Interval
2 hr to 3 hr	$P([2,3]) = \int_2^3 \tfrac{3}{117}x^2\,dx \approx 0.16$
3 hr to 4 hr	$P([3,4]) = \int_3^4 \tfrac{3}{117}x^2\,dx \approx 0.32$
4 hr to 5 hr	$P([4,5]) = \int_4^5 \tfrac{3}{117}x^2\,dx \approx 0.52$
2 hr to 5 hr	$P([2,5]) = \int_2^5 \tfrac{3}{117}x^2\,dx = 1.00$

It is certain (probability = 1) that a bus trip will take between 2 hr and 5 hr.

The results in the table lead us to the following definition of a probability density function.

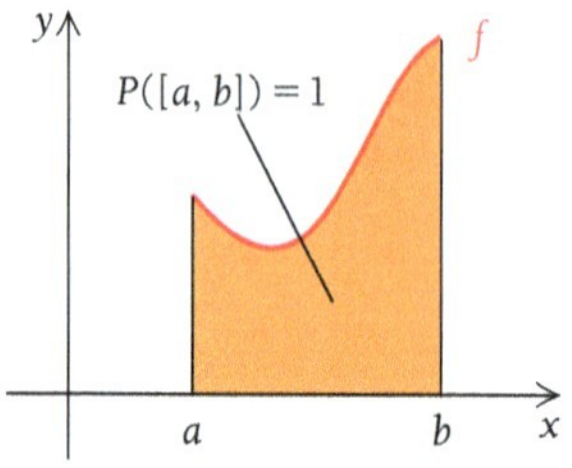

FIGURE 1

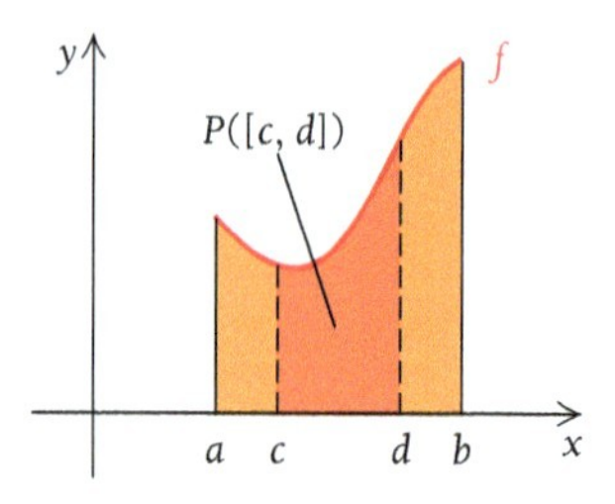

FIGURE 2

DEFINITION

Let x be a continuous random variable. A function f is said to be a **probability density function** for x if:

1. For all x in the domain of f, we have $f(x) \geq 0$.
2. The area under the graph of f is 1 (see Fig. 1).
3. For any subinterval $[c, d]$ in the domain of f (see Fig. 2), the probability that x will be in that subinterval is given by

$$P([c,d]) = \int_c^d f(x)\,dx.$$

EXAMPLE 3 Verify that Property 2 of the definition of a probability density function holds for

$$f(x) = \frac{3}{117}x^2, \quad \text{for } 2 \le x \le 5.$$

Solution We need to show that the area under f over $[2, 5]$ is 1.

$$\begin{aligned}\int_2^5 \frac{3}{117}x^2\,dx &= \frac{3}{117}\left[\frac{1}{3}x^3\right]_2^5 \\ &= \frac{1}{117}\left[x^3\right]_2^5 \\ &= \frac{1}{117}(5^3 - 2^3) \\ &= \frac{117}{117} = 1\end{aligned}$$

Quick Check 3 ✓

Assume that x is a continuous random variable. Verify that $g(x) = \frac{3}{14}\sqrt{x}$, for $1 \le x \le 4$, is a probability density function.

3 ✓

EXAMPLE 4 **Business: Life of a Product.** Luminox Corp. produces rechargeable LED batteries and determines that the life t of a battery is from 3 to 6 yr, with the probability density function for t given by

$$f(t) = \frac{24}{t^3}, \quad \text{for } 3 \le t \le 6.$$

a) Verify Property 2 of the definition of a probability density function.

b) Find the probability that a battery will last no more than 4 yr.

c) Find the probability that a battery will last at least 4 yr and at most 5 yr.

Solution

a) We must show that $\int_3^6 f(t)\,dt = 1$. We have

$$\begin{aligned}\int_3^6 \frac{24}{t^3}\,dt &= -12\left[\frac{1}{t^2}\right]_3^6 && \text{Integrating: } 24\left[\frac{t^{-2}}{-2}\right] = -12\left[\frac{1}{t^2}\right] \\ &= -12\left(\frac{1}{6^2} - \frac{1}{3^2}\right) && \text{Substituting} \\ &= -12\left(-\frac{3}{36}\right) = 1. && \text{Simplifying}\end{aligned}$$

Since the probability is 1, it is certain that the life of a battery is between 3 yr and 6 yr.

b) The probability that a battery will last no more than 4 yr is

$$\begin{aligned}P(3 \le t \le 4) &= \int_3^4 \frac{24}{t^3}\,dt \\ &= -12\left[\frac{1}{t^2}\right]_3^4 \\ &= -12\left(\frac{1}{4^2} - \frac{1}{3^2}\right) && \text{Substituting} \\ &= -12\left(-\frac{7}{144}\right) = \frac{7}{12} \approx 0.58. && \text{Simplifying}\end{aligned}$$

c) The probability that a battery will last at least 4 yr and at most 5 yr is

$$P(4 \le t \le 5) = \int_4^5 \frac{24}{t^3}\,dt$$
$$= -12\left[\frac{1}{t^2}\right]_4^5$$
$$= -12\left(\frac{1}{5^2} - \frac{1}{4^2}\right) \quad \text{Substituting}$$
$$= -12\left(-\frac{9}{400}\right)$$
$$= \frac{27}{100} = 0.27. \quad \text{Simplifying}$$

4 ✓

Quick Check 4 ✓

The time between arrivals of subway trains at a station is modeled by the probability density function

$$h(x) = \frac{10}{x^2}, \quad \text{for } 5 \le x \le 10,$$

where x is in minutes. Find the probability that:

a) the time between trains is between 5 and 7 min;

b) the time between trains is between 8 and 10 min.

Constructing Probability Density Functions

Suppose that $f(x)$ is nonnegative over $[a, b]$ and that

$$\int_a^b f(x)\,dx = K.$$

Multiplying both sides by $1/K$ gives

$$\frac{1}{K}\int_a^b f(x)\,dx = \frac{1}{K}\cdot K = 1, \quad \text{or} \quad \int_a^b \frac{1}{K}\cdot f(x)\,dx = 1.$$

Thus, when we multiply $f(x)$ by $1/K$, we have a function whose area over $[a, b]$ is 1. Such a function satisfies the definition of a probability density function.

EXAMPLE 5 Find k such that

$$f(x) = kx^2$$

is a probability density function over the interval $[1, 4]$. Then write the probability density function.

Solution Note that for $k \ge 0$, we have $kx^2 \ge 0$. For f to be a probability density function, we must also have $\int_1^4 kx^2\,dx = 1$. Since

$$\int_1^4 kx^2\,dx = k\left[\tfrac{1}{3}x^3\right]_1^4 = k\left[\tfrac{64}{3} - \tfrac{1}{3}\right] = k\cdot 21,$$

we have $21k = 1$, so $k = \frac{1}{21}$. Thus, the probability density function is

$$f(x) = \tfrac{1}{21}x^2, \quad \text{for } 1 \le x \le 4.$$

5 ✓

Quick Check 5 ✓

Find k such that $g(x) = \dfrac{k}{x}$ is a probability density function over the interval $[2, 7]$. Then write the probability density function.

Uniform Distributions

Consider again the probability density function given by $f(x) = \dfrac{1}{3}$ over $[2, 5]$, as shown below.

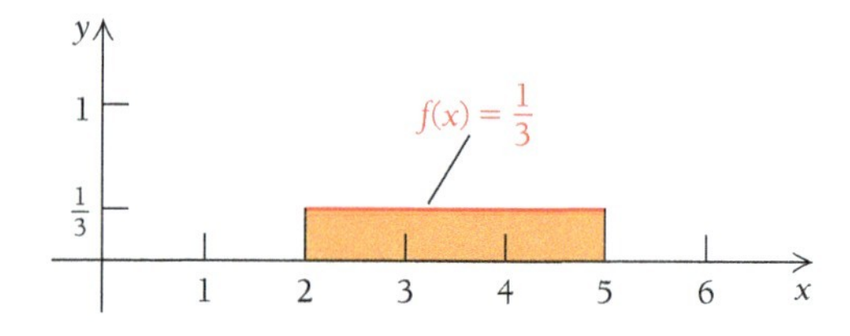

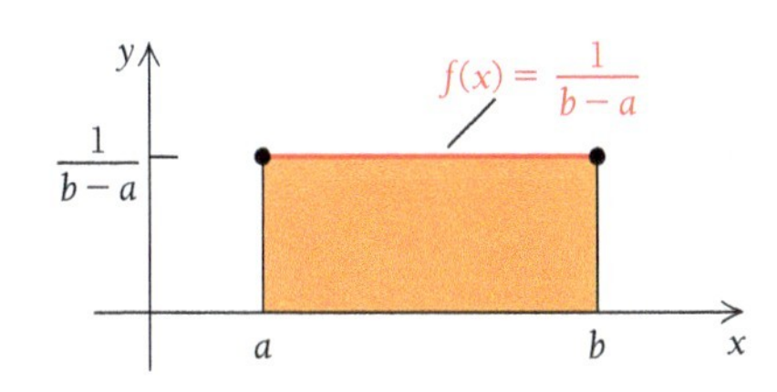

The length of the rectangle is the length of $[2, 5]$, which is 3, and the area is 1.

Generalizing, the length of the rectangle shown at the left is the length of $[a, b]$, or $b - a$. For the shaded area to be 1, the height of the rectangle must be $1/(b - a)$. Thus, $f(x) = 1/(b - a)$.

> **DEFINITION**
>
> A continuous random variable x is said to be **uniformly distributed** over an interval $[a, b]$ if it has a probability density function f given by
>
> $$f(x) = \frac{1}{b - a}, \quad \text{for } a \le x \le b.$$

EXAMPLE 6 **Business: Quality Control.** BlastOut Inc. produces sirens used for tornado warnings. The maximum loudness, L, of the sirens ranges from 70 to 100 decibels. The probability density function for L is

$$f(L) = \frac{1}{30}, \quad \text{for } 70 \le L \le 100.$$

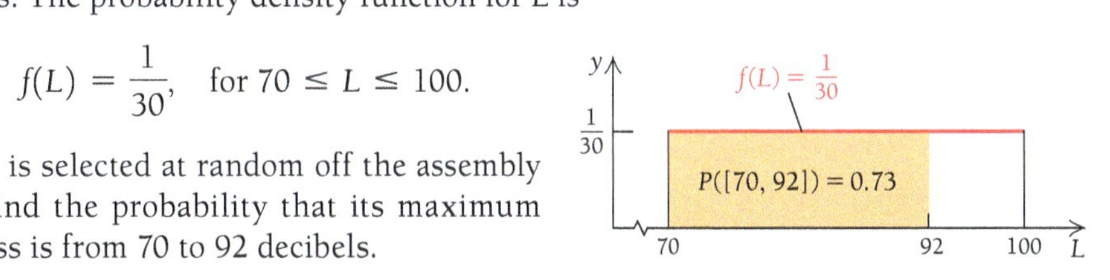

A siren is selected at random off the assembly line. Find the probability that its maximum loudness is from 70 to 92 decibels.

Solution The probability is

$$P(70 \le L \le 92) = \int_{70}^{92} \frac{1}{30}\, dL = \frac{1}{30}[L]_{70}^{92}$$

$$= \frac{1}{30}(92 - 70) = \frac{22}{30} = \frac{11}{15} \approx 0.73.$$

6 ✓

Quick Check 6 ✓

Business: Quality Control. The probability density function for the weight x, in pounds, of bags of feed sold at a feedstore is

$$f(x) = \frac{1}{8}, \quad \text{for } 45 \le x \le 53.$$

A bag is selected at random. Find the probability the bag weighs between 47.5 and 50.25 lb.

Exponential Distributions

The duration of a phone call, the distance between successive cars on a highway, and the amount of time required to learn a task are all examples of *exponentially distributed* random variables. That is, their probability density functions are exponential.

> **DEFINITION**
>
> A continuous random variable is **exponentially distributed** if it has a probability density function of the form
>
> $$f(x) = ke^{-kx}, \quad \text{over } [0, \infty).$$

To see that $f(x) = 2e^{-2x}$ is such a probability density function, first note that $f(x) \ge 0$ for all x in $[0, \infty)$. We have

$$\int_0^{\infty} 2e^{-2x}\, dx = \lim_{b \to \infty} \int_0^{b} 2e^{-2x}\, dx = \lim_{b \to \infty} \left[-e^{-2x}\right]_0^b = \lim_{b \to \infty} \left(\frac{-1}{e^{2b}} - (-1)\right) = 1.$$

The general case,

$$\int_0^{\infty} ke^{-kx}\, dx = 1,$$

can be verified in a similar way.

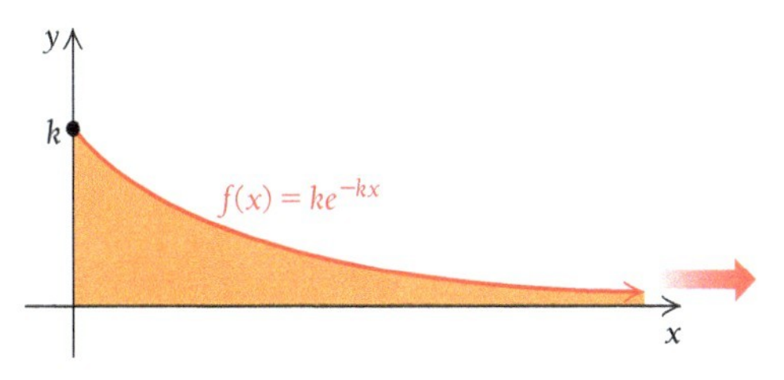

Why is it reasonable to assume that the distance between cars is

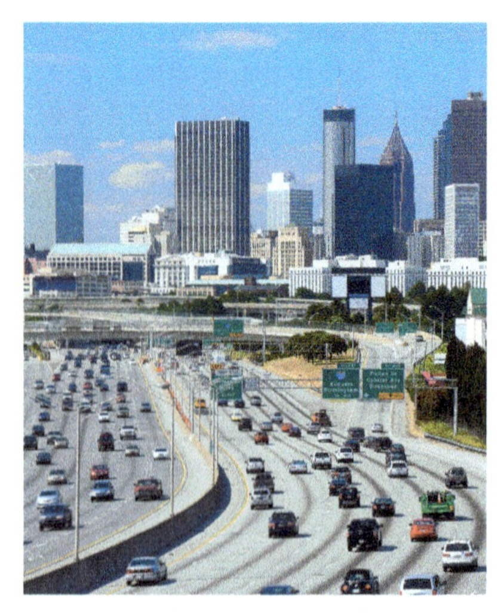

A transportation planner can determine the probabilities that cars are certain distances apart.

exponentially distributed? Part of the reason is that there are many more cases in which traffic is highly congested and involves many cars. Similarly for the duration of a phone call: that is, there are more short calls than long ones. Can you see how this is reflected in the graph of the exponential function?

EXAMPLE 7 **Business: Transportation Planning.** The distance x, in feet, between successive cars on a certain stretch of highway has a probability density function

$$f(x) = ke^{-kx}, \quad \text{for } 0 \leq x < \infty,$$

where $k = 1/a$ and a is the average distance between successive cars over some period of time. A transportation planner determines that the average distance between cars on a certain stretch of highway is 166 ft. What is the probability that the distance between two successive cars, chosen at random, is 50 ft or less?

Solution We first determine k:

$$k = \frac{1}{166} \approx 0.006024. \qquad \text{Using } k = \frac{1}{a} \text{ and substituting}$$

The probability density function for x is

$$f(x) = 0.006024e^{-0.006024x}, \quad \text{for } 0 \leq x < \infty.$$

The probability that the distance between the cars is 50 ft or less is

$$\begin{aligned} P(0 \leq x \leq 50) &= \int_0^{50} 0.006024e^{-0.006024x}\,dx \\ &= \left[\frac{0.006024}{-0.006024}e^{-0.006024x}\right]_0^{50} \\ &= \left[-e^{-0.006024x}\right]_0^{50} \\ &= (-e^{-0.006024 \cdot 50}) - (-e^{-0.006024 \cdot 0}) \\ &= -e^{-0.3012} + 1 \\ &= 1 - e^{-0.3012} \\ &= 1 - 0.739930 \approx 0.260. \end{aligned}$$

7 ✓

Quick Check 7 ✓

The response time for a paramedic unit has the probability density function

$$f(t) = 0.05e^{-0.05t}, \quad \text{for } 0 \leq t < \infty,$$

where t is in minutes. Find the probability of each response time:

a) between 5 and 10 min;

b) between 8 and 20 min;

c) between 1 and 45 min;

d) more than 60 min.

Section Summary

- The *probability* of an event is a number between 0 and 1, with 0 meaning that the event is certain *not* to occur and 1 meaning that the event is certain to occur.
- Probabilities are determined *experimentally* (by conducting trials) or *theoretically* (by mathematical reasoning).
- A *continuous random variable* is a quantity that can be observed (or measured) and whose possible values comprise an interval of real numbers.
- If x is a continuous random variable, then f is a *probability density function* for x if it meets the following criteria:
  (1) For all x in $[a, b]$, $f(x) \geq 0$.
  (2) The area under the graph of f over $[a, b]$ is 1; that is, $\int_a^b f(x)\,dx = 1$.
  (3) The probability that x is within the subinterval $[c, d]$ is given by $P([c, d]) = \int_c^d f(x)\,dx$.
- A continuous random variable x is *uniformly distributed* over $[a, b]$ if its probability density function has the form $f(x) = \dfrac{1}{b - a}$.
- A continuous random variable x is *exponentially distributed* over $[0, \infty)$ if its probability density function has the form $f(x) = ke^{-kx}$.

5.4 Exercise Set

In Exercises 1–10, verify Property 2 of the definition of a probability density function over the given interval.

1. $f(x) = \frac{1}{5}$, $[3, 8]$
2. $f(x) = 3$, $\left[0, \frac{1}{3}\right]$
3. $f(x) = \frac{1}{4}x$, $[1, 3]$
4. $f(x) = 2x$, $[0, 1]$
5. $f(x) = \frac{3}{64}x^2$, $[0, 4]$
6. $f(x) = \frac{3}{26}x^2$, $[1, 3]$
7. $f(x) = \frac{3}{2}x^2$, $[-1, 1]$
8. $f(x) = \frac{1}{3}x^2$, $[-2, 1]$
9. $f(x) = 4e^{-4x}$, $[0, \infty)$
10. $f(x) = 3e^{-3x}$, $[0, \infty)$

Find k such that each function in Exercises 11–22 is a probability density function over the given interval. Then write the probability density function.

11. $f(x) = kx$, $[2, 5]$
12. $f(x) = kx$, $[1, 4]$
13. $f(x) = kx^2$, $[-2, 2]$
14. $f(x) = kx^2$, $[-1, 1]$
15. $f(x) = k$, $[1, 4]$
16. $f(x) = k$, $[3, 9]$
17. $f(x) = k(2 - x)$, $[0, 2]$
18. $f(x) = k(4 - x)$, $[0, 4]$
19. $f(x) = \frac{k}{x}$, $[1, 3]$
20. $f(x) = \frac{k}{x}$, $[1, 2]$
21. $f(x) = ke^x$, $[0, 2]$
22. $f(x) = ke^x$, $[0, 3]$

23. A dart is thrown at a number line in such a way that it always lands in [0, 10]. Let x represent the number where the dart lands. Suppose the probability density function for x is given by

$$f(x) = \tfrac{1}{50}x, \quad \text{for } 0 \le x \le 10.$$

Find $P(2 \le x \le 6)$, the probability that the dart lands in [2, 6].

24. In Exercise 23, suppose the dart always lands in [0, 5], and the probability density function for x is given by

$$f(x) = \tfrac{3}{125}x^2, \quad \text{for } 0 \le x \le 5.$$

Find $P(1 \le x \le 4)$, the probability that the dart lands in [1, 4].

25. A number x is selected at random from [4, 20]. The probability density function for x is given by

$$f(x) = \tfrac{1}{16}, \quad \text{for } 4 \le x \le 20.$$

Find the probability that a number selected is in the subinterval [9, 20].

26. A number x is selected at random from [5, 29]. The probability density function for x is given by

$$f(x) = \tfrac{1}{24}, \quad \text{for } 5 \le x \le 29.$$

Find the probability that a number selected is in the subinterval [14, 29].

APPLICATIONS

Business and Economics

27. **Transportation planning.** Refer to Example 7. Roadway Design, Inc., determines that the average distance between cars on a certain highway is 200 ft. Find the probability that the distance between two successive cars, chosen at random, is at most 10 ft.

28. **Transportation planning.** Refer to Example 7. Traffic Tech, Inc., determines that the average distance between cars on a certain highway is 100 ft. Find the probability that the distance between two successive cars, chosen at random, is at most 40 ft.

29. **Duration of a phone call.** A cell phone provider determines that the duration t, in minutes, of a phone call is an exponentially distributed random variable with a probability density function

$$f(t) = 2e^{-2t}, \quad 0 \le t < \infty.$$

Find the probability that a phone call will last no more than 1 min.

30. **Duration of a phone call.** Referring to Exercise 29, find the probability that a phone call will last at least 2 min.

31. **Time to failure.** The *time to failure*, t, in hours, of a machine is often exponentially distributed with a probability density function

$$f(t) = ke^{-kt}, \quad 0 \le t < \infty,$$

where $k = 1/a$ and a is the average amount of time that will pass before a failure occurs. Suppose the average amount of time that will pass before a failure occurs is 100 hr. What is the probability that a failure will occur in 50 hr or less?

32. **Reliability of a machine.** The *reliability* of the machine (the probability that it will work) in Exercise 31 is defined as

$$R(T) = 1 - \int_0^T 0.01e^{-0.01t}\, dt,$$

where $R(T)$ is the reliability at time T. Write $R(T)$ without using an integral.

Life and Physical Sciences

33. **Wait time for 911 calls.** The wait time before a 911 call is answered in the state of California has a probability density function $f(t) = 0.23e^{-0.23t}$, for $0 \le t < \infty$, where t is in seconds. (*Source*: California Government Code.)
    a) The state standard is that 90% of 911 calls are to be answered within 10 sec. Verify that this standard is met using the probability density function f.
    b) What is the probability that a 911 call is answered within 15 to 25 sec after being made?

34. **Emergency room wait times.** The wait time at an emergency room has the probability density function $f(t) = 0.0259e^{-0.0259t}$, for $0 \le t < \infty$, where t is in minutes. (*Source*: www.cdc.gov.)
    a) Find the probability that a wait time is at most 1 hr.
    b) In 2014, 32.2% of patients had a wait time of at most 15 min. Verify this using the probability density function f.

Social Sciences

35. Time in a maze. In a psychology experiment, the time t, in seconds, that it takes a rat to learn the way through a maze is an exponentially distributed random variable with the probability density function

$$f(t) = 0.02e^{-0.02t}, \quad 0 \leq t < \infty.$$

Find the probability that a rat will learn the way through a maze in 150 sec or less.

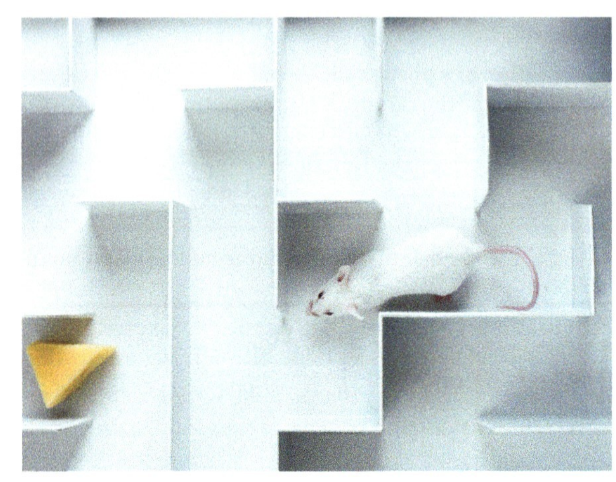

The time it takes a rat to learn the way through a maze is an exponentially distributed random variable.

36. Time in a maze. Using the equation in Exercise 35, find the probability that a rat will learn the way through the maze in 50 sec or less.

37. Use your answer to Exercise 35 to find the probability that a rat requires more than 150 sec to learn the way through the maze.

38. Using the equation in Exercise 35, find the probability that a rat will learn the way through the maze in exactly 125 sec.

39. Explain why the probability that a rat will learn the way through the maze in exactly k seconds is always 0. (See Exercise 38.)

SYNTHESIS

40. Let $f(x) = x^3$ be a probability density function over $[0, b]$. Find b.

41. Let $f(x) = 12x^2$ be a probability density function over $[-a, a]$. Find a.

42. Let $h(x) = x$ be a probability density function over $[a, 2a]$. Find a.

43. The wait times at an urgent care center are exponentially distributed. There is a 30% probability that a patient will have to wait up to 1 hr to see a doctor.

a) Find k, and then write the probability density function f.

b) Find the probability that a patient will have to wait between $\frac{1}{2}$ hr and 3 hr for a doctor.

44. The elapsed time between the arrivals of cars at a rural intersection is exponentially distributed. There is a 20% probability that 10 min will pass between the arrivals of cars at the intersection.

a) Find k, and then write the probability density function f.

b) Find the probability that two cars will come to the intersection within 5 min of one another.

45. The graph of f is a probability density function.

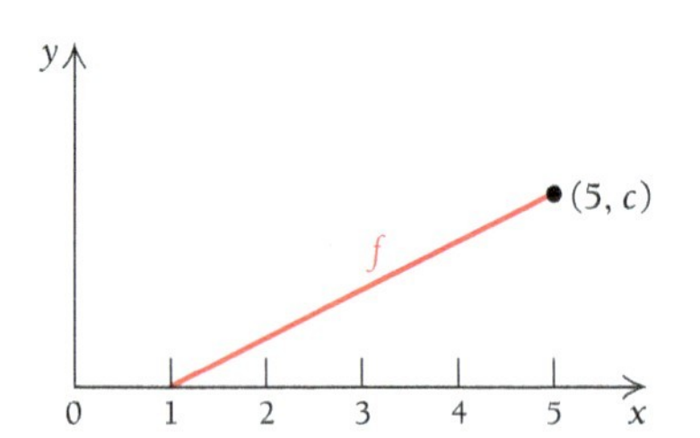

a) Find c.

b) Find f.

c) Find $P(2 \leq x \leq 3)$.

46. The graph of f is a probability density function.

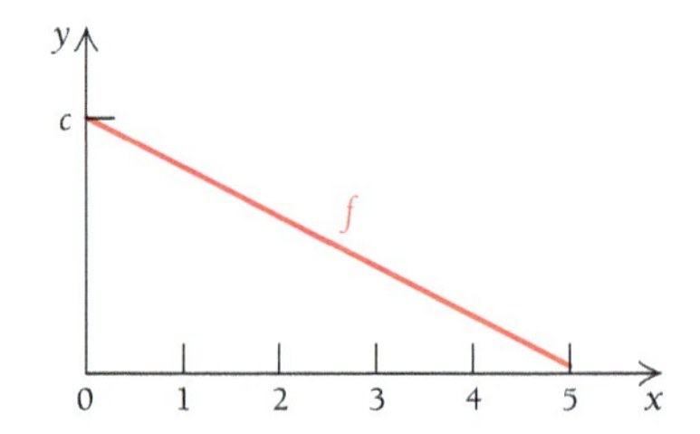

a) Find c.

b) Find f.

c) Find $P(1 \leq x \leq 4)$.

47. Find c such that $f(x) = cxe^{2x}$, for $1 \leq x \leq 2$, is a probability density function.

48. Find c such that $f(x) = cx\sqrt{1 + x}$, for $0 \leq x \leq 1$, is a probability density function.

Technology Connection

49–58. Use a calculator or algebra software to verify Property 2 of the definition of a probability density function for each of the functions in Exercises 1–10.

Answers to Quick Checks

1. (a) $\frac{4}{52}$, or $\frac{1}{13}$; **(b)** $\frac{13}{52}$, or $\frac{1}{4}$; **(c)** $\frac{1}{52}$
2. (a) $\frac{13}{20}$; **(b)** $\frac{16}{20}$, or $\frac{4}{5}$
3. $\int_1^4 \frac{3}{14}\sqrt{x}\,dx = \frac{3}{14}\left[\frac{2}{3}x^{3/2}\right]_1^4 = \frac{3}{14}\left(\frac{16}{3} - \frac{2}{3}\right) = 1$; $g(x) \geq 0$ on $[1, 4]$ **4. (a)** 0.57; **(b)** 0.25
5. $k = \dfrac{1}{\ln 7 - \ln 2}$; $g(x) = \dfrac{1}{x(\ln 7 - \ln 2)}$, for $2 \leq x \leq 7$ **6.** 0.34375 **7. (a)** 0.172; **(b)** 0.302; **(c)** 0.846; **(d)** 0.050

5.5

- Find $E(x)$, $E(x^2)$, the mean, the variance, and the standard deviation.
- Evaluate normal distribution probabilities using a table.
- Calculate percentiles for a normal distribution.

Probability: Expected Value; the Normal Distribution

Expected Value

Let's again consider a dart thrown at a number line so that it lands somewhere in the interval [3, 5]. We assume a uniform distribution, meaning that it is equally likely that the dart will land on any one point in the interval.

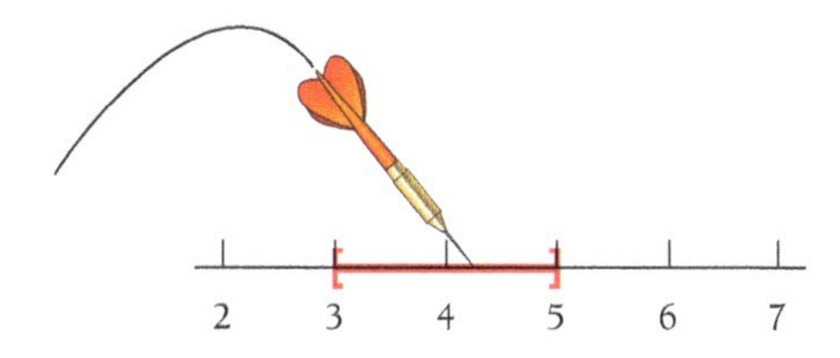

Suppose we throw the dart at the interval 100 times and keep track of the numbers where it lands. We can calculate the arithmetic mean, or average, $\bar{x}$ (read "x bar") of these numbers:

$$\bar{x} = \frac{x_1 + x_2 + x_3 + \cdots + x_{100}}{100} = \frac{\sum_{i=1}^{100} x_i}{100} = \sum_{i=1}^{100} x_i \cdot \frac{1}{100}.$$

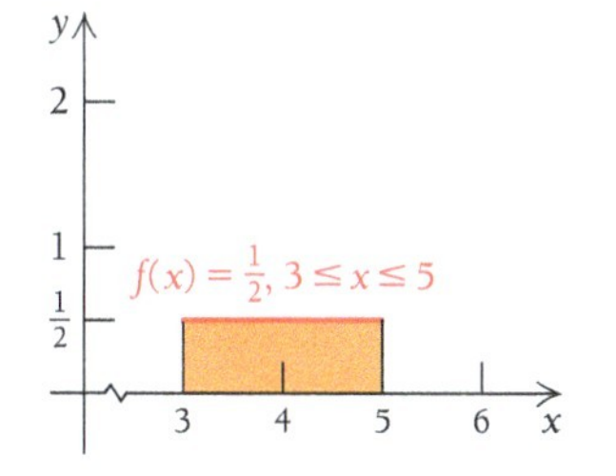

Assuming the x_i's are uniformly distributed over [3, 5], as shown to the left,

$$\sum_{i=1}^{n} x_i \cdot \frac{1}{n}, \quad \text{or} \quad \sum_{i=1}^{n} \left(x_i \cdot \frac{1}{2}\right) \frac{2}{n},$$

Note that the interval width is 2 and the height of the rectangle is $\frac{1}{2}$.

is analogous to

$$\int_3^5 x \cdot f(x)\, dx,$$

where $f(x) = \frac{1}{2}$ is a probability density function for x. Because the width of [3, 5] is 2, we can regard $\frac{2}{n}$ as Δx. The probability density function gives a "weight" to x. We add the values of

$$\left(x_i \cdot \frac{1}{2}\right)\left(\frac{2}{n}\right)$$

when we find $\sum_{i=1}^{n} \left(x_i \cdot \frac{1}{2}\right)\left(\frac{2}{n}\right)$. Similarly, we add all values of

$$(x \cdot f(x))(\Delta x)$$

when we find $\int_3^5 x \cdot f(x)\, dx$:

$$\int_3^5 x \cdot \frac{1}{2}\, dx = \frac{1}{2}\left[\frac{x^2}{2}\right]_3^5 = \frac{1}{4}[5^2 - 3^2] = 4.$$

This result, representing the average value of the distribution, is not surprising, since the distribution is uniform and centered around 4. The average of 100 dart throws may not be exactly 4, but as $n \to \infty$, we will have $\bar{x} \to 4$.

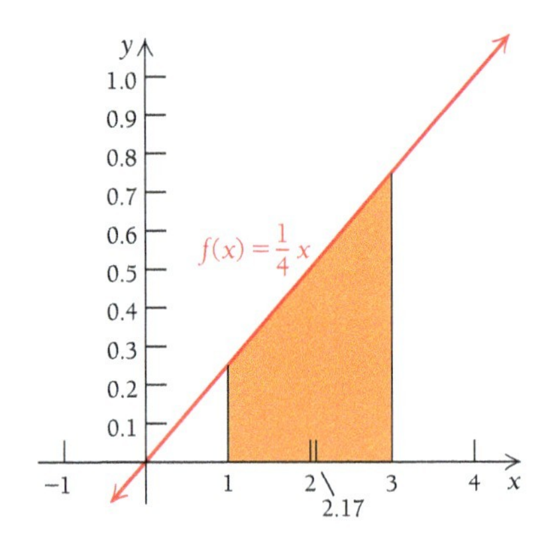

Consider the probability density function $f(x) = \frac{1}{4}x$ over $[1, 3]$. As we can see from the graph, this function gives more "weight" to the right side of the interval than to the left. We have

$$\begin{aligned}\int_1^3 x \cdot f(x)\,dx &= \int_1^3 x \cdot \frac{1}{4}x\,dx \\ &= \frac{1}{4}\int_1^3 x^2\,dx \\ &= \frac{1}{4}\left[\frac{x^3}{3}\right]_1^3 \\ &= \frac{1}{12}(3^3 - 1^3) = \frac{26}{12} \approx 2.17.\end{aligned}$$

Suppose we continue to throw the dart and compute averages. The more throws, the more we expect the average to approach 2.17.

DEFINITION

Let x be a continuous random variable over $[a, b]$ with probability density function f. The **expected value** of x is defined by

$$E(x) = \int_a^b x \cdot f(x)\,dx.$$

The concept of the expected value of a random variable can be generalized to functions of the random variable. Suppose $y = g(x)$ is a function of the random variable x. Then we have the following.

DEFINITION

The **expected value** of $g(x)$ is defined by

$$E(g(x)) = \int_a^b g(x) \cdot f(x)\,dx,$$

where f is a probability density function for x.

EXAMPLE 1 Given the probability density function

$$f(x) = \frac{1}{2}x - 2, \quad \text{over } [4, 6],$$

find $E(x)$ and $E(x^2)$.

Solution

$$\begin{aligned}E(x) &= \int_4^6 x \cdot \left(\frac{1}{2}x - 2\right)dx = \int_4^6 \left(\frac{1}{2}x^2 - 2x\right)dx \qquad \text{Using the definition of the expected value of } x \\ &= \left[\frac{1}{6}x^3 - x^2\right]_4^6 \\ &= \left[\frac{1}{6}(6^3) - 6^2\right] - \left[\frac{1}{6}(4^3) - 4^2\right] \\ &= \frac{16}{3}\end{aligned}$$

Using the definition of the expected value of $g(x)$, with $g(x) = x^2$, we have

$$E(x^2) = \int_4^6 x^2 \cdot \left(\frac{1}{2}x - 2\right) dx = \int_4^6 \left(\frac{1}{2}x^3 - 2x^2\right) dx$$
$$= \left[\frac{1}{8}x^4 - \frac{2}{3}x^3\right]_4^6$$
$$= \left[\frac{1}{8}(6^4) - \frac{2}{3}(6^3)\right] - \left[\frac{1}{8}(4^4) - \frac{2}{3}(4^3)\right]$$
$$= \frac{86}{3}.$$

1 ✓

Quick Check 1 ✓

Given the probability density function

$$f(x) = \frac{1}{2} - \frac{1}{8}x, \quad \text{over } [0, 4],$$

find $E(x)$ and $E(x^2)$.

DEFINITION

The **mean, μ,** of a continuous random variable x is defined to be $E(x)$. That is,

$$\mu = E(x) = \int_a^b x \cdot f(x)\, dx,$$

where f is a probability density function for x defined over $[a, b]$. (The symbol μ is the lowercase Greek letter *mu*, pronounced "mew.")

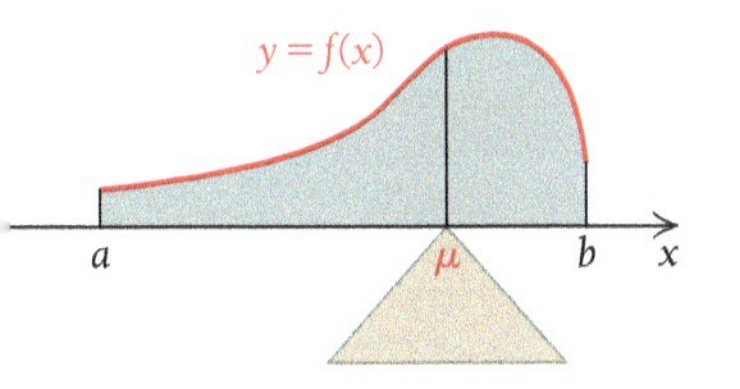

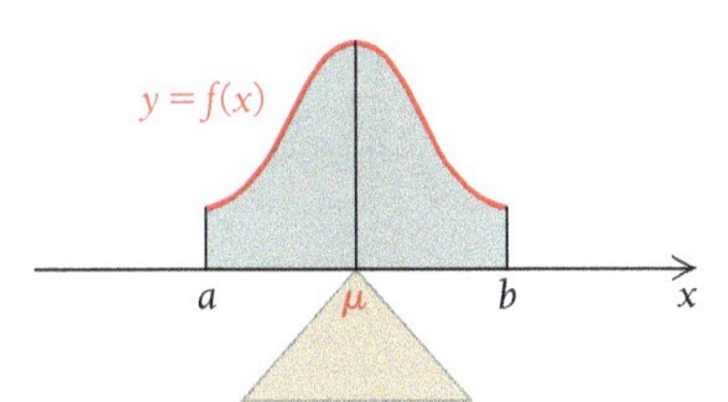

We can get a physical idea of the mean of a random variable by pasting the graph of the probability density function on cardboard and cutting out the area under the curve over the interval $[a, b]$. If we find a balance point on the x-axis, that balance point is the mean, μ.

Variance and Standard Deviation

Because two different distributions can have the same mean, it is useful to have a second statistic that serves as a measure of how the data in a distribution are spread out. Statistics that provide such a measure are the *variance* and (especially) the *standard deviation* of a distribution.

If μ is the mean of a distribution, then $x - \mu$ represents the deviation of a value x from the mean. The variance is the mean of the square of these deviations, or $E((x - \mu)^2)$.

DEFINITIONS

The **variance, σ^2,** of a continuous random variable x, defined on $[a, b]$, with probability density function f, is

$$\sigma^2 = E\left((x - \mu)^2\right) = E(x^2) - \mu^2$$
$$= E(x^2) - [E(x)]^2$$
$$= \int_a^b x^2 \cdot f(x)\, dx - \left[\int_a^b x \cdot f(x)\, dx\right]^2.$$

The **standard deviation, σ,** of a continuous random variable is defined as

$$\sigma = \sqrt{\text{variance}}.$$

(The symbol σ is the lowercase Greek letter *sigma*.)

EXAMPLE 2 Given the probability density function

$$f(x) = \frac{1}{2}x - 2, \quad \text{over } [4, 6],$$

find the mean, the variance, and the standard deviation.

Solution From Example 1, we have $E(x) = \frac{16}{3}$ and $E(x^2) = \frac{86}{3}$. Thus,

$$\text{mean} = \mu = E(x) = \tfrac{16}{3};$$

$$\begin{aligned}\text{variance} = \sigma^2 &= E(x^2) - [E(x)]^2 && \text{Using the definition of variance}\\ &= \tfrac{86}{3} - \left(\tfrac{16}{3}\right)^2 && \text{Substituting}\\ &= \tfrac{86}{3} - \tfrac{256}{9}\\ &= \tfrac{258}{9} - \tfrac{256}{9}\\ &= \tfrac{2}{9};\end{aligned}$$

$$\begin{aligned}\text{standard deviation} &= \sigma\\ &= \sqrt{\tfrac{2}{9}} && \text{The standard deviation is the square root of the variance.}\\ &= \tfrac{1}{3}\sqrt{2}\\ &\approx 0.47.\end{aligned}$$

2 ✓

Quick Check 2 ✓
Given the probability density function

$$f(x) = \frac{1}{2} - \frac{1}{8}x, \quad \text{over } [0, 4],$$

find the mean, the variance, and the standard deviation.

The standard deviation is a measure of the spread of a set of data, that is, how far the data points are, on average, from the line $x = \mu$, as indicated below.

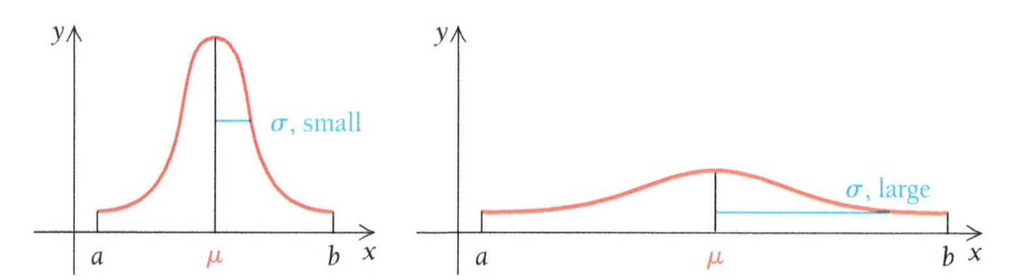

The Normal Distribution

Suppose the average speed of cars on a highway is 70 mi/hr. Usually there are about as many cars whose speeds are above the average as there are with speeds below the average; and the farther away from the average a particular speed is, the fewer cars on the highway traveling at that speed. Speeds on a highway are an example of a random variable that is often *normally* distributed.

Consider the function given by

$$g(x) = e^{-x^2/2}, \quad \text{over } (-\infty, \infty).$$

This function has the set of real numbers as its domain. Its graph is the bell-shaped curve shown below. We can find function values using a calculator:

x	$g(x)$
0	1
1	0.6
2	0.1
3	0.01
−1	0.6
−2	0.1
−3	0.01

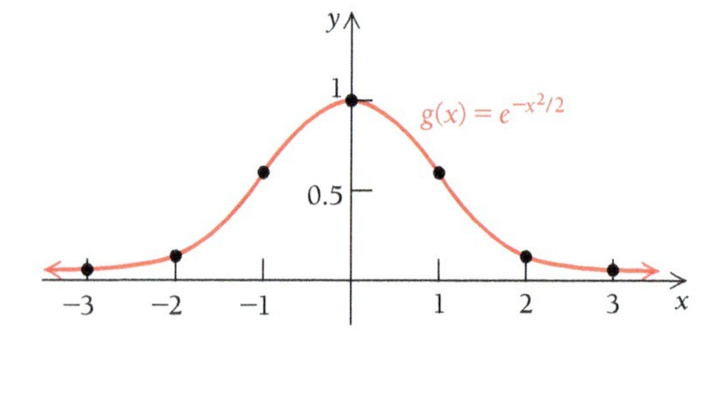

Technology Connection

Exploratory

Use a graphing calculator to confirm that

$$\int_{-\infty}^{\infty} e^{-x^2/2}\,dx = \sqrt{2\pi},$$

letting $y_1 = e^{-x^2/2}$.

1. Set the limits of integration at −2 and 2.
2. Repeat, setting the limits at −3 and 3.
3. Find $\sqrt{2\pi}$ and compare this number with the results from Exercises 1 and 2.

It can be shown that the improper integral that gives the area under the curve converges over $(-\infty, \infty)$ to the number

$$\int_{-\infty}^{\infty} e^{-x^2/2}\,dx = \sqrt{2\pi}.$$

Note that since the area is not 1, the function g is not a probability density function. However, the following function is:

$$f(x) = \frac{1}{\sqrt{2\pi}} e^{-x^2/2}, \quad \text{over } (-\infty, \infty).$$

DEFINITION

A continuous random variable x has a **standard normal distribution** if its probability density function is

$$f(x) = \frac{1}{\sqrt{2\pi}} e^{-x^2/2}, \quad \text{over } (-\infty, \infty).$$

Technology Connection 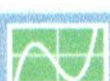

Exploratory

Use a graphing calculator to approximate

$$\int_{-b}^{b} \frac{1}{\sqrt{2\pi}} e^{-x^2/2}\,dx$$

for $b = 10$, 100, and 1000. What does this suggest about

$$\int_{-\infty}^{\infty} \frac{1}{\sqrt{2\pi}} e^{-x^2/2}\,dx?$$

This is a way to verify part of the assertion that

$$f(x) = \frac{1}{\sqrt{2\pi}} e^{-x^2/2}$$

is a probability density function. Use a similar approximation procedure to show that the mean is 0 and the standard deviation is 1.

This standard normal distribution has a mean of 0 and a standard deviation of 1. Its graph follows.

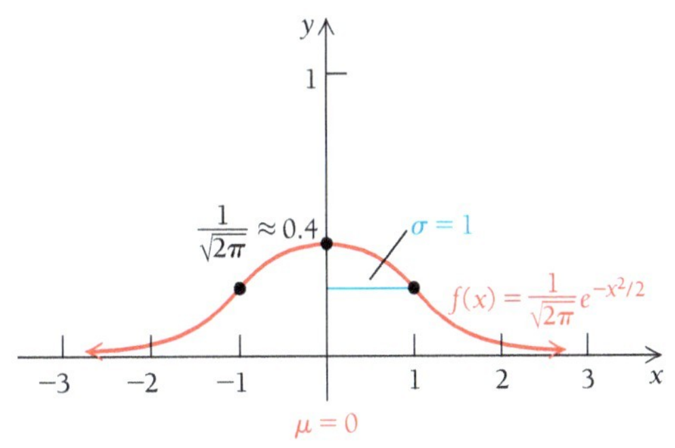

The general case is defined as follows.

DEFINITION

A continuous random variable x is **normally distributed** with mean μ and standard deviation σ if its probability density function is given by

$$f(x) = \frac{1}{\sigma\sqrt{2\pi}} e^{-(1/2)[(x-\mu)/\sigma]^2}, \quad \text{over } (-\infty, \infty).$$

The graph of any normal distribution is a transformation of the graph of the standard normal distribution. This can be visualized as translating the graph of a normal distribution along the x-axis and adjusting how tightly clustered the graph is about the mean. Some examples follow.

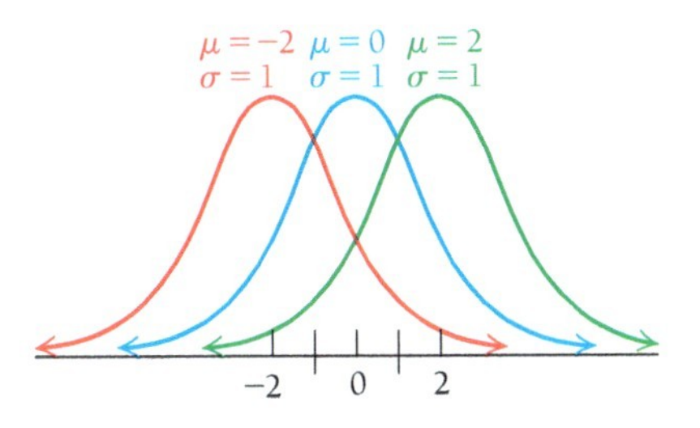

Normal distributions with same standard deviation but different means

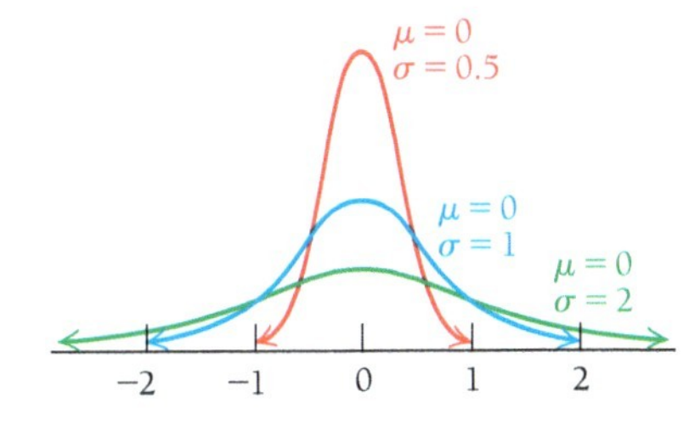

Normal distributions with same mean but different standard deviations

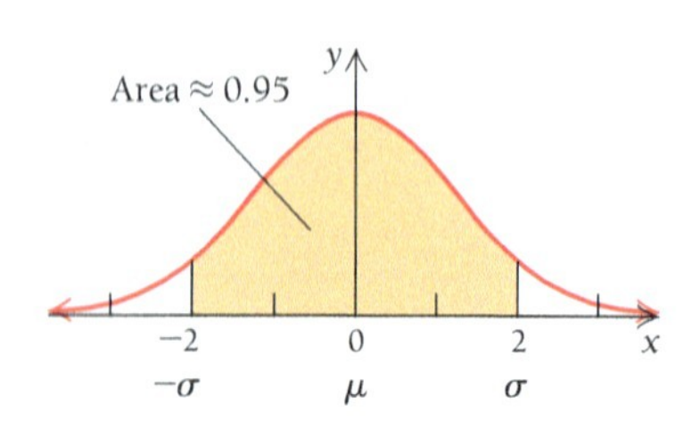

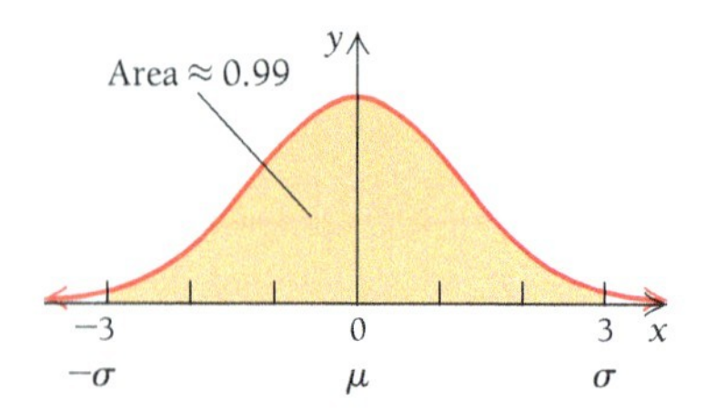

The 68-95-99 Rule: In a standard normal distribution, about 68% of the data is within one standard deviation of the mean, about 95% of the data is within two standard deviations of the mean, and about 99% of the data is within three standard deviations of the mean.

The normal distribution is important in statistics; it underlies research in the natural, behavioral, and social sciences. Because of this, tables of approximate values of the definite integral of the standard normal distribution have been prepared using numerical approximation methods like the Trapezoidal Rule given in Section 4.7. Appendix D at the back of the book (p. 639) presents such a table. It contains values of

$$P(0 \leq x \leq z) = \int_0^z \frac{1}{\sqrt{2\pi}} e^{-x^2/2}\, dx.$$

The symmetry of the graph of this function about the mean allows many types of probabilities to be computed from the table. Some involve addition or subtraction of areas.

EXAMPLE 3 Let x be a continuous random variable with a standard normal distribution. Using Appendix D at the back of the book, find each of the following.

a) $P(0 \leq x \leq 1.68)$
b) $P(-0.97 \leq x \leq 0)$
c) $P(-2.43 \leq x \leq 1.01)$
d) $P(0.90 \leq x \leq 1.74)$
e) $P(-1.98 \leq x \leq -0.42)$
f) $P(x \geq 0.61)$

Solution

a) $P(0 \leq x \leq 1.68)$ is the area bounded by the standard normal curve and the lines $x = 0$ and $x = 1.68$. We look this up in Appendix D by going down the left column to 1.6, then moving to the right to the column headed 0.08. There we read 0.4535. Thus,

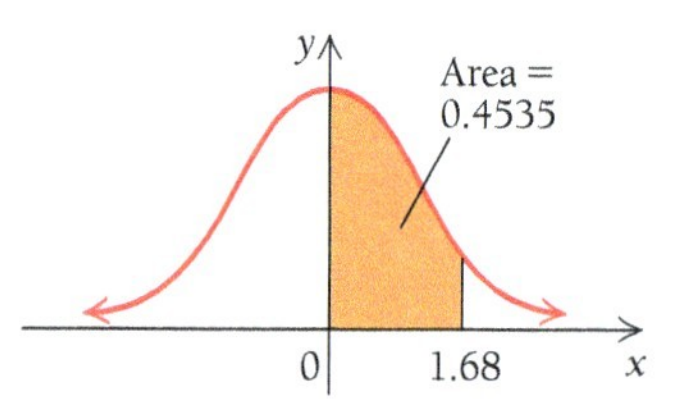

$$P(0 \leq x \leq 1.68) = 0.4535.$$

b) Because of the symmetry of the graph,

$$\begin{aligned} &P(-0.97 \leq x \leq 0) \\ &\quad = P(0 \leq x \leq 0.97) \quad \text{Using symmetry} \\ &\quad = 0.3340. \end{aligned}$$

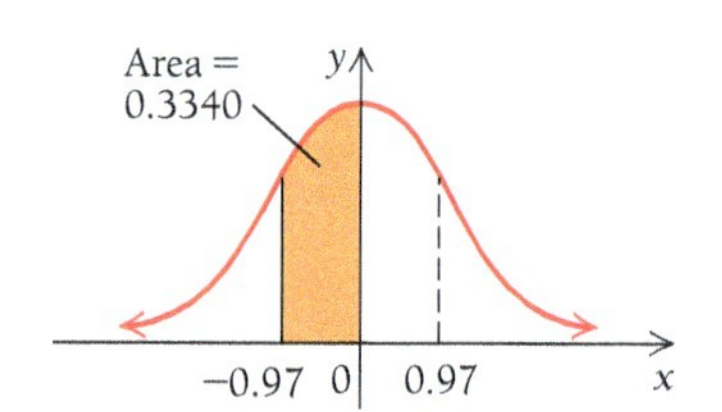

c)
$$\begin{aligned} &P(-2.43 \leq x \leq 1.01) \\ &\quad = P(-2.43 \leq x \leq 0) + P(0 \leq x \leq 1.01) \\ &\quad = P(0 \leq x \leq 2.43) + P(0 \leq x \leq 1.01) \\ &\quad = 0.4925 + 0.3438 \\ &\quad = 0.8363 \end{aligned}$$

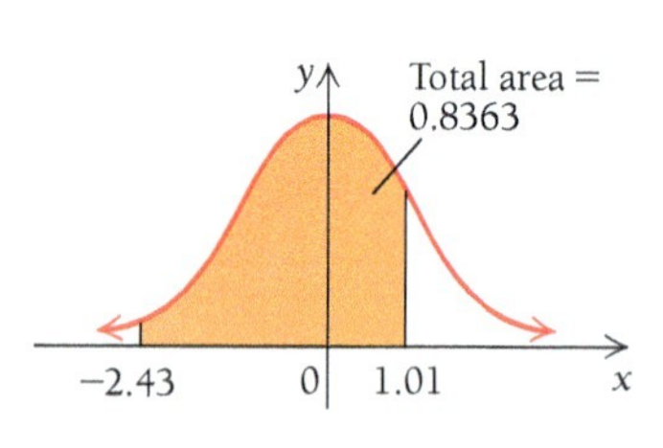

d)
$$\begin{aligned} &P(0.90 \leq x \leq 1.74) \\ &\quad = P(0 \leq x \leq 1.74) - P(0 \leq x \leq 0.90) \\ &\quad = 0.4591 - 0.3159 \\ &\quad = 0.1432 \end{aligned}$$

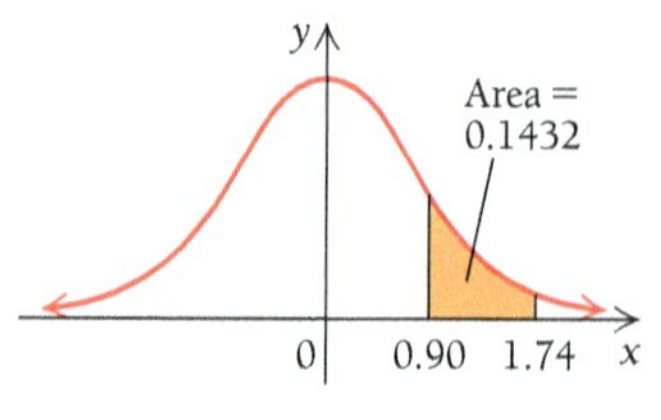

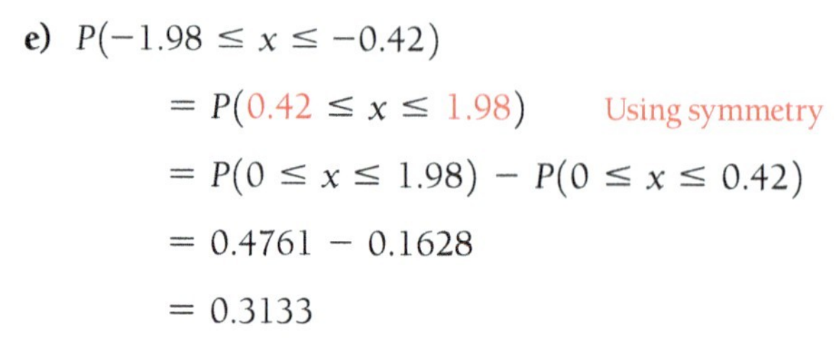

e)
$$\begin{aligned} &P(-1.98 \leq x \leq -0.42) \\ &\quad = P(0.42 \leq x \leq 1.98) \quad \text{Using symmetry} \\ &\quad = P(0 \leq x \leq 1.98) - P(0 \leq x \leq 0.42) \\ &\quad = 0.4761 - 0.1628 \\ &\quad = 0.3133 \end{aligned}$$

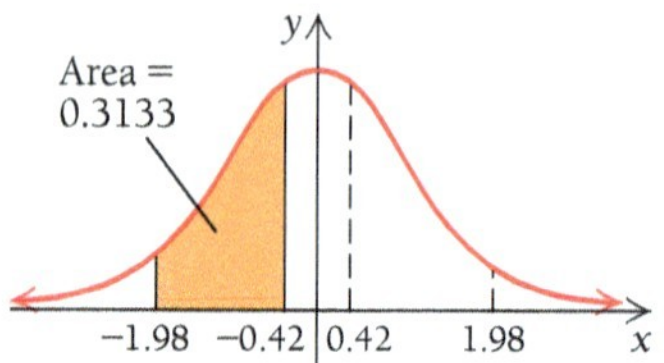

Quick Check 3 ✓
Let x be a continuous random variable with a standard normal distribution. Using Appendix D, find each of the following.

a) $P(-1 \le x \le \frac{1}{2})$
b) $P(x \le -0.77)$
c) $P(x \ge \frac{2}{5})$

f) $P(x \ge 0.61)$

$$= P(x \ge 0) - P(0 \le x \le 0.61)$$
$$= 0.5000 - 0.2291$$
$$= 0.2709$$

Because of symmetry, an area of 0.5 is on each side of $x = 0$ under the normal curve.

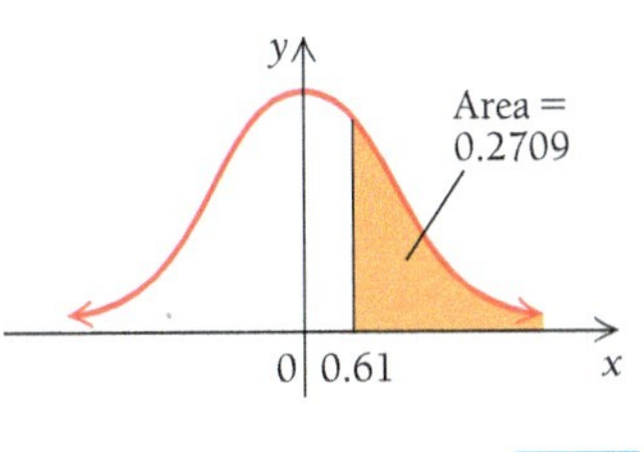

3 ✓

For most normal distributions, $\mu \neq 0$ and $\sigma \neq 1$. Thus, for any normal distribution, the transformation

$$z = \frac{x - \mu}{\sigma}$$

standardizes the distribution, so that we may use Appendix D. Such converted x-values are called *z-scores*, or *z-values*. Using z-scores, we have

$$P(a \le x \le b) = P\left(\frac{a - \mu}{\sigma} \le z \le \frac{b - \mu}{\sigma}\right),$$

and this last probability can be found using Appendix D.

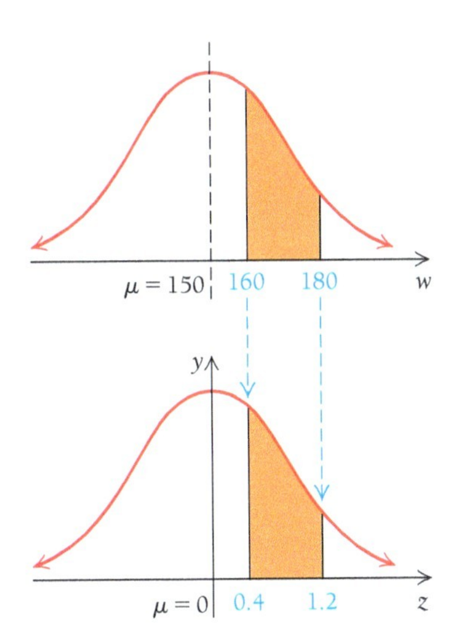

EXAMPLE 4 The weights, w, of the members of a cross-country track team are normally distributed with a mean, μ, of 150 lb and a standard deviation, σ, of 25 lb. Find the probability that the weight of a student on the team is between 160 lb and 180 lb.

Solution Letting $a = 160$ and $b = 180$, we first standardize the weights:

$$180 \text{ is standardized to } \frac{b - \mu}{\sigma} = \frac{180 - 150}{25} = 1.2;$$
$$160 \text{ is standardized to } \frac{a - \mu}{\sigma} = \frac{160 - 150}{25} = 0.4.$$

The z-scores measure the distance of w from μ in terms of σ.

We then have

$$P(160 \le w \le 180) = P(0.4 \le z \le 1.2)$$
$$= P(0 \le z \le 1.2) - P(0 \le z \le 0.4)$$
$$= 0.3849 - 0.1554$$
$$= 0.2295.$$

Now we can use Appendix D.

Thus, the probability that the weight of a randomly selected member of the team is 160 lb to 180 lb is 0.2295. That is, about 23% of the team members weigh between 160 lb and 180 lb.

4 ✓

Quick Check 4 ✓
Referring to Example 4, find the probability of each event.

a) The weight of a randomly selected member of the team is below 165 lb.
b) The weight of a randomly selected member of the team is between 135 lb and 155 lb.
c) The weight of a randomly selected member of the team is above 175 lb.

Percentiles of a Normal Distribution

Suppose you take an exam and score better than 85% of all students taking that exam. We say that your score is in the 85th *percentile*. For the standard normal distribution, the **percentile** for each z-value is the area under the standard normal curve to the left of z, multiplied by 100.

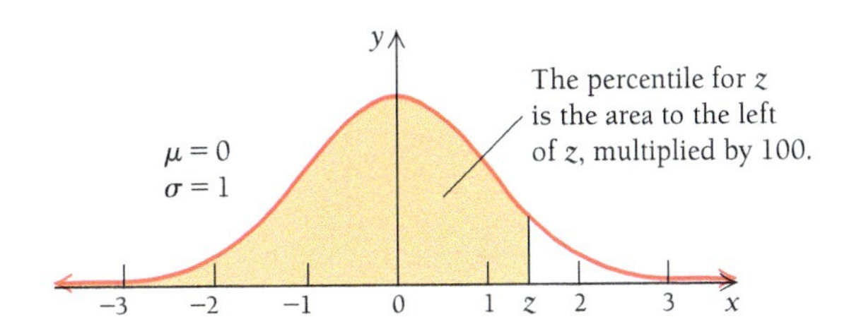

Technology Connection

Exploratory: Statistics on a Calculator

It is possible to use certain calculators to approximate the probability in Example 4 without performing a standard conversion, using Appendix D, or entering the normal probability density function. On most TI calculators, we can select an appropriate window, $[0, 300, -0.002, 0.02]$, with Xscl $= 50$ and Yscl $= 0.01$. Next, we use the ShadeNorm command, which we find by pressing 2ND DISTR ▷ ENTER. We then enter values as shown and press ENTER. (If necessary, the ClearDraw option on the DRAW menu can be used to clear the graph.)

Left endpoint of interval Right endpoint of interval

```
ShadeNorm(160,180,150,25)
```

Mean Standard deviation

```
Area = .229509
low = 160        up = 180
```

The area is shaded and given as 0.229509, or about 23%.

Alternatively, the probability can be calculated directly by pressing 2ND and DISTR and selecting normalcdf. The values are entered as shown:

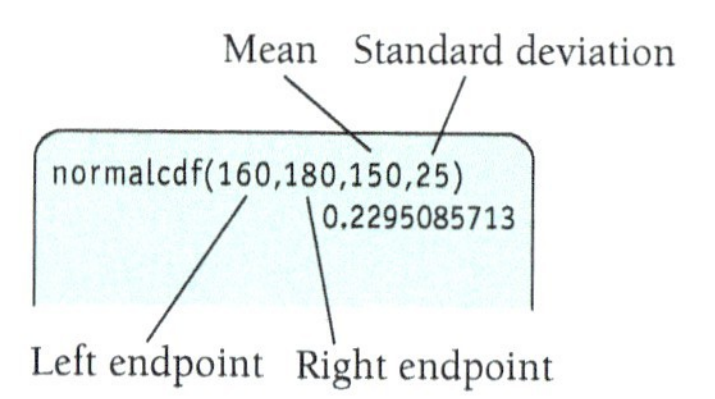

For cases involving an open-ended (infinite) bound, a rule of thumb is to set that bound at a value at least five standard deviations below or above the mean. This will give areas that are accurate to over six decimal places. For example, if we want to know the probability that a member of the cross-country track team weighs less than 145 lb, we can use 0 as the left endpoint:

```
normalcdf(0,145,150,25)
                0.4207403112
```

If we want to know the probability that a team member weighs more than 160 lb, we can use 300 as the right endpoint:

```
normalcdf(160,300,150,25)
                0.3445783019
```

EXAMPLE 5 For the standard normal distribution, with $\mu = 0$ and $\sigma = 1$, determine the percentile corresponding to each of the following z-values.

a) $z = 0$ **b)** $z = 2.25$ **c)** $z = -1.75$

Solution

a) The percentile corresponding to $z = 0$ is the area under the normal curve from $-\infty$ to 0 (to the left of 0). This is half of the total area of the standard normal distribution. Thus, a z-value of 0 corresponds to the 50th percentile: a score exactly at the mean is higher than 50% of all other scores.

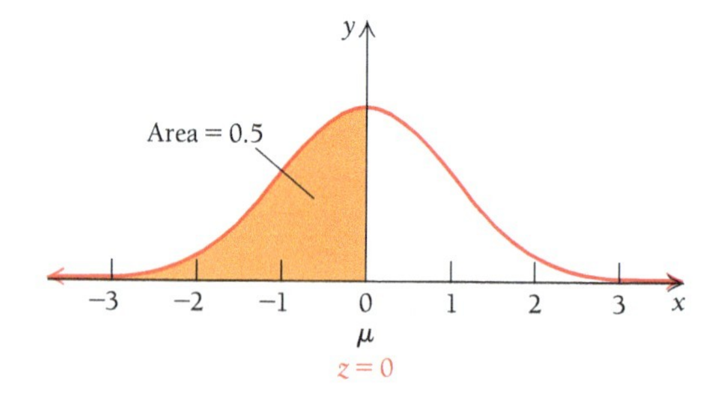

b) Appendix D shows that the area from 0 to 2.25 is 0.4878. We add this to 0.5, so the total area from $-\infty$ to 2.25 is 0.9878. A z-value of 2.25 corresponds to the 98.78th percentile.

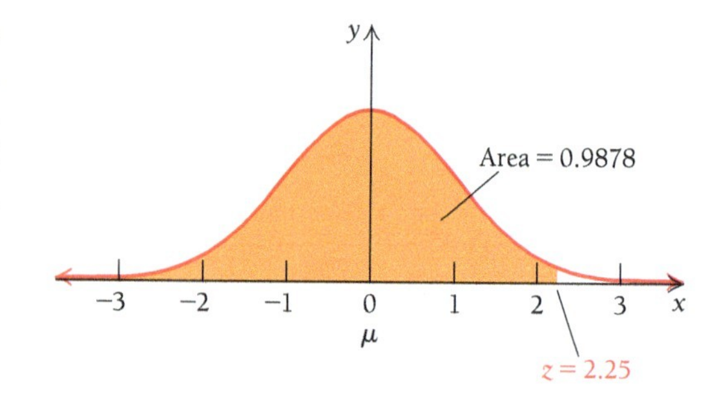

Quick Check 5 ✓
For the standard normal distribution, with $\mu = 0$ and $\sigma = 1$, determine the percentile corresponding to each of the following z-values.

a) $z = 0.25$
b) $z = 2.8$
c) $z = -1$

c) We use Appendix D to determine the area from 0 to 1.75, which is 0.4599. By symmetry, the area between -1.75 and 0 is also 0.4599. Since the area from $-\infty$ to 0 is 0.5, to find the area from $-\infty$ to -1.75, we subtract: $0.5 - 0.4599 = 0.0401$. Therefore, a z-value of -1.75 corresponds to the 4th percentile (rounded).

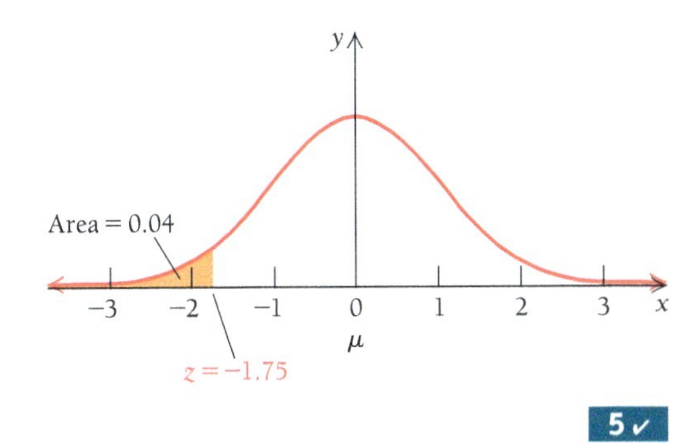

5 ✓

EXAMPLE 6 A large chemistry class takes an exam, and the scores are normally distributed; the mean score is $\mu = 72$, and the standard deviation is $\sigma = 9.1$. The professor gives any student scoring in the top 10% an A. What is the minimum score needed to get an A?

Solution The top 10% corresponds to the 90th percentile. We first determine the z-value that corresponds to the 90th percentile, noting in Appendix D that an area of 0.4 occurs at $z = 1.28$ (with rounding). When we include the area 0.5 for the left half of the distribution, we see that a z-value of 1.28 corresponds to the 90th percentile.

Quick Check 6 ✓
Speeds along a certain stretch of highway are normally distributed and have a mean of $\mu = 59$ mph with a standard deviation of $\sigma = 8$. The police will issue a speeding ticket to any driver whose speed is in the top 2% of this distribution. What is the minimum speed that will get a driver a ticket?

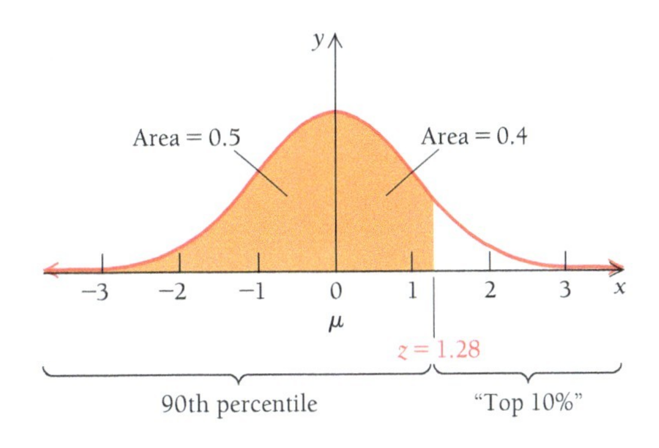

Next, we use the transformation formula to determine the x-value (test score) that corresponds to $z = 1.28$:

$$1.28 = \frac{x - 72}{9.1}$$

$$11.65 \approx x - 72 \quad \text{Multiplying both sides by 9.1 and rounding}$$

$$x = 83.65. \quad \text{Note that 83.65 is 1.28 standard deviations above the mean.}$$

Rounding gives a score of 84 as the minimum score needed to get an A. 6 ✓

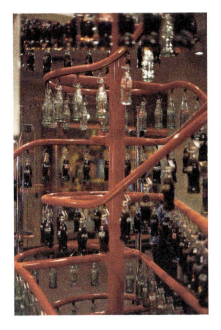

EXAMPLE 7 **Business: Quality Control.** Bottles of cola are to contain a volume with a mean of 591 mL, but some variation is expected. Any bottle at or below the 20th percentile of the volume distribution is rejected. Suppose we know that a bottle that contains 593 mL of cola is in the 60th percentile. What is the smallest volume that will be accepted? Assume that the volumes of cola in the bottles are normally distributed.

Solution We are not given the standard deviation, but we can determine it from the given information. Knowing that a bottle with 593 mL is in the 60th percentile, we want to find a z-value that corresponds to that percentile. Appendix D shows that the area from 0 to about 0.25 is 0.10, which gives 0.6 when added to the 0.5 from the left half of the

Technology Connection

Exploratory: Percentiles on a Calculator

On many calculators, z-values can be determined for percentiles of the standard normal distribution ($\mu = 0$ and $\sigma = 1$) by pressing 2ND and DISTR and selecting InvNorm. Enter the percentile as a decimal between 0 and 1, and press ENTER. The result is the z-value that corresponds to the given percentile. For example, the z-value that corresponds to the 70th percentile is 0.524.

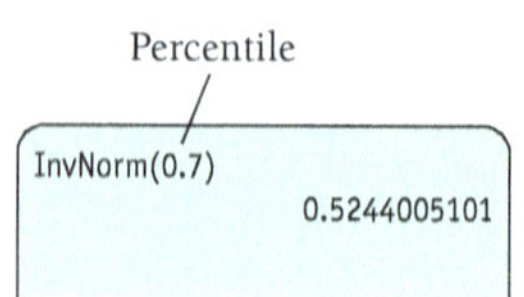

For any mean and standard deviation, the x-value can be found directly by entering the percentile, followed by the given mean and standard deviation, separated by commas. For example, if the mean is $\mu = 300$ and the standard deviation is $\sigma = 20$, then the x-value that corresponds to the 70th percentile is 310.488.

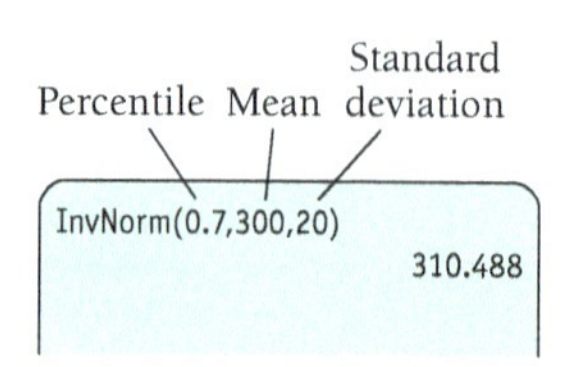

distribution. Thus, $z = 0.25$ corresponds to the 60th percentile. We can then use the transformation formula to solve for σ, with $x = 593$ and $\mu = 591$:

$$0.25 = \frac{593 - 591}{\sigma} \qquad \text{It is important to remember that } z = \frac{x - \mu}{\sigma}.$$

$$0.25 = \frac{2}{\sigma}$$

$$\sigma = \frac{2}{0.25} = 8. \qquad \text{Solving for } \sigma$$

We next determine the z-value that corresponds to the 20th percentile, and from that we can calculate the desired x-value. Appendix D shows that the area from 0 to 0.84 is about 0.3, so, by symmetry, the area from -0.84 to 0 is also about 0.3. Therefore, the area to the left of -0.84 is 0.2. The 20th percentile corresponds to a z-value of -0.84. We now solve for the x-value that corresponds to this z-value:

$$-0.84 = \frac{x - 591}{8}$$

$$-6.72 = x - 591 \qquad \text{Multiplying both sides by 8}$$

$$x = 584.3. \qquad \text{Adding 591}$$

We conclude that any bottle containing less than 584.3 mL of cola is rejected and any bottle containing 584.3 mL or more is accepted. 7 ✓

Quick Check 7 ✓

High school students take a statewide exam, and anyone scoring in the top 15% is awarded a scholarship for college. The scores are normally distributed, with a mean of $\mu = 79$. Your friend scored 87, which was in the 80th percentile, and did not get a scholarship. Your score was 91. Did you get a scholarship?

Section Summary

Assume that x is a continuous random variable and f is a probability density function for x over $[a, b]$.

- The *expected value* of x is
$$E(x) = \int_a^b x \cdot f(x)\, dx.$$
- If g is a function of x on the interval $[a, b]$, then the expected value of $g(x)$ is
$$E(g(x)) = \int_a^b g(x) \cdot f(x)\, dx.$$
- The mean, μ, is the expected value:
$$\mu = E(x) = \int_a^b x \cdot f(x)\, dx.$$
- The variance, σ^2, of x is
$$\sigma^2 = E([x - \mu]^2) = E(x^2) - \mu^2 = E(x^2) - [E(x)]^2$$
$$= \int_a^b x^2 f(x)\, dx - \left[\int_a^b x \cdot f(x)\, dx\right]^2.$$

- The *standard deviation* is the square root of the variance:

$$\sigma = \sqrt{\text{variance}}.$$

It is used to describe the "spread" of the data.

- The *standard normal distribution* of x is defined over $(-\infty, \infty)$ by the probability density function

$$f(x) = \frac{1}{\sqrt{2\pi}} e^{-x^2/2},$$

with mean $\mu = 0$ and standard deviation $\sigma = 1$.

- The general case of a normally distributed random variable x with mean μ and standard deviation σ over $(-\infty, \infty)$ has the probability density function

$$f(x) = \frac{1}{\sigma\sqrt{2\pi}} e^{-(1/2)[(x-\mu)/\sigma]^2}, \quad \text{over } (-\infty, \infty).$$

- For a normal distribution, data values x are converted into z-values by the transformation formula:

$$z = \frac{x - \mu}{\sigma}.$$

- For the standard normal distribution, the *percentile* for a z-value is the area under the standard normal curve to the left of z, multiplied by 100.

5.5 Exercise Set

For each probability density function, over the given interval, find $E(x)$, $E(x^2)$, the mean, the variance, and the standard deviation.

1. $f(x) = \frac{1}{4}$, $[3, 7]$

2. $f(x) = \frac{1}{5}$, $[3, 8]$

3. $f(x) = \frac{2}{9}x$, $[0, 3]$

4. $f(x) = \frac{1}{8}x$, $[0, 4]$

5. $f(x) = \frac{1}{4}x$, $[1, 3]$

6. $f(x) = \frac{2}{3}x$, $[1, 2]$

7. $f(x) = \frac{1}{3}x^2$, $[-2, 1]$

8. $f(x) = \frac{3}{2}x^2$, $[-1, 1]$

9. $f(x) = \frac{1}{\ln 5} \cdot \frac{1}{x}$, $[1.5, 7.5]$

10. $f(x) = \frac{1}{\ln 4} \cdot \frac{1}{x}$, $[0.8, 3.2]$

Let x be a continuous random variable with a standard normal distribution. Using Appendix D, find each of the following.

11. $P(0 \le x \le 2.13)$

12. $P(0 \le x \le 0.36)$

13. $P(-2.01 \le x \le 0)$

14. $P(-1.37 \le x \le 0)$

15. $P(-1.89 \le x \le 0.45)$

16. $P(-2.94 \le x \le 2.00)$

17. $P(0.76 \le x \le 1.45)$

18. $P(1.35 \le x \le 1.45)$

19. $P(-1.27 \le x \le -0.58)$

20. $P(-2.45 \le x \le -1.24)$

21. $P(x \ge 1.01)$

22. $P(x \ge 3.01)$

23. a) $P(-1 \le x \le 1)$

b) What percentage of the area is from -1 to 1?

24. a) $P(-2 \le x \le 2)$

b) What percentage of the area is from -2 to 2?

Let x be a continuous random variable that is normally distributed with mean $\mu = 22$ and standard deviation $\sigma = 5$. Using Appendix D, find each of the following.

25. $P(24 \le x \le 30)$

26. $P(22 \le x \le 27)$

27. $P(19 \le x \le 25)$

28. $P(18 \le x \le 26)$

29. $P(17.2 \le x \le 21.7)$

30. $P(20.3 \le x \le 27.5)$

31. $P(x \le 22.5)$

32. $P(x \ge 20)$

33. $P(x \le 18)$

34. $P(x \le 16)$

35. $P(x \ge 23.5)$

36. $P(x \ge 24.2)$

37. $P(x \ge 19.5)$

38. $P(x \ge 18.8)$

39. Find the z-value that corresponds to each percentile for a standard normal distribution.

a) 30th percentile
b) 50th percentile
c) 95th percentile

40. In a normal distribution with $\mu = 60$ and $\sigma = 7$, find the x-value that corresponds to the

a) 35th percentile
b) 75th percentile

41. In a normal distribution with $\mu = -15$ and $\sigma = 0.4$, find the x-value that corresponds to the

a) 46th percentile
b) 92nd percentile

42. In a normal distribution with $\mu = 0$ and $\sigma = 4$, find the x-value that corresponds to the

a) 50th percentile
b) 84th percentile

APPLICATIONS

Business and Economics

43. Mail orders. The number of orders, N, received daily by an online vendor of used video games is normally distributed with mean 250 and standard deviation 20. The company has to hire extra help or pay overtime on those days when the number of orders received is 300 or higher. On what percentage of days will the company have to hire extra help or pay overtime?

44. Bread baking. The number of loaves of bread, N, baked each day by Fireside Bakers is normally distributed with mean 1000 and standard deviation 50. The bakery pays bonuses to its employees on days when at least 1100 loaves are baked. On what percentage of days will the bakery have to pay a bonus?

Manufacturing. *In an automotive body-welding line, delays encountered during the process can be modeled by various probability distributions. (Source: R. R. Inman, "Empirical Evaluation of Exponential and Independence Assumptions in Queueing Models of Manufacturing Systems," Production and Operations Management, Vol. 8, 409–432 (1999).)*

45. The processing time for the robogate has a normal distribution with mean 38.6 sec and standard deviation 1.729 sec. Find the probability that the next operation of the robogate will take 40 sec or less.

46. The processing time for the automatic piercing station has a normal distribution with mean 36.2 sec and standard deviation 2.108 sec. Find the probability that the next operation of the piercing station will take between 35 and 40 sec.

General Interest

47. Test score distribution. In 2017, combined SAT scores were normally distributed with mean 1080 and standard deviation 190. Find the combined SAT scores that correspond to these percentiles. (*Source:* Based on data from www.collegeboard.com.)

a) 35th percentile
b) 60th percentile
c) 92nd percentile

48. Test score distribution. The scores on a biology test are normally distributed with mean 65 and standard deviation 20. A score from 80 to 89 is a B. What is the probability of getting a B?

49. Test score distribution. In a large class, student test scores had a mean of $\mu = 76$ and a standard deviation $\sigma = 7$.

a) The top 12% of students got an A. Find the minimum score needed to get an A (round to the appropriate integer).
b) The top 75% of students passed. Find the minimum score needed to pass (round to the appropriate integer).

50. Average temperature. Las Vegas, Nevada, has an average daily high temperature of 104°F in July, with a standard deviation of 4.5°F. (*Source:* www.weatherspark.com.)

a) In what percentile is a temperature of 112°F?
b) What temperature would be at the 67th percentile?
c) What temperature would be in the top 0.5% of all July temperatures for this location?

51. Heights of basketball players. Players in the National Basketball Association have a mean height of 6 ft 7 in. (79 in.). (*Source:* www.apbr.org.) If a basketball player who is 7 ft 2 in. (86 in.) tall is in the top 1% of players by height, in what percentile is a 6 ft 11 in. (83 in.) player?

52. Bowling scores. At the time this book was written, the bowling scores, S, of author Marv Bittinger were normally distributed with mean 201 and standard deviation 23.

a) Find the probability that one of Marv's scores is from 185 to 215.
b) Find the probability that one of his scores is from 160 to 175.
c) Find the probability that one of his scores is greater than 200.
d) Marv's best score is 299. Find the percentile that corresponds to this score, and explain what that number represents.

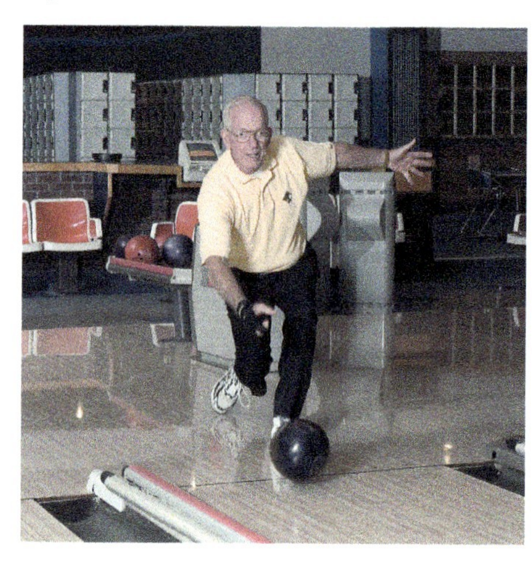

SYNTHESIS

For each probability density function, over the given interval, find $E(x)$, $E(x^2)$, the mean, the variance, and the standard deviation.

53. $f(x) = \dfrac{1}{b-a}$, over $[a, b]$

54. $f(x) = \dfrac{3a^3}{x^4}$, over $[a, \infty)$

Median. *Let x be a continuous random variable over $[a, b]$ with probability density function f. Then the median of the x-values is that number m for which*

$$\int_a^m f(x)\,dx = \frac{1}{2}.$$

Find each median.

55. $f(x) = \frac{1}{2}x$, $[0, 2]$

56. $f(x) = \frac{3}{2}x^2$, $[-1, 1]$

57. $f(x) = ke^{-kx}$, $[0, \infty)$

58. Business: coffee production. Suppose the amount of coffee beans loaded into a vacuum-packed bag has a mean weight of μ ounces, which can be adjusted on the filling machine. Also, the amount dispensed is normally distributed with $\sigma = 0.2$ oz. What should μ be set at to ensure that only 1 bag in 50 will have less than 16 oz?

59. Business: does thy cup overflow? Suppose the mean amount of cappuccino, μ, dispensed by a vending machine can be set. If a cup holds 8.5 oz and the amount dispensed is normally distributed with $\sigma = 0.3$ oz, what should μ be set at to ensure that only 1 cup in 100 will overflow?

Let x be a random variable with probability distribution function f over $[a, b]$ with mean $\mu = E(x)$. Use this information for Exercises 60–64.

60. Show that $E(kx) = kE(x)$, where k is any nonzero constant.

61. Show that $E(x^2 + x) = E(x^2) + E(x)$.

62. Show that $E(\mu) = E(E(x)) = E(x)$.

63. Show that $E(\mu^2) = E(x)^2$.

64. The following is an outline of a proof showing that $\sigma^2 = E((x - \mu)^2) = E(x^2) - \mu^2$. Supply a justification for each step of the proof. (*Hint*: Use the results from Exercises 60–63 to justify certain steps.)

a) $E((x - \mu)^2) = E(x^2 - 2\mu x + \mu^2)$

____

b) $E(x^2 - 2\mu x + \mu^2) = E(x^2) - E(2\mu x) + E(\mu^2)$

____

c) $E(x^2) - E(2\mu x) + E(\mu^2)$
$= E(x^2) - 2E(\mu)E(x) + E(x)^2$

____

d) $E(x^2) - 2E(\mu)E(x) + E(x)^2$
$= E(x^2) - 2E(x)^2 + E(x)^2$

____

e) $E(x^2) - 2E(x)^2 + E(x)^2 = E(x^2) - \mu^2$

____

65. Explain why a normal distribution may not apply if you are analyzing the distribution of weights of students in a classroom.

66. A professor gives an easy test worth 100 points. The mean is 94, and the standard deviation is 5. Is it possible to apply a normal distribution to this situation? Why or why not?

Technology Connection

67. For the probability density function $f(x) = -\frac{1}{50}x + \frac{1}{5}$, for $0 \leq x \leq 10$, find the x-value that corresponds to each percentile.

a) 20th percentile **b)** 50th percentile
c) 90th percentile

68. For the probability density function $g(x) = \frac{3}{117}x^2$, for $2 \leq x \leq 5$, find the x-value that corresponds to each percentile.

a) 25th percentile **b)** 62nd percentile
c) 97th percentile

Answers to Quick Checks

1. $E(x) = \frac{4}{3}$, $E(x^2) = \frac{8}{3}$ **2.** $\mu = \frac{4}{3}$, $\sigma^2 = \frac{8}{9}$, $\sigma = \frac{\sqrt{8}}{3} \approx 0.943$ **3. (a)** 0.5328; **(b)** 0.2206; **(c)** 0.3446 **4. (a)** 0.7257; **(b)** 0.3050; **(c)** 0.1587 **5. (a)** About the 59.9th percentile; **(b)** 99.7th percentile; **(c)** 15.9th percentile **6.** About 75.4 mph **7.** Yes, you were in the 89.7th percentile.

5.6

- Find the volume of a solid of revolution using disks.
- Find the volume of a solid of revolution using shells.

Volume

Volume by Disks

As Fig. 1 shows, the plane region bounded by the graph of $y = f(x)$, the x-axis, $x = a$, and $x = b$, when rotated about the x-axis, sweeps out a *solid of revolution*. To calculate the volume of this solid, we first approximate it as a finite sum of thin right circular cylinders, or **disks** (Fig. 2). We divide $[a, b]$ into equally sized subintervals, each of length Δx. Thus, the height h of each disk is Δx (Fig. 3). The radius of each disk is $f(x_i)$, where x_i is the right-hand endpoint of the subinterval that determines that disk.

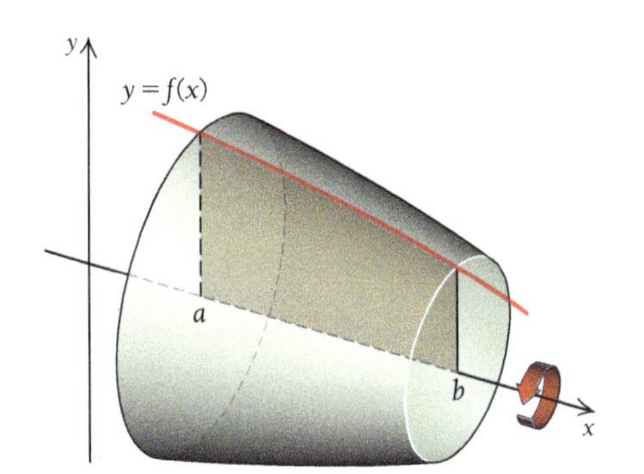

FIGURE 1

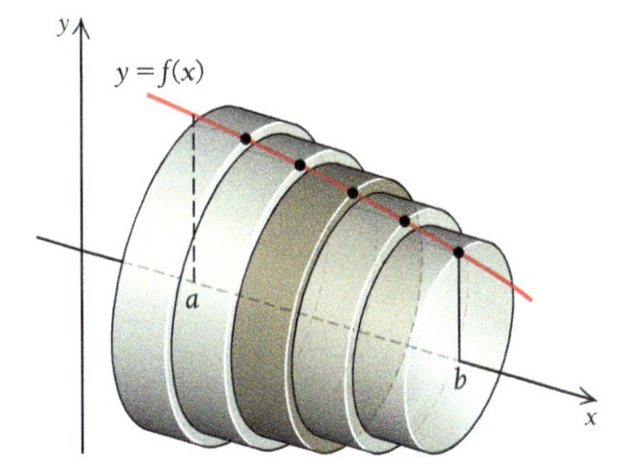

FIGURE 2

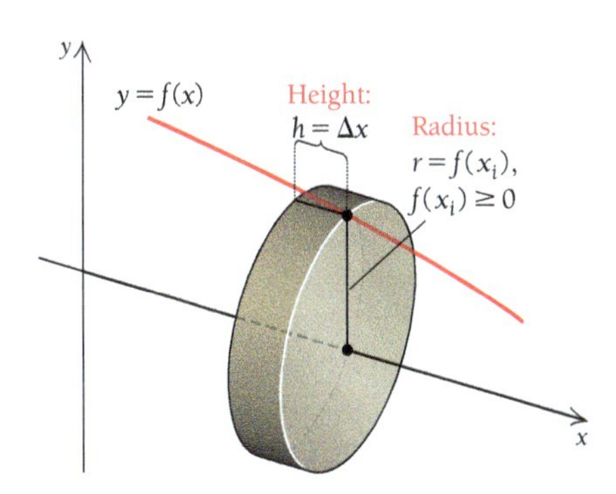

FIGURE 3

Since the volume of a right circular cylinder is given by

$$V = \pi r^2 h, \quad \text{or} \quad \text{Volume} = \text{area of the base} \cdot \text{height},$$

each of the approximating disks has volume

$$\pi[f(x_i)]^2 \Delta x.$$ Squaring allows for cases where $f(x) < 0$.

The volume of the solid of revolution is approximated by the sum of the volumes of all the disks:

$$V \approx \sum_{i=1}^{n} \pi[f(x_i)]^2 \Delta x.$$

The actual volume is the limit of this sum as the thickness (height) of each disk, Δx, approaches zero, and the number of disks approaches infinity:

$$V = \lim_{n \to \infty} \sum_{i=1}^{n} \pi[f(x_i)]^2 \Delta x = \pi \int_a^b [f(x)]^2 \, dx.$$

That is, the volume is the value of the definite integral of the function $y = \pi[f(x)]^2$ from a to b.

THEOREM 2 Volume by Disks

For a nonnegative continuous function f defined on $[a, b]$, the **volume**, V, of the solid of revolution obtained by rotating the area under the graph of f from a to b around the x-axis is given by

$$V = \pi \int_a^b [f(x)]^2 \, dx.$$

EXAMPLE 1 Find the volume of the solid of revolution generated by rotating the area under the graph of $y = \sqrt{x}$ from $x = 0$ to $x = 1$ around the x-axis.

Solution

$$V = \pi \int_a^b [f(x)]^2 \, dx$$

$$= \pi \int_0^1 [\sqrt{x}]^2 \, dx \quad \text{Substituting}$$

$$= \pi \int_0^1 x \, dx$$

$$= \pi \left[\frac{x^2}{2}\right]_0^1$$

$$= \frac{\pi}{2}\left[x^2\right]_0^1$$

$$= \frac{\pi}{2}(1^2 - 0^2) \quad \text{Evaluating}$$

$$= \frac{\pi}{2}$$

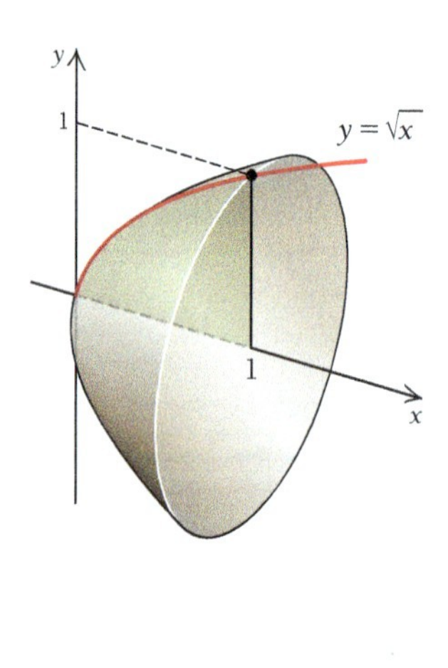

1 ✓

Quick Check 1 ✓
Find the volume of the solid of revolution generated by rotating the area under the graph of $y = x^3$ from $x = 0$ to $x = 2$ around the x-axis.

EXAMPLE 2 Find the volume of the solid of revolution generated by rotating the region under the graph of

$$y = e^x$$

from $x = -1$ to $x = 2$ around the x-axis.

Solution

$$
\begin{aligned}
V &= \pi \int_a^b [f(x)]^2 \, dx \\
&= \pi \int_{-1}^{2} [e^x]^2 \, dx && \text{Substituting} \\
&= \pi \int_{-1}^{2} e^{2x} \, dx \\
&= \left[\frac{\pi}{2} e^{2x} \right]_{-1}^{2} \\
&= \frac{\pi}{2} \left[e^{2x} \right]_{-1}^{2} \\
&= \frac{\pi}{2} \left(e^{2 \cdot 2} - e^{2(-1)} \right) && \text{Evaluating} \\
&= \frac{\pi}{2} \left(e^4 - e^{-2} \right) \\
&\approx 85.55
\end{aligned}
$$

Quick Check 2 ✓

Find the volume of the solid of revolution generated by rotating the area under the graph of $y = \frac{1}{x}$ from $x = 1$ to $x = 3$ around the x-axis.

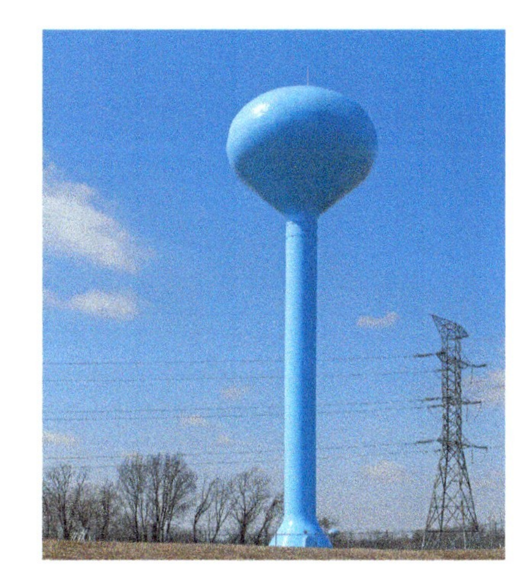

EXAMPLE 3 **Business: Water Storage.** The interior of a university's water storage tank has the shape of the solid of revolution generated by rotating the area under the graph of

$$f(x) = 50\sqrt{1 - \frac{x^2}{40^2}}$$

from $x = -40$ ft to $x = 40$ ft around the x-axis. What is the volume of this tank?

Solution The graph of f is shown in the margin. Rotating the graph of f about the x-axis gives the shape of the tank. The actual tank has this shape turned on its side.

If we rotate the portion of the graph from $x = 0$ to $x = 40$, we will get half of the solid. This has the advantage of using 0 as a bound of integration.

The volume for $0 \leq x \leq 40$ is

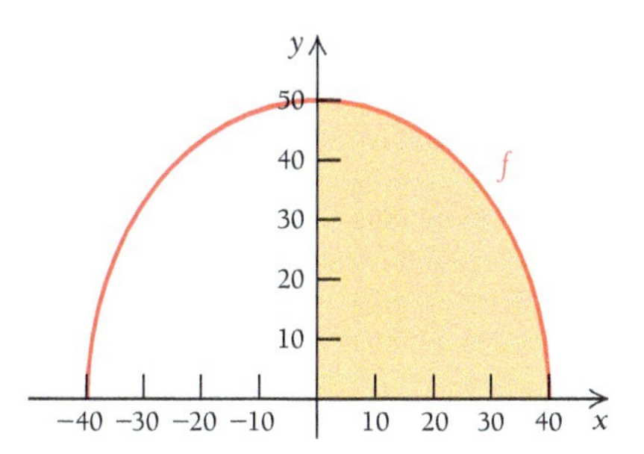

$$
\begin{aligned}
V &= \pi \int_0^{40} \left[50\sqrt{1 - \frac{x^2}{40^2}} \right]^2 dx && \text{This gives half of the tank's volume.} \\
&= \pi \int_0^{40} \left[2500 \left(1 - \frac{x^2}{1600} \right) \right] dx && \text{Simplifying} \\
&= \pi \int_0^{40} \left[2500 - \frac{25}{16} x^2 \right] dx && \text{Multiplying by 2500} \\
&= \pi \left[2500x - \frac{25}{48} x^3 \right]_0^{40} && \text{Antidifferentiating} \\
&= \frac{200{,}000}{3} \pi.
\end{aligned}
$$

Multiplying this result by 2 gives the tank's volume:

$$\frac{400{,}000}{3} \pi \approx 418{,}879 \text{ ft}^3.$$

Since 1 ft^3 holds 7.48 gal, this tank holds over 3.13 million gallons of water.

Quick Check 3 ✓

A tepee is a cone with a height of 15 ft at its center and a circular base with a radius of 8 ft. Determine the volume contained within this tepee. (*Hint:* Rotate the line $y = \frac{8}{15}x$ for $x = 0$ to $x = 15$ around the x-axis.)

Volume by Shells

Let R be the area bounded by the graph of $y = f(x)$, the x-axis, and the lines $x = a$ and $x = b$. Rotate R around the y-axis, as shown below.

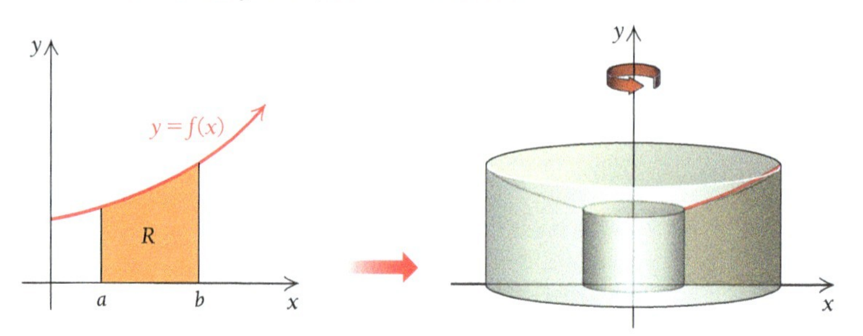

To find the volume of this solid of revolution, we divide $[a, b]$ into equally sized subintervals, each of width Δx. A rectangle, similar to those used in a Riemann sum, is drawn above each subinterval. When the area R is rotated around the y-axis, each rectangle sweeps out a **shell**, as shown below.

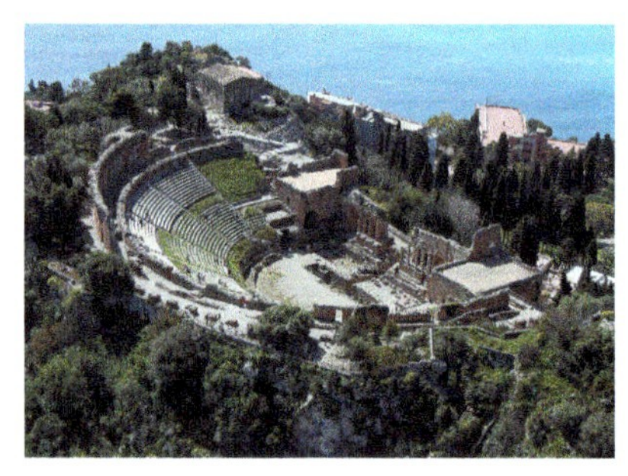

Explain how this amphitheater could be interpreted as a solid of revolution.

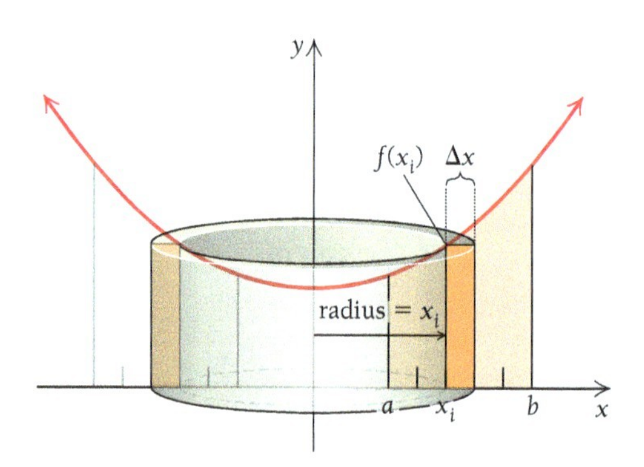

Let $f(x_i)$ be the height of the shell swept out by the rectangle above the ith subinterval. The radius of this shell is x_i, and its thickness is Δx. If we cut and flatten this shell, we can view it as a rectangular solid. Its width is Δx, its height is $f(x_i)$, and its length is the circumference, or $2\pi x_i$.

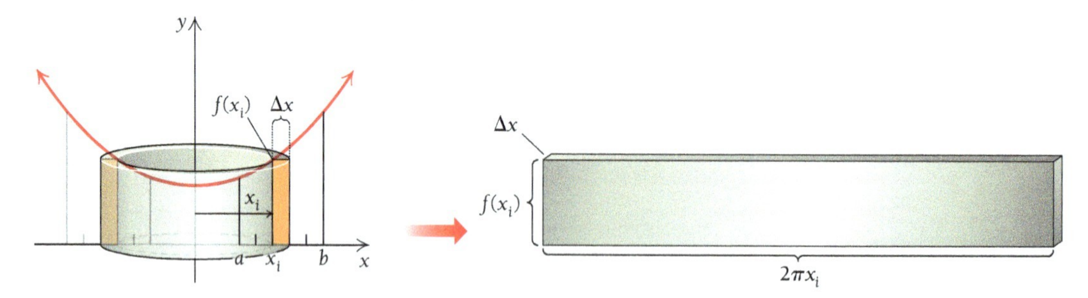

Therefore, the volume of the ith shell is

$$V_i = (\text{length})(\text{height})(\text{width})$$
$$= (2\pi x_i)(f(x_i))(\Delta x).$$

The volume of the solid of revolution is approximated by the sum of all such shells:

$$V \approx \sum_{i=1}^{n} (2\pi x_i)(f(x_i))(\Delta x).$$

As Δx approaches 0, the number of subdivisions, n, approaches ∞, and the volume of the solid of revolution is given by

$$V = \lim_{n \to \infty} \sum_{i=1}^{n} (2\pi x_i)(f(x_i))(\Delta x) = 2\pi \int_a^b x \cdot f(x)\, dx.$$

THEOREM 3 Volume by Shells

Let R be an area bounded by the graph of $y = f(x)$, the x-axis, and the lines $x = a$ and $x = b$. If R is rotated around the y-axis, the volume of the solid of revolution is given by

$$V = 2\pi \int_a^b x \cdot f(x)\, dx.$$

EXAMPLE 4 Find the volume of the solid of revolution formed by rotating the area under $y = x^2 + 1$ over $[0, 6]$ around the y-axis.

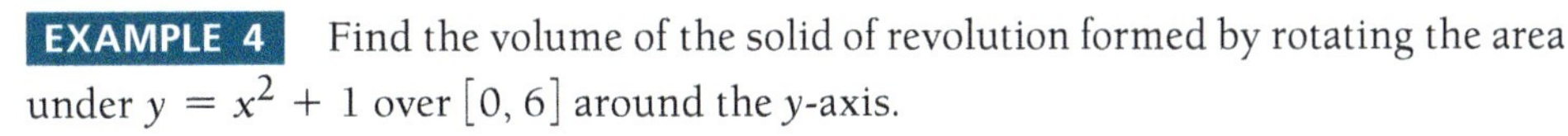

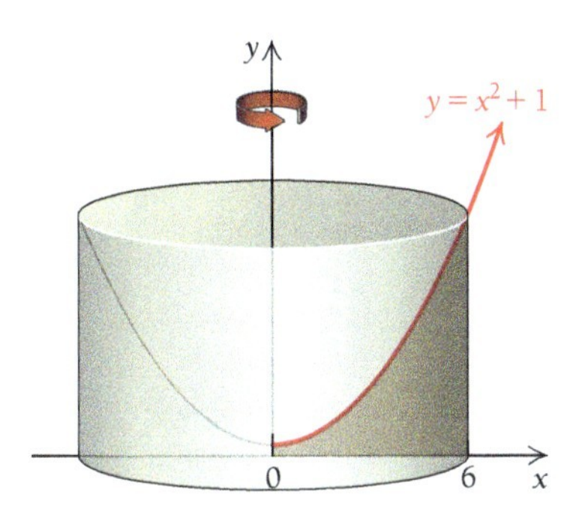

Solution We have

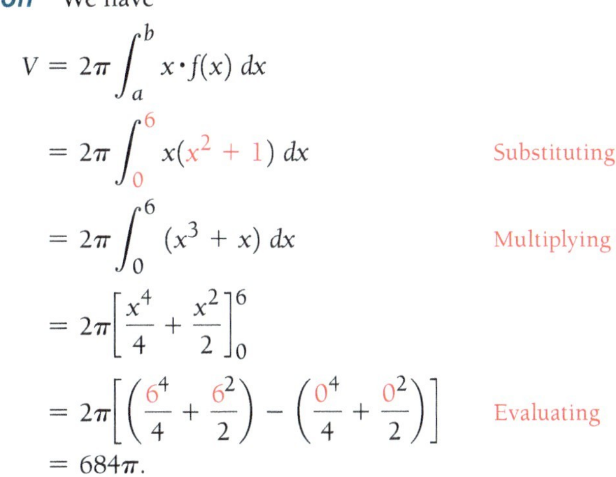

$$\begin{aligned} V &= 2\pi \int_a^b x \cdot f(x)\, dx \\ &= 2\pi \int_0^6 x(x^2 + 1)\, dx && \text{Substituting} \\ &= 2\pi \int_0^6 (x^3 + x)\, dx && \text{Multiplying} \\ &= 2\pi \left[\frac{x^4}{4} + \frac{x^2}{2}\right]_0^6 \\ &= 2\pi\left[\left(\frac{6^4}{4} + \frac{6^2}{2}\right) - \left(\frac{0^4}{4} + \frac{0^2}{2}\right)\right] && \text{Evaluating} \\ &= 684\pi. \end{aligned}$$

Quick Check 4 ✓
Find the volume of the solid of revolution formed by rotating the area under $y = \sqrt{x}$ over $[1, 4]$ around the y-axis.

Section Summary

- *Volume by disks*: If f is continuous over $[a, b]$, then the volume of the *solid of revolution* formed by rotating the area under the graph of f from a to b around the x-axis is given by

$$V = \pi \int_a^b [f(x)]^2\, dx.$$

- *Volume by shells*: If f is continuous over $[a, b]$, then the volume of the solid of revolution formed by rotating the area under the graph of f from a to b around the y-axis is given by

$$V = 2\pi \int_a^b x \cdot f(x)\, dx.$$

5.6 Exercise Set

Find the volume generated by rotating the area bounded by the graphs of each set of equations around the x-axis.

1. $y = x, x = 0, x = 1$

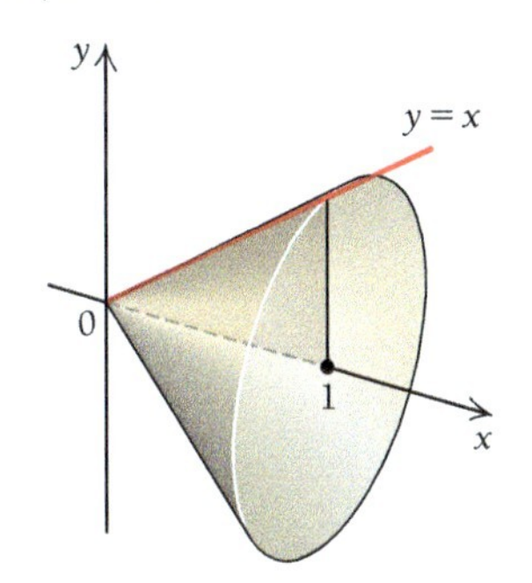

2. $y = x, x = 0, x = 2$

3. $y = \sqrt{x}, x = 1, x = 4$

4. $y = 2x, x = 1, x = 3$

5. $y = e^x, x = -2, x = 5$

6. $y = e^x, x = -3, x = 2$

7. $y = \frac{1}{x}, x = 1, x = 3$

8. $y = \frac{1}{x}, x = 1, x = 4$

9. $y = \frac{2}{\sqrt{x}}, x = 4, x = 9$

10. $y = \frac{1}{\sqrt{x}}, x = 1, x = 4$

11. $y = 4, x = 1, x = 3$

12. $y = 5, x = 1, x = 3$

13. $y = x^2, x = 0, x = 2$

14. $y = x + 1, x = -1, x = 2$

15. $y = \sqrt{1 + x}, x = 2, x = 10$

16. $y = 2\sqrt{x}, x = 1, x = 2$

17. $y = \sqrt{4 - x^2}, x = -2, x = 2$

18. $y = \sqrt{1 - x^2}, x = -1, x = 1$

Find the volume generated by rotating the area bounded by the graphs of each set of equations around the y-axis.

19. $y = 3x, x = 0, x = 5$

20. $y = 2x, x = 0, x = 3$

21. $y = x^2, x = 0, x = 3$

22. $y = x^3, x = 0, x = 3$

23. $y = \frac{1}{x^2}, x = 2, x = 4$

24. $y = \frac{1}{x}, x = 1, x = 5$

25. $y = x^2 + 3, x = 1, x = 2$

26. $y = x^3 + 1, x = 2, x = 5$

27. $y = \sqrt[3]{x}, x = 1, x = 8$

28. $y = \sqrt{x}, x = 4, x = 9$

29. $y = \sqrt{x^2 + 1}, x = 0, x = 3$

30. $y = \frac{1}{x^2 + 1}, x = 1, x = 7$

31. Let R be the area bounded by the graph of $y = 9 - x$ and the x-axis over $[0, 9]$.

a) Find the volume of the solid of revolution generated by rotating R around the x-axis.

b) Find the volume of the solid of revolution generated by rotating R around the y-axis.

c) Explain why the solids in parts (a) and (b) have the same volume.

32. Let R be the area bounded by the graph of $y = 9 - x^2$ and the x-axis over $[0, 3]$.

a) Find the volume of the solid of revolution generated by rotating R around the x-axis.

b) Find the volume of the solid of revolution generated by rotating R around the y-axis.

c) Explain why the solids in parts (a) and (b) do not have the same volume.

APPLICATIONS

33. Cooling tower volume. Cooling towers at nuclear power plants have a "pinched" chimney shape (which promotes cooling within the tower) formed by rotating a hyperbola around an axis. The function

$$y = 50\sqrt{1 + \frac{x^2}{22{,}500}}, \quad \text{for } -250 \le x \le 150,$$

where x and y are in feet, describes the shape of such a tower (lying on its side).

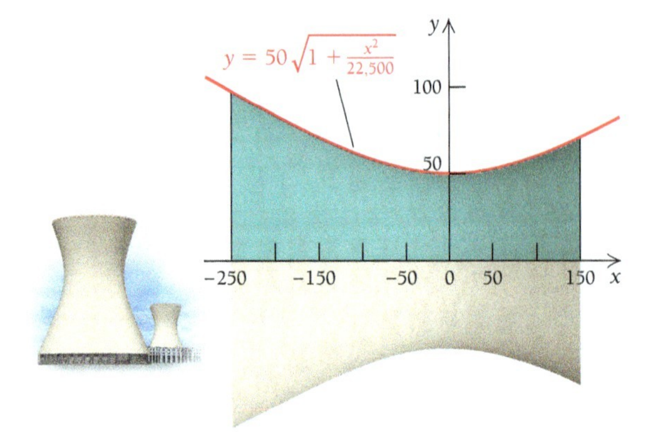

Determine the volume of the tower by rotating the area bounded by the graph of y around the x-axis.

34. Volume of a football. A regulation football used in the National Football League (NFL) is 11 in. from tip to tip and 7 in. in diameter at its thickest (the regulations allow for slight variation in these dimensions). (*Source:* NFL.) The shape of a football can be modeled by the function

$$f(x) = -0.116x^2 + 3.5, \quad \text{for } -5.5 \le x \le 5.5,$$

where x is in inches. Find the volume of an NFL football by rotating the area bounded by the graph of f around the x-axis.

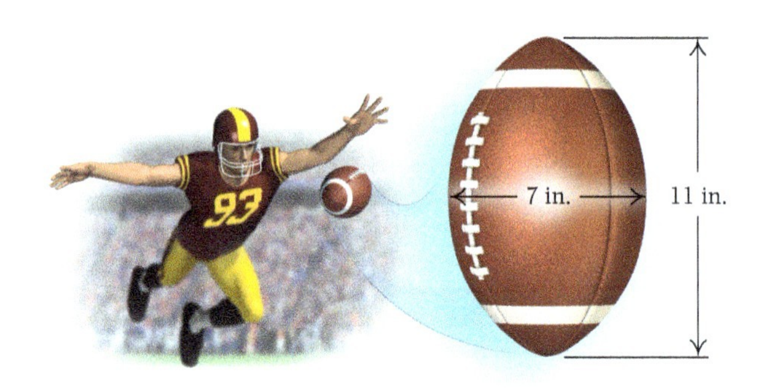

35. Volume of a hogan. A *hogan* is a circular shelter used by Native Americans in the Four Corners region of the southwestern United States. The volume of a hogan can be approximated if the graph of $y = -0.02x^2 + 12$, for $0 \le x \le 15$, where x and y are in feet and the x-axis represents ground level, is rotated around the y-axis. Find the volume.

36. Volume of a domed stadium. The volume of a stadium with a domed roof can be approximated if the graph of $y = -0.00025x^2 + 130$, for $0 \le x \le 400$, where x and y are in feet and the x-axis represents ground level, is rotated around the y-axis. Find the volume.

SYNTHESIS

37. Calculating volume using shells, prove that the volume of a right circular cone of height h and radius r is $V = \frac{1}{3}\pi r^2 h$.

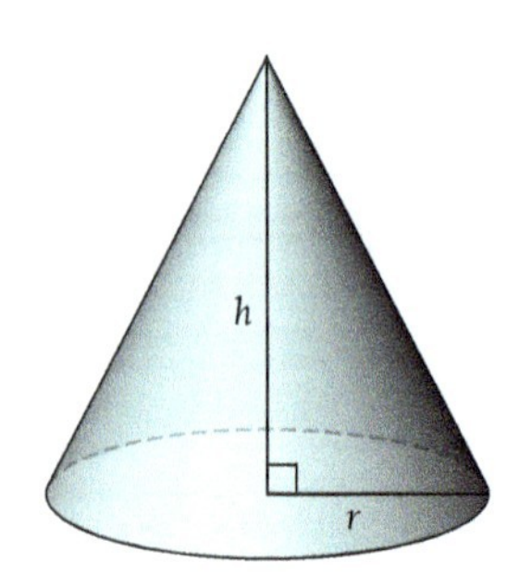

38. Calculating volume using disks, prove that the volume of a sphere of radius r is $\frac{4}{3}\pi r^3$.

Find the volume generated by rotating about the x-axis the area bounded by the graphs of each set of equations and the x-axis.

39. $y = \sqrt{\ln x}, x = e, x = e^3$

40. $y = \sqrt{xe^{-x}}, x = 1, x = 2$

In Exercises 41 and 42, the first quadrant is the region of the xy-plane in which $x > 0$ and $y > 0$.

41. Find the volume of the solid of revolution generated by rotating the area in the first quadrant between $y = -\frac{1}{3}x^3 + 3x$ and the x-axis around the y-axis.

42. Find the volume of the solid of revolution generated by rotating the area in the first quadrant between $y = x - x^3$ and the x-axis around the y-axis.

43. Let R be the area between $y = x + 1$ and the x-axis over $[0, a]$, where $a > 0$.

a) Find the volumes of the solids generated by rotating R, with $a = 1$, around the x-axis and around the y-axis. Which volume is larger?

b) Find the volumes of the solids generated by rotating R, with $a = 2$, around the x-axis and around the y-axis. Which volume is larger?

c) Find the value of a for which the two solids of revolution have the same volume.

44. Let R be the area between $y = kx$, the x-axis, and the line $x = 1$. Assume $k > 0$.

a) Find the value of k for which the volumes of the solids formed by rotating R around the x-axis and around the y-axis are the same.

b) Show that the answer to part (a) is true if the limits of integration are $[a, b]$, where $0 < a < b$.

45. Consider the function $y = 1/x$ over the interval $[1, \infty)$. We showed in Section 5.3 that the area under the curve is not finite; that is, $\int_1^\infty \frac{1}{x}\,dx$ diverges. Find the volume of the solid of revolution formed by rotating the area under the graph of $y = 1/x$ over $[1, \infty)$ around the x-axis. That is, find

$$\int_1^\infty \pi\left[\frac{1}{x}\right]^2 dx.$$

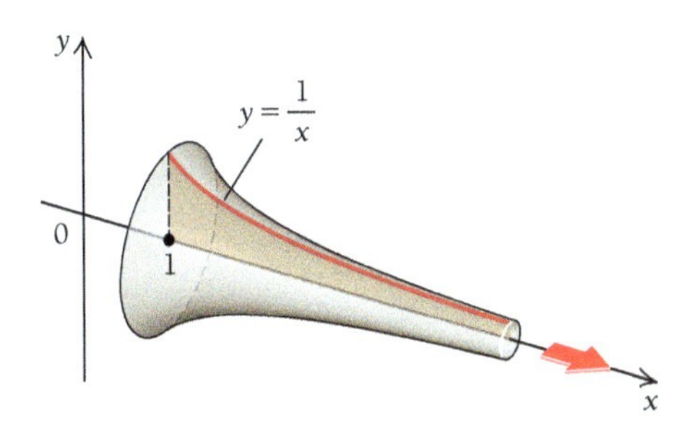

This solid is sometimes referred to as *Gabriel's horn*.

Technology Connection 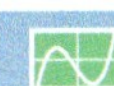

46. Paradox of Gabriel's horn or the infinite paint can. Though we cannot prove it here, the surface area of Gabriel's horn (see Exercise 45) is given by

$$S = \int_1^\infty \frac{2\pi}{x}\sqrt{1 + \frac{1}{x^4}}\,dx.$$

Show that the surface area of Gabriel's horn is infinite. The paradox is that the volume of the horn is finite, but the surface area is infinite. This is like a can of paint that has a finite volume but, when full, does not hold enough paint to paint the outside of the can.

47. Let R be the area between the graph of $y = \sqrt{x}$ and the x-axis. Find an upper bound a such that the volume generated by rotating R around the x-axis over $[0, a]$ is the same as the volume generated by rotating R around the y-axis.

48. Let R be the area between the graph of $y = x + x^2 - x^3$ and the x-axis, where $x \geq 0$.

a) Find the volume generated by rotating R around the x-axis.

b) Find the volume generated by rotating R around the y-axis.

49. A hemisphere of radius 1 ft is positioned with its open side up and holds a volume of water that is half the volume of the hemisphere. What is the maximum depth of the water?

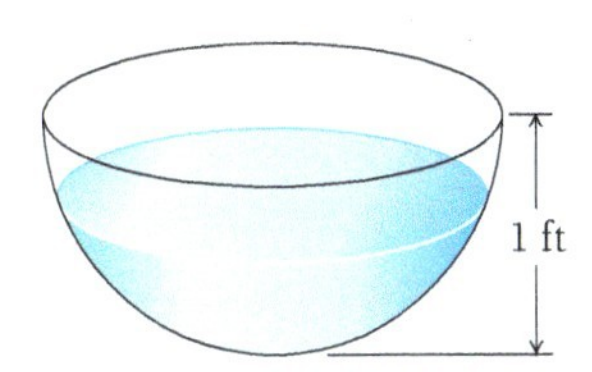

Answers to Quick Checks

1. $\frac{128\pi}{7}$ **2.** $\frac{2\pi}{3}$ **3.** 320π ft^3 **4.** $\frac{124\pi}{5}$

5.7 Differential Equations

- Determine general and particular solutions of a differential equation.
- Verify that a function is a solution of a differential equation.
- Solve differential equations using separation of variables.
- Solve differential equations using the uninhibited growth model.
- Solve applied problems using separation of variables.

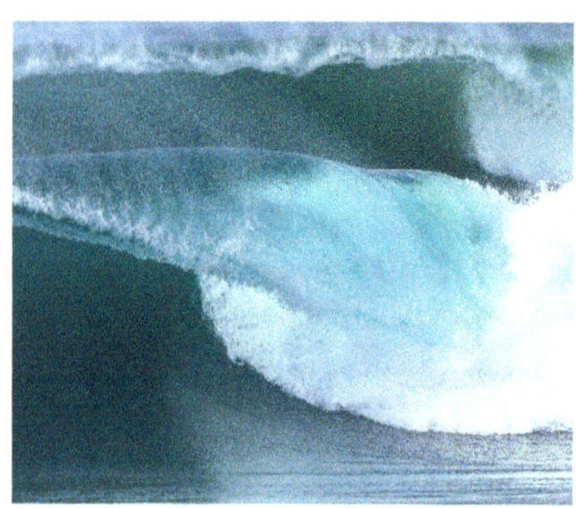

The motion of waves can be represented by differential equations.

In Chapter 2, we studied an important equation:

$$\frac{d}{dt}P(t) = k \cdot P(t) \quad \text{or} \quad \frac{dP}{dt} = kP.$$

We saw that the solution of this equation is a function,

$$P(t) = P_0 e^{kt}, \tag{1}$$

where P_0 is the initial quantity at time $t = 0$. Equations such as $dP/dt = kP$ are called *differential equations.*

DEFINITION

A **differential equation** is an equation that includes a derivative and has a function as a solution.

Solving Certain Differential Equations

In differential equations, P and $P(t)$ are often used interchangeably, as are dP/dt and $P'(t)$. We will also use the notation y' for a derivative. That is, if $y = f(x)$, then

$$y' = \frac{dy}{dx} = f'(x).$$

Certain differential equations are solved by finding the antiderivative. For example, the differential equation

$$\frac{dy}{dx} = f(x), \quad \text{or} \quad y' = f(x),$$

has the solution

$$y = \int f(x)\,dx = F(x) + C, \quad \text{where } \frac{d}{dx}F(x) = f(x).$$

Recall from Chapter 4 that an indefinite integral results in a set of functions, so there are infinitely many solutions. The set of all functions that solve a differential equation is called the **general solution**.

EXAMPLE 1 Find the general solution of $y' = 2x$.

Solution We find the solution by integrating both sides of the equation:

$$\frac{dy}{dx} = 2x \qquad \text{Using Leibniz notation for the derivative}$$

$$dy = 2x\,dx \qquad \text{Treating } dy/dx \text{ as a quotient, as in Sections 3.6 and 4.5}$$

$$\int dy = \int 2x\,dx \qquad \text{Integrating both sides}$$

$$y = x^2 + C.$$

As a check, note that $y' = \frac{d}{dx}(x^2 + C) = 2x + 0 = 2x$. **1✓**

Quick Check 1✓

Find the general solution of $y' = 3x^2 - x$.

The solution in Example 1, $y = x^2 + C$, is a general solution because substituting *all* values of C in it gives *all* of the solutions. Substituting a specific value of C gives a **particular solution** of the differential equation. For example, the following are particular solutions of $y' = 2x$:

$$y = x^2 + 3, \quad y = x^2, \quad y = x^2 - 3.$$

The graph shows the curves of these particular solutions. The general solution can be regarded as the set of all particular solutions.

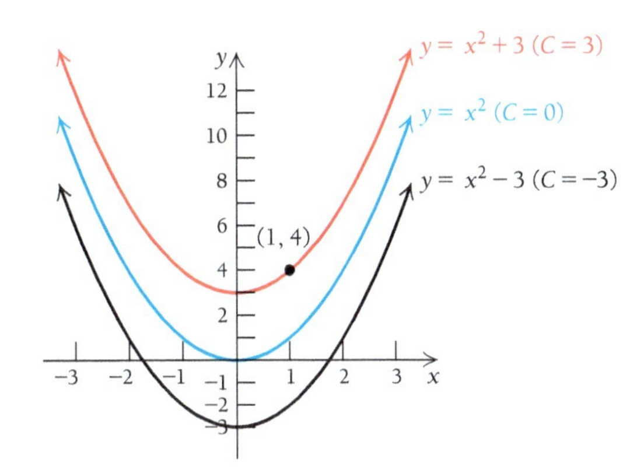

Knowing a specific function value often allows us to find a particular solution. For example, if the solution in Example 1 includes the ordered pair (1, 4), then a particular solution is $y = x^2 + 3$, since $4 = 1^2 + 3$. The requirement that (1, 4) must be included in the solution is called an **initial condition**. Often, an initial condition is given as $y(a) = b$. For example, the initial condition (1, 4) is expressed as $y(1) = 4$.

Verifying Solutions

To verify that a function is a solution of a differential equation, we find the necessary derivatives and substitute. For example, to verify that $P(t) = P_0e^{kt}$ is a solution of $dP/dt = kP$, we find the derivative of P, which is $P'(t) = P_0ke^{kt}$. We then substitute P_0ke^{kt} for dP/dt and P_0e^{kt} for P. Since

$$P_0ke^{kt} = k \cdot P_0e^{kt}$$

is true, we have confirmed that $P(t) = P_0e^{kt}$ is a solution of $dP/dt = kP$.

EXAMPLE 2 Consider the differential equation $y' = 2xy$.

a) Show that $y = e^{x^2}$ is a solution.

b) Show that $y = Ce^{x^2}$ is a solution, where C is a constant.

Solution For both parts (a) and (b), we find y' and then substitute.

a) If $y = e^{x^2}$, then $y' = 2xe^{x^2}$. Substituting, we have

$$\begin{array}{c|c} y' - 2xy & 0 \\ \hline 2xe^{x^2} - 2x \cdot e^{x^2} & ?\ 0 \\ 0 & 0 \quad \text{TRUE} \end{array}$$

Thus, $y = e^{x^2}$ is a solution of $y' - 2xy = 0$.

b) If $y = Ce^{x^2}$, then $y' = 2Cxe^{x^2}$. Substituting, we have

$$\begin{array}{c|c} y' - 2xy & 0 \\ \hline 2Cxe^{x^2} - 2x \cdot Ce^{x^2} & ?\ 0 \\ 0 & 0 \quad \text{TRUE} \end{array}$$

2 ✓

Quick Check 2 ✓
Let $y' - 2y = 0$.
a) Show that $y = e^{2x}$ is a solution.
b) Show that $y = Ce^{2x}$ is a solution.

In Example 2, $y = Ce^{x^2}$ is the general solution of $y' - 2xy = 0$, meaning that all solutions of this differential equation can be written in the form $y = Ce^{x^2}$. The solution $y = e^{x^2}$ is a particular solution, where $C = 1$.

A differential equation may include second- or higher-order derivatives. Recall that if $y = f(x)$, then $y' = \frac{d}{dx}f(x) = f'(x)$, $y'' = \frac{d}{dx}f'(x) = f''(x)$, and so on.

EXAMPLE 3 Show that $y = 4e^x + 5e^{3x}$ is a solution of $y'' - 4y' + 3y = 0$.

Solution We first find y' and y'':

$$y' = \frac{d}{dx}(4e^x + 5e^{3x}) = 4e^x + 15e^{3x};$$
$$y'' = \frac{d}{dx}y' = 4e^x + 45e^{3x}.$$

Then we substitute in the differential equation, as follows:

$y'' - 4y' + 3y$	$= 0$	
$(4e^x + 45e^{3x}) - 4(4e^x + 15e^{3x}) + 3(4e^x + 5e^{3x})$	? 0	
$4e^x + 45e^{3x} - 16e^x - 60e^{3x} + 12e^x + 15e^{3x}$	0	
$4e^x - 16e^x + 12e^x + 45e^{3x} - 60e^{3x} + 15e^{3x}$	0	Collecting
$0e^x + 0e^{3x}$	0	like terms
0	0	TRUE

Since a true statement, $0 = 0$, results, we have confirmed that $y = 4e^x + 5e^{3x}$ is a solution of the differential equation. **3 ✓**

Quick Check 3 ✓

Show that $y = x^2 + x$ is a solution of $y' + \frac{1}{x}y = 3x + 2$.

Separable Differential Equations

Consider the differential equation from Example 2:

$$\frac{dy}{dx} = 2xy. \quad (2)$$

Treating dy/dx as a quotient and multiplying both sides by dx and $1/y$, we get

$$\frac{1}{y}\,dy = 2x\,dx, \quad \text{or} \quad \frac{dy}{y} = 2x\,dx, \quad y \neq 0. \quad (3)$$

We have *separated the variables*, meaning that all expressions involving one of the variables appear on one side of the equation and all expressions involving the other variable are on the other, with both sides expressed as products. A differential equation in which the variables can be separated is called a *separable differential equation.*

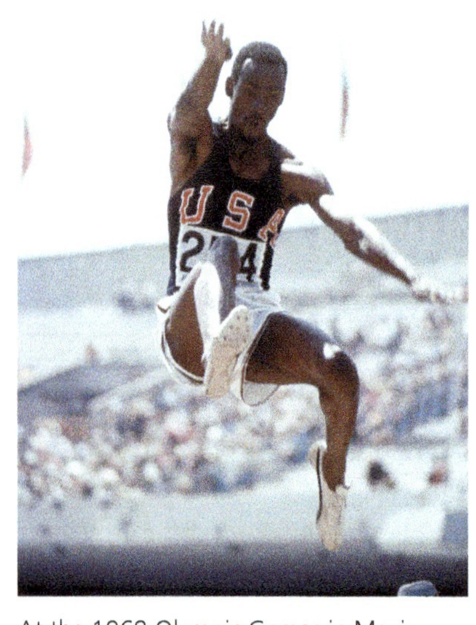

At the 1968 Olympic Games in Mexico City, Bob Beamon made a world-record long jump of 29 ft $2\frac{1}{2}$ in. Many believed that the jump's record length was due to the altitude, which was 7400 ft. Using differential equations for analysis, M. N. Bearley refuted the altitude theory in "The Long Jump Miracle of Mexico City" [*Mathematics Magazine*, Vol. 45, 241–246 (November 1972)]. Bearley argues that the world-record jump was a result of Beamon's exceptional speed (9.5 sec in the 100-yd dash) and the fact that he left the take-off board in perfect position.

DEFINITION

A **separable differential equation** is a differential equation that can be written in the form

$$f(y)\,dy = g(x)\,dx.$$

Equation (2) is an example of a separable differential equation, and equation (3) is equivalent to equation (2), but with the variables separated. To find a solution, we integrate both sides of equation (3):

$$\int \frac{dy}{y} = \int 2x\,dx$$
$$\ln|y| = x^2 + C_1.$$

We use only one constant because the two antiderivatives differ by, at most, a constant. Recall from Section R.6 that if $\log_a b = t$, then $b = a^t$. Since $\ln|y| = \log_e|y| = x^2 + C_1$, we have

$$|y| = e^{x^2 + C_1}, \quad \text{or} \quad y = \pm e^{x^2} \cdot e^{C_1}.$$

Thus, the solution of equation (2) is

$$y = Ce^{x^2}, \quad \text{where } C = \pm e^{C_1}.$$

Both C and $\pm e^{C_1}$ represent arbitrary constants.

As a check, we have $y' = \frac{dy}{dx} = 2Cxe^{x^2}$. Substituting y' and y into equation (2), we have

$$\frac{dy}{dx} = 2xy$$

$2Cxe^{x^2}$	? $2x \cdot Ce^{x^2}$	
$2Cxe^{x^2}$	$2Cxe^{x^2}$	TRUE

EXAMPLE 4 Find the particular solution of $3y^2 \frac{dy}{dx} + x = 0$, when $y(0) = 5$.

Solution We first separate the variables:

$$3y^2 \frac{dy}{dx} = -x \qquad \text{Adding } -x \text{ to both sides}$$

$$3y^2\, dy = -x\, dx. \qquad \text{Multiplying both sides by } dx$$

We then integrate both sides:

$$\int 3y^2\, dy = \int -x\, dx$$

$$y^3 = -\frac{x^2}{2} + C$$

$$y^3 = C - \frac{x^2}{2}. \tag{4}$$

Given that $y = 5$ when $x = 0$, we substitute to find C:

$$(5)^3 = C - \frac{(0)^2}{2} \qquad \text{Substituting}$$

$$125 = C.$$

Using this value for C and then taking the cube root of both sides of equation (4), we have the particular solution:

$$y = \sqrt[3]{125 - \frac{x^2}{2}}.$$

4 ✓

Quick Check 4 ✓

Solve $2\sqrt{y}\,\frac{dy}{dx} - 3x = 0$, when $y(0) = 9$.

EXAMPLE 5 Solve: $y' = x - xy$.

Solution We first replace y' with dy/dx:

$$\frac{dy}{dx} = x - xy.$$

Then we separate the variables:

$$dy = (x - xy)\, dx$$

$$dy = x(1 - y)\, dx$$

$$\frac{dy}{1 - y} = x\, dx, \quad y \neq 1.$$

Next, we integrate both sides:

$$\int \frac{dy}{1-y} = \int x\,dx$$

$$-\ln|1-y| = \frac{x^2}{2} + C_1$$

$$\ln|1-y| = -\frac{x^2}{2} - C_1$$

$$|1-y| = e^{-x^2/2-C_1} \qquad \text{Writing an equivalent exponential equation}$$

$$1-y = \pm e^{-x^2/2-C_1}$$

$$1-y = \pm e^{-x^2/2}e^{-C_1}. \qquad \text{Recalling that } a^{x+y} = a^x a^y$$

$$1-y = C_2 e^{-x^2/2} \qquad \text{Replacing } \pm e^{-C_1} \text{ with } C_2\text{; since } \pm e^{-C_1} \text{ is never zero, } C_2 \text{ cannot be zero.}$$

$$-y = C_2 e^{-x^2/2} - 1$$

$$y = 1 - C_2 e^{-x^2/2}. \qquad \text{Multiplying both sides by } -1$$

Quick Check 5 ✓
Solve
$(1 + x^2)y' = xy$.

If we replace $-C_2$ with C, we can replace the subtraction with addition. The general solution is

$$y = 1 + Ce^{-x^2/2}, \quad \text{where } C \neq 0.$$

5 ✓

In Example 5, we restricted y such that $y \neq 1$. Note that when $y = 1$, the differential equation is $\frac{dy}{dx} = x - x(1)$, or $\frac{dy}{dx} = 0$. This would imply that $y = C$, where C is *any* constant, is a solution, which contradicts the statement that $y \neq 1$.

The Uninhibited Growth Model

Recall from Section 2.4 that $dP/dt = kP$, with $k > 0$, is called the **uninhibited growth model** and is used when exponential growth continues forever, without constraints. The equation $dP/dt = kP$ is read "the rate of change of P is directly proportional to the amount P." Thus, as P increases, the rate of change dP/dt also increases. In simple terms, the larger P is, the faster P grows. The **constant of proportionality** k is also referred to as the **continuous growth rate**.

EXAMPLE 6 **Business: Growth of a Savings Account.** Darrell invests \$1000 in an account that earns interest at a rate of 4.5%, compounded continuously. Find the particular solution of the differential equation that describes the growth in value of this account.

Solution We let $A(t)$ be the amount, in dollars, in Darrell's account after t years. Because of continuous compounding, we have

$$\frac{dA}{dt} = kA$$

Separating variables, we have

$$\frac{dA}{A} = k\,dt, \quad A \neq 0.$$

Integrating both sides, we have

$$\int \frac{dA}{A} = \int k\,dt$$

$$\ln A = kt + C \qquad \text{Since } A \text{ is positive, we do not need to use absolute value.}$$

$$A = e^{kt+C} \qquad \text{Writing an equivalent exponential equation}$$

$$A = e^C e^{kt}$$

$$A(t) = Ce^{kt}. \qquad \text{Rewriting } e^C \text{ as } C$$

Technology Connection

Exploratory

Divide the value of $A'(t)$ by the value of $A(t)$ for each labeled point in the graph with Example 6. What is the result of each division?

The interest rate of 4.5% is expressed as $k = 0.045$, and since $A(0) = Ce^{k \cdot 0} = C \cdot 1 = 1000$, we have $C = 1000$.

Thus, the particular solution is $A(t) = 1000e^{0.045t}$. The graph of $A(t)$ shows the relationship between $A(t)$ and $A'(t)$. As $A(t)$ increases in value, so does the rate $A'(t)$.

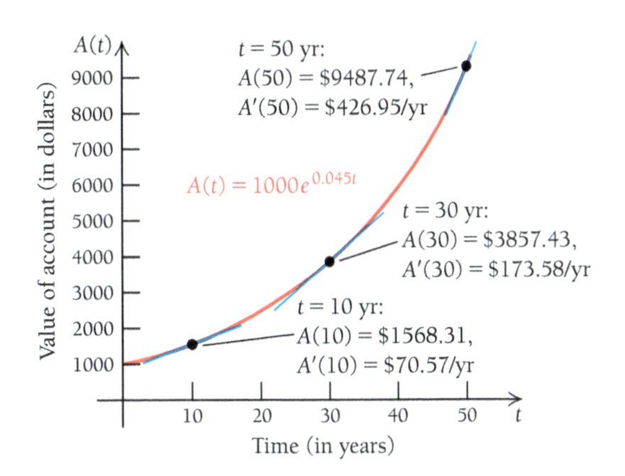

Quick Check 6 ✓

Find the particular solution of the differential equation $dA/dt = kA$, when $k = 0.032$ and $A_0 = \$2000$.

6 ✓

An Application to Economics: Elasticity

Technology Connection

Exploratory: Solutions to Differential Equations

At www.wolframalpha.com, you can solve differential equations and graph families of solutions. When given an initial condition, you can find the particular solution. For example, to solve $y' = x - xy$ (Example 5), key in y′=x-xy and press ENTER. Initial conditions are entered in the form y(a)=b and separated from the differential equation by a comma.

EXAMPLE 7 Suppose the elasticity of demand for a certain product (see Section 3.7) is 1 for all prices $x > 0$. That is, $E(x) = 1$ for $x > 0$. Find the demand function, $q = D(x)$.

Solution Recall that elasticity of demand is given by

$$E(x) = -\frac{xD'(x)}{D(x)}.$$

Since $E(x) = 1$ for all $x > 0$,

$$1 = -\frac{xD'(x)}{D(x)}$$ Setting $E(x)$ equal to 1

$$1 = -\frac{x}{q} \cdot \frac{dq}{dx}$$ Letting $D(x) = q$ and $D'(x) = \frac{dq}{dx}$

$$\frac{dx}{x} = -\frac{dq}{q}$$ Multiplying both sides by $\frac{dx}{x}$ to separate the variables

$$\int \frac{dx}{x} = -\int \frac{dq}{q}$$ Integrating both sides

$$\ln x = -\ln q + C_1$$ Both price, x, and quantity, q, are assumed to be positive, so using the absolute value is not necessary.

$$\ln x + \ln q = C_1$$

$$\ln (xq) = C_1$$ Using a property of logarithms

$$xq = e^{C_1}.$$ Rewriting as an equivalent exponential equation

We let $C = e^{C_1}$ so that $xq = C$:

$$q = \frac{C}{x}, \quad \text{or} \quad D(x) = \frac{C}{x}.$$

This result characterizes demand functions for which the elasticity is always 1. 7 ✓

Quick Check 7 ✓

Find the demand function $q = D(x)$ if the elasticity of demand is $E(x) = x$.

An Application to Psychology: Reaction to a Stimulus

In psychology, one model of stimulus-response asserts that the rate of change dR/dS of the reaction R with respect to a stimulus S is inversely proportional to the intensity of the stimulus. That is,

$$\frac{dR}{dS} = \frac{k}{S},$$

where k is a positive constant. This is known as the *Weber-Fechner Law.* To solve this equation for R, we separate variables and integrate both sides:

$$dR = k \cdot \frac{dS}{S}$$

$$\int dR = k \int \frac{dS}{S}$$

$$R = k \ln S + C. \quad \text{We assume } S > 0. \tag{5}$$

Let S_0 be the lowest level of a stimulus that can be detected. This is the *threshold value*, or the *detection threshold*. For example, the detection threshold for light is the flame of a candle 30 miles away on a clear, dark night. If S_0 is the lowest level of the stimulus that can be detected, we can assume that $R(S_0) = 0$. Substituting this condition into equation (5), we have

$$0 = k \ln S_0 + C, \quad \text{or} \quad -k \ln S_0 = C.$$

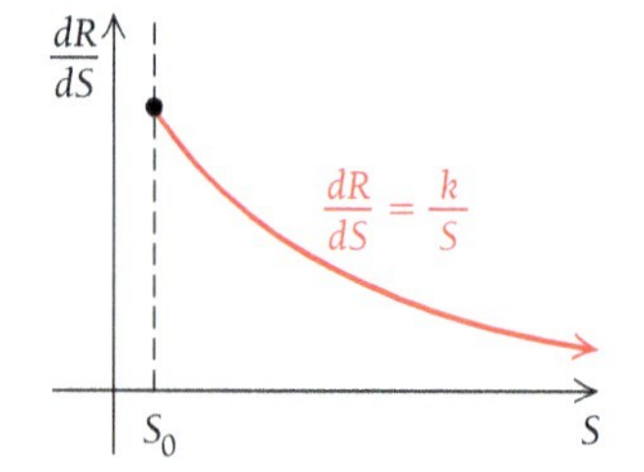

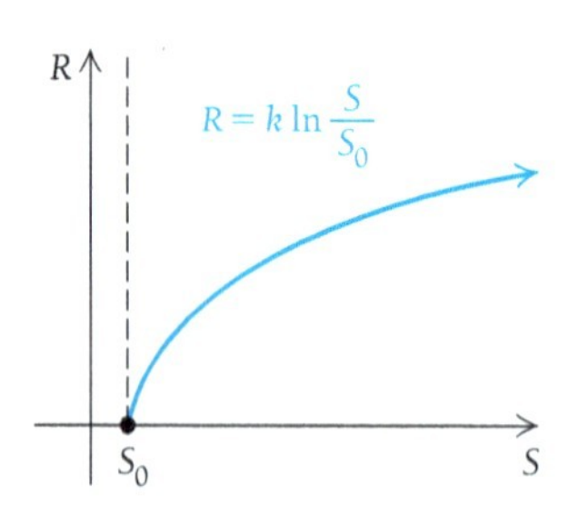

Replacing C in equation (5) with $-k \ln S_0$ gives us

$$R = k \ln S - k \ln S_0 \quad \text{As a check, note that } \frac{dR}{dS} = \frac{k}{S}.$$

$$= k(\ln S - \ln S_0)$$

$$= k \ln \frac{S}{S_0}. \quad \text{This is the solution of the original differential equation.}$$

Look at the graphs of dR/dS and R. Note that as the stimulus and the response get larger, the rate of change, dR/dS, decreases. For example, suppose a lamp has a 6-watt bulb in it. If the bulb were suddenly changed to an 8-watt one, you would probably be very aware of the difference. That is, your response would be strong. If the bulb were changed from 10 watts to 12 watts, your response would increase, but not as dramatically as it did for the change from 6 to 8 watts. A change from a 12-watt to a 14-watt bulb would cause even less increase in response, and so on.

The table lists some other detection thresholds you may find interesting.

Stimulus	Detection Threshold
Sound	The tick of a watch from 20 feet away in a quiet room
Taste	Water diluted with sugar in the ratio of 1 teaspoon to 2 gallons
Smell	One drop of perfume diffused into the volume of three average-size rooms
Touch	The wing of a bee dropped on your cheek at a distance of 1 centimeter (about $\frac{3}{8}$ of an inch)

Section Summary

- A *differential equation* is an equation that includes a derivative and has a function as a solution.
- The *general solution* of a differential equation of the form $y' = f(x)$ is a set of functions $y = F(x) + C$, where $\frac{d}{dx}F(x) = f(x)$. For other differential equations, the general solution may be of the form $y = Cf(x)$, where C is any constant.
- A requirement that a solution of a differential equation include a specific ordered pair is an *initial condition*. If an initial condition is given, then a *particular solution* in which the value of C is determined may be found.
- The differential equation $dP/dt = kP$, with $k > 0$, is called the *uninhibited growth model*, and its general solution is $P(t) = P_0e^{kt}$, where P_0 is the initial quantity at time $t = 0$. The value k is the *constant of proportionality*, also known as the *continuous growth rate*.
- A *separable differential equation* is a differential equation in which the variables can be isolated on opposite sides of the equation, in the form $f(y)\,dy = g(x)\,dx$.
- To solve a separable differential equation, the variables are separated, each side is integrated, and, if possible, the result is solved for one of the variables.

5.7 Exercise Set

In Exercises 1–6, find (a) *the general solution and* (b) *the particular solution for the given initial condition.*

1. $y' = 5x^6;\ y(0) = -3$

2. $y' = 10x^2;\ y(0) = 2$

3. $y' = e^{4x} - x + 2;\ y(0) = 4$

4. $y' = 2e^{-x} + x;\ y(1) = 1$

5. $y' = \frac{3}{x} + x^2 - x^4;\ y(1) = -4$

6. $y' = \frac{4}{x} - \frac{1}{x^2};\ y(1) = 5$

7. Let $y' + 4y = 0$.

a) Show that $y = e^{-4x}$ is a solution of this differential equation.

b) Show that $y = Ce^{-4x}$ is a solution, where C is a constant.

8. Let $y' - 3x^2y = 0$.

a) Show that $y = e^{x^3}$ is a solution of this differential equation.

b) Show that $y = Ce^{x^3}$ is a solution, where C is a constant.

9. Show that $y = x \ln x - 5x + 7$ is a solution of

$$y'' - \frac{1}{x} = 0.$$

10. Show that $y = x \ln x + 3x - 2$ is a solution of

$$y'' - \frac{1}{x} = 0.$$

11. Show that $y = -2e^x + xe^x$ is a solution of

$$y'' - 2y' + y = 0.$$

12. Show that $y = e^x + 3xe^x$ is a solution of

$$y'' - 2y' + y = 0.$$

13. Let $y'' - 7y' - 44y = 0$.

a) Show that $y = e^{11x}$ is a solution of this differential equation.

b) Show that $y = e^{-4x}$ is a solution.

c) Show that $y = C_1e^{11x} + C_2e^{-4x}$ is a solution, where C_1 and C_2 are constants.

14. Let $y'' - y' - 30y = 0$.

a) Show that $y = e^{6x}$ is a solution of this differential equation.

b) Show that $y = e^{-5x}$ is a solution.

c) Show that $y = C_1e^{6x} + C_2e^{-5x}$ is a solution, where C_1 and C_2 are constants.

In Exercises 15–20, (a) *find the general solution of each differential equation, and* (b) *check the solution by substituting into the differential equation.*

15. $\frac{dC}{dt} = 0.66C$

16. $\frac{dM}{dt} = 0.05M$

17. $\frac{dV}{dt} = -1.33V$

18. $\frac{dR}{dt} = -0.35R$

19. $\frac{dh}{dt} = 0.023h$

20. $\frac{dG}{dt} = 0.005G$

In Exercises 21–30, (a) *find the particular solution of each differential equation as determined by the initial condition, and* (b) *check the solution by substituting into the differential equation.*

21. $y' = x^2 + 2x - 3;\ y(0) = 4$

22. $y' = 3x^2 - x + 5;\ y(0) = 6$

23. $f'(x) = x^{2/3} - x;\ f(1) = -6$

24. $f'(x) = x^{2/5} + x;\ f(1) = -7$

25. $\frac{dB}{dt} = 0.03B$, where $B(0) = 500$

26. $\frac{dG}{dt} = 0.75G$, where $G(0) = 2000$

27. $\frac{dS}{dt} = -0.125S$, where $S = 750$ when $t = 0$

28. $\frac{dL}{dt} = -0.68L$, where $L = 1200$ when $t = 0$

29. $\frac{dT}{dt} = 0.015T$, where $T = 50$ when $t = 1$

30. $\frac{dP}{dt} = 0.024P$, where $P = 32$ when $t = 2$

Solve by separating variables.

31. $\frac{dy}{dx} = 5x^4y$

32. $\frac{dy}{dx} = 4x^3y$

33. $3y^2\frac{dy}{dx} = 5x$

34. $3y^2\frac{dy}{dx} = 8x$

35. $\frac{dy}{dx} = \frac{x}{2y}$

36. $\frac{dy}{dx} = \frac{2x}{y}$

37. $\frac{dy}{dx} = \frac{7}{y^2}$

38. $\frac{dy}{dx} = \frac{6}{y}$

Solve for y.

39. $y' = 3x + xy;\quad y = 5$ when $x = 0$

40. $y' = 2x - xy;\quad y = 9$ when $x = 0$

41. $y' = 5y^{-2};\quad y(2) = 3$

42. $y' = 7y^{-2};\quad y(1) = 3$

APPLICATIONS

Business and Economics

43. Growth of an account. Debra invests $A_0 = \$500$ in an account that earns interest at a rate of 3.75%, compounded continuously.

a) Write the differential equation, with the initial condition, that represents $A(t)$, the value of Debra's account after t years.
b) Find the particular solution of the differential equation from part (a).
c) Find $A(5)$ and $A'(5)$.
d) Find $A'(5)/A(5)$, and explain what this number represents.

44. Growth of an account. Jennifer invests $A_0 = \$1200$ in an account that earns 4.2% compounded continuously.

a) Write the differential equation, with the initial condition, that represents $A(t)$, the value of Jennifer's account after t years.
b) Find the particular solution of the differential equation from part (a).
c) Find $A(7)$ and $A'(7)$.
d) Find $A'(7)/A(7)$, and explain what this number represents.

45. Stock growth. The value of a share of stock of Leslie's Designs, Inc., is modeled by

$$\frac{dV}{dt} = k(L - V),$$

where V is the value of the stock, in dollars, after t months; k is a constant; $L = \$24.81$, the *limiting value* of the stock; and $V(0) = 20$. Find the solution of the differential equation in terms of t and k.

46. Total profit from marginal profit. Hanna's Hat Company's marginal profit, P, as a function of its total cost, C, is given by

$$\frac{dP}{dC} = \frac{-200}{(C + 3)^{3/2}}.$$

a) Find the profit function, $P(C)$, if $P = \$10$ when $C = \$61$.
b) At what cost will the firm break even ($P = 0$)?

47. Capital expansion. *Domar's capital expansion model* is

$$\frac{dI}{dt} = hkI,$$

where I is the initial investment, h is the investment productivity (constant), k is the marginal productivity to the consumer (constant), and t is the time.

a) Use separation of variables to solve the differential equation.
b) Rewrite the solution with $k = 0.4$, $h = 1.33$, and an initial investment of \$500,000.

48. Utility. The reaction R in pleasure units by a consumer receiving S units of a product can be modeled by the differential equation

$$\frac{dR}{dS} = \frac{k}{S + 1},$$

where k is a positive constant.

a) Use separation of variables to solve the differential equation.
b) Rewrite the solution in terms of the initial condition $R(0) = 0$.
c) Explain why the condition $R(0) = 0$ is reasonable.

Elasticity. *Find the demand function $q = D(x)$, given each set of elasticity conditions. Recall that elasticity of demand is given by $E(x) = -\frac{xD'(x)}{D(x)}$.*

49. $E(x) = \frac{4}{x}$; $q = 2$ when $x = 4$

50. $E(x) = \frac{x}{200 - x}$; $q = 190$ when $x = 10$

51. $E(x) = 2$, for all $x > 0$

52. $E(x) = n$, for some constant n and all $x > 0$

Life and Physical Sciences

53. Population growth. The city of New River had a population of 17,000 in 2012 ($t = 0$) with a continuous growth rate of 1.75% per year.

a) Write the differential equation, with the initial condition, that represents $P(t)$, the population of New River after t years.
b) Find the particular solution of the differential equation from part (a).
c) Find $P(10)$ and $P'(10)$.
d) Find $P'(10)/P(10)$, and explain what this number represents.

54. **Population growth.** An initial population of 70 bacteria is growing continuously at a rate of 2.5% per hour.

a) Write the differential equation, along with the initial condition, that represents $P(t)$, the population of bacteria after t hours.
b) Find the particular solution of the differential equation from part (a).
c) Find $P(24)$ and $P'(24)$.
d) Find $P'(24)/P(24)$, and explain what this number represents.

55. **Population growth.** Before 1859, rabbits did not exist in Australia. That year, a settler released 24 rabbits into the wild. Without natural predators, the growth of the Australian rabbit population can be modeled by the uninhibited growth model $dP/dt = kP$, where $P(t)$ is the population of rabbits t years after 1859. (*Source*: www.dpi.vic.gov.au/agriculture.)

a) When the rabbit population was estimated to be 8900, its rate of growth was about 2630 rabbits per year. Use this information to find k, and then find the particular solution of the differential equation.
b) Find the rabbit population in 1900 ($t = 41$) and the rate at which it was increasing in that year.
c) From the results of parts (a) and (b), find $P'(41)/P(41)$.

56. **Population growth.** Suppose 30 sparrows are released into a region where they have no natural predators. The growth of the region's sparrow population can be modeled by the uninhibited growth model $dP/dt = kP$, where $P(t)$ is the population of sparrows t years after their initial release.

a) When the sparrow population is estimated at 12,500, its rate of growth is about 1325 sparrows per year. Use this information to find k, and then find the particular solution of the differential equation.
b) Find the number of sparrows and the rate at which the population is increasing after 8 yr.
c) From the results of parts (a) and (b), find $P'(8)/P(8)$.

Social Sciences

57. **The Brentano-Stevens Law.** The validity of the Weber–Fechner Law has been the subject of great debate among psychologists. An alternative model,

$$\frac{dR}{dS} = k \cdot \frac{R}{S},$$

where k is a positive constant, has been proposed. Find the general solution of this equation. (This model has also been referred to as the *Power Law of Stimulus–Response*.)

58. **The simplified Stefan-Boltzmann equation for heat transfer.** When a hot object is placed in a colder surrounding medium, the object's temperature can be approximated by $\frac{dT}{dt} = -aT^4$, where $T(t)$ is the temperature of the object (in degrees Celsius) after t minutes.

a) Find the general solution of the differential equation.
b) An object with an initial temperature of 500°C is placed in a walk-in cooler where the temperature is 0°C. After 10 min, the object's temperature is 425°C. Find the particular solution of the differential equation.
c) After how many minutes will the object's temperature have dropped to 100°C?

SYNTHESIS

59. The amount of money, $A(t)$, in Ina's savings account after t years is modeled by $dA/dt = 0.0418A$.

a) What is the continuous growth rate?
b) Find the particular solution, $A(t)$, if Ina's account is worth $3479.02 after 2 yr.
c) Find the amount that Ina deposited initially.

60. The amount of money, $A(t)$, in Imani's savings account after t years is modeled by $dA/dt = 0.0325A$.

a) What is the continuous growth rate?
b) Find the particular solution, $A(t)$, if Imani's account is worth $2582.58 after 1 yr.
c) Find the amount that Imani deposited initially.

Solve.

61. $\frac{dy}{dx} = 5x^4y^2 + x^3y^2$

62. $e^{-1/x} \cdot \frac{dy}{dx} = x^{-2} \cdot y^2$

63. Explain the difference between a constant rate of growth and a constant percentage rate of growth.

64. What function is also its own derivative? Write a differential equation for which this function is a solution. Are there any other solutions to this differential equation? Why or why not?

Technology Connection

65. Charlie deposited a sum of money in a savings account. After 1 yr, the account was worth $4467.90, and after 3 yr, the account was worth $4937.80.

a) Use REGRESSION to find an exponential function of the form $y = ae^{bt}$ that models this situation.
b) Write a differential equation in the form $dA/dt = kA$, including the initial condition at time $t = 0$, to model this situation.

66. Solve $dy/dx = 5/y$. Graph the particular solutions for $C_1 = 5$, $C_2 = -200$, and $C_3 = 100$.

67. Solve $dy/dx = 2/y^2$. Graph the particular solutions for $C_1 = 0$, $C_2 = 4$, and $C_3 = -10$.

Answers to Quick Checks

1. $y = x^3 - \frac{1}{2}x^2 + C$ **2. (a)** $y' = 2e^{2x}$, so $2e^{2x} - 2e^{2x} = 0$; **(b)** $y' = 2Ce^{2x}$, so $2Ce^{2x} - 2(Ce^{2x}) = 0$ **3.** We have $y' = 2x + 1$, so $(2x + 1) + \frac{1}{x}(x^2 + x) = 2x + 1 + x + 1 = 3x + 2$. **4.** $y = \left(\frac{9}{8}x^2 + 27\right)^{2/3}$ **5.** $y = C\sqrt{1 + x^2}$ **6.** $A(t) = 2000e^{0.032t}$ **7.** $q = Ce^{-x}$

Chapter 5 Summary

KEY TERMS AND CONCEPTS

EXAMPLES

SECTION 5.1

If $p = D(x)$ is the demand function for x units of a product, then the **consumer surplus** for Q units, at price P per unit, is given by

$$\int_0^Q D(x)\,dx - QP.$$

If $p = S(x)$ is the supply function for x units of a product, then the **producer surplus** for Q units, at price P per unit, is given by

$$QP - \int_0^Q S(x)\,dx.$$

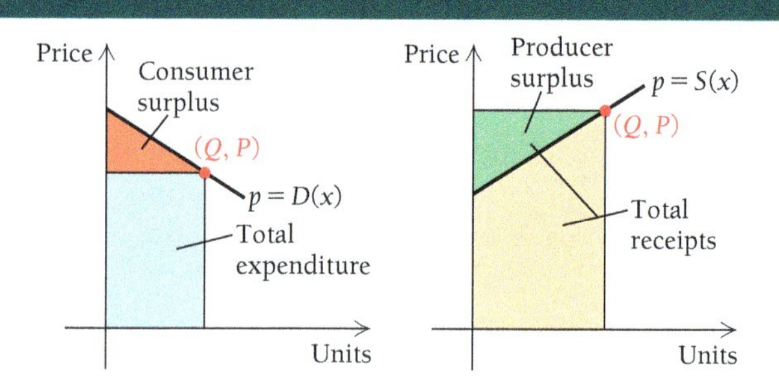

The **equilibrium point** (x_E, p_E) is the point at which the supply and demand curves intersect.

Let $p = D(x) = 12 - 1.5x$ be a demand function and $p = S(x) = 4 + 0.5x$ be a supply function, where p is the price, in dollars per unit, when x thousand units are sold. The two curves intersect at $(4, 6)$, the equilibrium point. At this point, the consumer surplus is

$$\int_0^4 (12 - 1.5x)\,dx - (4)(6) = 36 - 24 = 12, \text{ or } \$12{,}000,$$

and the producer surplus is

$$(4)(6) - \int_0^4 (4 + 0.5x)\,dx = 24 - 20 = 4, \text{ or } \$4000.$$

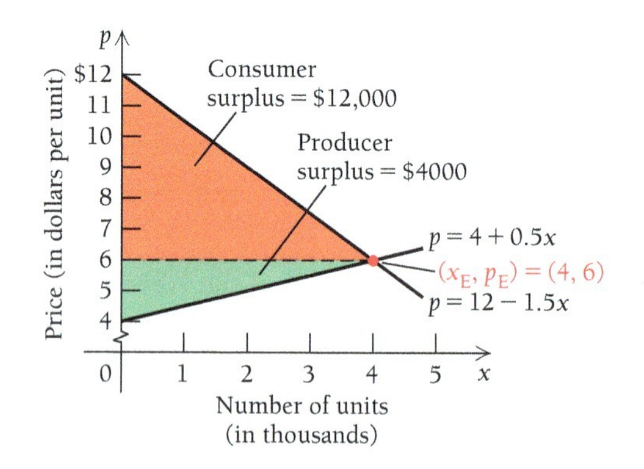

KEY TERMS AND CONCEPTS

EXAMPLES

SECTION 5.1 (continued)

A **price ceiling**, p_C, is an imposed maximum price such that $p_C < p_E$, where p_E is the equilibrium price.

The price ceiling p_C intersects the supply curve at (x_C, p_C), where $p_C = S(x_C)$, the supply price when x_C units are produced.

The new producer surplus is given by

$$(x_C)(p_C) - \int_0^{x_C} S(x)\,dx.$$

The new consumer surplus is given by

$$\int_0^{x_C} D(x)\,dx - (x_C)(p_C).$$

The **deadweight loss** is given by

$$\int_{x_C}^{x_E} (D(x) - S(x))\,dx.$$

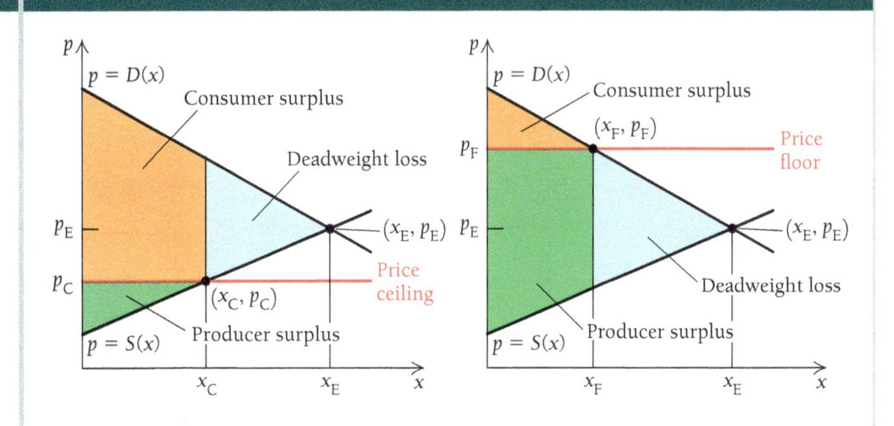

A **price floor**, p_F, is an imposed minimum price such that $p_F > p_E$, where p_E is the equilibrium price.

The price floor intersects the demand curve at (x_F, p_F), where $p_F = D(x_F)$.

The new consumer surplus is given by

$$\int_0^{x_F} D(x)\,dx - (x_F)(p_F).$$

The new producer surplus is given by

$$(x_F)(p_F) - \int_0^{x_F} S(x)\,dx.$$

The **deadweight loss** is given by

$$\int_{x_F}^{x_E} (D(x) - S(x))\,dx.$$

With the demand function $p = D(x) = 12 - 1.5x$ and the supply function $p = S(x) = 4 + 0.5x$, where p is the price, in thousands of dollars per unit, when x thousand units are produced and sold, a price floor of \$9000 is imposed.

- The price floor intersects the demand curve at (2, 9), where $x_F = 2$ and $p_F = 9$.
- The new consumer surplus is $\int_0^2 (12 - 1.5x)\,dx - (2)(9) = 3$, or \$3000.
- The new producer surplus is $(2)(9) - \int_0^2 (4 + 0.5x)\,dx = 9$, or \$9000.
- The deadweight loss is

$$\int_2^4 ((12 - 1.5x) - (4 + 0.5x))\,dx = \int_2^4 (8 - 2x)\,dx = 4, \text{ or } \$4000.$$

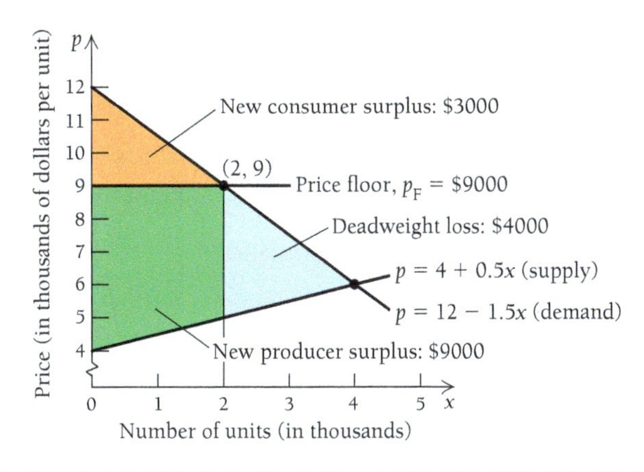

KEY TERMS AND CONCEPTS	EXAMPLES
SECTION 5.2	
The **future value** of P_0 dollars invested at interest rate k for t years, compounded continuously, is given by $P = P_0 e^{kt}$.	The future value of \$6000 invested at 3.75%, compounded continuously, for 5 yr is $P = 6000e^{0.0375(5)} = \$7237.38$.
The amount P_0 is called the **present value.** If a future value P is known, then $P_0 = Pe^{-kt}$.	Sue wants to have \$15,000 in 4 yr to make a down payment on a cabin by a lake. She opens a savings account that pays 4.5% interest, compounded continuously. The present value is the amount she needs to deposit now to have \$15,000 in 4 yr: $P = 15{,}000e^{-0.045(4)} = \$12{,}529.05$.
The **accumulated future value of a continuous income stream** is given by $A = e^{kT}\int_0^T R(t)e^{-kt}\,dt,$ where $R(t)$ is the rate of the continuous income stream, k is the interest rate, and T is the number of years. If $R(t)$ is a constant function, then $A = \frac{R(t)}{k}(e^{kT} - 1).$	A baseball pitcher signs a 6-yr contract and will be paid \$1,150,000 per year. The money will be invested at 5%, compounded continuously, for the 6-yr term. The accumulated future value is $A = \frac{1{,}150{,}000}{0.05}(e^{0.05(6)} - 1) = \$8{,}046{,}752.57.$
The **accumulated present value of a continuous income stream** is given by $B = \int_0^T R(t)e^{-kt}\,dt.$ If $R(t)$ is a constant, then $B = \frac{R(t)}{k}(1 - e^{-kT}).$ If $R(t)$ is not constant, the definite integral must be solved by an appropriate integration technique.	The accumulated present value of the pitcher's contract is $B = \int_0^6 1{,}150{,}000e^{-0.05t}\,dt = \frac{1{,}150{,}000}{0.05}(1 - e^{-0.05(6)}) = \$5{,}961{,}180.92.$
Consumption of a natural resource can be modeled by $\int_0^T P_0 e^{kt}\,dt = \frac{P_0}{k}(e^{kT} - 1),$ where $P(t) = P_0 e^{kt}$ is the annual consumption of the natural resource after t years and consumption is growing exponentially at growth rate k.	Suppose that a diamond mine produces diamonds according to the model $P(t) = 2.5e^{0.272t}$, where t is the number of years since 2010 and $P(t)$ is in millions of carats. Using this model, we can forecast the total production of diamonds between 2010 and 2026: $\int_0^{16} 2.5e^{0.272t}\,dt = \frac{2.5}{0.272}(e^{0.272(16)} - 1) = 704.353$ million carats.

KEY TERMS AND CONCEPTS

EXAMPLES

SECTION 5.3

An integral with infinity as a bound is called an **improper integral.** All improper integrals are evaluated as limits:

$$\int_a^\infty f(x)\,dx = \lim_{b\to\infty}\int_a^b f(x)\,dx,$$

$$\int_{-\infty}^b f(x)\,dx = \lim_{a\to-\infty}\int_a^b f(x)\,dx,$$

$$\int_{-\infty}^\infty f(x)\,dx = \int_{-\infty}^c f(x)\,dx + \int_c^\infty f(x)\,dx.$$

If the limit exists, an improper integral is **convergent.** Otherwise, it is **divergent.**

- $$\int_1^\infty \frac{1}{x^3}\,dx = \lim_{b\to\infty}\int_1^b \frac{1}{x^3}\,dx$$
$$= \lim_{b\to\infty}\left[-\frac{1}{2x^2}\right]_1^b$$
$$= \lim_{b\to\infty}\left[-\frac{1}{2(b)^2} - \left(-\frac{1}{2(1)^2}\right)\right]$$
$$= 0 - \left(-\frac{1}{2}\right) = \frac{1}{2}$$

- $$\int_{-\infty}^0 e^{4x}\,dx = \lim_{a\to-\infty}\int_a^0 e^{4x}\,dx$$
$$= \lim_{a\to-\infty}\left[\frac{1}{4}e^{4x}\right]_a^0$$
$$= \lim_{a\to-\infty}\left[\frac{1}{4}\left(e^{4(0)} - e^{4(a)}\right)\right]$$
$$= \frac{1}{4}(1-0) = \frac{1}{4}$$

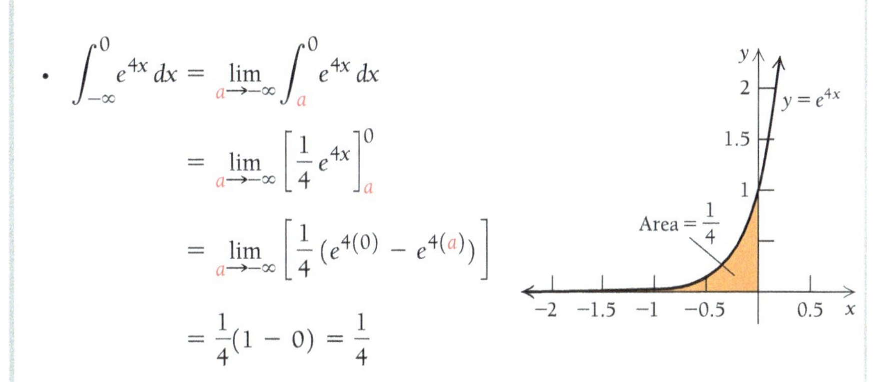

The **accumulated present value** of a continuous money flow into an investment at the rate of P dollars per year perpetually is

$$\int_0^\infty Pe^{-kt}\,dt = \frac{P}{k},$$

where k is the continuously compounded interest rate.

An investment of \$5000 per year perpetually at 7%, compounded continuously, has a present value of $\frac{5000}{0.07} = 71{,}428.57$.

SECTION 5.4

A **continuous random variable** is a quantity that can be observed (or measured) repeatedly and whose possible values comprise an interval of real numbers.

A function f is a **probability density function** for a continuous random variable x if it meets the following conditions:

- For all x in its domain, $f(x) \ge 0$.
- The area under the graph of f is 1.
- For any subinterval $[c, d]$ in the domain of f, the probability that x will be in that subinterval is $P([c,d]) = \int_c^d f(x)\,dx.$

The function $f(x) = \frac{2}{9}x$, for $0 \le x \le 3$, is a probability density function since

- $f(x) \ge 0$ for all x in $[0, 3]$.
- $$\int_0^3 \frac{2}{9}x\,dx = \left[\frac{1}{9}x^2\right]_0^3 = \frac{3^2}{9} - 0 = 1.$$

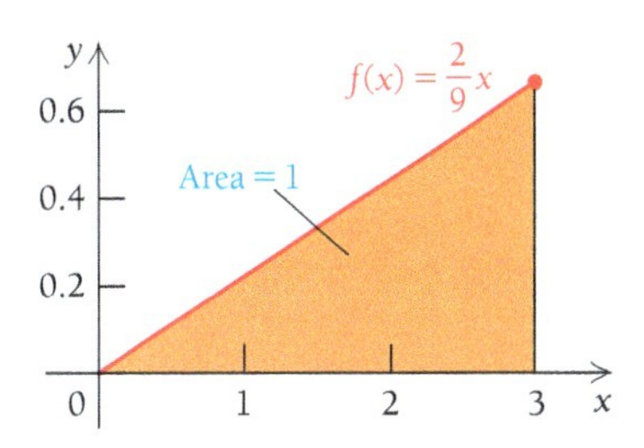

KEY TERMS AND CONCEPTS	EXAMPLES
SECTION 5.4 (*continued*)	
A probability density function is always stated with its domain.	The probability that x is between 1.5 and 2.3 is $$\int_{1.5}^{2.3} \frac{2}{9}x\,dx = \left[\frac{1}{9}x^2\right]_{1.5}^{2.3} = \frac{(2.3)^2}{9} - \frac{(1.5)^2}{9} \approx 0.338.$$ 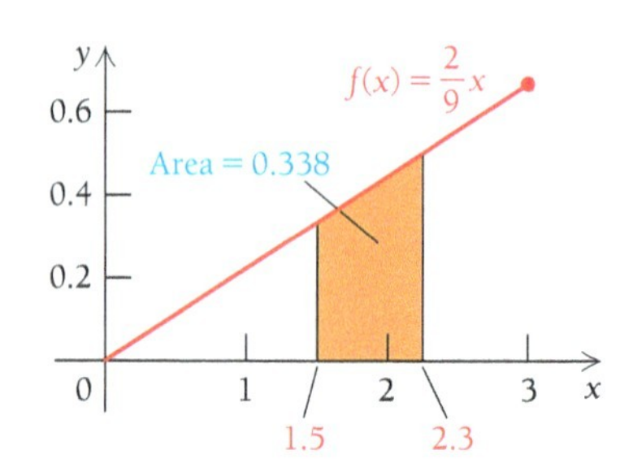
A continuous random variable is **uniformly distributed** over $[a, b]$ if it has a probability density function f given by $$f(x) = \frac{1}{b-a}, \quad \text{for } a \le x \le b.$$	Assume that helicopter tours over Hoover Dam last from 45 to 55 min, with the times uniformly distributed. If t is the time a tour lasts, in minutes, the probability density function f is $$f(t) = \frac{1}{10}, \quad \text{for } 45 \le t \le 55. \qquad \text{Note that } \frac{1}{10}(55-45) = 1.$$ The probability that a flight lasts between 48 and 53.5 min is $$\int_{48}^{53.5} \frac{1}{10}\,dx = \left[\frac{1}{10}x\right]_{48}^{53.5} = \frac{1}{10}(53.5-48) = 0.55.$$
A continuous random variable is **exponentially distributed** if it has a probability density function f of the form $$f(x) = ke^{-kx}, \quad \text{over } [0, \infty).$$	Suppose that the time t (in minutes) between shoppers entering a store is modeled by the probability density function $$f(x) = 3e^{-3t}, \quad \text{for } 0 \le t < \infty.$$ The probability that the time between shoppers entering is 30 sec or less is $$\int_0^{0.5} 3e^{-3t}\,dt = [-e^{-3t}]_0^{0.5} = (-e^{-1.5} - (-1)) \approx 0.78.$$
SECTION 5.5	
For x a continuous random variable over $[a, b]$ with probability density function f: the **mean** μ is the expected value of x, $$\mu = E(x) = \int_a^b x \cdot f(x)\,dx;$$ the **variance** σ^2 of x is $$\sigma^2 = E(x^2) - \mu^2 = \int_a^b x^2 \cdot f(x)\,dx - \left[\int_a^b x \cdot f(x)\,dx\right]^2;$$ and the **standard deviation** σ is the square root of the variance, $$\sigma = \sqrt{\text{variance}}.$$	Consider the probability density function $f(x) = \frac{2}{9}x$ over $[0, 3]$. • Its mean is $$\mu = \int_0^3 x \cdot \frac{2}{9}x\,dx = \int_0^3 \frac{2}{9}x^2\,dx = 2.$$ • Its variance is $$\sigma^2 = \left[\int_0^3 x^2 \cdot \frac{2}{9}x\,dx\right] - \mu^2 = 4.5 - 4 = 0.5.$$ • Its standard deviation is $$\sigma = \sqrt{0.5} \approx 0.71.$$

KEY TERMS AND CONCEPTS

EXAMPLES

SECTION 5.5 (continued)

A continuous random variable x has a **standard normal distribution** if it has a probability density function f given by

$$f(x) = \frac{1}{\sqrt{2\pi}}e^{-x^2/2}, \quad \text{over } (-\infty, \infty),$$

with $\mu = 0$ and $\sigma = 1$.

Tables or calculators are used to determine areas within the standard normal distribution.

To convert an x-value to a z-value for use with the standard normal distribution, we use the transformation formula

$$z = \frac{x - \mu}{\sigma}.$$

Weights of packages of gourmet coffee are normally distributed with mean $\mu = 3$ oz and standard deviation $\sigma = 0.5$. The probability that a package of coffee weighs between 2.75 oz and 3.15 oz is

$$P\left(\frac{2.75 - 3}{0.5} \le x \le \frac{3.15 - 3}{0.5}\right) = P(-0.5 \le z \le 0.3)$$
$$= 0.3094 = 30.94\%.$$

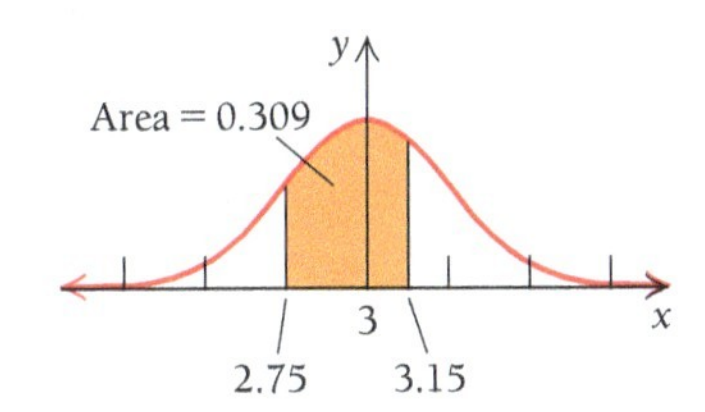

For the standard normal distribution, the *percentile* corresponding to a z-value is the area under the standard normal curve to the left of z, multiplied by 100.

In the standard normal distribution, the area to the left of $z = 1.5$ is 0.9332. Therefore, a z-value of 1.5 corresponds to the 93.32nd percentile.

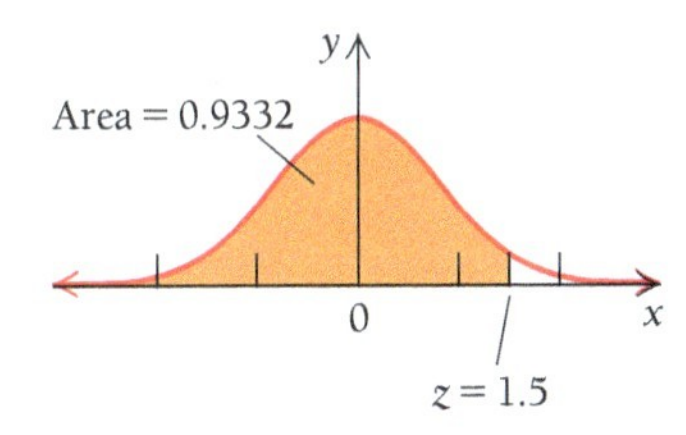

SECTION 5.6

Volume by disks: If f is continuous over $[a, b]$, the **volume of the solid of revolution** generated by rotating the area under the graph of f from a to b around the x-axis is given by

$$V = \pi\int_a^b [f(x)]^2\,dx.$$

Volume by shells: If f is continuous over $[a, b]$, the volume of the solid of revolution generated by rotating the area under the graph of f from a to b around the y-axis is given by

$$V = 2\pi\int_a^b xf(x)\,dx.$$

- The volume of the solid formed by rotating the area under the graph of $f(x) = \frac{1}{4}x^2$ from $x = -1$ to $x = 3$ around the x-axis is

$$V = \pi\int_{-1}^{3}\left(\frac{1}{4}x^2\right)^2 dx = \pi\int_{-1}^{3}\left(\frac{1}{16}x^4\right)dx = \frac{\pi}{16}\left[\frac{x^5}{5}\right]_{-1}^{3}$$
$$= \frac{\pi}{16}\left[\frac{243}{5} - \left(-\frac{1}{5}\right)\right] = \frac{244}{80}\pi = \frac{61}{20}\pi \approx 9.582.$$

- The volume of the solid of revolution formed by rotating the area under the graph of $f(x) = -\frac{1}{2}x^2 + 9$ from $x = 1$ to $x = 4$ around the y-axis is

$$V = 2\pi\int_1^4 x\left(-\frac{1}{2}x^2 + 9\right)dx$$
$$= 2\pi\int_1^4\left(-\frac{1}{2}x^3 + 9x\right)dx$$
$$= 2\pi\left[-\frac{1}{8}x^4 + \frac{9}{2}x^2\right]_1^4$$
$$= 2\pi\left[\left(-\frac{1}{8}(4)^4 + \frac{9}{2}(4)^2\right) - \left(-\frac{1}{8}(1)^4 + \frac{9}{2}(1)^2\right)\right]$$
$$= 2\pi\left[(-32 + 72) - \left(-\frac{1}{8} + \frac{9}{2}\right)\right]$$
$$= \frac{285}{4}\pi \approx 223.838.$$

KEY TERMS AND CONCEPTS	EXAMPLES
SECTION 5.7	
A **differential equation** is an equation that includes a derivative and has a function as a solution.	The equation $y' + 3y = 3x^2 + 2x$ is a differential equation since it involves the derivative of y. The function $y = x^2$ is a solution of this differential equation since $y' = 2x$ and $y' + 3y = 3x^2 + 2x$, $2x + 3x^2 = 3x^2 + 2x$.
The **general solution** of a differential equation of the form $y' = f(x)$ is a set of functions $F(x) + C$, where $\frac{d}{dx}F(x) = f(x)$. For other differential equations, the general solution may be of the form $y = Cf(x)$, where C is any constant.	• The general solution of $y' = 4x^2$ is $y = \int 4x^2\,dx = \frac{4}{3}x^3 + C.$ • The general solution of $y' = 7y$ is $y = Ce^{7x}$.
A **separable differential equation** is a differential equation for which the variables can be isolated on opposite sides of the equation. That is, a separable differential equation in x and y can be written in the form $f(y)\,dy = g(x)\,dx$. To solve a separable differential equation, the variables are separated, each side is integrated, and, if possible, the result is solved for one of the variables.	The differential equation $y' = \frac{x^2}{y}$ can be solved by separating variables: $\frac{dy}{dx} = \frac{x^2}{y}$ $y\,dy = x^2\,dx$ $\int y\,dy = \int x^2\,dx$ $\frac{y^2}{2} = \frac{x^3}{3} + C_1$ $y^2 = \frac{2}{3}x^3 + C, \quad \text{where } C = 2C_1.$ Therefore, the general solution is $y = \pm\sqrt{\frac{2}{3}x^3 + C}$.
If an initial condition is known, then a **particular solution** may be determined by solving for C.	If $(0, 2)$ is an initial condition, we can solve the general solution for C. We choose the positive root since the output, $y = 2$, is positive: $2 = \sqrt{\frac{2}{3}(0)^3 + C}$ $2 = \sqrt{C}$ $4 = C.$ Therefore, the particular solution that passes through the point $(0, 2)$ is $y = \sqrt{\frac{2}{3}x^3 + 4}$.

Chapter 5 Review Exercises

These review exercises are for test preparation. They can also be used as a practice test. Answers are at the back of the book. The red bracketed section references tell you what part(s) of the chapter to restudy if your answer is incorrect.

CONCEPT REINFORCEMENT

Match each term in column A with the most appropriate graph in column B.

Column A / **Column B**

1. Consumer surplus [5.1]

a) 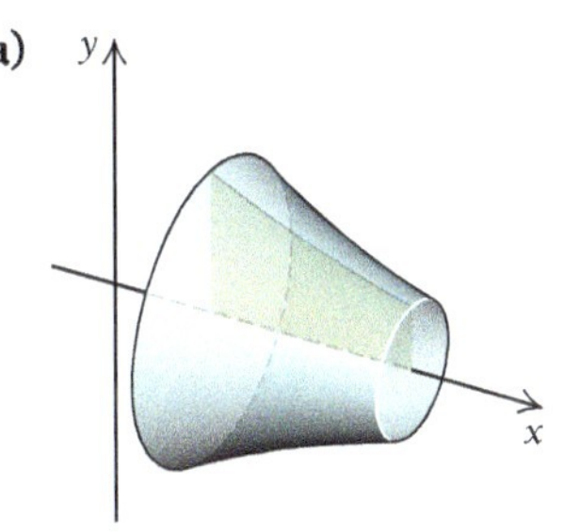

2. Producer surplus [5.1]

b) 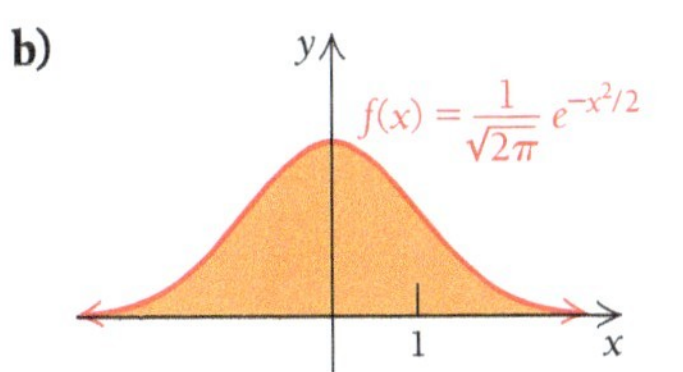

3. Deadweight loss [5.1]

c) 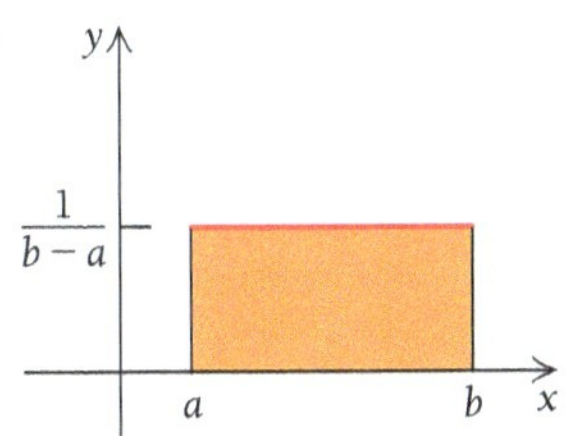

4. Standard normal distribution [5.5]

d) 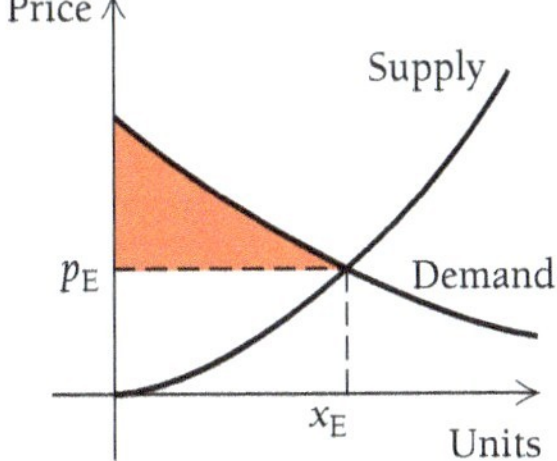

5. Uniform distribution [5.4]

e) 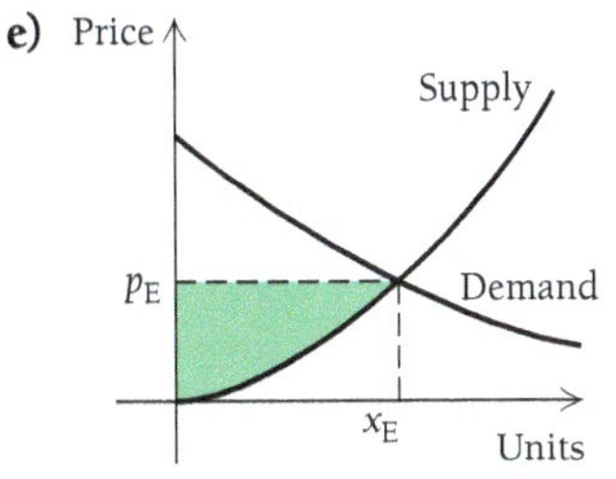

6. Solid of revolution [5.6]

f) 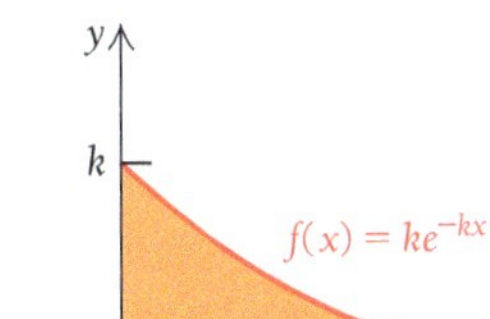

7. Exponential distribution [5.4]

g) 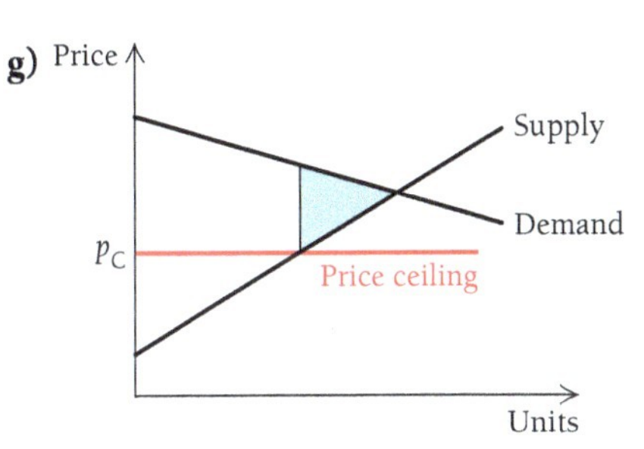

Classify each statement as either true or false.

8. The consumer surplus is the extra amount a consumer pays as a tax on a purchased product. [5.1]

9. A price floor is always less than a price ceiling. [5.1]

10. The accumulated present value of an investment is the value of the investment as a tax-deductible gift to a non-profit charity. [5.2]

11. If an integral has $-\infty$ or ∞ as a limit of integration, it is an improper integral. [5.3]

12. If f is a probability density function over $[a, b]$, then $f(x) \geq 0$ for all x in $[a, b]$. [5.4]

13. If f is a probability density function over $[a, b]$ and x is a continuous random variable over $[a, b]$, then the mean value of $f(x)$ is always $(b - a)/2$. [5.5]

14. If $y = e^{0.05t}$ is a solution of $y' = 0.05y$, then $y = Ce^{0.05t}$ is also a solution. [5.7]

REVIEW EXERCISES

Let $D(x) = (x - 6)^2$ be the price, in dollars per hundred units, that consumers are willing to pay for x hundred units of an item, and $S(x) = x^2 + 12$ be the price, in dollars per hundred units, that producers are willing to accept for x hundred units.

15. Find the equilibrium point. [5.1]

16. Find the consumer surplus at the equilibrium point. [5.1]

17. Find the producer surplus at the equilibrium point. [5.1]

18. A price ceiling of \$14 is imposed. [5.1]

a) Find the new consumer surplus.

b) Find the new producer surplus.

c) Find the deadweight loss.

19. Business: future value. Find the future value of $5000, at an annual percentage rate of 3.2%, compounded continuously, for 7 yr. [5.2]

20. Business: present value. Find the present value of $10,000 due in 5 yr, at an interest rate of 4.3%, compounded continuously. [5.2]

21. Business: future value of a continuous income stream. Find the accumulated future value of $2500 per year, at 4.25% compounded continuously, for 8 yr. [5.2]

22. Business: present accumulated value of a trust. The DeMars family welcomes a new baby, and the parents want to have $250,000 in 18 yr for the child's college education. Find the continuous money stream, at $R(t)$ dollars per year, they need to invest at 4.75% compounded continuously, to generate $250,000. [5.2]

23. Business: contract buyout. Cal Earl signs a 7-yr contract as a session drummer for a major recording company. His contract pays him $150,000 per year. After 3 yr, the company offers to buy out the remainder of his contract. What is the least amount Cal should accept, if the interest rate is 4.15%, compounded continuously? [5.2]

24. Physical science: iron ore production. In 2016 ($t = 0$), world production of iron ore was estimated at 2.23 billion metric tons, and production was growing exponentially at the rate of 0.5% per year. (*Source:* minerals.usgs.gov.) If production continues to grow at this rate, how much iron ore will be produced from 2020 to 2025? [5.2]

25. Physical science: depletion of iron ore. World reserves of iron ore in 2016 were estimated to be 82 billion metric tons. (*Source:* minerals.usgs.gov.) Assuming that the growth rate in Exercise 24 continues and no new reserves are discovered, when will world reserves of iron ore be depleted? [5.2]

Determine whether each improper integral is convergent or divergent, and find its value if it is convergent. [5.3]

26. $\displaystyle\int_1^{\infty} \frac{1}{x^2}\,dx$

27. $\displaystyle\int_1^{\infty} e^{4x}\,dx$

28. $\displaystyle\int_0^{\infty} e^{-2x}\,dx$

29. Find k such that $f(x) = k/x^3$ is a probability density function over $[1, 2]$. Then write the probability density function. [5.4]

30. Business: waiting time. Sharif arrives at a doctor's office where the waiting time t to see a doctor is no more than 25 min. The probability density function for t is $f(t) = \frac{1}{25}$, for $0 \leq t \leq 25$. Find the probability that Sharif will have to wait no more than 15 min to see a doctor. [5.4]

Given the probability density function

$$f(x) = 6x(1 - x), \quad \text{over } [0, 1],$$

find each of the following. [5.5]

31. $E(x^2)$

32. $E(x)$

33. The mean

34. The variance

35. The standard deviation

Let x be a continuous random variable with a standard normal distribution. Using Appendix D, find each of the following. [5.5]

36. $P(0 \leq x \leq 1.85)$

37. $P(-1.74 \leq x \leq 1.43)$

38. $P(-2.08 \leq x \leq -1.18)$

39. $P(x \geq 0)$

40. Business: pizza sales. The number of pizzas sold daily at Benito's Pizzeria is normally distributed with mean $\mu = 90$ and standard deviation $\sigma = 20$. What is the probability that at least 100 pizzas are sold during a day? [5.5]

41. Business: distribution of revenue. Benito's Pizzeria has daily mean revenues that are normally distributed, with $\mu = \$5500$ and $\sigma = \$425$. What daily revenue corresponds to the 95th percentile? [5.5]

Find the volume generated by rotating the area bounded by the graphs of each set of equations around the x-axis. [5.6]

42. $y = x^3, x = 1, x = 2$

43. $y = \dfrac{1}{x + 2}, x = 0, x = 1$

Find the volume generated by rotating the area bounded by the graphs of each set of equations around the y-axis. [5.6]

44. $y = 12 - x^2, x = 0, x = 2$

45. $y = e^{x^2}, x = 1, x = 3$

46. $y = x \ln x, x = 1, x = 5$

Solve each differential equation. [5.7]

47. $\dfrac{dy}{dx} = 11x^{10}y$

48. $\dfrac{dy}{dx} = \dfrac{2}{y}$

49. $\dfrac{dy}{dx} = 4y; \quad y = 5 \text{ when } x = 0$

50. $\dfrac{dv}{dt} = 5v^{-2}; \quad v = 4 \text{ when } t = 3$

51. $y' = \dfrac{3x}{y}$

52. $y' = 8x - xy$

53. Economics: elasticity. Find the demand function $q = D(x)$, given the elasticity condition

$$E(x) = \frac{x}{100 - x}; \quad q = 70 \text{ when } x = 30. \quad [5.7]$$

54. Business: stock growth. The growth rate of the stock of Greenwich Corp., in dollars per month, can be modeled by

$$\frac{dV}{dt} = k(L - V),$$

where V is the value of a share, in dollars, after t months; k is a constant; L is $36.37, the limiting value of the stock; and $V(0) = 30$. Express the solution of the differential equation in terms of t and k. [5.7]

SYNTHESIS

55. The function $f(x) = \frac{1}{3}x^2$ is a probability density function over $[0, c]$. Find c. [5.4]

Determine whether each improper integral is convergent or divergent, and find its value if it is convergent. [5.3]

56. $\int_{-\infty}^{0} x^4 e^{-x^5}\,dx$

57. $\int_{0}^{\infty} \frac{dx}{(x+1)^{4/3}}$

Technology Connection 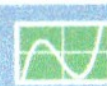

Evaluate:

58. $\int_{1}^{\infty} \frac{\ln x}{x^2}\,dx$ [5.3]

59. $\int_{-\infty}^{\infty} \frac{2}{1+4x^2}\,dx$ [5.3]

60. Let R be the area under the curve $y = 6x - e^x$ and above the x-axis. Find the volume generated by rotating R around the x-axis. [5.6]

Chapter 5 Test

Let $D(x) = (x - 7)^2$ be the price, in dollars per dozen units, that consumers are willing to pay for x dozen units of an item, and let $S(x) = x^2 + x + 4$ be the price, in dollars per dozen units, that producers are willing to accept for x dozen units. Assume $x \le 7$. Find:

1. The equilibrium point
2. The consumer surplus at the equilibrium point
3. The producer surplus at the equilibrium point
4. A price floor of \$20 is imposed.
   a) Find the new consumer surplus.
   b) Find the new producer surplus.
   c) Find the deadweight loss.
5. **Business: future value.** Find the future value of \$12,000 invested for 10 yr at an annual percentage rate of 3.75%, compounded continuously.
6. **Business: future value of a continuous income stream.** Find the accumulated future value of \$8000 per year, at an interest rate of 3.78%, compounded continuously, for 6 yr.
7. **Physical science: production of potash.** In 2016 ($t = 0$), world production of potash was approximately 19.4 million metric tons, and demand was increasing at the rate of 1.6% a year. (*Source:* minerals.usgs.gov.) If demand continues to grow at this rate, how much potash will be produced from 2020 to 2030?
8. **Physical science: depletion of potash.** See Exercise 7. The world reserves of potash in 2016 were approximately 720 million metric tons. (*Source:* minerals.usgs.gov.) Assuming demand for potash continues to grow at the rate of 1.6% per year and no new reserves are discovered, when will world reserves be depleted?
9. **Business: accumulated present value of a continuous income stream.** Bruce Kent wants to have \$50,000 in 5 yr for a down payment on a house. Find the amount he needs to save, at $R(t)$ dollars per year, at 2.125%, compounded continuously, to achieve the desired future value.
10. **Business: contract buyout.** Guy Laplace signs a 6-yr contract to play professional hockey at a salary of \$800,000 per year. After 2 yr, his team offers to buy out the remainder of his contract. What is the least amount Guy should accept, assuming an interest rate of 3.1%, compounded continuously?
11. **Business: future value of a noncontinuous income stream.** Sonia signs a contract that will pay her an income of $R(t) = 100{,}000 + 10{,}000t$, where t is in years and $0 \le t \le 8$. If she invests this money at 5%, compounded continuously, what is the future value of the income stream?

Determine whether each improper integral is convergent or divergent, and find its value if it is convergent.

12. $\int_{1}^{\infty} \frac{dx}{x^5}$
13. $\int_{0}^{\infty} \frac{4}{1+3x}\,dx$
14. Find k such that $f(x) = kx^3$ is a probability density function over $[0, 2]$. Then write the probability density function.
15. **Business: times of phone calls.** A cell-phone carrier determines that the length of a phone call, t, in minutes, is an exponentially distributed random variable with probability density function

$$f(t) = 2e^{-2t}, \quad 0 \le t < \infty.$$

Find the probability that a randomly selected call lasts between 1 min and 2 min.

Given the probability density function $f(x) = \frac{1}{4}x$ over $[1, 3]$, find each of the following.

16. $E(x)$
17. $E(x^2)$
18. The mean
19. The variance
20. The standard deviation

Let x be a continuous random variable with a standard normal distribution. Using Appendix D, find each of the following.

21. $P(0 \le x \le 1.3)$
22. $P(-2.31 \le x \le -1.05)$
23. $P(-1.61 \le x \le 1.76)$

24. Business: price distribution. The price per pound p of wild salmon at various stores in a certain city is normally distributed with mean $\mu = \$16$ and standard deviation $\sigma = \$2.50$. What is the probability that the price at a randomly selected store is at least $17.25 per pound?

25. Business: price distribution. If the price per pound p of haddock is normally distributed with mean $\mu = \$12$ and standard deviation $\sigma = \$2.50$, what price corresponds to the 85th percentile?

Find the volume generated by rotating the area bounded by the graphs of each set of equations around the x-axis.

26. $y = \frac{1}{\sqrt{x}}, \quad x = 1, x = 5$

27. $y = \sqrt{2 + x}, \quad x = 0, x = 1$

28. Find the volume generated by rotating the portion of the graph of $y = 4 - (x - 5)^2$ that lies above the x-axis around that axis.

29. Find the volume generated by rotating the area bounded by $y = x^2 + x, x = 1, x = 4$, and the x-axis, around the y-axis.

30. Business: grain storage. A grain silo is a circular cylinder with a conical roof. The roof can be modeled by rotating the area under the graph of $y = 30 - 0.5x$, where $0 \leq x \leq 10$, around the y-axis. Find the volume of the silo, assuming the floor of the cylinder lies on the x-axis and both x and y are measured in feet.

Solve each differential equation.

31. $\frac{dy}{dx} = 8x^7y$

32. $\frac{dy}{dx} = \frac{9}{y}; \quad y(2) = 3$

33. $\frac{dy}{dt} = 6y; \quad y = 11$ when $t = 0$

34. $y' = 5x^2 - x^2y$

35. $\frac{dv}{dt} = 2v^{-3}; \quad v(0) = 10$

36. $y' = 4y + xy$

37. Economics: elasticity. Find the demand function $q = D(x)$, given the elasticity condition

$$E(x) = 4 \quad \text{for all } x > 0.$$

38. Business: stock growth. The growth rate of Fabric Industries stock, in dollars per month, can be modeled by

$$\frac{dV}{dt} = k(L - V),$$

where V is the value of a share, in dollars, after t months; L is $36, the limiting value of the stock; k is a constant; and $V(0) = 0$.

a) Express the solution $V(t)$ in terms of L and k.

b) If $V(6) = 18$, determine k to the nearest hundredth.

c) In how many months will the value of a share be $30?

SYNTHESIS

39. If $f(x) = x^3$ is a probability density function over $[0, b]$, what is b?

40. Determine whether the following improper integral is convergent or divergent, and find its value if it is convergent:

$$\int_{-\infty}^{0} x^3 e^{-x^4}\, dx.$$

Technology Connection 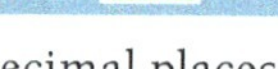

41. Approximate to three decimal places:

$$\int_{-\infty}^{\infty} \frac{2}{1 + 3x^2}\, dx.$$

42. Let R be the region between the graph of $y = 2x + 1$ and the x-axis, where $0 \leq x < b$. Find b if the volume generated by rotating R around the x-axis is 275π cubic units.

EXTENDED TECHNOLOGY APPLICATION 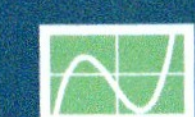

Curve Fitting and Volumes of Containers

Consider the vase shown at the right. To estimate the volume of its interior, we can turn it on its side, as shown below, and take a series of vertical measurements of the radius of the vase. Using REGRESSION, we can fit a curve to the data and then generate a solid of revolution by rotating the regression curve around the x-axis. Finally, we can use integration to find the volume.

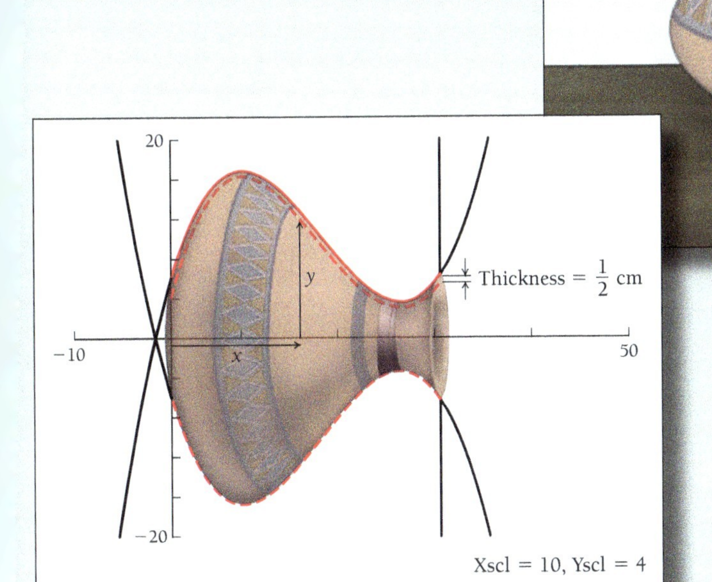

Let's assume that the wall of the vase is $\frac{1}{2}$-cm thick. In the following table, the inner radius, y, is given for several values of the distance x from the base of the vase.

x (in centimeters)	y (in centimeters)
0	4
2	10
7	17
12	16
17	10
22	5
25	3.5
31	7

Exercises

1. Using REGRESSION, fit a cubic function to the data.
2. Using the function found in Exercise 1, find the inside volume of the vase over [0, 31]. (*Hint:* If the function in Exercise 1 is Y1, find the volume by using the VARS key to enter πY1^2 as Y2. Then use the CALC option to integrate.)

Now consider the bottle shown at the right. To find the bottle's volume in a similar manner, we turn it on its side, use a measuring device to take vertical measurements of the radii, and proceed as we did with the vase.

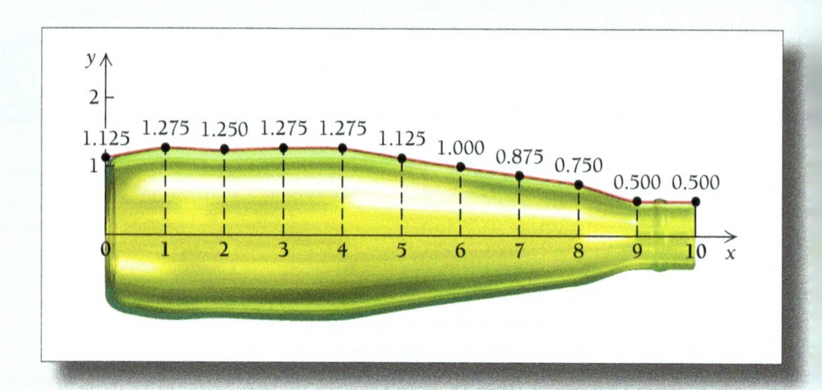

The table of measurements is as follows.

x (in inches)	y (in inches)
0	1.125
1	1.275
2	1.250
3	1.275
4	1.275
5	1.125
6	1.000
7	0.875
8	0.750
9	0.500
10	0.500

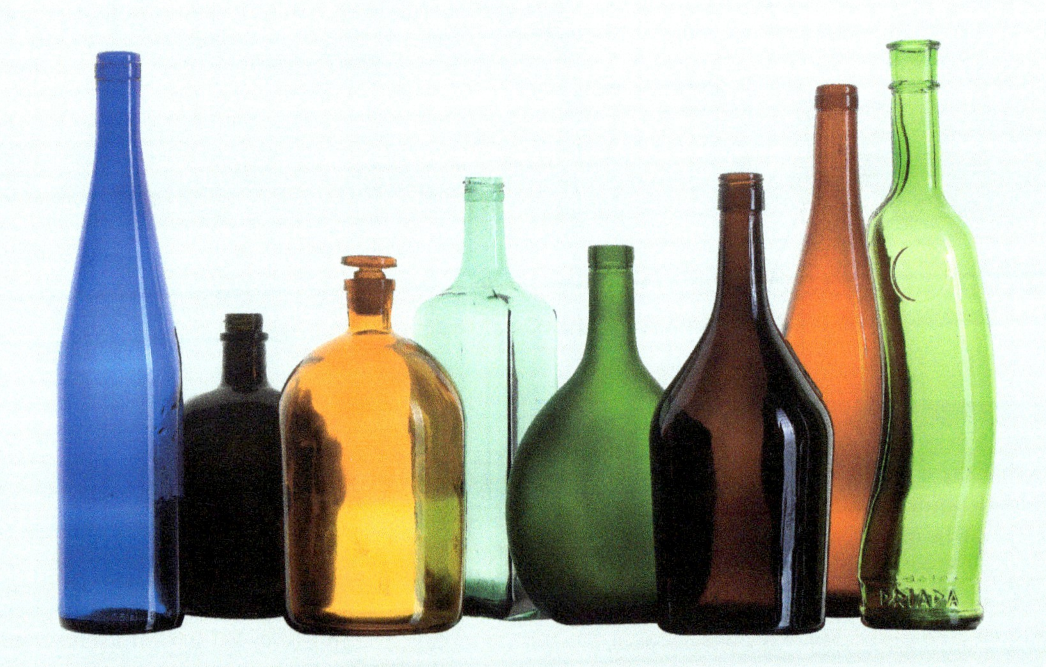

Exercises

3. Using REGRESSION, fit a quartic function to the data. Label this function y_1.

4. Using the function found in Exercise 3, find the volume of the bottle in cubic inches.

5. Find the volume of the bottle in fluid ounces, using the conversion 1 $\text{in}^3 = 0.55424$ fl oz. Will the bottle hold 20 oz of fluid?

6. Suppose the bottle is made of plastic that is 0.015-in. thick. Add 0.015 to each measurement in the table, and find a regression curve for these adjusted radii. Fit a quartic polynomial function to the data, and label this curve y_2.

7. To determine the volume of the bottle's base, extend the x-axis 0.015 unit to the left of 0. The total volume of the plastic that forms the bottle can then be found by first integrating $y_3 = \pi(y_2)^2$ over $[-0.015, 0]$ to find the volume of the base and then integrating $y_4 = \pi(y_2 - y_1)^2$ over $[0, 10]$ to find the volume of the side. What is the total volume of plastic used to form the bottle?

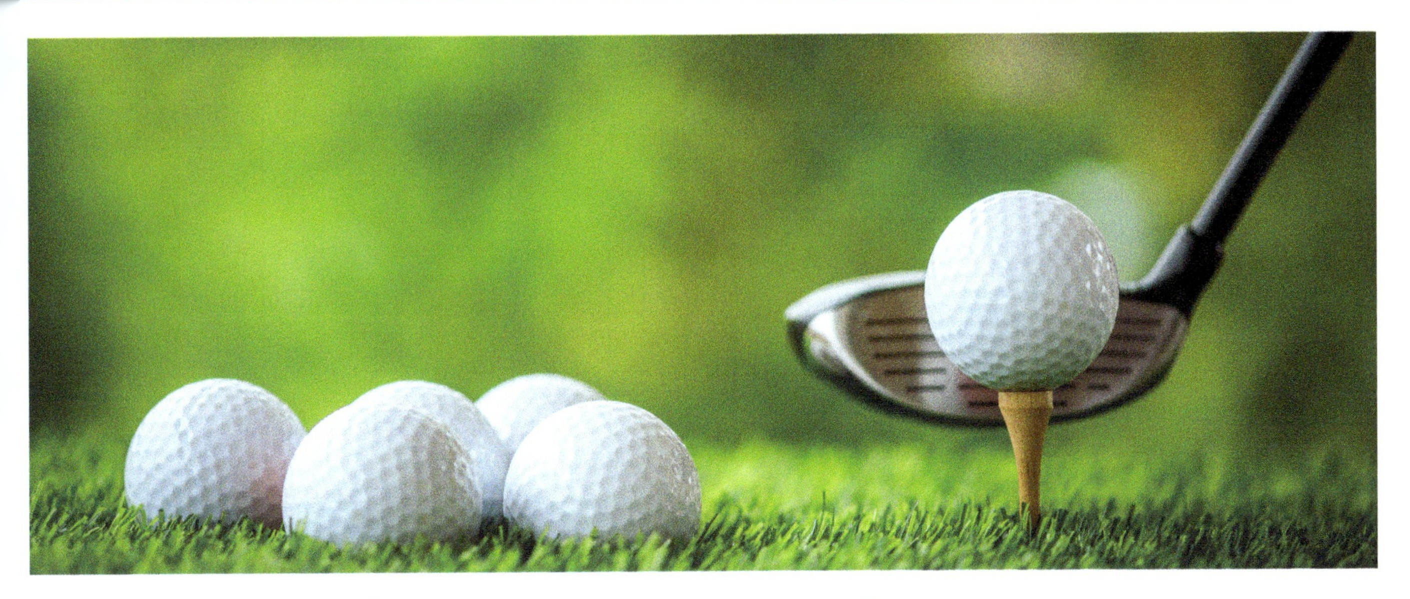

6 Functions of Several Variables

What You'll Learn

Why It's Important

Functions that have more than one input are called *functions of several variables*. We introduce these functions in this chapter and learn to differentiate them to find *partial derivatives*. Then we use such functions to find regression lines and solve maximum–minimum problems. Finally, we study the integration of functions of several variables.

Where It's Used

Maximizing Profit: Fly Straight, Inc., produces two types of golf balls: one type sells for \$3 each and the other sells for \$2 each. The total profit from manufacturing and selling x thousand \$3 balls and y thousand \$2 balls is given by

$$P(x, y) = -2x^2 + 2xy - y^2 + 12x - 4y - 7.$$

How many golf balls of each type must be produced and sold to maximize the company's profit?

(*This problem appears as Example 3 in Section 6.3.*)

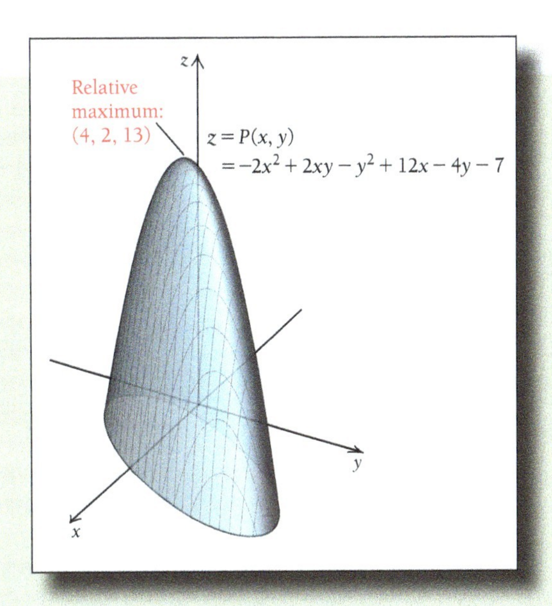

6.1

- Find a function value for a function of several variables.

Functions of Several Variables

Suppose that a souvenir stand at a community theater sells programs for \$5 each, tee-shirts for \$12 each, and caps for \$20 each. If x programs are sold, then the revenue, in dollars, is given by

$$R(x) = 5x.$$

This is a function of one variable.

If x programs and y tee-shirts are sold, then the revenue, in dollars, is given by

$$R(x, y) = 5x + 12y.$$

This is a *function of two variables*.

Similarly, if x programs, y tee-shirts, and z caps are sold, then the revenue, in dollars, is given by

$$R(x, y, z) = 5x + 12y + 20z.$$

This is a *function of three variables*.

These functions suggest the following.

> **DEFINITION**
>
> A **function of n variables** assigns to each input of n ordered inputs, $(x_1, x_2, \ldots, x_n)$, called an **n-tuple**, exactly one output, $f(x_1, x_2, \ldots, x_n)$. Any function of two or more input variables is called a **function of several variables**.

For example, we can regard a function of two variables as a machine that has two inputs. When such a function is given by a formula, the domain normally consists of all ordered pairs (x, y) that are meaningful replacements in the formula.

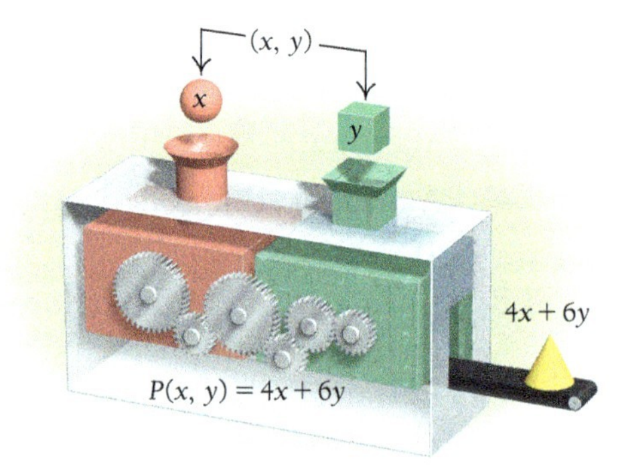

EXAMPLE 1 For the souvenir stand's revenue function in three variables, $R(x, y, z) = 5x + 12y + 20z$, find $R(2, 1, 4)$, and interpret the meaning of this number.

Solution The number $R(2, 1, 4)$ is the value of the revenue function found by substituting 2 for x, 1 for y, and 4 for z:

$$\begin{aligned} R(2, 1, 4) &= 5(2) + 12(1) + 20(4) \quad \text{Substituting} \\ &= 10 + 12 + 80 \\ &= 102. \end{aligned}$$

When 2 programs, 1 tee-shirt, and 4 caps are sold, the souvenir stand takes in a total of \$102. 1✓

Quick Check 1✓

Bellview Craft's cost function for x mugs and y vases is given by $C(x, y) = 6.5x + 7.25y$, where $C(x, y)$ is in dollars. Find $C(10, 15)$, and interpret the meaning of this number.

EXAMPLE 2 **Future Value with Compound Interest.** The future value, in dollars, of an investment of P dollars at an annual interest rate r, compounded c times per year for t years, is given by

$$A(P, r, c, t) = P\left(1 + \frac{r}{c}\right)^{ct}.$$

Find $A(3000, 0.023, 12, 5)$, and interpret the meaning of this number.

Quick Check 2 ✓

In basketball, a player's total points is a statistic given by $P(t, u, v) = t + 2u + 3v$, where t is the number of free throws made, u is the number of two-point field goals made, and v is the number of three-point field goals made. Find $P(5, 8, 3)$, and interpret the meaning of this number.

Solution Substituting 3000 for P, 0.023 for r, 12 for c, and 5 for t, we have

$$A(3000, 0.023, 12, 5) = 3000\left(1 + \frac{0.023}{12}\right)^{12 \cdot 5} \quad \text{Substituting}$$

$$\approx 3365.25. \quad \text{Using a calculator}$$

An investment of \$3000 in an account with an annual percentage rate of 2.3%, compounded monthly for 5 yr, has a future value of \$3365.25. **2 ✓**

EXAMPLE 3 **Business: Monthly Payment on Amortized Loan.** The monthly payment per thousand dollars borrowed is a function of r, the annual percentage rate (APR), and t, the term of the loan (in years), and is given by

$$P(r, t) = \frac{1000r\left(1 + \frac{r}{12}\right)^{12t}}{12\left(1 + \frac{r}{12}\right)^{12t} - 12}.$$

How much per month will a borrower pay per thousand dollars borrowed at an APR of 6.5% for a 6-yr term?

Solution We let $r = 0.065$ and $t = 6$ and evaluate $P(0.065, 6)$:

$$P(0.065, 6) = \frac{1000(0.065)\left(1 + \frac{0.065}{12}\right)^{12(6)}}{12\left(1 + \frac{0.065}{12}\right)^{12(6)} - 12} \approx \$16.81.$$

The monthly payment is \$16.81 per thousand dollars borrowed. **3 ✓**

Quick Check 3 ✓

Determine the monthly payment per thousand dollars borrowed at an APR of 7.25% for a term of 8 yr.

EXAMPLE 4 **Business: Payment Tables.** The formula in Example 3 is used to generate a table of payments that shows borrowers the combined effects of r (the APR) and the term t (in years).

Monthly Payment per \$1000 Borrowed

Annual Percentage Rate, r	Term, t (in years)				
	4	5	6	7	8
0.05	\$23.03	\$18.87	\$16.10	\$14.13	\$12.66
0.055	\$23.26	\$19.10	\$16.34	\$14.37	\$12.90
0.06	\$23.49	\$19.33	\$16.57	\$14.61	\$13.14
0.065	\$23.71	\$19.57	\$16.81	\$14.85	\$13.39
0.07	\$23.95	\$19.80	\$17.05	\$15.09	\$13.63
0.075	\$24.18	\$20.04	\$17.29	\$15.34	\$13.88

a) What can a borrower expect to pay per month with an APR of 5.5% for a 7-yr term?

b) What can a borrower expect to pay per month with the same APR as in part (a) but for a 6-yr term?

c) Assuming that the borrower makes the monthly payments for the entire term of the loan, which option, the 7-yr term or the 6-yr term, results in less total interest paid?

Solution The monthly payments are read directly from the table.

a) We see that $P(0.055, 7) = \$14.37$ per month.

b) From the table, $P(0.055, 6) = \$16.34$ per month.

c) With the 6-yr term, the borrower pays \$16.34 per month for 72 months, for a total of \$1176.48, of which \$1176.48 − \$1000 = \$176.48 is interest. With the 7-yr term, the borrower pays \$14.37 per month for 84 months, for a total of \$1207.08, of which \$1207.08 − \$1000 = \$207.08 is interest. Although the monthly payment is less with the longer term, the total amount of interest paid is more. The 6-yr term results in less total interest paid. 4 ✓

Quick Check 4 ✓

a) What is the monthly payment per thousand dollars borrowed at an APR of 7% for a 5-yr term?

b) How much less per month would the payment be with the same APR but a term of 6 yr?

c) Assuming that the borrower makes the payment each month for the entire term, which term results in lower total interest paid, per thousand dollars borrowed? How much lower?

EXAMPLE 5 **Business: Cost of Storage Equipment.** Sunny & Soy purchases a storage tank that costs C_1 dollars and has capacity V_1. Later it wishes to replace the tank with a new one that costs C_2 dollars and has capacity V_2. Industrial economists have found that in such cases, the cost of the new piece of equipment can be estimated by the function of three variables

$$C_2 = \left(\frac{V_2}{V_1}\right)^{0.6} C_1.$$

For \$45,000, Sunny & Soy buys a storage tank that has a capacity of 10,000 gal. Later it decides to buy a tank with double that capacity. Estimate the cost of the new tank.

Solution We substitute 20,000 for V_2, 10,000 for V_1, and 45,000 for C_1:

$$C_2 = \left(\frac{20{,}000}{10{,}000}\right)^{0.6}(45{,}000)$$
$$= 2^{0.6}(45{,}000)$$
$$\approx \$68{,}207.25.$$

Note that a 100% increase in capacity was achieved by about a 52% increase in cost. This is independent of any increase in the costs of labor, management, or other equipment resulting from the purchase of the tank. 5 ✓

Quick Check 5 ✓

a) Repeat Example 5 assuming that the company buys a tank with a capacity of 2.75 times that of the original.

b) What is the percentage increase in cost for this tank compared to the cost of the original tank?

Quick Check 6 ✓

Suppose that the cost, in dollars per copy, of printing Q copies of a book that contains P photographs and has R pages is given by

$$C(Q, P, R) = \frac{4.57QP}{R^{1.88}}.$$

Find the cost, in dollars per copy, of printing 500 copies of a book that contains 25 photographs and has 175 pages.

EXAMPLE 6 **Social Science: The Gravity Model.** As the populations of two cities grow, the number of telephone calls between the cities increases, much like the gravitational pull increases between two objects in space that are gaining mass. The average number of telephone calls per day between two cities is given by

$$N(d, P_1, P_2) = \frac{2.8P_1P_2}{d^{2.4}},$$

where d is the distance, in miles, between the cities and P_1 and P_2 are their populations. The cities of Dallas and Fort Worth are 30 mi apart and have populations of 1,138,000 and 854,000, respectively. (*Sources:* Population Division, U.S. Census Bureau, 2016 estimates, and Rand McNally.) Find the average number of calls per day between the two cities.

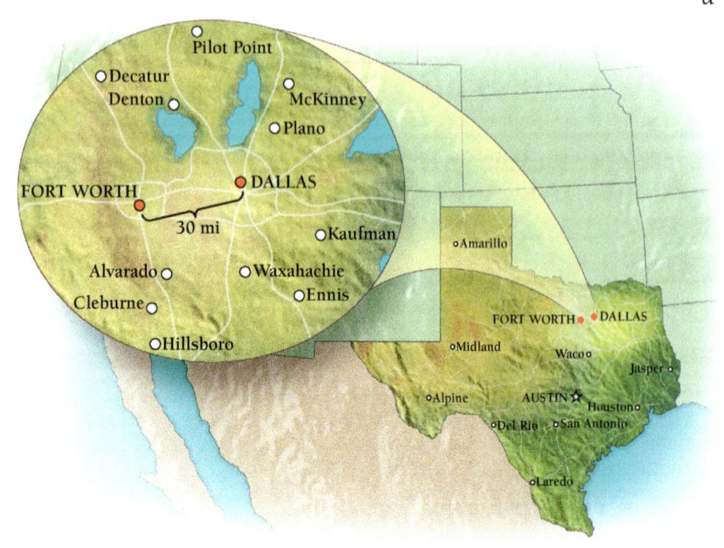

Solution We evaluate the function with the aid of a calculator:

$$N(30, 1{,}138{,}000, 854{,}000) = \frac{2.8(1{,}138{,}000)(854{,}000)}{30^{2.4}}$$
$$\approx 775{,}652{,}422.$$

6 ✓

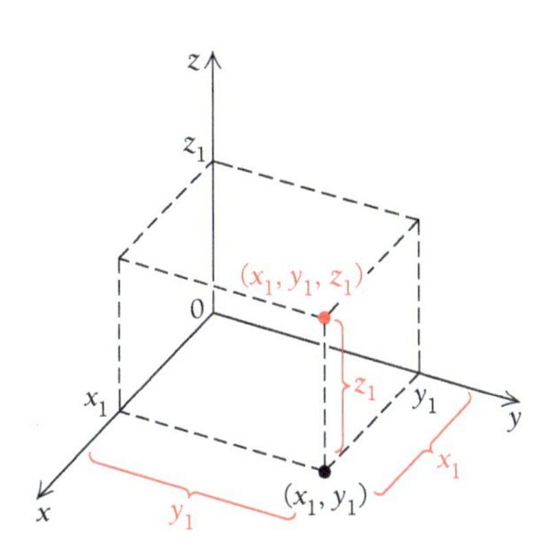

Geometric Interpretations

Visually, a function of two variables, $z = f(x, y)$, can be thought of as matching a point (x_1, y_1) in the xy-plane with the number z_1 on a number line. Thus, to graph a function of two variables, we need a three-dimensional coordinate system. The axes are generally oriented as shown to the left. The line z, called the z-axis, is perpendicular to the xy-plane at the origin.

To help visualize this, think of looking into the corner of a room, where the floor is the xy-plane and the z-axis is the intersection of the two walls. To plot a point (x_1, y_1, z_1), we locate the point (x_1, y_1) in the xy-plane and move up or down in space according to the value of z_1.

EXAMPLE 7 Plot these points:

$P_1(2, 3, 5)$,
$P_2(2, -2, -4)$,
$P_3(0, 5, 2)$,
and $P_4(2, 3, 0)$.

Solution The solution is shown at right.

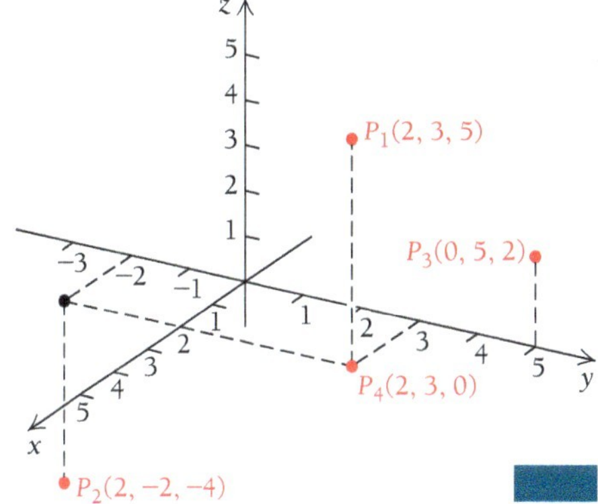

The *graph* of a function of two variables, $z = f(x, y)$, consists of ordered triples (x_1, y_1, z_1), where $z_1 = f(x_1, y_1)$. This graph may be a **surface**, S. The **domain**, D, of a two-variable function is the set of points in the xy-plane for which f is defined.

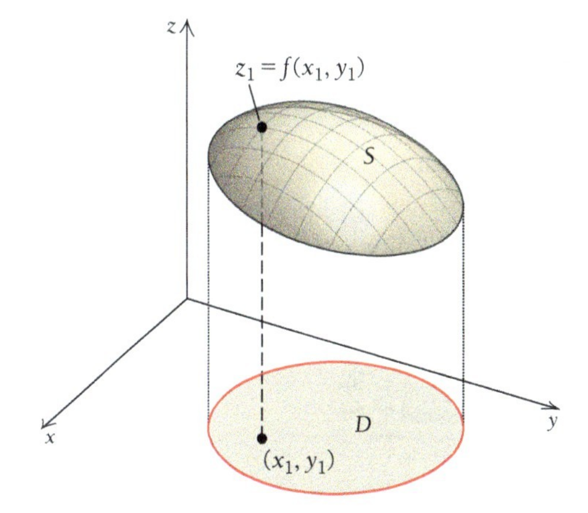

EXAMPLE 8 Find the domain of each two-variable function.

a) $f(x, y) = x^2 + y^2$

b) $g(x, y) = \sqrt{1 - x^2 - y^2}$

c) $h(x, y) = x^2 + y^2 + \dfrac{1}{x^2 + y^2}$

Solution

a) Since we can square any real number and add any two squares, the function f is defined for all x and all y. Therefore, the domain of f is

$$D = \{(x, y) | -\infty < x < \infty, \quad -\infty < y < \infty\}.$$

The graph of f is a surface called an *elliptic paraboloid*. A satellite dish is an example of an elliptic paraboloid: the weak incoming signals bounce off the interior surface of the paraboloid and collect at a single point, called the *focus*, thus amplifying the signal.

Elliptic paraboloid: $z = x^2 + y^2$

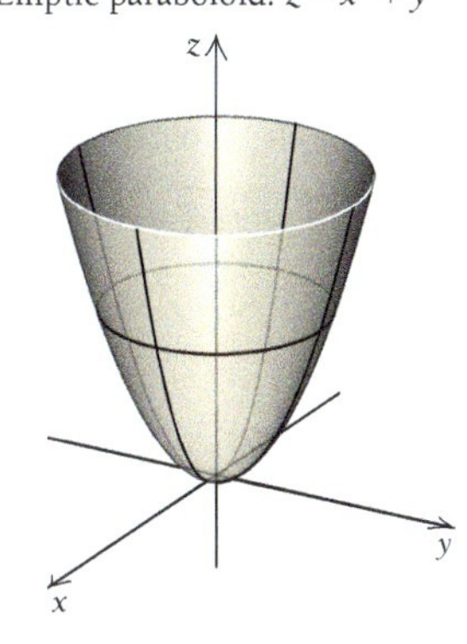

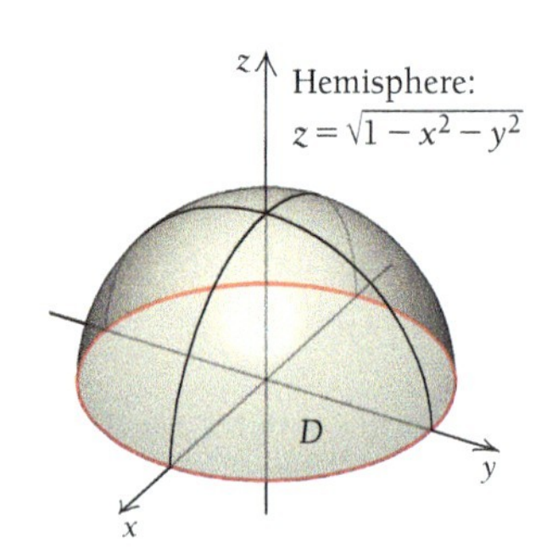

Quick Check 7 ✓

Find the domain of each two-variable function.

a) $f(x, y) = \dfrac{x + y}{x - y}$

b) $g(x, y) = \dfrac{1}{x - 2} + \dfrac{2}{3 + y}$

c) $h(x, y) = \ln(y - x^3)$

b) The expression within the radical must be nonnegative. Therefore, $1 - x^2 - y^2 \geq 0$, which is equivalent to $x^2 + y^2 \leq 1$. The domain of g is

$$D = \{(x, y) | x^2 + y^2 \leq 1\}.$$

The graph of g, shown to the left, is a surface called a *hemisphere*, of radius 1. Its domain is a filled-in circle of radius 1 on the xy-plane. We can think of the domain of g as the "shadow" it casts on the xy-plane.

c) Since zero cannot be in the denominator, we must have $x^2 + y^2 \neq 0$. Therefore, x and y cannot be 0 simultaneously. The domain of h is

$$D = \{(x, y) | (x, y) \neq (0, 0)\}.$$

The graph of h is shown to the right.

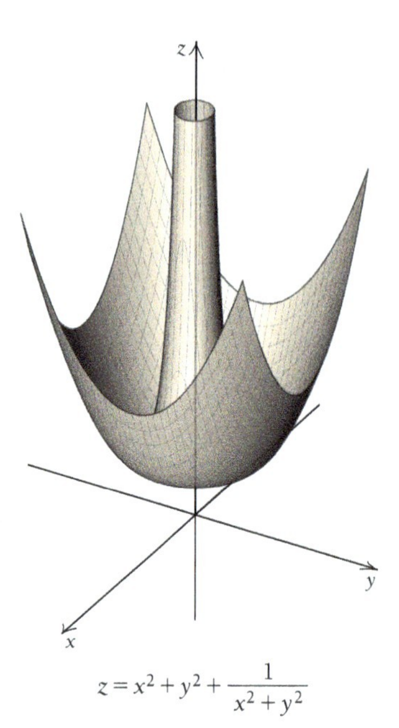

$z = x^2 + y^2 + \dfrac{1}{x^2 + y^2}$

7 ✓

Technology Connection

Exploratory

Graphs of surfaces can be generated using software such as *Maple, Mathematica, MATLAB*, or *GeoGebra* or at websites such as www.wolframalpha.com. There are also inexpensive or free apps that can graph surfaces, and many of these offer touch-based zoom and the ability to view a graph from any angle.

Some surfaces and their graphs are presented here.

EXAMPLE 1 Graph:

$(1 - \sqrt{x^2 + y^2})^2 + z^2 = 0.2.$

This is entered as follows:

```
(1-sqrt(x^2+y^2))^2+z^2=0.2
```

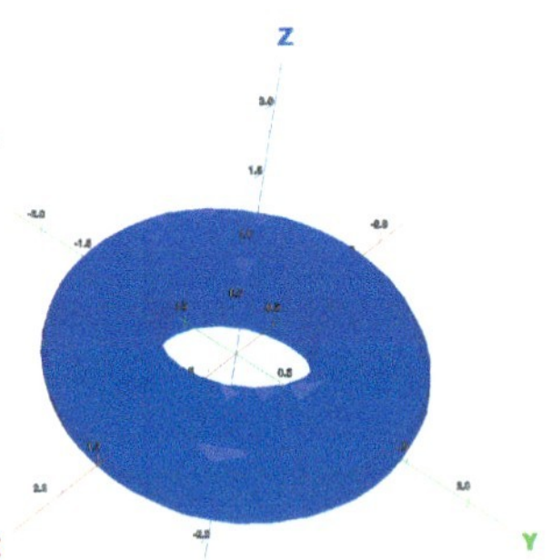

EXAMPLE 2 Graph:

$|(2x^2 + 2y^2)^{0.25}| + \sqrt{|z|} = 1.$

This is entered as follows:

```
abs((2x^2+2y^2)^0.25)+(abs(z))^0.5=1
```

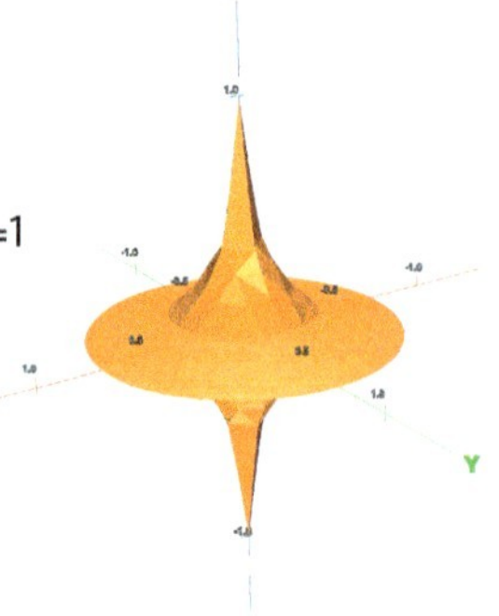

EXAMPLE 3 Graph:

$z = e^{-4(x^2+y^2)}.$

This is entered as follows:

```
z=e^(-4(x^2+y^2))
```

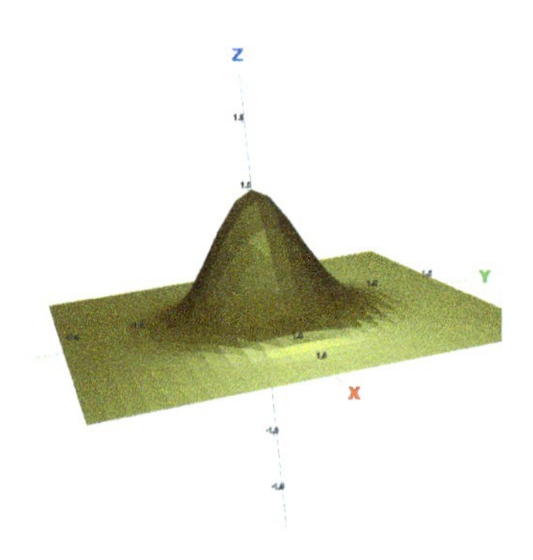

EXAMPLE 4 Graph:

$4x^2 + 2y^2 + z^2 = 1.$

This is entered as follows:

```
4x^2+2y^2+z^2=1
```

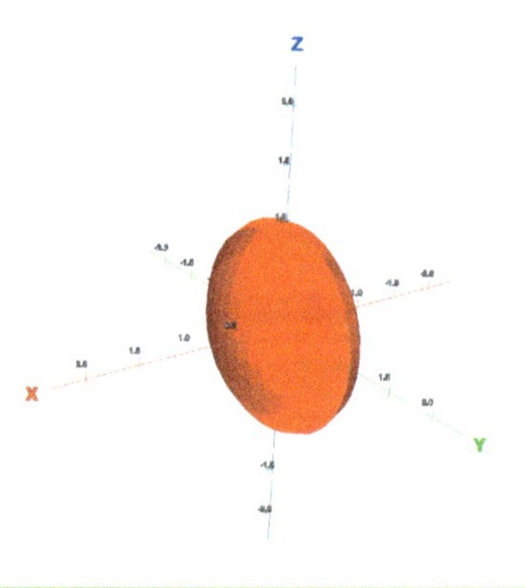

Section Summary

- A *function of n variables* assigns to each input of n ordered inputs, $(x_1, x_2, \ldots, x_n)$, called an *n-tuple*, exactly one output, $f(x_1, x_2, \ldots, x_n)$. Any function of two or more input variables is called a *function of several variables*.
  - A *function of two variables* assigns to each input pair, (x, y), exactly one output, $f(x, y)$.
  - A function of two variables generates points (x, y, z), where $z = f(x, y)$.
  - The graph of a function of two variables is a *surface* and requires a three-dimensional coordinate system.
- The *domain* of a function of several variables is the set of n-tuples for which the function is defined.

6.1 Exercise Set

1. For $f(x, y) = (y^2 + 2xy)^3$, find $f(-2, 0)$, $f(3, 2)$, and $f(-5, 10)$.

2. For $f(x, y) = x^2 - 3xy$, find $f(0, -2)$, $f(2, 3)$, and $f(10, -5)$.

3. For $f(x, y) = \log(x + y) + 3x^2$, find $f(3, 7)$, $f(1, 99)$, and $f(2, -1)$.

4. For $f(x, y) = 3^x + 7xy$, find $f(0, -2)$, $f(-2, 1)$, and $f(2, 1)$.

5. For $f(x, y) = 2^x - 3^y$, find $f(0, 2)$, $f(3, 1)$, and $f(2, 3)$.

6. For $f(x, y) = \ln x + y^3$, find $f(e, 2)$, $f(e^2, 4)$, and $f(e^3, 5)$.

7. For $f(x, y, z) = 2^x + 5zy - x$, find $f(0, 1, -3)$ and $f(1, 0, -3)$.

8. For $f(x, y, z) = x^2 - y^2 + z^2$, find $f(-1, 2, 3)$ and $f(2, -1, 3)$.

In Exercises 9–12, determine the domain of each function of two variables.

9. $h(x, y) = xe^{\sqrt{y}}$

10. $k(x, y) = \dfrac{1}{x} + \dfrac{y}{x - 1}$

11. $f(x, y) = \sqrt{y - 3x}$

12. $g(x, y) = \dfrac{1}{y + x^2}$

APPLICATIONS

Business and Economics

13. Yield. The *yield* of a stock is given by

$$Y(D, P) = \frac{D}{P},$$

where D is the dividend per share of stock and P is the price per share. On October 18, 2018, the price per share of Texas Instruments (TI) stock was \$99.54, and the dividend per share was \$0.62. (*Source:* finance.yahoo.com, October 19, 2018.) Find the yield. Use percent notation rounded to the nearest hundredth of a percent.

14. Price–earnings ratio. The *price–earnings ratio* of a stock is given by

$$R(P, E) = \frac{P}{E},$$

where P is the price per share of the stock and E is the earnings per share. On October 18, 2018, the price per share of Hewlett-Packard Enterprises (HPE) stock was \$15.33, and the earnings per share were \$0.43. (*Source:* finance.yahoo.com, October 19, 2018.) Find the price–earnings ratio. Use decimal notation rounded to the nearest hundredth.

15. Cost of storage equipment. Consider the cost model in Example 5. For \$100,000, Tonopah Storage buys a storage tank that has a capacity of 80,000 gal. Later it replaces the tank with a new one that has triple that capacity. Estimate the cost of the new tank.

16. Savings and interest. A sum of \$1000 is deposited in a savings account for which interest is compounded monthly. The future value, $A(r, t)$, in dollars, is a function of the annual percentage rate r and the term t, in months, and is given by

$$A(r, t) = 1000\left(1 + \frac{r}{12}\right)^{12t}.$$

a) Determine $A(0.05, 10)$.

b) What is the interest earned for the rate and term in part (a)?

c) How much more interest can be earned over the same term as in part (a) if the APR is increased to 5.75%?

17. Monthly car payments. Ashley wants to buy a 2019 Chevrolet Bolt electric car and finance \$20,000 of the cost through a loan. Use the table in Example 4 to answer the following questions.

a) SouthBank will lend Ashley \$20,000 at an APR of 5.0% for 7 yr. What will her monthly payment be?

b) Find Ashley's total payments, assuming that she pays the amount found in part (a) every month for the full term of the loan.

c) Valley Credit Union offers a 5-yr term on a loan of \$20,000. What is the highest APR that Ashley can accept if she wants to pay less overall than what she would with the loan from SouthBank?

d) If she accepts Valley Credit Union's offer of a 5-yr term with an APR of 6.5% and makes every monthly payment, how much less overall will she pay?

18. Monthly car payments. Kim is shopping for a car. She will finance \$10,000 through a lender. Use the table in Example 4 to answer the following questions.

a) One lender offers Kim an APR of 6% for a 6-yr term. What would Kim's monthly payment be?

b) A competing lender offers an APR of 5.5% but for a 7-yr term. What would Kim's monthly payment be?

c) Assume that Kim makes the minimum payment each month for the entire term of the loan. Calculate her total payments for both options described in parts (a) and (b). Which option costs Kim less overall?

Life and Physical Sciences

19. Poiseuille's Law. The speed of blood in a vessel is given by

$$V(L, p, R, r, v) = \frac{p}{4Lv}(R^2 - r^2),$$

where R is the radius of the vessel, r is the distance of the blood from the center of the vessel, L is the length of the blood vessel, p is the blood pressure, and v is the viscosity of the blood. Find

$$V(1, 100, 0.0075, 0.0025, 0.05).$$

20. Body surface area. The Haycock formula for approximating the surface area S, in square meters (m^2), of a human is given by

$$S(h, w) = 0.024265h^{0.3964}w^{0.5378},$$

where h is the person's height in centimeters and w is the person's weight in kilograms. (*Source:* www.halls.md.) Use the Haycock approximation to estimate the surface area of a person whose height is 165 cm and whose weight is 80 kg.

21. Body surface area. The Mosteller formula for approximating the surface area S, in square meters (m^2), of a human is given by

$$S(h, w) = \frac{\sqrt{hw}}{60},$$

where h is the person's height in centimeters and w is the person's weight in kilograms. (*Source:* www.halls.md.) Use the Mosteller approximation to estimate the surface area of a person whose height is 165 cm and whose weight is 80 kg.

22. Torricelli's Law. The speed, v, in meters per second, of a fluid flowing out of a hole in a container h meters above the base of the container is given by

$$v(g, h) = \sqrt{2gh},$$

where g is the gravitational constant, $g = 9.8$ m/s^2. Find the speed of a fluid that is flowing from a hole 2 m above the base of a vat.

General Interest

23. Baseball: total bases. A batter's *total bases* is a statistic given by

$$B(s, d, t, h) = s + 2d + 3t + 4h,$$

where s is the number of singles, d the number of doubles, t the number of triples, and h the number of home runs hit by the batter. During the 2017 season, Arizona's Paul Goldschmidt hit 93 singles, 34 doubles, 3 triples, and 36 home runs. (*Source:* retrosheet.org.)

a) Find $B(93, 34, 3, 36)$.

b) Interpret the meaning of this number.

24. Soccer: point system. A point system is used to rank each club in Major League Soccer. (*Source:* MLS.com.) A club's ranking in points, P, is given by

$$P(w, t) = 3w + t,$$

where w is the number of games won and t is the number of games tied. Clubs receive no points for a loss.

a) The Chicago Fire had a record of 16 wins, 11 losses, and 7 ties for the 2017 season. How many points did the Chicago Fire earn?

b) The Atlanta United FC had a record of 16 wins, 9 losses, and 10 ties for the 2017 season. How many points did Atlanta United FC earn?

25. Dewpoint. The *dewpoint* is the temperature at which moisture in the air condenses into liquid (dew). It is a function of air temperature t and relative humidity h. The table below shows the dewpoints for select values of t and h.

Air Temperature, t (°F)	Relative Humidity (%)				
	20	40	60	80	100
70	29	44	55	63	70
80	35	53	65	73	80
90	43	62	74	83	90
100	52	71	84	93	100

(*Source:* medschools.info.)

a) What is the dewpoint when the air temperature is 80°F with a relative humidity of 60%?

b) What is the dewpoint when the air temperature is 90°F with a relative humidity of 40%?

c) Air feels humid when the dewpoint reaches about 60. If the air temperature is 100°F, at what approximate relative humidity will the air feel humid?

d) Explain why the dewpoint is equal to the air temperature when the relative humidity is 100%.

26. Heat index. The heat index, $n(h, t)$, is the temperature perceived by the human skin at relative humidity h and air temperature t. Below is a table showing heat index values for select values of h and t.

Relative Humidity (%)	Temperature (°F)					
	80	84	88	92	96	100
40	80	83	88	94	101	109
50	81	85	91	99	108	118
60	82	88	95	105	116	129
70	83	90	100	112	126	
80	84	94	106	121		
90	86	98	113	131		
100	87	103	121			

(*Source:* National Weather Service.)

a) What is the heat index when the air temperature is 96°F with a relative humidity of 60%?

b) What is the heat index when the air temperature is 88°F with a relative humidity of 80%?

c) Suppose the heat index one afternoon is 100°F with a relative humidity of 70%. What is the air temperature?

d) For an air temperature of 92°F, use regression and the data in the above table to find a linear function that gives the heat index at 92°F as a function of the humidity.

SYNTHESIS

27. Using the formula for speed of fluid flow in Exercise 22, find the height above the base of a container of a hole from which fluid is exiting at 9 m/sec.

28. According to the Mosteller formula in Exercise 21, if a person's weight drops 19%, by what percentage does his or her surface area change?

29. Explain the difference between a function of two variables and a function of one variable.

30. Find some examples of functions of several variables not considered in the text, including at least one that does not have a formula.

Technology Connection

General Interest

Wind chill temperature. *Because wind speed enhances the loss of heat from the skin, we feel colder when there is wind than when there is not. The wind chill temperature is what the temperature would have to be with no wind in order to give the same chilling effect. The wind chill temperature, W, is given by*

$$W(v, T) = 91.4 - \frac{(10.45 + 6.68\sqrt{v} - 0.447v)(457 - 5T)}{110},$$

where T is the temperature measured by a thermometer, in degrees Fahrenheit, and v is the speed of the wind, in miles per hour. Find the wind chill temperature in each case. Round to the nearest degree.

31. $T = 30°\text{F}, v = 25$ mph

32. $T = 20°\text{F}, v = 20$ mph

33. $T = 20°\text{F}, v = 40$ mph

34. $T = -10°\text{F}, v = 30$ mph

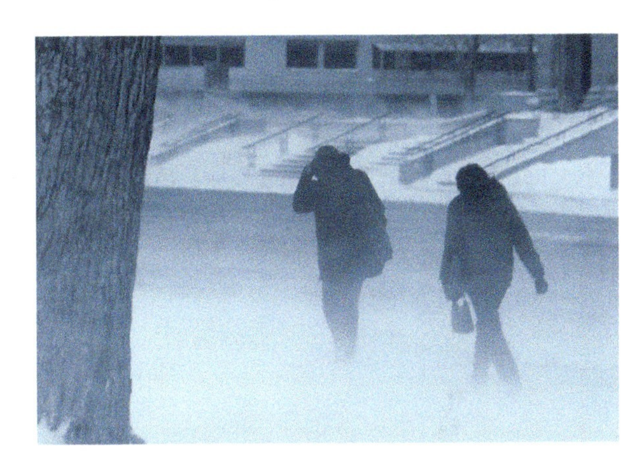

35. Use a graphics program such as *Maple* or *Mathematica*, a website such as www.wolframalpha.com, a graphing calculator, or an online app to view the graph of each function given in Exercises 1–6.

Use a 3D graphics program to generate the graph of each function.

36. $f(x, y) = y^2$

37. $f(x, y) = x^2 + y^2$

38. $f(x, y) = (x^4 - 16x^2)e^{-y^2}$

39. $f(x, y) = 4(x^2 + y^2) - (x^2 + y^2)^2$

40. $f(x, y) = x^3 - 3xy^2$

41. $f(x, y) = \dfrac{1}{x^2 + 4y^2}$

Answers to Quick Checks

1. 173.75; it costs \$173.75 to produce 10 mugs and 15 vases. **2.** $P(5, 8, 3) = 30$. A basketball player who makes 5 free throws, 8 two-point field goals, and 3 three-point field goals will score a total of 30 points. **3.** \$13.76 **4. (a)** \$19.80; **(b)** \$2.75 per month; **(c)** 5-yr term, lower by \$39.60 **5. (a)** \$82,568.07 **(b)** 83.5% increase **6.** \$3.47/copy **7. (a)** $D = \{(x, y) | y \neq x\}$; **(b)** $D = \{(x, y) | x \neq 2, y \neq -3\}$; **(c)** $D = \{(x, y) | y > x^3\}$

6.2

- Find the partial derivatives of a given function.
- Evaluate partial derivatives.
- Use differentials of a multivariable function to estimate the change in the function.
- Find the four second-order partial derivatives of a function in two variables.

Partial Derivatives

Finding Partial Derivatives

Consider the function f given by

$$z = f(x, y) = x^2y^3 + xy + 4y^2.$$

Suppose we fix y at 3. Then

$$f(x, 3) = x^2(3^3) + x(3) + 4(3^2) = 27x^2 + 3x + 36.$$

Note that we now have a function of only one variable. Taking the first derivative with respect to x, we have

$$54x + 3.$$

In general, without replacing y with a specific number, let's regard y as fixed. Then f becomes a function of x alone, and we can calculate its derivative with respect to x. This is called the *partial derivative of f with respect to x*, denoted by

$$\frac{\partial f}{\partial x} \quad \text{or} \quad \frac{\partial z}{\partial x}.$$

Now, let's again consider the function

$$z = f(x, y) = x^2y^3 + xy + 4y^2.$$

The color blue indicates the variable x when we fix y and treat it as a constant. The expressions y^3, y, and y^2 are then also treated as constants. We have

$$\frac{\partial f}{\partial x} = \frac{\partial}{\partial x}(x^2 y^3 + xy + 4y^2)$$

$$= 2xy^3 + (1)y + 0 \qquad \text{Differentiating with respect to } x$$

$$= 2xy^3 + y.$$

Similarly, we find $\partial f/\partial y$ or $\partial z/\partial y$ by fixing x (treating it as a constant) and calculating the derivative with respect to y. From

$$z = f(x, y) = x^2y^3 + xy + 4y^2, \qquad \text{The color blue indicates the variable.}$$

we get

$$\frac{\partial f}{\partial y} = \frac{\partial}{\partial y}(x^2 y^3 + xy + 4y^2)$$

$$= x^2(3y^2) + x(1) + 8y \qquad \text{Differentiating with respect to } y$$

$$= 3x^2y^2 + x + 8y.$$

A definition of partial derivatives follows.

DEFINITION

For $z = f(x, y)$, the **partial derivatives with respect to x and y** are

$$\frac{\partial z}{\partial x} = \lim_{h \to 0} \frac{f(x + h, y) - f(x, y)}{h} \quad \text{and} \quad \frac{\partial z}{\partial y} = \lim_{h \to 0} \frac{f(x, y + h) - f(x, y)}{h}.$$

We can find partial derivatives of functions of any number of variables. Since the earlier theorems for finding derivatives apply, we rarely need to use the above definition to find a partial derivative.

EXAMPLE 1 For $w = x^2 - xy + y^2 + 2yz + 2z^2 + z$, find

$$\frac{\partial w}{\partial x}, \quad \frac{\partial w}{\partial y}, \quad \text{and} \quad \frac{\partial w}{\partial z}.$$

Solution In order to find $\partial w/\partial x$, we regard x as the variable and treat y and z as constants. From

$$w = x^2 - xy + y^2 + 2yz + 2z^2 + z,$$

we have

$$\frac{\partial w}{\partial x} = 2x - y. \qquad \text{Differentiating with respect to } x$$

To find $\partial w/\partial y$, we regard y as the variable and treat x and z as constants. We have

$$\frac{\partial w}{\partial y} = -x + 2y + 2z. \qquad \text{Differentiating with respect to } y$$

To find $\partial w/\partial z$, we regard z as the variable and treat x and y as constants. We have

$$\frac{\partial w}{\partial z} = 2y + 4z + 1. \qquad \text{Differentiating with respect to } z$$

1 ✓

Quick Check 1 ✓

For $u = x^2y^3z^4$, find

$$\frac{\partial u}{\partial x}, \frac{\partial u}{\partial y}, \text{ and } \frac{\partial u}{\partial z}.$$

We often write $f_x(x, y)$ or f_x for the partial derivative of f with respect to x and $f_y(x, y)$ or f_y for the partial derivative of f with respect to y. Similarly, if $z = f(x, y)$, then z_x represents the partial derivative of z with respect to x, and z_y represents the partial derivative of z with respect to y.

EXAMPLE 2 For $f(x, y) = 3x^2y + xy^2$, find $f_x(x, y)$ and $f_y(x, y)$.

Solution We have

$$f_x(x, y) = \frac{\partial}{\partial x}(3x^2y + xy^2) = 6xy + y^2,$$

$$f_y(x, y) = \frac{\partial}{\partial y}(3x^2y + xy^2) = 3x^2 + 2xy.$$

2 ✓

Quick Check 2 ✓

For $f(x, y) = 7x^3y^2 - \frac{x}{y}$, find $f_x(x, y)$ and $f_y(x, y)$.

For the function in Example 2, let's evaluate f_x at $(2, -3)$:

$$f_x(2, -3) = -27.$$

If we use the notation $\partial f/\partial x = 6xy + y^2$, where $f = 3x^2y + xy^2$, the value of the partial derivative at $(2, -3)$ can be written as

$$\frac{\partial}{\partial x}f(2, -3) = 6 \cdot 2 \cdot (-3) + (-3)^2$$
$$= -27.$$

EXAMPLE 3 For $f(x, y) = e^{xy} + y \ln x$, find f_x and f_y.

Solution We have

$$f_x = y \cdot e^{xy} + y \cdot \frac{1}{x} \qquad \text{Treating } y \text{ as a constant}$$

$$= ye^{xy} + \frac{y}{x},$$

and $$f_y = x \cdot e^{xy} + \ln x. \qquad \text{Treating } x \text{ and } \ln x \text{ as constants}$$

3 ✓

Quick Check 3 ✓

For $g(x, y) = \ln(x^2 + xy^4)$, find g_x and g_y.

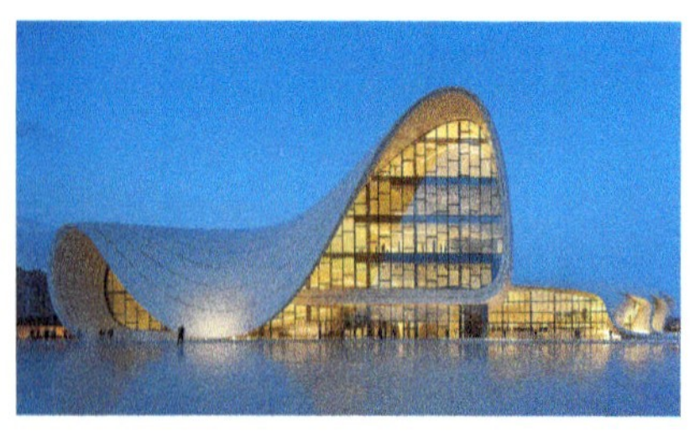
The roof of this building is a smooth continuous surface. The slope at a point on the surface depends on the direction in which the tangent line is oriented.

The Geometric Interpretation of Partial Derivatives

Suppose that the graph of $z = f(x, y)$ is a surface S, similar to the one shown to the right. Here each input pair (x, y) in the domain D has the output $z = f(x, y)$.

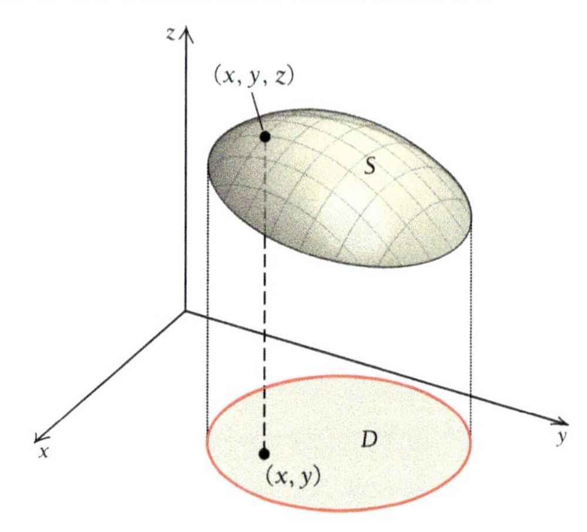

Now suppose we hold x fixed at the value a. The set of all points with $x = a$ is a plane parallel to the yz-plane; thus, when x is fixed at a, y and z vary along that plane, as shown to the right. The plane $x = a$ in the figure cuts the surface along the curve C_1. The partial derivative f_y gives the slope of tangent lines to this curve, in the positive y-direction.

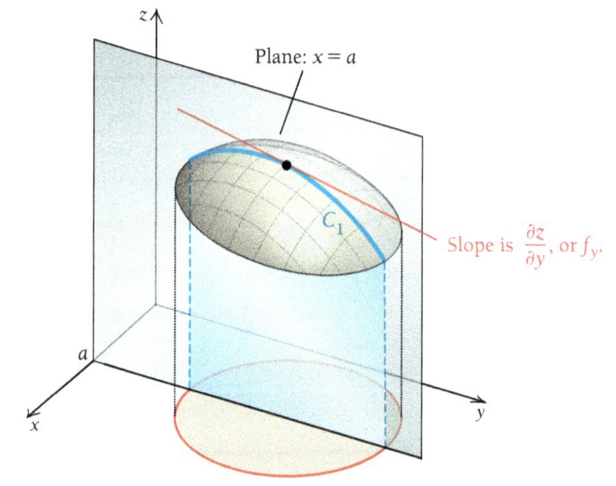

Similarly, if we fix y at the value b, we obtain a curve C_2, as shown to the right. The partial derivative f_x gives the slope of tangent lines to this curve, in the positive x-direction.

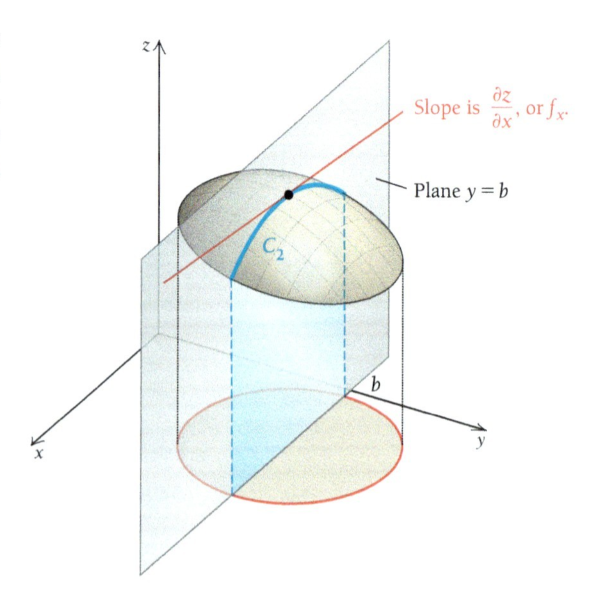

Application: Productivity and Differentials

One model of production that is frequently applied in business and economics is the *Cobb–Douglas production function:*

$$p(x, y) = Ax^a y^{1-a}, \quad \text{for} \quad A > 0 \quad \text{and} \quad 0 < a < 1,$$

where p is the number of units produced with x units of labor and y units of capital. (Capital is the cost of machinery, buildings, tools, and other supplies.) The partial derivatives

$$\frac{\partial p}{\partial x} \quad \text{and} \quad \frac{\partial p}{\partial y}$$

are called, respectively, the *marginal productivity of labor* and the *marginal productivity of capital.*

EXAMPLE 4 MyTell Cellular has the following production function for a smartphone:

$$p(x, y) = 50x^{2/3}y^{1/3},$$

where p is the number of units produced with x units of labor and y units of capital.

a) Find the number of units produced with 125 units of labor and 64 units of capital.

b) Find the marginal productivities.

c) Evaluate the marginal productivities at $x = 125$ and $y = 64$.

Solution

a) $p(125, 64) = 50(125)^{2/3}(64)^{1/3} = 50(25)(4) = 5000$ units

b) Marginal productivity of labor $= \dfrac{\partial p}{\partial x} = p_x = 50\left(\dfrac{2}{3}\right)x^{-1/3}y^{1/3} = \dfrac{100y^{1/3}}{3x^{1/3}}$

Marginal productivity of capital $= \dfrac{\partial p}{\partial y} = p_y = 50\left(\dfrac{1}{3}\right)x^{2/3}y^{-2/3} = \dfrac{50x^{2/3}}{3y^{2/3}}$

c) For 125 units of labor and 64 units of capital, we have

Marginal productivity of labor $= p_x(125, 64)$

$$= \frac{100(64)^{1/3}}{3(125)^{1/3}} = \frac{100(4)}{3(5)} = 26\tfrac{2}{3},$$

Marginal productivity of capital $= p_y(125, 64)$

$$= \frac{50(125)^{2/3}}{3(64)^{2/3}} = \frac{50(25)}{3(16)} = 26\tfrac{1}{24}.$$

4 ✓

Quick Check 4 ✓

A publisher's production function for textbooks is given by $p(x, y) = 72x^{0.8}y^{0.2}$, where p is the number of books produced, x is units of labor, and y is units of capital. Determine the marginal productivity of labor and the marginal productivity of capital at $x = 90$ and $y = 50$.

Let's interpret the marginal productivities of Example 4. To visualize the marginal productivity of labor, suppose capital is fixed at 64 units. Then a one-unit change in labor, from 125 to 126, will cause production to increase by about $26\frac{2}{3}$ units. To visualize the marginal productivity of capital, suppose the amount of labor is fixed at 125 units. Then a one-unit change in capital from 64 to 65 will cause production to increase by about $26\frac{1}{24}$ units.

A Cobb–Douglas production function is consistent with the law of diminishing returns. That is, if one input (either labor or capital) is held fixed while the other increases infinitely, then production will eventually increase at a decreasing rate.

Partial derivatives can also be used to approximate small changes in a function. Recall from Section 3.6 that dx and dy are *differentials*, representing changes in x and y, respectively, with $y = f(x)$ and $dx \approx \Delta x$ and $dy \approx \Delta y$. When these changes are small, we have

$$\frac{\Delta y}{\Delta x} \approx \frac{dy}{dx}, \quad \text{so} \quad \Delta y \approx f'(x)\,\Delta x.$$

For functions of several variables, the differentials of each variable are similarly related. For example, if $z = f(x, y)$, then we have

$$dz \approx f_x(x, y)\,dx + f_y(x, y)\,dy.$$

EXAMPLE 5 **General Interest: Tolerances.** A circular swimming pool has a radius of 12 ft and a depth of 4 ft. Both measurements have a tolerance of ± 3 in. $\left(\pm\frac{1}{4}\text{ ft}\right)$.

a) Find the volume of this pool assuming a radius of 12 ft and a depth of 4 ft.

b) Use differentials to estimate the change in volume, assuming that both measurements include the extra 3 in.

c) Compare the result in part (b) to the actual change in volume, assuming that both measurements include the extra 3 in.

Solution The formula for the volume of a right circular cylinder of radius r and depth h is

$$V(r, h) = \pi r^2 h.$$

a) We have

$$V(12, 4) = \pi(12)^2(4) \qquad \text{Substituting}$$
$$= 576\pi, \quad \text{or about } 1809.6 \text{ ft}^3.$$

b) To approximate the change in V, we first determine $\frac{\partial V}{\partial r}$ and $\frac{\partial V}{\partial h}$:

$$\frac{\partial V}{\partial r} = 2\pi rh \quad \text{and} \quad \frac{\partial V}{\partial h} = \pi r^2.$$

We then have

$$\Delta V \approx V_r(r, h)\,dr + V_h(r, h)\,dh$$
$$= 2\pi rh \cdot dr + \pi r^2 \cdot dh. \qquad \text{Substituting}$$

Thus, for $r = 12$, $h = 4$, and $\Delta r = \Delta h = \frac{1}{4}$, we have

$$\Delta V \approx 2\pi(12)(4)\left(\frac{1}{4}\right) + \pi(12)^2\left(\frac{1}{4}\right) \qquad \text{Substituting}$$
$$= 60\pi, \quad \text{or about } 188.5 \text{ ft}^3.$$

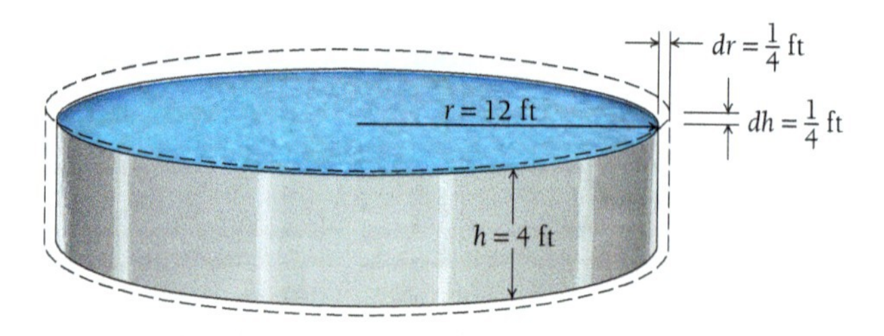

The dashed lines show the increase in volume with the tolerance of 3 in. $\left(\frac{1}{4}\text{ ft}\right)$ added to the pool's radius and depth. The approximate increase in volume is $dV = 188.5 \text{ ft}^3$.

Quick Check 5 ✓

Consider the swimming pool of Example 5.

a) Find the surface area of the empty pool (side and base only), assuming a radius of 12 ft and a depth of 4 ft.

b) Use differentials to estimate the change in surface area of the empty pool, assuming that both measurements include the extra 3 in.

c) Compare the result in part (b) to the actual change in surface area, assuming that both measurements include the extra 3 in.

c) The actual change in V is found by evaluating $V(r + \Delta r, h + \Delta h) - V(r, h)$. We have

$$\begin{aligned}\Delta V &= V(r + \Delta r, h + \Delta h) - V(r, h)\\ &= V\left(12 + \frac{1}{4}, 4 + \frac{1}{4}\right) - V(12, 4) && \text{Substituting}\\ &= \pi(12.25)^2(4.25) - \pi(12)^2(4)\\ &\approx 194 \text{ ft}^3. && \text{Using a calculator and rounding}\end{aligned}$$

5 ✓

Higher-Order Partial Derivatives

Consider

$$z = f(x, y) = 3xy^2 + 2xy + x^2.$$

Then $\dfrac{\partial z}{\partial x} = \dfrac{\partial f}{\partial x} = 3y^2 + 2y + 2x.$

Suppose we now find the first partial derivative of $\partial z/\partial x$ with respect to y. This will be a **second-order partial derivative** of the original function z, denoted by

$$\begin{aligned}\frac{\partial}{\partial y}\left(\frac{\partial z}{\partial x}\right) &= \frac{\partial}{\partial y}\left(\frac{\partial f}{\partial x}\right)\\ &= \frac{\partial}{\partial y}(3y^2 + 2y + 2x) && \text{Substituting}\\ &= 6y + 2.\end{aligned}$$

The notation $\dfrac{\partial}{\partial y}\left(\dfrac{\partial z}{\partial x}\right)$ is often expressed as

$$\frac{\partial^2 z}{\partial y\,\partial x} \quad \text{or} \quad \frac{\partial^2 f}{\partial y\,\partial x} \quad \text{or} \quad f_{xy}.$$

In the notation f_{xy}, it is important to note that x and y are in the order (left to right) in which the differentiation is done. In the notation

$$\frac{\partial^2 f}{\partial y\,\partial x},$$

the order of x and y is reversed. In each case, the differentiation with respect to x is done first, followed by differentiation with respect to y.

Notation for the four second-order partial derivatives is as follows.

DEFINITION Second-Order Partial Derivatives

1. $\dfrac{\partial^2 z}{\partial x\,\partial x} = \dfrac{\partial^2 f}{\partial x\,\partial x} = \dfrac{\partial^2 z}{\partial x^2} = \dfrac{\partial^2 f}{\partial x^2} = f_{xx}$ Take the partial derivative with respect to x, and then with respect to x again.
2. $\dfrac{\partial^2 z}{\partial y\,\partial x} = \dfrac{\partial^2 f}{\partial y\,\partial x} = f_{xy}$ Take the partial derivative with respect to x, and then with respect to y.
3. $\dfrac{\partial^2 z}{\partial x\,\partial y} = \dfrac{\partial^2 f}{\partial x\,\partial y} = f_{yx}$ Take the partial derivative with respect to y, and then with respect to x.
4. $\dfrac{\partial^2 z}{\partial y\,\partial y} = \dfrac{\partial^2 f}{\partial y\,\partial y} = \dfrac{\partial^2 z}{\partial y^2} = \dfrac{\partial^2 f}{\partial y^2} = f_{yy}$ Take the partial derivative with respect to y, and then with respect to y again.

EXAMPLE 6 For

$$z = f(x, y) = x^2y^3 + x^4y + xe^y,$$

find the four second-order partial derivatives.

Solution

a) $\dfrac{\partial^2 f}{\partial x^2} = f_{xx} = \dfrac{\partial}{\partial x}(2xy^3 + 4x^3y + e^y)$ — Differentiate f with respect to x.

$= 2y^3 + 12x^2y$ — Differentiate f_x with respect to x.

b) $\dfrac{\partial^2 f}{\partial y\, \partial x} = f_{xy} = \dfrac{\partial}{\partial y}(2xy^3 + 4x^3y + e^y)$ — Differentiate f with respect to x.

$= 6xy^2 + 4x^3 + e^y$ — Differentiate f_x with respect to y.

c) $\dfrac{\partial^2 f}{\partial x\, \partial y} = f_{yx} = \dfrac{\partial}{\partial x}(3x^2y^2 + x^4 + xe^y)$ — Differentiate f with respect to y.

$= 6xy^2 + 4x^3 + e^y$ — Differentiate f_y with respect to x.

d) $\dfrac{\partial^2 f}{\partial y^2} = f_{yy} = \dfrac{\partial}{\partial y}(3x^2y^2 + x^4 + xe^y)$ — Differentiate f with respect to y.

$= 6x^2y + xe^y$ — Differentiate f_y with respect to y. **6 ✓**

Quick Check 6 ✓

For

$$z = g(x, y) = 6x^2 + 3xy^4 - y^2,$$

find the four second-order partial derivatives.

Comparing parts (b) and (c) of Example 5, we see that

$$\frac{\partial^2 f}{\partial y\, \partial x} = \frac{\partial^2 f}{\partial x\, \partial y} \quad \text{and} \quad f_{xy} = f_{yx}.$$

Although this will be true for virtually all functions that we consider in this text, it is *not* true for all functions. One function for which it is not true is given in Exercise 67.

In Section 6.3, we will see how higher-order partial derivatives are used in applications to find extrema for functions of two variables.

Section Summary

- For $z = f(x, y)$, the *partial derivatives with respect to x and y* are, respectively:

$$\frac{\partial z}{\partial x} = \lim_{h \to 0} \frac{f(x + h, y) - f(x, y)}{h} \quad \text{and}$$

$$\frac{\partial z}{\partial y} = \lim_{h \to 0} \frac{f(x, y + h) - f(x, y)}{h}.$$

- Alternative notations for partial derivatives are $f_x(x, y)$ or f_x, $f_y(x, y)$ or f_y, and z_x for $\dfrac{\partial z}{\partial x}$ and z_y for $\dfrac{\partial z}{\partial y}$.
- For a surface $z = f(x, y)$ and a point (x_0, y_0, z_0) on this surface, the partial derivative of f with respect to x gives the slope of the tangent line at (x_0, y_0, z_0) in the positive x-direction. Similarly, the partial derivative of f with respect to y gives the slope of the tangent line at (x_0, y_0, z_0) in the positive y-direction.
- If $z = f(x, y)$, then the differential of z is

$$dz \approx f_x(x, y)\, dx + f_y(x, y)\, dy.$$

- For $z = f(x, y)$, the *second-order partial derivatives* are

$$f_{xx} = \frac{\partial^2 f}{\partial x^2}, f_{xy} = \frac{\partial^2 f}{\partial y\, \partial x}, f_{yx} = \frac{\partial^2 f}{\partial x\, \partial y}, \text{ and } f_{yy} = \frac{\partial^2 f}{\partial y^2}.$$

Often (but not always), $f_{xy} = f_{yx}$.

6.2 Exercise Set

Find $\dfrac{\partial z}{\partial x}, \dfrac{\partial z}{\partial y}, \dfrac{\partial}{\partial x}z(-2, -3)$, *and* $\dfrac{\partial}{\partial y}z(0, -5)$.

1. $z = 2x - 3y$

2. $z = 7x - 5y$

3. $z = 2x^3 + 3xy - x$

4. $z = 3x^2 - 2xy + y$

Find $f_x(x, y)$, $f_y(x, y)$, $f_x(-2, 4)$, *and* $f_y(4, -3)$.

5. $f(x, y) = 5x + 7y$

6. $f(x, y) = 2x - 5xy$

Find f_x, f_y, $f_x(-2, 1)$, and $f_y(-3, -2)$.

7. $f(x, y) = \sqrt{x^2 - y^2}$

8. $f(x, y) = \sqrt{x^2 + y^2}$

Find f_x and f_y.

9. $f(x, y) = e^{2x-y}$

10. $f(x, y) = e^{3x-2y}$

11. $f(x, y) = e^{2xy}$

12. $f(x, y) = e^{xy}$

13. $f(x, y) = y \ln(x + 2y)$

14. $f(x, y) = x \ln(x - y)$

15. $f(x, y) = y \ln(xy)$

16. $f(x, y) = x \ln(xy)$

17. $f(x, y) = \frac{x}{y} - \frac{y}{3x}$

18. $f(x, y) = \frac{x}{y} + \frac{y}{5x}$

19. $f(x, y) = 3(2x + y - 5)^2$

20. $f(x, y) = 4(3x + y - 8)^2$

Find $\frac{\partial f}{\partial b}$ and $\frac{\partial f}{\partial m}$.

21. $f(b, m) = 5m^2 - mb^2 - 3b + (2m + b - 8)^2 + (3m + b - 9)^2$

22. $f(b, m) = m^3 + 4m^2b - b^2 + (2m + b - 5)^2 + (3m + b - 6)^2$

Find f_x, f_y, and f_λ. (The symbol λ is the Greek letter lambda.)

23. $f(x, y, \lambda) = 5xy - \lambda(2x + y - 8)$

24. $f(x, y, \lambda) = x^2 + y^2 - \lambda(10x + 2y - 4)$

25. $f(x, y, \lambda) = 9xy - \lambda(3x - y + 7)$

26. $f(x, y, \lambda) = x^2 - y^2 - \lambda(4x - 7y - 10)$

Find the four second-order partial derivatives.

27. $f(x, y) = 3x^2y - 2xy + 4y$

28. $f(x, y) = 7xy^2 + 5xy - 2y$

29. $f(x, y) = x^4y^3 - x^2y^3$

30. $f(x, y) = x^5y^4 + x^3y^2$

Find f_{xx}, f_{xy}, f_{yx}, and f_{yy}. (Remember that f_{yx} means to differentiate with respect to y and then with respect to x.)

31. $f(x, y) = 3x + 5y$

32. $f(x, y) = 2x - 3y$

33. $f(x, y) = e^{xy}$

34. $f(x, y) = e^{2xy}$

35. $f(x, y) = x \ln y$

36. $f(x, y) = y \ln x$

37. Let $z = f(x, y) = x^2 + y^3$.

a) Use differentials to estimate Δz for $x = 3$, $y = 4$, $\Delta x = 0.02$, and $\Delta y = 0.03$.

b) Find Δz by evaluating $f(x + \Delta x, y + \Delta y) - f(x, y)$.

38. Let $z = f(x, y) = \frac{x}{y}$.

a) Use differentials to estimate Δz for $x = 4$, $y = 2$, $\Delta x = 0.01$, and $\Delta y = 0.04$.

b) Find Δz by evaluating $f(x + \Delta x, y + \Delta y) - f(x, y)$.

39. Let $z = f(x, y) = \sqrt{2x + y^2}$.

a) Use differentials to estimate Δz for $x = 6$, $y = 3$, $\Delta x = 0.5$, and $\Delta y = 0.2$.

b) Find Δz by evaluating $f(x + \Delta x, y + \Delta y) - f(x, y)$.

40. Let $z = f(x, y) = e^{xy}$.

a) Use differentials to estimate Δz for $x = 2$, $y = 4$, $\Delta x = -0.03$, and $\Delta y = 0.01$.

b) Find Δz by evaluating $f(x + \Delta x, y + \Delta y) - f(x, y)$.

APPLICATIONS

Business and Economics

41. The Cobb–Douglas model. Lincolnville Sporting Goods has the following production function for a certain product:

$$p(x, y) = 2400x^{2/5}y^{3/5},$$

where p is the number of units produced with x units of labor and y units of capital.

a) Find the number of units produced with 32 units of labor and 1024 units of capital.

b) Find the marginal productivities.

c) Evaluate the marginal productivities at $x = 32$ and $y = 1024$.

d) Interpret the meanings of the marginal productivities found in part (c).

42. The Cobb–Douglas model. Riverside Appliances has the following production function for a certain product:

$$p(x, y) = 1800x^{0.621}y^{0.379},$$

where p is the number of units produced with x units of labor and y units of capital.

a) Find the number of units produced with 2500 units of labor and 1700 units of capital.

b) Find the marginal productivities.

c) Evaluate the marginal productivities at $x = 2500$ and $y = 1700$.

d) Interpret the meanings of the marginal productivities found in part (c).

43. Business: tolerance. The four walls of a square banquet room are to be painted. Each wall is 120 ft long and 15 ft high. Assume that the measurements have a tolerance of ± 6 in.

a) Find the surface area of the four walls, assuming that the given measurements are exact.

b) Use differentials to approximate the change in surface area, assuming that the measurements include the extra 6 in.

c) Find the actual change in surface area, assuming that the measurements include the extra 6 in.

d) If one can of paint covers 300 ft^2, how many extra cans of paint are needed to ensure that the job is completed?

44. Business: tolerance. A large aquarium is rectangular, measuring 6 ft long by 4 ft wide by 3 ft high. Assume that the measurements have a tolerance of ± 1 in.

a) Find the volume of the aquarium assuming that the given measurements are exact.

b) Use differentials to approximate the change in volume, assuming that the measurements include the extra 1 in.

c) Find the actual change in volume, assuming that the measurements include the extra 1 in.

d) One cubic foot of water weighs 62.4 lb. Find the extra weight of water in the aquarium, assuming that the measurements include the extra 1 in.

Nursing facilities. *A study of Texas nursing homes found that the annual profit P (in dollars) of profit-seeking, independent nursing homes in urban locations is modeled by*

$$P(w, r, s, t) = 0.007955w^{-0.638}r^{1.038}s^{0.873}t^{2.468},$$

where w is the average hourly wage of nurses and aides (in dollars), r is the occupancy rate (as a percentage), s is the total square footage of the facility, and t is the Texas Index of Level of Effort (TILE), a number between 1 and 11 that measures state Medicaid reimbursement. [Source: K. J. Knox, E. C. Blankmeyer, and J. R. Stutzman, "Relative Economic Efficiency in Texas Nursing Facilities," Journal of Economics and Finance, Vol. 23, 199–213 (1999).] Use this information for Exercises 45 and 46.

45. A profit-seeking, independent Texas nursing home in an urban setting has nurses and aides with an average hourly wage of \$40 an hour, a TILE of 8, an occupancy rate of 80%, and 400,000 ft^2 of space.

a) Estimate the nursing home's annual profit.

b) Find the four partial derivatives of P.

c) Interpret the meaning of the partial derivatives found in part (b).

46. The change in P due to a change in w when the other variables are held constant is approximately

$$\Delta P \approx \frac{\partial P}{\partial w}\Delta w.$$

Use the values of w, r, s, and t in Exercise 45 and assume that the nursing home gives its nurses and aides a small raise so that the average hourly wage is now \$40.25 an hour. By approximately how much does profit change?

Life and Physical Sciences

Temperature–humidity heat index. *In summer, higher humidity interacts with the outdoor temperature, making a person feel hotter because of reduced heat loss from the skin. The temperature–humidity index, T_h, is what the temperature would have to be with no humidity in order to give the same heat effect. One index often used is given by*

$$T_h = 1.98T - 1.09(1 - H)(T - 58) - 56.9,$$

where T is the air temperature, in degrees Fahrenheit, and H is the relative humidity, expressed as a decimal. Find the temperature–humidity index in each case. Round to the nearest tenth of a degree.

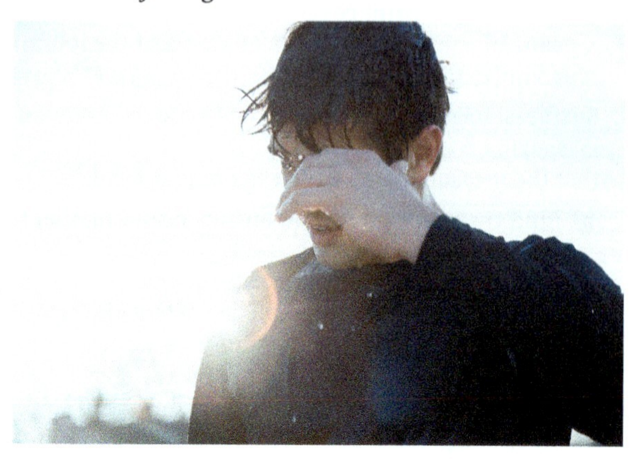

47. $T = 90°F$ and $H = 90\%$

48. $T = 78°F$ and $H = 100\%$

Use the equation for T_h given above for Exercises 49 and 50.

49. Find $\frac{\partial T_h}{\partial H}$, and interpret its meaning.

50. Find $\frac{\partial T_h}{\partial T}$, and interpret its meaning.

51. Body surface area. The Mosteller formula for approximating the surface area, S, in m^2, of a human is

$$S = \frac{\sqrt{hw}}{60},$$

where h is the person's height in centimeters and w is the person's weight in kilograms. (*Source:* www.halls.md.)

a) Compute $\frac{\partial S}{\partial h}$.

b) Compute $\frac{\partial S}{\partial w}$.

c) The change in S due to a change in w when h is constant is approximately

$$\Delta S \approx \frac{\partial S}{\partial w}\Delta w.$$

Use this formula to approximate the change in someone's surface area given that the person is 170 cm tall, weighs 80 kg, and loses 2 kg.

52. Body surface area. The Haycock formula for approximating the surface area, S, in m^2, of a human is

$$S = 0.024265h^{0.3964}w^{0.5378},$$

where h is the person's height in centimeters and w is the person's weight in kilograms. (*Source:* www.halls.md.)

a) Compute $\frac{\partial S}{\partial h}$.

b) Compute $\frac{\partial S}{\partial w}$.

c) The change in S due to a change in w when h is constant is approximately

$$\Delta S \approx \frac{\partial S}{\partial w}\Delta w.$$

Use this formula to approximate the change in someone's surface area given that the person is 170 cm tall, weighs 80 kg, and loses 2 kg.

Social Sciences

Reading ease. *The following formula is used by psychologists and educators to predict the reading ease, E, of a passage of words:*

$$E = 206.835 - 0.846w - 1.015s,$$

where w is the number of syllables in a 100-word section and s is the average number of words per sentence. Use this information for Exercises 53–56.

53. Find E when $w = 146$ and $s = 5$.

54. Find E when $w = 180$ and $s = 6$.

55. Find $\frac{\partial E}{\partial w}$.

56. Find $\frac{\partial E}{\partial s}$.

SYNTHESIS

Find f_x and f_t.

57. $f(x, t) = \dfrac{x^2 + t^2}{x^2 - t^2}$

58. $f(x, t) = \sqrt[4]{x^3 t^5}$

59. $f(x, t) = 6x^{2/3} - 8x^{1/4}t^{1/2} - 12x^{-1/2}t^{3/2}$

60. $f(x, t) = \left(\dfrac{x^2 + t^2}{x^2 - t^2}\right)^5$

In Exercises 61 and 62, find f_{xx}, f_{xy}, f_{yx}, and f_{yy}.

61. $f(x, y) = \dfrac{x}{y^2} - \dfrac{y}{x^2}$

62. $f(x, y) = \dfrac{xy}{x - y}$

63. Let $w = f(x, y, z) = xyz$.
   a) Use differentials to estimate Δw when $x = 6$, $y = 3$, $z = 5$, $\Delta x = 0.5$, $\Delta y = 0.2$, and $\Delta z = -0.3$.
   b) Find Δw by evaluating $f(x + \Delta x, y + \Delta y, z + \Delta z) - f(x, y, z)$.

64. Let $w = f(x, y, z) = xy + 2yz + 3xz$.
   a) Use differentials to estimate Δw when $x = 2$, $y = 4$, $z = 1$, $\Delta x = -0.3$, $\Delta y = 0.1$, and $\Delta z = -0.1$.
   b) Find Δw by evaluating $f(x + \Delta x, y + \Delta y, z + \Delta z) - f(x, y, z)$.

In Exercises 65 and 66, find f_{xx}, f_{yy}, f_{zz}, f_{xy}, f_{yx}, f_{xz}, f_{zx}, f_{yz}, and f_{zy}.

65. $f(x, y, z) = 2x^2y^3z^4$

66. $f(x, y, z) = \dfrac{x}{y + z}$

67. Consider the function f defined as follows:

$$f(x, y) = \begin{cases} \dfrac{xy(x^2 - y^2)}{x^2 + y^2}, & \text{for } (x, y) \neq (0, 0), \\ 0, & \text{for } (x, y) = (0, 0). \end{cases}$$

   a) Find $f_x(0, y)$ by evaluating the limit

$$\lim_{h \to 0} \frac{f(h, y) - f(0, y)}{h}.$$

   b) Find $f_y(x, 0)$ by evaluating the limit

$$\lim_{h \to 0} \frac{f(x, h) - f(x, 0)}{h}.$$

   c) Now find and compare $f_{yx}(0, 0)$ and $f_{xy}(0, 0)$.

68. Do some research on the Cobb–Douglas production function, and explain how it was developed.

69. Explain the meaning of the first partial derivatives of a function of two variables in terms of slopes of tangent lines.

Answers to Quick Checks

1. $\dfrac{\partial u}{\partial x} = 2xy^3z^4$, $\dfrac{\partial u}{\partial y} = 3x^2y^2z^4$, $\dfrac{\partial u}{\partial z} = 4x^2y^3z^3$
2. $f_x(x, y) = 21x^2y^2 - \dfrac{1}{y}$, $f_y(x, y) = 14x^3y + \dfrac{x}{y^2}$
3. $g_x = \dfrac{2x + y^4}{x^2 + xy^4}$, $g_y = \dfrac{4xy^3}{x^2 + xy^4} = \dfrac{4y^3}{x + y^4}$
4. $p_x(90, 50) = 51.21$ textbooks/unit of labor, $p_y(90, 50) = 23.05$ textbooks/unit of capital
5. **(a)** $A(12, 4) = 240\pi$, or about 753.98 ft^2; **(b)** $\Delta V \approx 14\pi$, or about 43.982 ft^2; **(c)** $A(12.25, 4.25) - A(12, 4) = \dfrac{227}{16}\pi \approx 44.571\ \text{ft}^2$
6. $g_{xx} = 12$, $g_{yy} = 36xy^2 - 2$, $g_{xy} = 12y^3$, $g_{yx} = 12y^3$

6.3 Maximum–Minimum Problems

- Find relative extrema of a function of two variables.
- Solve applied problems by finding the minimum or maximum value for a function of two variables.

We will now find maximum and minimum values for functions of two variables.

DEFINITION

A function f of two variables:

1. has a **relative maximum** at (a, b) if

$$f(x, y) \leq f(a, b)$$

   for all points (x, y) in a region containing (a, b);

2. has a **relative minimum** at (a, b) if

$$f(x, y) \geq f(a, b)$$

   for all points (x, y) in a region containing (a, b).

This definition is illustrated in Figs. 1 and 2.

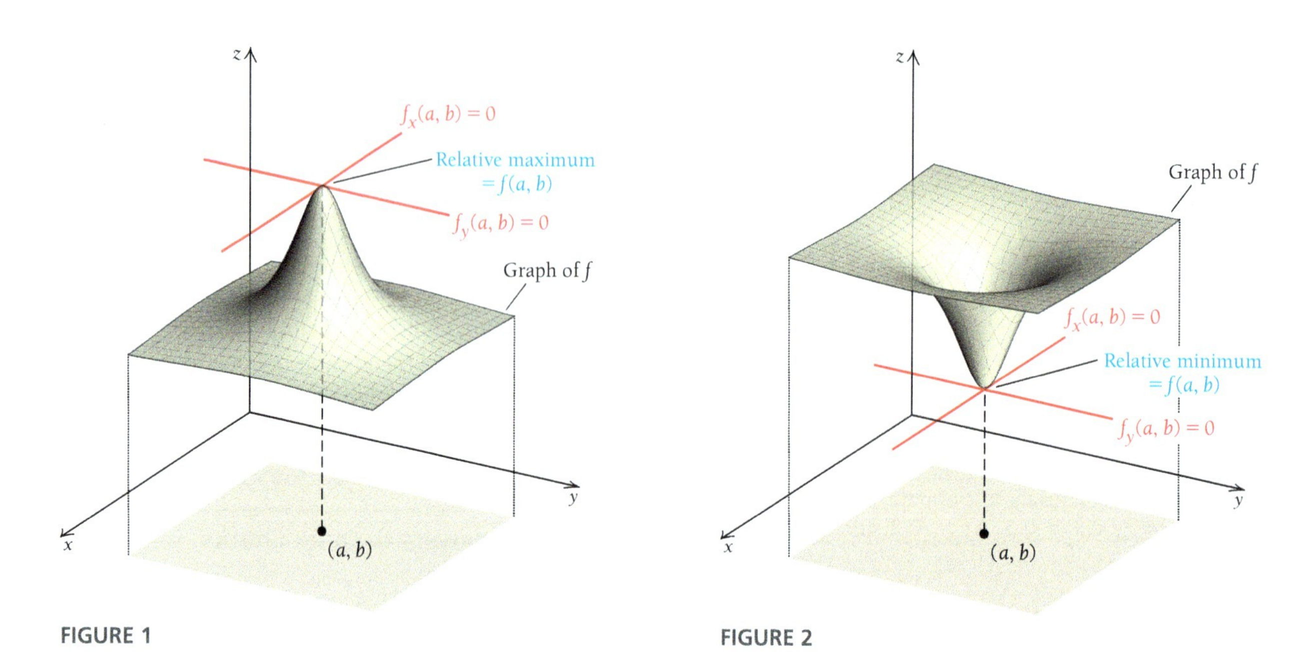

FIGURE 1

FIGURE 2

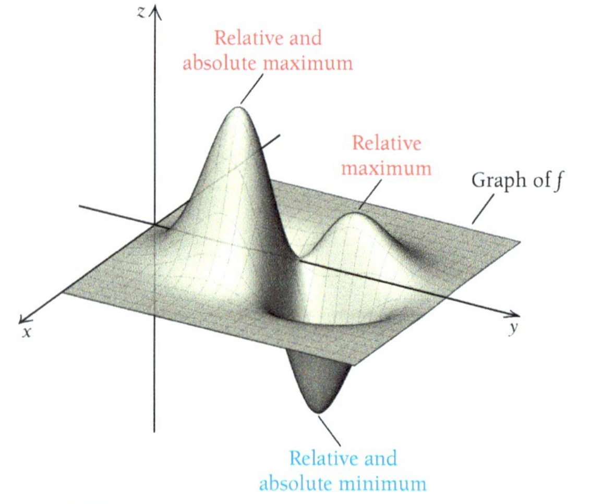

FIGURE 3

Note that a relative maximum (or minimum) may not be an "absolute" maximum (or minimum), as illustrated in Fig. 3.

Determining Maximum and Minimum Values

Suppose a differentiable function f has a relative extremum at (a, b). If we fix y at the value b, then $f(x, b)$ can be regarded as a function of x. Because a relative maximum or minimum occurs at (a, b), we know that $f(x, b)$ achieves a maximum or minimum at (a, b), and therefore $f_x = 0$. Similarly, if we fix x at a, then $f(a, y)$ can be regarded as a function of y that achieves a relative extremum at (a, b), and thus $f_y = 0$. In short, since an extremum exists at (a, b), we must have

$$f_x(a, b) = 0 \quad \text{and} \quad f_y(a, b) = 0. \tag{1}$$

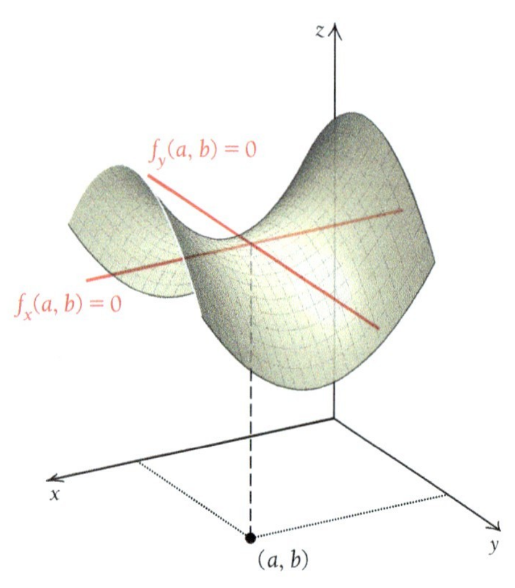

FIGURE 4

We call a point (a, b) at which both partial derivatives are 0 a **critical point.** This is comparable to a critical value for functions of one variable. Thus, one strategy for finding relative maximum or minimum values is to solve a system of equations like (1) to find critical points. Just as for functions of one variable, this strategy does *not* guarantee that we will have a relative maximum or minimum value. We have argued only that *if* a continuous, differentiable function f has a maximum or minimum value at (a, b), *then* both partial derivatives must be 0 at that point. Look at Figs. 1 and 2 and then at Fig. 4, which illustrates a case in which both partial derivatives are 0 but the function does not have a relative maximum or minimum value at (a, b).

In Fig. 4, suppose we fix y at b. Then $f(x, b)$ has a minimum at a, but $f(x, y)$ does not (see the blue curve in Fig. 5). Similarly, if we fix x at a, then $f(a, y)$ has a maximum at b, but $f(x, y)$ does not (see the red curve in Fig. 5). The point $(a, b, f(a, b))$ is called a **saddle point.** At this point, $f_x(a, b) = 0$ and $f_y(a, b) = 0$ [the point (a, b) is a critical point], but f has no extremum at (a, b).

A test that uses first- and second-order partial derivatives to find relative maximum and minimum values is stated in the following theorem, which we will not prove.

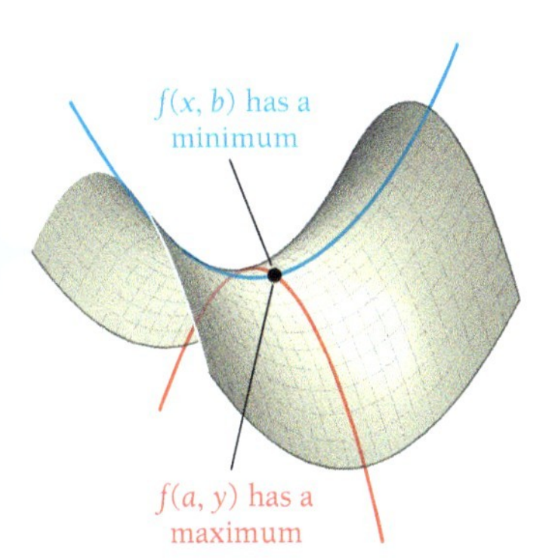

FIGURE 5

THEOREM 1 The *D*-Test

Let f be a differentiable function of x and y, let (a, b) represent a solution of the system of equations $f_x = 0, f_y = 0$, and let

$$D = f_{xx}(a, b) \cdot f_{yy}(a, b) - [f_{xy}(a, b)]^2.$$

Then

if $D > 0$ and $f_{xx}(a, b) < 0$, it follows that f has a relative maximum at (a, b);
if $D > 0$ and $f_{xx}(a, b) > 0$, if follows that f has a relative minimum at (a, b);
if $D < 0$, it follows that f has neither a maximum nor a minimum at (a, b); and
if $D = 0$, this test is not applicable.

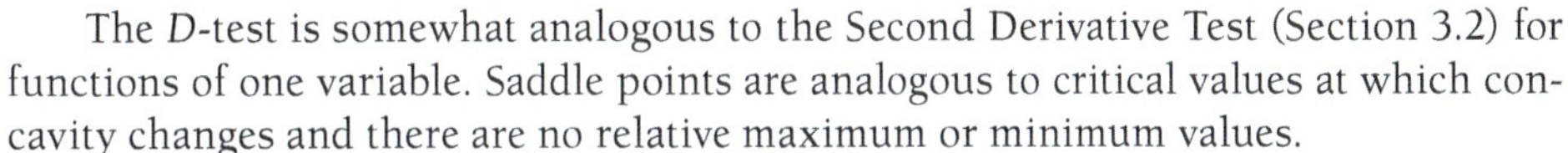

The *D*-test is somewhat analogous to the Second Derivative Test (Section 3.2) for functions of one variable. Saddle points are analogous to critical values at which concavity changes and there are no relative maximum or minimum values.

Relative extrema *may or may not be absolute extrema*. Testing for absolute extrema can be complicated. We will restrict our attention to finding *relative* extrema, and in most of the applications that we consider, relative extrema turn out to be absolute as well.

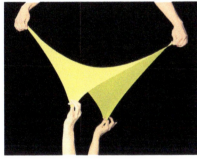

The shape of a perfect tent. To give a tent roof the maximum strength possible, designers draw the fabric into a three-dimensional shape that resembles a horse's saddle and that mathematicians call an *anticlastic curve*. Two people stretching a rectangular piece of cloth can duplicate the shape, as shown above. One person pulls up and out on two diagonal corners; the other person pulls down and out on the other corners. The opposing tensions draw each point of the fabric's surface into rigid equilibrium. The more pronounced the curve, the stiffer the surface.

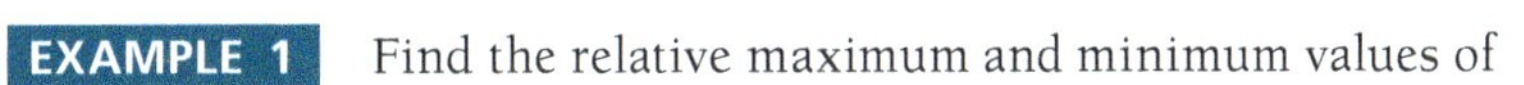

EXAMPLE 1 Find the relative maximum and minimum values of

$$f(x, y) = x^2 + xy + 2y^2 - 7x.$$

Solution We find f_x, f_y, f_{xx}, f_{yy}, and f_{xy}:

$$f_x = 2x + y - 7, \qquad f_y = x + 4y,$$
$$f_{xx} = 2; \qquad f_{yy} = 4;$$
$$f_{xy} = 1.$$

Now we solve the system of equations $f_x = 0, f_y = 0$:

$$2x + y - 7 = 0, \qquad (2)$$
$$x + 4y = 0. \qquad (3)$$

Solving equation (3) for x, we get $x = -4y$. Substituting $-4y$ for x in equation (2) and solving, we get

$$2(-4y) + y - 7 = 0$$
$$-8y + y - 7 = 0$$
$$-7y = 7$$
$$y = -1.$$

To find x when $y = -1$, we substitute -1 for y in equation (2) or equation (3). We choose equation (3):

$$x + 4(-1) = 0$$
$$x = 4.$$

Thus, $(4, -1)$ is the only critical point, and $f(4, -1)$ is our candidate for a maximum or minimum value. We check to see whether $f(4, -1)$ is a maximum or minimum value:

$$D = f_{xx}(4, -1) \cdot f_{yy}(4, -1) - [f_{xy}(4, -1)]^2$$
$$= 2 \cdot 4 - [1]^2 \qquad \text{Substituting}$$
$$= 7.$$

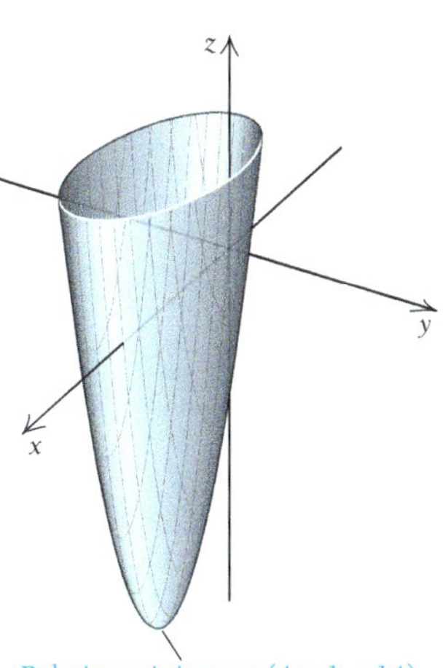

Relative minimum: $(4, -1, -14)$

$z = f(x, y) = x^2 + xy + 2y^2 - 7x$

Technology Connection 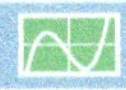

Exploratory

Examine the graph of the equation in Example 1 using a 3D graphing utility to visualize the relative minimum.

Thus, $D = 7$ and $f_{xx}(4, -1) = 2$. Since $D > 0$ and $f_{xx}(4, -1) > 0$, it follows from the D-test that f has a relative minimum at $(4, -1)$. That minimum value is found as follows:

$$f(4, -1) = 4^2 + 4(-1) + 2(-1)^2 - 7 \cdot 4$$
$$= 16 - 4 + 2 - 28$$
$$= -14. \quad \text{This is the relative minimum.}$$

1 ✓

Quick Check 1 ✓

Find the relative maximum and minimum values of

$$f(x, y) = x^2 + xy + y^2 - 3x.$$

EXAMPLE 2 Find the relative maximum and minimum values of

$$f(x, y) = xy - x^3 - y^2.$$

Solution We find f_x, f_y, f_{xx}, f_{yy}, and f_{xy}:

$$f_x = y - 3x^2, \qquad f_y = x - 2y,$$
$$f_{xx} = -6x; \qquad f_{yy} = -2;$$
$$f_{xy} = 1.$$

Next, we solve the system of equations $f_x = 0, f_y = 0$:

$$y - 3x^2 = 0, \quad (4)$$
$$x - 2y = 0. \quad (5)$$

Solving equation (4) for y, we get $y = 3x^2$. Substituting $3x^2$ for y in equation (5) and solving, we get

$$x - 2(3x^2) = 0$$
$$x - 6x^2 = 0$$
$$x(1 - 6x) = 0 \quad \text{Factoring}$$
$$x = 0 \quad or \quad 1 - 6x = 0$$
$$x = 0 \quad or \quad x = \tfrac{1}{6}.$$

To find y when $x = 0$, we substitute 0 for x in equation (4) or equation (5):

$$0 - 2y = 0 \quad \text{Substituting into equation (5)}$$
$$-2y = 0$$
$$y = 0.$$

Thus, $(0, 0)$ is a critical point, and $f(0, 0)$ is a possible extremum. To find another candidate, we substitute $\frac{1}{6}$ for x in equation (4) or equation (5):

$$\tfrac{1}{6} - 2y = 0 \quad \text{Substituting into equation (5)}$$
$$-2y = -\tfrac{1}{6}$$
$$y = \tfrac{1}{12}.$$

Thus, $(\frac{1}{6}, \frac{1}{12})$ is another critical point, and $f(\frac{1}{6}, \frac{1}{12})$ is another possible extremum.

Using the D-test, we check both $(0, 0)$ and $(\frac{1}{6}, \frac{1}{12})$ to see whether they yield maximum or minimum values.

For $(0, 0)$: $D = f_{xx}(0, 0) \cdot f_{yy}(0, 0) - [f_{xy}(0, 0)]^2$

$$= (-6 \cdot 0) \cdot (-2) - [1]^2 \quad \text{Substituting}$$
$$= -1.$$

Technology Connection

Exploratory

Examine the graph of the equation in Example 2 with a 3D graphing utility to visualize the relative maximum and the saddle point.

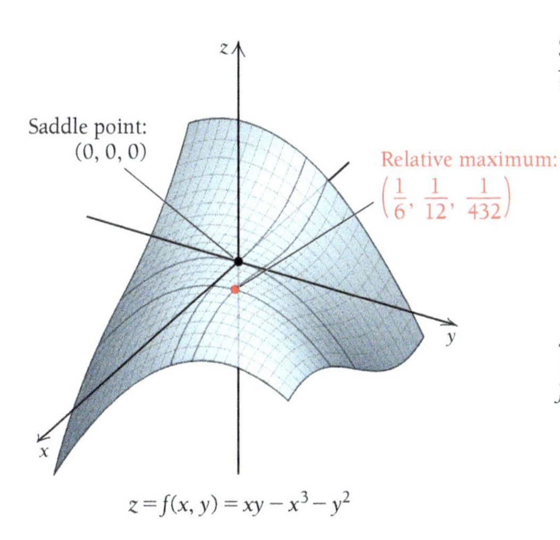

Since $D < 0$, it follows that $f(0, 0)$ is neither a maximum nor a minimum value, but is instead a saddle point.

$$\text{For } \left(\tfrac{1}{6}, \tfrac{1}{12}\right): \quad D = f_{xx}\left(\tfrac{1}{6}, \tfrac{1}{12}\right) \cdot f_{yy}\left(\tfrac{1}{6}, \tfrac{1}{12}\right) - \left[f_{xy}\left(\tfrac{1}{6}, \tfrac{1}{12}\right)\right]^2$$

$$= \left(-6 \cdot \tfrac{1}{6}\right) \cdot (-2) - [1]^2 \qquad \text{Substituting}$$

$$= -1(-2) - 1$$

$$= 1.$$

Thus, $D = 1$ and $f_{xx}\left(\frac{1}{6}, \frac{1}{12}\right) = -1$. Since $D > 0$ and $f_{xx}\left(\frac{1}{6}, \frac{1}{12}\right) < 0$, it follows that f has a relative maximum at $\left(\frac{1}{6}, \frac{1}{12}\right)$; that maximum value is

$$f\left(\tfrac{1}{6}, \tfrac{1}{12}\right) = \tfrac{1}{6} \cdot \tfrac{1}{12} - \left(\tfrac{1}{6}\right)^3 - \left(\tfrac{1}{12}\right)^2$$

$$= \tfrac{1}{72} - \tfrac{1}{216} - \tfrac{1}{144} = \tfrac{1}{432}. \qquad \text{This is the relative maximum.}$$

2 ✓

Quick Check 2 ✓

Find the critical points of

$$g(x, y) = x^3 + y^2 - 3x - 4y + 3.$$

Then use the D-test to determine if each point has a relative maximum or a relative minimum or is a saddle point.

EXAMPLE 3 **Business: Maximizing Profit.** Fly Straight, Inc., produces two types of golf balls: one type sells for \$3 each and the other sells for \$2 each. The total revenue, in thousands of dollars, from the sale of x thousand \$3 balls and y thousand \$2 balls is given by

$$R(x, y) = 3x + 2y.$$

The company determines that the total cost, in thousands of dollars, of producing x thousand of the \$3 ball and y thousand of the \$2 ball is given by

$$C(x, y) = 2x^2 - 2xy + y^2 - 9x + 6y + 7.$$

How many golf balls of each type must be produced and sold to maximize the company's profit?

Solution The total profit $P(x, y)$ is given by

$$P(x, y) = R(x, y) - C(x, y)$$

$$= 3x + 2y - (2x^2 - 2xy + y^2 - 9x + 6y + 7) \qquad \text{Substituting}$$

$$P(x, y) = -2x^2 + 2xy - y^2 + 12x - 4y - 7. \qquad \text{Simplifying}$$

We find P_x, P_y, P_{xx}, P_{yy}, and P_{xy}:

$$P_x = -4x + 2y + 12, \qquad P_y = 2x - 2y - 4,$$

$$P_{xx} = -4; \qquad P_{yy} = -2;$$

$$P_{xy} = 2.$$

Next, we solve the system of equations $P_x = 0$, $P_y = 0$:

$$-4x + 2y + 12 = 0, \qquad (6)$$

$$2x - 2y - 4 = 0. \qquad (7)$$

Adding the left and right sides of equations (6) and (7), we get

$$-2x + 8 = 0$$

$$-2x = -8$$

$$x = 4.$$

To find y when $x = 4$, we substitute 4 for x in equation (6) or equation (7):

$$2 \cdot 4 - 2y - 4 = 0 \quad \text{Substituting in equation 7}$$
$$-2y + 4 = 0$$
$$-2y = -4$$
$$y = 2.$$

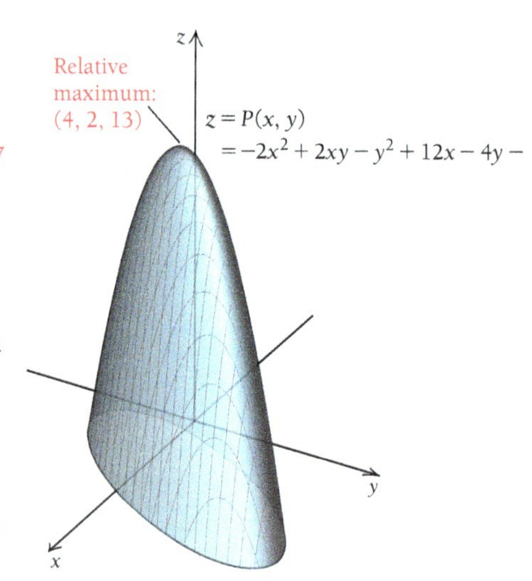

Thus, (4, 2) is the only critical point, and $P(4, 2)$ is a candidate for a maximum or minimum value.

To see whether $P(4, 2)$ is a maximum or minimum value, we use the D-test:

$$D = P_{xx}(4, 2) \cdot P_{yy}(4, 2) - [P_{xy}(4, 2)]^2$$
$$= (-4)(-2) - 2^2 \quad \text{Substituting}$$
$$= 4.$$

Quick Check 3 ✓

Repeat Example 3 using the same cost function and assuming that the company's total revenue, in thousands of dollars, comes from the sale of x thousand balls at \$3.50 each and y thousand at \$2.75 each.

Thus, $D = 4$ and $P_{xx}(4, 2) = -4$. Since $D > 0$ and $P_{xx}(4, 2) < 0$, it follows that P has a relative maximum at (4, 2). Therefore, to maximize profit, the company must produce and sell 4 thousand of the \$3 golf balls and 2 thousand of the \$2 golf balls. The maximum profit will be

$$P(4, 2) = -2 \cdot 4^2 + 2 \cdot 4 \cdot 2 - 2^2 + 12 \cdot 4 - 4 \cdot 2 - 7 = 13,$$

or \$13 thousand.

3 ✓

Constrained Optimization

We saw in Section 3.5 that some maximum–minimum problems have constraints on the variables. In such a case, we can often express one variable in terms of the other and use substitution to reduce the number of independent variables by one. The same is true of multivariable functions. For example, if $f(x, y, z)$ is a function of three variables such that $z = g(x, y)$ represents a constraint, we can treat f as a function of two variables, $f(x, y, g(x, y))$, and use various techniques to find possible extrema. One such method, shown below, uses substitution. In Section 6.5, we consider an alternative method called the method of Lagrange multipliers.

EXAMPLE 4 **Optimization with Constraints.** Express Shipping requires that the sum of the length, width, and height of a large rectangular shipping box be 90 in. What is the maximum volume of such a box?

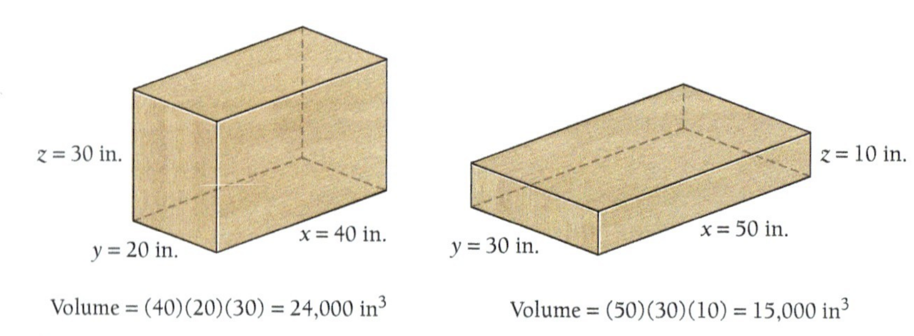

Two shipping boxes for which the length, width, and height measurements add to 90 in., with their corresponding volumes.

Solution We let x, y, and z be, respectively, the length, width, and height of the box, in inches. Thus, the volume of the box is given by the function of three variables

$$V(x, y, z) = xyz.$$

The sum of the box's length, width, and height is 90 in. This is a constraint:

$$x + y + z = 90$$
$$z = 90 - x - y. \quad \text{Solving for } z$$

Substituting, we now treat V as a function of two variables x and y:

$$V(x, y, 90 - x - y) = xy(90 - x - y) \quad \text{Substituting}$$
$$V(x, y) = 90xy - x^2y - xy^2.$$

To find possible critical points, we find the first- and second-order partial derivatives:

$$V_x = 90y - 2xy - y^2, \quad V_y = 90x - x^2 - 2xy,$$
$$V_{xx} = -2y, \quad V_{yy} = -2x,$$
$$V_{xy} = 90 - 2x - 2y.$$

We solve the system $V_x = 0$, $V_y = 0$:

$$90y - 2xy - y^2 = 0, \quad (8)$$
$$90x - x^2 - 2xy = 0. \quad (9)$$

Since these are measurements, we can assume that x, y, and z are all positive. This allows us to simplify equation (8) by dividing both sides by y and equation (9) by dividing both sides by x:

$$90 - 2x - y = 0, \quad (10)$$
$$90 - x - 2y = 0. \quad (11)$$

We solve for y in equation (10), getting $y = 90 - 2x$, and then substitute this for y in equation (11).

$$90 - x - 2(90 - 2x) = 0 \quad \text{Substituting}$$
$$90 - x - 180 + 4x = 0 \quad \text{Multiplying}$$
$$-90 + 3x = 0 \quad \text{Simplifying}$$
$$3x = 90$$
$$x = \frac{90}{3}, \text{ or } 30.$$

Using either equation (10) or (11), we find y:

$$90 - 30 - 2y = 0 \quad \text{Substituting 30 for } x \text{ in equation (11)}$$
$$60 - 2y = 0$$
$$y = \frac{60}{2}, \text{ or } 30.$$

Thus, (30, 30) is a critical point. To determine if this gives a maximum or minimum, we use the D-test:

$$D = V_{xx}(30, 30) \cdot V_{yy}(30, 30) - [V_{xy}(30, 30)]^2$$
$$= (-2(30)) \cdot (-2(30)) - [90 - 2(30) - 2(30)]^2 \quad \text{Substituting}$$
$$= (-60)(-60) - (-30)^2$$
$$= 2700.$$

Since $D > 0$ and $V_{xx}(30, 30) < 0$, we conclude that $V(30, 30)$ is a maximum. We find $V(30, 30)$:

$$\begin{aligned} V(30, 30) &= 90(30)(30) - (30)^2(30) - (30)(30)^2 \quad \text{Substituting} \\ &= 81{,}000 - 27{,}000 - 27{,}000 \\ &= 27{,}000 \text{ in}^3. \end{aligned}$$

Quick Check 4 ✓

Maximize $V(x, y, z) = xyz$, where $2x + 3y + z = 30$.

Note that when $x = 30$ and $y = 30$, we have $z = 90 - 30 - 30 = 30$. Thus, the box will have a maximum volume of 27,000 in^3 when each side measures 30 in.; the box is a cube.

4 ✓

Section Summary

- A two-variable function f has a *relative maximum* at (a, b) if $f(x, y) \leq f(a, b)$ for all points in a region containing (a, b) and has a *relative minimum* at (a, b) if $f(x, y) \geq f(a, b)$ for all points in a region containing (a, b).
- The *D-test* is used to determine if a *critical point* has a relative minimum or a relative maximum or is a *saddle point*.

6.3 Exercise Set

Find the relative maximum or minimum value.

1. $f(x, y) = x^2 + xy + y^2 - 5y$
2. $f(x, y) = x^2 + xy + 3y^2 + 11x$
3. $f(x, y) = 4xy - x^3 - 2y^2$
4. $f(x, y) = 2xy - x^3 - y^2$
5. $f(x, y) = x^3 + y^3 - 3xy$
6. $f(x, y) = x^3 + y^3 - 6xy$
7. $f(x, y) = x^2 + 2xy + 2y^2 - 6y + 2$
8. $f(x, y) = x^2 + y^2 - 4x + 2y - 5$
9. $f(x, y) = 4y + 6x - x^2 - y^2$
10. $f(x, y) = x^2 + y^2 + 8x - 10y$
11. $f(x, y) = x^2 - y^2$
12. $f(x, y) = 4x^2 - y^2$
13. $f(x, y) = e^{x^2-2x+y^2-4y+2}$
14. $f(x, y) = e^{x^2+y^2+1}$
15. Maximize $f(x, y, z) = xyz$, where $2x + y + 5z = 10$.
16. Maximize $f(x, y, z) = xyz$, where $x + 6y + 2z = 12$.
17. Minimize $d(x, y, z) = x^2 + y^2 + z^2$, where $x + 2y + z = 8$.
18. Minimize $d(x, y, z) = x^2 + y^2 + z^2$, where $x + y + 3z = 12$.

APPLICATIONS

Business and Economics

In Exercises 19–28, assume that relative maximum and minimum values are absolute maximum and minimum values.

19. **Maximizing profit.** A concert promoter produces two kinds of souvenir shirt. Total revenue from the sale of x thousand shirts at \$18 each and y thousand at \$25 each is given by
$$R(x, y) = 18x + 25y.$$
The company determines that the total cost, in thousands of dollars, of producing x thousand of the \$18 shirt and y thousand of the \$25 shirt is
$$C(x, y) = 4x^2 - 6xy + 3y^2 + 20x + 19y - 12.$$
How many shirts of each type must be produced and sold to maximize profit?

20. **Maximizing profit.** Safe Shades produces two kinds of sunglasses. The total revenue in thousands of dollars from the sale of x thousand sunglasses at \$17 each and y thousand at \$21 each is given by
$$R(x, y) = 17x + 21y.$$
The company determines that the total cost, in thousands of dollars, of producing x thousand of the \$17 sunglasses and y thousand of the \$21 sunglasses is given by
$$C(x, y) = 4x^2 - 4xy + 2y^2 - 11x + 25y - 3.$$
How many of each type of sunglasses must be produced and sold to maximize profit?

21. **Maximizing profit.** Humphrey's Medical Supply finds that its profit, P, in millions of dollars, is given by
$$P(a, n) = -5a^2 - 3n^2 + 48a - 4n + 2an + 290,$$
where a is the amount spent on advertising, in millions of dollars, and n is the number of items sold, in thousands. Find the maximum value of P and the values of a and n at which it occurs.

22. **Maximizing profit.** McLeod Corp. finds that its profit, P, in millions of dollars, is given by
$$P(a, p) = 2ap + 80p - 15p^2 - \tfrac{1}{10}a^2p - 80,$$

where a is the amount spent on advertising, in millions of dollars, and p is the price charged per unit, in dollars. Find the maximum value of P and the values of a and p at which it occurs.

23. Two-variable revenue maximization. Rad Designs sells two kinds of sweatshirts that compete with one another. Their demand functions are expressed by the following relationships:

$$q_1 = 78 - 6p_1 - 3p_2, \quad (1)$$

$$q_2 = 66 - 3p_1 - 6p_2, \quad (2)$$

where p_1 and p_2 are the prices of the sweatshirts, in multiples of $10, and q_1 and q_2 are the quantities of the sweatshirts demanded, in hundreds of units.

a) Find a formula for the total-revenue function, R, in terms of the variables p_1 and p_2. [*Hint:* $R = p_1q_1 + p_2q_2$; then substitute expressions from equations (1) and (2) to find $R(p_1, p_2)$.]
b) What prices p_1 and p_2 should be charged for each product in order to maximize total revenue?
c) How many units will be demanded?
d) What is the maximum total revenue?

24. Two-variable revenue maximization. Repeat Exercise 23, using

$$q_1 = 64 - 4p_1 - 2p_2$$

and

$$q_2 = 56 - 2p_1 - 4p_2.$$

25. Maximizing the volume of a container. A crawlspace in a warehouse can hold a rectangular container provided that the sum of its length, width, and height does not exceed 270 in. Find the volume of the largest possible container that will fit in this crawlspace.

26. Maximizing the volume of a container. A closet underneath a stairway can hold a rectangular container provided that its length x, width y, and height z, all in feet, satisfies the constraint $2x + 4y + 3z = 12$. Find the volume of the largest possible container that will fit in the closet.

27. Minimizing the cost of a container. ProHauling Services is designing an open-top, rectangular container that will have a volume of 320 ft^3. The cost of making the bottom of the container is $5 per square foot, and the cost of the sides is $4 per square foot. Find the dimensions of the container that will minimize total cost. (*Hint:* Make a substitution using the formula for volume.)

28. Minimizing the cost of a container. Danni's Designs manufactures rectangular jewelry boxes that have a volume of 40 in^3. If the material for the top and bottom costs $1.25 per square inch, and the material for the sides costs $1.75 per square inch, find the dimensions that minimize the cost of materials for one jewelry box.

Life and Physical Sciences

29. Temperature. A flat metal plate is mounted on a coordinate plane. The temperature of the plate, in degrees Fahrenheit, at point (x, y) is given by

$$T(x, y) = x^2 + 2y^2 - 8x + 4y.$$

Find the minimum temperature and where it occurs. Is there a maximum temperature?

30. Population density. The population density of a city is given by

$$P(x, y) = -25x^2 - 30y^2 + 250x + 420y + 180,$$

where x and y are miles from the southwest corner of the city limits and P is the number of people per square mile. Find the maximum population density, and specify where it occurs.

SYNTHESIS

In Exercises 31–34, find the relative maximum and minimum values as well as any saddle points.

31. $f(x, y) = e^x + e^y - e^{x+y}$

32. $f(x, y) = xy + \dfrac{2}{x} + \dfrac{4}{y}$

33. $f(x, y) = 2y^2 + x^2 - x^2y$

34. $S(b, m) = (m + b - 72)^2 + (2m + b - 73)^2 + (3m + b - 75)^2$

35. The surface given by $f(x, y) = x^4 + y^4$ has a critical point at (0, 0, 0), but the D-test does not classify that point as a minimum, maximum, or saddle point. Explain how you would classify this critical point using other means.

36. Explain the difference between a relative minimum and an absolute minimum for a function of two variables.

Technology Connection

Use a 3D graphics program to graph each of the following functions. Then estimate any relative extrema.

37. $f(x, y) = \dfrac{-5}{x^2 + 2y^2 + 1}$

38. $f(x, y) = x^3 + y^3 + 3xy$

39. $f(x, y) = \dfrac{3xy(x^2 - y^2)}{x^2 + y^2}$

40. $f(x, y) = \dfrac{y + x^2y^2 - 8x}{xy}$

Answers to Quick Checks

1. $(2, -1, -3)$, relative minimum **2.** $(1, 2, -3)$, relative minimum; $(-1, 2, 1)$, saddle point
3. Maximum profit is $17.031 thousand when $x = \$4.625$ thousand and $y = \$3$ thousand
4. $V = \dfrac{500}{3}$, when $x = 5$, $y = \dfrac{10}{3}$, and $z = 10$

6.4 An Application: The Least-Squares Technique

- Find the equation of a regression line.
- Solve applied problems involving regression lines.
- Find an exponential regression curve.

We often use a graphing calculator to perform regression. In this section, we develop an understanding of regression by using the method for finding the minimum value for a function of two variables. An equation found by regression models data, which allows predictions to be made. For example, in business, one might want to predict future sales on the basis of past data. In environmental studies, one might want to predict future demand for a resource on the basis of past usage. Suppose we wish to find a linear equation,

$$y = mx + b,$$

that provides the best fit to some data. To determine this equation is to determine the values of m and b. Let's do this with an example.

EXAMPLE 1 Sky Blue Car Rentals offers hybrid (gas-electric) vehicles and charts its revenue as shown in Fig. 1 and the table below. We can use the data to predict the company's revenue for the year 2021.

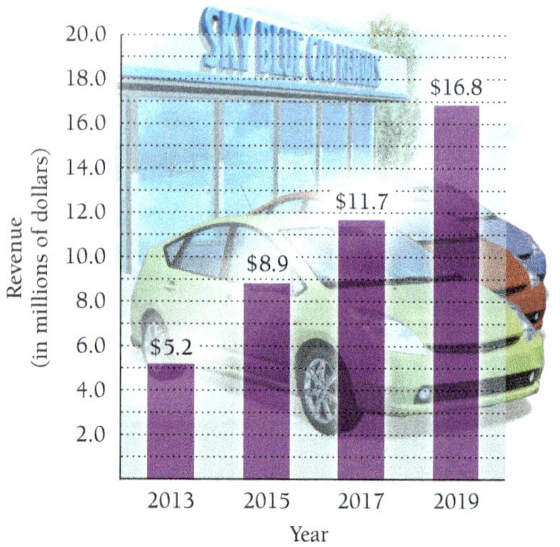

FIGURE 1

Year, x	2013	2015	2017	2019	2021
Yearly Revenue, y (in millions of dollars)	5.2	8.9	11.7	16.8	?

Solution When we have plotted these points, there are several ways in which we might draw a line through them (see Figs. 2 and 3). Each would give a different estimate of the company's total revenue for 2021.

Note that the years for which revenue is given follow 2-yr increments. Thus, computations can be simplified if we use the data points (1, 5.2), (2, 8.9), (3, 11.7), and (4, 16.8), as plotted in Fig. 3, where each horizontal unit represents 2 yr and $x = 1$ is 2013.

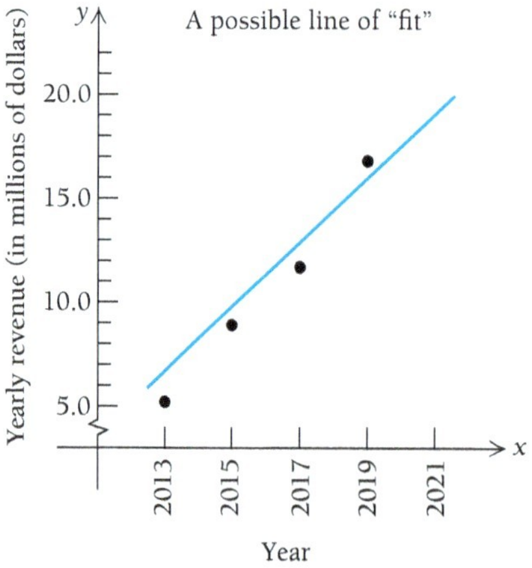

A possible line of "fit"

FIGURE 2

Another possible line of "fit"

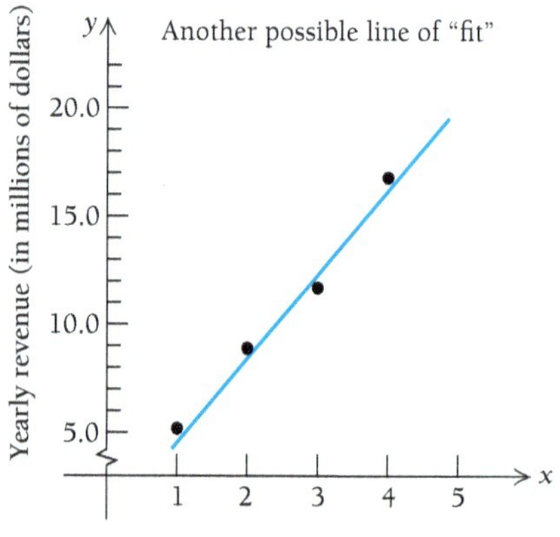

FIGURE 3

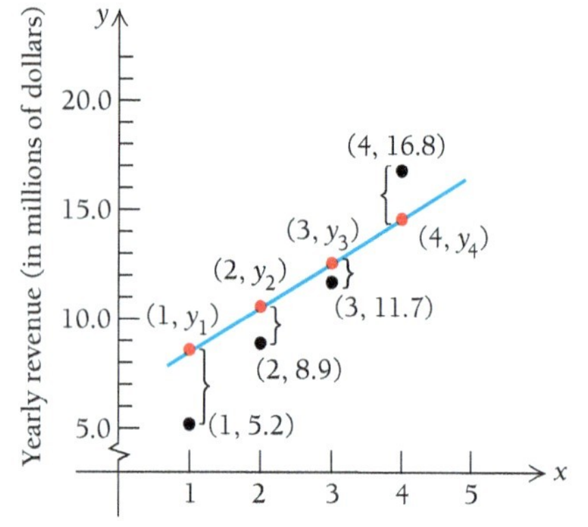

FIGURE 4

To determine the equation of the line that "best" fits the data, we note that for each data point there is a *deviation*, or error, between its y-value and the y-value at the point on the line directly above or below the data point. Those deviations, in this case, $y_1 - 5.2$, $y_2 - 8.9$, $y_3 - 11.7$, and $y_4 - 16.8$, are positive or negative, depending on the location of the line (see Fig. 4).

We wish to fit these data points with a line,

$$y = mx + b,$$

such that the values of m and b minimize the y-deviations. To minimize the deviations, we use the *least-squares assumption*.

The Least-Squares Assumption

The line of best fit is the line for which the sum of the squares of the vertical deviations, or y-deviations, is a minimum. This is called the **regression line.**

Note that squaring each y-deviation gives us a series of nonnegative terms that we can add.

Using the least-squares assumption with the yearly revenue data, we want to minimize

$$(y_1 - 5.2)^2 + (y_2 - 8.9)^2 + (y_3 - 11.7)^2 + (y_4 - 16.8)^2. \qquad (1)$$

Also, since the points $(1, y_1)$, $(2, y_2)$, $(3, y_3)$, and $(4, y_4)$ must be solutions of $y = mx + b$, it follows that

$$y_1 = m(1) + b = m + b,$$
$$y_2 = m(2) + b = 2m + b,$$
$$y_3 = m(3) + b = 3m + b,$$
$$y_4 = m(4) + b = 4m + b.$$

Substituting $m + b$ for y_1, $2m + b$ for y_2, $3m + b$ for y_3, and $4m + b$ for y_4 in equation (1), we form a function of two variables:

$$S(m, b) = (m + b - 5.2)^2 + (2m + b - 8.9)^2 + (3m + b - 11.7)^2 + (4m + b - 16.8)^2.$$

To find the regression line for the given data, we must find the values of m and b that minimize $S(m, b)$.

To apply the D-test, we first find the partial derivatives:

$$\frac{\partial S}{\partial b} = 2(m + b - 5.2) + 2(2m + b - 8.9) + 2(3m + b - 11.7) + 2(4m + b - 16.8)$$
$$= 20m + 8b - 85.2, \quad \text{Simplifying}$$

and

$$\frac{\partial S}{\partial m} = 2(m + b - 5.2) + 2(2m + b - 8.9)2 + 2(3m + b - 11.7)3 + 2(4m + b - 16.8)4$$
$$= 60m + 20b - 250.6. \quad \text{Simplifying}$$

We set these derivatives equal to 0 and solve the resulting system:

$$20m + 8b - 85.2 = 0, \qquad 5m + 2b = 21.3, \qquad (2)$$

or

$$60m + 20b - 250.6 = 0, \qquad 15m + 5b = 62.65. \qquad (3)$$

To solve this system, we solve for b in equation (2), and then substitute:

$$b = -\frac{5}{2}m + \frac{21.3}{2}, \quad \text{or} \quad b = -2.5m + 10.65.$$

Using equation (3), we have

$$15m + 5(-2.5m + 10.65) = 62.65 \quad \text{Substituting}$$
$$15m - 12.5m + 53.25 = 62.65 \quad \text{Multiplying}$$
$$2.5m = 9.4 \quad \text{Simplifying}$$
$$m = \frac{9.4}{2.5} = 3.76.$$

Now, we can find b:

$$b = -2.5(3.76) + 10.65 \quad \text{Using the above equation for } b$$
$$= 1.25. \quad \text{Using a calculator}$$

We leave it to the student to complete the D-test to verify that (3.76, 1.25) does, in fact, yield the minimum of S. There is no need to compute $S(3.76, 1.25)$.

The values of m and b are enough to determine $y = mx + b$. The regression line is

$$y = 3.76x + 1.25. \quad \text{Substituting for } m \text{ and } b$$

The graph of this "best-fit" regression line, together with the data points, is shown in Fig. 5. Compare it to Figs. 2, 3, and 4.

Using this regression line, we can now predict Sky Blue Car Rentals' yearly revenue in 2021:

$$y = 3.76(5) + 1.25 = 20.05.$$

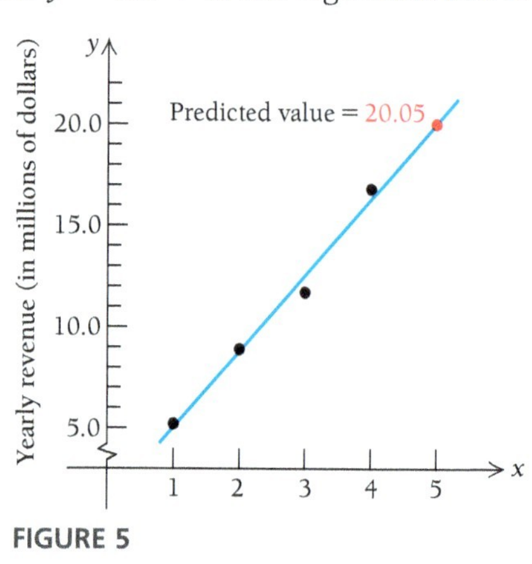

FIGURE 5

The yearly revenue in 2021 is predicted to be about \$20.05 million.

The method of least squares is demonstrated here with only four data points in order to simplify the explanation. Most researchers would want more than four data points to get a "good" regression line. Furthermore, making predictions too far into the future from any mathematical model may not be valid. The further into the future a prediction is made, the more skeptical one should be about the prediction. **1 ✓**

Quick Check 1 ✓

Use the method of least squares to determine the regression line for the data points (1, 25), (2, 48), (3, 76.7), and (4, 104.8).

Exponential Regression

This process can be expanded for other forms of regression that we often consider in this text. In the following example, we show how an exponential regression model can be developed from a set of data.

EXAMPLE 2 The table below gives the yearly revenue of Helman Insurance for 2016 through 2019.

Number of Years since 2016, x	0	1	2	3
Revenue, y (in thousands of dollars)	150	235	480	815

Find the exponential model that best fits the data, and use it to predict the revenue of Helman Insurance in 2022.

Solution We plot the given data points and note that they appear to lie on an exponential curve.

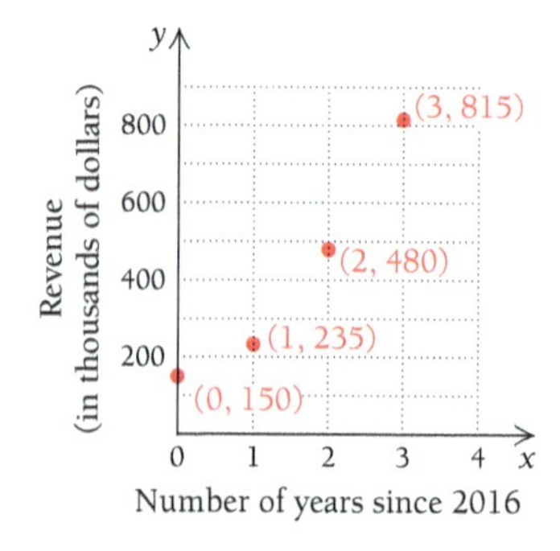

To find a function of the form $y = a \cdot b^x$, we first find the natural logarithm of both sides:

$$\ln y = \ln(a \cdot b^x)$$

$$\ln y = \ln a + \ln b^x \quad \text{Recalling that } \ln(uv) = \ln u + \ln v$$

$$\ln y = \ln a + x \ln b \quad \text{Recalling that } \ln(u^x) = x \ln u$$

If we relabel $\ln y$ as $\widetilde{y}$ (read "y-tilde"), $\ln b$ as $\widetilde{b}$, and $\ln a$ as $\widetilde{a}$, the equation $\ln y = \ln a + x \ln b$ can be treated as a linear equation in terms of x and $\widetilde{y}$:

$$\widetilde{y} = \widetilde{b}x + \widetilde{a}.$$

We find the natural logarithms of the given y-values:

x	0	1	2	3
y	150	235	480	815
$\widetilde{y} = \ln y$	$\ln 150 \approx 5.0106$	$\ln 235 \approx 5.4596$	$\ln 480 \approx 6.1738$	$\ln 815 \approx 6.7032$

Plotting the ordered pairs $(x, \widetilde{y})$, we see that they appear to have a linear relationship.

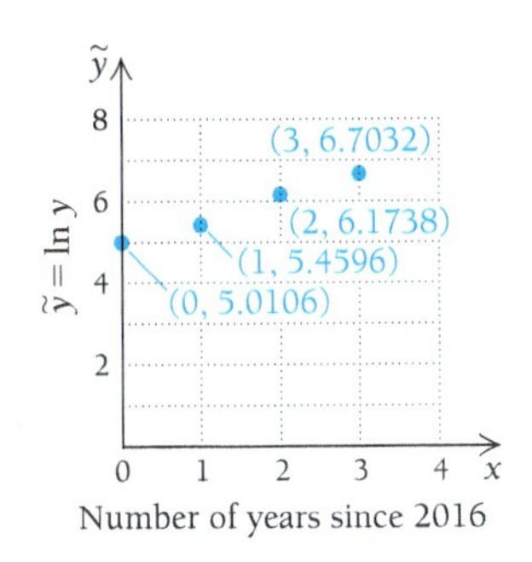

The method outlined in Example 1 yields a regression line, $\widetilde{y} = \widetilde{b}x + \widetilde{a}$, using the values in the table. We find that

$$\widetilde{b} \approx 0.579 \text{ and } \widetilde{a} \approx 4.968.$$

Since $\ln b = \widetilde{b}$, we have $b = e^{\widetilde{b}} = e^{0.579}$, and since $\ln a = \widetilde{a}$, we have $a = e^{\widetilde{a}} = e^{4.968} = 143.74$. The exponential regression model is

$$\begin{aligned} y &= a \cdot b^x \\ &= 143.74 \cdot (e^{0.579})^x \quad \text{Substituting} \\ &= 143.74e^{0.579x}. \end{aligned}$$

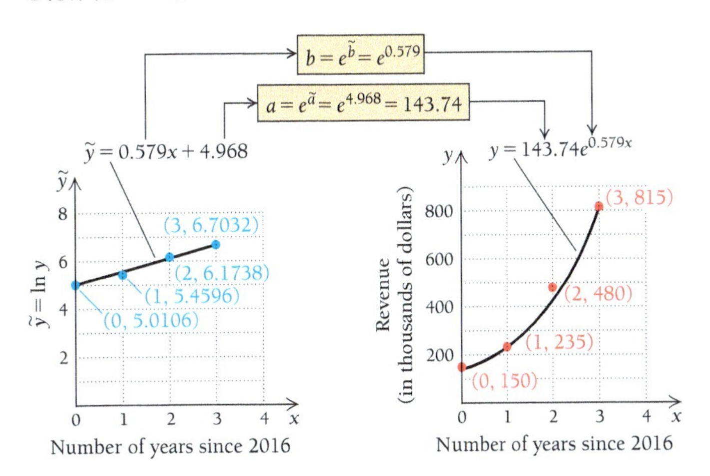

Using this model, the estimated revenue of Helman Insurance in 2022 is found by substituting 6 for x:

$$y = 143.74e^{0.579(6)} \approx 4637.85.$$

Helman Insurance can expect a revenue of about \$4,637,850 in 2022, if growth continues according to the trend observed between 2016 and 2019. 2 ✓

Quick Check 2 ✓
Use the method outlined in Example 2 to find an exponential regression curve for the data points (0, 3), (2, 5), and (4, 9).

Section Summary

- Regression is a technique for determining a continuous function that "best fits" a set of data points.
- According to the least-squares assumption, the line of best fit is that for which the sum of the squares of the y-deviations is a minimum.
- For linear regression, calculus is used to find the values m and b that determine the *regression line* $y = mx + b$, the line of best fit.
- For exponential regression, calculus is used to find values of a and b that determine the exponential regression curve, $y = a \cdot b^x$, that best fits the data. The equation of this curve can also be written in the form $y = ae^{\widetilde{b}x}$, where $e^{\widetilde{b}} = b$.

6.4 Exercise Set

In Exercises 1–4, find the regression line for each data set.

1.

x	1	3	5
y	2	4	7

2.

x	1	2	4	5
y	1	3	3	4

3.

x	1	2	4
y	3	5	8

4.

x	1	2	3	5
y	0	1	3	4

In Exercises 5–8, find an exponential regression curve for each data set.

5.

x	1	3	7
y	8	4	1.5

6.

x	0	1	2
y	10	19	42

7.

x	2	4	6	8
y	13	7	3.7	1

8.

x	1	2	3	4
y	8	25	72	225

All of the following exercises can be done with a graphing calculator if your instructor so directs. The calculator can also be used to check your work.

APPLICATIONS

Business and Economics

9. Hourly wage. The minimum hourly wage in California has grown over the years, as shown in the following table.

Number of Years, x, since 2014	Minimum Hourly Wage (in dollars)
0	9.00
2	10.00
3	10.50
4	11.00
5	12.00

(*Source:* www.dir.ca.gov/iwc/minimumwagehistory.htm.)

a) For the data in the table, find the regression line, $y = mx + b$.

b) Use the regression line to predict the minimum hourly wage in 2022.

c) By 2024, the minimum hourly wage in California will be \$15.00. Is the estimate of this future value provided by the regression line accurate?

10. Football ticket prices. Ticket prices for NFL football games have experienced steady growth, as shown in the table below.

Number of Years, x, since 2012	Average Ticket Price (in dollars)
0	78.38
1	81.54
2	84.43
3	85.83
4	92.98

(*Source:* Team Marketing Report.)

a) Find the regression line, $y = mx + b$.

b) Use the regression line to predict the average ticket price for an NFL game in 2020 and 2025.

Life and Physical Sciences

11. Life expectancy of women. Consider the data in the following table showing the average life expectancy of women in various years.

Number of Years, x, since 2004	Life Expectancy of Women, y (in years)
0	79.96
2	80.21
5	80.81
7	80.95
10	81.11

(*Source:* www.ssa.gov.)

a) Find the regression line, $y = mx + b$.
b) Use the regression line to predict the life expectancy of women in 2025.

12. Life expectancy of men. Consider the following data showing the average life expectancy of men in various years.

Number of Years, x, since 2004	Life Expectancy of Men, y (in years)
0	74.83
2	75.10
5	75.90
7	76.18
10	76.33

(*Source:* www.ssa.gov.)

a) Find the regression line, $y = mx + b$.
b) Use the regression line to predict the life expectancy of men in 2025.

General Interest

13. Social network users. The number of social network users, in billions, for several years after 2012, is shown in the table below. (*Source*: Based on data from eMarketer.)

Number of Years, x, since 2012	Number of Social Network Users (in billions)
0	1.4
1	1.69
2	1.91
3	2.14
4	2.34

a) Find the regression line, $y = mx + b$.
b) Use the regression line to predict the number of social network users in 2022.
c) In what year will the number of social network users first exceed 4 billion?

14. Grade predictions. Professor Suarez wants to predict students' final examination scores on the basis of their midterm test scores. An equation was determined using data consisting of the scores of three students in the same course the previous semester (see the following table).

Midterm Score, x	Final Exam Score, y
70%	75%
60	62
85	89

a) Find the regression line, $y = mx + b$. (*Hint:* The y-deviations are $70m + b - 75$, $60m + b - 62$, and so on.)
b) The midterm score of a student was 81%. Use the regression line to predict the student's final exam score.

15. Predicting the world record in the high jump. It has been established that most world records in track and field can be modeled by a linear function. The table below shows world high-jump records for various years.

Number of Years, x, since 1912	World Record in High Jump, y (in inches)
0 (George Horme)	78.0
44 (Charles Dumas)	84.5
61 (Dwight Stones)	90.5
77 (Javier Sotomayer)	96.0
81 (Javier Sotomayer)	96.5

(*Source:* www.topendsports.com.)

a) Find the regression line, $y = mx + b$.
b) Use the regression line to predict the world record in the high jump in 2020 and in 2050.
c) Does your answer in part (b) for 2050 seem realistic? Explain why estimating so far into the future could be a problem.

16. Population. The data in the following table give the population of Detroit since 1970 (see Exercise 18, Section R.7). (*Source*: www.census.gov.)

Number of Years, x, since 1970	Population (in millions)
0	1.5
10	1.2
20	1.0
30	0.95
40	0.71
45	0.68

a) Find the exponential regression curve, $y = ae^{kx}$.
b) Use the regression curve to estimate when the population of Detroit will be 500,000.

17. Stock prices. The data in the following table give the price of one share of Microsoft stock on January 1 of various years (see Exercise 20, Section R.7). (*Sources*: yahoo.finance and NASDAQ.)

Number of Years, x, since 2012	Price of One Share of Microsoft Stock on January 1
0	\$29.53
1	\$27.45
2	\$37.84
3	\$40.40
4	\$55.09
5	\$64.65

a) Find the exponential regression curve, $y = ae^{kx}$.
b) Use the regression curve to estimate when the price of one share of Microsoft stock will first exceed \$90.

18. Discuss the idea of linear regression with a professor from another discipline in which regression is used. Explain how it is used in that field.

Technology Connection 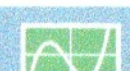

19. General interest: predicting the world record for the 100-m sprint. The following table shows the world-record times for the men's 100-m sprint.

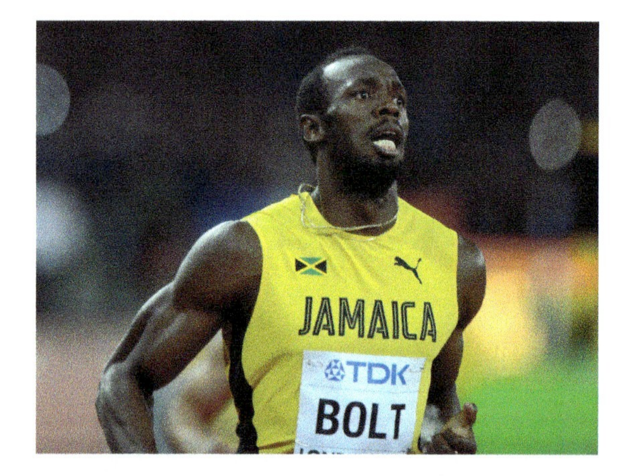

Number of Years since 1968, x	World-Record Time (in seconds)
0 (Jim Hines, United States)	9.95
15 (Calvin Smith, United States)	9.93
22 (Leroy Burrell, United States)	9.90
26 (Leroy Burrell, United States)	9.85
28 (Donovan Bailey, Canada)	9.84
31 (Maurice Greene, United States)	9.79
37 (Asafa Powell, Jamaica)	9.77
40 (Usain Bolt, Jamaica)	9.69
41 (Usain Bolt, Jamaica)	9.58

(*Source:* Based on data from IAAF.)

a) Find the regression line, $y = mx + b$, that fits the data in the table.
b) Use the regression line to predict the world-record time in 2030.
c) Use the regression line to predict the year in which the world-record in the 100-m sprint will be set at 9.40 sec.

20. Power regression. The data in the following table can be modeled by a *power regression curve* of the form $y = ax^b$.

x	1	3	5
y	3.05	43.1	147

a) Find the natural logarithm of both sides of $y = ax^b$, and use laws of logarithms to simplify the right side.
b) Relabel $\ln y$ as $\tilde{y}$, $\ln a$ as $\tilde{a}$, and $\ln x$ as $\tilde{x}$, and find a regression line that expresses $\tilde{y}$ as a function of $\tilde{x}$.
c) Use the results from part (b) to write the power regression equation, $y = ax^b$.
d) Use the power regression equation to estimate y when $x = 7$.

Answers to Quick Checks
1. $y = 26.81x - 3.4$ **2.** $y = 2.9617e^{0.27465x}$

6.5

- Find minimum and maximum values using Lagrange multipliers.
- Solve constrained optimization problems involving Lagrange multipliers.
- Use the Extreme-Value Theorem for Two-Variable Functions to find absolute minimum and maximum values.

Constrained Optimization: Lagrange Multipliers and the Extreme-Value Theorem

In Section 6.3, we discussed a method for determining maximum and minimum values of a two-variable function, $z = f(x, y)$. If restrictions are placed on the input variables x and y, we can determine the maximum and minimum values of f subject to the restrictions. This process is called **constrained optimization.**

Lagrange Multipliers

Suppose you are hiking up a mountain. If there are no constraints on your movement, you may seek out the mountain's summit—its "maximum point." The figure at the right shows a relief map of a mountaintop; its unconstrained maximum point occurs at •, labeled with an elevation of 6903 ft. A hiking trail, marked as a black dashed line, bypasses the summit. If you were constrained to this path, you would not reach the summit. You could, however, achieve a maximum elevation along the path. This constrained maximum point is approximated at M.

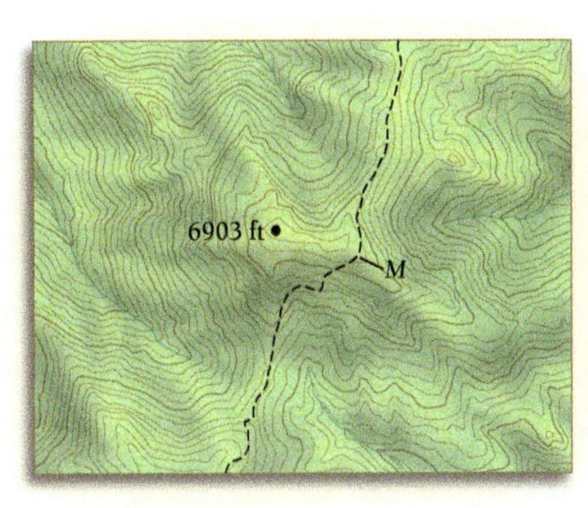

(*Source*: USGS maps at www.mytopo.com.)

In many applications modeled by multivariable functions, constraints on the input variables are necessary. If the input variables are related to one another by an equation, that equation is called a **constraint.**

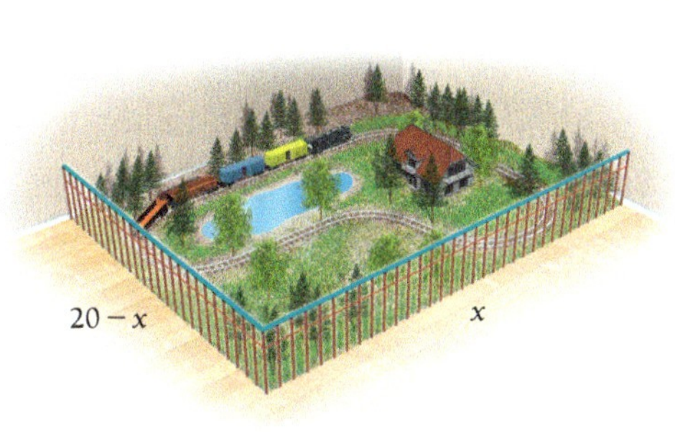

Let's return to a problem from Chapter 3: A hobby store has 20 ft of fencing to fence off a rectangular electric-train area in a corner of its display room. The two sides up against the wall require no fence. What dimensions of the rectangle will maximize the area?

We wish to maximize the two-variable function

$$A = xy$$

subject to the condition, or *constraint*, $x + y = 20$.

By itself, the function of two variables

$$A(x, y) = xy, \quad \text{where } x \geq 0 \text{ and } y \geq 0,$$

has no maximum value. With the constraint $x + y = 20$, the function does have a maximum. We see this in the following graph.

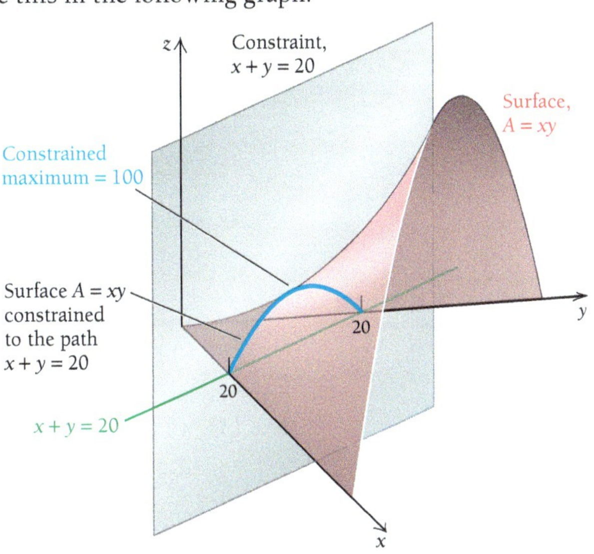

In Section 3.5, we solved the constraint equation for y, getting $y = 20 - x$. Substituting this for y in $A(x, y) = xy$, we expressed A as a function of a single variable:

$$A(x, 20 - x) = x(20 - x) \quad \text{Substituting}$$
$$A(x) = 20x - x^2. \quad \text{Simplifying}$$

Sometimes it can be difficult to isolate a variable in the constraint equation. The method outlined below allows us to proceed without doing so. The proof of why this method works is beyond the scope of this text.

The Method of Lagrange Multipliers

To find a maximum or minimum value of a function $f(x, y)$ subject to the constraint $g(x, y) = 0$:

1. Form a new function, called the **Lagrange function**:

$$F(x, y, \lambda) = f(x, y) - \lambda g(x, y).$$

The variable λ (lambda) is called a **Lagrange multiplier**.

2. Find the first partial derivatives F_x, F_y, and F_λ.

3. Solve the system

$$F_x = 0, \quad F_y = 0, \quad \text{and} \quad F_\lambda = 0.$$

Let (a, b, λ) represent a solution of this system. We then must determine whether (a, b) yields a maximum or minimum of the function f.

The method of Lagrange multipliers also applies to functions of three or more variables.

We illustrate the method of Lagrange multipliers by solving the electric-train area problem.

EXAMPLE 1 Find the extremum of

$$A(x, y) = xy$$

subject to the constraint $x + y = 20$.

Solution Note first that $x + y = 20$ is equivalent to $x + y - 20 = 0$.

1. We form the Lagrange function F, given by

$$F(x, y, \lambda) = xy - \lambda \cdot (x + y - 20)$$
$$= xy - \lambda x - \lambda y + 20\lambda.$$

2. We find the first partial derivatives:

$$F_x = y - \lambda,$$
$$F_y = x - \lambda,$$
$$F_\lambda = 20 - x - y.$$

3. We set each derivative equal to 0 and solve the resulting system:

$$y - \lambda = 0, \quad (1)$$
$$x - \lambda = 0, \quad (2)$$
$$20 - x - y = 0. \quad (3)$$

From equations (1) and (2), it follows that $x = y = \lambda$. Substituting x for y in equation (3), we get

$$20 - x - x = 0$$
$$x = 10.$$

Quick Check 1✓

Find the extremum of $A(x, y) = 3xy$ subject to the constraint $2x + y = 8$. State whether it is a maximum or a minimum value.

Thus, $y = x = 10$. The extreme value of A subject to the constraint occurs at $(10, 10)$ and is

$$A(10, 10) = 10 \cdot 10 = 100.$$

Test points can be used to check that this value is a maximum. For example, $A(11, 9) = 99$, $A(9, 11) = 99$, $A(8, 12) = 96$, and so on. These results support our assertion that $A(10, 10) = 100$ is a maximum value. **1✓**

EXAMPLE 2 **Business: The Beverage-Can Problem.** The standard beverage can holds 12 fl. oz and has a volume of 21.66 in^3. What dimensions yield the minimum surface area? Find the minimum surface area, assuming that the can is a right-circular cylinder.

Solution We want to minimize s, the surface area of a right circular cylinder, given by

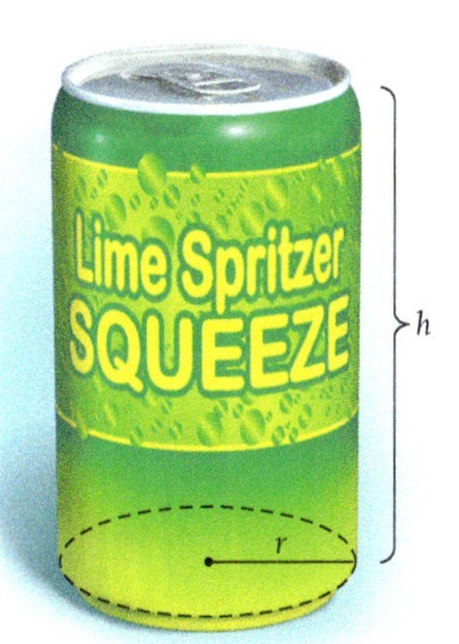

$$s(h, r) = 2\pi rh + 2\pi r^2$$

subject to the volume constraint

$$\pi r^2 h = 21.66,$$

or $$\pi r^2 h - 21.66 = 0.$$

Note that $s(h, r)$ has no minimum without the constraint.

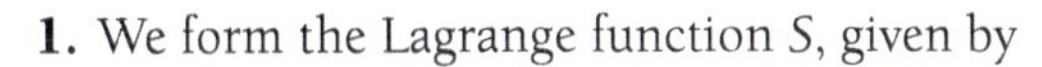

1. We form the Lagrange function S, given by

$$\begin{aligned} S(h, r, \lambda) &= 2\pi rh + 2\pi r^2 - \lambda(\pi r^2 h - 21.66). \\ &= 2\pi rh + 2\pi r^2 - \lambda\pi r^2 h + 21.66\lambda. \end{aligned}$$

2. We find the first partial derivatives:

$$\frac{\partial S}{\partial h} = 2\pi r - \lambda\pi r^2,$$

$$\frac{\partial S}{\partial r} = 2\pi h + 4\pi r - 2\lambda\pi rh,$$

$$\frac{\partial S}{\partial \lambda} = 21.66 - \pi r^2 h.$$

3. We set each derivative equal to 0 and solve the resulting system:

$$2\pi r - \lambda\pi r^2 = 0, \quad (4)$$

$$2\pi h + 4\pi r - 2\lambda\pi rh = 0, \quad (5)$$

$$21.66 - \pi r^2 h = 0. \quad (6)$$

We can solve equation (4) for r:

$$\pi r(2 - \lambda r) = 0$$

$$\pi r = 0 \quad \text{or} \quad 2 - \lambda r = 0$$

$$r = 0 \quad \text{or} \quad r = \frac{2}{\lambda}. \quad \text{We assume } \lambda \neq 0.$$

Since $r = 0$ cannot be a solution to the original problem, we solve for h by substituting $2/\lambda$ for r in equation (5):

$$2\pi h + 4\pi \cdot \frac{2}{\lambda} - 2\lambda\pi \cdot \frac{2}{\lambda} \cdot h = 0$$

$$2\pi h + \frac{8\pi}{\lambda} - 4\pi h = 0$$

$$\frac{8\pi}{\lambda} - 2\pi h = 0$$

$$\frac{8\pi}{\lambda} = 2\pi h,$$

so

$$\frac{4}{\lambda} = h.$$

Since $h = 4/\lambda$ and $r = 2/\lambda$, it follows that $h = 2r$. Substituting $2r$ for h in equation (6) yields

$$21.66 - \pi r^2(2r) = 0 \qquad \text{Using equation (6)}$$

$$21.66 = 2\pi r^3$$

$$\frac{10.83}{\pi} = r^3$$

$$r = \sqrt[3]{\frac{10.83}{\pi}} \approx 1.51 \text{ in.}$$

Thus, when $r = 1.51$ in., we have $h = 3.02$ in. The surface area is then a minimum and is approximately

$$2\pi(1.51)(3.02) + 2\pi(1.51)^2, \quad \text{or about } 42.98 \text{ in}^2.$$

Test points can be used to support our assertion that this value is a minimum. 2 ✓

Quick Check 2 ✓

Repeat Example 2 for a right circular cylinder with no top and a volume of 500 cm^3.

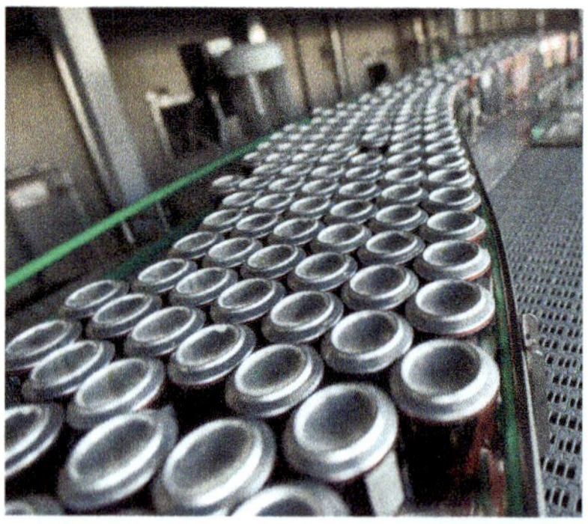

The actual dimensions of a standard 12-oz beverage can are $r = 1.25$ in. and $h = 4.875$ in. A natural question is, "Why don't beverage companies make cans using the dimensions found in Example 2?" Doing so would mean an enormous cost for retooling. New machines, including vending machines, would have to be designed. Market research has also shown that a can with the dimensions found in Example 2 is not as comfortable for consumers to hold. A partial response to the desire to save aluminum has been found in recycling and in manufacturing cans with beveled edges. These cans require less aluminum. As a result of many engineering advances, the amount of aluminum required to make 1000 cans has been reduced over the years from 36.5 lb to 28.1 lb.

In the next example, we show how the method of Lagrange multipliers is used for a function of three variables by revisiting Example 4 from Section 6.3.

EXAMPLE 3 Find the maximum volume of a rectangular box if the sum of its length, width, and height has to be 90 in.

Solution We let x, y, and z be the length, width, and height, respectively, of the box, in inches. Thus, the volume of the box is given by the function of three variables

$$V(x, y, z) = xyz.$$

The sum of the length, width, and height must be 90 in., so we have a constraint, $x + y + z = 90$, which is the same as $x + y + z - 90 = 0$. Note that for the volume of the box to be nonzero, we must have $x > 0$, $y > 0$, and $z > 0$.

1. We form the Lagrange function F:

$$F(x, y, z) = xyz - \lambda(x + y + z - 90)$$
$$= xyz - \lambda x - \lambda y - \lambda z + 90\lambda.$$

2. We then find the first partial derivatives:

$$F_x = yz - \lambda$$
$$F_y = xz - \lambda$$
$$F_z = xy - \lambda$$
$$F_\lambda = -x - y - z + 90.$$

3. We set each partial derivative equal to 0 and solve the resulting system:

$$yz - \lambda = 0 \quad (7)$$
$$xz - \lambda = 0 \quad (8)$$
$$xy - \lambda = 0 \quad (9)$$
$$-x - y - z + 90 = 0 \quad (10)$$

From equations (7) and (8), we have $\lambda = yz$ and $\lambda = xz$, so $yz = xz$. Since $z > 0$, we can divide both sides by z, giving $y = x$. From equations (7) and (9), we have $\lambda = yz$ and $\lambda = xy$, so $yz = xy$. Since $y > 0$, we can divide both sides by y, giving $z = x$.

Substituting x for y and z in equation (10), we have

$$-x - x - x + 90 = 0 \qquad \text{Substituting}$$
$$-3x = -90$$
$$x = 30.$$

Since $z = x$ and $y = x$, it follows that $z = 30$ and $y = 30$. Thus, the box with the maximum volume has a length of 30 in., a width of 30 in., and a height of 30 in., for a volume of $V(30, 30, 30) = 30^3 = 27{,}000 \text{ in}^3$. 3 ✓

Quick Check 3 ✓

Use the method of Lagrange multipliers to maximize $V(x, y, z) = xyz$, where $2x + 3y + z = 30$.

Closed and Bounded Regions: The Extreme-Value Theorem

Constraints may also be expressed as inequalities. Suppose we want to maximize or minimize $f(x, y)$. Multiple constraints on x and y can be plotted on the xy-plane to form a *region of feasibility*, containing all (x, y) pairs that satisfy all the constraints simultaneously. If the constraints form a closed and bounded region (*closed* meaning it includes the boundaries, and *bounded* meaning it has finite area, with no portions tending to infinity), then the Extreme-Value Theorem can be adapted for the two-variable function.

THEOREM Extreme-Value Theorem for Two-Variable Functions

If $f(x, y)$ is continuous for all (x, y) within a region of feasibility that is closed and bounded, then f has both an absolute maximum value and an absolute minimum value over that region.

Recall from Section 3.4 that a continuous function f defined on a closed interval $[a, b]$ must have an absolute maximum value and an absolute minimum value over $[a, b]$. In such cases, it is possible that the absolute maximum or minimum value occurs at an endpoint of the interval. Similarly, absolute maximum or minimum values may occur on the boundaries of a region of feasibility.

EXAMPLE 4 **Business: Maximizing Revenue.** Kim creates embroidered knit caps: one style has a script x on the front, the other a script y on the front. She sells them to raise funds for the Math Team, and her weekly revenue is modeled by the two-variable function

$$R(x, y) = -x^2 - xy - y^2 + 20x + 22y - 25,$$

where x is the number of x-caps produced and sold and y is the number of y-caps produced and sold. Kim spends 2 hr working on each x-cap, and 4 hr on each y-cap, and she works no more than 40 hr per week. How many of each style should she produce and sell in order to maximize her weekly revenue? Assume $x \geq 0$ and $y \geq 0$.

Solution The number of hours that Kim works is a constraint:

$$2x + 4y \leq 40.$$

Along with $x \geq 0$ and $y \geq 0$, we sketch these constraints and shade the region of feasibility.

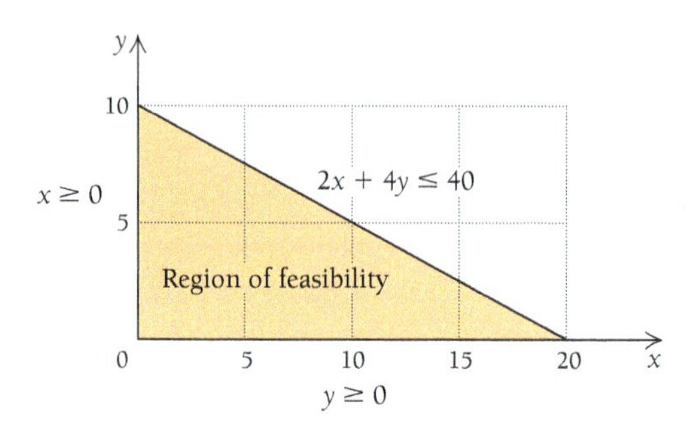

The region of feasibility is closed and bounded. Since R is continuous for all x and y in this region, by the Extreme-Value Theorem for Two-Variable Functions, R has an absolute maximum value.

We first check for possible critical points within the interior of the region using techniques from Section 6.3. Differentiating R with respect to x and to y, we have

$$R_x = -2x - y + 20,$$
$$R_y = -x - 2y + 22.$$

Setting these expressions equal to 0, we solve the system for x and y:

$$-2x - y + 20 = 0,$$
$$-x - 2y + 22 = 0;$$
$$\left.\begin{aligned} 2x + y &= 20 \\ x + 2y &= 22 \end{aligned}\right\} \text{After simplification}$$

The solution of this system is $(6, 8)$. However, this point lies outside the region of feasibility, since $2(6) + 4(8) = 44$, which is greater than 40. Thus, this point is ignored.

The boundaries must also be checked for possible critical points. Points at which two constraints intersect will also be considered as critical points.

- Along the y-axis, we have $x = 0$ for $0 \leq y \leq 10$:

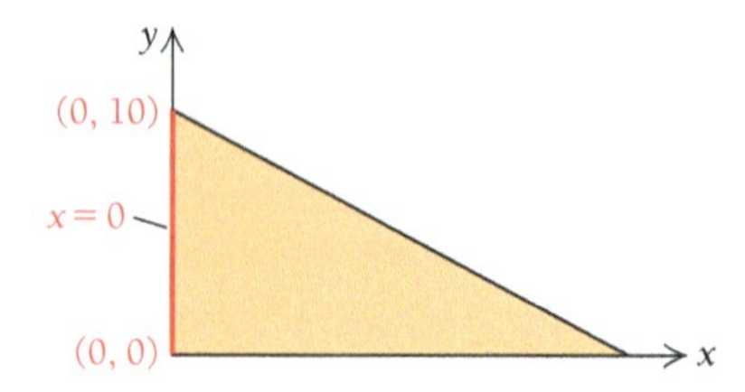

To find possible critical points, we substitute $x = 0$ into R:

$$R(0, y) = 0^2 - 0 \cdot y - y^2 + 20 \cdot 0 + 22y - 25$$
$$= -y^2 + 22y - 25.$$

The first derivative is $R_y(0, y) = -2y + 22$. Setting $-2y + 22$ equal to 0, we obtain $y = 11$. However, $y = 11$ lies outside the region of feasibility and is ignored. The two endpoints of the interval, $(0, 0)$ and $(0, 10)$, remain possibilities for critical points.

- Along the x-axis, we have $y = 0$ for $0 \leq x \leq 20$:

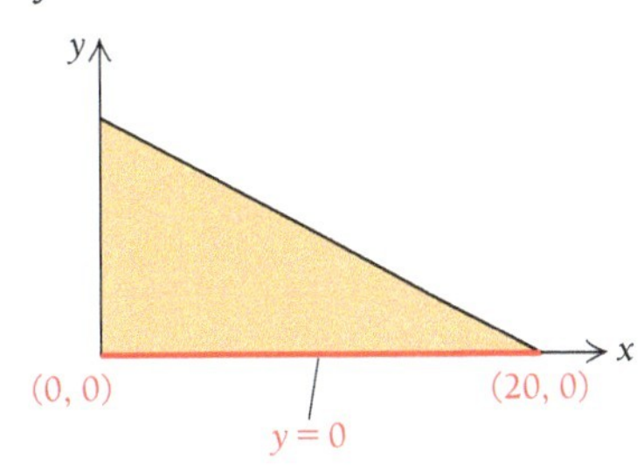

To find possible critical points, we substitute $y = 0$ into R:

$$\begin{aligned} R(x, 0) &= -x^2 - x \cdot 0 - 0^2 + 20x + 22 \cdot 0 - 25 \\ &= -x^2 + 20x - 25. \end{aligned}$$

The first derivative is $R_x(x, 0) = -2x + 20$. Setting $-2x + 20$ equal to 0, we obtain $x = 10$. This lies within the region of feasibility, so $(10, 0)$ is a critical point. The two endpoints of the interval, $(0, 0)$ and $(20, 0)$, are also considered possible critical points.

- Along the line $2x + 4y = 40$, we have $0 \leq x \leq 20$ and $0 \leq y \leq 10$. The endpoints, $(0, 10)$ and $(20, 0)$, are critical points, identified earlier.

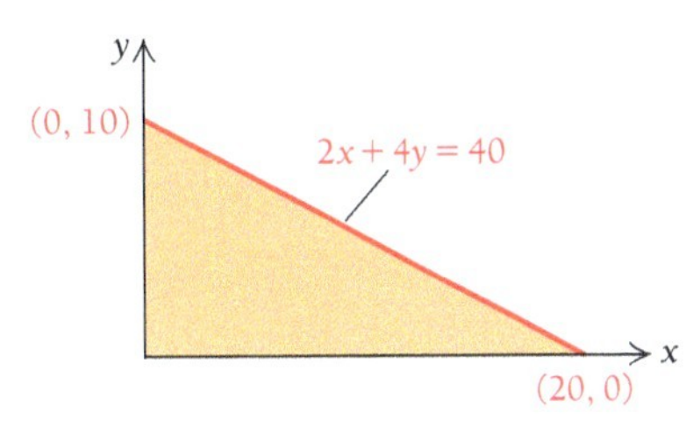

To check for critical points along the line $2x + 4y = 40$, we can use the method of Lagrange multipliers. The constraint is written as $2x + 4y - 40 = 0$, and we have

$$\begin{aligned} F(x, y, \lambda) &= R(x, y) - \lambda(2x + 4y - 40) \\ &= -x^2 - xy - y^2 + 20x + 22y - 25 - 2\lambda x - 4\lambda y + 40\lambda. \end{aligned}$$

The first derivatives are

$$\begin{aligned} F_x &= -2x - y + 20 - 2\lambda \\ F_y &= -x - 2y + 22 - 4\lambda \\ F_\lambda &= -2x - 4y + 40. \end{aligned}$$

We set each partial derivative equal to 0:

$$-2x - y + 20 - 2\lambda = 0 \quad (11)$$

$$-x - 2y + 22 - 4\lambda = 0 \quad (12)$$

$$-2x - 4y + 40 = 0. \quad (13)$$

We solve equations (11) and (12) for λ:

$$\lambda = -x - \tfrac{1}{2}y + 10 \quad \text{and} \quad \lambda = -\tfrac{1}{4}x - \tfrac{1}{2}y + \tfrac{11}{2}.$$

Because both equations include the term $-\frac{1}{2}y$, let's equate their right-hand sides and solve for x:

$$\begin{aligned} -x - \tfrac{1}{2}y + 10 &= -\tfrac{1}{4}x - \tfrac{1}{2}y + \tfrac{11}{2} \\ -\tfrac{3}{4}x &= -\tfrac{9}{2} && \text{Adding } \tfrac{1}{2}y + \tfrac{1}{4}x - 10 \text{ to both sides} \\ x &= 6. && \text{Multiplying both sides by } -\tfrac{4}{3} \end{aligned}$$

We now substitute 6 for x in an equation that is equivalent to equation (13):

$$2(6) + 4y = 40$$
$$12 + 4y = 40$$
$$4y = 28$$
$$y = 7.$$

Since (6, 7) is in the region of feasibility, it is a critical point.

We now have five critical points, which we evaluate in the revenue function $R(x, y)$:

Critical Point (x, y)	$R(x, y)$
(0, 0)	−25
(0, 10)	95
(10, 0)	75
(20, 0)	−25
(6, 7)	122 ← Maximum

Thus, revenue is maximized when Kim produces 6 of the x-caps and 7 of the y-caps, for a weekly revenue of \$122. If there were no constraints, the maximum weekly revenue of \$123 would occur at $x = 6$ and $y = 8$. Kim might think it is not worth working an extra 4 hr for one more dollar in revenue. 4✓

Quick Check 4✓

Repeat Example 4, using the same revenue function but assuming that each x-cap requires 4 hr to create, each y-cap requires 2 hr to create, and Kim is willing to work at most 36 hr per week. How many of each style of cap should she produce to maximize her weekly revenue?

Section Summary

- If input variables x and y for a function $f(x, y)$ are related by another equation, that equation is a *constraint*.
- *Constrained optimization* is a method of determining maximum and minimum points on a surface represented by $z = f(x, y)$, subject to restrictions (constraints) on the input variables x and y.
- The *method of Lagrange multipliers* allows us to find a maximum or minimum value of $f(x, y)$ subject to the constraint $g(x, y) = 0$. This method can also be used on functions of three or more variables.
- If the constraints are inequalities, the set of points that satisfy all the constraints simultaneously is called the *region of feasibility*.
- If the region of feasibility is closed and bounded and the surface $z = f(x, y)$ is continuous over the region, then the *Extreme-Value Theorem* guarantees that f will have both an absolute maximum and an absolute minimum value over that region.
- Critical points may be located at vertices, along a boundary, or in the interior of a region of feasibility.

6.5 Exercise Set

Find the extremum of $f(x, y)$ subject to the given constraint, and state whether it is a maximum or a minimum.

1. $f(x, y) = 2xy;\ 4x + y = 16$

2. $f(x, y) = xy;\ 3x + y = 10$

3. $f(x, y) = x^2 + y^2;\ x + 4y = 17$

4. $f(x, y) = x^2 + y^2;\ 2x + y = 10$

5. $f(x, y) = 3 - x^2 - y^2;\ x + 6y = 37$

6. $f(x, y) = 4 - x^2 - y^2;\ x + 2y = 10$

7. $f(x, y) = 2x^2 + y^2 - xy;\ x + y = 8$

8. $f(x, y) = 2y^2 - 6x^2;\ 2x + y = 4$

9. $f(x, y, z) = xyz;\ 3x + 4y + 6z = 12$

10. $f(x, y, z) = xyz;\ 5x + 2y + z = 10$

11. $f(x, y, z) = x^2 + y^2 + z^2;\ x + y + z = 2$

12. $f(x, y, z) = x^2 + y^2 + z^2;\ y + 2x - z = 3$

Use the method of Lagrange multipliers to solve each of the following.

13. Of all numbers whose sum is 70, find the two that have the maximum product.

14. Of all numbers whose sum is 50, find the two that have the maximum product.

15. Of all numbers whose difference is 4, find the two that have the minimum product.

16. Of all numbers whose difference is 6, find the two that have the minimum product.

17. Of all points (x, y, z) that satisfy $3x + 4y + 2z = 52$, find the one that minimizes

$$(x - 1)^2 + (y - 4)^2 + (z - 2)^2.$$

18. Of all points (x, y, z) that satisfy $x + 2y + 3z = 13$, find the one that minimizes

$$(x - 1)^2 + (y - 1)^2 + (z - 1)^2.$$

19. Find the point on the line $-2x + 5y = 10$ that is closest to the origin.

20. Find the point on the line $3x + y = 6$ that is closest to the origin.

21. Find the point on the plane $x + 2y + z = 8$ that is closest to the origin.

22. Find the point on the plane $2x + y + 3z = 6$ that is closest to the origin.

APPLICATIONS

Business and Economics

23. **Maximizing typing area.** A standard piece of printer paper has a perimeter of 39 in. Find the dimensions of the paper that will give the most area. What is that area? Does standard $8\frac{1}{2} \times 11$ in. paper have the maximum area for its perimeter?

24. **Maximizing room area.** A carpenter is building a rectangular room with a fixed perimeter of 80 ft. What are the dimensions of the largest room that can be built? What is its area?

25. **Minimizing surface area.** An oil drum of standard size has a volume of 200 gal, or 27 ft^3. What dimensions yield the minimum surface area? Find the minimum surface area.

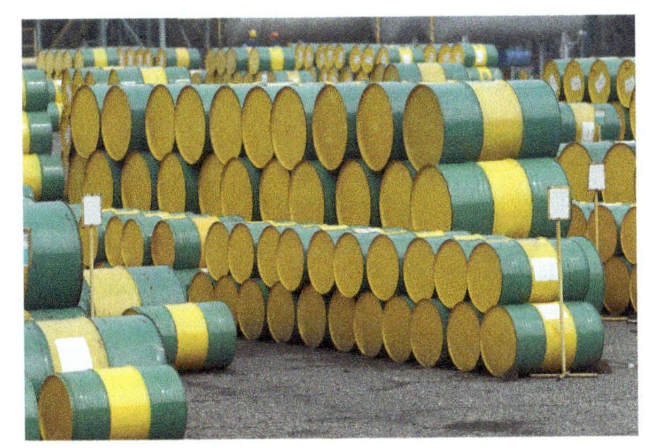

Do these drums appear to be made in such a way as to minimize surface area?

26. **Juice-can problem.** A large juice can has a volume of 99 in^3. What dimensions yield the minimum surface area? Find the minimum surface area.

27. **Maximizing total sales.** Total sales, S, of Cre-Tech are given by

$$S(L, M) = ML - L^2,$$

where M is the cost of materials and L is the cost of labor. Find the maximum value of this function subject to the budget constraint

$$M + L = 90.$$

28. **Maximizing total sales.** Total sales, S, of Sea Change, Inc., are given by

$$S(L, M) = ML - L^2,$$

where M is the cost of materials and L is the cost of labor. Find the maximum value of this function subject to the budget constraint

$$M + L = 70.$$

29. **Minimizing construction costs.** Denney Construction is building a warehouse with an interior volume of 252,000 ft^3. Construction costs per square foot are as follows:

Walls:	\$3.00
Floor:	\$4.00
Ceiling:	\$3.00

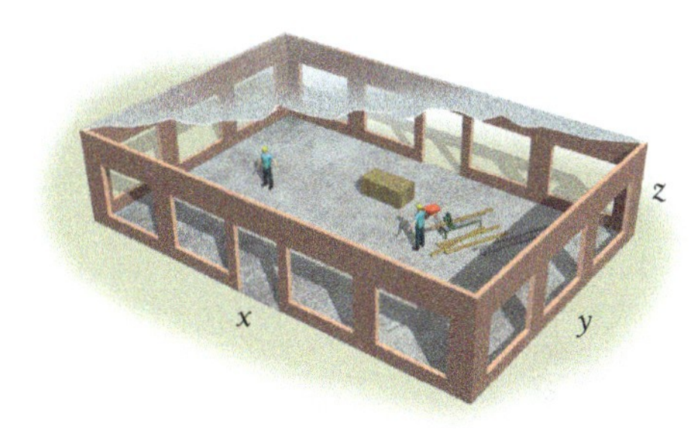

a) The total cost of the building is $C(x, y, z)$, where x is the length, y is the width, and z is the height, all in feet. Find a formula for $C(x, y, z)$.

b) What dimensions of the building will minimize the total cost? What is the minimum cost?

30. **Minimizing the costs of container construction.** Northside Nursery is designing a 12-ft^3 shipping crate with a square bottom and top. The cost of the top and the sides is \$2 per square foot, and the cost of the bottom is \$3 per square foot. What dimensions will minimize the cost of the crate?

31. **Minimizing total cost.** Each unit of a product can be made on either machine A or machine B. The nature of the machines makes their cost functions differ:

Machine A: $\quad C_A(x) = 10 + \dfrac{x^2}{6},$

Machine B: $\quad C_B(y) = 200 + \dfrac{y^3}{9}.$

Total cost is given by $C(x, y) = C_A(x) + C_B(y)$. How many units should be made on each machine in order to minimize total costs if $x + y = 10{,}100$ units are required?

32. Minimizing distance and cost. A highway passes near the small town of Las Cienegas. From Las Cienegas, the highway is 5 miles to the north and 3 miles to the east. Assume that the highway is straight as it passes through this region. The town wants to build an access road, at a cost of \$250,000 per mile, to connect to the highway. What is the shortest possible distance (to three decimal places) from Las Cienegas to the highway, and what would be the minimum cost, to the nearest dollar, of constructing such a road?

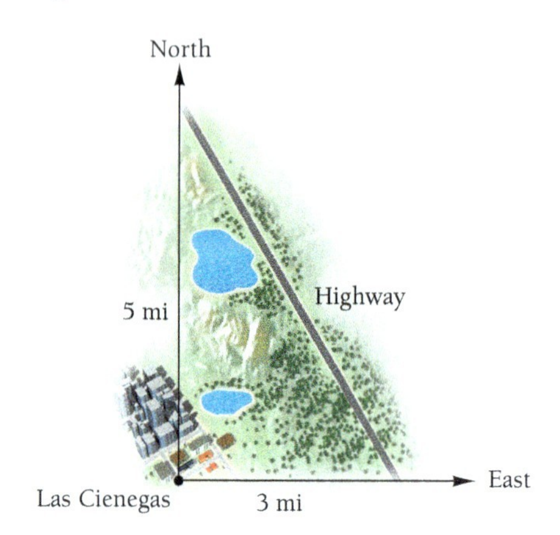

33. Minimizing distance and cost. From the center of Bridgeton, a water main runs northwest at a 45° angle relative to due north and due west. A new house is being built at a point 2 miles west and 1 mile north of the center of town. The cost to connect the house to the water main is \$8,000 per mile. What is the shortest possible distance (to three decimal places) from the house to the water main, and what would be the minimum cost, to the nearest dollar, of connecting the house to the water main?

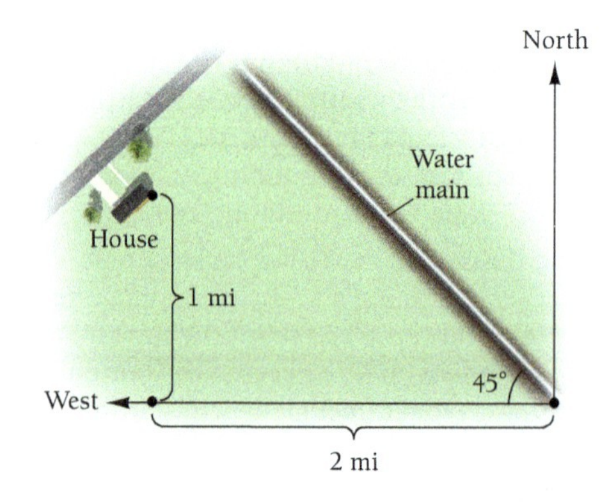

In Exercises 34–37, find the absolute maximum and minimum values of each function, subject to the given constraints.

34. $f(x, y) = x^2 + y^2 - 2x - 2y;\quad x \geq 0, y \geq 0, x \leq 4$, and $y \leq 3$

35. $g(x, y) = x^2 + 2y^2;\quad -1 \leq x \leq 1$ and $-1 \leq y \leq 2$

36. $h(x, y) = x^2 + y^2 - 4x - 2y + 1;\quad x \geq 0, y \geq 0$, and $x + 2y \leq 5$

37. $k(x, y) = -x^2 - y^2 + 4x + 4y;\quad 0 \leq x \leq 3, y \geq 0$, and $x + y \leq 6$

38. Business: maximizing profits with constraints. Lancaster Artisans produces two models of decorative end tables, basic and large. Its weekly profit function is modeled by

$$P(x, y) = -x^2 - 2y^2 - xy + 140x + 210y - 4300,$$

where x is the number of basic models sold each week and y is the number of large models sold each week. The warehouse can hold at most 90 tables. Assume that x and y are nonnegative. How many of each model should be produced to maximize weekly profit, and what will the maximum profit be?

39. Business: minimizing costs with constraints. Farmer Frank grows two crops: celery and lettuce. He has determined that the cost of planting these crops is modeled by

$$C(x, y) = x^2 + 3xy + 3.5y^2 - 775x - 1600y + 250{,}000,$$

where x is the number of acres of celery and y is the number of acres of lettuce. Suppose Farmer Frank has 300 acres available for planting and must plant more acres of lettuce than of celery. Find the number of acres of celery and of lettuce he should plant to minimize the cost, and state the cost.

General Interest

40. Find the maximum volume of a rectangular box that is contained within the sphere $x^2 + y^2 + z^2 = 4$.

41. Find the maximum volume of a rectangular box that is contained within the sphere $x^2 + y^2 + z^2 = 16$.

SYNTHESIS

Find the maximum or minimum value, as indicated, of $f(x, y)$ subject to the given constraint.

42. Minimum: $f(x, y) = 2x^2 + y^2 + 2xy + 3x + 2y$; $y^2 = x + 1$

43. Minimum: $f(x, y) = xy$; $x^2 + y^2 = 9$

44. Maximum: $f(x, y, z) = x^2y^2z^2$; $x^2 + y^2 + z^2 = 2$

45. Maximum: $f(x, y, z) = x + y + z$; $x^2 + y^2 + z^2 = 1$

46. Maximum: $f(x, y, z, t) = x + y + z + t$; $x^2 + y^2 + z^2 + t^2 = 1$

47. Maximum: $f(x, y, z) = x + 2y - 2z$; $x^2 + y^2 + z^2 = 4$

48. Minimum: $f(x, y, z) = x^2 + y^2 + z^2$; $x - 2y + 5z = 1$

49. Find the absolute maximum and absolute minimum points of $f(x, y) = x^2 + y^2 - 2x + 4y$ such that $x^2 + y^2 \leq 25$.

50. Find the absolute maximum and absolute minimum points of $f(x, y) = x^2 + y^2 + 6x + 2y$ such that $x^2 + y^2 \leq 16$.

51. Find the absolute maximum and absolute minimum points of $g(x, y) = 4x + 2y + 5$ such that $x^3 + y^3 \leq 8$, where $x \geq 0$ and $y \geq 0$.

52. Find the absolute maximum and absolute minimum points of $g(x, y) = 8x - 4y + 6$ such that $x^4 + y^4 \leq 16$.

53. Find the absolute maximum and absolute minimum points of $h(x, y) = xy$ such that $2x^2 + y^2 \leq 4$.

54. Find the absolute maximum and absolute minimum points of $h(x, y) = -xy$ such that $x^2 + 3y^2 \leq 6$.

55. **Economics: the Law of Equimarginal Productivity.** Suppose $p(x, y)$ represents the production of a two-product firm. The company produces x units of the first product at a cost of c_1 each and y units of the second product at a cost of c_2 each. The budget constraint, B, is

$$B = c_1x + c_2y.$$

Use the method of Lagrange multipliers to find the value of λ in terms of p_x, p_y, c_1, and c_2. The resulting equation holds for any production function p and is called the *Law of Equimarginal Productivity.*

56. **Business: maximizing production.** A computer company has the following Cobb–Douglas production function for a certain product:

$$p(x, y) = 800x^{3/4}y^{1/4},$$

where x is the cost of labor and y is the cost of capital, both measured in dollars. Suppose the company can make a total investment in labor and capital of $1,000,000. How should it allocate the investment between labor and capital in order to maximize production?

57. Discuss the difference between solving a maximum–minimum problem using the method of Lagrange multipliers and the method of Section 6.3.

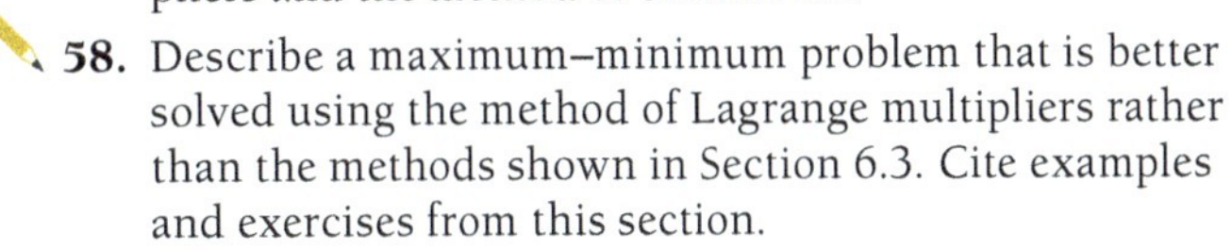

58. Describe a maximum–minimum problem that is better solved using the method of Lagrange multipliers rather than the methods shown in Section 6.3. Cite examples and exercises from this section.

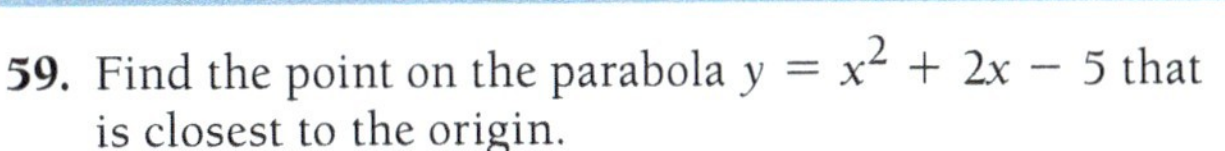

Technology Connection

59. Find the point on the parabola $y = x^2 + 2x - 5$ that is closest to the origin.

60. Find the point on the circle $x^2 + y^2 = 1$ that is closest to the point $(2, 1)$.

Answers to Quick Checks

1. Maximum: 24, when $x = 2$ and $y = 4$
2. $r \approx 5.419$ cm, $h = 5.419$ cm, $s \approx 276.76$ cm^2
3. $V = \frac{500}{3}$, when $x = 5$, $y = \frac{10}{3}$, and $z = 10$
4. $x = 5$, $y = 8$, maximum revenue = $122

6.6 Double Integrals

- Evaluate a double integral.
- Solve applied problems involving double integrals.
- Find the average value of a two-variable function over a given region.

In this section, we consider integration of a function of two variables, in a process called *iterated integration.*

The following is an example of a *double iterated integral,* or more simply, a *double integral:*

$$\int_3^6 \int_{-1}^2 10xy^2\,dx\,dy, \quad \text{or} \quad \int_3^6 \left(\int_{-1}^2 10xy^2\,dx \right) dy.$$

To evaluate a double integral, we first evaluate the inside integral, with respect to the innermost differential (here dx), and treat the other variable (here y) as a constant:

$$\int_{-1}^2 10xy^2\,dx = 10y^2\left[\frac{x^2}{2}\right]_{-1}^2 = 5y^2\left[x^2\right]_{-1}^2 = 5y^2\left[2^2 - (-1)^2\right] = 15y^2.$$

Color indicates the variable of integration.

Then we evaluate the outside integral, associated with the differential dy:

$$\begin{aligned}\int_3^6 15y^2\,dy &= 15\left[\frac{y^3}{3}\right]_3^6 \quad \text{Using } 15y^2 \text{ as the integrand}\\ &= 5\left[y^3\right]_3^6\\ &= 5(6^3 - 3^3)\\ &= 945.\end{aligned}$$

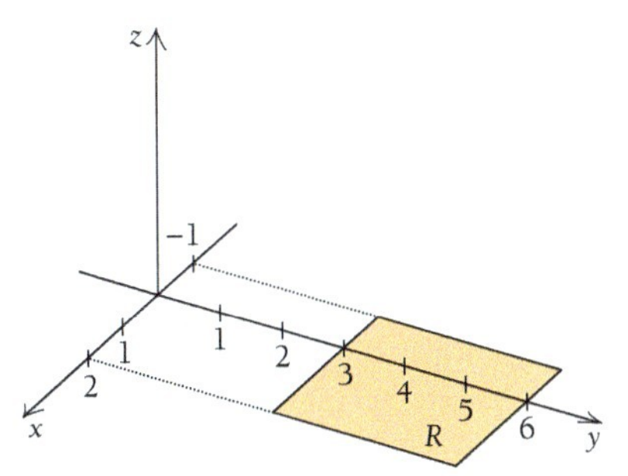

The region of integration, R, $-1 \leq x \leq 2$ and $3 \leq y \leq 6$, is a rectangle in the xy-plane.

If dx and dy, as well as the limits of integration, are interchanged, we have

$$\int_{-1}^2 \int_3^6 10xy^2\,dy\,dx.$$

We first evaluate the inside integral with respect to y, treating x as a constant:

$$\int_3^6 10xy^2\,dy = 10x\left[\frac{y^3}{3}\right]_3^6 \qquad \text{Treating } y \text{ as the variable}$$
$$= \frac{10x}{3}\left[y^3\right]_3^6$$
$$= \frac{10}{3}x(6^3 - 3^3) = 630x.$$

Then we evaluate the outside integral with respect to x:

$$\int_{-1}^2 630x\,dx = 630\left[\frac{x^2}{2}\right]_{-1}^2$$
$$= 315\left[x^2\right]_{-1}^2$$
$$= 315\left[2^2 - (-1)^2\right] = 945.$$

Note that we get the same result as before.

DEFINITION

If $f(x, y)$ is defined over the rectangular region R bounded by $a \le x \le b$ and $c \le y \le d$, then the **double integral** of $f(x, y)$ over R is given by

$$\int_c^d \int_a^b f(x, y)\,dx\,dy \quad \text{or} \quad \int_a^b \int_c^d f(x, y)\,dy\,dx.$$

In a more technical definition of the double integral, Riemann sums are used. However, for the functions in this text, the above definition is sufficient.

Sometimes double integrals are defined over a nonrectangular region, in which case the bounds of integration may contain variables.

EXAMPLE 1 Evaluate

$$\int_0^1 \int_{x^2}^x xy^2\,dy\,dx.$$

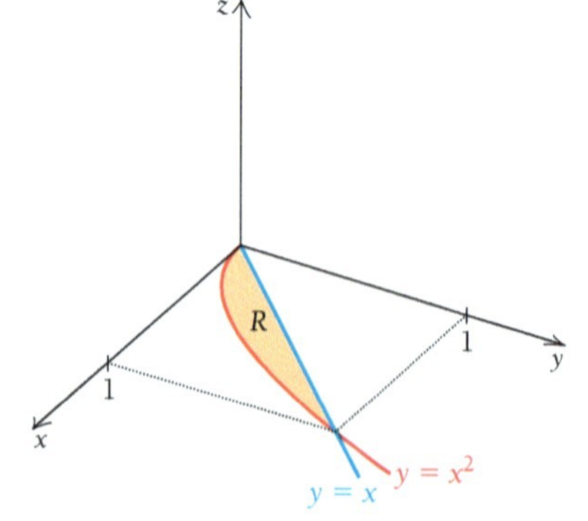

The region of integration, R, for the double integral in Example 1 is shown above.

Solution We first evaluate the inside integral with respect to y, treating x as a constant:

$$\int_{x^2}^x xy^2\,dy = x\left[\frac{y^3}{3}\right]_{x^2}^x$$
$$= \frac{1}{3}x\left[x^3 - (x^2)^3\right]$$
$$= \frac{1}{3}(x^4 - x^7).$$

Then we substitute this result into the original double integral and evaluate the outside integral:

$$\frac{1}{3}\int_0^1 (x^4 - x^7)\,dx = \frac{1}{3}\left[\frac{x^5}{5} - \frac{x^8}{8}\right]_0^1$$
$$= \frac{1}{3}\left[\left(\frac{1^5}{5} - \frac{1^8}{8}\right) - \left(\frac{0^5}{5} - \frac{0^8}{8}\right)\right] = \frac{1}{40}.$$

Thus, $\displaystyle\int_0^1 \int_{x^2}^x xy^2\,dy\,dx = \frac{1}{40}.$

1 ✓

Quick Check 1 ✓

Evaluate

$$\int_0^4 \int_{x/2}^{\sqrt{x}} 2xy\,dy\,dx.$$

The Geometric Interpretation of Multiple Integrals

Suppose region D in the xy-plane is bounded by the graphs of $y_1 = g(x)$ and $y_2 = h(x)$ and the lines $x_1 = a$ and $x_2 = b$. We want to find the volume, V, of the solid between D and the surface $z = f(x, y)$. We can think of the solid as composed of many vertical columns, one of which is shown in Fig. 1 in red.

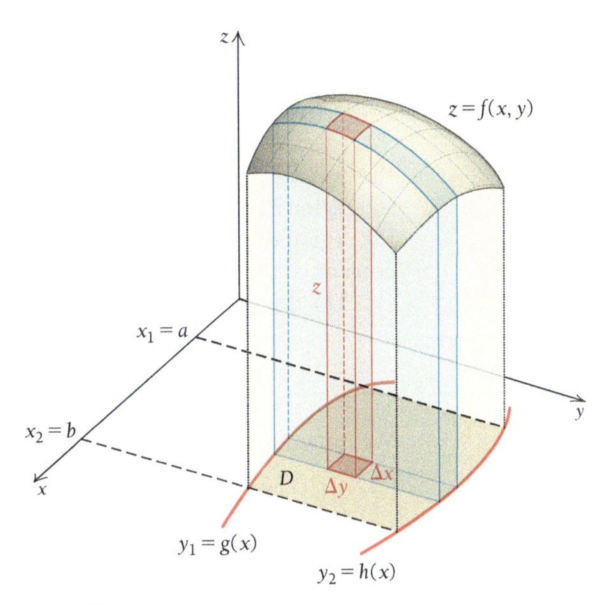

FIGURE 1

The volume of this column can be thought of as $l \cdot w \cdot h$, or $z \cdot \Delta y \cdot \Delta x$. Integrating such columns in the y-direction, we obtain

$$\int_{y_1}^{y_2} z\,dy, \quad \text{so} \left[\int_{y_1}^{y_2} z\,dy\right]\Delta x$$

can be pictured as a "slab," or slice, outlined in blue in Fig. 1. Integrating such slices in the x-direction, we obtain the entire volume:

$$V = \int_a^b \left[\int_{y_1}^{y_2} z\,dy\right] dx,$$

This can be thought of as a collection of slices that fills the volume.

$$\text{or} \quad V = \int_a^b \int_{g(x)}^{h(x)} z\,dy\,dx,$$

where $z = f(x, y)$.

In Example 1, the region of integration R is the plane region between the graphs of $y = x^2$ and $y = x$.

When we evaluated the double integral in Example 1, we found the volume of the solid based on R and capped by the surface $z = xy^2$, as shown in Fig. 2.

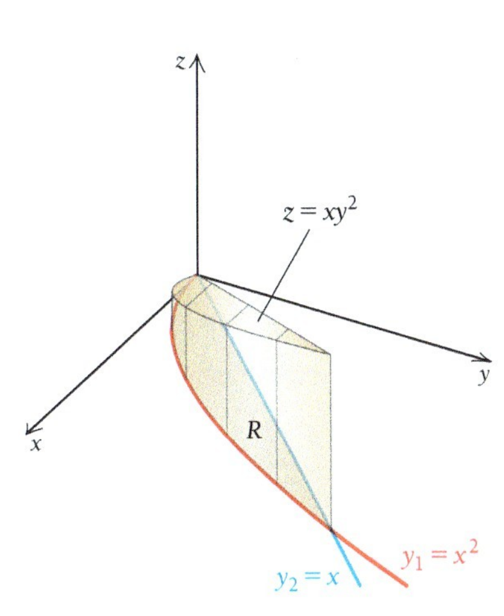

FIGURE 2

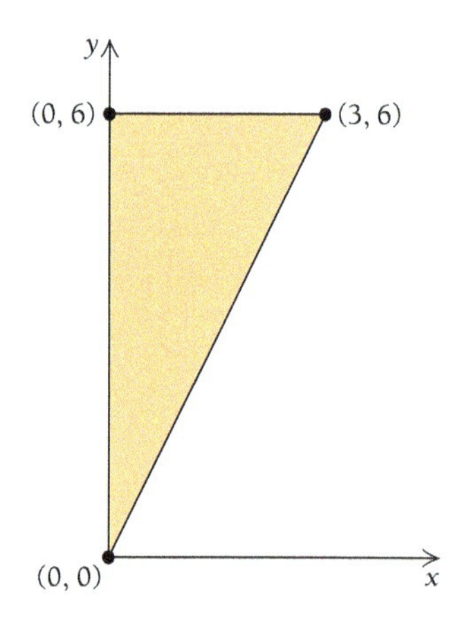

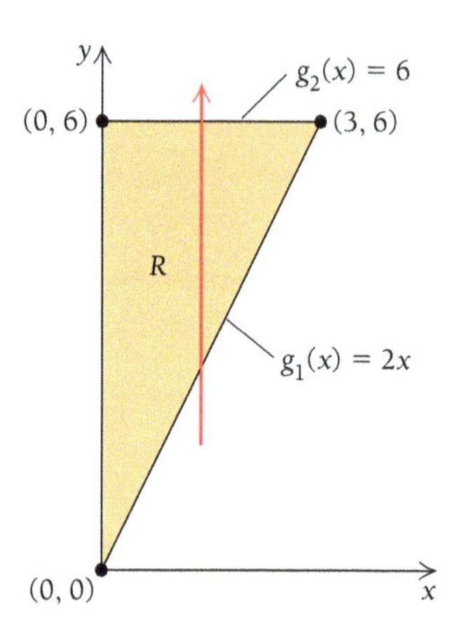

EXAMPLE 2 **Business: Demographics and Vehicle Ownership.** The density of privately owned vehicles in Leatonville is given by $p(x, y) = \frac{1}{8}xy$, where x is the number of miles from the southwest corner of town in the east–west direction, y is the number of miles from that corner in the north–south direction, and p is the number of privately owned vehicles per square mile, in thousands. If the city limits are as shown in the figure to the left, what is the total number of privately owned vehicles in Leatonville?

Solution If we choose to integrate with respect to y first and x second, the double integral is

$$\int_a^b \int_{g_1(x)}^{g_2(x)} \frac{1}{8}xy\,dy\,dx.$$

See below for clarification of $g_1(x)$ and $g_2(x)$.

Since we are integrating with respect to y first, a helpful visual method for determining the bounds of integration is to draw an arrow in the positive y-direction, intersecting the region R, representing the city. The arrow enters the region at $g_1(x) = 2x$ and exits the region through $g_2(x) = 6$. The bounds for the outer integral, with respect to x, are constants: the region extends from $x = 0$ to $x = 3$.

The double integral is

$$\int_0^3 \int_{2x}^{6} \frac{1}{8}xy\,dy\,dx.$$

We integrate the inside integral first, with respect to y:

$$\begin{aligned}\int_{2x}^{6} \frac{1}{8}xy\,dy &= \frac{1}{8}x\left[\frac{1}{2}y^2\right]_{2x}^{6}\\ &= \frac{1}{8}x\left[\frac{1}{2}(6)^2 - \frac{1}{2}(2x)^2\right]\\ &= \frac{1}{8}x(18 - 2x^2)\\ &= \frac{9}{4}x - \frac{1}{4}x^3.\end{aligned}$$

We substitute this result into the original double integral and evaluate:

$$\begin{aligned}\int_0^3 \left(\frac{9}{4}x - \frac{1}{4}x^3\right)dx &= \left[\frac{9}{8}x^2 - \frac{1}{16}x^4\right]_0^3\\ &= \frac{9}{8}(3)^2 - \frac{1}{16}(3)^4 - 0\\ &= \frac{81}{16}, \quad \text{or } 5.0625.\end{aligned}$$

Therefore, since $\int_0^3 \int_{2x}^{6} \frac{1}{8}xy\,dy\,dx = 5.0625$, Leatonville has about 5063 privately owned vehicles. As a partial check, we can examine the units: Region R is measured in miles • miles, or square miles, and $p(x, y)$ is in vehicles per square mile. Thus, the units for the double integral are miles^2 • vehicles/miles^2, or simply vehicles. **2 ✓**

Quick Check 2 ✓

Write the double integral in Example 2 using the reverse order of integration, that is, integrating first with respect to x and then with respect to y.

Average Value of a Multivariable Function

Recall from Section 4.4 that the average value of a continuous single-variable function $y = f(x)$ over $[a, b]$ is given by

$$y_{av} = \frac{1}{b-a}\int_a^b f(x)\,dx.$$

The average value of a continuous two-variable function $z = f(x, y)$ is found in a similar way.

DEFINITION

Let $z = f(x, y)$ be a continuous function over a region of integration R in the xy-plane. The **average value**, z_{av}, over R is given by

$$z_{av} = \frac{1}{A(R)} \iint_R f(x, y)\, dy\, dx,$$

where $A(R)$ is the area of the region of integration and R is used to determine the limits of integration.

EXAMPLE 3 **Business: Average Vehicle Ownership.** Find the average number of privately owned vehicles per square mile in Leatonville (see Example 2).

Solution Since the region of integration R is a triangle with vertices (0, 0), (0, 6), and (3, 6), its area can be found using the formula for the area of a triangle, $A = \frac{1}{2}bh$. Thus, we have

$$A(R) = \tfrac{1}{2}(3)(6) = 9.$$

Therefore, the average number of privately owned vehicles per square mile in the city is

$$p_{av} = \frac{1}{A(R)} \int_0^3 \int_{2x}^6 \frac{1}{8} xy\, dy\, dx$$

$$\approx \frac{1}{9} \cdot 5.0625 \qquad \text{Using the result from Example 2}$$

$$\approx 0.5625.$$

Leatonville has an average of about 563 privately owned vehicles per square mile. 3 ✓

Quick Check 3 ✓

Find the average value of $g(x, y) = 2x + y$, where $0 \le x \le 4$ and $-2 \le y \le 1$.

Section Summary

- The *double integral* of a two-variable function $f(x, y)$ over a rectangular region R bounded by $a \le x \le b$ and $c \le y \le d$ is written

$$\int_c^d \int_a^b f(x, y)\, dx\, dy \quad \text{or} \quad \int_a^b \int_c^d f(x, y)\, dy\, dx.$$

- If the region of integration is not rectangular, the double integral may have variables in its bounds.
- The *average value* of a continuous two-variable function $z = f(x, y)$ over a region R is given by

$$z_{av} = \frac{1}{A(R)} \iint_R f(x, y)\, dy\, dx,$$

where $A(R)$ is the area of the region of integration and R is used to determine the limits of integration.

6.6 Exercise Set

In Exercises 1–16, evaluate the double integral.

1. $\int_0^3 \int_0^2 2y\, dx\, dy$

2. $\int_0^4 \int_0^3 3x\, dx\, dy$

3. $\int_1^4 \int_{-2}^1 x^3 y\, dy\, dx$

4. $\int_{-1}^3 \int_1^2 x^2 y\, dy\, dx$

5. $\int_0^5 \int_{-2}^{-1} (3x + y)\, dx\, dy$

6. $\int_{-4}^{-1} \int_1^3 (x + 5y)\, dx\, dy$

7. $\int_{-1}^1 \int_x^2 (x^2 + y)\, dy\, dx$

8. $\int_0^1 \int_x^1 xy\, dy\, dx$

9. $\int_0^1 \int_1^{e^x} \frac{1}{y}\,dy\,dx$

10. $\int_0^1 \int_{x^2}^{x} (x + y)\,dy\,dx$

11. $\int_0^1 \int_{-1}^{x} (x^2 + y^2)\,dy\,dx$

12. $\int_0^2 \int_0^{x} (x + y^2)\,dy\,dx$

13. $\int_0^5 \int_0^{\ln 2} 2xe^{3y}\,dy\,dx$

14. $\int_1^3 \int_0^{\ln 4} (4x - e^{2y})\,dy\,dx$

15. $\int_1^6 \int_0^{\ln x} xe^{y}\,dy\,dx$

16. $\int_2^5 \int_0^{\ln x} x^2e^{2y}\,dy\,dx$

17–32. For each double integral in Exercises 1–16, find the average value of the function in the integrand over the region defined by the bounds of integration.

33. Find the volume of the solid capped by the surface $z = 1 - y - x^2$ over the region bounded on the xy-plane by $y = 1 - x^2$, $y = 0$, $x = 0$, and $x = 1$, by evaluating

$$\int_0^1 \int_0^{1-x^2} (1 - y - x^2)\,dy\,dx.$$

34. Find the volume of the solid capped by the surface $z = x + y$ over the region bounded on the xy-plane by $y = 1 - x$, $y = 0$, $x = 0$, and $x = 1$, by evaluating

$$\int_0^1 \int_0^{1-x} (x + y)\,dy\,dx.$$

35. Find the average value of $f(x, y) = 2x - y$, where $0 \le x \le 2$ and $2 \le y \le 3$.

36. Find the average value of $g(x, y) = 4 - x - y$, where $-1 \le x \le 1$ and $-2 \le y \le 3$.

37. Find the average value of $f(x, y) = x^2 y$, where the region of integration is a triangle with vertices $(0, 0)$, $(6, 0)$, and $(6, 3)$.

38. Find the average value of $g(x, y) = 2 + xy$, where the region of integration is a triangle with vertices $(0, 0)$, $(4, 4)$, and $(4, -4)$.

39. Life sciences: population. The population density of fireflies in a field is given by $p(x, y) = \frac{1}{100}x^2y$, where $0 \le x \le 30$ and $0 \le y \le 20$, x and y are in yards, and p is the number of fireflies per square yard. Let $(0, 0)$ be the southwest corner of the field.

a) Determine the total population of fireflies in this field.
b) Determine the average number of fireflies per square yard of the field.

40. Life sciences: population. The population density of Gladstone City is given by $p(x, y) = 2x^2 + 5y$, where x and y are in miles and p is the number of people per square mile, in hundreds. The city limits are as shown in the graph below.

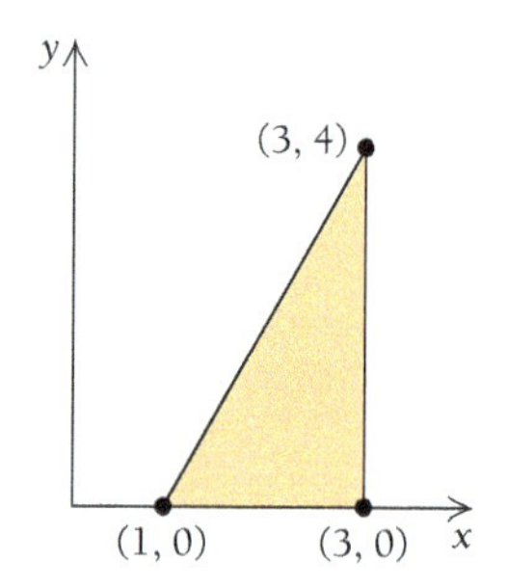

a) Determine the city's population.
b) Determine the average number of people per square mile of the city.

SYNTHESIS

A triple iterated integral such as

$$\int_r^s \int_c^d \int_a^b f(x, y, z)\,dx\,dy\,dz$$

is evaluated in much the same way as a double iterated integral. We first evaluate the inside x-integral, treating y and z as constants. Then we evaluate the middle y-integral, treating z as a constant. Finally, we evaluate the outside z-integral. Evaluate the following triple integrals.

41. $\int_0^1 \int_1^3 \int_{-1}^2 (2x + 3y - z)\,dx\,dy\,dz$

42. $\int_0^2 \int_1^4 \int_{-1}^2 (8x - 2y + z)\,dx\,dy\,dz$

43. $\int_0^1 \int_0^{1-x} \int_0^{2-x} xyz\,dz\,dy\,dx$

44. $\int_0^2 \int_{2-y}^{6-2y} \int_0^{\sqrt{4-y^2}} z\,dz\,dx\,dy$

A function $z = f(x, y)$ is a joint probability density function over a region R in the xy-plane if $f(x, y) \geq 0$ for all x and y in R and if $\iint_R f(x, y)\,dx\,dy = 1$. Use this information in Exercises 45 and 46.

45. Suppose a dart is thrown at a region R in the xy-plane for which $1 \le x \le 2$ and $3 \le y \le 5$, with a joint probability density function given by

$$f(x, y) = x^2 - 3x + \tfrac{1}{3}xy - \tfrac{1}{3}y + 2.$$

a) Verify that $\iint_R f(x, y)\,dx\,dy = 1$.

b) Find the probability that the dart lands at a point in R for which $1 \le x \le 2$ and $3 \le y \le 4$.

c) Find the probability that the dart lands at a point in R for which $1 \le x \le 2$ and $4 \le y \le 5$.

d) Find the probability that the dart lands at a point in R for which $y \le x + 2$.

46. Suppose a dart is thrown at a square region R for which $-1 \le x \le 1$ and $-1 \le y \le 1$, and the joint probability density function g is uniform over R.

a) Find $g(x, y)$.

b) Find the probability that the dart lands at a point where both x and y are nonnegative.

c) Use the result from part (b) to find the probability that the dart lands at a point where at least one of x and y is negative.

d) Explain why the probability of the dart landing on the origin is 0.

In Exercises 47–50, rewrite each double integral by reversing the order of integration.

47. $\int_0^3 \int_0^{4x} f(x, y)\, dy\, dx$

48. $\int_0^7 \int_1^{2x+1} f(x, y)\, dy\, dx$

49. $\int_0^4 \int_{x^2}^{16} g(x, y)\, dy\, dx$

50. $\int_0^2 \int_{x^3}^{8} g(x, y)\, dy\, dx$

Center of mass. *For a density function $d(x, y)$ defined over a region R in the xy-plane, the center of mass, $(\bar{x}, \bar{y})$, is given by*

$$\bar{x} = \frac{\iint_R x \cdot d(x, y)\, dy\, dx}{\iint_R d(x, y)\, dy\, dx} \text{ and } \bar{y} = \frac{\iint_R y \cdot d(x, y)\, dy\, dx}{\iint_R d(x, y)\, dy\, dx}.$$

51. Find the center of mass of the density function $d(x, y) = x + 2y$ over the rectangle with vertices $(0, 0)$, $(5, 0)$, $(5, 3)$, and $(0, 3)$.

52. Find the center of mass of the density function $d(x, y) = 3x + y$ over the rectangle with vertices $(1, 2)$, $(5, 2)$, $(5, 8)$, and $(1, 8)$.

53. Find the center of mass of the density function $d(x, y) = xy$ over the triangle with vertices $(3, 3)$, $(7, 3)$, and $(7, 11)$.

54. Find the center of mass of the density function $d(x, y) = -xy$ over the triangle with vertices $(0, 0)$, $(4, 0)$, and $(0, 4)$.

55. Life sciences: population. The researcher in Exercise 39 wants to place a camera at the center of the firefly population. Determine where she should place the camera in terms of the distribution of fireflies in the field.

If a distribution function is constant, meaning that there is uniform distribution of mass throughout the region R, then the center of mass is the same as the region's physical center.

56. Find the physical center of the triangle with vertices $(0, 0)$, $(0, 10)$, and $(8, 0)$.

57. Find the physical center of the triangle with vertices $(0, 0)$, $(4, 4)$, and $(4, -4)$.

58. Find the physical center of the region enclosed by the circle $x^2 + y^2 = 1$ such that $x \ge 0$ and $y \ge 0$. (*Hint:* Use geometry and symmetry to develop your answer.)

59. Find the physical center of the region enclosed by the circle $x^2 + y^2 = 4$ such that $y \ge 0$.

Technology Connection

60. Find the average value of $f(x, y) = x + 2y$ bounded above by $y = e^{x^2}$ and below by $y = 1$, such that $0 \le x \le 2$.

61. Find the center of the region bounded above by $y = \sqrt{x^2 + 1}$ and below by $y = 1$, such that $0 \le x \le 5$.

Answers to Quick Checks

1. $\frac{16}{3}$ **2.** $\int_0^6 \int_0^{y/2} \frac{1}{8} xy\, dx\, dy$ **3.** $\frac{7}{2}$

Chapter 6 Summary

KEY TERMS AND CONCEPTS	EXAMPLES
SECTION 6.1	
A **function of n variables** assigns to each input, $(x_1, x_2, \ldots, x_n)$, called an **n-tuple**, exactly one output, $f(x_1, x_2, \ldots, x_n)$. Thus, a **function of two variables** assigns to each input pair, (x, y), exactly one output, $f(x, y)$.	**Business.** Lenny's Lids produces two styles of baseball cap. The first style costs \$5.25 per unit to produce, and the second costs \$7.50 per unit to produce. If x is the number of units of the first style of cap and y is the number of units of the second, the cost function C is given by this function of two variables: $C(x, y) = 5.25x + 7.50y.$ If the company produces 30 units of the first style and 45 units of the second, the total cost of producing the caps is $C(30, 45) = 5.25(30) + 7.50(45) = \$495.$
The graph of a function of two variables is a **surface**; graphing such a function requires a three-dimensional coordinate system. Points on the surface are expressed as ordered triples (x, y, z), where $z = f(x, y)$.	The graph of $g(x, y) = \sqrt{4 - x^2 - y^2}$ is a hemisphere of radius 2. Examples of points on the surface of this hemisphere are $(0, 0, 2)$, $(2, 0, 0)$, $(1, 1, \sqrt{2})$, and $\left(-\frac{1}{2}, -\frac{2}{3}, \frac{\sqrt{119}}{6}\right)$. 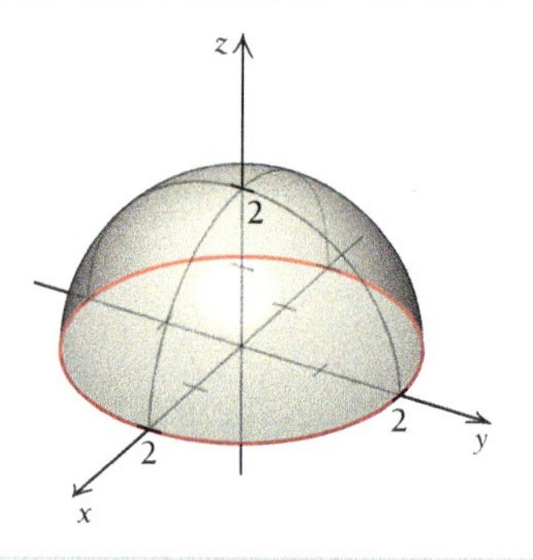
The **domain** of a function of two variables is the set of points in the xy-plane for which f is defined.	• The function $f(x, y) = x^3 + y^3 - 3x - 27y - 2$ is defined for all x and for all y. Therefore, the domain of f is $D = \{(x, y) \mid -\infty < x < \infty, -\infty < y < \infty\}.$ • The function $g(x, y) = \sqrt{4 - x^2 - y^2}$ is defined provided that $4 - x^2 - y^2 \geq 0$, or $x^2 + y^2 \leq 4$. Therefore, the domain of g is $D = \{(x, y) \mid x^2 + y^2 \leq 4\}.$ • For the cost function $C(x, y) = 5.25x + 7.50y$ considered above, x and y represent quantities of hats. Thus, the domain of C is $D = \{(x, y) \mid x \geq 0, y \geq 0\}$, where x and y are integers.
SECTION 6.2	
Let f be a function of two variables, x and y. The **partial derivative of f with respect to x** is defined as $\frac{\partial f}{\partial x} = \lim_{h \to 0} \frac{f(x + h, y) - f(x, y)}{h}.$ The variable y is treated as a constant during this differentiation.	Let $f(x, y) = x^2 + 2xy^3 + \sqrt{y}$. The partial derivative of f with respect to x is $\frac{\partial f}{\partial x} = 2x + 2y^3.$
The **partial derivative of f with respect to y** is defined as $\frac{\partial f}{\partial y} = \lim_{h \to 0} \frac{f(x, y + h) - f(x, y)}{h}.$ The variable x is treated as a constant during this differentiation.	The partial derivative of f with respect to y is $\frac{\partial f}{\partial y} = 6xy^2 + \frac{1}{2\sqrt{y}}.$

KEY TERMS AND CONCEPTS	EXAMPLES
SECTION 6.2 (*continued*)	
Other common notations for partial derivatives are f_x for the partial derivative of f with respect to x and f_y for the partial derivative of f with respect to y. The partial derivative $\partial f/\partial x$ is interpreted as the slope of the tangent line at a point (x, y, z) on the surface representing the graph of f in the positive x-direction. Similarly, $\partial f/\partial y$ is interpreted as the slope of the tangent line at a point (x, y, z) on the surface in the positive y-direction.	When $x = 2$ and $y = 1$, the slope of the tangent line in the positive x-direction at $(2, 1, 9)$ on the surface representing the graph of f is $$f_x(2, 1) = 2(2) + 2(1)^3 = 6.$$ The slope of the tangent line at $(2, 1, 9)$ on the surface in the positive y-direction is $$f_y(2, 1) = 6(2)(1)^2 + \frac{1}{2\sqrt{(1)}} = 12.5.$$
For functions of many variables, the partial derivative with respect to one of the variables is found by treating all the other variables as constants and differentiating using previously developed techniques.	Let $w(x, y, z) = 3x^2y^3z^7$. The partial derivatives of w are $$w_x = 6xy^3z^7,$$ $$w_y = 9x^2y^2z^7,$$ $$w_z = 21x^2y^3z^6.$$
Let f be a function of two variables, x and y. Its **second-order partial derivatives** are $$f_{xx} = \frac{\partial^2 f}{\partial x^2}, \quad f_{xy} = \frac{\partial^2 f}{\partial y\, \partial x},$$ $$f_{yx} = \frac{\partial^2 f}{\partial x\, \partial y}, \quad \text{and} \quad f_{yy} = \frac{\partial^2 f}{\partial y^2}.$$ For the functions considered in this text, $f_{xy} = f_{yx}$.	Let $f(x, y) = x^2 + 2xy^3 + \sqrt{y}$. Its first partial derivatives are $$f_x = \frac{\partial f}{\partial x} = 2x + 2y^3 \quad \text{and} \quad f_y = \frac{\partial f}{\partial y} = 6xy^2 + \frac{1}{2\sqrt{y}}.$$ Its second-order partial derivatives are $$f_{xx} = 2, \quad f_{xy} = 6y^2, \quad f_{yx} = 6y^2, \quad \text{and} \quad f_{yy} = 12xy - \frac{1}{4\sqrt{y^3}}.$$
If $z = f(x, y)$, then the **differential** of z is $$dz = f_x(x, y)\, dx + f_y(x, y)\, dy.$$ If Δx and Δy are small, then the above formula offers a good estimation of $$\Delta z = f(x + \Delta x, y + \Delta y) - f(x, y).$$	Let $f(x, y) = x^2y^4$. When $x = 2$, $y = 3$, $\Delta x = 0.1$, and $\Delta y = 0.05$, we have $$\begin{aligned} dz &= (2xy^4)\, dx + (4x^2y^3)\, dy \\ &= 2(2)(3)^4(0.1) + 4(2)^2(3)^3(0.05) \\ &= 32.4 + 21.6 \\ &= 54. \end{aligned}$$ Note that $$\begin{aligned} \Delta z &= f(x + \Delta x, y + \Delta y) - f(x, y) \\ &= f(2.1, 3.05) - f(2, 3) \\ &= (2.1)^2(3.05)^4 - (2)^2(3)^4 \\ &\approx 381.626 - 324 = 57.626. \quad \text{Rounding} \end{aligned}$$

KEY TERMS AND CONCEPTS	EXAMPLES
SECTION 6.3	
If f is a function of two variables, x and y, it has a **relative maximum** at (a, b) if $$f(x, y) \leq f(a, b)$$ for all points (x, y) in a region containing (a, b). Similarly, f has a **relative minimum** at (a, b) if $$f(x, y) \geq f(a, b)$$ for all points (x, y) in a region containing (a, b). For a differentiable function f, a **critical point** occurs at $(a, b, f(a, b))$ if both partial derivatives of f at (a, b) are 0; that is, if $f_x(a, b) = 0$ and $f_y(a, b) = 0$.	Let $f(x, y) = x^3 + y^3 - 3x - 27y - 2$. The first partial derivatives are $f_x(x, y) = 3x^2 - 3$ and $f_y(x, y) = 3y^2 - 27$. When $f_x = 0$, we have $x = \pm 1$. Similarly, when $f_y = 0$, we have $y = \pm 3$. This gives four critical points: $(1, 3, -58)$, where $f(1, 3) = -58$, $(1, -3, 50)$, where $f(1, -3) = 50$, $(-1, 3, -54)$, where $f(-1, 3) = -54$, and $(-1, -3, 54)$, where $f(-1, -3) = 54$. The four second-order partial derivatives are $f_{xx} = 6x$, $f_{yy} = 6y$, and $f_{xy} = f_{yx} = 0$. Therefore, $D = (6x)(6y) - 0^2 = 36xy$.
The **D-test** is used to determine whether critical points are relative maxima or minima. If $(a, b, f(a, b))$ is a critical point, then $$D = f_{xx}(a, b) \cdot f_{yy}(a, b) - [f_{xy}(a, b)]^2.$$ And: If $D > 0$ and $f_{xx}(a, b) < 0$, then it follows that f has a **maximum** at (a, b). If $D > 0$ and $f_{xx}(a, b) > 0$, then it follows that f has a **minimum** at (a, b). If $D < 0$, then it follows that f has a **saddle point** at (a, b). The D-test is not applicable if $D = 0$.	• At $(1, 3)$, we have $D = 108 > 0$, and $f_{xx}(1, 3) = 6 > 0$. Therefore, $(1, 3, -58)$ is a relative minimum. • At $(1, -3)$ and at $(-1, 3)$, we have $D = -108 < 0$. Therefore, $(1, -3, 50)$ and $(-1, 3, -54)$ are saddle points. • At $(-1, -3)$, we have $D = 108 > 0$, and $f_{xx}(-1, -3) = -6 < 0$. Therefore, $(-1, -3, 54)$ is a relative maximum. 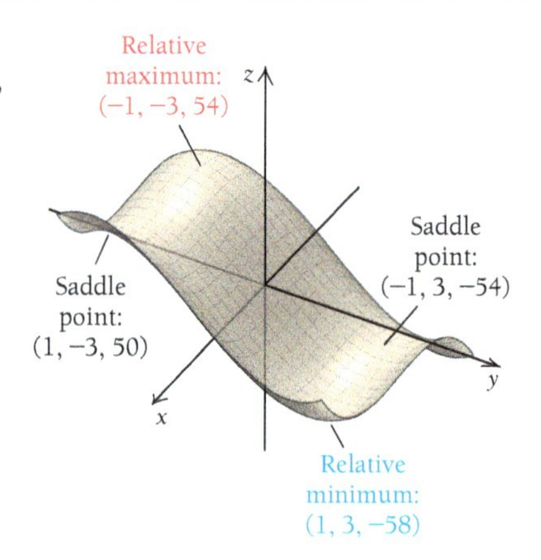
If the input variables x and y of a function $f(x, y)$ are themselves related by an equation $g(x, y) = 0$, then $g(x, y) = 0$ is a **constraint**. The process of determining maximum and minimum values of f subject to the constraint g is called **constrained optimization.**	Maximize $f(x, y) = xy$, subject to the constraint $x + 2y = 1$. We can substitute $x = 1 - 2y$ into f: $$f(1 - 2y, y) = (1 - 2y)y = y - 2y^2.$$ Differentiating f with respect to y, we get $f_y = 1 - 4y$. Setting this equal to 0, we get $y = \frac{1}{4}$. Therefore, $x = 1 - 2(\frac{1}{4}) = \frac{1}{2}$. Since $f_{yy} = -4 < 0$, the function f has a maximum value of $\frac{1}{8}$ at $x = \frac{1}{2}$ and $y = \frac{1}{4}$, which lies on the line given by the constraint.

KEY TERMS AND CONCEPTS

EXAMPLES

SECTION 6.4

Regression is a technique for determining a continuous function that "best fits" a set of data.

For linear regression, calculus can be used to find the values m and b that determine the **regression line**, $y = mx + b$, the line of best fit.

For exponential regression, calculus can be used to find values of a and b that determine the exponential regression curve, $y = a \cdot b^x$, that best fits the data. This equation can also be written in the form $y = ae^{\tilde{b}x}$, where $e^{\tilde{b}} = b$.

A researcher obtains the data points $(1, 3)$, $(4, 5)$, and $(6, 7)$. Find the regression line.

The method of least squares is used to minimize

$$(y_1 - 3)^2 + (y_2 - 5)^2 + (y_3 - 7)^2,$$

where
$$y_1 = m(1) + b = m + b,$$
$$y_2 = m(4) + b = 4m + b,$$
$$y_3 = m(6) + b = 6m + b.$$

After substitution, this results in a function of two variables:

$$S(m, b) = (m + b - 3)^2 + (4m + b - 5)^2 + (6m + b - 7)^2.$$

The partial derivatives are (after simplification):

$$S_m = 106m + 22b - 130,$$
$$S_b = 22m + 6b - 30.$$

Setting each partial derivative equal to 0 and solving the system gives

$$m = \frac{15}{19} \quad \text{and} \quad b = \frac{40}{19}.$$

Therefore, the regression line is $y = \frac{15}{19}x + \frac{40}{19}$.

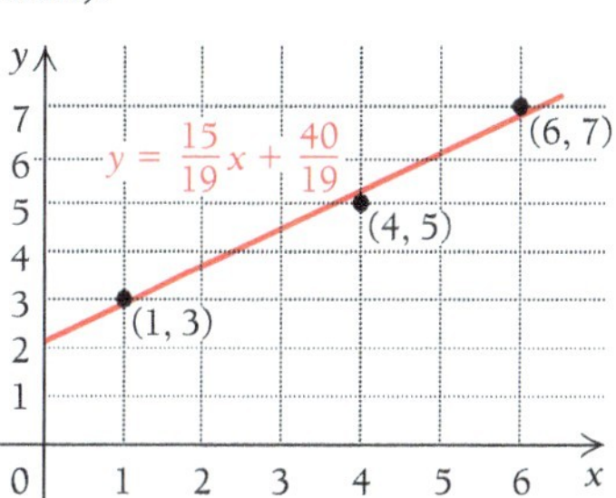

SECTION 6.5

The method of **Lagrange multipliers** is one way to determine an extreme value of a function f subject to a constraint g.

1. Form the **Lagrange function**
$$F(x, y, \lambda) = f(x, y) - \lambda g(x, y).$$
The variable λ is a *Lagrange multiplier.*
2. Find the first partial derivatives F_x, F_y, and F_λ.
3. Solve the system
$$F_x = 0, \quad F_y = 0, \quad \text{and} \quad F_\lambda = 0.$$

A suggested method of solution is to isolate λ in the equations $F_x = 0$ and $F_y = 0$, substitute for λ, and solve the resulting equation for x or y. Make another substitution into $F_\lambda = 0$, and determine the values of x and y.

Find the extremum of $f(x, y) = xy$, subject to the constraint $x + 2y = 1$.

1. Write the constraint as $x + 2y - 1 = 0$ and form the Lagrange function:
$$F(x, y, \lambda) = xy - \lambda(x + 2y - 1).$$
2. Differentiate F with respect to each of the three input variables:
$$F_x = y - \lambda, \quad F_y = x - 2\lambda, \quad \text{and} \quad F_\lambda = -x - 2y + 1.$$
3. Set all three expressions equal to 0. From $F_x = 0$ and $F_y = 0$, isolate λ:
$$\lambda = y \text{ and } \lambda = \tfrac{1}{2}x.$$
Thus, $y = \frac{1}{2}x$. Substituting $\frac{1}{2}x$ for y in F_λ and setting the expression equal to 0 gives
$$-x - 2(\tfrac{1}{2}x) + 1 = 0.$$
Solving for x gives $x = \frac{1}{2}$. Therefore, $y = \frac{1}{2}(\frac{1}{2}) = \frac{1}{4}$, and f has a constrained maximum value of $\frac{1}{8}$ at $(\frac{1}{2}, \frac{1}{4})$.
Choosing test points (x, y) such that $x + 2y = 1$ and evaluating $f(x, y)$ with them supports the assertion that the value $\frac{1}{8}$ is a maximum.

If $f(x, y)$ is continuous over a region of feasibility that is closed and bounded, then the **Extreme-Value Theorem** guarantees the existence of an absolute maximum value and an absolute minimum value of f over that region.

Find the absolute maximum and minimum values of $f(x, y) = x^2 + y^2 - 2x - 2y$, subject to the constraints $0 \le x \le 2$ and $0 \le y \le 3$.

Since f is continuous on $0 \le x \le 2$ and on $0 \le y \le 3$, check for critical points at all boundaries and vertices and in the interior. In this case, f has an absolute maximum of 3 at both $(0, 3)$ and $(2, 3)$ and an absolute minimum of -2 at $(1, 1)$.

KEY TERMS AND CONCEPTS	EXAMPLES
SECTION 6.6	
If $f(x, y)$ is defined over a rectangular region R bounded by $a \le x \le b$ and $c \le y \le d$, then the **double iterated integral** of $f(x, y)$ over R is $$\int_c^d \int_a^b f(x, y)\, dx\, dy$$ or $$\int_a^b \int_c^d f(x, y)\, dy\, dx.$$ If the region is not rectangular, then the bounds of integration may contain variables. Iterated integrals are evaluated by first integrating the inside integral, indicated by the innermost differential, and then integrating the outer integral.	To evaluate $$\int_0^2 \int_1^3 x^2 y\, dy\, dx,$$ the inside integral is integrated first. Integrate with respect to y, treating x as a constant: $$\int_1^3 x^2 y\, dy = x^2\left[\frac{1}{2}y^2\right]_1^3 = x^2\left(\frac{9}{2} - \frac{1}{2}\right) = 4x^2.$$ The result is then integrated with respect to x: $$\int_0^2 4x^2\, dx = \left[\frac{4}{3}x^3\right]_0^2 = \frac{4}{3}(8 - 0) = \frac{32}{3}.$$
The **average value** of a continuous two-variable function $z = f(x, y)$ over a region of integration R is given by $$z_{av} = \frac{1}{A(R)} \iint_R f(x, y)\, dy\, dx,$$ where $A(R)$ is the area of the region of integration.	The average value of $f(x, y) = 2xy$ over a region R that is a triangle with vertices $(-2, 0)$, $(2, 0)$, and $(2, 8)$ is $$z_{av} = \frac{1}{A(R)} \int_{-2}^{2} \int_0^{2x+4} 2xy\, dy\, dx = \frac{1}{16} \cdot \frac{256}{3} = \frac{16}{3}.$$

Chapter 6 Review Exercises

These review exercises are for test preparation. They can also be used as a practice test. Answers are at the back of the book. The red bracketed section references tell you what part(s) of the chapter to restudy if your answer is incorrect.

CONCEPT REINFORCEMENT

Match each expression in column A with an equivalent expression in column B. Assume that $z = f(x, y)$. [6.2, 6.6]

Column A	Column B
1. $\frac{\partial z}{\partial y}$	**a)** $\int_2^3 \frac{1}{2} x\, dx$
2. $\frac{\partial z}{\partial x}$	**b)** f_{yx}
3. $\frac{\partial}{\partial x}(5x^3y^7)$	**c)** f_{xy}
4. $\frac{\partial}{\partial y}(5x^3y^7)$	**d)** $\int_2^3 y^3\, dy$
5. $\frac{\partial^2 z}{\partial y\, \partial x}$	**e)** f_x
6. $\frac{\partial^2 z}{\partial x\, \partial y}$	**f)** $15x^2y^7$
7. $\int_2^3 \int_0^1 2xy^3\, dx\, dy$	**g)** $35x^3y^6$
8. $\int_2^3 \int_0^1 2xy^3\, dy\, dx$	**h)** f_y

REVIEW EXERCISES

Given $f(x, y) = e^y + 3xy^3 + 2y$, find each of the following. [6.1, 6.2]

9. $f(2, 0)$ **10.** f_x **11.** f_y

12. f_{xy} **13.** f_{yx} **14.** f_{xx}

15. f_{yy}

16. State the domain of $f(x, y) = \dfrac{2}{x - 1} + \sqrt{y - 2}$. [6.1]

Given $z = 2x^3 \ln y + xy^2$, find each of the following. [6.2]

17. $\dfrac{\partial z}{\partial x}$ **18.** $\dfrac{\partial z}{\partial y}$ **19.** $\dfrac{\partial^2 z}{\partial x\, \partial y}$

20. $\dfrac{\partial^2 z}{\partial y\, \partial x}$ **21.** $\dfrac{\partial^2 z}{\partial x^2}$ **22.** $\dfrac{\partial^2 z}{\partial y^2}$

23. Let $z = f(x, y) = 2x^4 - y^2$. [6.2]

a) Use differentials to estimate Δz when $x = 3, y = 2, \Delta x = 0.01$, and $\Delta y = 0.02$.

b) Find Δz by evaluating $f(x + \Delta x, y + \Delta y) - f(x, y)$.

Find any relative maximum and minimum values, identify the ordered pair that gives each one's location, and state whether it is a relative maximum or relative minimum. [6.3]

24. $f(x, y) = x^3 - 6xy + y^2 + 6x + 3y - \frac{1}{5}$

25. $f(x, y) = 3x - 6y - x^2 - y^2$

26. $f(x, y) = x^4 + y^4 + 4x - 32y + 80$

27. Consider the data in the following table regarding enrollment in colleges and universities, where x is the number of years since 2014. [6.4]

Number of Years, x, since 2014	Enrollment, y (in millions)
0	23.2
1	22.7
2	22.4

(*Source:* Based on data from the U.S. Department of Education.)

a) Find the regression line, $y = mx + b$.

b) Use the regression line to predict enrollment in 2018.

c) Use the regression line to estimate when enrollment will be 21 million.

28. The table below lists the amount of the monthly payment to a homeowners' association, where x is the number of years since 2005. [6.4]

Number of Years, x, since 2005	Monthly Payment to Homeowners' Association
0	\$129
6	\$226
12	\$360
13	\$380

a) Find the regression line, $y = mx + b$.

b) Use the regression line to predict the amount of the monthly payment in 2020.

c) Find the exponential regression curve, $y = ae^{kx}$.

d) Use the exponential regression curve to estimate the amount of the monthly payment in 2020.

29. Find the extremum of

$$f(x, y) = x^2 - 2xy + 2y^2 + 20$$

subject to the constraint $2x - 6y = 15$. State where it occurs and whether it is a maximum or a minimum. [6.5]

30. Find the extremum of $f(x, y) = 6xy$ subject to the constraint $2x + y = 20$. State where it occurs and whether it is a maximum or a minimum. [6.5]

31. Find the point on the plane $4x + y + 2z = 12$ that is closest to the origin. [6.5]

32. Find the absolute maximum and minimum values of $f(x, y) = x^2 - y^2$ subject to the constraints $-1 \le x \le 3$ and $-1 \le y \le 2$, and state where each occurs. [6.5]

Evaluate. [6.6]

33. $\displaystyle\int_0^1 \int_1^2 x^2 y^3\, dy\, dx$ **34.** $\displaystyle\int_0^1 \int_{x^2}^{x} (x - y)\, dy\, dx$

35. **Business: demographics.** The density of students living in a region near a university is modeled by

$$p(x, y) = 9 - x^2 - y^2,$$

where x and y are in miles and p is the number of students per square mile, in hundreds. Assume the university is located at $(0, 0)$ in the following graph representing the region. [6.6]

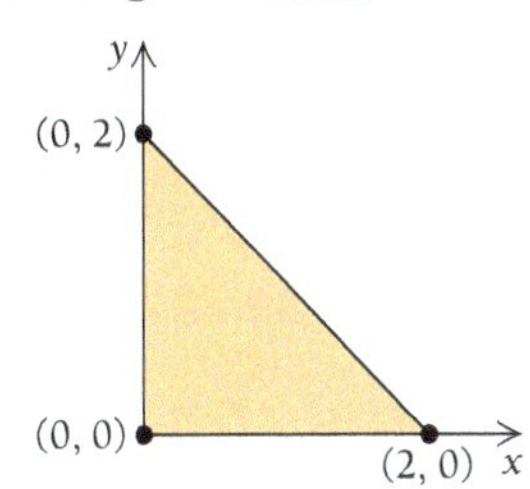

a) Find the number of students who live in the region.

b) Find the average number of students per square mile of the region.

SYNTHESIS

36. Evaluate $\displaystyle\int_0^2 \int_{1-2x}^{1-x} \int_0^{\sqrt{2-x^2}} z\, dz\, dy\, dx$. [6.6]

37. **Business: minimizing surface area.** A beverage can be packaged in either a rectangular container with a square top and bottom or a cylindrical can. Each container is designed to have the minimum surface area for its shape. For a volume of 26 in^3, which container will have the smaller surface area and by how much? [6.3, 6.5]

38. Nature uses spheres, such as oranges and grapefruits, to "package" juices. How does the surface area of a spherical container compare to that of a cylindrical container of the same volume (see Exercise 37)?

Technology Connection

39. Find the average value of $f(x, y) = x + y$ over the region bounded by $0 \le y \le \sqrt{2 - x}$ and $0 \le x \le 2$.

Chapter 6 Test

Given $f(x, y) = 2x^3y + y$, find each of the following.

1. $f(-1, 2)$
2. $\frac{\partial f}{\partial x}$
3. $\frac{\partial f}{\partial y}$
4. $\frac{\partial^2 f}{\partial x^2}$
5. $\frac{\partial^2 f}{\partial x\, \partial y}$
6. $\frac{\partial^2 f}{\partial y\, \partial x}$
7. $\frac{\partial^2 f}{\partial y^2}$

8. Let $z = f(x, y) = y - x^2$.
   a) Use differentials to estimate Δz when $x = 1, y = 5, \Delta x = 0.03$, and $\Delta y = 0.1$.
   b) Find Δz by evaluating $f(x + \Delta x, y + \Delta y) - f(x, y)$.

9. Find the relative maximum and minimum values of $f(x, y) = x^3 + y^3 - 3x - 12y$, and specify where each occurs.

10. **Business: predicting total sales.** Consider the data in the following table regarding the total sales of Miracle Fashions during the first three years of operation.

Year, x	Sales, y (in millions)
1	$10
2	15
3	19

   a) Find the regression line, $y = mx + b$.
   b) Use the regression line to estimate sales in the fourth year.
   c) Find the exponential regression curve, $y = ae^{kx}$.
   d) Use the exponential regression curve to estimate sales in the fourth year.

11. Find the maximum value of
$$f(x, y) = 6xy - 4x^2 - 3y^2$$
subject to the constraint $x + 3y = 19$, and specify where it occurs.

12. Evaluate $\int_0^3 \int_1^3 4x^3y^2\, dx\, dy$, and determine the average value of the integrand over the region R defined by the bounds of integration.

13. Evaluate $\int_{-1}^2 \int_{x^2}^{x+2} xy\, dy\, dx$.

SYNTHESIS

14. **Business: maximizing production.** Southwest Appliances has the following Cobb–Douglas production function for a certain product:
$$p(x, y) = 50x^{2/3}y^{1/3},$$
where x is the amount spent on labor and y is capital, both measured in dollars. Suppose Southwest can make a total investment in labor and capital of $600,000. How should it allocate the investment between labor and capital in order to maximize production?

15. Find the largest possible volume of a rectangular box for which the length x, width y, and height z (all in inches) satisfy $x + y + 3z = 120$.

Technology Connection 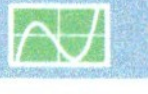

16. Find the average value of $f(x, y) = \sqrt{x + 2y}$ over the region R in the xy-plane defined by $0 \le x \le 3$ and $0 \le y \le 5$.

EXTENDED TECHNOLOGY APPLICATION 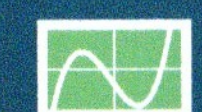

Minimizing Employees' Travel Time in a Building

If employees spend considerable time moving between offices, a building designed to minimize travel time can save a company money. To minimize travel time between the most remote points in a square multilevel building, we can use Lagrange multipliers to help design the building.

Assume that each floor has a square grid of hallways, as shown in the figure at the lower right, and suppose that you are at point P in the top northeast corner of the twelfth floor of this building. How long will it take you to reach point Q, the most remote point at the southwest corner on the first floor?

Let's call the time t, measured in seconds. We find a formula for t in two steps:

1. You have to go from the twelfth floor to the first floor. This is a move in a vertical direction.
2. You need to cross horizontally from one corner of the building to the other corner.

Let h represent the height, in feet, of point P above the ground floor and a represent the speed at which you can travel in a vertical direction (elevator speed), in feet per second. Your vertical travel time is h/a.

The horizontal travel time is the time required to navigate one level of the square grid of hallways (from R to Q in the figure). If each floor is a square with side of length k, then the distance from R to Q is $2k$. If the walking speed is b, in feet per second, then the horizontal time is $2k/b$.

Thus, the time it takes to go from P to Q is a function of h and k, given by

$$\begin{aligned} t(h, k) &= \text{vertical time} + \text{horizontal time} \\ &= \frac{h}{a} + \frac{2k}{b}, \end{aligned}$$

where a and b, the elevator speed and the walking speed, are constants.

Suppose we must choose between two (or more) building plans with the same total floor area, but with different dimensions.

Will the travel time differ for the two buildings? First, what is the total floor area of a given building?

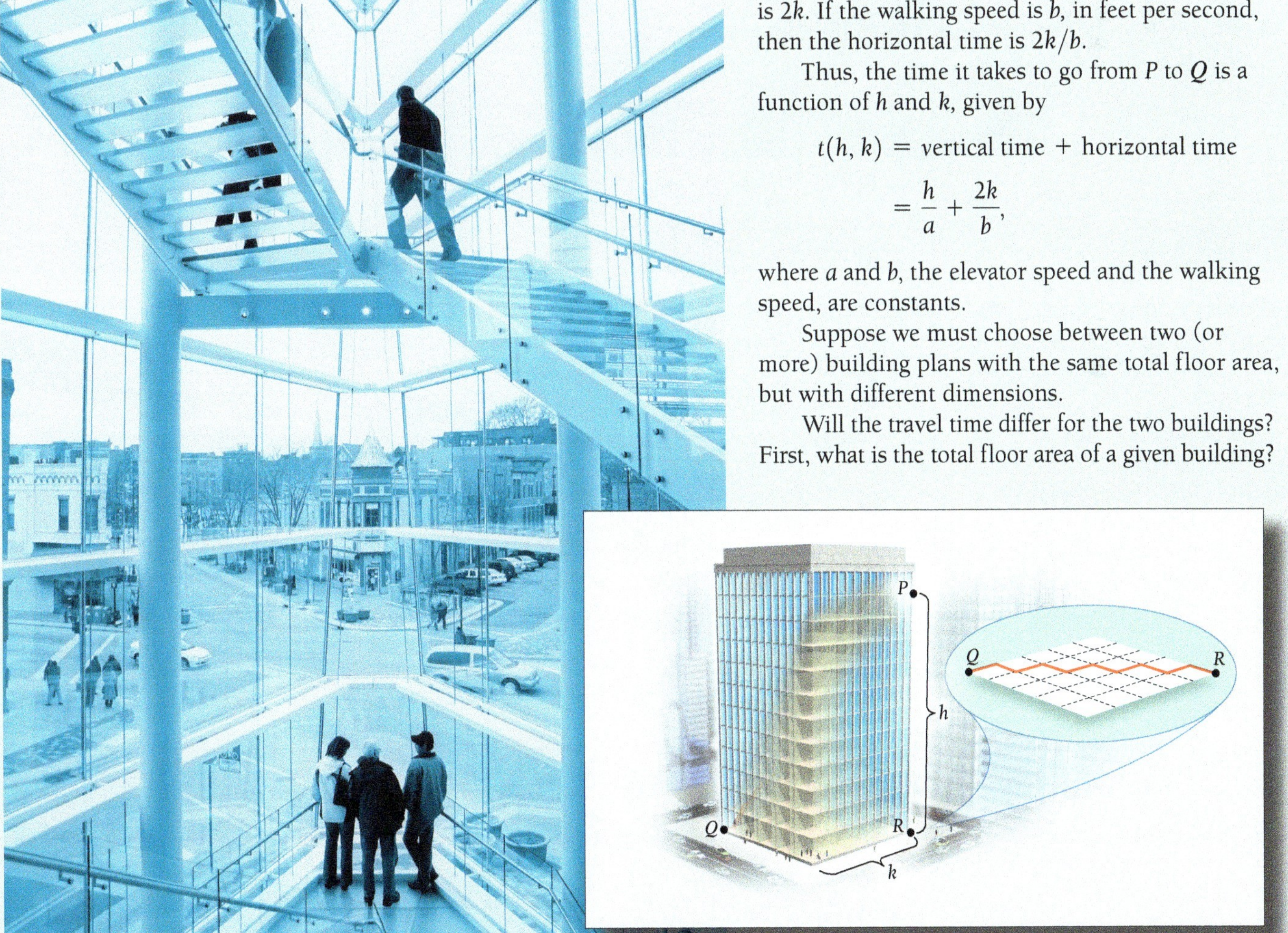

Suppose the building has n floors, each a square with sides k feet long. Then the total floor area is given by

$$A = nk^2.$$

If h is the height of point P and c is the height of each floor—that is, the distance from the carpeting on one floor to the carpeting on the floor above—then $n = 1 + h/c$, and we have the constraint

$$A = (1 + h/c)k^2.$$

Let's return to the problem of two buildings with the same total floor area, but with different dimensions, and see what happens to the travel time, $t(h, k)$.

Exercises

1. Using the TABLE feature of a calculator or spreadsheet software, complete the table below. For each case, let the elevator speed $a = 10$ ft/sec, the walking speed $b = 4$ ft/sec, and the height of each floor $c = 15$ ft. Each case in the table covers two situations, with the total floor area essentially the same.

2. Do different dimensions, with a fixed floor area, yield different travel times?

In Exercises 3–5, assume that you are finding the dimensions of a multilevel building with a square base that will minimize travel time t between the most remote points in the building. Each floor has a square grid of hallways. The height of point P is h, and the length of a side of each floor is k. The elevator speed is 10 ft/sec and the average speed of a person walking is 4 ft/sec. The total floor area of the building is 40,000 ft^2. The height of each floor is 12 ft.

3. Use the information given to find a formula for the function $t(h, k)$.

4. Find a formula for the constraint.

5. Use the method of Lagrange multipliers to find the dimensions of the building that minimizes travel time t between the most remote points in the building.

6. Use a 3D graphics program to graph the equation in Exercise 3 subject to the constraint in Exercise 4. Then visually check the results you found analytically.

Case	Building	n	k	A	h	$t(h, k)$
1	B1	2	40	3200	15	21.5
	B2	3	32.66	3200	30	19.4
2	B1	2	60	7200		
	B2	3	48.99			
3	B1	4	40			
	B2	5	35.777			
4	B1	5	60			
	B2	10	42.426			
5	B1	5	150			
	B2	10	106.066			
6	B1	10	40			
	B2	17	30.679			
7	B1	10	80			
	B2	17	61.357			
8	B1	17	40			
	B2	26	32.344			
9	B1	17	50			
	B2	26	40.43			
10	B1	26	77			
	B2	50	55.525			

Cumulative Review

1. For $f(x) = x^2 - 5$, find $f(x + h)$ and $\frac{f(x+h) - f(x)}{h}$. [1.3]

2. a) Graph:
$$f(x) = \begin{cases} 5 - x, & \text{for } x \neq 2, \\ -3, & \text{for } x = 2. \end{cases}$$
b) Find $\lim_{x\to 2} f(x)$.
c) Find $f(2)$.
d) Is f continuous at 2? [1.2]

3. a) Graph: $g(x) = \begin{cases} 9 - x^2, & x \leq 1, \\ x + 7, & x > 1. \end{cases}$
b) Find $\lim_{x\to 1} g(x)$.
c) Find $g(1)$.
d) Is g continuous at 1? [1.2]

Find each limit, if it exists. If a limit does not exist, state that fact. [1.1], [1.2]

4. $\lim_{x\to 1} \sqrt{x^3 + 8}$

5. $\lim_{x\to -4} \frac{x^2 - 16}{x + 4}$

6. $\lim_{x\to 3} \frac{4}{x - 3}$

7. $\lim_{x\to\infty} \frac{12x - 7}{3x + 2}$

8. $\lim_{x\to\infty} \frac{2x^3 - x}{8x^5 - x^2 + 1}$

9. If $f(x) = x^2 + 3$, find $f'(x)$ by determining $\lim_{h\to 0} \frac{f(x+h) - f(x)}{h}$. [1.4]

For Exercises 10–12, refer to the following graph of $y = g(x)$.

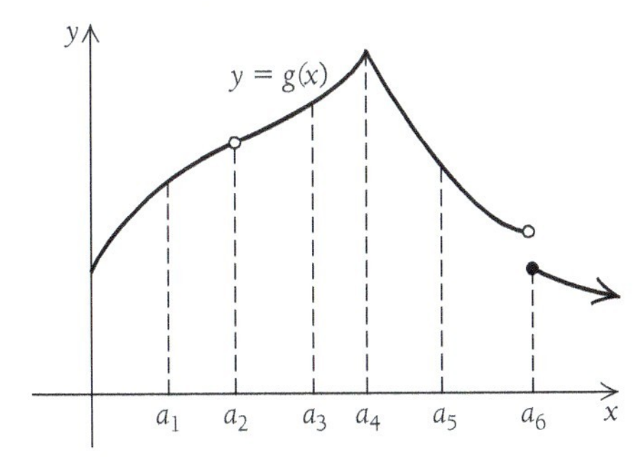

10. For what members of the domain does g have no limit? [1.1]

11. For what members of the domain is g discontinuous? [1.2]

12. For what members of the domain does g' not exist? [1.4]

Differentiate.

13. $y = x^2 - 7x + 3$ [1.5]

14. $y = x^{1/4}$ [1.5]

15. $f(x) = x^{-6}$ [1.5]

16. $f(x) = \sqrt[3]{2x^5 - 8}$ [1.7]

17. $f(x) = \frac{5x^3 + 4}{2x - 1}$ [1.6]

18. $y = \ln(x^2 + 5)$ [2.3]

19. $y = e^{3x}(x^2 + 4x)$ [1.6], [1.7]

20. $y = e^{3x} + x^2$ [2.2]

21. $y = e^{\sqrt{x-3}}$ [1.7], [2.2]

22. $f(x) = \ln(e^x - 4)$ [1.7], [2.3]

23. For $y = x^2 - \frac{2}{x}$, find d^2y/dx^2. [1.5], [1.8]

24. **Business: average cost.** Doubletake Clothing finds that the cost, in dollars, of producing x pairs of jeans is given by $C(x) = 320 + 9\sqrt{x}$. Find the rate at which the average cost is changing, to the nearest cent, when 100 pairs of jeans have been produced. [1.5]

25. Find an equation of the line tangent to the graph of $y = e^x - x^2 - 3$ at the point $(0, -2)$. [1.4], [2.2]

26. Find the x-value(s) at which the line tangent to $f(x) = x^3 - 2x^2$ has a slope of -1. [1.4]

Sketch the graph of each function. List and label the coordinates of any extrema and points of inflection. State where the function is increasing or decreasing, where it is concave up or concave down, and where any asymptotes occur. [3.2–3.4]

27. $f(x) = x^3 - 3x + 1$

28. $f(x) = \ln(x^2 + 2x + 5)$

29. $f(x) = \frac{8x}{x^2 + 1}$

30. $f(x) = 4xe^{-3x}$

Find the absolute maximum and minimum values, if they exist, over the indicated interval. If no interval is indicated, consider the entire real number line. [3.4]

31. $f(x) = 3x^2 - 6x - 4$

32. $f(x) = xe^{1-x}$

33. $f(x) = \frac{1}{3}x^3 - x^2 - 3x + 5;\quad [-2, 0]$

34. Business: maximizing profit. Detailed Clothing's total revenue, $R(x)$, and total cost, $C(x)$, in dollars, from the sale of x custom sweatshirts are given by

$$R(x) = 4x^2 + 11x + 110,$$
$$C(x) = 4.2x^2 + 5x + 10.$$

Find the number of sweatshirts, x, that must be produced and sold in order to maximize profit. [3.5]

35. Business: minimizing inventory costs. Smash Electronics sells 450 sets of headphones each year. It costs $4 to store a set for a year. When placing an order, there is a fixed cost of $1 plus $0.75 for each set. How many times per year should the store reorder headphones, and in what lot size, in order to minimize inventory costs? [3.5]

36. Let $y = 3x^2 - 2x + 1$. Use differentials to find the approximate change in y when $x = 2$ and $\Delta x = 0.05$. [3.6]

37. Let $f(x) = x^3$. [3.6]

a) Find the linearization, $L(x)$, of f at $a = 4$.
b) Use the result from part (a) to estimate $f(4.2)$.

38. Economics: elasticity of demand. Consider the demand function given by

$$q = D(x) = 240 - 20x,$$

where q is the quantity of coffee mugs demanded at a price of x dollars per mug. [3.7]

a) Find the elasticity.
b) Find the elasticity at $x = 2$, and state whether the demand is elastic or inelastic.
c) Find the elasticity at $x = 9$, and state whether the demand is elastic or inelastic.
d) At a price of $2, will a small increase in price cause total revenue to increase or decrease?
e) Find the value of x for which the total revenue is a maximum.

39. Business: approximating cost overage. A square plot of ground measures 75 ft by 75 ft, with a tolerance of ± 4 in. Landscapers are going to cover the plot with grass sod. Each slab of sod costs $8 and covers 9 ft^2. [3.6]

a) Use differentials to estimate the change in area when the measurement tolerance is taken into acount.
b) How many extra slabs of sod should be bought and how much extra will this cost?

Differentiate. [3.8]

40. $f(x) = \dfrac{x^5 e^{2x}}{\sqrt{x+4}}$

41. $f(x) = \dfrac{(x^3 + 2x + 5)\sqrt{3x - e^{3x}}}{e^{4x^2 - 3x}}$

42. Differentiate implicitly to find dy/dx if $x^3 + x/y = 7$. [3.8]

43. Related rates. Landscapers have raked leaves into a large circular pile of constant height. As they bag the leaves, the pile shrinks in size at a rate of 10 ft^2 per minute. What is the rate of change in the radius when the pile is 20 ft in diameter? [3.9]

Evaluate.

44. $\int_{-1}^{0} (2e^x + 1)\, dx$ [4.3]

45. $\int (x^2 + 1)(2x - 3)\, dx$ [4.1]

46. $\int x^3 e^{x^4}\, dx$ [4.5]

47. $\int 2xe^{-5x}\, dx$ [4.6]

48. $\int_{-1}^{2} 3x(x^2 + 1)^4\, dx$ [4.5]

49. Let $f(x) = x^3 + x + 6$. [4.4]

a) Find the area between the graph of f and the x-axis, over $[1, 5]$.
b) Find the average value of f over $[1, 5]$.

50. Find the area between the graphs of $y = x^2 + 2$ and $y = 3x + 6$. [4.4]

51. The table below shows Julia's speeds (in mi/hr) at 1-min intervals during the first 10 min of her morning run. Approximate the total distance Julia traveled (in miles) by finding L_{10} and R_{10} and their average. (*Hint:* 1 min $= \frac{1}{60}$ hr.) [4.7]

Time (1-min intervals)	Speed (mi/hr)
0	0
1	8
2	9
3	9
4	10
5	9.5
6	8.5
7	6
8	6
9	7
10	8

52. Approximate the value of $\int_0^3 \sqrt{e^x + 1}\, dx$ to three decimal places by finding T_6. [4.7]

53. Rent control. Demand for apartments in Hoover Estates is given by $D(x) = 1800 - 4x$, and supply is given by $S(x) = 750 + 20x$, where x is in hundreds of apartments and $D(x)$ and $S(x)$ give the rent, in dollars per month per apartment. [5.1]

a) Find the equilibrium point.
b) Find the consumer surplus and the producer surplus.
c) Suppose a maximum rent of $1450 per month is imposed by the city council. Find the point (x_C, p_C) where the price ceiling intersects the supply function.
d) Find the new consumer surplus and new producer surplus at (x_C, p_C).
e) Find the deadweight loss.

54. Business: value of a fund. Leigh Ann wants to have \$50,000 in 10 yr. [5.2]

a) She makes a one-time deposit at an APR of 5.45%, compounded continuously. Find the amount she should deposit.
b) Calculate the interest earned in part (a).

55. Business: contract buyout. An athlete has an 8-yr contract that pays her \$200,000 per year. She invests the money at an APR of 4.85%, compounded continuously. After 5 yr, the team offers to buy out the remainder of her contract. What is the lowest amount she should accept? [5.2]

56. Determine whether the following improper integral is convergent or divergent, and calculate its value if it is convergent:

$$\int_2^\infty \frac{3}{x^2}\,dx. \text{ [5.3]}$$

57. A jar contains 12 yellow candies, 15 red candies, and 20 green candies. A single candy is chosen at random. [5.4]

a) Find the probability that a yellow candy is chosen.
b) Find the probability that a green candy is not chosen.
c) Find the probability that a red or green candy is chosen.
d) Find the probability that a blue candy is chosen.

58. Business: distribution of weights. The weight, in pounds, of an economy-size bag of a certain cereal is uniformly distributed between 2 lb and 2.25 lb. Find the probability that a randomly chosen bag of this cereal weighs between 2.07 lb and 2.1 lb. [5.4]

59. Business: wait times. The wait time t, in minutes, between customers at Teri's Book Nook can be modeled by the probability density function $f(t) = 0.45e^{-0.45t}$, for $0 \le t < \infty$. [5.5]

a) What is the probability that the wait time is at most 2 min?
b) What is the probability that the wait time is greater than 5 min?

60. Business: distribution of salaries. The salaries paid by a high-tech start-up are normally distributed with mean $\mu = \$75{,}000$ and standard deviation $\sigma = \$6000$. [5.5]

a) Find the probability that a randomly chosen employee earns between \$72,000 and \$85,000.
b) An executive at the start-up earns \$90,000 per year. In what percentile does this salary place the executive?
c) A new employee insists on a salary in the top 2%. What is the minimum salary that this employee would accept?

61. Find the volume of the solid of revolution generated by rotating the region under the graph of $y = e^{-x}$, from $x = 0$ to $x = 5$, around the x-axis. [5.6]

62. Find the volume of the solid of revolution generated by rotating the region under the graph of $y = (x^2 + 1)^2$, from $x = 0$ to $x = 2$, around the y-axis. [5.6]

63. Solve the differential equation $y' + 4xy = 3x$, where $y = 3$ when $x = -1$. [5.7]

64. Suppose the rate of change of y with respect to x is directly proportional to the square root of y, where $y \ge 0$. [5.7]

a) Write a differential equation that models this situation.
b) Find the general solution of the equation from part (a).

Given $f(x, y) = e^y + 4x^2y^3 + 3x$, find each of the following. [6.2]

65. f_x

66. f_{yy}

67. Find the relative maximum and minimum values of $f(x, y) = x^2 + y^2 - xy - 8x + 7y + 9$. [6.3]

68. Maximize $f(x, y) = 4x + 2y - x^2 - y^2 + 4$, subject to the constraint $x + 2y = 9$. [6.5]

69. Consider the data in the following table. [6.4]

Age of Business (in years)	1	3	5
Profit (in tens of thousands of dollars)	4	7	12

a) Find the regression line, $y = mx + b$.
b) Use the regression line to predict the profit when the business is 10 years old.
c) Find the exponential regression curve, $y = ae^{bx}$.
d) Use the exponential regression curve to predict the profit when the business is 10 years old.

70. Evaluate $\int_0^3 \int_{-1}^2 e^x\,dy\,dx$. [6.6]

71. Let $f(x, y) = 2xy$. [6.6]

a) Evaluate $\iint_R 2xy\,dA$, where R is the region bounded by $-1 \le x \le 3$ and $0 \le y \le 5$.
b) Find the average value of f over the region R.

72. Business: demographics. The number of shoppers, in hundreds per square mile, who frequent a mall is modeled by $f(x, y) = 10 - x - y^2$, where x is miles from the mall to the east and y is miles from the mall to the north. The graph below shows a shaded region to the northeast of the mall, which is at (0, 0). Find the total number of shoppers in the region who frequent the mall. [6.6]

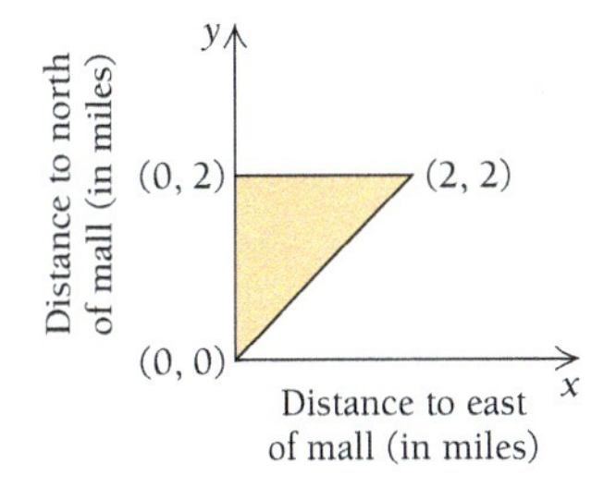

APPENDIX A
Review of Basic Algebra

- Manipulate exponential expressions.
- Multiply and factor algebraic expressions.
- Solve equations, inequalities, and applied problems.

This appendix covers most of the algebraic topics essential to a study of calculus. It can be used in conjunction with Chapter R or as needed throughout the book.

Exponential Notation

Let's review the meaning of

$$a^n,$$

where a is any real number and n is an integer; that is, n is a number in the set $\{\ldots, -3, -2, -1, 0, 1, 2, 3, \ldots\}$. The number a is the **base** and n is the **exponent**.

> For an integer n greater than or equal to 1,
>
> $$a^n = \underbrace{a \cdot a \cdot a \cdots a}_{n \text{ factors}}.$$

In other words, a^n is the product of n **factors**, each of which is a.

EXAMPLE 1 Write equivalent expressions without exponents.

a) 4^3 **b)** $(-2)^5$ **c)** $(-2)^4$ **d)** -2^4 **e)** $\left(\frac{1}{2}\right)^3$

Solution

a) $4^3 = 4 \cdot 4 \cdot 4 = 64$

b) $(-2)^5 = (-2)(-2)(-2)(-2)(-2) = -32$

c) $(-2)^4 = (-2)(-2)(-2)(-2) = 16$

d) $-2^4 = -(2^4) = -(2)(2)(2)(2) = -16$ The base is 2, not -2.

e) $\left(\frac{1}{2}\right)^3 = \frac{1}{2} \cdot \frac{1}{2} \cdot \frac{1}{2} = \frac{1}{8}$

1 ✓

Quick Check 1 ✓
Write equivalent expressions without exponents.
a) 3^5
b) $(-5)^2$
c) $\left(\frac{2}{3}\right)^4$

We define an exponent of 1 as follows:

> For any real number a, $a^1 = a$.

In other words, any real number to the first power is that number itself.

We define an exponent of 0 as follows:

> For any nonzero real number a, $a^0 = 1$.

EXAMPLE 2 Write equivalent expressions without exponents.

a) $(-2x)^0$ **b)** $(-2x)^1$ **c)** $\left(\frac{1}{2}\right)^0$ **d)** $-e^0$ **e)** e^1 **f)** $\left(\frac{1}{2}\right)^1$

Quick Check 2 ✓

Write equivalent expressions without exponents.

a) $\left(\frac{2}{5}\right)^0$

b) $\left(\frac{2}{5}\right)^1$

c) -4^0

Solution

a) $(-2x)^0 = 1$ b) $(-2x)^1 = -2x$ c) $\left(\frac{1}{2}\right)^0 = 1$

d) $-e^0 = -1$ e) $e^1 = e$ f) $\left(\frac{1}{2}\right)^1 = \frac{1}{2}$ **2 ✓**

The meaning of a negative integer as an exponent is as follows:

> For any nonzero real number a, $a^{-n} = \left(\frac{1}{a}\right)^n = \frac{1}{a^n}$.

Any nonzero real number a to the $-n$ power is the reciprocal of a^n.

EXAMPLE 3 Write equivalent expressions without negative exponents.

a) 2^{-5} b) $\left(\frac{3}{4}\right)^{-2}$ c) $2x^{-5}$ d) e^{-k} e) $\frac{1}{t^{-1}}$

Quick Check 3 ✓

Write equivalent expressions without negative exponents.

a) 3^{-2}

b) $\frac{1}{4^{-3}}$

c) $8x^{-5}$

Solution

a) $2^{-5} = \frac{1}{2^5} = \frac{1}{2 \cdot 2 \cdot 2 \cdot 2 \cdot 2} = \frac{1}{32}$ b) $\left(\frac{3}{4}\right)^{-2} = \left(\frac{4}{3}\right)^2 = \frac{4^2}{3^2} = \frac{16}{9}$

c) $2x^{-5} = \frac{2}{x^5}$ The base is x, not $2x$.

d) $e^{-k} = \frac{1}{e^k}$ e) $\frac{1}{t^{-1}} = \left(\frac{1}{t}\right)^{-1} = t^1 = t$ **3 ✓**

Properties of Exponents

Note the result when we multiply two expressions that have the same base:

$$\begin{aligned} b^5 \cdot b^3 &= (b \cdot b \cdot b \cdot b \cdot b) \cdot (b \cdot b \cdot b) \\ &= b \cdot b \cdot b \cdot b \cdot b \cdot b \cdot b \cdot b \\ &= b^8. \end{aligned}$$

We can obtain the same result by adding the exponents.

> **THEOREM 1**
>
> For any nonzero real number a and any integers n and m,
>
> $$a^n \cdot a^m = a^{n+m}.$$
>
> (To multiply when the bases are the same, add the exponents.)

EXAMPLE 4 Multiply:

a) $x^5 \cdot x^6$ b) $x^{-5} \cdot x^6$ c) $2x^{-3} \cdot 5x^{-4}$ d) $r^2 \cdot r$ e) $x^3 \cdot x^7 \cdot x^{-2}$

Quick Check 4 ✓

Multiply.

a) $t^5 \cdot t^3$

b) $4x^2 \cdot 7x^{-5}$

c) $y^4 y^{-9} y$

Solution

a) $x^5 \cdot x^6 = x^{5+6} = x^{11}$ b) $x^{-5} \cdot x^6 = x^{-5+6} = x$

c) $2x^{-3} \cdot 5x^{-4} = 10x^{-3+(-4)} = 10x^{-7}$, or $\frac{10}{x^7}$ d) $r^2 \cdot r = r^{2+1} = r^3$

e) $x^3 \cdot x^7 \cdot x^{-2} = x^{3+7+(-2)} = x^8$ **4 ✓**

Note the result when one expression is divided by another expression with the same base:

$$b^5 \div b^2 = \frac{b^5}{b^2} = \frac{b \cdot b \cdot b \cdot b \cdot b}{b \cdot b}$$
$$= \frac{b \cdot b}{b \cdot b} \cdot b \cdot b \cdot b$$
$$= 1 \cdot b \cdot b \cdot b = b^3.$$

We can obtain the same result by subtracting the exponents.

THEOREM 2

For any nonzero real number a and any integers n and m,

$$\frac{a^n}{a^m} = a^{n-m}.$$

(To divide when the bases are the same, subtract the exponent in the denominator from the exponent in the numerator.)

EXAMPLE 5 Divide:

a) $\frac{a^3}{a^2}$ **b)** $\frac{x^7}{x^7}$ **c)** $\frac{e^3}{e^{-4}}$ **d)** $\frac{e^{-4}}{e^{-1}}$ **e)** $\frac{c^2c^8}{c^{12}}$

Quick Check 5 ✓

Divide.

a) $\frac{d^7}{d^2}$

b) $\frac{t^3}{t^{-5}}$

c) $\frac{u^5u^{12}}{u^3}$

Solution

a) $\frac{a^3}{a^2} = a^{3-2} = a^1 = a$

b) $\frac{x^7}{x^7} = x^{7-7} = x^0 = 1$

This result explains why a base raised to the 0 power is 1.

c) $\frac{e^3}{e^{-4}} = e^{3-(-4)} = e^{3+4} = e^7$

d) $\frac{e^{-4}}{e^{-1}} = e^{-4-(-1)} = e^{-4+1} = e^{-3}$, or $\frac{1}{e^3}$

e) $\frac{c^2c^8}{c^{12}} = c^{2+8-12} = c^{-2}$, or $\frac{1}{c^2}$

5 ✓

Note the result when an expression raised to a power is raised to another power:

$$(b^2)^3 = b^2 \cdot b^2 \cdot b^2 = b^{2+2+2} = b^6.$$

We can obtain the same result by multiplying the exponents. The other results in Theorem 3 can be similarly motivated.

THEOREM 3

For any nonzero real numbers a and b and any integers n and m,

$$(a^n)^m = a^{nm}, \quad (ab)^n = a^nb^n, \quad \text{and} \quad \left(\frac{a}{b}\right)^n = \frac{a^n}{b^n}.$$

EXAMPLE 6 Simplify:

a) $(x^{-2})^3$ **b)** $(e^x)^2$ **c)** $(2x^4y^{-5}z^3)^{-3}$ **d)** $\left(\frac{x^2}{p^4q^5}\right)^3$

Solution

a) $(x^{-2})^3 = x^{-2 \cdot 3} = x^{-6}$, or $\frac{1}{x^6}$

b) $(e^x)^2 = e^{2x}$

Quick Check 6 ✓
Simplify.

a) $(x^5)^7$

b) $(z^{-2})^8$

c) $\left(\frac{4x}{y^2z^{-1}}\right)^4$

c) $(2x^4y^{-5}z^3)^{-3} = 2^{-3}(x^4)^{-3}(y^{-5})^{-3}(z^3)^{-3}$

$$= \frac{1}{2^3}x^{-12}y^{15}z^{-9}, \quad \text{or} \quad \frac{y^{15}}{8x^{12}z^9}$$

d) $\left(\frac{x^2}{p^4q^5}\right)^3 = \frac{(x^2)^3}{(p^4q^5)^3} = \frac{x^6}{(p^4)^3(q^5)^3} = \frac{x^6}{p^{12}q^{15}}$ 6 ✓

Multiplication: The Distributive Law

The distributive law is important when multiplying.

The Distributive Law

For any numbers a, b, and c,

$$a(b + c) = ab + ac.$$

Because subtraction can be regarded as addition of an additive inverse, it follows that

$$a(b - c) = ab - ac.$$

EXAMPLE 7 Multiply:

a) $3(x - 5)$ **b)** $P(1 + r)$ **c)** $(x - 5)(x + 3)$ **d)** $(a + b)(a + b)$

Solution

a) $3(x - 5) = 3 \cdot x - 3 \cdot 5 = 3x - 15$

b) $P(1 + r) = P \cdot 1 + P \cdot r = P + Pr$

c) $(x - 5)(x + 3) = (x - 5)x + (x - 5)3$
$= x \cdot x - 5x + 3x - 5 \cdot 3$
$= x^2 - 2x - 15$

d) $(a + b)(a + b) = (a + b)a + (a + b)b$
$= a \cdot a + ba + ab + b \cdot b$
$= a^2 + 2ab + b^2$ 7 ✓

Quick Check 7 ✓
Multiply.

a) $-4(x - 3)$

b) $x(y + 3z)$

c) $(x + 1)(2x - 7)$

The following formulas, which are obtained using the distributive law, are also useful. All three are used in Example 8.

$$(a + b)^2 = a^2 + 2ab + b^2$$
$$(a - b)^2 = a^2 - 2ab + b^2$$
$$(a - b)(a + b) = a^2 - b^2$$

EXAMPLE 8 Multiply:

a) $(x + h)^2$ **b)** $(2x - t)^2$ **c)** $(3c + d)(3c - d)$

Solution

a) $(x + h)^2 = x^2 + 2xh + h^2$

b) $(2x - t)^2 = (2x)^2 - 2(2x)t + t^2 = 4x^2 - 4xt + t^2$

c) $(3c + d)(3c - d) = (3c)^2 - d^2 = 9c^2 - d^2$ 8 ✓

Quick Check 8 ✓
Multiply.

a) $(2x + 3)^2$

b) $(3x - 1)^2$

c) $(y - 5z)(y + 5z)$

Factoring

To factor an expression, we find an equivalent expression that is a product of two or more expressions.

EXAMPLE 9 Factor:

a) $P + Pi$ **b)** $2xh + h^2$ **c)** $x^2 - 6xy + 9y^2$
d) $x^2 - 5x - 14$ **e)** $6x^2 + 7x - 5$ **f)** $x^2 - 9t^2$

Solution

a) $P + Pi = P \cdot 1 + P \cdot i = P(1 + i)$
b) $2xh + h^2 = h(2x + h)$
} Check by using the distributive law.

c) $x^2 - 6xy + 9y^2 = (x - 3y)^2$

d) $x^2 - 5x - 14 = (x - 7)(x + 2)$ Finding factors of -14 whose sum is -5

e) $6x^2 + 7x - 5 = (2x - 1)(3x + 5)$ Considering ways of factoring the first term—for example, $(2x\ \ )(3x\ \ )$; then looking for factors of -5 that yield the desired product

f) $x^2 - 9t^2 = (x - 3t)(x + 3t)$ Using the formula $(a - b)(a + b) = a^2 - b^2$

9 ✓

Quick Check 9 ✓
Factor.
a) $2m^2n + 4mn^2$
b) $x^2 - 10x + 25$
c) $3x^2 + 10x + 3$
d) $16t^2 - 81u^2$

Some expressions with four terms can be factored by first looking for a common factor that is a binomial (an expression with two terms). This is called **factoring by grouping.**

EXAMPLE 10 Factor:

a) $t^3 + 6t^2 - 2t - 12$ **b)** $x^3 - 7x^2 - 4x + 28$

Solution

a) $t^3 + 6t^2 - 2t - 12 = t^2(t + 6) - 2(t + 6)$ Factoring the first two terms and then the second two terms

$= (t + 6)(t^2 - 2)$ Factoring the common binomial, $(t + 6)$

b) $x^3 - 7x^2 - 4x + 28 = x^2(x - 7) - 4(x - 7)$ Factoring the first two terms and then the second two terms

$= (x - 7)(x^2 - 4)$ Factoring the common binomial, $(x - 7)$

$= (x - 7)(x - 2)(x + 2)$ Using $(a - b)(a + b) = a^2 - b^2$

10 ✓

Quick Check 10 ✓
Factor.
a) $u^3 + 4u^2 + 3u + 12$
b) $x^3 + 2x^2 - x - 2$

Solving Equations

The *Addition Principle* and the *Multiplication Principle* are often used to find solutions to equations. We can add (or subtract) the same number on both sides of an equation and obtain an equivalent equation, that is, a new equation that has the same solutions as the original equation. We can also multiply (or divide) by a nonzero number on both sides of an equation and obtain an equivalent equation.

The Addition Principle

For any real numbers a, b, and c, $a = b$ is equivalent to $a + c = b + c$.

The Multiplication Principle

For any real numbers a, b, and c, with $c \neq 0$, $a = b$ is equivalent to $a \cdot c = b \cdot c$.

When solving a linear equation, we use these principles and other properties of real numbers to get the variable alone on one side. Then it is easy to determine the solution.

EXAMPLE 11 Solve: $-\frac{5}{6}x + 10 = \frac{1}{2}x + 2$.

Solution We first multiply by 6 on both sides to clear the fractions:

$$6\left(-\tfrac{5}{6}x + 10\right) = 6\left(\tfrac{1}{2}x + 2\right)$$

$$6\left(-\tfrac{5}{6}x\right) + 6\cdot 10 = 6\left(\tfrac{1}{2}x\right) + 6\cdot 2 \qquad \text{Using the distributive law}$$

$$-5x + 60 = 3x + 12 \qquad \text{Simplifying}$$

$$60 = 8x + 12 \qquad \text{Using the Addition Principle: adding } 5x \text{ on both sides}$$

$$48 = 8x \qquad \text{Adding } -12\text{, or subtracting 12, on both sides}$$

$$\tfrac{1}{8}\cdot 48 = \tfrac{1}{8}\cdot 8x \qquad \text{Using the Multiplication Principle}$$

$$6 = x.$$

The variable is now isolated on one side, and we see that 6 is the solution. You can check by substituting 6 into the original equation. **11 ✓**

Quick Check 11 ✓
Solve:
$3x - 15 = \frac{1}{2}x + 4$.

Another principle for solving equations is the *Principle of Zero Products.*

The Principle of Zero Products

For any numbers a and b, if $ab = 0$, then $a = 0$ or $b = 0$; and if $a = 0$ or $b = 0$, then $ab = 0$.

To solve an equation using this principle, we must have 0 on one side and the other side must be a product. Solutions are then obtained by setting each factor equal to 0 and solving the resulting equations.

EXAMPLE 12 Solve: $3x(x - 2)(5x + 4) = 0$.

Solution We have

$$3x(x - 2)(5x + 4) = 0$$

$$3x = 0 \quad \text{or} \quad x - 2 = 0 \quad \text{or} \quad 5x + 4 = 0 \qquad \text{Using the Principle of Zero Products}$$

$$\tfrac{1}{3}\cdot 3x = \tfrac{1}{3}\cdot 0 \quad \text{or} \quad x = 2 \quad \text{or} \quad 5x = -4 \qquad \text{Solving each equation separately}$$

$$x = 0 \quad \text{or} \quad x = 2 \quad \text{or} \quad x = -\tfrac{4}{5}.$$

The solutions are 0, 2, and $-\frac{4}{5}$. **12 ✓**

Quick Check 12 ✓
Solve:
$2x(3x - 1)(x + 5) = 0$.

Note that the Principle of Zero Products applies ***only*** when a product is 0.

EXAMPLE 13 Solve: $4x^3 = x$.

Solution We have

$$4x^3 = x$$

$$4x^3 - x = 0 \qquad \text{Adding } -x \text{ to both sides to get 0 on one side}$$

$$x(4x^2 - 1) = 0$$

$$x(2x - 1)(2x + 1) = 0 \qquad \text{Factoring}$$

$$x = 0 \quad \text{or} \quad 2x - 1 = 0 \quad \text{or} \quad 2x + 1 = 0 \qquad \text{Using the Principle of Zero Products}$$

$$x = 0 \quad \text{or} \quad 2x = 1 \quad \text{or} \quad 2x = -1$$

$$x = 0 \quad \text{or} \quad x = \tfrac{1}{2} \quad \text{or} \quad x = -\tfrac{1}{2}.$$

The solutions are 0, $\frac{1}{2}$, and $-\frac{1}{2}$. **13 ✓**

Quick Check 13 ✓
Solve: $9x^3 = 4x$.

Rational Equations

Expressions like the following are polynomials in one variable:

$$x^2 - 4, \qquad x^3 + 7x^2 - 8x + 9, \qquad t - 19.$$

The **least common multiple, LCM,** of two polynomials is found by factoring and using each factor the greatest number of times that it occurs in any one factorization.

EXAMPLE 14 Find the LCM: $x^2 + 2x + 1$, $5x^2 - 5x$, and $x^2 - 1$.

Solution

$$\left.\begin{aligned} x^2 + 2x + 1 &= (x+1)(x+1); \\ 5x^2 - 5x &= 5x(x-1); \\ x^2 - 1 &= (x+1)(x-1) \end{aligned}\right\} \text{Factoring}$$

$$\text{LCM} = 5x(x+1)(x+1)(x-1)$$

14 ✓

Quick Check 14 ✓
Find the LCM:
$x^2 + 2x + 1$, $x^2 - 9$, and $x^2 + 4x + 3$.

A **rational expression** is a ratio of polynomials. Each of the following is a rational expression:

$$\frac{x^2 - 6x + 9}{x^2 - 4}, \quad \frac{x - 2}{x - 3}, \quad \frac{a + 7}{a^2 - 16}, \quad \frac{5}{5t - 15}.$$

A **rational equation** is an equation containing one or more rational expressions, such as

$$\frac{2}{3} - \frac{5}{6} = \frac{1}{x}, \quad x + \frac{6}{x} = 5, \quad \text{or} \quad \frac{2x}{x - 3} - \frac{6}{x} = \frac{18}{x^2 - 3x}.$$

To solve a rational equation, we clear the equation of fractions by multiplying both sides by the LCM of all the denominators. The resulting equation might have solutions that are *not* solutions of the original equation. Thus, we check all possible solutions in the original equation.

EXAMPLE 15 Solve: $\dfrac{2x}{x - 3} - \dfrac{6}{x} = \dfrac{18}{x^2 - 3x}$.

Solution Note that $x^2 - 3x = x(x - 3)$. The LCM of the denominators is $x(x - 3)$. We multiply by $x(x - 3)$.

$$x(x-3)\left(\frac{2x}{x-3} - \frac{6}{x}\right) = x(x-3)\left(\frac{18}{x^2 - 3x}\right) \qquad \text{Multiplying by the LCM on both sides}$$

$$x(x-3)\cdot\frac{2x}{x-3} - x(x-3)\cdot\frac{6}{x} = x(x-3)\left(\frac{18}{x^2 - 3x}\right) \qquad \text{Using the distributive law}$$

$$\begin{aligned} 2x^2 - 6(x-3) &= 18 \qquad \text{Simplifying} \\ 2x^2 - 6x + 18 &= 18 \\ 2x^2 - 6x &= 0 \\ 2x(x-3) &= 0 \end{aligned}$$

$$2x = 0 \quad or \quad x - 3 = 0$$
$$x = 0 \quad or \quad x = 3$$

The numbers 0 and 3 are possible solutions. But each makes a denominator in the original equation 0. Since division by 0 is not allowed, we see that $x \neq 0$ and $x \neq 3$.

We can also carry out a check, as follows.

Check

For 0: $\dfrac{2x}{x-3} - \dfrac{6}{x} = \dfrac{18}{x^2 - 3x}$

$$\frac{2(0)}{0-3} - \frac{6}{0} \stackrel{?}{=} \frac{18}{0^2 - 3(0)}$$

$$0 - \frac{6}{0} \;\Big|\; \frac{18}{0} \quad \text{UNDEFINED; FALSE}$$

For 3: $\dfrac{2x}{x-3} - \dfrac{6}{x} = \dfrac{18}{x^2 - 3x}$

$$\frac{2(3)}{3-3} - \frac{6}{3} \stackrel{?}{=} \frac{18}{3^2 - 3(3)}$$

$$\frac{6}{0} - 2 \;\Big|\; \frac{18}{0} \quad \text{UNDEFINED; FALSE}$$

The original equation has *no solution*.

EXAMPLE 16 Solve: $\dfrac{x^2}{x-2} = \dfrac{4}{x-2}$.

Solution Note that $x \neq 2$. The LCM of the denominators is $x - 2$. We multiply both sides by $x - 2$.

$$(x-2) \cdot \frac{x^2}{x-2} = (x-2) \cdot \frac{4}{x-2}$$

$$x^2 = 4 \qquad \text{Simplifying}$$

$$x^2 - 4 = 0$$

$$(x+2)(x-2) = 0$$

$$x = -2 \quad or \quad x = 2 \qquad \text{Using the Principle of Zero Products}$$

Check

For 2: $\dfrac{x^2}{x-2} = \dfrac{4}{x-2}$

$$\frac{2^2}{2-2} \stackrel{?}{=} \frac{4}{2-2}$$

$$\frac{4}{0} \;\Big|\; \frac{4}{0} \quad \text{UNDEFINED; FALSE}$$

For -2: $\dfrac{x^2}{x-2} = \dfrac{4}{x-2}$

$$\frac{(-2)^2}{-2-2} \stackrel{?}{=} \frac{4}{-2-2}$$

$$\frac{4}{-4} \;\Big|\; \frac{4}{-4}$$

$$-1 \;\Big|\; -1 \quad \text{TRUE}$$

The number -2 is a solution, but 2 is not. **15 ✓**

Quick Check 15 ✓

Solve: $\dfrac{t^2}{t+3} = \dfrac{9}{t+3}$.

Square Roots and Equations of the Type $x^2 = a$

When we raise a number to the second power, we say that we have *squared* the number. Sometimes, we may need to find the number that was squared. We call this process *finding the square root* of a number.

> **DEFINITION**
>
> The number c is a **square root** of a if $c^2 = a$. The positive square root of a is written $\sqrt{a}$.

For example, 5 is a square root of 25 since $5^2 = 25$, and -5 is also a square root of 25 since $(-5)^2 = 25$. Thus, we can write $\sqrt{25} = 5$ and $\sqrt{25} = -5$. However, -4 does not have a real-number square root since there is no real number c such that $c^2 = -4$. That is, $\sqrt{-4}$ is not a real number.

Properties of the Square Root

- Every positive real number a has two real-number square roots. For $a > 0$, the square roots of a are $\sqrt{a}$ and $-\sqrt{a}$. We often represent the two square roots using the plus-minus symbol: $\pm\sqrt{a}$.
- The number 0 has just one square root, 0.
- Negative numbers do not have real-number square roots.

Consider the equation $x^2 = 25$. The solutions are the two square roots of 25, so $x = \pm 5$. In general, we conclude that if $x^2 = a$, then its solutions are $x = \pm\sqrt{a}$. This is the *Principle of Square Roots.*

The Principle of Square Roots

The solutions of $x^2 = a$ are $x = \pm\sqrt{a}$.

- When $a > 0$, the solutions are two real numbers.
- When $a = 0$, the solution is 0.
- When $a < 0$, there are no real-number solutions.

EXAMPLE 17 Use the Principle of Square Roots to solve each equation.

a) $x^2 = 81$ **b)** $x^2 = 7$ **c)** $x^2 = -16$ **d)** $3x^2 = 12$ **e)** $(2x + 1)^2 = 36$

Solution

a) We have

$$x^2 = 81$$
$$x = \pm\sqrt{81} \quad \text{Using the Principle of Square Roots}$$
$$x = \pm 9. \quad \text{Simplifying}$$

b) We have

$$x^2 = 7$$
$$x = \pm\sqrt{7} \quad \text{Using the Principle of Square Roots}$$
$$x \approx \pm 2.646. \quad \text{Using a calculator}$$

c) Since $-16 < 0$, there is no real-number solution of $x^2 = -16$.

d) We have

$$3x^2 = 12$$
$$\tfrac{1}{3} \cdot 3x = \tfrac{1}{3} \cdot 12 \quad \text{Multiplying both sides by } \tfrac{1}{3}$$
$$x^2 = 4 \quad \text{Simplifying}$$
$$x = \pm\sqrt{4} \quad \text{Using the Principle of Square Roots}$$
$$x = \pm 2. \quad \text{Simplifying}$$

The solutions are 2 and -2.

e) We have

$$(2x + 1)^2 = 36$$
$$2x + 1 = 6 \quad or \quad 2x + 1 = -6 \quad \text{Using the Principle of Square Roots}$$
$$2x = 5 \qquad 2x = -7 \quad \text{Simplifying}$$
$$x = \tfrac{5}{2} \qquad x = -\tfrac{7}{2}.$$

The solutions are $\frac{5}{2}$ and $-\frac{7}{2}$. **16 ✓**

Quick Check 16 ✓
Use the Principle of Square Roots to solve each equation.

a) $x^2 = 121$

b) $t^2 = 13$

c) $4(3 - 5r)^2 = 100$

Solving Inequalities

Two inequalities are **equivalent** if they have the same solutions. For example, the inequalities $x > 4$ and $4 < x$ are equivalent. Principles for solving inequalities are similar to those for solving equations. We can add the same number to both sides of an inequality. We can also multiply on both sides by the same nonzero number, but if that number is negative, we must reverse the inequality sign. The following are the inequality-solving principles.

The Inequality-Solving Principles

For any real numbers a, b, and c,

$$a < b \quad \text{is equivalent to} \quad a + c < b + c.$$

For any real numbers a, b, and any *positive* number c,

$$a < b \quad \text{is equivalent to} \quad ac < bc.$$

For any real numbers a, b, and any *negative* number c,

$$a < b \quad \text{is equivalent to} \quad ac > bc.$$

Similar statements hold for $\leq$ and $\geq$.

EXAMPLE 18 Solve: $17 - 8x \geq 5x - 9$.

Solution We have

$$17 - 8x \geq 5x - 9$$
$$-8x \geq 5x - 26 \qquad \text{Adding } -17 \text{ to both sides}$$
$$-13x \geq -26 \qquad \text{Adding } -5x \text{ to both sides}$$
$$-\tfrac{1}{13}(-13x) \leq -\tfrac{1}{13}(-26) \qquad \text{Multiplying both sides by } -\tfrac{1}{13} \text{ and } \textit{reversing} \text{ the inequality sign}$$
$$x \leq 2.$$

Any number less than or equal to 2 is a solution. 17 ✓

Quick Check 17 ✓
Solve: $3x + 4 < 5x - 2$.

Applications and Problem-Solving Strategies

To solve applied problems, we first translate to mathematical language, usually an equation. Then we solve the equation and check to see whether the solution of the equation is a solution of the problem.

EXAMPLE 19 **Life Science: Weight Gain.** After a 5% gain in weight, a grizzly bear weighs 693 lb. What was its original weight?

Solution We first translate to an equation:

$$\underbrace{\textit{Original weight}}_{w} + \underbrace{5\% \textit{ of the}}_{0.05\ \cdot} \underbrace{\textit{original weight}}_{w} = 693$$
$$w + 0.05 \cdot w = 693.$$

Now we solve the equation:

$$1 \cdot w + 0.05 \cdot w = 693$$
$$w(1 + 0.05) = 693$$
$$1.05w = 693$$
$$w = \frac{693}{1.05} = 660.$$

Check: $660 + 5\% \cdot 660 = 660 + 0.05 \cdot 660 = 660 + 33 = 693$

The original weight of the bear was 660 lb. 18 ✓

Quick Check 18 ✓
Including a sales tax of 6%, the cost of a set of dinner plates is \$132.50. What is the price of the plates without the tax?

EXAMPLE 20 **Business: Total Sales.** Raggs, Ltd., a clothing firm, determines that its total revenue, in dollars, from the sale of x suits is given by

$$200x + 50.$$

Determine the number of suits that the firm must sell to ensure that its total revenue will be more than \$70,050.

Solution We translate to an inequality and solve:

$$200x + 50 > 70{,}050$$
$$200x > 70{,}000 \quad \text{Adding } -50 \text{ to both sides}$$
$$x > 350. \quad \text{Multiplying both sides by } \tfrac{1}{200}$$

Thus, the company's total revenue will exceed \$70,050 when it sells more than 350 suits. **19 ✓**

Quick Check 19 ✓
Shoe Express determines that its total revenue, in dollars, from the sale of x pairs of shoes is given by

$$85x + 120.$$

How many pairs of shoes must the store sell to ensure that its total revenue will be more than \$30,000?

A Exercise Set

Express as an equivalent expression without exponents.

1. 5^3
2. 7^2
3. $(-7)^2$
4. $(-5)^3$
5. $(1.01)^2$
6. $(1.01)^3$
7. $\left(\frac{1}{2}\right)^4$
8. $\left(\frac{1}{4}\right)^3$
9. $(6x)^0$
10. $(6x)^1$
11. $-t^1$
12. $-t^0$
13. $\left(\frac{1}{3}\right)^0$
14. $\left(\frac{1}{3}\right)^1$

Express as an equivalent expression without negative exponents.

15. 3^{-2}
16. 4^{-2}
17. $\left(\frac{1}{2}\right)^{-3}$
18. $\left(\frac{7}{2}\right)^{-2}$
19. $\frac{1}{3^{-2}}$
20. $\frac{1}{4^{-1}}$
21. 10^{-1}
22. 10^{-4}
23. e^{-b}
24. t^{-k}
25. b^{-1}
26. h^{-1}

Multiply.

27. $x^2 \cdot x^3$
28. $t^3 \cdot t^4$
29. $x^{-7} \cdot x$
30. $x^5 \cdot x$
31. $5x^2 \cdot 7x^3$
32. $4t^3 \cdot 2t^4$
33. $x^{-4} \cdot x^7 \cdot x$
34. $x^{-3} \cdot x \cdot x^3$
35. $e^{-t} \cdot e^t$
36. $e^k \cdot e^{-k}$

Divide.

37. $\frac{x^8}{x^2}$
38. $\frac{x^7}{x^3}$
39. $\frac{x^2}{x^5}$
40. $\frac{x^3}{x^7}$
41. $\frac{e^k}{e^k}$
42. $\frac{t^k}{t^k}$
43. $\frac{e^t}{e^4}$
44. $\frac{e^k}{e^3}$
45. $\frac{t^6}{t^{-8}}$
46. $\frac{t^5}{t^{-7}}$
47. $\frac{t^{-9}}{t^{-11}}$
48. $\frac{t^{-11}}{t^{-7}}$
49. $\frac{ab(a^2b)^3}{ab^{-1}}$
50. $\frac{x^2y^3(xy^3)^2}{x^{-3}y^2}$

Simplify.

51. $(t^{-2})^3$
52. $(t^{-3})^4$
53. $(e^x)^4$
54. $(e^x)^5$
55. $(2x^2y^4)^3$
56. $(2x^2y^4)^5$
57. $(3x^{-2}y^{-5}z^4)^{-4}$
58. $(5x^3y^{-7}z^{-5})^{-3}$
59. $(-3x^{-8}y^7z^2)^2$
60. $(-5x^4y^{-5}z^{-3})^4$
61. $\left(\frac{cd^3}{2q^2}\right)^4$
62. $\left(\frac{4x^2y}{a^3b^3}\right)^3$

Multiply.

63. $5(x - 7)$
64. $x(1 + t)$
65. $(x - 5)(x - 2)$
66. $(x - 4)(x - 3)$
67. $(a - b)(a^2 + ab + b^2)$
68. $(x^2 - xy + y^2)(x + y)$
69. $(2x + 5)(x - 1)$
70. $(3x + 4)(x - 1)$
71. $(a - 2)(a + 2)$
72. $(3x - 1)(3x + 1)$
73. $(5x + 2)(5x - 2)$
74. $(t - 1)(t + 1)$
75. $(a - h)^2$
76. $(a + h)^2$
77. $(5x + t)^2$
78. $(7a - c)^2$
79. $5x(x^2 + 3)^2$
80. $-3x^2(x^2 - 4)(x^2 + 4)$

Use the following equation for Exercises 81–84.

$$\begin{aligned}(x + h)^3 &= (x + h)(x + h)^2\\ &= (x + h)(x^2 + 2xh + h^2)\\ &= (x + h)x^2 + (x + h)2xh + (x + h)h^2\\ &= x^3 + x^2h + 2x^2h + 2xh^2 + xh^2 + h^3\\ &= x^3 + 3x^2h + 3xh^2 + h^3\end{aligned}$$

81. $(a + b)^3$
82. $(a - b)^3$
83. $(x - 5)^3$
84. $(2x + 3)^3$

Factor.

85. $x - xt$
86. $x + xh$
87. $x^2 + 6xy + 9y^2$
88. $x^2 - 10xy + 25y^2$
89. $x^2 - 2x - 15$
90. $x^2 + 8x + 15$
91. $x^2 - x - 20$
92. $x^2 - 9x - 10$
93. $49x^2 - t^2$
94. $9x^2 - b^2$
95. $36t^2 - 16m^2$
96. $25y^2 - 9z^2$
97. $a^3b - 16ab^3$
98. $2x^4 - 32$
99. $a^8 - b^8$
100. $36y^2 + 12y - 35$
101. $10a^2x - 40b^2x$
102. $x^3y - 25xy^3$
103. $2 - 32x^4$
104. $2xy^2 - 50x$
105. $9x^2 + 17x - 2$
106. $6x^2 - 23x + 20$
107. $x^3 + 8$ (*Hint*: See Exercise 68.)
108. $a^3 - 27$ (*Hint*: See Exercise 67.)
109. $y^3 - 64t^3$
110. $m^3 + 1000p^3$
111. $3x^3 - 6x^2 - x + 2$
112. $5y^3 + 2y^2 - 10y - 4$
113. $x^3 - 5x^2 - 9x + 45$
114. $t^3 + 3t^2 - 25t - 75$

Solve.

115. $-7x + 10 = 5x - 11$
116. $-8x + 9 = 4x - 70$
117. $5x - 17 - 2x = 6x - 1 - x$
118. $5x - 2 + 3x = 2x + 6 - 4x$
119. $x + 0.8x = 216$
120. $x + 0.5x = 210$
121. $x + 0.08x = 216$
122. $x + 0.05x = 210$
123. $2x(x + 3)(5x - 4) = 0$
124. $7x(x - 2)(2x + 3) = 0$
125. $x^2 + 1 = 2x + 1$
126. $2t^2 = 9 + t^2$
127. $t^2 - 2t = t$
128. $6x - x^2 = x$
129. $6x - x^2 = -x$
130. $2x - x^2 = -x$
131. $9x^3 = x$
132. $16x^3 = x$
133. $(x - 3)^2 = x^2 + 2x + 1$
134. $(x - 5)^2 = x^2 + x + 3$
135. $\frac{4x}{x + 5} + \frac{20}{x} = \frac{100}{x^2 + 5x}$
136. $\frac{x}{x + 1} + \frac{3x + 5}{x^2 + 4x + 3} = \frac{2}{x + 3}$
137. $\frac{50}{x} - \frac{50}{x - 2} = \frac{4}{x}$
138. $\frac{60}{x} = \frac{60}{x - 5} + \frac{2}{x}$
139. $0 = 2x - \frac{250}{x^2}$
140. $5 - \frac{35}{x^2} = 0$
141. $x^2 = 64$
142. $x^2 = 144$
143. $u^2 = 30$
144. $w^2 = 97$
145. $4t^2 = 49$
146. $100k^2 = 169$
147. $9x^2 = 20$
148. $25y^2 = 3$
149. $5z^2 = 4$
150. $3b^2 = 144$
151. $(3x - 2)^2 = 1$
152. $(6x + 5)^2 = 400$
153. $(2 - 5x)^2 = 10$
154. $(1 - 4y)^2 = 2$
155. $3 - x \le 4x + 7$
156. $x + 6 \le 5x - 6$
157. $5x - 5 + x > 2 - 6x - 8$
158. $3x - 3 + 3x > 1 - 7x - 9$
159. $-7x < 4$
160. $-5x \ge 6$
161. $5x + 2x \le -21$
162. $9x + 3x \ge -24$
163. $2x - 7 < 5x - 9$
164. $10x - 3 \ge 13x - 8$
165. $8x - 9 < 3x - 11$
166. $11x - 2 \ge 15x - 7$
167. $8 < 3x + 2 < 14$
168. $2 < 5x - 8 \le 12$
169. $3 \le 4x - 3 \le 19$
170. $9 \le 5x + 3 < 19$
171. $-7 \le 5x - 2 \le 12$
172. $-11 \le 2x - 1 < -5$

APPLICATIONS

Business and Economics

173. Investment increase. An investment is made at $4\frac{1}{2}\%$, compounded annually. It grows to \$679.25 at the end of 1 yr. How much was invested originally?

174. Investment increase. An investment is made at 7%, compounded annually. It grows to \$856 at the end of 1 yr. How much was invested originally?

175. Total revenue. Sunshine Products determines that the total revenue, in dollars, from the sale of x flowerpots is $3x + 1000$. Determine the number of flowerpots that must be sold so that the total revenue will be more than \$22,000.

176. Total revenue. Beeswax Inc. determines that the total revenue, in dollars, from the sale of x candles is $5x + 1000$. Determine the number of candles that must be sold so that the total revenue will be more than \$22,000.

Life and Physical Sciences

177. Weight gain. After a 6% gain in weight, an elk weighs 508.8 lb. What was its original weight?

178. Weight gain. After a 7% gain in weight, a deer weighs 363.8 lb. What was its original weight?

Social Sciences

179. Population increase. After a 2% increase, the population of Burnside City is 826,200. What was the city's former population?

180. Population increase. After a 3% increase, the student population of Glen Oaks College is 5356. What was the former student population?

General Interest

181. **Grade average.** To get a B in a course, a student's average must be greater than or equal to 80% (at least 80%) and less than 90%. On the first three tests, Claudia scores 78%, 90%, and 92%. Determine the scores on the fourth test that will guarantee her a B.

182. **Grade average.** To get a C in a course, a student's average must be greater than or equal to 70% and less than 80%. On the first three tests, Horace scores 65%, 83%, and 82%. Determine the scores on the fourth test that will guarantee him a C.

183. **Auditorium seating.** The seats at Ardon Auditorium are arranged in a square, with n rows, each containing n seats. If the auditorium can seat 324 people, how many people can be seated in one row?

184. **Tiling a room.** The conference room at the Fireside Hotel is square, and the floor is covered by 5625 equal-size square tiles. How many tiles run along each edge of the room?

185. **Finding one's age.** Gina is 10 years older than her brother Dave. In 4 years, she'll be twice Dave's age. How old are Gina and Dave now?

186. **Inheritance.** Frank gave his eldest child half of his estate, his second-eldest child one-fifth of his estate, and his third-eldest child the remainder. If the second-eldest child received $50,000, how much did the third-eldest child receive?

187. Three consecutive integers sum to 177. What are the three integers?

188. When the same number is subtracted from both the numerator and the denominator of a fraction, the result is $\frac{1}{2}$. What was the original fraction?

189. **Right triangles.** The lengths of the two legs, a and b, of a right triangle are related to the length of its hypotenuse, c, by the Pythagorean formula: $a^2 + b^2 = c^2$. If a right triangle has one leg of length 12 and a hypotenuse of length 13, find the length of the other leg.

190. **Right triangles.** One leg of a right triangle is 3 more than 3 times the length of the other leg. If the hypotenuse has length 25, find the lengths of the two legs.

Answers to Quick Checks

1. **(a)** 243; **(b)** 25; **(c)** $\frac{16}{81}$ **2.** **(a)** 1; **(b)** $\frac{2}{5}$; **(c)** -1
3. **(a)** $\frac{1}{9}$; **(b)** 64; **(c)** $\frac{8}{x^5}$ **4.** **(a)** t^8; **(b)** $\frac{28}{x^3}$; **(c)** $\frac{1}{y^4}$
5. **(a)** d^5; **(b)** t^8; **(c)** u^{14} **6.** **(a)** x^{35}; **(b)** $\frac{1}{z^{16}}$;
(c) $\frac{256x^4z^4}{y^8}$ **7.** **(a)** $-4x + 12$; **(b)** $xy + 3xz$;
(c) $2x^2 - 5x - 7$ **8.** **(a)** $4x^2 + 12x + 9$;
(b) $9x^2 - 6x + 1$; **(c)** $y^2 - 25z^2$ **9.** **(a)** $2mn(m + 2n)$;
(b) $(x - 5)^2$; **(c)** $(x + 3)(3x + 1)$;
(d) $(4t + 9u)(4t - 9u)$ **10.** **(a)** $(u + 4)(u^2 + 3)$;
(b) $(x + 2)(x - 1)(x + 1)$ **11.** $x = \frac{38}{5}$ **12.** $0, \frac{1}{3}, -5$
13. $0, \frac{2}{3}, -\frac{2}{3}$ **14.** $(x + 1)^2(x^2 - 9)$ **15.** $t = 3$
16. **(a)** $x = \pm 11$; **(b)** $t = \pm\sqrt{13}$; **(c)** $r = -\frac{2}{5}, \frac{8}{5}$
17. $x > 3$ **18.** $125 **19.** $x \geq 352$

APPENDIX B
Indeterminate Forms and l'Hôpital's Rule

- Find the limit of the indeterminate form $0/0$ or ∞/∞ using l'Hôpital's Rule.
- Find the limit of the indeterminate form 0^0, 1^∞, or ∞^0 using l'Hôpital's Rule.
- Find the limit of the indeterminate form $\infty - \infty$ using l'Hôpital's Rule.

Indeterminate Forms $0/0$ and ∞/∞ and l'Hôpital's Rule

In Example 3 of Section 1.1, we showed that

$$\lim_{x \to 1} \left(\frac{x^2 - 1}{x - 1} \right) = 2.$$

Note that as x approaches 1, both the numerator and the denominator approach 0. The expression $0/0$ is an *indeterminate form*. Another common indeterminate form, ∞/∞, arises when x approaches some value a and both the numerator and the denominator increase (or decrease) without bound.

When we attempt to evaluate a limit by substitution and get an indeterminate form such as $0/0$ or ∞/∞, the limit may exist, but we must use a method other than direct evaluation to find it. In Chapter 1, we used numerical methods. Here, we use differentiation to find the limit (if it exists) using l'Hôpital's Rule.

L'Hôpital's Rule is named for the French mathematician and author Guillaume de l'Hôpital (1661–1704). The name is pronounced "low-pee-tall."

THEOREM l'Hôpital's Rule

Let f and g be differentiable over an open interval containing $x = a$ (although not necessarily differentiable at a itself). If

$$\lim_{x \to a} \left(\frac{f(x)}{g(x)} \right) = \frac{0}{0} \quad \text{or} \quad \lim_{x \to a} \left(\frac{f(x)}{g(x)} \right) = \frac{\pm\infty}{\pm\infty},$$

and if $\lim_{x \to a} \left(\frac{f'(x)}{g'(x)} \right)$ exists, then

$$\lim_{x \to a} \left(\frac{f(x)}{g(x)} \right) = \lim_{x \to a} \left(\frac{f'(x)}{g'(x)} \right).$$

A simplified proof of l'Hôpital's Rule for the case of the indeterminate form $0/0$ is outlined in Exercise 37.

When using l'Hôpital's Rule, we first check whether $f(x)/g(x)$ gives an indeterminate form by substituting $x = a$. If we obtain an indeterminate form, we differentiate the numerator and the denominator of the original expression separately. We then evaluate $\lim_{x \to a} [f'(x)/g'(x)]$.

EXAMPLE 1 Evaluate

$$\lim_{x \to -3} \left(\frac{x^2 - x - 12}{x + 3} \right).$$

(This is Example 5 in Section 1.2.)

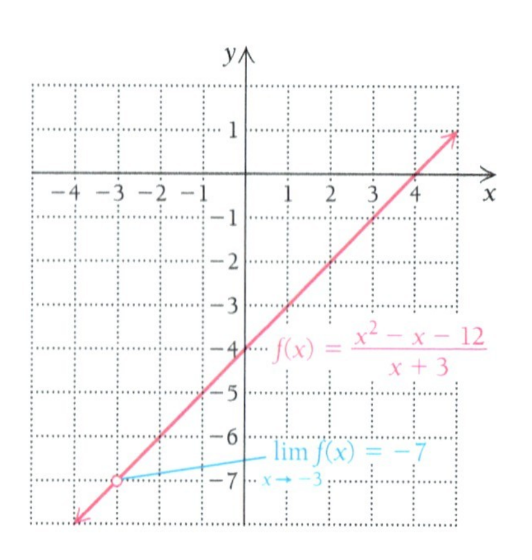

Solution We attempt to evaluate the limit by substituting $x = -3$ into the given expression:

$$\lim_{x \to -3} \left(\frac{x^2 - x - 12}{x + 3} \right) = \frac{(-3)^2 - (-3) - 12}{(-3) + 3}$$

$$= \frac{9 + 3 - 12}{-3 + 3} \quad \text{Simplifying}$$

$$= \frac{0}{0}. \quad \text{This is an indeterminate form.}$$

Using l'Hôpital's Rule, we differentiate the numerator and the denominator, and then find the limit:

$$\lim_{x \to -3} \left(\frac{x^2 - x - 12}{x + 3} \right) = \lim_{x \to -3} \frac{2x - 1}{1} \quad \text{Differentiating the numerator and the denominator}$$

$$= \frac{2(-3) - 1}{1} \quad \text{Substituting}$$

$$= -7.$$

1 ✓

Quick Check 1 ✓

Evaluate $\lim_{x \to 2} \left(\frac{x^3 - 8}{x - 2} \right)$.

EXAMPLE 2 Evaluate $\lim_{x \to \infty} \left(\frac{x^2}{e^{3x}} \right)$.

Solution As x approaches ∞, the expression x^2/e^{3x} approaches the indeterminate form ∞/∞. To use l'Hôpital's Rule, we differentiate the numerator and the denominator of the expression, and then evaluate the limit:

$$\lim_{x \to \infty} \left(\frac{x^2}{e^{3x}} \right) = \lim_{x \to \infty} \left(\frac{2x}{3e^{3x}} \right) \quad \text{Differentiating the numerator and the denominator}$$

$$= \frac{\infty}{\infty}. \quad \lim_{x \to \infty} 2x = \infty \text{ and } \lim_{x \to \infty} 3e^{3x} = \infty$$

Since we obtain the same indeterminate form, ∞/∞, we use l'Hôpital's Rule again:

$$\lim_{x \to \infty} \left(\frac{2x}{3e^{3x}} \right) = \lim_{x \to \infty} \left(\frac{2}{9e^{3x}} \right) \quad \text{Differentiating the numerator and the denominator}$$

$$= \frac{2}{\infty} \quad \lim_{x \to \infty} 2 = 2 \text{ and } \lim_{x \to \infty} 9e^{3x} = \infty$$

$$= 0.$$

Thus, as x approaches ∞, the expression x^2/e^{3x} approaches 0. This indicates that the graph of $y = x^2/e^{3x}$ has a horizontal asymptote at $y = 0$ (the x-axis).

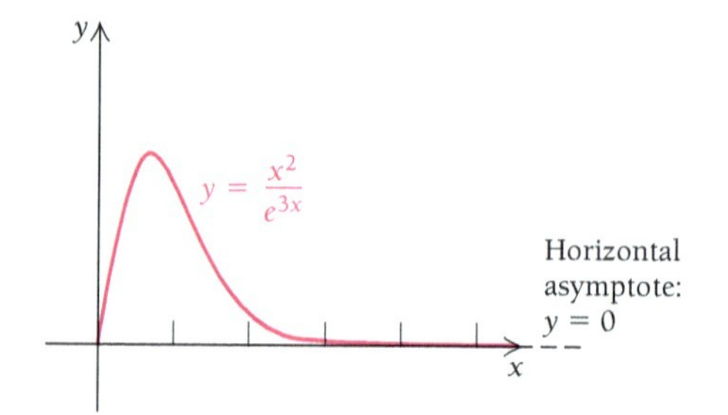

2 ✓

Quick Check 2 ✓

Evaluate $\lim_{x \to \infty} \left(\frac{e^{4x}}{x^4} \right)$.

Indeterminate Forms 0^0, 1^∞, and ∞^0

The expressions 0^0, 1^∞, and ∞^0 are also indeterminate forms. We use logarithms to rewrite such a form as a ratio so that we may use l'Hôpital's Rule. Suppose $y = f(x)^{g(x)}$ and $\lim_{x\to a} f(x)^{g(x)}$ is indeterminate. Using natural logarithms, we have $\ln y = \ln f(x)^{g(x)} = g(x)\ln f(x)$. Although we do not prove it here, if

$$\lim_{x\to a}\left[g(x)\ln f(x)\right] = L,$$

then

$$\lim_{x\to a} f(x)^{g(x)} = e^L.$$

EXAMPLE 3 Evaluate

$$\lim_{h\to 0}(1+h)^{1/h}.$$

Solution As h approaches 0, the base $1 + h$ approaches 1, and the exponent $1/h$ approaches ∞. Thus, we have the indeterminate form 1^∞. We let $y = (1 + h)^{1/h}$ and find the natural logarithm of both sides:

$$y = (1+h)^{1/h}$$

$$\ln y = \ln(1+h)^{1/h}$$

$$\ln y = \frac{1}{h}\ln(1+h) \qquad \text{Using a property of logarithms}$$

$$\ln y = \frac{\ln(1+h)}{h}.$$

As h approaches 0, we have for the numerator, $\ln(1 + h) = \ln(1 + 0) = \ln 1 = 0$, and for the denominator, $h = 0$. Thus, the expression $\ln(1 + h)/h$ approaches the indeterminate form $0/0$, and we use l'Hôpital's Rule:

$$\lim_{h\to 0}(\ln y) = \lim_{h\to 0}\left(\frac{\ln(1+h)}{h}\right)$$

$$= \lim_{h\to 0}\left(\frac{\frac{1}{1+h}}{1}\right) \qquad \text{Differentiating the numerator and the denominator}$$

$$= \lim_{h\to 0}\left(\frac{1}{1+h}\right) \qquad \text{Simplifying}$$

$$= \frac{1}{1+0} = 1. \qquad \text{Evaluating the limit}$$

Since $\lim_{h\to 0}(\ln y) = 1$, we have $\lim_{h\to 0} y = e^1 = e$. Therefore,

$$\lim_{h\to 0}(1+h)^{1/h} = e.$$

3 ✓

Quick Check 3 ✓

Evaluate $\lim_{x\to\infty}\left(1 + \frac{2}{x}\right)^x$.

Indeterminate Form $\infty - \infty$

We can use L'Hôpital's Rule in cases where the limit is of the indeterminate form $\infty - \infty$. The expression is first rewritten as a ratio, and then, if possible, l'Hôpital's Rule is applied.

EXAMPLE 4 Evaluate

$$\lim_{x \to \infty} (\sqrt{x^2 + x} - x).$$

Solution As x approaches ∞, the expression $\sqrt{x^2 + x} - x$ approaches $\infty - \infty$, which is an indeterminate form. Before we can use l'Hôpital's Rule, we must rewrite $\sqrt{x^2 + x} - x$ as a ratio:

$$\begin{aligned}
\sqrt{x^2 + x} - x &= \sqrt{x^2\left(1 + \frac{1}{x}\right)} - x && \text{Factoring} \\
&= x\sqrt{1 + \frac{1}{x}} - x && \text{Assuming } x > 0 \\
&= x\left(\sqrt{1 + \frac{1}{x}} - 1\right) && \text{Factoring} \\
&= \frac{\sqrt{1 + \frac{1}{x}} - 1}{\frac{1}{x}} && \text{Rewriting } x \text{ as } 1/(1/x)
\end{aligned}$$

The expression is now a ratio. Note that as x approaches ∞, both the numerator and the denominator approach 0. Thus, the expression approaches the indeterminate form $0/0$, and we can use l'Hôpital's Rule:

$$\begin{aligned}
\lim_{x \to \infty} \frac{\sqrt{1 + \frac{1}{x}} - 1}{\frac{1}{x}} &= \lim_{x \to \infty} \frac{\frac{1}{2\sqrt{1 + \frac{1}{x}}} \cdot \left(-\frac{1}{x^2}\right)}{-\frac{1}{x^2}} && \text{Differentiating} \\
&= \lim_{x \to \infty} \frac{1}{2\sqrt{1 + \frac{1}{x}}} && \text{Simplifying} \\
&= \frac{1}{2}. && \text{Evaluating the limit}
\end{aligned}$$

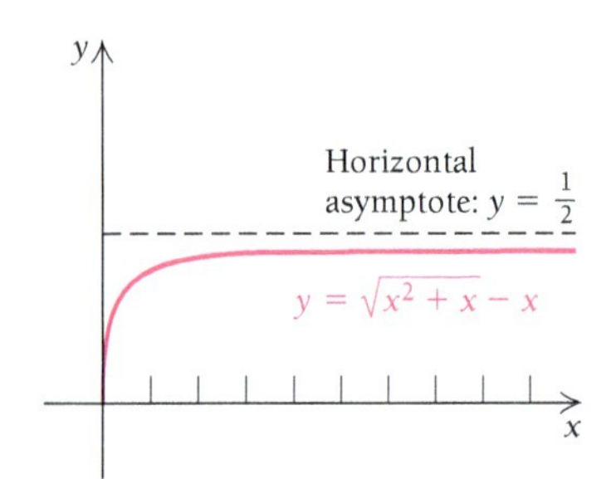

Thus, $\lim_{x \to \infty} (\sqrt{x^2 + x} - x) = \frac{1}{2}$. This indicates that the graph of $y = \sqrt{x^2 + x} - x$ has a horizontal asymptote at $y = \frac{1}{2}$. **4 ✓**

Quick Check 4 ✓

Evaluate $\lim_{x \to \infty} (\sqrt{x^2 + 3x} - x)$.

B Exercise Set

Evaluate each limit. Use l'Hôpital's Rule when necessary.

1. $\lim_{x \to 5} \left(\frac{x^2 - 25}{2x - 10}\right)$
2. $\lim_{x \to -2} \left(\frac{x^2 - 4}{x + 2}\right)$
3. $\lim_{x \to 1} \left(\frac{x^3 + 2x - 3}{x^2 - 1}\right)$
4. $\lim_{x \to 3} \left(\frac{x^3 - x - 24}{x^2 - 9}\right)$
5. $\lim_{x \to -3} \left(\frac{x^2 - 9}{x - 3}\right)$
6. $\lim_{x \to -4} \left(\frac{x^2 + x - 12}{x - 2}\right)$
7. $\lim_{x \to 2} \left(\frac{x^3 + 5x + 1}{2x^2 - 6}\right)$
8. $\lim_{x \to 10} \left(\frac{x^2 + x - 120}{x + 10}\right)$
9. $\lim_{x \to \infty} \left(\frac{4x^2 + x - 3}{2x^2 + 1}\right)$
10. $\lim_{x \to -\infty} \left(\frac{3x^3 + x + 11}{6x^3 + x + 2}\right)$
11. $\lim_{x \to 0} \left(\frac{e^{2x} - 1}{3x}\right)$
12. $\lim_{x \to 0} \left(\frac{e^{4x} + x - 1}{5x}\right)$
13. $\lim_{x \to 0} \left(\frac{2e^{-3x} + x - 2}{4x}\right)$
14. $\lim_{x \to 0} \left(\frac{5e^{-2x} + x - 5}{2x}\right)$
15. $\lim_{x \to 0} \left(\frac{x^2 + x}{e^{3x} - 1}\right)$
16. $\lim_{x \to 0} \left(\frac{4x}{e^{2x} - 1}\right)$
17. $\lim_{x \to 2} \left(\frac{x - 2}{\ln(x - 1)}\right)$
18. $\lim_{x \to -3} \left(\frac{x + 3}{\ln(x + 4)}\right)$

19. $\lim_{x\to 0}(1+2x)^{1/x}$

20. $\lim_{x\to 0}(1-3x)^{1/x}$

21. $\lim_{x\to\infty}\left(1-\frac{4}{x}\right)^x$

22. $\lim_{x\to\infty}\left(1+\frac{5}{x}\right)^x$

23. $\lim_{x\to 0^+} x^x$

24. $\lim_{x\to\infty} \sqrt[x]{x}$

25. $\lim_{x\to\infty}(\sqrt{x^2-x}-x)$

26. $\lim_{x\to\infty}(\sqrt{x^2+5x}-x)$

27. $\lim_{x\to\infty}(\sqrt[3]{x^3+x^2}-x)$

28. $\lim_{x\to\infty}(\sqrt[3]{8x^3+x^2}-2x)$

29. Show that for all k, $\lim_{x\to\infty}\left(1+\frac{k}{x}\right)^x = e^k$.

30. Show that for all k, $\lim_{x\to\infty}(\sqrt{x^2+kx}-x) = \frac{k}{2}$.

31. Evaluate $\lim_{x\to\infty}\left(\frac{1}{\sqrt{x^2+4x}-x}\right)$.

32. Evaluate $\lim_{x\to\infty}\left(\frac{1}{\sqrt{x^2-6x}-x}\right)$.

33. Evaluate $\lim_{x\to\infty}\left(\frac{\sqrt{x^2-4x}-x}{\sqrt{x^2+10x}-x}\right)$.

34. Evaluate $\lim_{x\to\infty}\left(\frac{\sqrt{x^2+7x}-x}{\sqrt{x^2-3x}-x}\right)$.

SYNTHESIS

35. Consider $\lim_{x\to\infty}\left(\frac{x^n}{e^x}\right)$.

a) Evaluate this limit for $n = 3, 4, 5$, and 6.

b) Predict the limit when $n = 100$, and explain how you would demonstrate this using l'Hôpital's Rule.

c) Is there a positive integer n for which this limit is not zero? Why or why not?

36. Consider $\lim_{x\to\infty}\left(\frac{e^{2x}}{e^{3x}}\right)$.

a) Use algebra to simplify the expression; then evaluate the limit.

b) Explain why l'Hôpital's Rule is not needed to find this limit.

37. The proof of l'Hôpital's Rule for the indeterminate form $0/0$ is outlined below. Assume that f and g are differentiable at $x = a$ and that $f(a) = 0$ and $g(a) = 0$, and recall that the derivative of f at $x = a$ can be defined as $f'(a) = \lim_{x\to a}\left(\frac{f(x)-f(a)}{x-a}\right)$. Give a reason that justifies each step.

a) $\lim_{x\to a}\frac{f(x)}{g(x)} = \lim_{x\to a}\frac{f(x)-f(a)}{g(x)-g(a)}$

____

b) $\lim_{x\to a}\frac{f(x)-f(a)}{g(x)-g(a)} = \lim_{x\to a}\frac{\left(\frac{f(x)-f(a)}{x-a}\right)}{\left(\frac{g(x)-g(a)}{x-a}\right)}$

____

c) $\lim_{x\to a}\frac{\left(\frac{f(x)-f(a)}{x-a}\right)}{\left(\frac{g(x)-g(a)}{x-a}\right)} = \frac{\lim_{x\to a}\left(\frac{f(x)-f(a)}{x-a}\right)}{\lim_{x\to a}\left(\frac{g(x)-g(a)}{x-a}\right)}$

____

d) $\frac{\lim_{x\to a}\left(\frac{f(x)-f(a)}{x-a}\right)}{\lim_{x\to a}\left(\frac{g(x)-g(a)}{x-a}\right)} = \frac{f'(a)}{g'(a)}$

____

e) $\frac{f'(a)}{g'(a)} = \lim_{x\to a}\frac{f'(x)}{g'(x)}$

____

38. Find and correct the error in the following limit calculation.

$$\lim_{x\to 2}\left(\frac{x^2-4}{x+2}\right) = \lim_{x\to 2}\left(\frac{2x}{1}\right) = 4.$$

Answers to Quick Checks

1. 12 **2.** ∞ **3.** e^2 **4.** $\frac{3}{2}$

APPENDIX C
Regression and Microsoft Excel

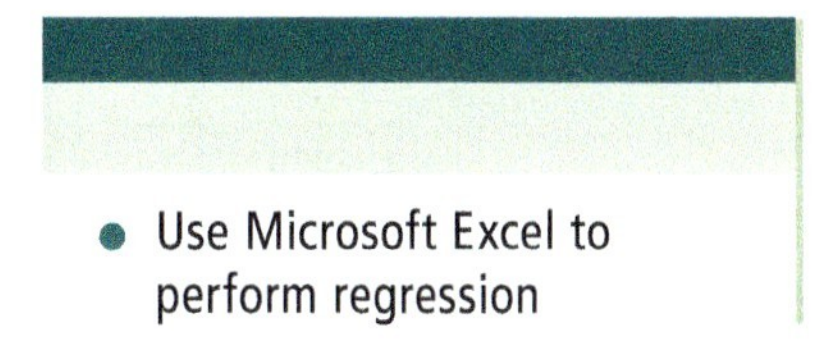

- Use Microsoft Excel to perform regression

Using Excel 2016

Microsoft Excel can be used to enter and plot data and to find lines of best fit using regression. Suppose you are given the following data:

x	0	2	4	5	6
y	3	4.7	6	6.8	8

Step 1: Open a blank workbook and enter the data into two columns, as shown in Fig. 1.

Step 2: Highlight the columns of data (see Fig. 2). Then within the Insert tab, select Scatter in Charts. Next, choose the first option that appears, with the markers shown as distinct points.

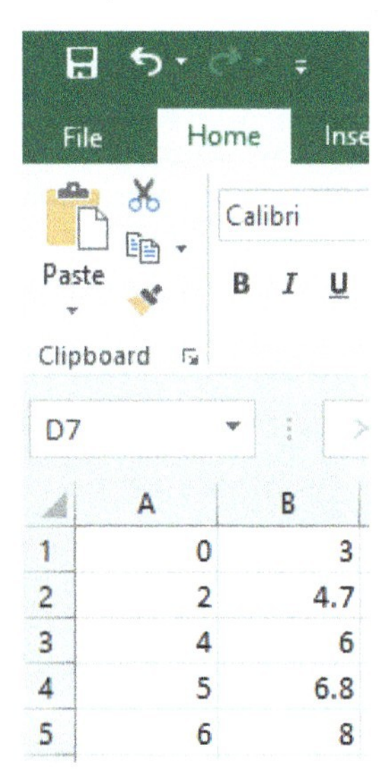

FIGURE 1

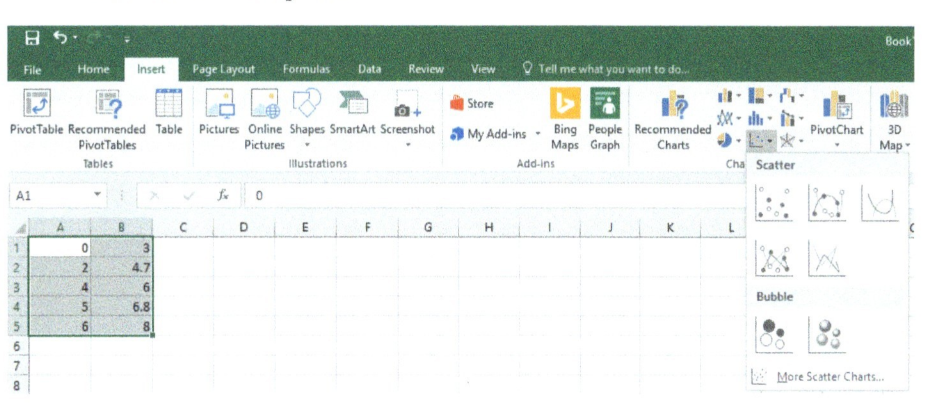

FIGURE 2

Step 3: A scatterplot of the data appears, as shown in Fig. 3. Click on ⊞ near the upper-right corner of the graph.

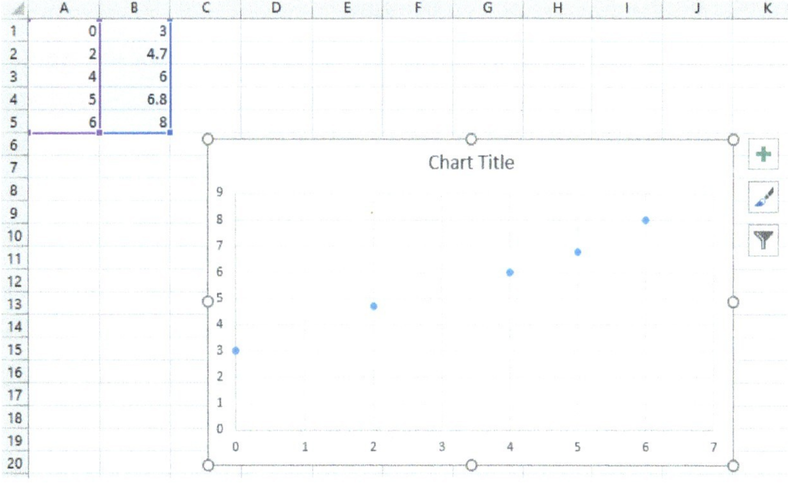

FIGURE 3

Select Trendline, then click on the pointer and choose More Options... (see Fig. 4).

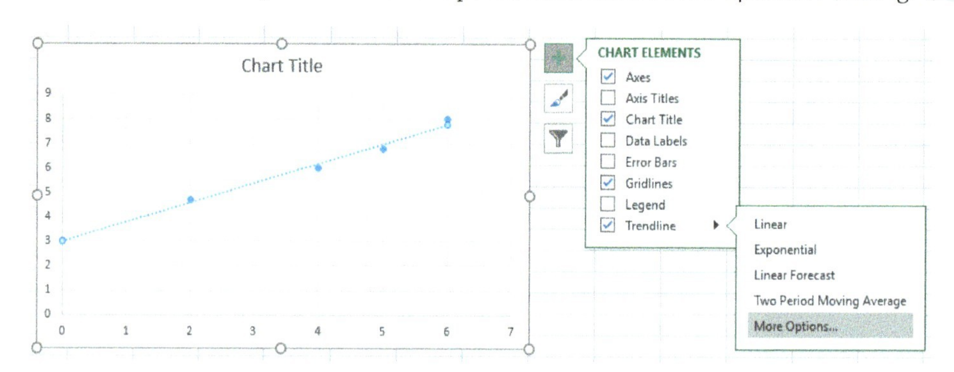

FIGURE 4

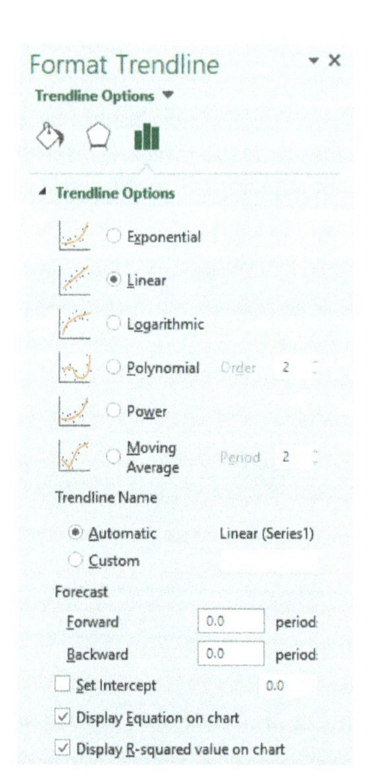

FIGURE 5

Step 4: A Format Trendline box opens (Fig. 5), with Linear selected as the default. At the bottom, check the box next to Display Equation on chart, as well as the box next to Display R-squared value on chart.

The line of best fit is now displayed on the scatterplot, along with its equation and the R^2 value, as shown in Fig. 6. The R^2 value is called the *squared correlation coefficient*. An R^2 value close to 1 indicates that the data have a strong linear trend.

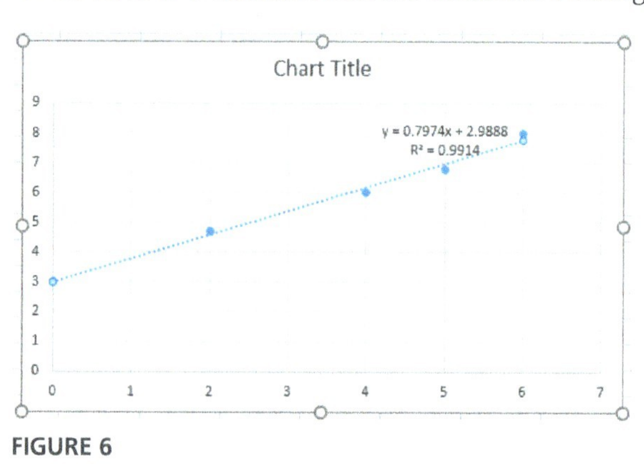

FIGURE 6

In this book, regression is also used to fit exponential and polynomial functions to data. The student can experiment with the various regression options under Format Trendline.

Using Excel for Mac 2016

The steps for finding the line of best fit using Excel for Mac 2016 are given below. There are two toolbar levels in Excel for Mac: the primary toolbar across the top of the screen, and a secondary toolbar with icons below the primary toolbar.

Step 1: Open Excel, and choose the Workbook option (default).

Step 2: Enter the data into two columns.

Step 3: Highlight the data. Then select Insert from the primary toolbar, followed by Recommended Charts in the secondary toolbar. Select the first option, Scatter. A scatterplot of the data appears on the screen.

Step 4: Click on the points to "activate" them. They will appears as X's.

Step 5: Select Chart Design from the primary toolbar, and then choose Add Chart Element from the secondary toolbar. From the drop-down menu, select Trendline, and then choose More Trendline Options.

Step 6: Select Linear from the list of curves, and also select Display Equation on chart and Display R-squared value on chart. The equation and the R^2 value will appear on the scatterplot, along with the trendline.

C Exercise Set

1. Use Excel to find the line of best fit for the following data.

x	4	6	8	10	12
y	15	22	27	33	44

2. Use Excel to find the line of best fit for the following data.

x	−5	−1	3	8
y	2	10	19	35

3. Use Excel to find a quadratic function (polynomial of power 2) that best fits the data in Exercise 2.

APPENDIX D
Areas for a Standard Normal Distribution

Entries in the table represent area under the curve between $z = 0$ and a positive value of z. Because of the symmetry of the curve, area under the curve between $z = 0$ and a negative value of z is found in a similar manner.

$$\text{Area} = \text{Probability} = P(0 \leq x \leq z) = \int_0^z \frac{1}{\sqrt{2\pi}} e^{-x^2/2}\, dx$$

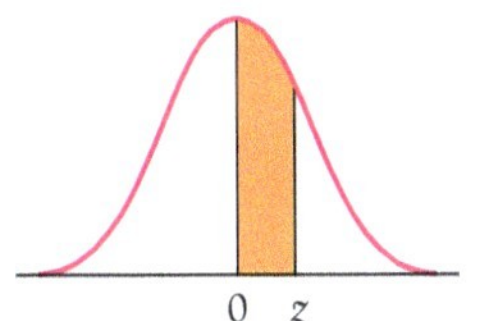

z	0.00	0.01	0.02	0.03	0.04	0.05	0.06	0.07	0.08	0.09
0.0	.0000	.0040	.0080	.0120	.0160	.0199	.0239	.0279	.0319	.0359
0.1	.0398	.0438	.0478	.0517	.0557	.0596	.0636	.0675	.0714	.0753
0.2	.0793	.0832	.0871	.0910	.0948	.0987	.1026	.1064	.1103	.1141
0.3	.1179	.1217	.1255	.1293	.1331	.1368	.1406	.1443	.1480	.1517
0.4	.1554	.1591	.1628	.1664	.1700	.1736	.1772	.1808	.1844	.1879
0.5	.1915	.1950	.1985	.2019	.2054	.2088	.2123	.2157	.2190	.2224
0.6	.2257	.2291	.2324	.2357	.2389	.2422	.2454	.2486	.2517	.2549
0.7	.2580	.2611	.2642	.2673	.2704	.2734	.2764	.2794	.2823	.2852
0.8	.2881	.2910	.2939	.2967	.2995	.3023	.3051	.3078	.3106	.3133
0.9	.3159	.3186	.3212	.3238	.3264	.3289	.3315	.3340	.3365	.3389
1.0	.3413	.3438	.3461	.3485	.3508	.3531	.3554	.3577	.3599	.3621
1.1	.3643	.3665	.3686	.3708	.3729	.3749	.3770	.3790	.3810	.3830
1.2	.3849	.3869	.3888	.3907	.3925	.3944	.3962	.3980	.3997	.4015
1.3	.4032	.4049	.4066	.4082	.4099	.4115	.4131	.4147	.4162	.4177
1.4	.4192	.4207	.4222	.4236	.4251	.4265	.4279	.4292	.4306	.4319
1.5	.4332	.4345	.4357	.4370	.4382	.4394	.4406	.4418	.4429	.4441
1.6	.4452	.4463	.4474	.4484	.4495	.4505	.4515	.4525	.4535	.4545
1.7	.4554	.4564	.4573	.4582	.4591	.4599	.4608	.4616	.4625	.4633
1.8	.4641	.4649	.4656	.4664	.4671	.4678	.4686	.4693	.4699	.4706
1.9	.4713	.4719	.4726	.4732	.4738	.4744	.4750	.4756	.4761	.4767
2.0	.4772	.4778	.4783	.4788	.4793	.4798	.4803	.4808	.4812	.4817
2.1	.4821	.4826	.4830	.4834	.4838	.4842	.4846	.4850	.4854	.4857
2.2	.4861	.4864	.4868	.4871	.4875	.4878	.4881	.4884	.4887	.4890
2.3	.4893	.4896	.4898	.4901	.4904	.4906	.4909	.4911	.4913	.4916
2.4	.4918	.4920	.4922	.4925	.4927	.4929	.4931	.4932	.4934	.4936
2.5	.4938	.4940	.4941	.4943	.4945	.4946	.4948	.4949	.4951	.4952
2.6	.4953	.4955	.4956	.4957	.4959	.4960	.4961	.4962	.4963	.4964
2.7	.4965	.4966	.4967	.4968	.4969	.4970	.4971	.4972	.4973	.4974
2.8	.4974	.4975	.4976	.4977	.4977	.4978	.4979	.4979	.4980	.4981
2.9	.4981	.4982	.4982	.4983	.4984	.4984	.4985	.4985	.4986	.4986
3.0	.4987	.4987	.4987	.4988	.4988	.4989	.4989	.4989	.4990	.4990

APPENDIX E
Using Tables of Integration Formulas

- Evaluate integrals using a table of integration formulas.

Table 1 is a table of integration formulas. Such tables are usually organized by the form of the integrand. The idea is to match the integral to be evaluated with a formula in the table. Sometimes algebra or a technique such as substitution or integration by parts may be needed in order to use a formula from a table.

TABLE 1 Integration Formulas

1. $\displaystyle\int x^n\,dx = \frac{x^{n+1}}{n+1} + C, \quad n \neq -1$

2. $\displaystyle\int \frac{dx}{x} = \ln|x| + C, \quad \text{or, for } x > 0, \int \frac{dx}{x} = \ln x + C$

3. $\displaystyle\int u\,dv = uv - \int v\,du$

4. $\displaystyle\int e^{ax}\,dx = \frac{1}{a}e^{ax} + C$

5. $\displaystyle\int xe^{ax}\,dx = \frac{1}{a^2}e^{ax}(ax - 1) + C$

6. $\displaystyle\int x^n e^{ax}\,dx = \frac{x^n e^{ax}}{a} - \frac{n}{a}\int x^{n-1}e^{ax}\,dx + C$

7. $\displaystyle\int \ln x\,dx = x\ln x - x + C, \quad x > 0$

8. $\displaystyle\int (\ln x)^n\,dx = x(\ln x)^n - n\int (\ln x)^{n-1}\,dx + C, \quad n \neq -1, x > 0$

9. $\displaystyle\int x^n \ln x\,dx = x^{n+1}\left[\frac{\ln x}{n+1} - \frac{1}{(n+1)^2}\right] + C, \quad n \neq -1, x > 0$

10. $\displaystyle\int a^x\,dx = \frac{a^x}{\ln a} + C, \quad a > 0, a \neq 1$

11. $\displaystyle\int \frac{1}{\sqrt{x^2 + a^2}}\,dx = \ln|x + \sqrt{x^2 + a^2}| + C$

12. $\displaystyle\int \frac{1}{\sqrt{x^2 - a^2}}\,dx = \ln|x + \sqrt{x^2 - a^2}| + C$

(continued)

13. $$\int \frac{1}{x^2 - a^2}\, dx = \frac{1}{2a} \ln \left| \frac{x - a}{x + a} \right| + C$$

14. $$\int \frac{1}{a^2 - x^2}\, dx = \frac{1}{2a} \ln \left| \frac{a + x}{a - x} \right| + C$$

15. $$\int \frac{1}{x\sqrt{a^2 + x^2}}\, dx = -\frac{1}{a} \ln \left| \frac{a + \sqrt{a^2 + x^2}}{x} \right| + C$$

16. $$\int \frac{1}{x\sqrt{a^2 - x^2}}\, dx = -\frac{1}{a} \ln \left| \frac{a + \sqrt{a^2 - x^2}}{x} \right| + C$$

17. $$\int \frac{x}{a + bx}\, dx = \frac{x}{b} - \frac{a}{b^2} \ln|a + bx| + C$$

18. $$\int \frac{x}{(a + bx)^2}\, dx = \frac{a}{b^2(a + bx)} + \frac{1}{b^2} \ln|a + bx| + C$$

19. $$\int \frac{1}{x(a + bx)}\, dx = \frac{1}{a} \ln \left| \frac{x}{a + bx} \right| + C$$

20. $$\int \frac{1}{x(a + bx)^2}\, dx = \frac{1}{a(a + bx)} + \frac{1}{a^2} \ln \left| \frac{x}{a + bx} \right| + C$$

21. $$\int \sqrt{x^2 + a}\, dx = \frac{1}{2}\left[x\sqrt{x^2 + a} + a \ln\left|x + \sqrt{x^2 + a}\right|\right] + C, \quad a > 0$$

22. $$\int \sqrt{x^2 - a}\, dx = \frac{1}{2}\left[x\sqrt{x^2 - a} - a \ln\left|x + \sqrt{x^2 - a}\right|\right] + C, \quad a > 0$$

23. $$\int x\sqrt{a + bx}\, dx = \frac{2}{15b^2}(3bx - 2a)(a + bx)^{3/2} + C$$

24. $$\int x^2\sqrt{a + bx}\, dx = \frac{2}{105b^3}(15b^2x^2 - 12abx + 8a^2)(a + bx)^{3/2} + C$$

25. $$\int \frac{x\, dx}{\sqrt{a + bx}} = \frac{2}{3b^2}(bx - 2a)\sqrt{a + bx} + C$$

26. $$\int \frac{x^2\, dx}{\sqrt{a + bx}} = \frac{2}{15b^3}(3b^2x^2 - 4abx + 8a^2)\sqrt{a + bx} + C$$

EXAMPLE 1 Find: $\displaystyle\int \frac{dx}{x(3 - x)}$.

Solution The integral $\displaystyle\int \frac{dx}{x(3 - x)}$ is in the form of formula 19 in Table 1:

$$\int \frac{1}{x(a + bx)}\, dx = \frac{1}{a} \ln \left| \frac{x}{a + bx} \right| + C.$$

In the given integral, $a = 3$ and $b = -1$, so we have, by the formula,

$$\int \frac{dx}{x(3 - x)} = \frac{1}{3} \ln \left| \frac{x}{3 + (-1)x} \right| + C$$

$$= \frac{1}{3} \ln \left| \frac{x}{3 - x} \right| + C.$$

We check our answer by differentiation:

$$\frac{d}{dx}\left(\frac{1}{3}\ln\left|\frac{x}{3-x}\right| + C\right) = \frac{1}{3}\cdot\frac{d}{dx}(\ln|x| - \ln|3-x|)$$

Recalling that $\ln\left(\frac{a}{b}\right) = \ln a - \ln b$

$$= \frac{1}{3}\left(\frac{d}{dx}\ln|x| - \frac{d}{dx}\ln|3-x|\right)$$

$$= \frac{1}{3}\left(\frac{1}{x} - \frac{1}{3-x}(-1)\right)$$ Differentiating

$$= \frac{1}{3}\left(\frac{1}{x} + \frac{1}{3-x}\right)$$ Simplifying

$$= \frac{1}{3}\left(\frac{1}{x}\cdot\left(\frac{3-x}{3-x}\right) + \frac{1}{3-x}\cdot\left(\frac{x}{x}\right)\right)$$ Using a common denominator

$$= \frac{1}{3}\left(\frac{3-x+x}{x(3-x)}\right)$$

$$= \frac{1}{3}\left(\frac{3}{x(3-x)}\right)$$

$$= \frac{1}{x(3-x)}.$$

1 ✓

Quick Check 1 ✓

Find: $\int \frac{2x}{(3-5x)^2}\,dx.$

EXAMPLE 2 Find: $\int \frac{5x}{7x-8}\,dx.$

Solution We first factor 5 from the integrand. The integral is then in the form of formula 17 in Table 1:

$$\int \frac{x}{a+bx}\,dx = \frac{x}{b} - \frac{a}{b^2}\ln|a+bx| + C.$$

In the given integral, $a = -8$ and $b = 7$, so we have, by the formula,

$$\int \frac{5x}{7x-8}\,dx = 5\int \frac{x}{-8+7x}\,dx$$

$$= 5\left[\frac{x}{7} - \frac{-8}{7^2}\ln|-8+7x|\right] + C$$ Substituting

$$= 5\left[\frac{x}{7} + \frac{8}{49}\ln|7x-8|\right] + C$$

$$= \frac{5x}{7} + \frac{40}{49}\ln|7x-8| + C.$$

2 ✓

Quick Check 2 ✓

Find: $\int \frac{3}{2x(7-3x)^2}\,dx.$

EXAMPLE 3 Find: $\int \sqrt{16x^2+3}\,dx.$

Solution This integral is *almost* in the form of formula 21 in Table 1:

$$\int \sqrt{x^2+a}\,dx = \tfrac{1}{2}\left[x\sqrt{x^2+a} + a\ln\left|x+\sqrt{x^2+a}\right|\right] + C.$$

To change the coefficient of x^2 to 1, we factor 16. We then use formula 21:

$$\int \sqrt{16x^2 + 3}\, dx = \int \sqrt{16\left(x^2 + \tfrac{3}{16}\right)}\, dx \quad \text{Factoring}$$

$$= \int 4\sqrt{x^2 + \tfrac{3}{16}}\, dx$$

$$= 4\int \sqrt{x^2 + \tfrac{3}{16}}\, dx \quad \text{We have } a = \tfrac{3}{16} \text{ in formula 21.}$$

$$= 4 \cdot \tfrac{1}{2}\left[x\sqrt{x^2 + \tfrac{3}{16}} + \tfrac{3}{16} \ln \left|x + \sqrt{x^2 + \tfrac{3}{16}}\right|\right] + C$$

$$= 2\left[x\sqrt{x^2 + \tfrac{3}{16}} + \tfrac{3}{16} \ln \left|x + \sqrt{x^2 + \tfrac{3}{16}}\right|\right] + C.$$

3 ✓

Quick Check 3 ✓

Find: $\int x^2\sqrt{8 + 3x}\, dx$.

EXAMPLE 4 Find: $\displaystyle\int \frac{dx}{x^2 - 25}$.

Solution This integral is in the form of formula 13 in Table 1, with $a^2 = 25$. Then $a = 5$, and we have

$$\int \frac{1}{x^2 - a^2}\, dx = \frac{1}{2a} \ln \left|\frac{x - a}{x + a}\right| + C.$$

$$\int \frac{dx}{x^2 - 25} = \frac{1}{2 \cdot 5} \ln \left|\frac{x - 5}{x + 5}\right| + C$$

$$= \frac{1}{10} \ln \left|\frac{x - 5}{x + 5}\right| + C.$$

Note that $a = -5$ yields an equivalent result. 4 ✓

Quick Check 4 ✓

Find: $\displaystyle\int \frac{4}{x^2 - 11}\, dx$.

EXAMPLE 5 Find: $\int (\ln x)^3\, dx$. Assume $x > 0$.

Solution This integral is in the form of formula 8 in Table 1:

$$\int (\ln x)^n\, dx = x(\ln x)^n - n\int (\ln x)^{n-1}\, dx + C, \quad n \neq -1.$$

We apply the formula three times:

$$\int (\ln x)^3\, dx = x(\ln x)^3 - 3\int (\ln x)^2\, dx + C \quad \text{Formula 8, with } n =$$

$$= x(\ln x)^3 - 3\left[x(\ln x)^2 - 2\int \ln x\, dx\right] + C \quad \text{Applying formula 8 again, with } n = 2$$

$$= x(\ln x)^3 - 3\left[x(\ln x)^2 - 2\left(x \ln x - \int dx\right)\right] + C \quad \text{Applying formula 8 for the third time, with } n = 1$$

$$= x(\ln x)^3 - 3x(\ln x)^2 + 6x \ln x - 6x + C.$$

5 ✓

Quick Check 5 ✓

Find: $\int x^4 \ln x\, dx$. Assume $x > 0$.

Section Summary

- We can use tables of integration formulas to evaluate many integrals.
- Some algebraic manipulation may be required before a corresponding integral form from a table can be identified.

E Exercise Set

Solve each integral using Table 1.

1. $\int xe^{-3x}\,dx$

2. $\int 2xe^{3x}\,dx$

3. $\int 6^x\,dx$

4. $\int \frac{1}{\sqrt{x^2-9}}\,dx$

5. $\int \frac{1}{25-x^2}\,dx$

6. $\int \frac{1}{x\sqrt{4+x^2}}\,dx$

7. $\int \frac{x}{3-x}\,dx$

8. $\int \frac{x}{(1-x)^2}\,dx$

9. $\int \frac{1}{x(8-x)^2}\,dx$

10. $\int \sqrt{x^2+9}\,dx$

11. $\int \ln(3x)\,dx,\quad x>0$

12. $\int \ln\left(\frac{4}{5}x\right)dx,\quad x>0$

13. $\int x^4\ln x\,dx,\quad x>0$

14. $\int x^3e^{-2x}\,dx$

15. $\int x^3\ln x\,dx,\quad x>0$

16. $\int 5x^4\ln x\,dx,\quad x>0$

17. $\int \frac{dx}{\sqrt{x^2+7}}$

18. $\int \frac{3\,dx}{x\sqrt{1-x^2}}$

19. $\int \frac{10\,dx}{x(5-7x)^2}$

20. $\int \frac{2}{5x(7x+2)}\,dx$

21. $\int \frac{-5}{4x^2-1}\,dx$

22. $\int \sqrt{9t^2-1}\,dt$

23. $\int \sqrt{4m^2+16}\,dm$

24. $\int \frac{3\ln x}{x^2}\,dx$

25. $\int \frac{-5\ln x}{x^3}\,dx,\quad x>0$

26. $\int (\ln x)^4\,dx,\quad x>0$

27. $\int \frac{e^x}{x^{-3}}\,dx$

28. $\int \frac{3}{\sqrt{4x^2+100}}\,dx$

29. $\int x\sqrt{1+2x}\,dx$

30. $\int x\sqrt{2+3x}\,dx$

APPLICATIONS

Business and Economics

31. **Supply from marginal supply.** Stellar Lawn Care introduces a new kind of lawn seeder. It finds that its marginal supply for the seeder satisfies

$$S'(x) = \frac{100x}{(20-x)^2},\quad 0 \le x \le 19,$$

where $S(x)$ is the quantity purchased when the price is x thousand dollars per seeder. Find $S(x)$, given that the company sells 2000 seeders when the price is 19 thousand dollars.

Social Sciences

32. **Learning rate.** The rate of change of the probability that an employee learns a task on a new assembly line is

$$p'(t) = \frac{1}{t(2+t)^2},$$

where $p(t)$ is the probability of learning the task after t months. Find $p(t)$ given that $p(2) = 0.8267$.

SYNTHESIS

Evaluate using Table 1.

33. $\int \frac{8}{3x^2-2x}\,dx$

34. $\int \frac{x\,dx}{4x^2-12x+9}$

35. $\int \frac{dx}{x^3-4x^2+4x}$

36. $\int e^x\sqrt{e^{2x}+1}\,dx$

37. $\int \frac{-e^{-2x}\,dx}{9-6e^{-x}+e^{-2x}}$

38. $\int \frac{\sqrt{(\ln x)^2+49}}{2x}\,dx$

39. In Example 4, we used $a = 5$, since $a^2 = 25$. Show that $a = -5$ yields an equivalent result.

40. Prove formula 17 in Table 1 using the substitution $u = a + bx$.

41. Prove formula 5 in Table 1 using integration by parts.

Answers to Quick Checks

1. Using formula 18: $\frac{6}{25(3-5x)} + \frac{2}{25}\ln|3-5x| + C$

2. Using formula 20: $\frac{3}{14(7-3x)} + \frac{3}{98}\ln\left|\frac{x}{7-3x}\right| + C$

3. Using formula 24: $\frac{2}{2835}(135x^2 - 288x + 512)(8+3x)^{3/2} + C$

4. Using formula 13: $\frac{2}{11}\sqrt{11}\ln\left|\frac{x-\sqrt{11}}{x+\sqrt{11}}\right| + C$

5. Using formula 9: $\frac{x^5}{5}\ln x - \frac{x^2}{25} + C$

Credits

p. 1: Mike Kuhlman/Shutterstock. p. 11: ZUMA Press, Inc./Alamy Stock Photo. p. 57: Kyslynskyy/Fotolia. p. 78: Brian Jackson/Fotolia. p. 99: Stephen Coburn/Shutterstock. p. 101: Olegdudko/123RF. p. 138: Oliver Hausen/Fotolia. p. 156: Kushnirov Avraham/Fotolia. p. 161: Shawn Goldberg/Shutterstock. p. 166: Brian Spurlock. p. 181: Dotshock/Shutterstock. p. 192: sirtravelalot/Shutterstock. p. 193: New York Daily News Archive/Getty Images. p. 195: PA Images/Alamy Stock Photo. p. 204: MinDof/Shutterstock. p. 220: Dragon Images/Shutterstock. p. 222: PA Images/Alamy Stock Photo. p. 227: (left) Vladimir Mucibabic/Fotolia; (right) EZIO PETERSEN/UPI/Newscom. p. 228: Edelweiss/Fotolia. p. 229: (left) Pictorial Press Ltd/Alamy Stock Photo; (right) Sean Lema/Shutterstock. p. 234: alefbet/Shutterstock. p. 239: Josemaria Toscano/Fotolia. p. 243: Ethan Daniels/Shutterstock. p. 259: Creative Family/Shutterstock. p. 260: Moviestore Collection Ltd/Alamy Stock Photo. p. 261: Pictorial Press Ltd/Alamy Stock Photo. p. 263: artstock/Alamy Stock Photo. p. 292: gpointstudio/Shutterstock. p. 306: ZUMA Press, Inc./Alamy Stock Photo. p. 319: artstock/Alamy Stock Photo. p. 331: Nicholas Rous/Alamy Stock Photo. p. 362: SergiiAfonin/Shutterstock. p. 365: francesco de marco/Shutterstock. p. 366: Konstantin Inozemtcev/123RF. p. 381: Otvalo/Fotolia. p. 382: (left) njsphotography/Fotolia; (right) mattjeppson/Fotolia. p. 383: Catalin Petolea/Shutterstock. p. 385: Pavel Byrkin/123RF. p. 390: Pavel Byrkin/123RF. p. 392: Josep Suria/Shutterstock. p. 393: michaeljung/Shutterstock. p. 398: Sira Anamwong/Shutterstock. p. 410: martinkay78/123RF. p. 416: Karichs/Fotolia. p. 435: Tero Vesalainen/Shutterstock. p. 466: Shao-Chun Wang/123RF. p. 468: andersphoto/Shutterstock. p. 469: rawpixel/123RF. p. 471: Yvette Cardozo/Alamy Stock Photo. p. 481: Strahil Dimitrov/123RF. p. 492: anekoho/Fotolia. p. 506: SeanPavonePhoto/Fotolia. p. 508: Tetra Images/Alamy Stock Photo. p. 517: LOOK Die Bildagentur der Fotografen GmbH/Alamy Stock Photo. p. 520: Brian Spurlock. p. 523: dvande/Shutterstock. p. 524: fotogrammi3/Fotolia. p. 528: ChrisVanLennepPhoto/Fotolia. p. 530: Rolls Press/Popperfoto/Getty Images. p. 550: vladimir salman/Shutterstock. p. 551: Pongphan Ruengchai/123RF. p. 556: KZ Labs. p. 559: Corbis/VCG/Getty Images. p. 562: Hufton+Crow-VIEW/Alamy Stock Photo. p. 568: Maisie Paterson/Getty Images. p. 571: Rick Hanston/Latent Images. p. 584: Mariano Garcia/Alamy Stock Photo. p. 588: Igor Akimov/123RF. p. 593: picsfive/Fotolia. p. 609: Suzanne Tucker/Shutterstock.

Answers

DIAGNOSTIC TEST, p. xvii

Part A

The red bracketed references indicate where worked-out solutions can be found in Appendix A: Review of Basic Algebra. For example, [Ex. 1] means that the problem is worked out in Example 1 of the appendix.

1. 64 [Ex. 1] **2.** -32 [Ex. 1] **3.** $\frac{1}{8}$ [Ex. 1]
4. $-2x$ [Ex. 2] **5.** 1 [Ex. 2] **6.** $\dfrac{1}{x^5}$ [Ex. 3]
7. 16 [Ex. 3] **8.** $\dfrac{1}{t}$ [Ex. 3] **9.** x^{11} [Ex. 4]
10. x^7 [Ex. 4] **11.** $40x^3$ [Ex. 4] **12.** a [Ex. 5]
13. b^8 [Ex. 5] **14.** $\dfrac{1}{x^6}$ [Ex. 6] **15.** $\dfrac{y^{15}}{8x^{12}z^9}$ [Ex. 6]
16. $3x - 15$ [Ex. 7] **17.** $x^2 - 2x - 15$ [Ex. 7]
18. $a^2 + 2ab + b^2$ [Ex. 7] **19.** $4x^2 - 4xt + t^2$ [Ex. 8]
20. $9c^2 - d^2$ [Ex. 8] **21.** $h(2x + h)$ [Ex. 9]
22. $(x - 3y)^2$ [Ex. 9] **23.** $(x + 2)(x - 7)$ [Ex. 9]
24. $(2x - 1)(3x + 5)$ [Ex. 9]
25. $(x - 7)(x + 2)(x - 2)$ [Ex. 10]
26. $x = 6$ [Ex. 11] **27.** $x = 0, 2, -\frac{4}{5}$ [Ex. 12]
28. $x = 0, \frac{1}{2}, -\frac{1}{2}$ [Ex. 13] **29.** No solution [Ex. 15]
30. $x \leq \frac{21}{13}$ or $\left(-\infty, \frac{21}{13}\right]$ [Ex. 17] **31.** 660 lb [Ex. 19]
32. 199 suits [Ex. 20]

Part B

The red bracketed references indicate where worked-out solutions can be found in Chapter R. For example, [Ex. R.2.5] means that the problem is worked out in Example 5 of Section R.2.

1.

$y = 2x + 1$

[Ex. R.1.1]

2.

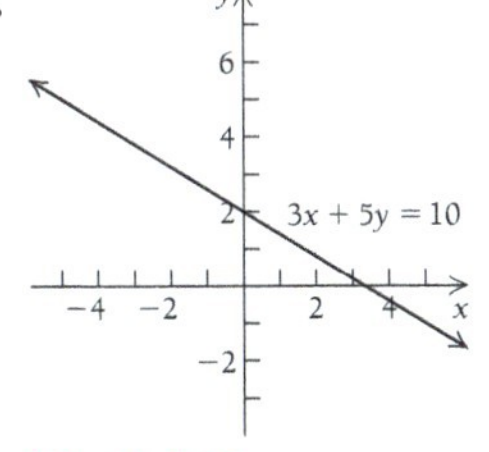

[Ex. R.1.2]

3.

$y = x^2 - 1$

[Ex. R.1.3]

4.

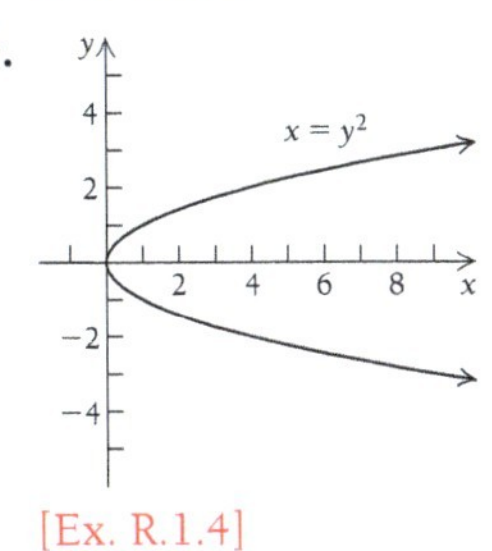

[Ex. R.1.4]

5. $g(0) = 8$; $g(-5) = 143$; $g(7a) = 147a^2 - 14a + 8$ [Ex. R.2.4] **6.** $x = 4$ [Ex. R.2.4]

7.

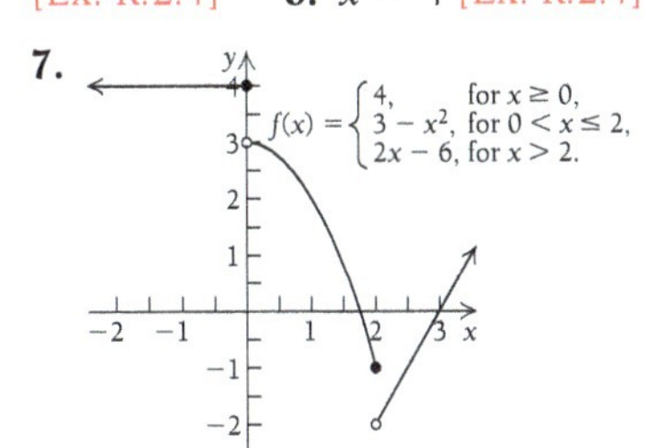

[Ex. R.2.8]

8. $(-4, 5)$ [Ex. R.3.1a] **9.** $\{x \mid x \text{ is any real number } and\ x \neq \frac{5}{2}\}$ or $\left(-\infty, \frac{5}{2}\right) \cup \left(\frac{5}{2}, \infty\right)$ [Ex. R.3.5] **10.** Slope $m = \frac{1}{2}$; y-intercept: $\left(0, -\frac{7}{4}\right)$ [Ex. R.4.6] **11.** $y = 3x - 2$ [Ex. R.4.7]
12. $m = -\frac{3}{2}$ [Ex. R.4.1] **13.** $x = 5$ [Ex. R.6.7]
14. $x = -2$ [Ex. R.6.7]

15. $f(x) = x^2 - 2x - 3$ [Ex. R.5.1]

16. $g(x) = x^3$ [Ex. R.5.4]

17. $f(x) = \dfrac{1}{x}$ [Ex. R.5.5]

18. $f(x) = |x|$ [Ex. R.5.7]

19. $f(x) = -\sqrt{x}$ [Ex. R.5.8]

20. \$1102.50 [Ex. R.1.6]

CHAPTER R

Technology Connection, p. 7

1. Left to the student

Exercise Set R.1, p. 10

1.

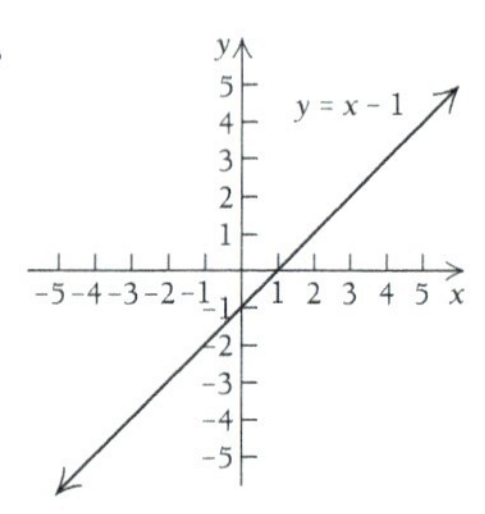

3.

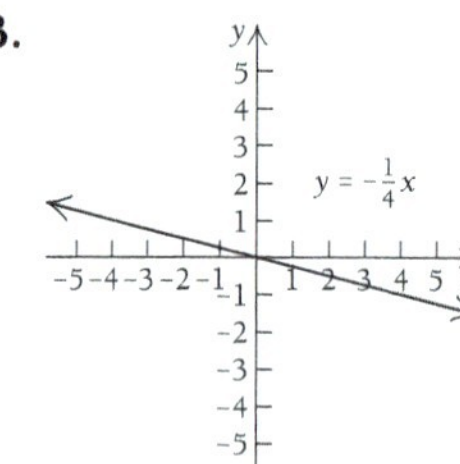

5.

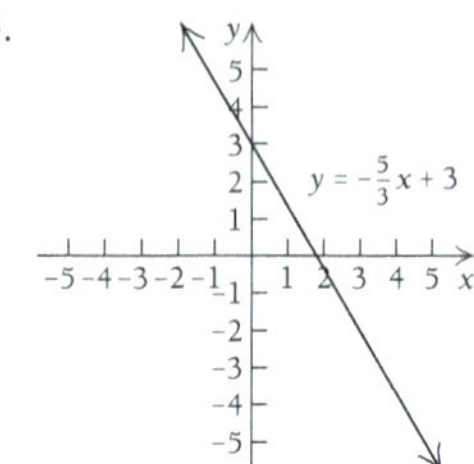

7.

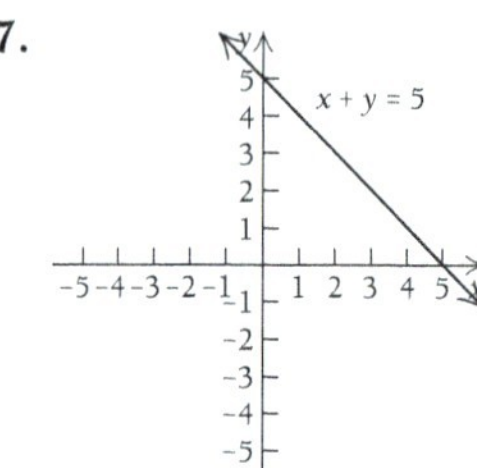

9.

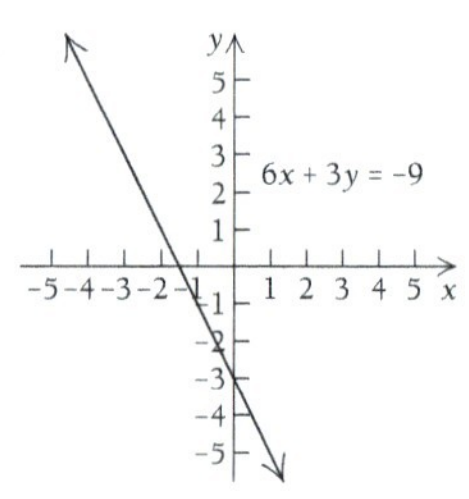

11.

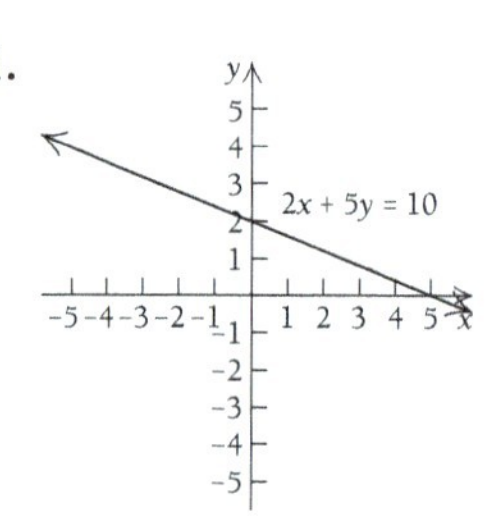

13.

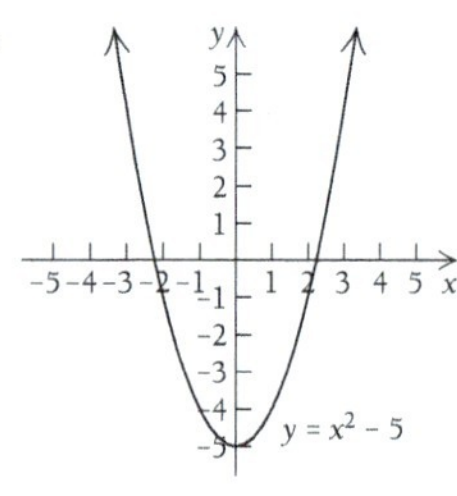

15.

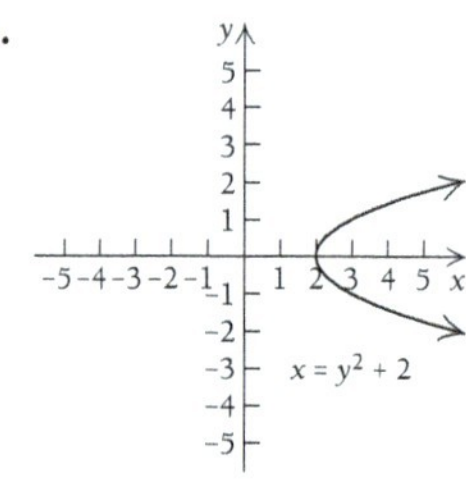

17.

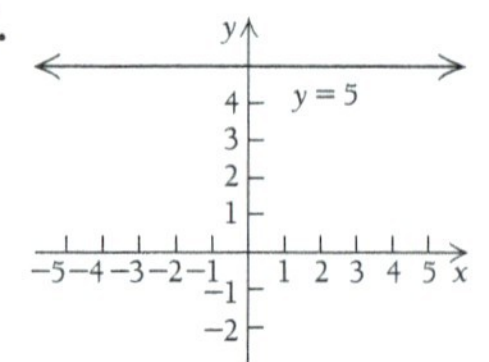

19.

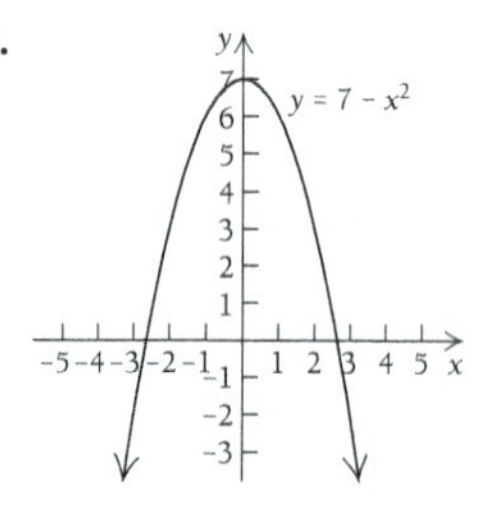

21.

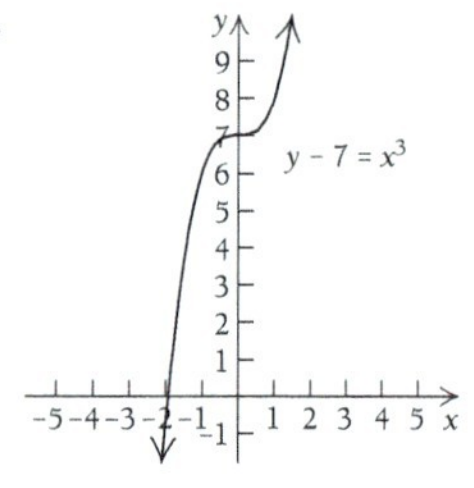

23. 344.4 mg **25.** **(a)** 18.62°; **(b)** 32.92°; **(c)** 43.56° **27.** **(a)** 3.50 million; **(b)** 2024 **29.** About 27.25 mi/hr **31.** **(a)** \$102,800; **(b)** \$102,819.60; **(c)** \$102,829.54; **(d)** \$102,839.46; **(e)** \$102,839.56 **33.** **(a)** \$33,745.92; **(b)** \$33,784.87; **(c)** \$33,804.75; **(d)** \$33,824.68; **(e)** \$33,824.90 **35.** \$536.25 **37.** \$70,561.01 **39.** **(a)** 2008–2014; **(b)** 2006–2008 and 2014–2016; **(c)** 2010, 9.6%; **(d)** 2006–2007, 4.6% **41.** **(a)** \$88,382.67; **(b)** \$42,000, \$46,382.67 **43.** 5.43% **45.** 3.82% **47.** **(a)** Western 2.5%, Commonwealth 2.46%; **(b)** Western's account **49.** 2.179%

51.

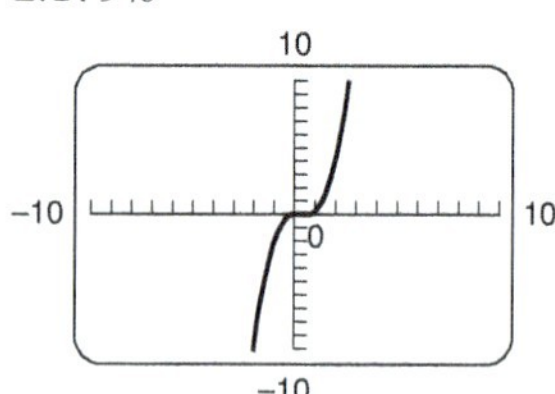

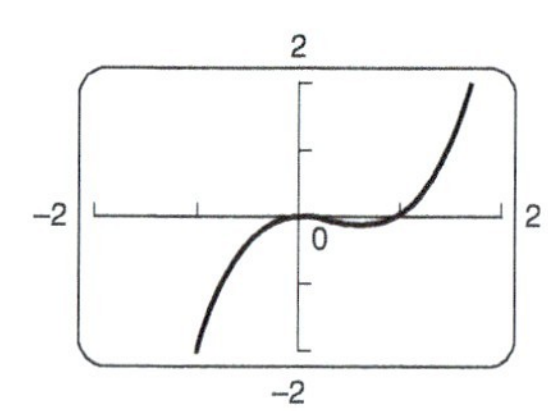

The window $[-2, 2, -2, 2]$ shows better detail around the origin.

Technology Connection, p. 16

1. 951; 42,701 **2.** 21,813

Exercise Set R.2, p. 20

1. Yes **3.** Yes **5.** Yes **7.** Yes **9.** Yes **11.** No **13.** Yes **15.** Yes **17.** No **19.** Yes **21.** No **23.** **(a)** 17.4, 17.04, 17.004, 17; **(b)** 13, 9, −11, $4k - 3$, $4x + 4h - 3$ **25.** −2, −3, −2, 22, $a^2 + 2ah + h^2 - 3$, $2x + h$, for $h \neq 0$ **27.** $\frac{1}{49}, \frac{1}{9}, \frac{1}{(a+3)^2}, \frac{1}{(x+h+3)^2}, \frac{-2x-h-6}{(x+h+3)^2(x+3)^2}$

29. **(a)** $f(x) = 4x + 2$; **(b)**

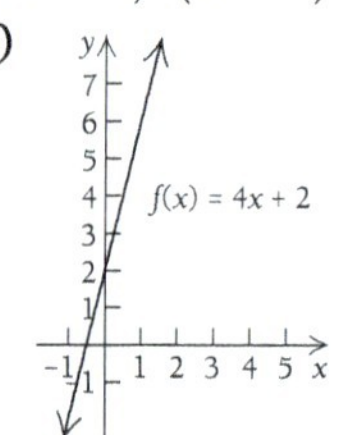

31. **(a)** $h(x) = x^2 + x$; **(b)**

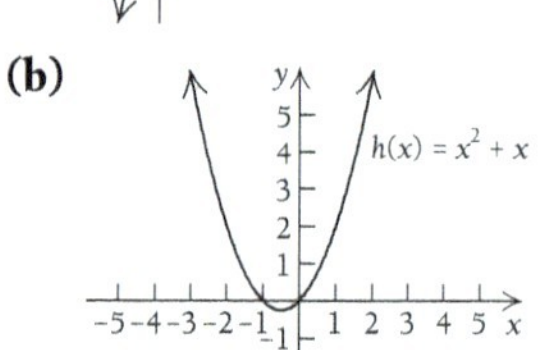

33.

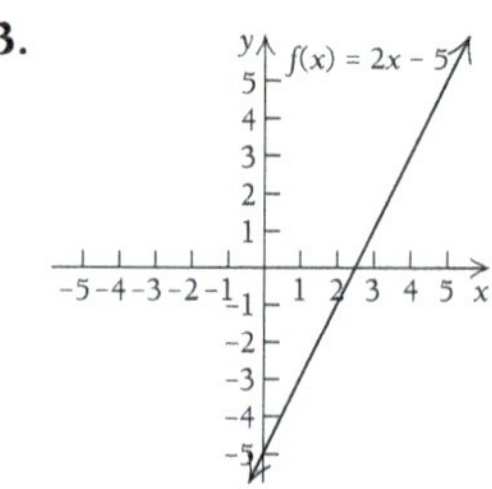

35.

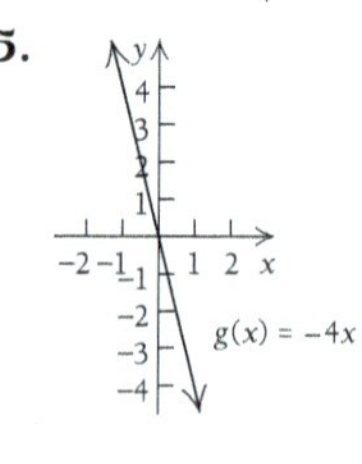

37.

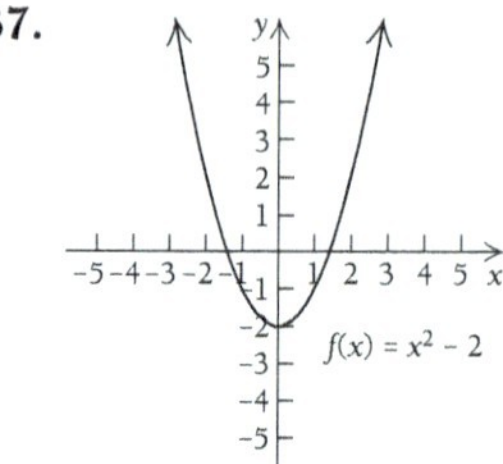

39.

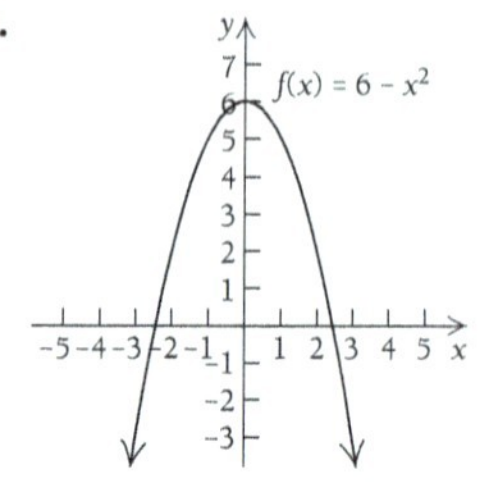

41.

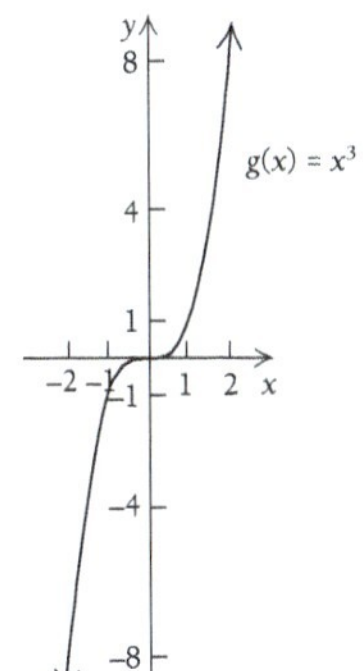

43. Yes **45.** No **47.** Yes **49.** Yes **51.** Yes
53. Yes **55.** No

57. (a)

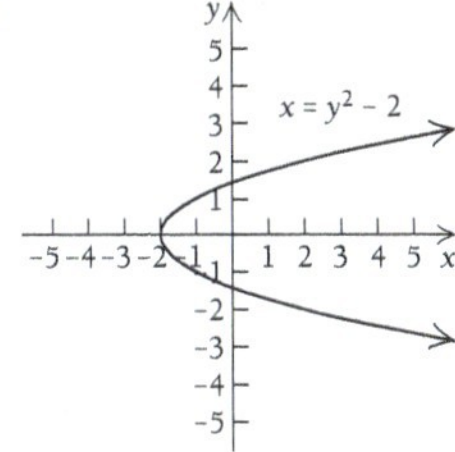

(b) No, the graph fails the vertical-line test.
59. $2x + h - 3$, for $h \neq 0$ **61.** 3, −2 **63.** 17, 6

65.

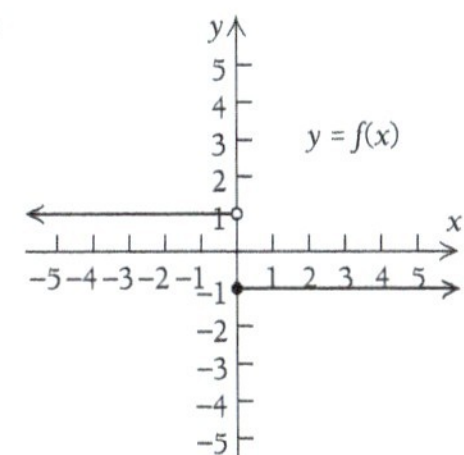

67.

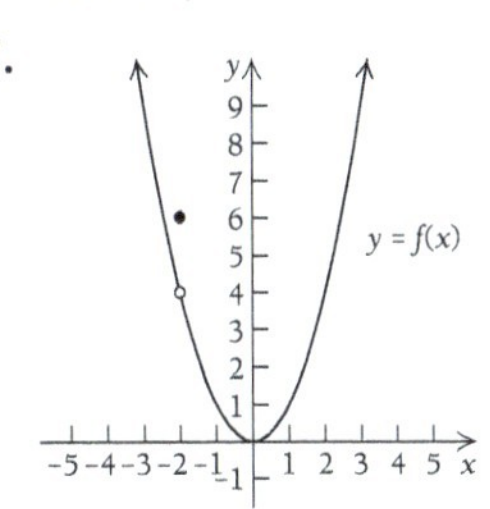

69.

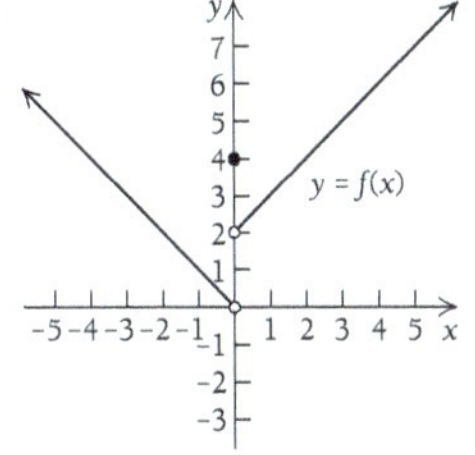

71.

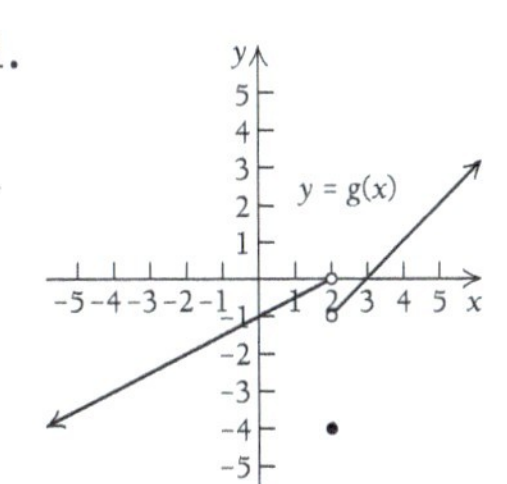

73.

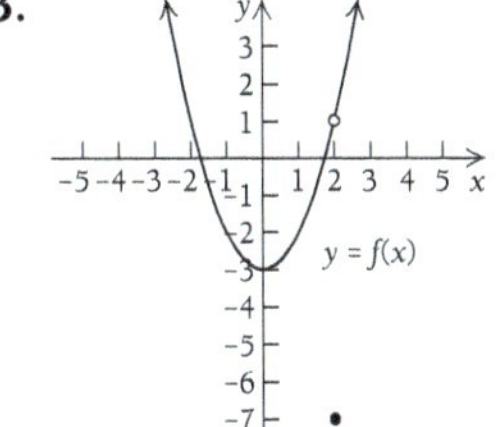

75. \$530.80 **77. (a)** 1.818 m^2; **(b)** 2.173 m^2; **(c)** 1.537 m^2
79. (a) Yes; **(b)** yes; **(c)** no; **(d)** yes **81.** $y = 5$; yes
83. $y = \pm\sqrt{x}$; no **85.** Answers may vary.

87.

X	Y1
−3	−10
−1	−8
1	−14
3	20
5	142
7	400
9	842
X = −3	

89. Left to the student

91. (a) $f(x) = 5(x + 2)$, $g(x) = 5x + 2$;
(b)

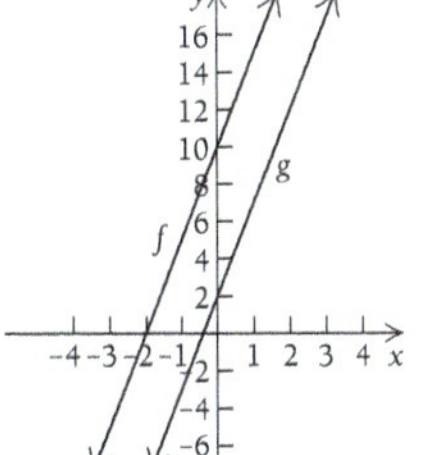

(c) no **93.** $h = 2$

Exercise Set R.3, p. 31

1. $(-1, 3)$ **3.** $(0, 5)$ **5.** $(-9, -5]$ **7.** $[x, x + h]$
9. $[-4, -1) \cup (2, 3]$ **11.** $[-2, 2]$
13. $(6, 20]$
15. $(-3, \infty)$
17. $(-2, 3]$
19. $[-4, -3) \cup (0, 5]$
21. (a) 3; **(b)** $\{-3, -1, 1, 3, 5\}$; **(c)** 3; **(d)** $\{-2, 0, 2, 3, 4\}$
23. (a) 4; **(b)** $\{-5, -3, 1, 2, 3, 4, 5\}$; **(c)** −5, −3, 4;
(d) $\{-3, 2, 4, 5\}$ **25. (a)** −1; **(b)** $[-2, 4]$ **(c)** 3;
(d) $[-3, 3]$ **27. (a)** −2; **(b)** $[-4, 2]$; **(c)** −2; **(d)** $[-3, 3]$
29. (a) 3; **(b)** $[-3, 3]$; **(c)** at about −1.4 and 1.4; **(d)** $[-5, 4]$
31. (a) 1; **(b)** $[-5, 5)$; **(c)** $[3, 5)$; **(d)** $\{-2, -1, 0, 1, 2\}$
33. $(-\infty, 2) \cup (2, \infty)$
35. $[0, \infty)$
37. $\mathbb{R}$ $(-\infty, \infty)$
39. $(-\infty, 2) \cup (2, \infty)$
41. $\mathbb{R}$ $(-\infty, \infty)$
43. $\left(-\infty, \frac{7}{2}\right) \cup \left(\frac{7}{2}, \infty\right)$
45. $\left[-\frac{4}{5}, \infty\right)$
47. $\mathbb{R}$ $(-\infty, \infty)$
49. $(-\infty, -5) \cup (-5, 5) \cup (5, \infty)$
51. $\mathbb{R}$ $(-\infty, \infty)$ **53.** $[-1, 3]$
55. $[-1, 2]$ **57.** 1 **59.** $\{-3, 4\}$
61. Domain: [0, 80], range: [0, 3200] **63. (a)** [25, 102]; **(b)** [0, 455]; **(c)** answers may vary. **65. (a)** $f(4) = 15.5$; the charge for the first mile is \$5, and then the charge for the next 3 mi is \$3.50 each, giving a fare of \$15.50 for a 4-mi trip; **(b)** $f(4.25) = \$19$; the 0.25 mi is considered part of a fourth additional mile after the first mile is charged at the \$5 rate, so the total fare is \$19.00 for a trip of at least 4 mi up to and including 5 mi. **(c)** The fares will be \$5, \$8.50, \$12, and so on, in increments of \$3.50, up to \$36.50. Thus, the range is $\{5, 8.5, 12, 15.5, 19, 22.5, 26, 29.5, 33, 36.5\}$.

67. $[0, 5)$ **69.** $(-\infty, -3) \cup (-3, 0) \cup (0, 3) \cup (3, \infty)$

71. Answers may vary. One example is $f(x) = \dfrac{1}{x(x^2 - 4)}$.

73. Answers may vary. **75.** $(-\infty, -1] \cup [4, \infty)$

Technology Connection, p. 40

1. Graphs are left to the student. The two lines are parallel; $y = x - 5$ is shifted down 5 units from $y = x$. **2.** Left to the student

Exercise Set R.4, p. 44

1.

$m = -2$, y-intercept $= (0, 0)$

3.

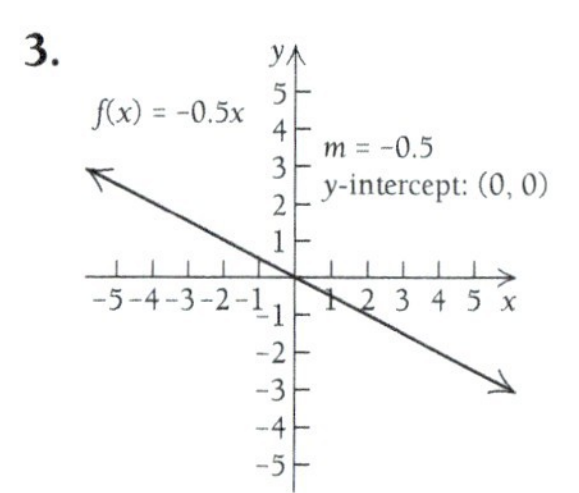

$m = -0.5$, y-intercept $= (0, 0)$

5.

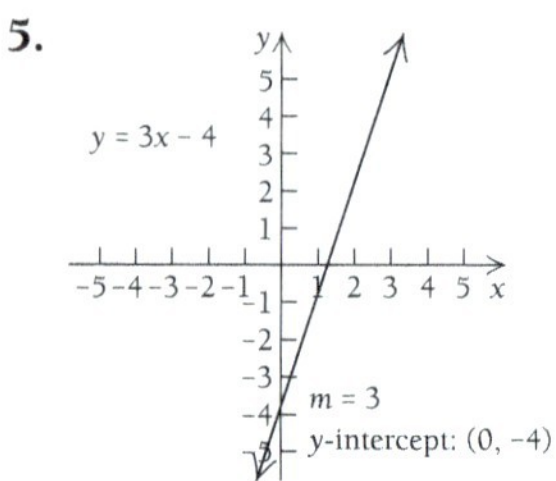

$m = 3$, y-intercept $= (0, -4)$

7.

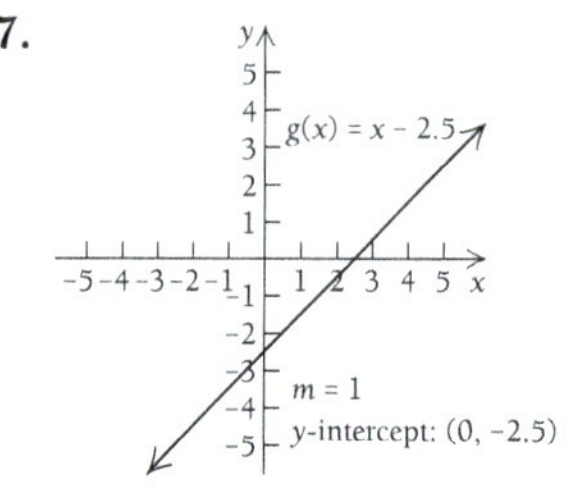

$m = 1$, y-intercept $= (0, -2.5)$

9.

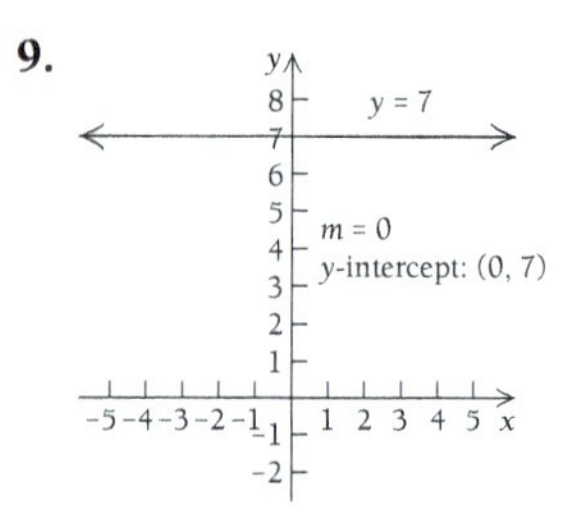

$m = 0$, y-intercept $= (0, 7)$

11. $m = 4$, y-intercept $= (0, 1)$

13. $m = -2$, y-intercept $= (0, 3)$

15. $m = 1$, y-intercept $= (0, 2)$

17. $m = \frac{1}{3}$, y-intercept $= \left(0, -\frac{7}{3}\right)$

19. **(a)** $y - 7 = 7(x - 1)$; **(b)** $y = 7x$

21. **(a)** $y - 3 = -2(x - 2)$; **(b)** $y = -2x + 7$

23. **(a)** $y - 0 = -5(x - 5)$; **(b)** $y = -5x + 25$

25. **(a)** $y + 6 = \frac{1}{2}(x - 0)$; **(b)** $y = \frac{1}{2}x - 6$

27. **(a)** $y - 8 = 0 \cdot (x - 4)$; **(b)** $y = 8$

29. **(a)** $m = 2$; **(b)** $y = 2x + 3$; **(c)** $(0, 3)$

31. **(a)** $m = 1$; **(b)** $y = x + 4$; **(c)** $(0, 4)$

33. **(a)** $m = \frac{2}{5}$; **(b)** $y = \frac{2}{5}x - \frac{19}{5}$ **(c)** $\left(0, -\frac{19}{5}\right)$

35. **(a)** $m = -\frac{9}{5}$; **(b)** $y = -\frac{9}{5}x - \frac{87}{5}$; **(c)** $\left(0, -\frac{87}{5}\right)$

37. **(a)** $m = 0$; **(b)** $y = 6$; **(c)** $(0, 6)$; horizontal line

39. **(a)** $m = 0$; **(b)** $y = 0$; **(c)** $(0, 0)$; horizontal line

41. **(a)** Undefined; **(b)** $x = 4$; **(c)** no y-intercept; vertical line

43. **(a)** Undefined; **(b)** $x = 0$; **(c)** all points on the y-axis are on this line, which is vertical.

45. **(a)** $m = \frac{1}{3}$; **(b)** $y = \frac{1}{3}x - 1$; **(c)** $(0, -1)$

47. **(a)** $m = \frac{8}{15}$; **(b)** $y = \frac{8}{15}x + \frac{1}{15}$; **(c)** $\left(0, \frac{1}{15}\right)$

49. **(a)** $m = \frac{3}{2}$; **(b)** $y = \frac{3}{2}x + k - \frac{3}{2}h$; **(c)** $\left(0, k - \frac{3}{2}h\right)$

51. $\frac{0.4}{5} = 0.08$, or 8% **53.** $\frac{43.33}{1238} = 0.035$, or 3.5%

55. $\frac{55}{100} = 0.55$, or 55% **57.** **(a)** $T(w) = 0.000806w$; **(b)** \$2.98 **59.** **(a)** $C(x) = 3x + 1{,}000{,}000$; **(b)** $R(x) = 75x$; **(c)** $P(x) = 72x - 1{,}000{,}000$; **(d)** profit of \$9,800,000; **(e)** 13,889 calculators

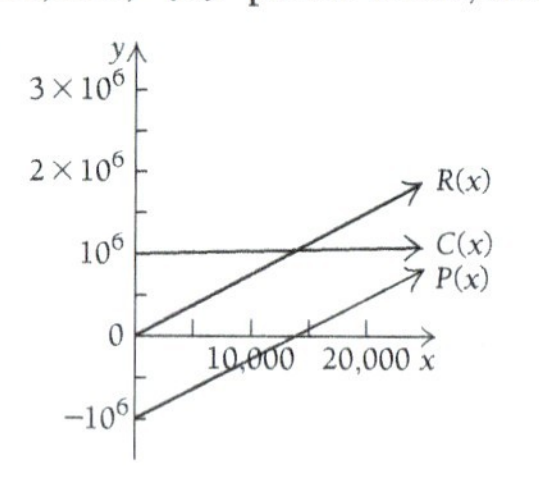

61. **(a)** $C(x) = 4x + 250$; **(b)** $R(x) = 20x$; \$20 **(c)** 16 lawns

63. **(a)** $V(t) = 5200 - 512.5t$; **(b)** $V(0) = \$5200$, $V(1) = \$4687.50$, $V(2) = \$4175$, $V(3) = \$3662.50$, $V(4) = \$3150$, $V(7) = \$1612.50$, $V(8) = \$1100$ **65.** \$25,200 **67.** About 91% (don't round up for legal reasons!) **69.** \$682.75 **71.** \$161.89/yr

73. **(a)** $R = 4.17T$; **(b)** 25 **75.** **(a)** $M = 0.4W$; **(b)** $M = 40\%W$, which indicates that muscle weight is 40% of body weight; **(c)** 48 lb **77.** **(a)** 115 ft, 75 ft, 135 ft, 179 ft. **(b)** For every increase of 1°F in the air temperature, the stopping distance increases by 2 ft. **(c)** Answers may vary.

79. **(a)** 145.78 cm; **(b)** 142.98 cm

81. **(a)** $y = 289.75x + 3143$; **(b)** 4882; **(c)** answers may vary. **83.** **(a)** 19.7, 19.78, 20.5, 23.7, 24.5; **(b)** 25.3; **(c)**

85. Answers may vary. **87.** $[0, 15]$

Technology Connection, p. 51

1. **(a)** 2, 4; **(b)** left to the student

Technology Connection, p. 53

1. $-2, 1$ **2.** $0, -1.414, 1.414$ **3.** 0, 700 **4.** $-2.079, 0.463, 3.116$ **5.** $-0.387, 1.721$ **6.** $-1.414, 1.414, 1, -2$

Technology Connection, p. 55

1. Left to the student **2.** Left to the student

Exercise Set R.5, p. 60

1.

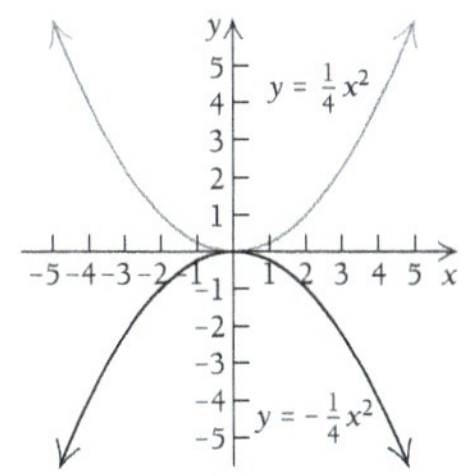

Domain: $(-\infty, \infty)$, or $\mathbb{R}$, for both

3.

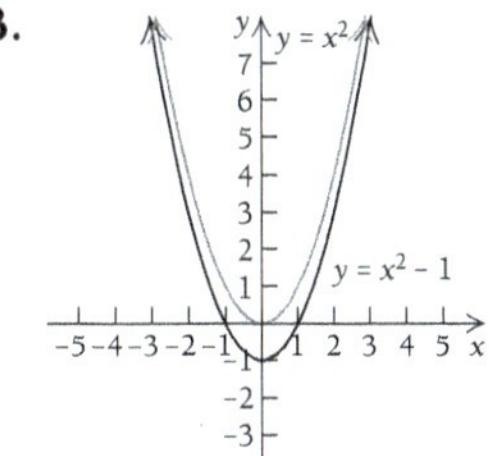

Domain: $(-\infty, \infty)$, or $\mathbb{R}$, for both

5.

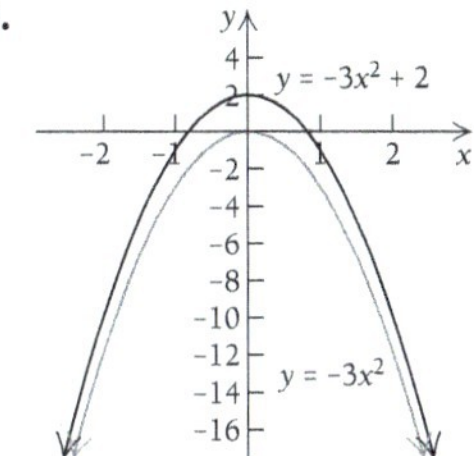

Domain: $(-\infty, \infty)$, or $\mathbb{R}$, for both

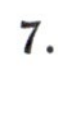

7.

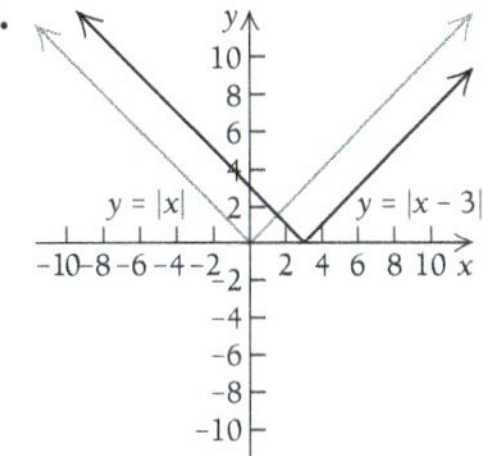

Domain: $(-\infty, \infty)$, or $\mathbb{R}$, for both

9.

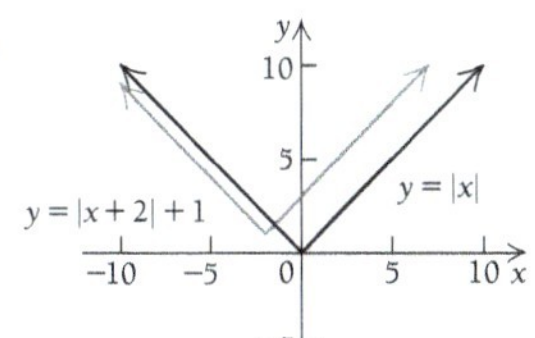

Domain: $(-\infty, \infty)$, or $\mathbb{R}$, for both

11.

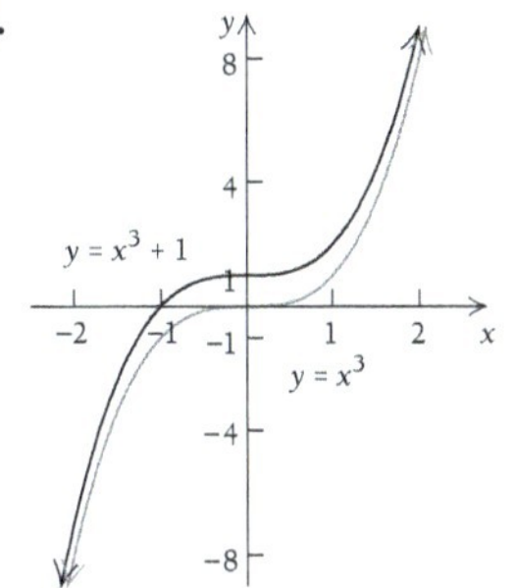

Domain: $(-\infty, \infty)$, or $\mathbb{R}$, for both

13.

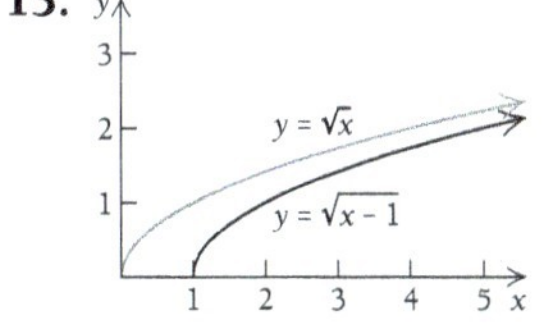

Domains: $[0, \infty)$ and $[1, \infty)$

15.

$y = \sqrt{x}$

$y = \sqrt{x + 2} - 1$

Domains: $[0, \infty)$ and $[-2, \infty)$

17. (a) $(-2, -1)$, $x = -2$; **(b)** opens upward; **(c)** $(-3, 0)$, $(-1, 0)$ **19. (a)** $(-4, -16)$, $t = -4$; **(b)** opens upward; **(c)** $(-8, 0)$, $(0, 0)$

21. (a) $\left(\frac{1}{4}, \frac{33}{8}\right)$, $s = \frac{1}{4}$; **(b)** opens downward; **(c)** $\left(\frac{1 - \sqrt{33}}{4}, 0\right)$, $\left(\frac{1 + \sqrt{33}}{4}, 0\right)$

23. (a) $\left(-\frac{6}{5}, -\frac{121}{50}\right)$, $x = -\frac{6}{5}$; **(b)** opens upward; **(c)** $\left(-\frac{17}{5}, 0\right)$, $(1, 0)$

25.

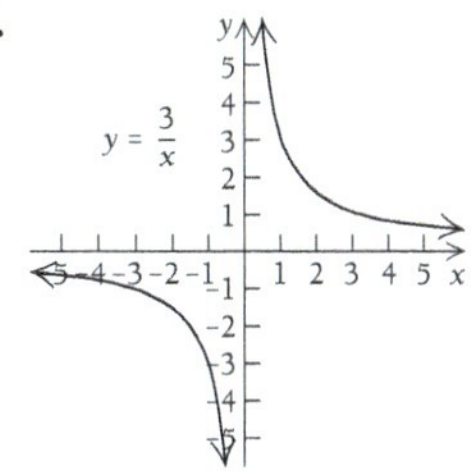

Domain: $(-\infty, 0) \cup (0, \infty)$

27.

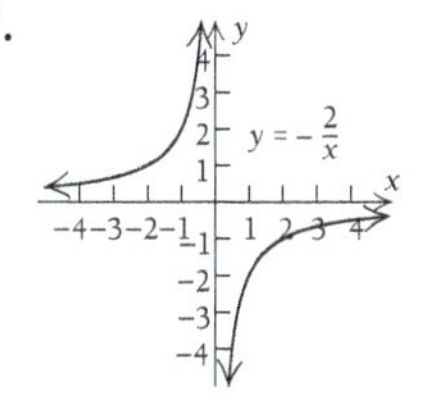

Domain: $(-\infty, 0) \cup (0, \infty)$

29.

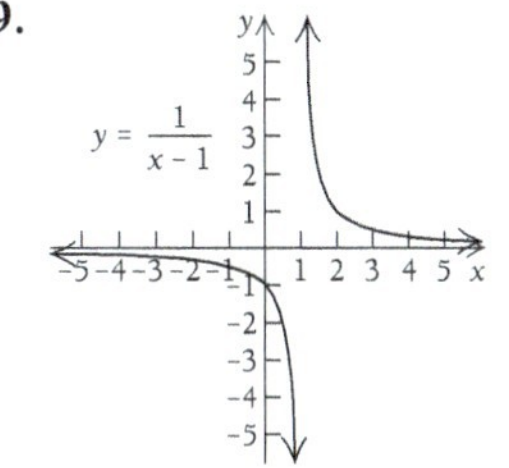

Domain: $(-\infty, 1) \cup (1, \infty)$

31.

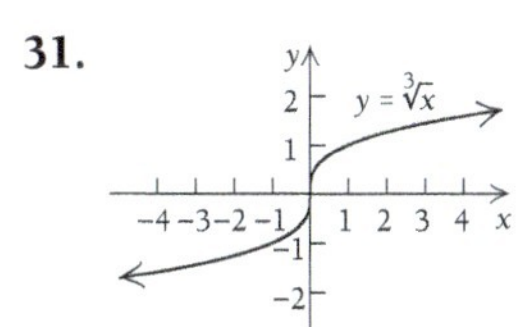

Domain: $(-\infty, \infty)$, or $\mathbb{R}$

33.

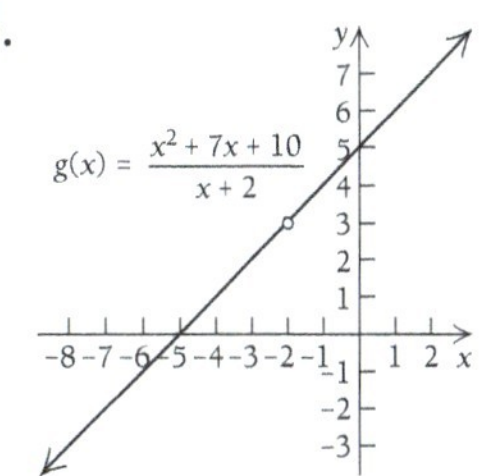

Domain: $(-\infty, -2) \cup (-2, \infty)$

35. $x = 1 \pm \sqrt{3}$ **37.** $x = -3 \pm \sqrt{10}$

39. $x = \frac{1 \pm \sqrt{2}}{2}$ **41.** $y = \frac{-4 \pm \sqrt{10}}{3}$

43. $x = \frac{-7 \pm \sqrt{13}}{2}$ **45.** $\sqrt[5]{x}$ **47.** $\sqrt[3]{y^2}$

49. $\frac{1}{\sqrt[5]{t^2}}$ **51.** $\frac{1}{\sqrt[3]{b}}$ **53.** $\frac{1}{\sqrt{x^2 + 3}}$

55. $x^{3/2}, x \geq 0$ **57.** $a^{3/5}$ **59.** $x^3, x \geq 0$

61. $t^{-5/2}, t \neq 0$ **63.** $(x^2 + 7)^{-1/2}$ **65.** 27 **67.** 16

69. $(-\infty, 5) \cup (5, \infty)$ **71.** $(-\infty, 2) \cup (2, 3) \cup (3, \infty)$

73. $\left[-\frac{4}{5}, \infty\right)$ **75.** $(-\infty, 7]$

77. (50, 500); quantity = 50, price = \$500

79. (5, 1); quantity = 5000, price = \$100

81. (1, 4); quantity = 100, price = \$4

83. (2, 3); quantity = 2000, price = \$3000

85. 140 tickets

87. (a) 166 mi, 176 mi, 184 mi; **(b)**

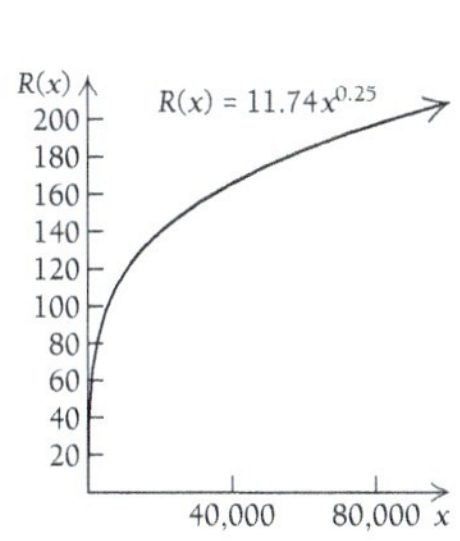

89. **(a)** 10.43 μg/m^3; 10.20 μg/m^3; 10.03 μg/m^3;
(b)

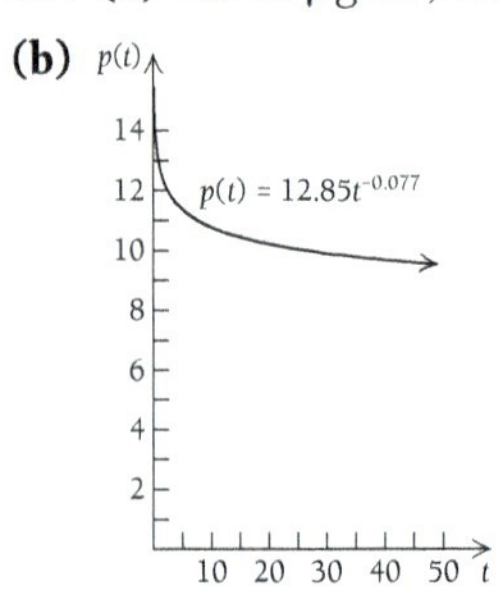

91. 26, 51 **93.** Answers may vary.
95. −1.831, −0.856, 3.188 **97.** 1.489, 5.673
99. −2, 3 **101.** [−1, 2] **103.** $\frac{1 + \sqrt{5}}{2}$ **105.** $\frac{1 + \sqrt{5}}{2}$

Exercise Set R.6, p. 72

1. **(a)**

x	−3	−2	−1	0	1	2	3
$f(x) = 4^x$	0.0156	0.0625	0.25	1	4	16	64

(b) 300%; **(c)** (0, 1); **(d)**

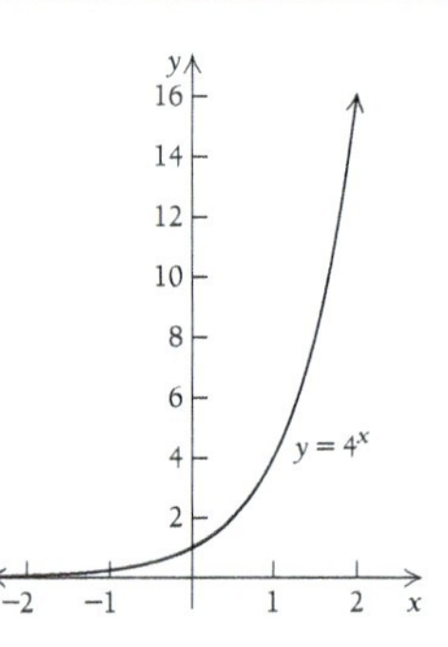

3. **(a)**

x	−3	−2	−1	0	1	2	3
$h(x) = 2 \cdot 1.5^x$	0.5926	0.8889	1.3333	2	3	4.5	6.75

(b) 50%; **(c)** (0, 2); **(d)**

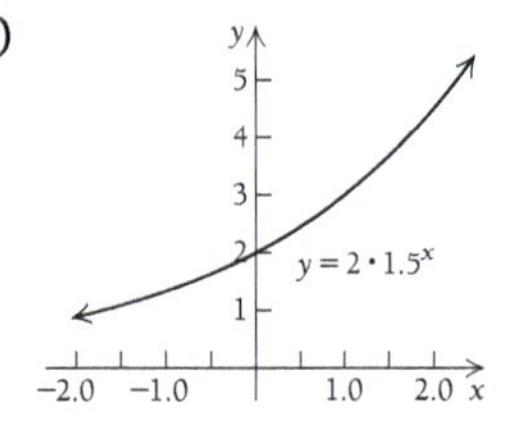

5. **(a)**

x	$m(x) = -3 \cdot 2.15^x$
−3	−0.3019
−2	−0.649
−1	−1.3953
0	−3
1	−6.45
2	−13.8675
3	−29.8151

(b) 115%; **(c)** (0, −3); **(d)**

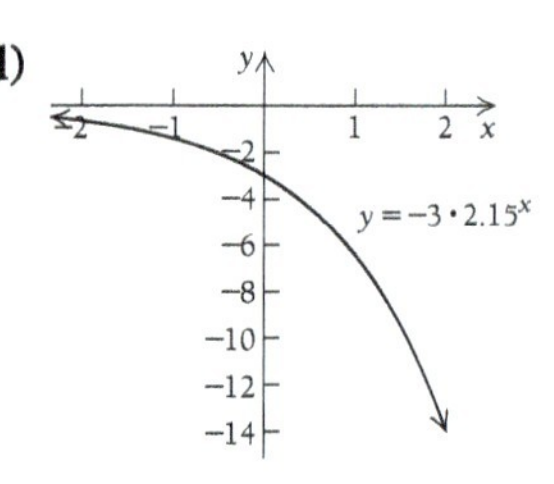

7. **(a)**

x	$p(x) = 12{,}000(0.95)^x$
−3	13,996.2094
−2	13,296.3989
−1	12,631.579
0	12,000
1	11,400
2	10,830
3	10,288.5

(b) −5%; **(c)** (0, 12,000); **(d)**

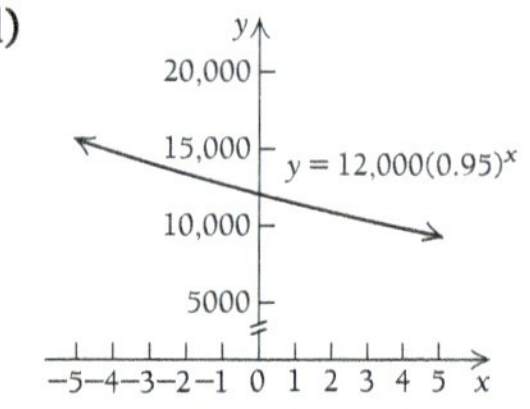

9. **(a)**

x	$r(x) = r_0(0.233)^x$
−3	$79.0555r_0$
−2	$18.4199r_0$
−1	$4.2918r_0$
0	r_0
1	$0.233r_0$
2	$0.0543r_0$
3	$0.0126r_0$

(b) −76.7%; **(c)** $(0, r_0)$; **(d)**

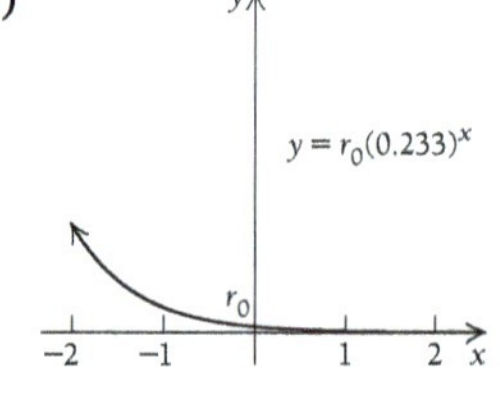

11. $\log_4 64 = 3$ **13.** $\log_{10} 0.01 = -2$, or $\log 0.01 = -2$
15. $\log_{25} 5 = \frac{1}{2}$ **17.** $\log_{216} 6 = \frac{1}{3}$ **19.** $\log_P Q = n$
21. $2^7 = 128$ **23.** $10^7 = 10{,}000{,}000$ **25.** $16^{1/2} = 4$
27. $7^{1/3} = \sqrt[3]{7}$ **29.** $9^0 = 1$ **31.** 256 **33.** 5 **35.** 1
37. −2 **39.** π **41.** 2.80735 **43.** 2.52372 **45.** 2.32193
47. 1.73249 **49.** 0.61315 **51.** 1.71241 **53.** 2.43068
55. 10.76961 **57.** 1.89620 **59.** 1.03018 **61.** 1.449
63. 1.732 **65.** 0.283 **67.** 1.966 **69.** −0.483

71.

$\{x | x > 0\}$

73.

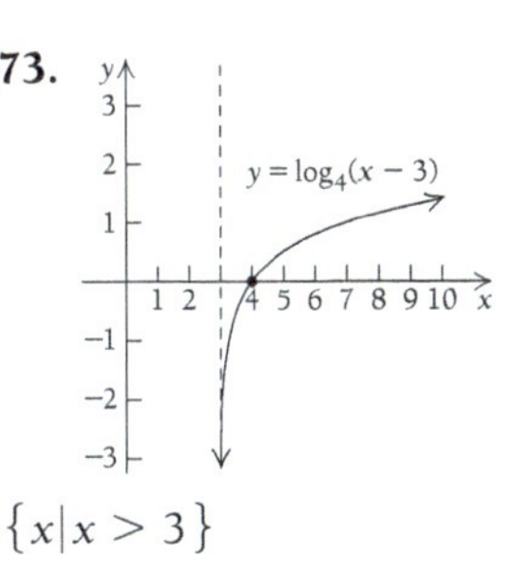

$\{x | x > 3\}$

75.

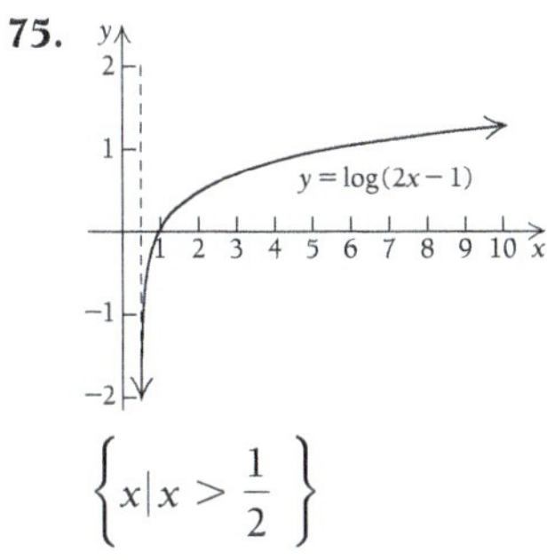

$\left\{x \middle| x > \frac{1}{2}\right\}$

77. **(a)** $A(t) = 900(1.045)^t$; **(b)** $A(5) = 1121.56$, which means that in 2020 the student population will be about 1122; **(c)** after 6.54 yr (or in 2021) **79.** **(a)** $M(t) = 50(0.9875)^t$; **(b)** $M(15) = 41.4$, which means that after 15 days the mass of the sample is 41.4 mg; **(c)** after 72.8 days **81.** **(a)** $E(t) = 550(1.471)^t$; **(b)** $E(10) = 26{,}090.92$, which means that in 10 years there will be about 26,091 students enrolled in the online program; **(c)** after 5.72 yr (in the 6th year) **83.** In 28.1 yr **85.** After 10.5 weeks **87.** Left to the student **89.** Left to the student **91.** $80^{90} > 90^{80}$ **93.** $(-\infty, -1) \cup (1, \infty)$

Technology Connection, p. 79

1. **(a)** Left to the student; **(b)** 93.5; **(c)** left to the student

Technology Connection, p. 81

1. $y = 0.0016278847x^4 - 0.1814259451x^3 + 6.716198092x^2 - 91.87760958x + 397.9916923$; the fit of this equation is slightly better. **2.** Graphs are left to the student. **(a)** $y = -58.21428571x^2 + 5258.214286x - 45{,}399.19643$; **(b)** $y = -0.3055555555x^3 - 17.42261905x^2 + 3597.290675x - 25{,}339.89435$; **(c)** $y = 0.00416666666x^4 - 1.047222222x^3 + 29.25625x^2 + 2380.242163x - 14{,}388.75272$; **(d)** quartic; **(e)** \$48,667, \$73,624

Exercise Set R.7, p. 82

1. Linear **3.** Quadratic with $a < 0$ **5.** Quadratic with $a > 0$ **7.** Linear **9.** Exponential with $0 < a < 1$ **11.** **(a)** $y = 0.933x + 63.2$; **(b)** \$71.6 billion **13.** **(a)** $y = 237.5x^2 - 1400x + 54{,}762.5$ **(b)** \$64,512.50 **15.** **(a)** $y = 1.491x - 33.549$; **(b)** 41%; **(c)** the estimate is higher than the actual value. **17.** **(a)** $y = 11.42(1.02)^x$; **(b)** 33.9 million **19.** **(a)** $y = 108.708(1.03)^x$; **(b)** \$354.62; **(c)** answers may vary. **21.** Answers may vary. **23.** **(a)** $2, \frac{3}{2}, 1$, so the average slope is 1.5; **(b)** $y = 1.5x - 1.166666\ldots$; **(c)** they are the same. **25.** **(a)** $y = 0.00648x^2 - 0.884x + 33.217$; **(b)** 5.2; **(c)** $y = 24.068(0.975)^x$, which gives an estimate of about 6.9; **(d)** answers may vary. **27.** **(a)** Equation (4) is $-24a - 2b = 495$; **(b)** equation (5) is $32a + 2b = 341$; **(c)** $a = \frac{836}{8} = 104.5$; **(d)** $b = -\frac{3003}{2} = -1501.5$; **(e)** $c = 6016$

Chapter R Review Exercises, p. 93

1. (d) **2.** (b) **3.** (f) **4.** (a) **5.** (e) **6.** (g) **7.** (h) **8.** (c) **9.** True **10.** False **11.** True **12.** True **13.** False **14.** False **15.** True **16.** **(a)** 4.1 million; **(b)** 32 and 85; **(c)** [0, 92.3] **17.** \$4177.94 **18.** \$13,402.43 **19.** No. Elizabeth (input) has three outputs. **20.** **(a)** −6; **(b)** −30; **(c)** $-a^2 + a$; **(d)** $-x^2 - 2xh - h^2 + x + h$

21.

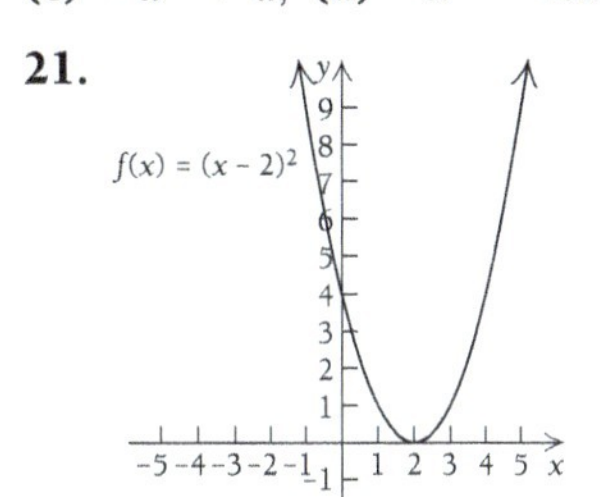

22.

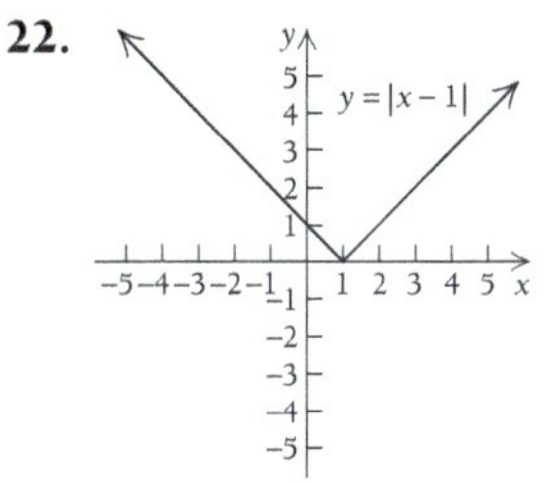

23.

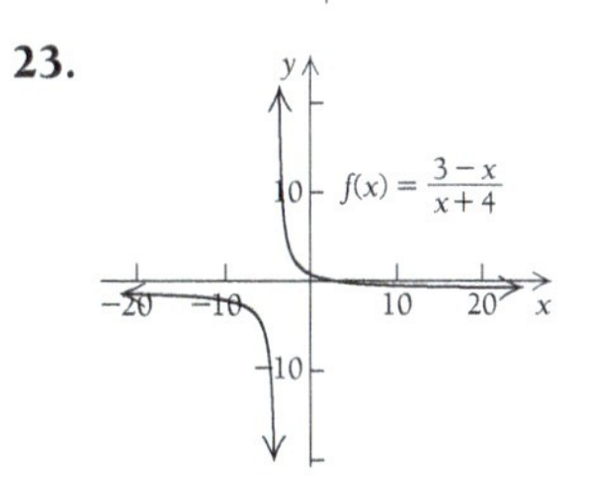

24.

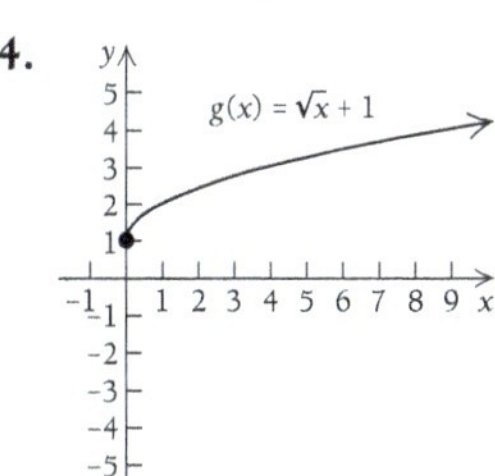

25. No **26.** Yes **27.** Yes **28.** No **29.** **(a)** 1; **(b)** $[-4, 4]$; **(c)** −3; **(d)** $[-1, 3]$

30. **(a)** 1, 4, 3; **(b)**

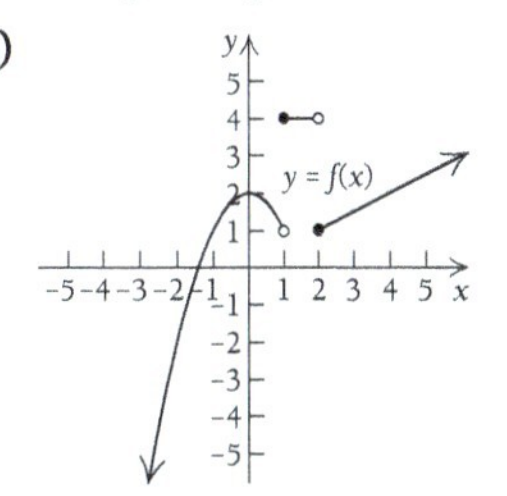

31. **(a)** $[-2, 5]$; **(b)** $(-1, 3]$; **(c)** $(-\infty, a)$; **(d)** $(-\infty, -1] \cup [3, 4)$ **32.** **(a)** $[-4, 5)$ **(b)** $(2, \infty)$ **33.** **(a)** −2; **(b)** $\{-3, -2, -1, 0, 1, 2, 3\}$; **(c)** $\{-1, 3\}$; **(d)** $\{-2, 1, 2, 3, 4\}$ **34.** **(a)** $(-\infty, 5) \cup (5, \infty)$; **(b)** $[-6, \infty)$; **(c)** $(2, \infty)$; **(d)** [0, 5] **35.** Slope: −3, y-intercept: (0, 2) **36.** $y = \frac{1}{4}x - 7$ **37.** −3 **38.** −\$350/yr **39.** 75 pages/day **40.** $A = 0.1V$

41. **(a)** $C(x) = 0.5x + 4000$; **(b)** $R(x) = 10x$; **(c)** $P(x) = 9.5x - 4000$; **(d)** 422 CDs

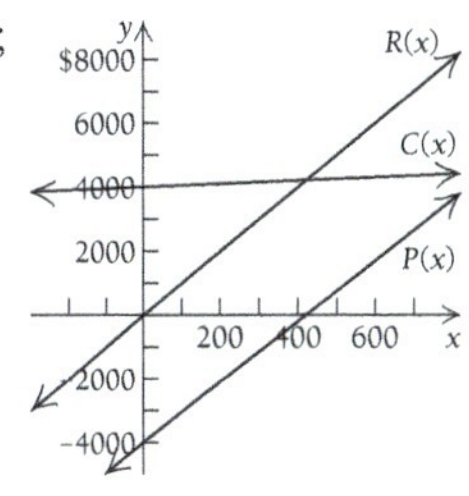

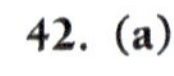

42. **(a)**

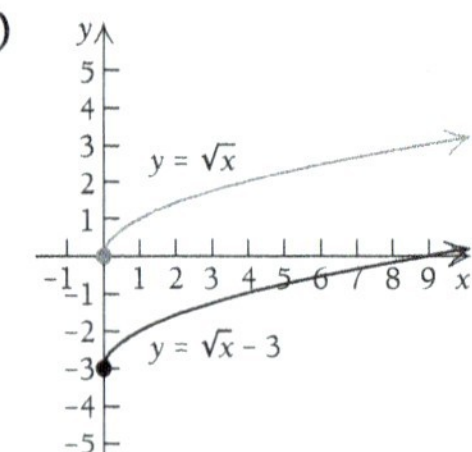

(b)

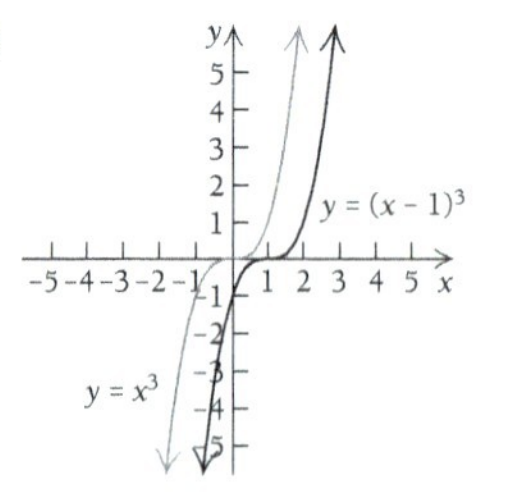

43. **(a)**

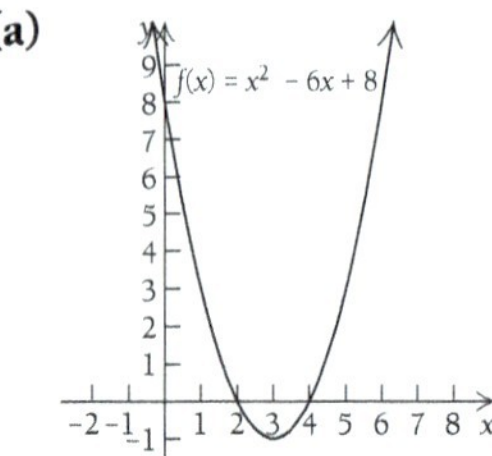

vertex: $(3, -1)$

(b)

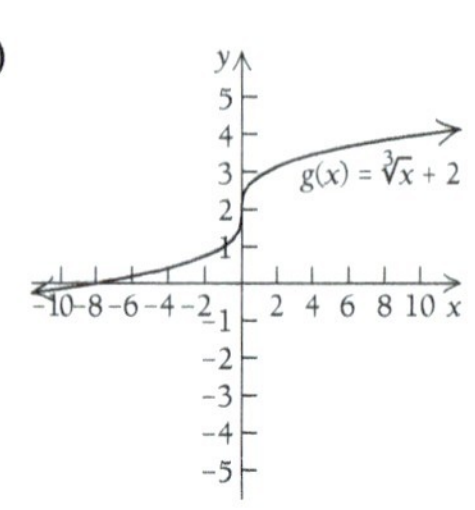

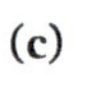

(c)

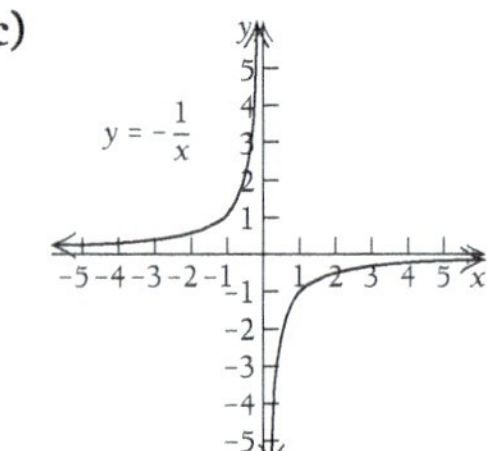

(d)

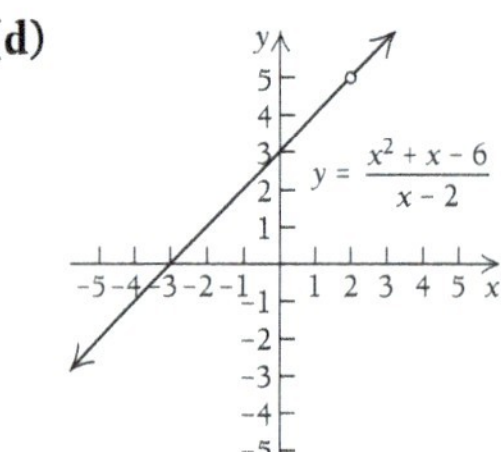

44. **(a)** $x = 1, x = 3$; **(b)** $x = \frac{2 \pm \sqrt{10}}{2}$ **45.** **(a)** $x^{4/5}$; **(b)** t^4; **(c)** $m^{-2/3}$; **(d)** $(x^2 - 9)^{-1/2}$ **46.** **(a)** $\sqrt[5]{x^2}$; **(b)** $\frac{1}{\sqrt[5]{m^3}}$; **(c)** $\sqrt{x^2 - 5}$; **(d)** $\sqrt[3]{t}$ **47.** $\left[\frac{9}{2}, \infty\right)$

48. **(a)**

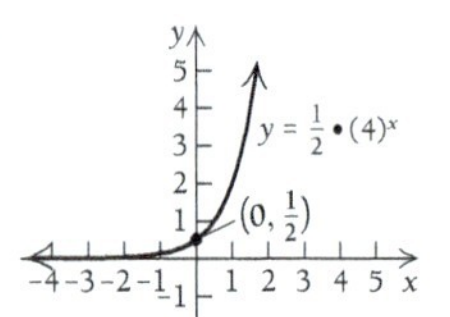

(b)

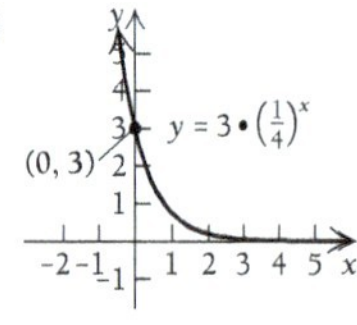

49. **(a)** 2.3%; **(b)** 25,209, which means that in 2023 the population of Arvon Hill will be 25,209; **(c)** after 19.4 yr, or in 2037 **50.** **(a)** $M(t) = 125(0.986)^t$; **(b)** -1.4%/week; **(c)** after 65 weeks **51.** **(a)** 1.256; **(b)** 0.183; **(c)** 1.497 **52.** 4, which is the power to which 3 must be raised to give 81 **53.** (3, 16); quantity = 300, price = \$16 **54.** About 3.3 hr **55.** **(a)** $M = 0.2r + 160$

(b)

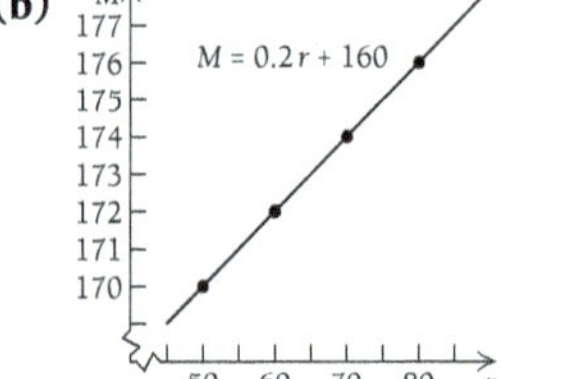
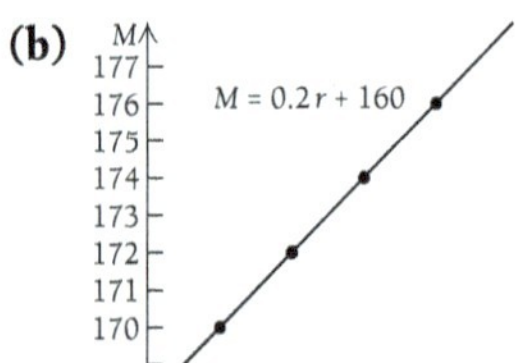

(c) 173.4 beats/min

56. **(a)** Left to the student; **(b)** yes; **(c)** $P = 1.9975x^2 - 89.8444x + 870$; **(d)** about $-\$27.56$; **(e)** answers may vary. **57.** **(a)** 525,375 lb; **(b)** \$4.31/lb

58. $[-5, 5]$ **59.** $[1, 2]$ **60.** $a = -\frac{1}{2}$

61. $y = x^3 - 9x^2 + 27x + 50$

$x = -1.25$; domain and range: $(-\infty, \infty)$

62.

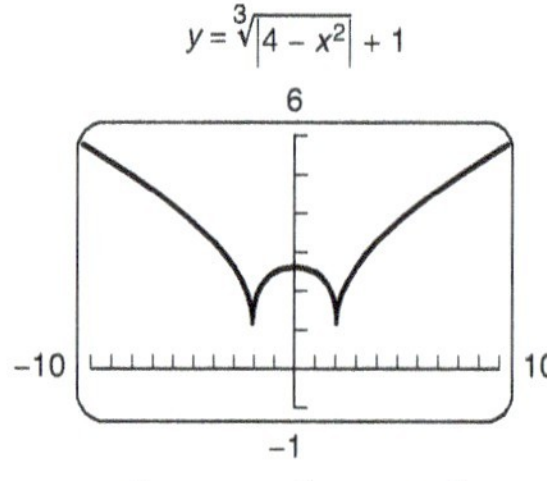

no zeros; domain: $(-\infty, \infty)$, range: $[1, \infty)$

63. $(-1.21, 2.36)$ **64.** **(a)** $P = 1.86x^2 - 84.18x + 943.86$; **(b)** \$95.46; **(c)** answers may vary.

65. **(a)** Linear: $A = -9.190819894x + 697.05481$; quadratic: $A = 0.0757317559x^2 - 15.51100944x + 801.4311225$; cubic: $A = 0.0052352573x^3 - 0.5849501976x^2 + 9.082584281x + 545.8186828$;
exponential: $A = 1014.883046(0.9677603597)^x$;

(b)

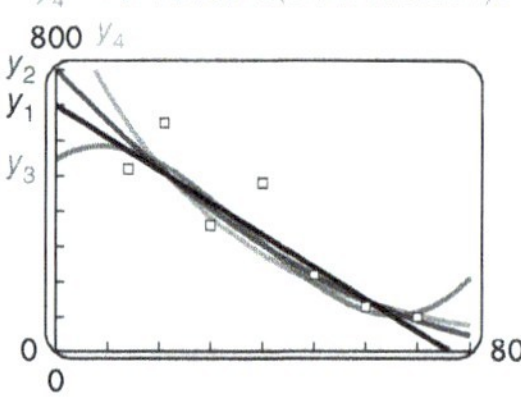

(c) Answers may vary.

Chapter R Test, p. 97

1. \$750 **2.** **(a)** -4; **(b)** $-x^2 - 2xh - h^2 + 5$

3. $m = \frac{4}{5}$; y-intercept: $\left(0, -\frac{2}{3}\right)$ **4.** $y = \frac{1}{4}x + \frac{31}{4}$

5. $-\frac{1}{2}$ **6.** $-\$700$/yr; **7.** $\frac{1}{2}$ lb/bag **8.** $F = \frac{2}{3}W$

9. **(a)** $C(x) = 0.08x + 8000$; **(b)** $R(x) = 0.50x$; **(c)** $P(x) = 0.42x - 8000$; **(d)** 19,048 cards **10.** (3, 25); quantity = 3000, price = \$25 **11.** Yes **12.** No

13. **(a)** -4; **(b)** $(-\infty, \infty)$; **(c)** $\{-3, 3\}$; **(d)** $[-5, \infty)$

14.

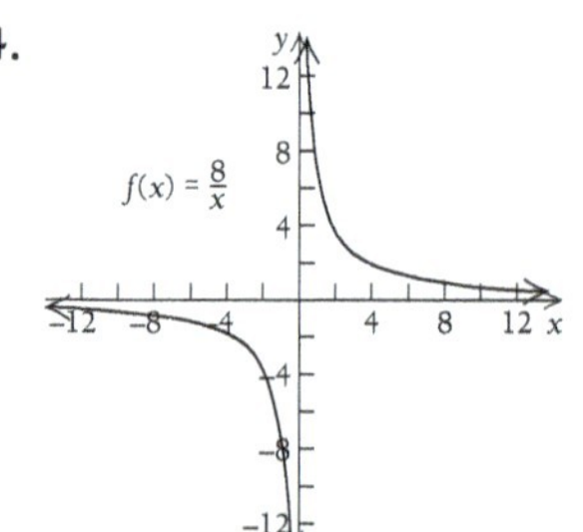

15. $t^{-1/2}$

16. $\frac{1}{\sqrt[5]{t^3}}$

17. $-\frac{1}{2}$

18.

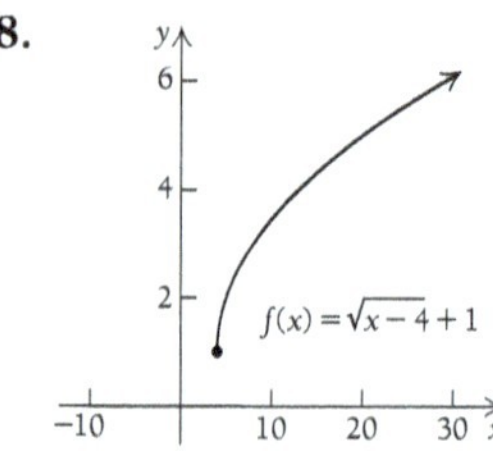

19. $[c, d)$

20. $(-2, \infty)$

21. $(-\infty, -7) \cup (-7, 2) \cup (2, \infty)$

22.

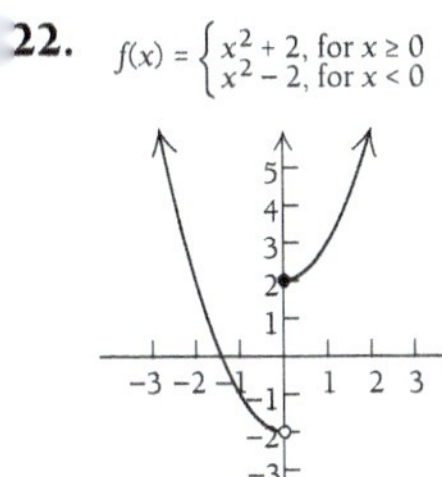

$f(x) = \begin{cases} x^2 + 2, \text{ for } x \geq 0 \\ x^2 - 2, \text{ for } x < 0 \end{cases}$

23.

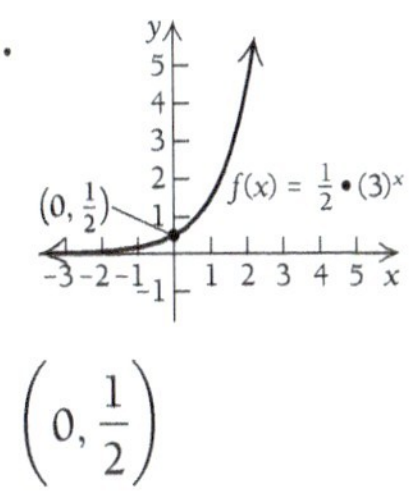

$\left(0, \frac{1}{2}\right)$

24. **(a)** 4.1%/yr; **(b)** after 10.09 yr

25. **(a)**

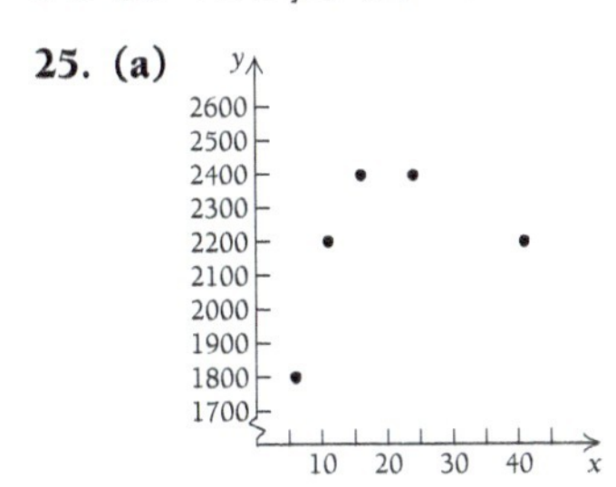

(b) Yes; **(c)** $y = -1.94x^2 + 102.74x + 1253.49$; **(d)** About 2590 calories; **(e)** answers may vary.

26. $\frac{1}{16}$ **27.** Domain: $\left(-\infty, \frac{5}{3}\right]$, x-intercept: $\left(-798\frac{2}{3}, 0\right)$

28. One possible equation is $y = (x + 3)(x - 1)(x - 4)$. **29.** $\frac{51}{7}$

30.

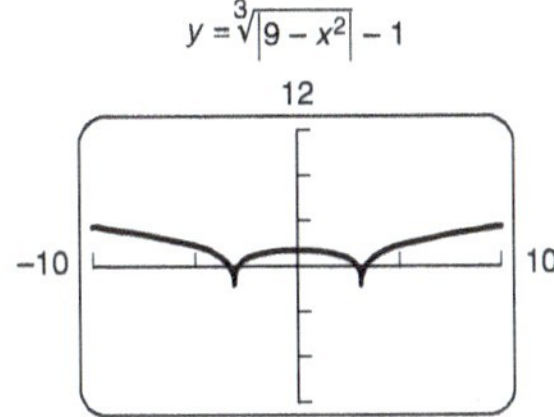

Zeros: $\pm\sqrt{8}, \pm\sqrt{10}$; domain: $(-\infty, \infty)$; range: $[-1, \infty)$

31. **(a)** $y = -1.51x^2 + 79.98x + 1436.93$; **(b)** about 2480 calories; **(c)** answers may vary.

Extended Technology Application, p. 99

1. **(a)** $P(t) = 0.1267032967t - 0.5842857143$;

(b) **(c)** \$8.28, \$8.92, answers may vary; **(d)** 2112, which seems too far into the future.

2. **(a)** $P(t) = 0.0014796703t^2 + 0.0305247253t + 0.3775$;

(b) **(c)** \$9.76, \$10.99, answers may vary; **(d)** 2055, which is plausible.

3. **(a)** $P(t) = -0.00000183t^3 + 0.0016588147t^2 + 0.0260369288t + 0.3972058824$;

(b)

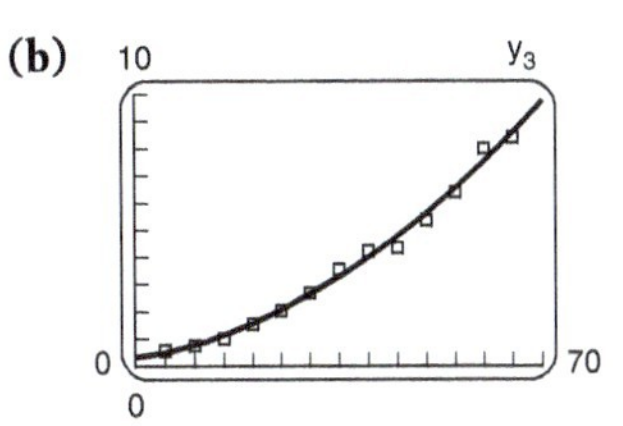

(c) \$9.72, \$10.91, answers may vary; **(d)** 2057, which is also plausible.

4. **(a)** $P(t) = 0.00000046249829t^4 - 0.00006196216t^3 + 0.004115011t^2 - 0.006602236t + 0.4680672269$;

(b)

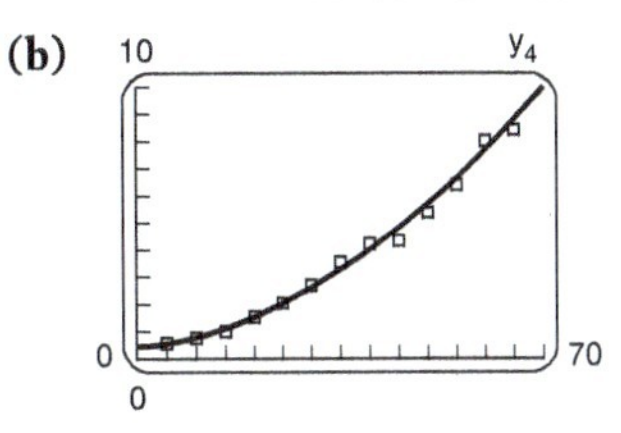

(c) \$10.02, \$11.61, answers may vary; **(d)** 2042, which is plausible, but may be too soon.

5. **(a)** $P(t) = 0.5430389024(1.047332533)^t$;

(b)

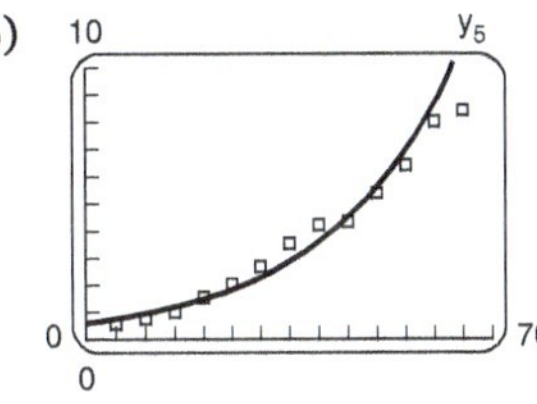

(c) \$13.83, \$17.43, answers may vary; **(d)** 2028, which is probably too soon.

6. Answers may vary.

CHAPTER 1

Exercise Set 1.1, p. 112

1. $0.3, x \to 0.3^-$ **3.** $-3, x \to -3^-$ **5.** $\frac{2}{3}, x \to \left(\frac{2}{3}\right)^-$ **7.** $0.3, x \to 0.3^-$ **9.** $1, x \to 1^+$ **11.** -2 **13.** $\lim_{x \to 2^+}$ **15.** $\lim_{x \to 5}$ **17.** "the limit, as x approaches 4, of $f(x)$" or "the limit of $f(x)$ as x approaches 4" **19.** "the limit, as x approaches 5 from the left, of $F(x)$" or "the limit of $F(x)$ as x approaches 5 from the left" **21.** **(a)** -3; **(b)** -3; **(c)** -3 **23.** **(a)** -1; **(b)** -1; **(c)** -1 **25.** 5 **27.** Does not exist **29.** 2 **31.** 2 **33.** 1 **35.** 4 **37.** 0 **39.** 0 **41.** 0 **43.** 1 **45.** 4 **47.** 1 **49.** 1 **51.** -1 **53.** 2 **55.** Does not exist **57.** 0 **59.** 2

61.

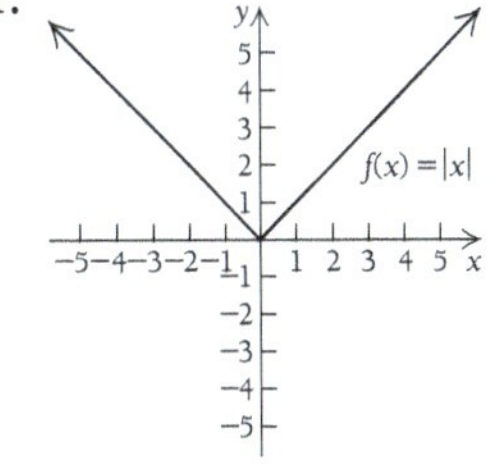

0, 2

63.

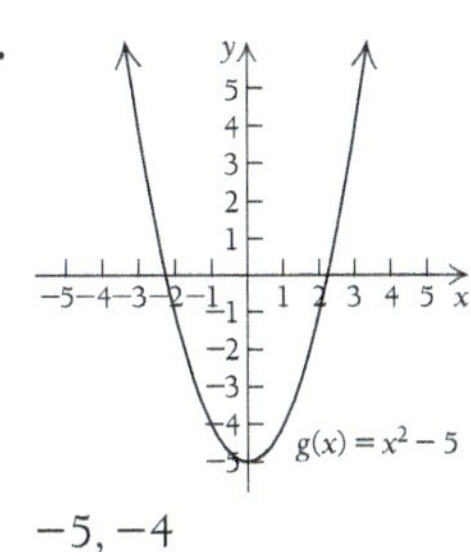

$-5, -4$

65.

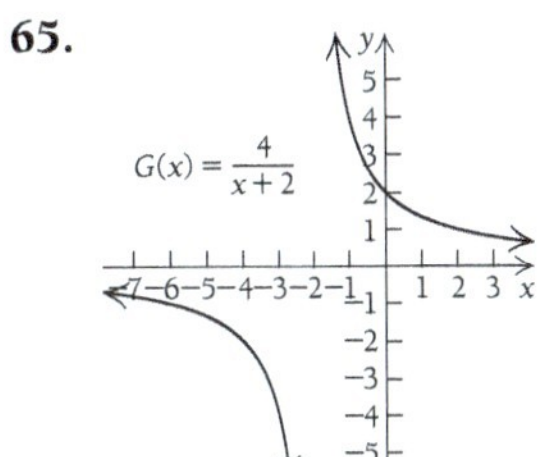

4, does not exist

67.

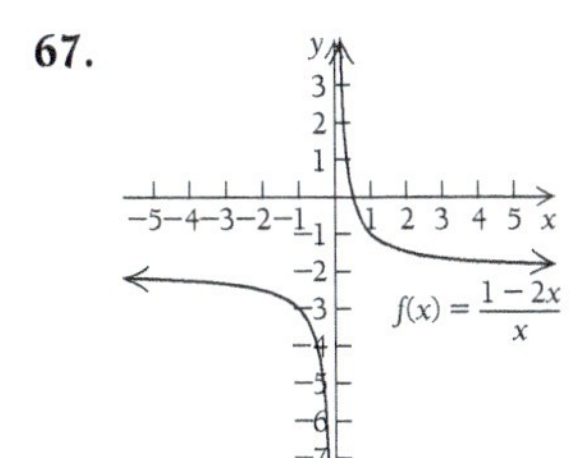

-2, does not exist

69.
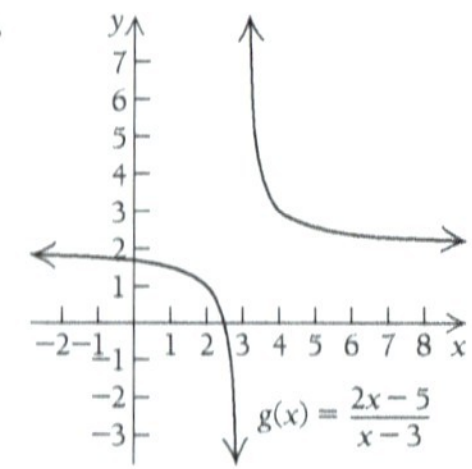

2, does not exist

71.
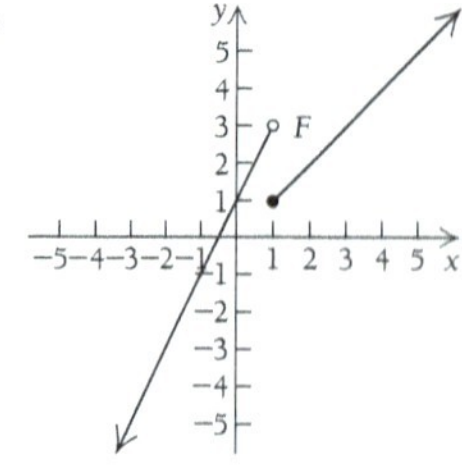

3, 1, does not exist

73.
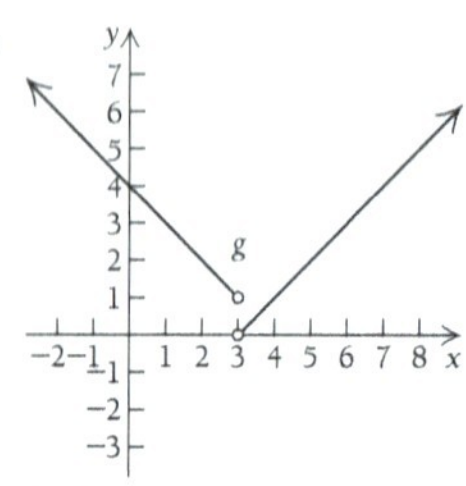

1, 0, does not exist

75.
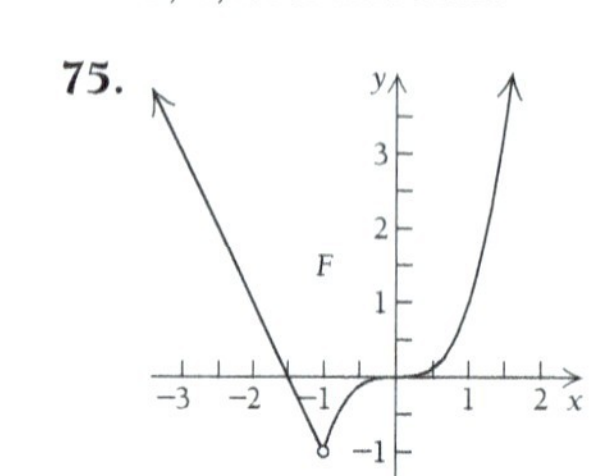

-1

77.
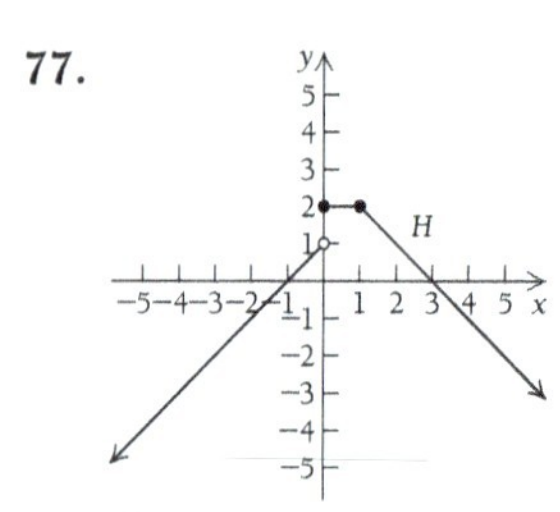

does not exist, 2

79. \$3.50, \$3.50, \$3.50 **81.** \$4.00, \$4.50, does not exist **83.** \$1.21, \$1.42, does not exist **85.** Does not exist **87.** 10%, 12%, does not exist **89.** 22%, does not exist **91.** 12%, 22%, does not exist **93.** 3 **95.** -1 **97.** **(a)** 4; **(b)** 4, **(c)** 4; **(d)** 4; **(e)** 4; **(f)** no; **(g)** yes **99.** 0, 0

Exercise Set 1.2, p. 124

1. True **3.** True **5.** True **7.** False **9.** 5 **11.** -3 **13.** 4 **15.** 15 **17.** 1 **19.** 10 **21.** $\frac{7}{2}$ **23.** $-\frac{13}{6}$ **25.** 3 **27.** -6 **29.** Does not exist **31.** $\frac{5}{4}$ **33.** $\frac{1}{6}$ **35.** $\frac{1}{3}$ **37.** 0 **39.** Does not exist **41.** 3 **43.** Does not exist **45.** 0 **47.** Not continuous **49.** Continuous **51.** Not continuous **53.** **(a)** -1, 2, does not exist; **(b)** -1; **(c)** no, the limit does not exist; **(d)** 3; **(e)** 3; **(f)** yes, the limit exists and equals the function value. **55.** **(a)** 2; **(b)** does not exist; **(c)** no, the function value does not exist; **(d)** -2; **(e)** -2; **(f)** yes, the limit exists and equals the function value. **57.** **(a)** 3; **(b)** 1; **(c)** does not exist; **(d)** 1; **(e)** no, the limit does not exist; **(f)** yes, the limit exists and equals the function value; **(g)** yes, the limit exists and equals the function value.
59. Yes, the limit exists and equals the function value at 4.
61. No, the limit does not exist and G is not defined at 0.
63. Yes, the limit exists and equals the function value at 4.
65. No, the limit does not exist at 3. **67.** No, g is not defined at 4.
69. No, the limit value does not equal the function value at 2.
71. Yes, the limit exists and equals the function value at 4.
73. No, the limit does not exist and the function is not defined at 5.
75. No, the limit does not exist and the function is not defined at 2.
77. Yes, because $\lim_{x\to a} g(x) = g(a)$ for all a such that $-4 < a < 4$ **79.** Yes, because $\lim_{x\to a} g(x) = g(a)$ for all a such that $1 < a < \infty$, and $\lim_{x\to 1^+} g(x) = g(1)$
81. Yes, because $\lim_{x\to a} F(x) = F(a)$ for all a such that $-5 < a < 5$, and $\lim_{x\to -5^+} F(x) = F(-5)$ and $\lim_{x\to 5^-} F(x) = F(5)$ **83.** 30, 25, does not exist **85.** 120, 120, 120 **87.** Yes **89.** Yes **91.** No **93.** Yes **95.** 2 **97.** $a = \frac{19}{4}, b = -3$ **99.** $\frac{1}{2}$ **101.** $\frac{1}{2}$ **103.** $\frac{1}{\sqrt{7}}$ **105.** 0

Exercise Set 1.3, p. 133

1. The temperature rose 3 degrees/hr. **3.** Marcus delivered 7 packages/hr. **5.** Tanya scored 25 points/game.
7. Burnham Industries had 5,000,000 dollars/month in revenue.
9. Unemployment changed by -0.333 percentage point/month.
11. 3 **13.** 2 **15.** $-\frac{1}{32}$ **17.** 8 **19.** 4.25
21. **(a)** $10x + 5h$; **(b)** 60, 55, 50.5, 50.05
23. **(a)** $-10x - 5h$; **(b)** $-60, -55, -50.5, -50.05$
25. **(a)** $2x + h - 1$; **(b)** 11, 10, 9.1, 9.01 **27.** **(a)** $-\frac{9}{x(x+h)}$; **(b)** $-\frac{9}{35}, -\frac{3}{10}, -\frac{6}{17}, -\frac{60}{167}$ **29.** **(a)** 2; **(b)** 2, 2, 2, 2
31. **(a)** $36x^2 + 36xh + 12h^2$; **(b)** 1308, 1092, 918.12, 901.8012
33. **(a)** $2x + h - 4$; **(b)** 8, 7, 6.1, 6.01 **35.** **(a)** $2x + h - 3$; **(b)** 9, 8, 7.1, 7.01 **37.** 0.36 percentage point/yr, -0.3 percentage point/yr, 0.09 percentage point/yr
39. 0.66 percentage point/yr, -0.15 percentage point/yr, 0.21 percentage point/yr **41.** 0.1 percentage point/yr, -0.04 percentage point/yr, 0.03 percentage point/yr
43. 2.1 percentage points/yr, -4.3 percentage points/yr, -1.5 percentage points/yr **45.** $-\$450$/yr, \$1266.67/yr, \$580/yr
47. **(a)** 70, 39, 29, 23; **(b)** answers may vary.
49. **(a)** \$26.62; **(b)** \$31.16; **(c)** \$4.54; **(d)** 0.7567, which means that prices increased by an average of about \$0.76 per year
51. The average cost of production of between 300 and 305 holders is \$19.75 per unit. **53.** 17.62; the average rate of change in Amazon's revenue between 2014 and 2017 was \$17.62 billion per year.
55. **(a)** 1.49 hectares/g; **(b)** home range increases by 1.0902 hectares per gram as the animal's weight grows from 200 g to 300 g.
57. **(a)** 1.25, 1.25, 0.625, 0, 0; **(b)** answers may vary.
59. **(a)** 256 ft; **(b)** 128 ft/sec **61.** **(a)** 125 thousand people/yr; **(b)** answers may vary; **(c)** **A:** 290 thousand people/year, -40 thousand people/yr, -50 thousand people/yr, 300 thousand people/yr; **B:** 125 thousand people/yr, 125 thousand people/yr, 125 thousand people/yr, 125 thousand people/yr **(d)** answers may vary.
63. 825.46; Harbor University's undergraduate population was increasing at the rate of 825.46 students per year between the 2nd and 6th years. **65.** $2ax + b + ah$ **67.** $4x^3 + 6x^2h + 4xh^2 + h^3$
69. $5ax^4 + 10ax^3h + 10ax^2h^2 + 5axh^3 + ah^4 + 4bx^3 + 6bx^2h + 4bxh^2 + bh^3$ **71.** $\frac{1}{(1-x-h)(1-x)}$
73. $\frac{2}{\sqrt{2(x+h)+1} + \sqrt{2x+1}}$

Exercise Set 1.4, p. 144

1. **(a)** and **(b)**

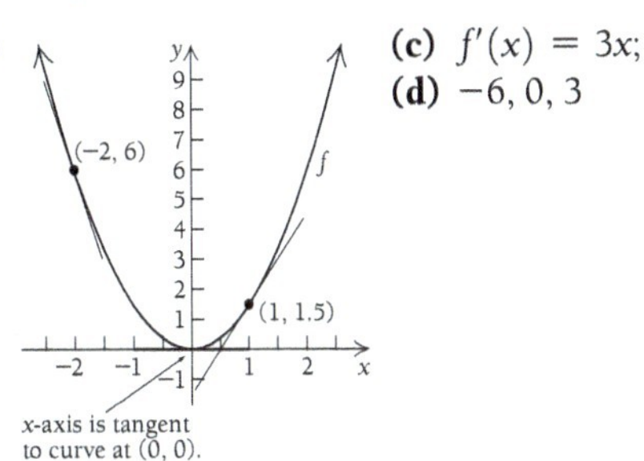

(c) $f'(x) = 3x$; **(d)** $-6, 0, 3$

3. **(a)** and **(b)**

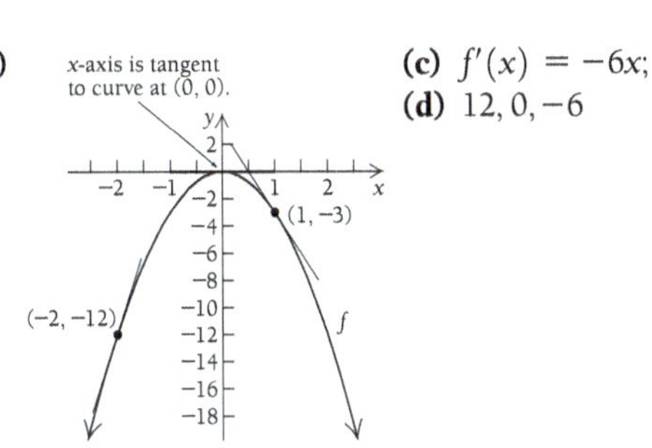

(c) $f'(x) = -6x$; **(d)** $12, 0, -6$

5. **(a)** and **(b)**

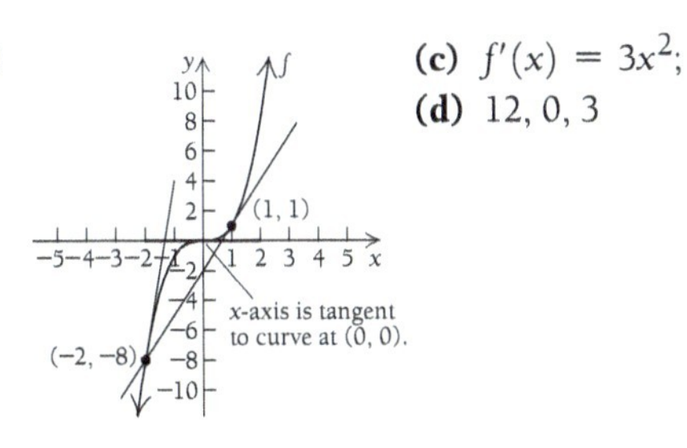

(c) $f'(x) = 3x^2$; **(d)** $12, 0, 3$

7. **(a)** and **(b)**

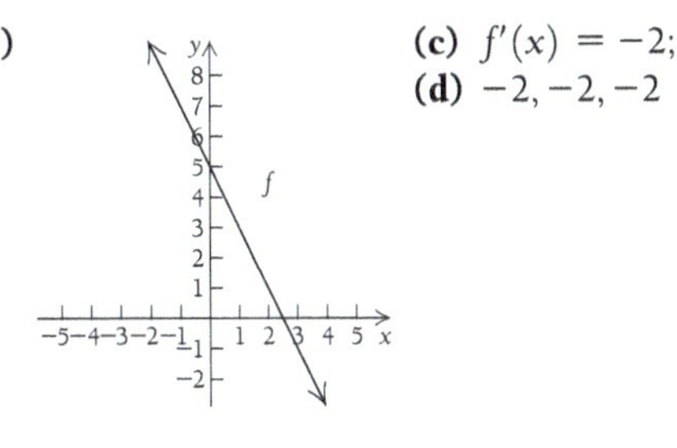

(c) $f'(x) = -2$; **(d)** $-2, -2, -2$

9. **(a)** and **(b)**

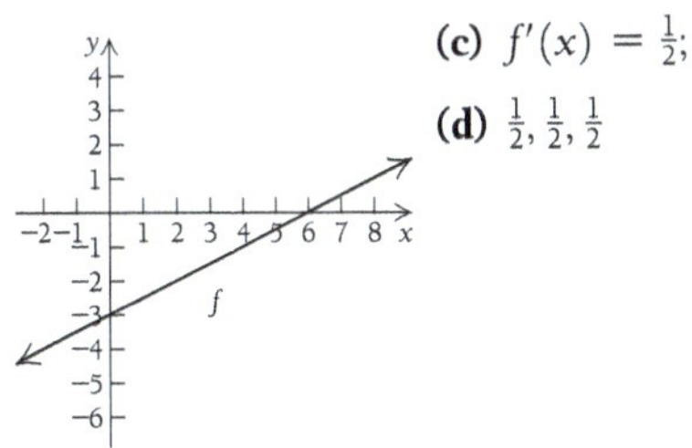

(c) $f'(x) = \frac{1}{2}$; **(d)** $\frac{1}{2}, \frac{1}{2}, \frac{1}{2}$

11. **(a)** and **(b)**

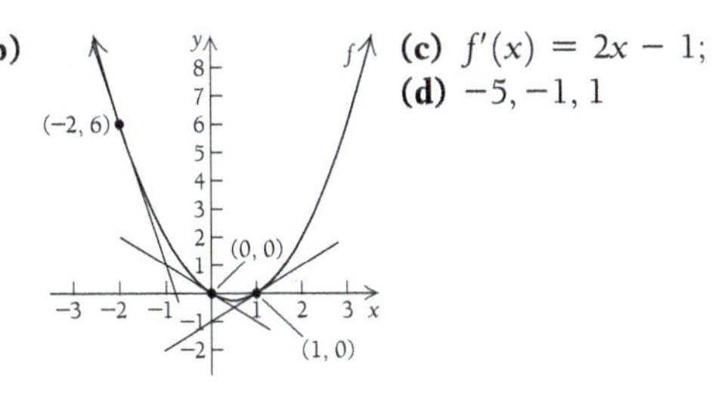

(c) $f'(x) = 2x - 1$; **(d)** $-5, -1, 1$

13. **(a)** and **(b)**

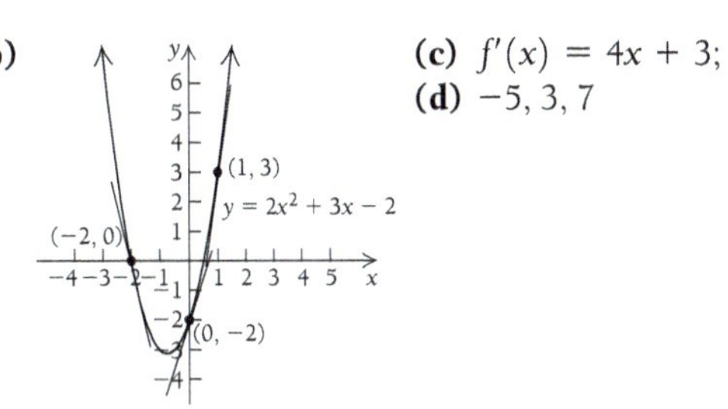

(c) $f'(x) = 4x + 3$; **(d)** $-5, 3, 7$

15. **(a)** and **(b)**

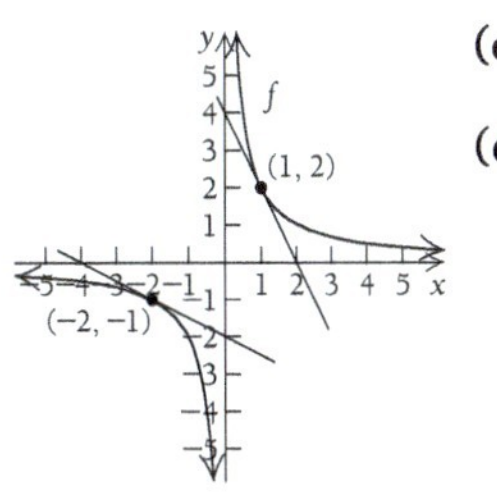

(c) $f'(x) = -\dfrac{2}{x^2}$; **(d)** $-\frac{1}{2}$, not defined, -2

17. **(a)** $y = 12x + 16$; **(b)** $y = 0$; **(c)** $y = 48x - 128$
19. **(a)** $y = -2x + 4$; **(b)** $y = -2x - 4$; **(c)** $y = -0.0002x + 0.04$
21. **(a)** $y = -6x - 4$; **(b)** $y = -1$; **(c)** $y = 6x - 16$
23. $f'(x) = m$ **25.** x_1, x_3, x_4, x_5, x_7 **27.** $x_0, x_3, x_4, x_6, x_{12}$
29. x_1, x_2, x_3, x_4 **31–37.** Left to the student **39.** False
41. False **43.** Answers may vary. **45.** $f'(x) = \dfrac{1}{(1 - x)^2}$
47. $f'(x) = -\dfrac{2}{x^3}$ **49.** $f'(x) = \dfrac{1}{\sqrt{2x + 1}}$
51. $f'(x) = 2ax + b$ **53.** **(a)** $x = -3$; **(b)** answers may vary; **(c)** 1 **55.** **(a)** $x = 3$; **(b)** answers may vary; **(c)** $-1, -1, 1, 1$
57. Answers may vary. **59.** **(a)** Limit is 1 and $G(1) = 1$, so G is continuous at $x = 1$. **(b)** Yes, the graph is a smooth nonvertical curve at $x = 1$. **61.** $\frac{3}{2}$ **63.** The trucker's average speed was $290/4 = 72.5$, and his distance function is differentiable for the entire 4-hr drive, so he must have driven 72.5 miles per hour at least once in that 4-hr period.

Exercise Set 1.5, p. 154

1. The derivative of u with respect to v is $f'(v)$; the derivative of u with respect to v is u'; the derivative of u with respect to v is $\dfrac{du}{dv}$, the derivative of u with respect to v is $\dfrac{d}{dv}f(v)$. **3.** The derivative of p with respect to q is $R'(q)$; the derivative of p with respect to q is p'; the derivative of p with respect to q is $\dfrac{dp}{dq}$; the derivative of p with respect to q is $\dfrac{d}{dq}R(q)$. **5.** The derivative of h with respect to k is $m'(k)$; the derivative of h with respect to k is h'; the derivative of h with respect to k is $\dfrac{dh}{dk}$; the derivative of h with respect to k is $\dfrac{d}{dk}m(k)$. **7.** $7x^6$ **9.** -3 **11.** 0 **13.** $30x^{14}$
15. $-6x^{-7}$ **17.** $-8x^{-3}$ **19.** $3x^2 + 6x$ **21.** $\dfrac{4}{\sqrt{x}}$
23. $0.9x^{-0.1}$ **25.** $\dfrac{2}{5}x^{-1/5}$ **27.** $-\dfrac{21}{x^4}$ **29.** $\dfrac{1}{4\sqrt[4]{x^3}} + \dfrac{3}{x^2}$
31. $-\dfrac{10}{3}\sqrt[3]{x^2}$ **33.** $\dfrac{5}{11}$ **35.** $-\dfrac{12}{5x^7}$ **37.** $-\dfrac{4}{x^2} - \dfrac{3}{5}x^{-2/5}$
39. 7 **41.** $\dfrac{1}{2}\sqrt{x}$ **43.** $-0.02x + 0.4$

45. $-\frac{3}{4}x^{-7/4} - 2x^{-1/3} + \frac{5}{4}x^{1/4} - \frac{8}{x^5}$ **47.** $\frac{1}{7} - \frac{7}{x^2}$ **49.** $\frac{1}{4}$

51. -5 **53.** $\frac{1}{12}$ **55.** $-\frac{3}{640}$ **57.** **(a)** $y = \frac{3}{2}x - \frac{3}{2}$; **(b)** $y = \frac{31}{4}x - 17$; **(c)** $y = \frac{107}{6}x - \frac{165}{2}$

59. **(a)** $y = -\frac{2}{3}x + \frac{1}{3}$; **(b)** $y = \frac{2}{3}x + \frac{1}{3}$; **(c)** $y = \frac{1}{3}x + \frac{4}{3}$

61. $(0, 4)$ **63.** $(0, -2)$ **65.** $(0.3, 7.55)$ **67.** $(20, 54)$

69. None **71.** All points (the graph is a horizontal line)

73. $\left(1, -55\frac{1}{3}\right), \left(11, 111\frac{1}{3}\right)$ **75.** $(-\sqrt{2}, 1 + 4\sqrt{2})$, $(\sqrt{2}, 1 - 4\sqrt{2})$ **77.** $(3, 0)$ **79.** $(2.5, 8.75)$ **81.** $(50, 75)$

83. $\left(1 + \sqrt{6}, -\frac{11}{3} - 3\sqrt{6}\right), \left(1 - \sqrt{6}, -\frac{11}{3} + 3\sqrt{6}\right)$

85. $\left(-\frac{1}{8}, -\frac{11}{24}\right), \left(\frac{1}{8}, \frac{11}{24}\right)$

87. **(a)** $w'(t) = 1.82 - 0.1192t + 0.002274t^2$; **(b)** 21.148 lb; **(c)** 0.855 pound per month **89.** **(a)** $R'(v) = -\frac{6000}{v^2}$; **(b)** 75 beats per minute; **(c)** -0.9375 beat per minute

91. **(a)** $\frac{dP}{dt} = 4000t$; **(b)** 300,000 people **(c)** 40,000 people per year **(d)** answers will vary. **93.** **(a)** $\frac{dv}{dh} = \frac{0.61}{\sqrt{h}}$; **(b)** 244 mi; **(c)** 0.00305 mile per foot gained; **(d)** answers will vary.

95. **(a)** About \$1490; **(b)** $\frac{dp}{dt} = 1.716t - 18.864$; **(c)** about \$72.08 per year **97.** $(-\infty, -1) \cup (3, \infty)$

99. $(0, -2), \left(\frac{1}{\sqrt{3}}, -\frac{55}{27}\right), \left(-\frac{1}{\sqrt{3}}, -\frac{55}{27}\right)$

101. $g'(x) = -2 - 3x^2$ is always negative for all x.

103. $f'(x) = 3x^2 + a$; when $a \geq 0$, then the derivative is always nonnegative for all x, but when $a < 0$, the derivative changes sign at least twice. **105.** $2x$ **107.** $3x^2 - \frac{1}{x^2}\ (x \neq 0)$

109. $\frac{2}{3\sqrt[3]{x^2}}$ **111.** $3x^2 + 6x + 3$

113.

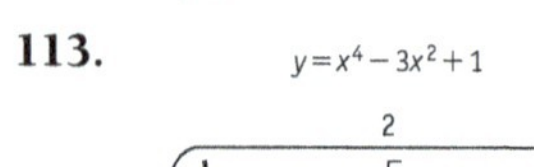

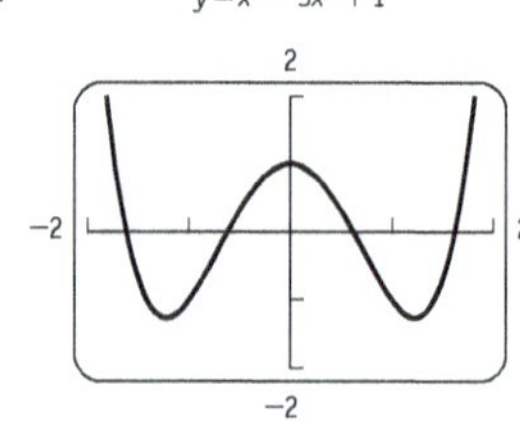

$x = -1.225, x = 0, x = 1.225$

115. $x \approx 0.432$

117.

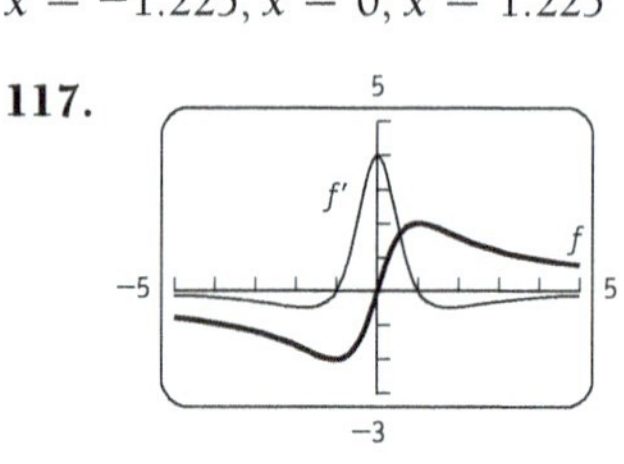

$f'(1) = 0$

Technology Connection, p. 160

1. (c) **2–4.** Left to the student

Exercise Set 1.6, p. 162

1. $11x^{10}$ **3.** $12x + 7$ **5.** $20x^4 + 60x^2$ **7.** $\frac{15}{2}x^{3/2} + 4x$

9. $24x^2 + 12x + 11$ **11.** $\frac{9\sqrt{t}}{2} - \frac{1}{2\sqrt{t}} + 2$ **13.** $4x^3\ (x \neq 0)$

15. $18x^5 - 2x\ (x \neq 0)$ **17.** $2x - 3\ (x \neq -3)$

19. $1\ (t \neq -4)$ **21.** $48x^3 + 3x^2 + 22x + 17$

23. $\frac{-10x^4 + 6x^2 + 30x}{(2x^3 + 3)^2}$ **25.** $120x^2 + \frac{25}{2}x^{3/2} + \frac{3}{2}x^{-1/2} + 24$

27. $\frac{3}{(3 - t)^2} + 15t^2$ **29.** $2x + 6$

31. $2x(x^2 - 4)(3x^2 - 4)$ **33.** $5 - 100x^{-3} + 30x^{-4}$

35. $3t^2 - 1 + \frac{6}{t^2}$ **37.** $-\frac{x^4 + 3x^2 + 2x}{(x^3 - 1)^2} - 10x$

39. $\frac{-\sqrt{x} + 21x^{1/6} + 6}{6x^{2/3}(\sqrt{x} + 3)^2}$ **41.** $\frac{x(x + 2)}{(x + 1)^2}$ **43.** $-\frac{1}{(t - 4)^2}$

45. $\frac{-2x^2 + 6x + 2}{(x^2 + 1)^2}$ **47.** $-\frac{t^2 + 18t - 22}{(t^2 - 2t + 4)^2}$ **49.** **(a)** $y = \frac{1}{2}$; **(b)** $y = \frac{12}{25}x + \frac{7}{25}$ **51.** **(a)** $y = 4x$; **(b)** $y = -2$

53. $-\$0.0925$/belt **55.** $-\$0.0153$/belt **57.** \$0.0772/belt

59. \$1.64/vase **61.** **(a)** $P'(t) = -\frac{1000t^2 - 4500}{(2t^2 + 9)^2}$; **(b)** 133,824 residents; **(c)** 1730 residents/yr; **(d)** 95,202 residents; **(e)** -1581 residents/yr **63.** **(a)** 0; **(b)** $\frac{3}{4}$; **(c)** -2; **(d)** $-\frac{4}{3}$ **65.** $\frac{15x^2 + 112x - 12}{2(5x^2 + 4)^2}$

67. $72x^7 + 108x^5 - 30x^4 + 84x^3 + 84x - 14$

69. **(a)** $\frac{1}{(x + 1)^2}$; **(b)** $\frac{1}{(x + 1)^2}$; **(c)** answers may vary.

71. Answers may vary. **73.** **(a)** $\frac{dR}{dQ} = -Q^2 + kQ$; **(b)** answers may vary. **75.** \$0.79/bottle; \$0.0024/bottle at $x = 328$

77. $(0, 0), (-1.414, -4), (1.414, -4)$,

79.

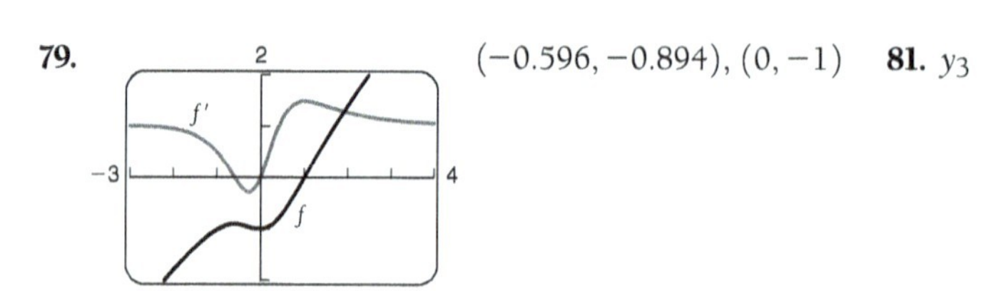

$(-0.596, -0.894), (0, -1)$ **81.** y_3

Exercise Set 1.7, p. 171

1. $8x - 12$ **3.** $-55(7 - x)^{54}$ **5.** $\dfrac{3x}{\sqrt{3x^2 - 4}}$ **7.** $-\dfrac{1}{2\sqrt{1 - x}}$
9. $-400x(4x^2 + 1)^{-51}$ **11.** $4(x - 4)^7(2x + 3)^5(7x - 6)$
13. $-\dfrac{8}{(4x + 5)^3}$ **15.** $\dfrac{4x(5x + 14)}{(7 - 5x)^4}$
17. $-5(2x - 3)^3(10x - 3)$ **19.** $4(5x + 2)^3(2x - 3)^7(30x - 7)$
21. $\dfrac{2x(5x - 1)}{\sqrt{4x - 1}}$ **23.** $\dfrac{2x - 5}{4(x^2 - 5x + 2)^{3/4}}$ **25.** $\dfrac{44(3x - 1)^3}{(5x + 2)^5}$
27. $-\dfrac{5(7x - 2)^4}{(3x - 1)^6}$ **29.** $\dfrac{(5x - 4)^6(120x + 107)}{(6x + 1)^4}$
31. $\dfrac{13}{2\sqrt{(2x + 3)(5 - x)^3}}$ **33.** $-\dfrac{45}{u^4}, 2, -\dfrac{90}{(2x + 1)^4}$
35. $50u^{49}, 12x^2 - 4x, 200x(4x^3 - 2x^2)^{49}(3x - 1)$
37. $3x^2(10x^3 + 13)$ **39.** $\dfrac{-6t - 11}{3(t + 2)^2(3t + 5)^2}$ **41.** $y = 0$
43. $y = 4x - 3$ **45.** **(a)** $-\dfrac{64(6x + 1)}{(2x - 5)^3}$; **(b)** same as in part (a); **(c)** answers may vary. **47.** -216 **49.** $\dfrac{4}{\sqrt[3]{169}}$, or about 0.72
51. **(a)** $f(x) = x^5, g(x) = 3x^2 + 2x$; **(b)** 4,587,520
53. **(a)** $f(x) = \dfrac{x + 1}{x + 4}$; $g(x) = x^3$; **(b)** $\frac{9}{25}$
55. $6(2x^3 + (4x - 5)^2)^5(6x^2 + 8(4x - 5))$
57. $\dfrac{1}{2\sqrt{x^2 + \sqrt{1 - 3x}}}\left(2x - \dfrac{3}{2\sqrt{1 - 3x}}\right)$
59. \$1,000,000/airplane **61.** \$510,429/airplane
63. **(a)** $\dfrac{dA}{dr} = 5000\left(1 + \dfrac{r}{4}\right)^{19}$; units are dollars per interest rate. **(b)** It is the rate of change in the amount as the interest rate r changes.
65. **(a)** $P(t) = 2t^2 + 400.8t + 80.08$; **(b)** \$592.80/month
67. **(a)** $D(c) = 4.25c + 106.25$, $c(w) = \dfrac{95w}{43.2} = 2.199w$; **(b)** 4.25 mg/unit of creatine clearance; **(c)** 2.199 units of creatine clearance/kg; **(d)** 9.35 mg/kg; **(e)** it is the rate of change in dosage as the patient's weight, in kilograms, varies.
69. **(a)** $(F \circ C)(3000) = F(C(3000)) = F(86.67) = 188$, which means that water at 3000 m boils at 188°F; **(b)** -0.008, which means that at 3000 m in altitude, the boiling point of water drops by 0.008°F/m as altitude increases. **71.** $4x(x^2 + 1)$
73. $8x((x^2 + 1)^2 + 1)(x^2 + 1)$ **75.** $\dfrac{6x^7 + 32x^5 + 5x^4}{(x^3 + 6x + 1)^{2/3}}$
77. $\dfrac{1}{(1 - x)\sqrt{1 - x^2}}$ **79.** $\dfrac{x^2 + x - 2}{\sqrt{(2x + 1)^3(x^2 - 4x)}}$
81. $-72(6x(3 - x)^5 + 2)^3(3 - x)^4(2x - 1)$
83. Left to the student
85.

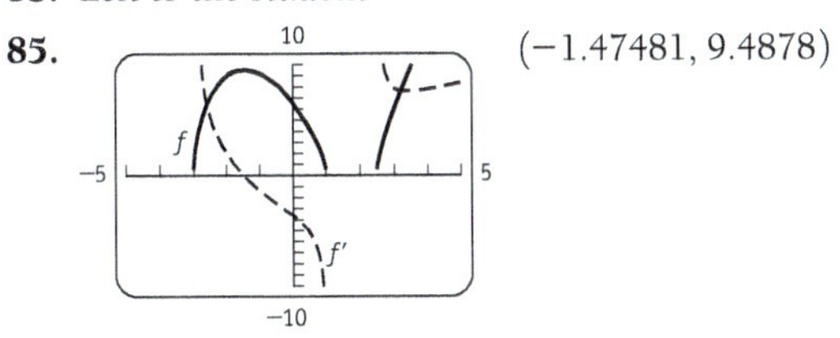

$(-1.47481, 9.4878)$

Exercise Set 1.8, p. 179

1. $20x^3$ **3.** $30x$ **5.** 8 **7.** 0 **9.** $\dfrac{6}{x^4}$ **11.** $-\dfrac{3}{16x^{7/4}}$
13. $12x^2 + \dfrac{6}{x^3}$ **15.** $-\dfrac{2}{9x^{5/3}}$ **17.** $\dfrac{48}{x^5}$
19. $6(x^3 + 2x)^4(51x^4 + 72x^2 + 20)$ **21.** $\dfrac{3(x^2 + 2)}{4(x^2 + 1)^{5/4}}$
23. $\dfrac{3}{4\sqrt{x}}$ **25.** $\dfrac{45x^4 - 54x^2 - 3}{16(x^3 - x)^{5/4}}$ **27.** $\dfrac{44}{(2x - 3)^3}$
29. $120x$ **31.** $720x$ **33.** $-\dfrac{2520}{x^8} + \dfrac{1760}{243x^{14/3}}$
35. **(a)** $v(t) = 3t^2 + 1$; **(b)** $a(t) = 6t$; **(c)** 49 ft/sec, 24 ft/sec^2
37. **(a)** $v(t) = 2t - \dfrac{1}{2}$; **(b)** $a(t) = 2$; **(c)** 1.5 m/sec, 2 m/sec^2
39. **(a)** 144 ft; **(b)** 96 ft/sec; **(c)** 32 ft/sec^2 **41.** 19.6 m/sec, 9.8 m/sec^2 **43.** **(a)** At a time t near 0, since the slope is steepest there; **(b)** negative, since the slopes of the tangent lines are decreasing **45.** **(a)** $(7, 11)$; **(b)** $(2, 4)$, $(7, 11)$, and $(13, 15)$; **(c)** $(0, 2)$ and $(11, 13)$; **(d)** $(4, 7)$; **(e)** answers may vary.
47. **(a)** \$146,000/month, \$84,000/month, $-$\$4000/month; **(b)** $-$\$68,000/month^2, $-$\$56,000/month^2, $-$\$32,000/month^2; **(c)** answers may vary. **49.** **(a)** 11.34, 1.98, 0.665; **(b)** $-0.789, -0.0577, -0.0112$; **(c)** answers may vary.
51. **(a)** Height: 74.7 m, horizontal distance: 54.5 m; **(b)** vertical: 2.55 m/sec, horizontal: 27.25 m/sec; **(c)** vertical: -9.8 m/sec^2, horizontal: 0; **(d)** it is moving upward, since $v(2) > 0$; **(e)** and **(f)** answers may vary.
53. Graph I **55.** Graph II **57.** False **59.** False
61. $f'(x) = \dfrac{3}{(x + 2)^2}$, $f''(x) = -\dfrac{6}{(x + 2)^3}$, $f'''(x) = \dfrac{18}{(x + 2)^4}$, $f''''(x) = -\dfrac{72}{(x + 2)^5}$ **63.** **(a)** 3.24 m; **(b)** 3.24 m/sec; **(c)** 1.62 m/sec^2; **(d)** it is the gravitational constant on the moon.
65. 42.33 ft/sec **67.** **(a)** $6 < x < 8$; **(b)** $3 < x < 6$; **(c)** $10 < x < 12$; **(d)** $8 < x < 10$; **(e)** $8 < x < 12$; **(f)** answers may vary.
69.

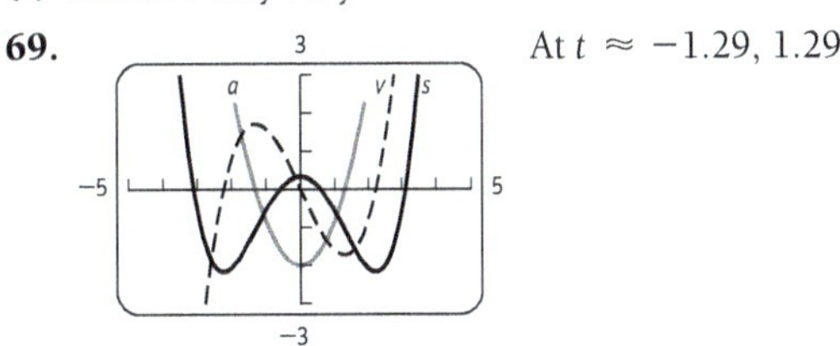

At $t \approx -1.29, 1.29$

71.

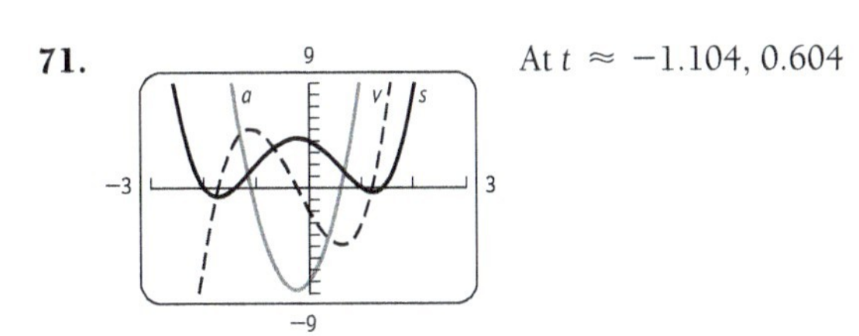

At $t \approx -1.104, 0.604$

Chapter 1 Review Exercises, p. 188

1. False **2.** False **3.** True **4.** False **5.** True **6.** True **7.** False **8.** True **9.** (e) **10.** (c) **11.** (a) **12.** (f) **13.** (b) **14.** (d) **15.** **(a)** $-10.1, -10.01, -10.001$ and $-9.9, -9.99, -9.999$; **(b)** $-10, -10, -10$

16.

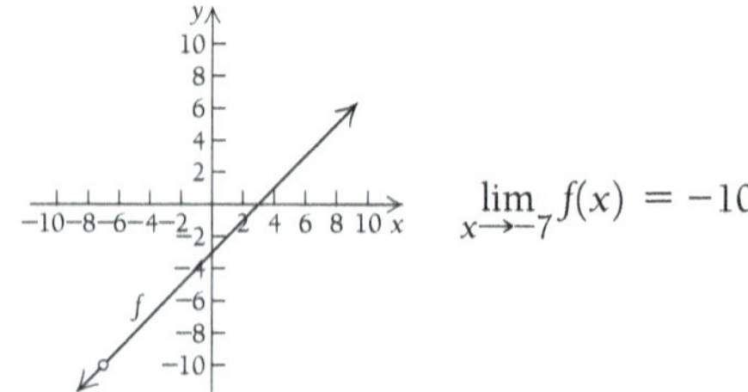

$\lim_{x \to -7} f(x) = -10$

17. $\dfrac{x^2 + 4x - 21}{x + 7} = \dfrac{(x + 7)(x - 3)}{x + 7} = x - 3$, for $x \neq -7$. Thus, $\lim_{x \to -7} (x - 3) = -10$. **18.** -4 **19.** 10 **20.** -12 **21.** 3 **22.** 4 **23.** Does not exist **24.** -4 **25.** -4 **26.** Yes, since $\lim_{x \to 1} g(x) = g(1)$ **27.** Does not exist **28.** -2 **29.** No, since $\lim_{x \to -2} g(x)$ does not exist **30.** No **31.** $-\frac{2}{3}$ **32.** 0 **33.** Not defined at $x = -2$, since g is discontinuous there **34.** Not defined at $x = -2$, since there is a corner there **35.** -2 **36.** -3 **37.** Yes, since $\lim_{x \to -2} f(x) = f(-2)$ **38.** Yes **39.** 2 **40.** $-6x - 3h, h \neq 0$ **41.** $y = x - 1$ **42.** $(4, 5)$ **43.** $45x^4$ **44.** $\frac{8}{3}x^{-2/3}$ **45.** $\frac{24}{x^9}$ **46.** $6x^{-3/5}$ **47.** $0.7x^6 - 12x^3 - 3x^2$ **48.** $\frac{5}{2}x^5 + 32x^3 - 2$ **49.** $(x^3 + 5)\left(\dfrac{1}{2\sqrt{x}} + 4\right) + (\sqrt{x} + 4x)(3x^2)$ **50.** $\dfrac{-x^2 + 16x + 8}{(8 - x)^2}$ **51.** $2(5 - x)(2x - 1)^4(26 - 7x)$ **52.** $35x^4(x^5 - 3)^6$ **53.** $\dfrac{11x^2 + 4x}{(4x + 2)^{1/4}}$ **54.** $-48x^{-5}$ **55.** $3x^5 - 60x + 26$ **56.** **(a)** $P'(t) = 100t$; **(b)** 30,000 people; **(c)** 2000 people/yr **57.** $(3, 5), (7, 8), (9, 13), (15, 18)$ **58.** $(7, 8), (15, 18)$ **59.** $(0, 3), (8, 9)$ **60.** $(5, 7), (13, 15)$ **61.** **(a)** 656 ft; **(b)** -96 ft/sec; **(c)** -32 ft/sec^2; **(d)** -226.27 ft/sec; **(e)** answers may vary. **62.** **(a)** $\overline{C} = \dfrac{5\sqrt{x} + 100}{x}, \overline{R} = 40, \overline{P} = 40 - \dfrac{5\sqrt{x} + 100}{x}$; **(b)** $-\$1.33$/lamp **63.** $\dfrac{d}{dx}(f \circ g)(x) = -4(1 - 2x)$; $\dfrac{d}{dx}(g \circ f)(x) = -4x$ **64.** $\dfrac{-9x^4 - 4x^3 + 9x + 2}{2\sqrt{1 + 3x}(1 + x^3)^2}$ **65.** $\dfrac{1}{243}x^{-242/243}$ **66.** -0.25 **67.** $\frac{1}{6}$

68.

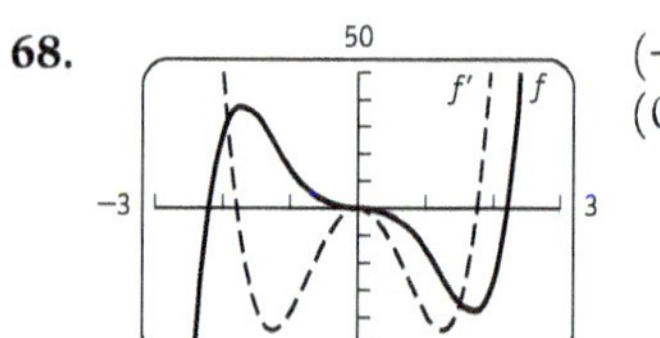

$(-1.7137, 37.445)$, $(0, 0)$, $(1.7137, -37.445)$

Chapter 1 Test, p. 190

1. **(a)** 11.9, 11.99, 11.999 and 12.1, 12.01, 12.001; **(b)** 12, 12, 12

2. $\lim_{x \to 6} f(x) = 12$

3. $\dfrac{x^2 - 36}{x - 6} = \dfrac{(x + 6)(x - 6)}{x - 6} = x + 6, x \neq 6$. Thus, $\lim_{x \to 6} (x + 6) = 12$ **4.** Does not exist **5.** 0 **6.** Does not exist **7.** 2 **8.** 4 **9.** 1 **10.** 1 **11.** 2 **12.** 0 **13.** 0 **14.** $-5, -3, -2, 1, 4$ **15.** $-5, -3, -2, -1, 1, 3, 4$ **16.** Continuous **17.** Not continuous, since $\lim_{x \to 3} f(x)$ does not exist **18.** **(a)** Does not exist; **(b)** 1; **(c)** no **19.** 3 **20.** 6 **21.** $\frac{1}{8}$ **22.** Does not exist, since the left-hand limit does not equal the right-hand limit **23.** $4x + 3 + 2h$ **24.** $y = \frac{3}{4}x + 2$ **25.** $(0, 0), (2, -4)$ **26.** $23x^{22}$ **27.** $\frac{4}{3}x^{-2/3} + \frac{5}{2}x^{-1/2}$ **28.** $\dfrac{10}{x^2}$ **29.** $\frac{5}{4}x^{1/4}$ **30.** $-x + 0.61$ **31.** $x^2 - 2x + 2$ **32.** $(3\sqrt{x} + 1)(2x - 1) + (x^2 - x)\left(\dfrac{3}{2\sqrt{x}}\right)$ **33.** $\dfrac{5}{(5 - x)^2}$ **34.** $(x + 3)^3(7 - x)^4(13 - 9x)$ **35.** $-5(x^5 - 4x^3 + x)^{-6}(5x^4 - 12x^2 + 1)$ **36.** $\dfrac{2x^2 + 5}{\sqrt{x^2 + 5}}$ **37.** $24x$ **38.** **(a)** $M'(t) = -0.003t^2 + 0.2t$; **(b)** 9 words; **(c)** 1.7 words/min **39.** **(a)** $\overline{R} = 50, \overline{C} = \dfrac{x^{2/3} + 750}{x}$, $\overline{P} = 50 - \dfrac{x^{2/3} + 750}{x}$; **(b)** $-\$11.74$/speaker **40.** $24x^5 - 6x^2$ **41.** $6(x^2 - x)^2(2x - 1)$ **42.** Graph A **43.** $-\dfrac{1 + 9x}{2(1 - 3x)^{2/3}(1 + 3x)^{5/6}}$ **44.** 27

45.

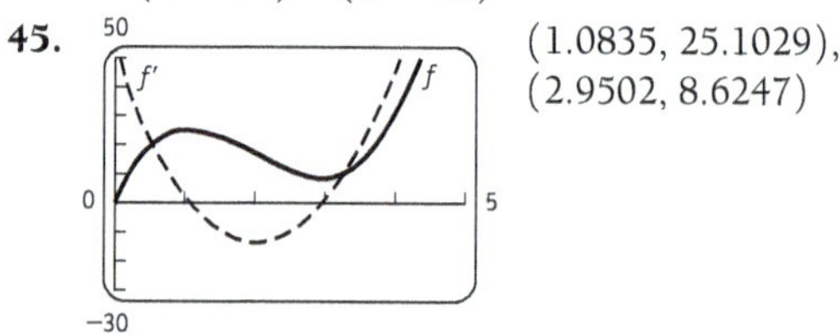

$(1.0835, 25.1029)$, $(2.9502, 8.6247)$

46. 0.5

Extended Technology Application, p. 192

1.

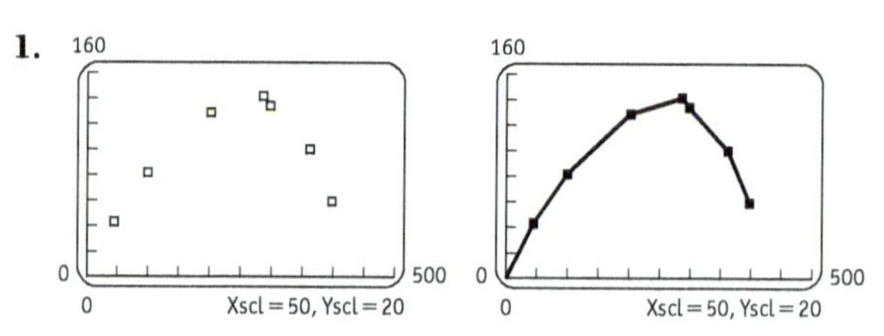

2. **(a)** $y = -0.0000045x^3 + 0.000204x^2 + 0.7806x + 4.6048$;

(b)

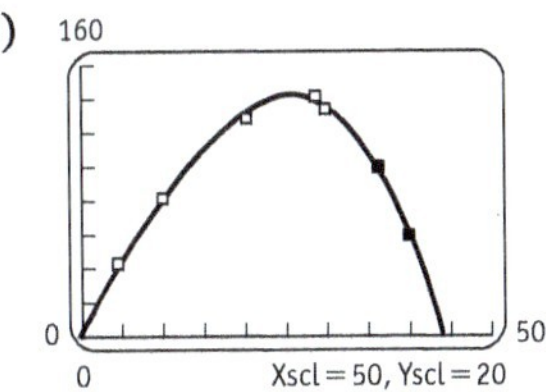

(c) acceptable fit; **(d)** about 441 ft; **(e)** $y' = -0.0000135x^2 + 0.000408x + 0.7806$; **(f)** at about (256, 142), meaning that the ball reached a maximum height of 142 ft at 256 ft from home plate.
3. (a) $y = -0.0000000024x^4 - 0.0000026x^3 - 0.00026x^2 + 0.815x + 4.3026$; **(b)**

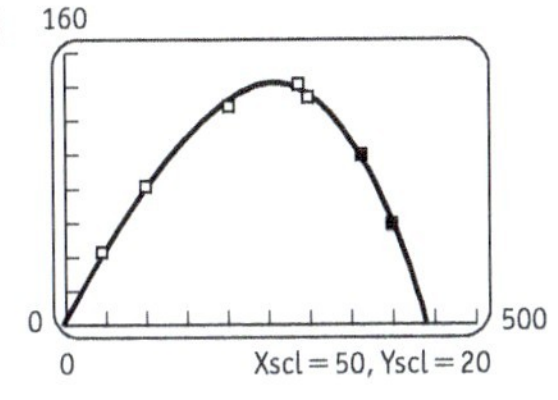

(c) acceptable fit; **(d)** about 440 feet; **(e)** $y' = -0.0000000096x^3 - 0.0000078x^2 - 0.00053x + 0.815$; **(f)** at about (257, 142), meaning that the ball reached a maximum height of 142 ft at 257 ft from home plate.
4. (a)

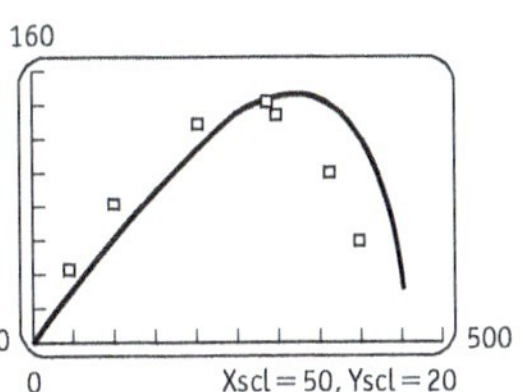

(b) 450 ft; **(c)** $y' = \dfrac{303.75 - 0.003x^2}{\sqrt{202{,}500 - x^2}}$; **(d)** at about (318, 152), meaning that the ball reached a maximum height of 152 ft at 318 ft from home plate. **5.** The two models are similar; the main difference is that the maximum height is reached farther from home plate using the model in Exercise 4. **6.** 466 ft, 442 ft, 430 ft **7.** Left to the student **8. (a)** 523 ft; **(b)** 490 ft, 450 ft; **(c)** 551 ft

CHAPTER 2

Exercise Set 2.1, p. 203

1.

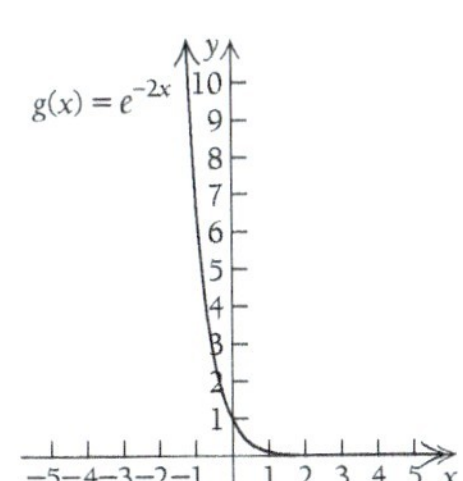

Domain: $(-\infty, \infty)$; range: $(0, \infty)$; y-intercept: (0, 1); decreasing

3.

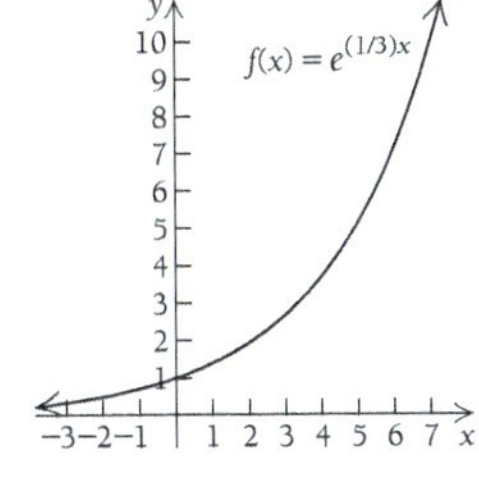

Domain: $(-\infty, \infty)$; range: $(0, \infty)$; y-intercept: (0, 1); increasing

5.

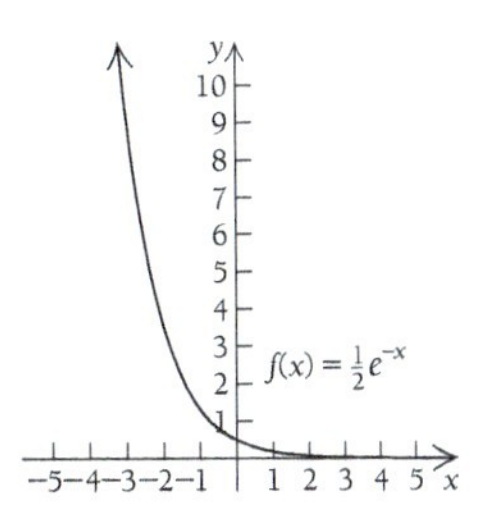

Domain: $(-\infty, \infty)$; range: $(0, \infty)$; y-intercept: $(0, \frac{1}{2})$; decreasing

7.

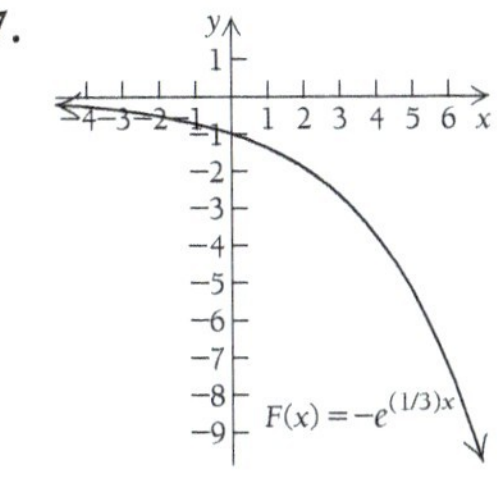

Domain: $(-\infty, \infty)$; range: $(-\infty, 0)$; y-intercept: $(0, -1)$; decreasing

9. (a) \$1698.12; **(b)** \$1701.14; **(c)** \$1701.41; **(d)** \$1701.42; **(e)** 22 yr **11. (a)** \$85,587.46; **(b)** \$85,818.59; **(c)** \$85,839.54; **(d)** \$85,840.26; **(e)** 15.4 yr **13. (a)** \$304.45; **(b)** \$305.00; **(c)** \$305.04; **(d)** \$305.05; **(e)** 34.8 yr **15. (a)** \$10,621.26; **(b)** \$10,633.19; **(c)** \$10,634.27; **(d)** \$10,634.30; **(e)** 16.9 yr
17. 0.693; $e^{0.693} = 1.9997\ldots \approx 2$
19. 1.504; $e^{1.504} = 4.4996\ldots \approx 4.5$
21. −2.957; $e^{-2.957} = 0.05197\ldots \approx 0.052$
23. −0.288; $e^{-0.288} = 0.74976\ldots \approx 0.75$
25. 5; $e^5 = e^5$ **27.** 4.382 **29.** −1.6094
31. 2.3863 **33.** 4 **35.** −0.2231 **37.** 0.3863
39. 2.079 **41.** 2.267 **43.** 4.605 **45.** 140.671
47. 0.549 **49.** 24.414

51. $(-\frac{4}{3}, \infty)$

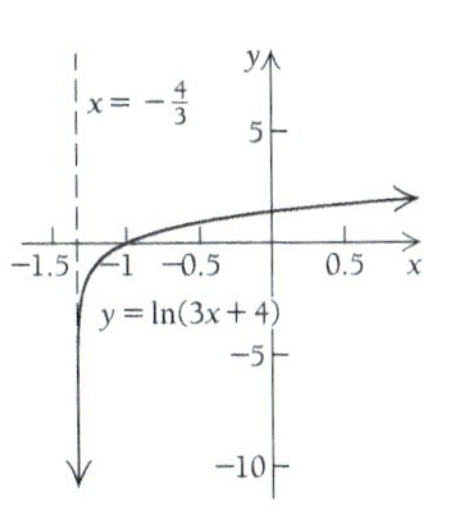

53. $(-\infty, 4)$

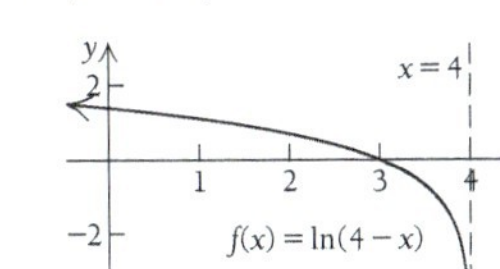

55. $(-3, 5)$

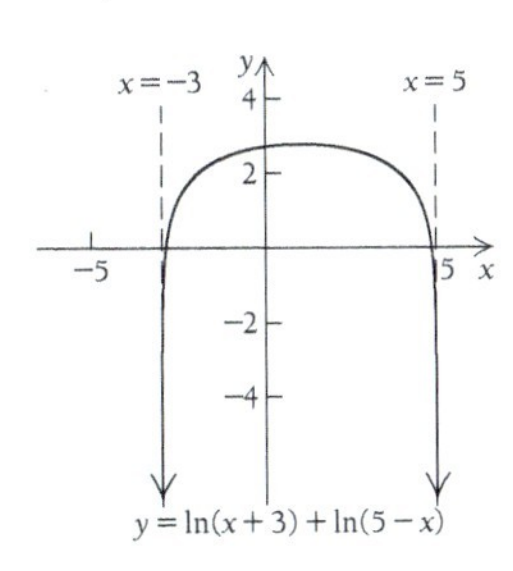

57. $(0, \infty)$

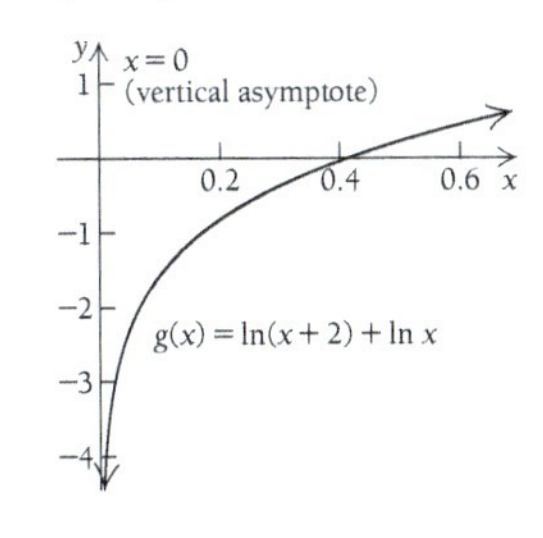

59. $(-\infty, \infty)$

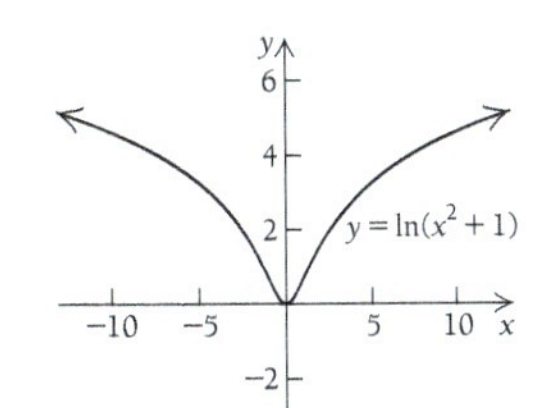

61. $e^{10} \approx 22{,}026.466$
63. $e^{4.5} \approx 90.017$
65. $\frac{1}{2}(e^{1.5} - 1) \approx 1.741$
67. 4
69. (a) 2018: \$222.7 billion, 2020: \$268.7 billion; **(b)** in 2.8 yr; **(c)** in 7.37 yr
71. (a) $A(t) = 10{,}000e^{0.0288t}$; **(b)** \$11,548.84; **(c)** in 14.1 yr; **(d)** in 24.1 yr

73. **(a)** \$52.53; **(b)** \$25; **(c)** after 30.1 weeks
75. **(a)** \$594.43; **(b)** about 2136 thousand units
77. **(a)** $A(t) = 45{,}000e^{0.03t}$; **(b)** about 60,744; **(c)** in 6.7 yr; **(d)** in 23.1 yr **79.** **(a)** $A(t) = 2e^{0.045t}$; **(b)** 3.14 mm^2; **(c)** after 71.5 hr; **(d)** after 15.4 hr **81.** **(a)** 75°C; **(b)** 58.4°C; **(c)** in 95.5 min; **(d)** 30, meaning that the coffee will decrease in temperature toward 30°C **83.** **(a)** 3.87 mg; **(b)** 6.26 days; **(c)** 2.7 days; **(d)** 0, which means that the sample will eventually decay toward zero. **85.** $x = 0, x = \ln 4$
87. $x = \ln 4, x = \ln 8$ **89.** $x = \ln 4$
91. $x = e^{e^2-1} \approx 595.29$ **93.** $x = e, x = e^3$
95. 6.077%; 11.4 yr **97.** 3.45 hr **99.** Answers may vary.
101. 20 yr **103.** Answers may vary. **105.** $x = 0.933$
107. $x = 0.27$

Exercise Set 2.2, p. 210

1. $2e^{2x}$ **3.** $15e^{5x}$ **5.** $3x^2 - 10e^{2x}$ **7.** $5x^4e^{2x} + 2x^5e^{2x}$
9. $\frac{2e^{2x}(x-2)}{x^5}$ **11.** x^2e^x **13.** $(8 - 2x)e^{-x^2+8x}$ **15.** $\frac{e^x}{2\sqrt{e^x - 1}}$
17. $3x^2 - xe^x$ **19.** $(8x^3 - 22x^2 - 13x + 3)e^{x^2-7x}$ **21.** $\frac{1-2t}{e^{2t}}$
23. $-\frac{2t^3 + 4t^2 - 2t - 2}{e^{t^2}}$ **25.** $4e^{2x}$ **27.** $\frac{1}{4}e^{(-1/2)x}$
29. $2e^{x^2}(2x^2 + 1)$ **31.** $4e^{2x+1}$ **33.** $\frac{e^{\sqrt{x}}(\sqrt{x} - 1)}{4x\sqrt{x}}$
35. $e^x(x + 2)$ **37.** $3e^{3t}(6t + 13)$ **39.** $8e^{2x}(2e^{2x} + 1)$
41. $e^{5t}(25t^2 + 70t + 97)$ **43.** $\frac{3e^{3x}(3x^2 - 4x + 2)}{x^4}$
45. $\frac{9e^{3t}(e^{3t} - 2)}{4(e^{3t} - 1)^{3/2}}$ **47.** **(a)** $dC/dx = 50e^{-x}$; **(b)** \$50 million/yr; **(c)** \$916,000/yr; **(d)** 100 and 0 **49.** **(a)** \$29,289.59; **(b)** \$1596.28/yr **51.** **(a)** −\$2355.35/yr; **(b)** \$20,019
53. **(a)** 0, 3.7, 5.4, 4.5, 0.05 (all in ppm);
(b)

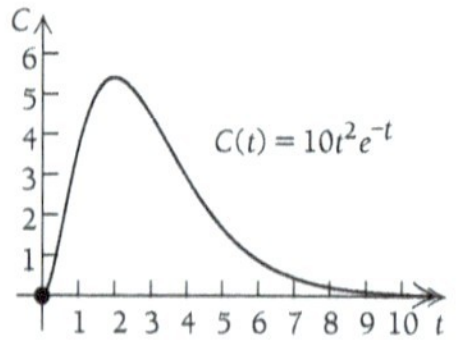

(c) $C(5) = 1.68$ ppm, $C'(5) = -1.01$ ppm/hr. After 5 hr, the concentration of the medication is about 1.68 ppm, and it is decreasing by about 1.01 ppm/hr.
55. **(a)** 443.5, 370.4, 274.4 (all in mm^2);
(b)

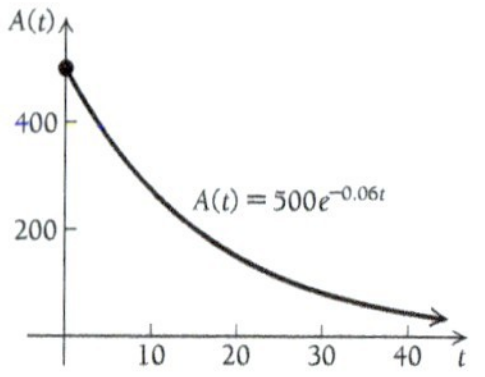

(c) $A(12) = 243.4\ \text{mm}^2$, $A'(12) = -14.6\ \text{mm}^2/\text{hr}$. After 12 hr, the area of the colony is about 243.4 mm^2, and it is decreasing by about 14.6 mm^2/hr. **57.** **(a)** 100%, 69.8%, 54.8%, 40.9%, 40.1%; **(b)** 40%;
(c)

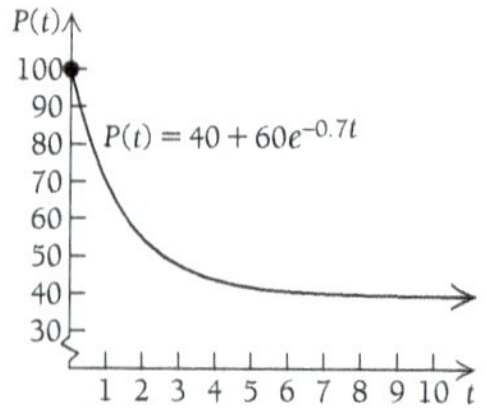

(d) $P'(t) = -42e^{-0.7t}$; **(e)** answers may vary.
59. $\frac{xe^{(1/2)x}}{2\sqrt{x-1}}$ **61.** $\frac{4}{(e^x + e^{-x})^2}$ **63.** ex^{e-1}
65. $g^{(7)}(x) = 128e^{2x}$ **67.** $y = -8x + 2$ **69.** $(1, e)$
71.

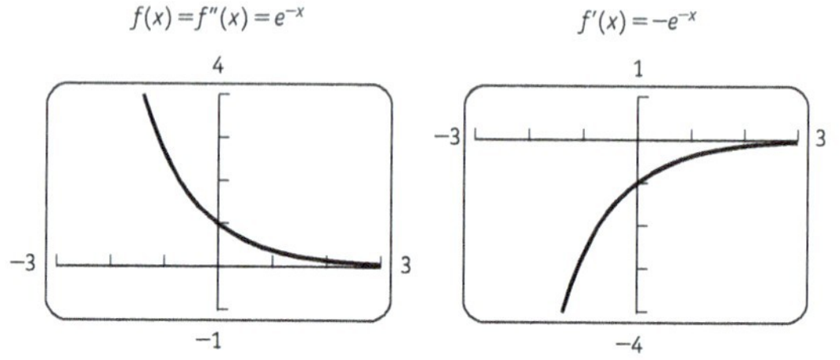

73.

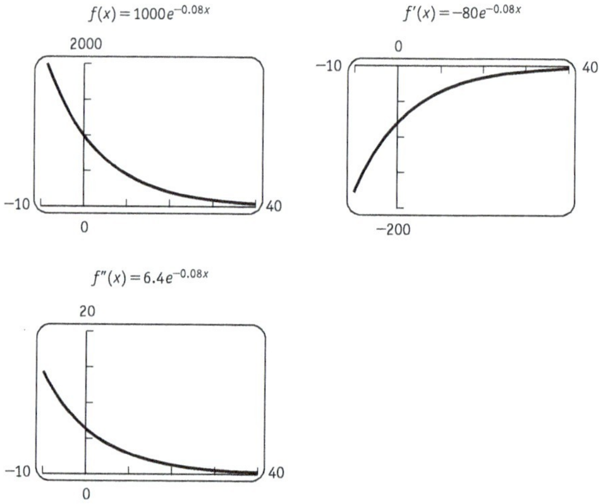

75. **(a)** 1.0517, 1.005, 1.0005, 0.95163, 0.999502, 0.99995; **(b)** 1

Exercise Set 2.3, p. 216

1. $-\frac{9}{x}$ **3.** $\frac{1}{x}$ **5.** $\frac{1}{x}$ **7.** $x^5(1 + 6\ln x)$ **9.** $\frac{1 - 5\ln x}{x^6}$
11. $\frac{2}{x}$ **13.** $\frac{6x + 2}{3x^2 + 2x - 1}$ **15.** $\frac{2x}{x^2 + 5} - \frac{1}{x}$ **17.** $\frac{4(\ln x)^3}{x}$
19. $\frac{2}{x} + \frac{3x^2}{x^3 + 1} - 2$ **21.** $y = 0.732x - 0.990$
23. $y = 4.329x - 6.75$ **25.** **(a)** 2000; **(b)** $N'(a) = \frac{500}{a}$, $N'(10) = 50$; **(c)** \$7390; **(d)** answers may vary.
27. **(a)** $R(x) = 53.5x - 8x\ln x$; **(b)** $R'(x) = 45.5 - 8\ln x$; **(c)** 5400 **29.** **(a)** 78%; **(b)** 53.9%; **(c)** 29.7%; **(d)** $S'(t) = -\frac{15}{t+1}$; **(e)** $S'(4) = -3$, which means that, after 4 months, the average score is decreasing by 3 percentage points per month; $S'(24) = -0.6$, which means that, after 24 months, the average score is decreasing by 0.6 percentage point per month.
31. **(a)** $t(15) = 20.27$ min and $t'(15) = 5$ min/°C, which mean that it takes 20.27 min to warm the water to 15°C, at which time

the time needed for the water to warm by 1°C is changing by 5 min/degree; **(b)** 20.48°C **33. (a)** $t(5000) = 22.34$ months, $t'(p) = 0.0152$ month/bird. It takes about 22.34 months for the population to reach 5000 birds, and the time needed for the population to increase by one bird is about 0.0152 month/bird (about one new bird born every 10.9 hr); **(b)** 6570 birds
35. $\frac{1}{x}$ **37.** $\frac{1}{(w-1)^2} - \frac{1}{w^2}$ **39. (a)** $T(t) = 25 - 15e^{-0.02t}$;
(b) 25, meaning that the water's temperature approaches 25°C as a limit. **41. (a)** $p(t) = 7500 - 4500e^{-0.0263t}$; **(b)** 7500, meaning that the population of birds approaches 7500 as a limit.
43. (1.35, 0.3) **45.** $a = e^{-1}$

Technology Connection, p. 221

1. 1.85 trillion **2.** 2.1 quadrillion **3.** 8.52×10^{22} (85.2 sextillion) **4.** Left to the student

Exercise Set 2.4, p. 226

1. $f(x) = ce^{4x}$ **3.** $A(t) = ce^{-9t}$ **5.** $Q(t) = ce^{kt}$
7. (a) $N(t) = 453{,}000e^{0.039t}$; **(b)** 782,000; **(c)** about 30,499 applications/yr **9. (a)** $P(t) = P_0e^{0.059t}$; **(b)** \$1060.78, \$1125.24; **(c)** \$62.59/yr, \$66.39/yr **11. (a)** $G(t) = 11.8e^{0.085t}$; **(b)** 27.6 billion gallons; **(c)** 2.347 billion gallons/yr
13. (a) $k = 0.151$ (or 15.1%), $V(t) = 30{,}000e^{0.151t}$; **(b)** \$2,486,000,000; **(c)** \$375,000,000/yr; **(d)** 78 yr
15. (a) $F(t) = 2.77e^{0.055314t}$; **(b)** \$4.08 trillion; **(c)** after 23.2 yr, or in 2036 **17. (a)** $y = 7.384736154(1.472630104)^x$, $y = 7.384736154e^{0.3870499885x}$; **(b)** 38.7%; **(c)** 163.3 EB; **(d)** after 8.5 yr; **(e)** about 77 EB/yr **19.** About \$11 billion
21. (a) $S(t) = 4e^{0.0451t}$; **(b)** 4.5%/yr; **(c)** 60 cents, 66 cents; **(d)** \$10,000; **(e)** answers may vary. **23. (a)** 2%; **(b)** 3.8%, 7%, 21.6%, 50.2%, 93.1%, 98%;
(c) $P'(x) = \frac{637e^{-0.13x}}{(1 + 49e^{-0.13x})^2}$;
(d)

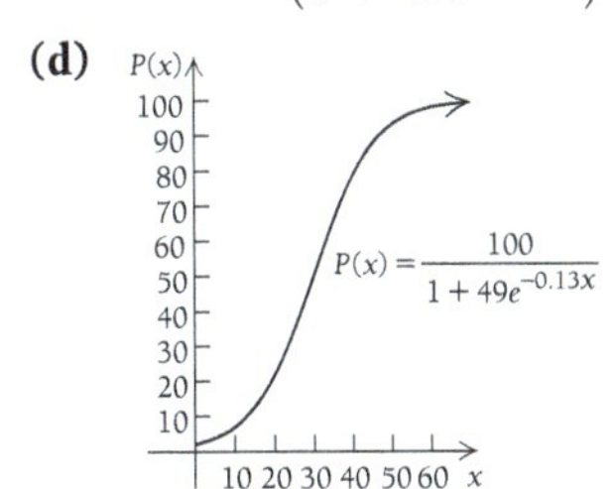

25. (a) $V(t) = 0.10e^{0.227t}$; **(b)** about \$12,132,700; **(c)** after 86 yr, or in 2024 **27.** After 80.8 yr, in 2019
29. (a) 40, 185, 199; **(b)** $P'(t) = \frac{61{,}100e^{-0.0982t}}{(17 + 183e^{-0.0982t})^2}$
(c) 3.13 people/yr, 1.34 people/yr, 0.13 people/yr; **(d)** 200 **31. (a)** 400, 520, 1214, 2059, 2396, 2478;
(b) $P'(t) = \frac{4200e^{-0.32t}}{(1 + 5.25e^{-0.32t})^2}$;
(c)

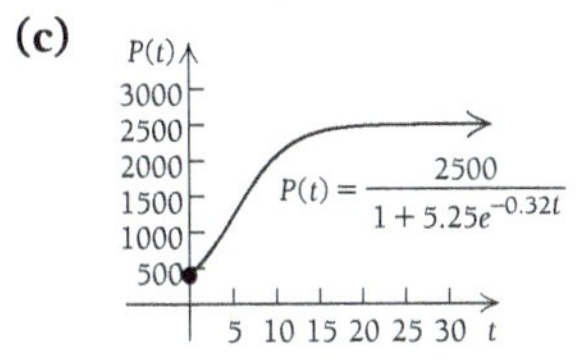

33. (a) 0.244, 0.429, 0.753, 0.954, 0.989, 0.996; **(b)** $p'(t) = 0.28e^{-0.28t}$;
(c)

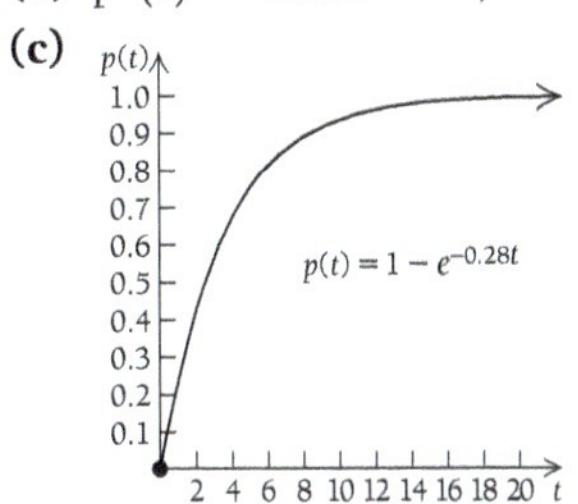

35. (a) 0%, 33%, 55%, 70%, 86%, 99.2%, 99.8%; **(b)** 2.43, which means that after 7 months, the percentage of physicians prescribing the new drug is increasing by 2.43 percentage points per month;
(c)

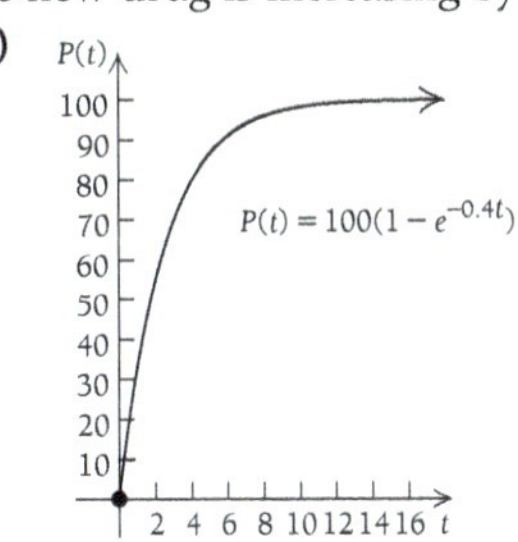

37–49. Answers may vary.
51. $P'(t) = -kCe^{-kt}$, and $k(L - P) = k(L - (L + Ce^{-kt})) = k(-Ce^{-kt}) = P'(t)$

Exercise Set 2.5, p. 237

1. (a) $N(t) = N_0e^{-0.096t}$; **(b)** 341 g; **(c)** -32.7 g/day; **(d)** 7.2 days **3. (a)** $N(t) = N_0e^{-0.000081547t}$; **(b)** 53.1 mg; **(c)** -0.00433 mg/yr; **(d)** 8500 yr **5. (a)** $N(t) = N_0e^{-0.2572t}$; **(b)** 1.65 mg; **(c)** -0.425 mg/day; **(d)** 2.69 days; **(e)** 7.38 days
7. (a) $P(t) = 116{,}646e^{-0.0187t}$; **(b)** 60,621; **(c)** -1134 people/yr; **(d)** 37 yr **9. (a)** $A(t) = A_0e^{-kt}$; **(b)** 11 hr **11. (a)** $A(t) = 35e^{-0.034t}$; **(b)** 47.34 min
13. (a) $P(t) = 5000e^{-0.116t}$; **(b)** 10.38 yr **15.** 5.78 yr
17. 86.64 months **19.** 23.1 yr **21.** 36.48 weeks
23. 23.1%/min **25.** 22 yr **27.** 42.9 g **29.** 4223 yr
31. 25 days **33.** 3965 yr **35.** \$13,858.23 **37.** \$6,788,463
39. \$42,863.76 **41. (a)** \$40,000; **(b)** \$5413.41; **(c)** answers may vary. **43. (a)** \$23,500; **(b)** \$14,541; **(c)** answers may vary.
45. (a) \$2600; **(b)** \$2171.70; **(c)** left to the student
47. (a) 0.022, 0.031, 0.069;
(b)

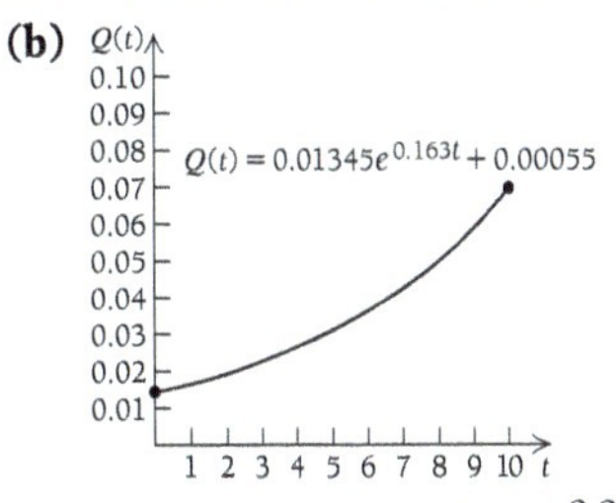

49. (a) $N(t) = 5{,}650{,}000e^{-0.0153t}$; **(b)** 1,790,000; **(c)** in about 2063 **51. (a)** $P(t) = 3.81e^{-0.00623t}$; **(b)** 3.36 million; **(c)** in 2028 **53. (a)** 60; **(b)** 0.01740; **(c)** 90°F; **(d)** 235 min; **(e)** answers may vary. **55.** At about 8 p.m. on the previous evening **57. (a)** 112 lb; **(b)** -1 lb/day
59. (a) 14.0 lb/in^2; **(b)** 5.4 lb/in^2; **(c)** 0 ft; **(d)** answers may vary.

61. **(a)** $N(t) = 69{,}895e^{-0.0336t}$; **(b)** 8138, 7115; **(c)** after 78 yr, or in 2034 **63.** (a) **65.** (c) **67.** (b) or (d)
69. (f) **71.** (b) **73.** **(a)** 4.27 yr; **(b)** 5.64 yr
75. Answers may vary. **77.** Answers may vary.

Exercise Set 2.6, p. 248

1. $P(t) = 450 \cdot 2^{t/5}$; $P(t) = 450e^{0.1386t}$
3. $P(t) = 5000 \cdot 3^{t/8}$; $P(t) = 5000e^{0.1373t}$
5. $P(t) = 100 \cdot 7^{t/12}$; $P(t) = 100e^{0.1622t}$
7. $P(t) = 1200(0.9)^{t/2}$; $P(t) = 1200e^{-0.05268t}$
9. $P(t) = 60{,}000(0.6)^{t/8}$; $P(t) = 60{,}000e^{-0.0639t}$
11. $P(t) = 6500 \cdot 1.5^{t/6}$; $P(t) = 6500e^{0.06758t}$
13. $\ln 6 \cdot 6^x$ **15.** $\ln 15 \cdot 15^t$ **17.** $\ln 12.5 \cdot 12.5^x$
19. $3 \ln 5 \cdot 5^x$ **21.** $4x^3 \cdot \ln 7 \cdot 7^{x^4+2}$ **23.** $100 \ln 0.52 \cdot 0.52^t$
25. $\frac{1}{x \ln 6}$ **27.** $\frac{3}{x \ln 4}$ **29.** $\frac{3}{(3x - 1)\ln 2}$ **31.** $\frac{10x + 5}{(x^2 + x)\ln 6}$
33. $\frac{4^x}{x \ln 5} + \ln 4 \cdot 4^x \cdot \log_5 x$ **35.** $3^x x(x \ln 3 + 2)$
37. $x^2\left(\frac{1}{\ln 7} + 3 \log_7 x\right)$ **39.** $\frac{9^x((2x + 1)\ln 9 - 2)}{(2x + 1)^2}$
41. **(a)** $P(t) = 10{,}000 \cdot 2^{t/9}$; **(b)** $P(t) = 10{,}000e^{0.07702t}$; **(c)** 7.702%/yr; **(d)** 80,000 people; **(e)** by 3081 people/yr
43. **(a)** $F(t) = 50 \cdot 3^{t/7}$; **(b)** $F(t) = 50e^{0.1569t}$; **(c)** 15.69%/month; **(d)** 450 followers; **(e)** by 212 people/month
45. **(a)** $V(t) = 100(0.5)^{t/5}$; **(b)** $V(t) = 100e^{-0.1386t}$; **(c)** −13.86%/day; **(d)** \$12.50; **(e)** by −\$3.47/day
47. **(a)** $A(t) = 50{,}000 \cdot 1.2^{t/4}$; **(b)** $A(8) = 72{,}000$, which means that after 8 yr, the account is worth \$72,000; **(c)** $A'(8) = 3281.79$, which means that after 8 yr, the account is growing by \$3281.79/yr **49.** **(a)** After 5 yr, the value of the machine is \$1703.94; **(b)** after 5 yr, the value is changing by −\$380.22/yr; **(c)** after 3.11 yr **51.** **(a)** After 4 yr, there are 5408.51 lb of glass still in use; **(b)** after 4 yr, the amount of glass in use is changing by −5818.87 lb/yr; **(c)** after 2.78 yr
53. **(a)** $I(7) = I_0 10^7$; **(b)** $I(8) = I_0 10^8$; **(c)** a magnitude 8 quake is 10 times more powerful than a magnitude 7 quake; **(d)** $I'(R) = I_0 10^R(\ln 10)$; **(e)** answers may vary.
55. **(a)** $R'(I) = \frac{1}{I \ln 10}$; **(b)** answers may vary.
57. **(a)** $P(t) = 35{,}000 \cdot 2^{t/16.233}$; **(b)** $P(t) = 35{,}000 \cdot 4^{t/32.466}$; **(c)** with base 4, the value of T is double that with base 2;
(d) 48.699 **59.** **(a)** $P(t) = 100{,}000\left(\frac{1}{3}\right)^{t/33.291}$;
(b) $P(t) = 100{,}000\left(\frac{1}{9}\right)^{t/66.582}$; **(c)** with base $\frac{1}{9}$, the value of T is double that with base $\frac{1}{3}$; **(d)** 99.873 **61.** **(a)** 7.925 yr;
(b) 800% **63.** **(a)** 37.6 hr; **(b)** 75% **65.** $\ln a$ **67.** $\ln 7$

Chapter 2 Review Exercises, p. 255

1. (b) **2.** (e) **3.** (f) **4.** (c) **5.** (a) **6.** (d)
7. False **8.** False **9.** False **10.** False **11.** True
12. True **13.** False **14.** True **15.** False **16.** False
17. $\frac{1}{x}$ **18.** e^x **19.** $\frac{4x^3}{x^4 + 5}$ **20.** $\frac{e^{2\sqrt{x}}}{\sqrt{x}}$ **21.** $\frac{1}{2x}$
22. $3x^4e^{3x} + 4x^3e^{3x}$ **23.** $\frac{1 - 3 \ln x}{x^4}$ **24.** $\frac{e^{x^2}}{x} + 2xe^{x^2}(\ln 4x)$
25. $4e^{4x} - \frac{1}{x}$ **26.** $\frac{1 - x}{e^x}$ **27.** $(\ln 9)9^x$ **28.** $\frac{1}{x \ln 2}$
29. $\frac{2 \cdot 3^x}{(2x + 1)\ln 4} + 3^x(\ln 3)(\log_4(2x + 1))$
30. No x-intercept, y-intercept at $(0, e^{-2}) \approx (0, 0.135)$, domain: $\{x|-\infty < x < \infty\}$, range: $\{y|0 < y < \infty\}$

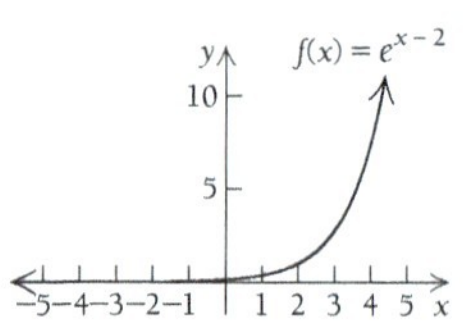

31. x-intercept at $(\frac{3}{2}, 0)$, y-intercept at $(0, \ln 4)$, domain: $\{x|-\infty < x < 2\}$, range: $\{y|-\infty < y < \infty\}$

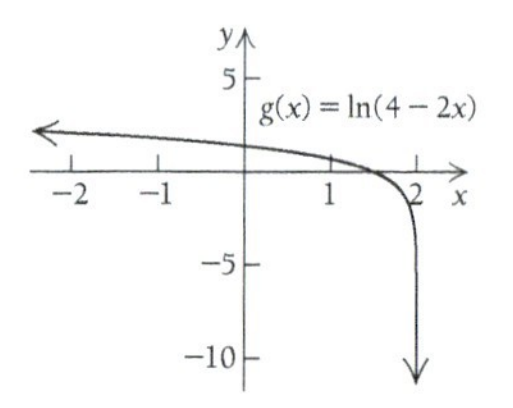

32. 2.639 **33.** −1.253 **34.** 3.332 **35.** 1.253 **36.** 0.973
37. −1.386 **38.** $Q(t) = 25e^{7t}$ **39.** **(a)** $r = 0.0433$, or 4.33%; **(b)** $P(t) = 4000e^{0.0433t}$; **(c)** 5416; **(d)** 235 people/yr
40. \$411.51/yr **41.** **(a)** $C(t) = 15.81e^{0.0206t}$; **(b)** \$34.59; **(c)** \$0.71/yr **42.** **(a)** $C(t) = 2.69e^{0.0039t}$; **(b)** \$3.14; **(c)** \$0.012/yr **43.** **(a)** $P(t) = 120 - 40e^{-0.0406t}$; **(b)** 0.721, meaning that the stock is increasing in value by about \$0.72/week after 20 weeks; **(c)** after about 34 weeks
44. **(a)** $N(t) = \frac{1000}{1 + 49e^{-0.0604t}}$; **(b)** after about 64.4 hr
45. **(a)** $N(t) = 60e^{0.12t}$; **(b)** 157; **(c)** about 19 franchises/yr
46. **(a)** $N(t) = 24e^{0.07t}$; **(b)** about 74; **(c)** about 5.15 franchises/yr
47. **(a)** $N(t) = 10e^{-0.13t}$; **(b)** 6.77 mg; **(c)** −0.88 mg/yr
48. **(a)** −18.2%/day; **(b)** $N(t) = 50e^{-0.182t}$; **(c)** −3.05 mg/day
49. **(a)** $A(t) = 800e^{-0.07t}$; **(b)** 197 g; **(c)** −13.81 g/day
50. **(a)** 0.5, 0.75, 0.97, 0.999; **(b)** $p'(t) = 0.7e^{-0.7t}$; **(c)** answers may vary;
(d)

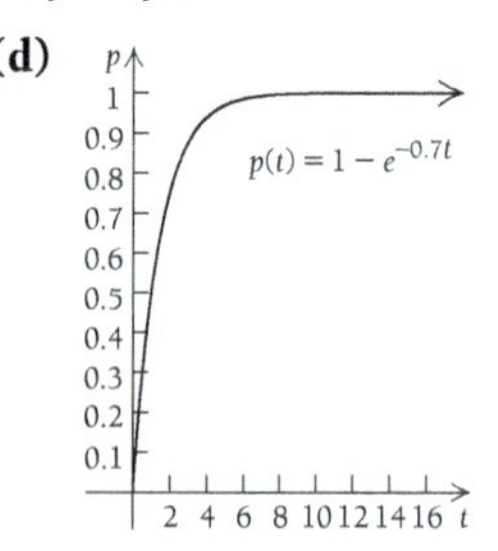

51. \$186,373.98 **52.** **(a)** $P(t) = 2500 \cdot 2^{t/6.5}$; **(b)** $P(t) = 2500e^{0.1066t}$; **(c)** 10.66%; **(d)** \$10,000
53. **(a)** $P(t) = 15{,}000 \cdot 1.25^{t/5}$; **(b)** 23,438 people; **(c)** 1045.99, meaning that Oak Fork was growing by about 1046 people/yr in 2000 **54.** $\ln 4 \cdot 4^{x^3+2x+1}[6x + \ln 4(9x^4 + 12x^2 + 4)]$
55. 19.02 yr **56.** 18.68 yr **57.** 0
58. **(a)** $y = 989.9661965(1.033223777)^x$, $y = 989.9661965e^{0.0326837949t}$, 3.27%; **(b)** \$1616.4 billion; **(c)** after about 21.5 yr; **(d)** 21.2 yr

Chapter 2 Test, p. 257

1. $6e^{3x}$ **2.** $\frac{4(\ln x)^3}{x}$ **3.** $-2xe^{-x^2}$ **4.** $\frac{1}{x}$ **5.** $e^x - 15x^2$
6. $\frac{3e^x}{x} + 3e^x \ln x$ **7.** $(\ln 7)7^x + (\ln 3)3^x$ **8.** $\frac{1}{x \ln 14}$
9. (a) 9.5427; **(b)** 0.2746 **10.** 2.302 **11.** 3.218
12. −0.916 **13.** $M(t) = 2e^{6t}$ **14.** 23.1%/hr
15. (a) $A(t) = 10{,}000e^{0.06931t}$; **(b)** $13,194.83; **(c)** $914.53/yr
16. (a) $C(t) = 3.22e^{0.0028t}$; **(b)** $3.39; **(c)** $0.009/yr
17. (a) $A(t) = 3e^{-0.1t}$; **(b)** 1.1 cc; **(c)** −0.11 cc/hr; **(d)** after 6.9 hr **18.** About 16.47 centuries, or 1647 yr
19. (a) $A(t) = 14e^{-0.04077t}$; **(b)** 1.21 mg; **(c)** −0.049 mg/s
20. (a) 4%; **(b)** 5.2%, 14.5%, 40.7%, 91.8%, 99.5%;
(c) $P'(t) = \frac{672e^{-0.28t}}{(1 + 24e^{-0.28t})^2}$; **(d)** answers may vary;
(e)

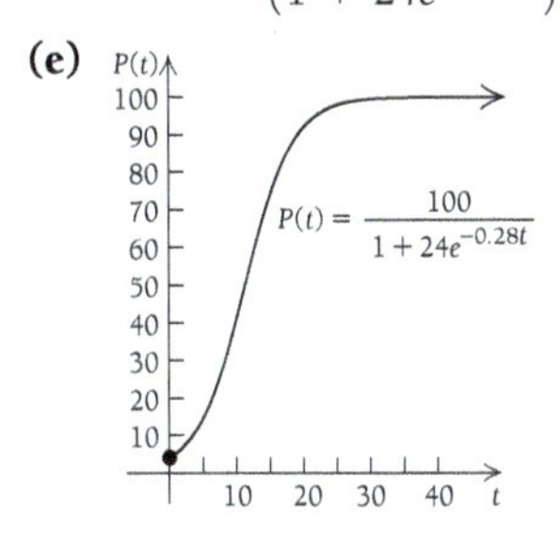

21. (a) $A(t) = 10{,}000 \cdot 2^{t/8.25}$; **(b)** $A(t) = 10{,}000e^{0.084t}$; **(c)** 8.4%; **(d)** 2301.70, which means that the value of Andres's account is growing by about $2301.70 per year after 12 yr
22. (a) $P(t) = 7500 \cdot (0.8)^{t/3}$; **(b)** 9.32 yr; **(c)** −307.68, which means that after 8 yr, the population is decreasing by about 308 people/yr **23.** $(\ln x)^2$ **24.** $\frac{24 - 18x^2}{(3x^2 + 4)^2 \ln 3}$
25. 2 **26. (a)** $y = 740336.2908(1.073657297)^x$, $y = 740336.2908e^{0.071070855t}$; **(b)** $7.2 million; **(c)** 101 yr; **(d)** about 9.8 yr

Extended Technology Application, p. 259

1. Linear: $G = -0.455t + 5.035$

$G = -0.455t + 5.035$

Quadratic: $G = -0.2546428571t^2 + 1.836785714t + 1.215357143$

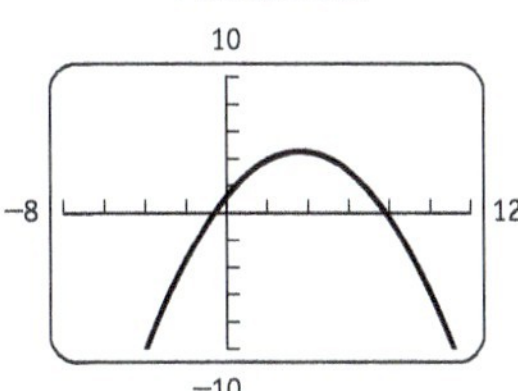

Cubic: $G = 0.122979798t^3 - 1.91487013t^2 + 8.17024531t - 4.872142857$

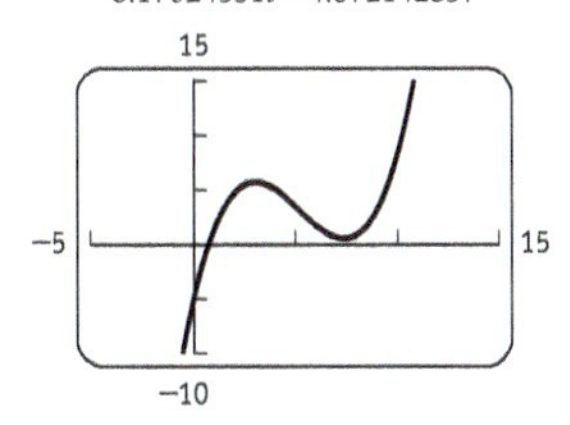

Exponential: $G = 5.58938024(0.8225245267)^t$

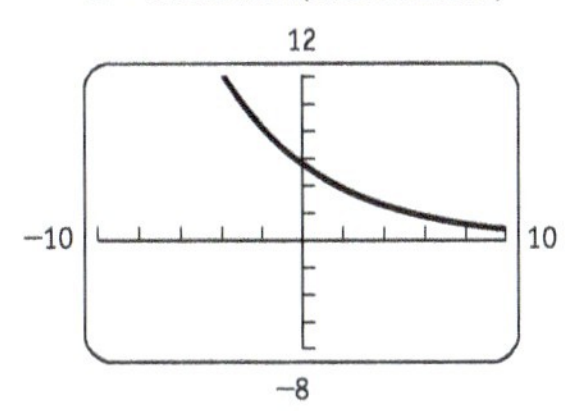

The cubic function fits well, but rises at higher values of t, which is not appropriate since weekly revenues are expected to fall as t increases. The exponential function also fits well and is better suited for forecasting future revenue. **2.** Week 9: $0.96 million; week 10: $0.79 million; week 11: $0.65 million; week 12: $0.54 million; week 13: $0.44 million **3.** Week 9: $24.86 million; week 10: $25.65 million; week 11: $26.3 million; week 12: $26.84 million; week 13: $27.28 million **4.** $R(t) = \frac{23.38497984}{1 + 23.62209015e^{-1.055833743t}}$. The limiting value is about $23.4 million, which seems too low.
5. $R(t) = \frac{24.31102164}{1 + 8.994071065e^{-0.7582056951t}}$. The limiting value is about $24.3 million, which agrees better with the actual data.
6. Left to the student
7. Linear: $G = -3.689404762t + 35.60107143$

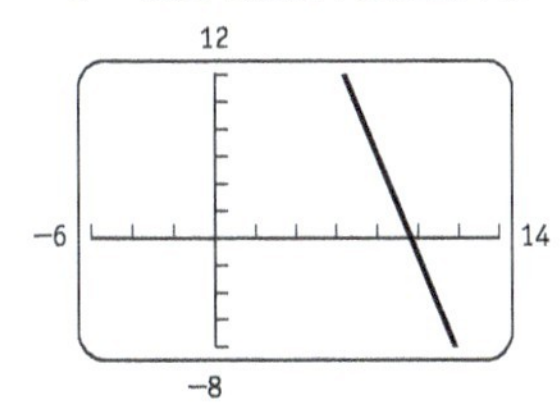

Quadratic: $G = 0.307797619t^2 - 6.459583333t + 40.21803571$

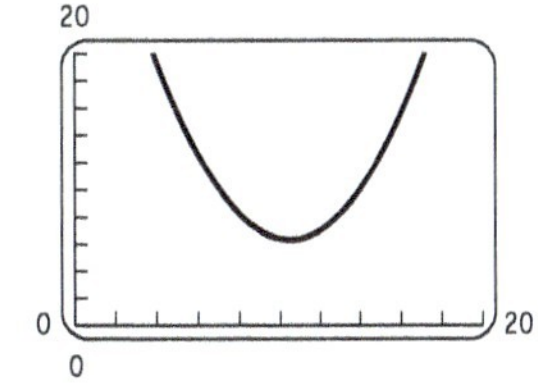

Cubic: $G = 0.0810858586t^3 - 0.7868614719t^2 - 2.283661616t + 36.20428571$

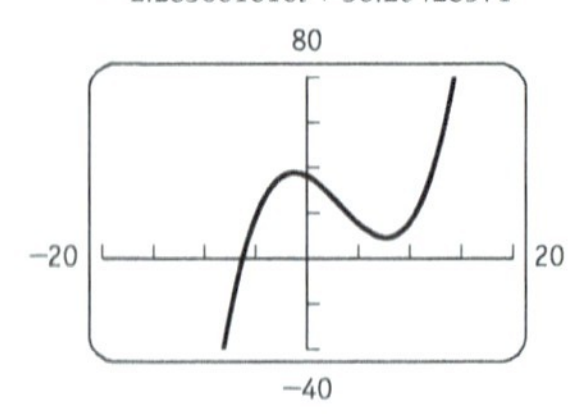

Exponential: $G = 42.47474076(0.8159645734)^t$

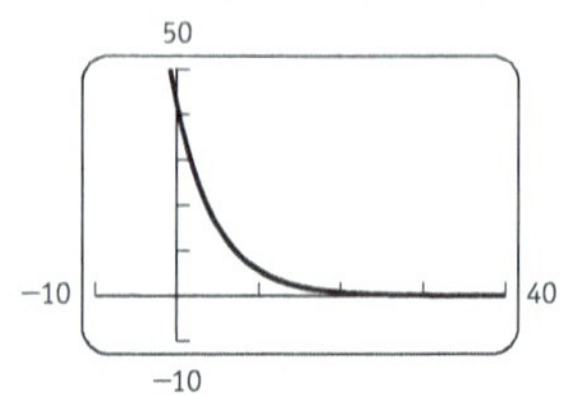

The exponential function is an excellent fit. **8.** Week 9: \$6.81 million; week 10: \$5.56 million; week 11: \$4.53 million; week 12: \$3.7 million; week 13: \$3.02 million; week 14: \$2.46 million

9. $R(t) = \dfrac{153.2872607}{1 + 5.563261043e^{-0.6327045804t}}$. The limiting value is about \$153.29 million, which seems too low.

10. $R(t) = \dfrac{169.4506888}{1 + 3.215356463e^{-0.4138102809t}}$. The limiting value is about \$169.45 million. This seems to be a better estimation.

11. In the 9th week **12.** Answers may vary.

CHAPTER 3

Technology Connection, p. 274

1.

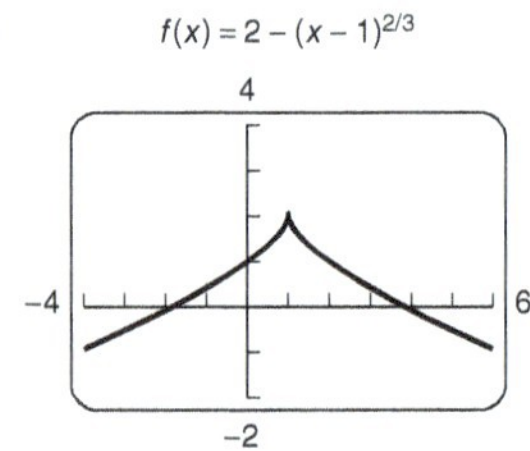

2.

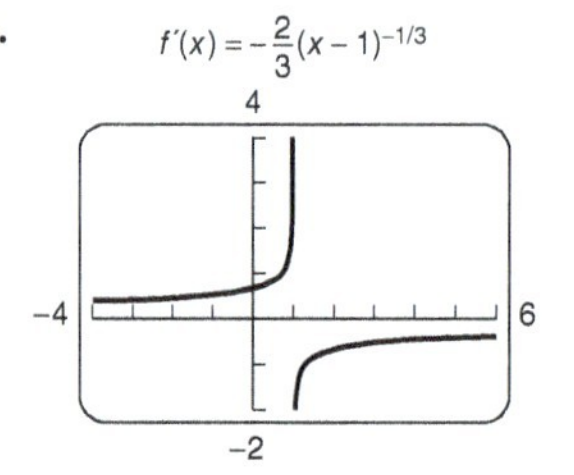

The derivative is not defined at $(1, 2)$.

Technology Connection, p. 275

1. Relative maximum at $(-1, 42)$; relative minimum at $\left(\frac{5}{2}, -\frac{175}{4}\right)$

Exercise Set 3.1, p. 276

1. **(a)** $x = 1, x = 3$; **(b)** relative minimum 1; **(c)** relative maximum 4; **(d)** relative minimum point $(1, 1)$; **(e)** relative maximum point $(3, 4)$ **3.** **(a)** $x = -2, x = 2$; **(b)** relative minimum -3; **(c)** relative maximum -1; **(d)** relative minimum point $(2, -3)$; **(e)** relative maximum point $(-2, -1)$ **5–15.** Answers may vary. **17.** **(a)** $x = -1$; **(b)** relative minimum $(-1, 1)$ **19.** **(a)** $x = -2, x = 2$; **(b)** relative maximum $(-2, 21)$, relative minimum $(2, -11)$ **21.** **(a)** $x = -1, x = 5$; **(b)** relative minimum $(5, -99)$, relative maximum $(-1, 9)$ **23.** **(a)** $x = 2$; **(b)** relative minimum $(2, 0)$ **25.** **(a)** $x = 2$; **(b)** relative minimum $(2, 5)$ **27.** **(a)** No critical values; **(b)** no relative extrema **29.** **(a)** $x = -\frac{1}{4}$; **(b)** relative minimum $\left(-\frac{1}{4}, -0.092\right)$ **31.** **(a)** $x = -1$; **(b)** relative minimum $(-1, 1.609)$

33. Relative minimum $(-3, -12)$, decreasing on $(-\infty, -3)$, increasing on $(-3, \infty)$

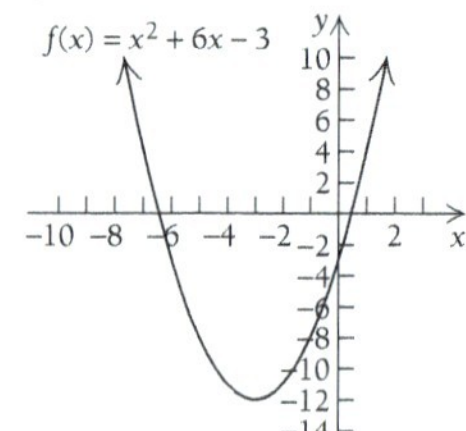
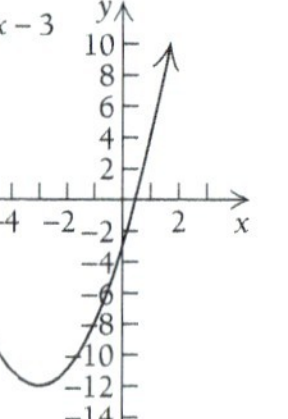

35. Relative minimum $(-2, -13)$, decreasing on $(-\infty, -2)$, increasing on $(-2, \infty)$

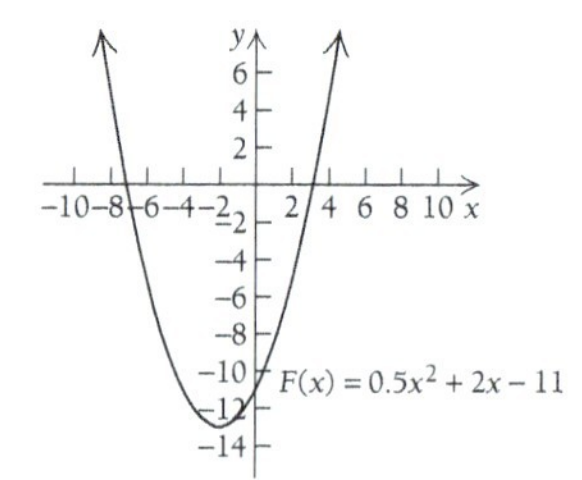

37. Relative minimum $\left(\frac{2}{3}, \frac{113}{27}\right)$, relative maximum $\left(-1, \frac{13}{2}\right)$, decreasing on $\left(-1, \frac{2}{3}\right)$, increasing on $(-\infty, -1)$ and on $\left(\frac{2}{3}, \infty\right)$

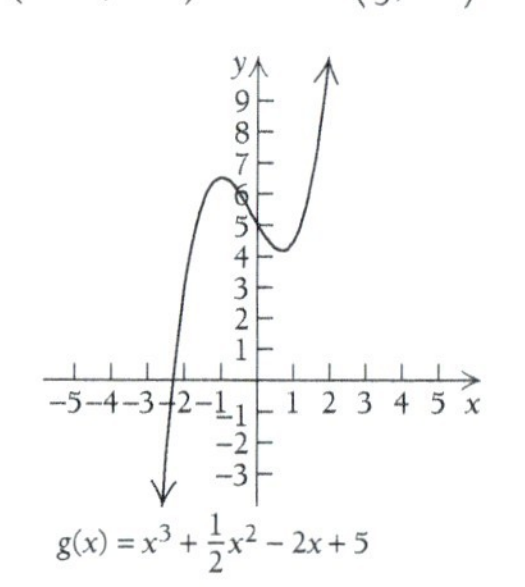

39. Relative minimum $(2, -4)$, relative maximum $(0, 0)$, decreasing on $(0, 2)$, increasing on $(-\infty, 0)$ and on $(2, \infty)$

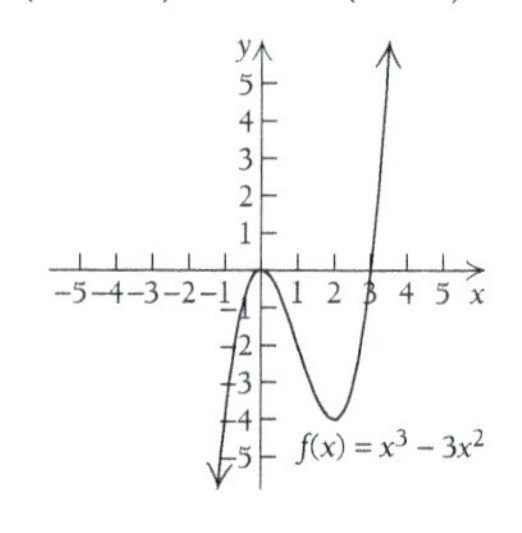

41. No relative extrema, decreasing on $(-\infty, \infty)$

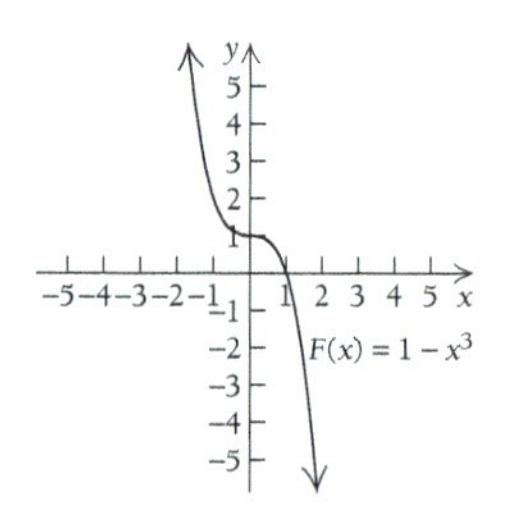

43. Relative minimum $\left(-\dfrac{1}{2}, -\dfrac{1}{2e}\right)$, decreasing on $\left(-\infty, -\frac{1}{2}\right)$, increasing on $\left(-\frac{1}{2}, \infty\right)$

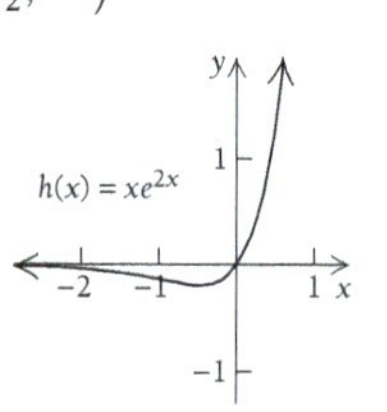

45. Relative minimum $\left(\ln\left(\frac{1}{2}\right), -\frac{1}{4}\right)$, decreasing on $\left(-\infty, \ln\left(\frac{1}{2}\right)\right)$, increasing on $\left(\ln\left(\frac{1}{2}\right), \infty\right)$

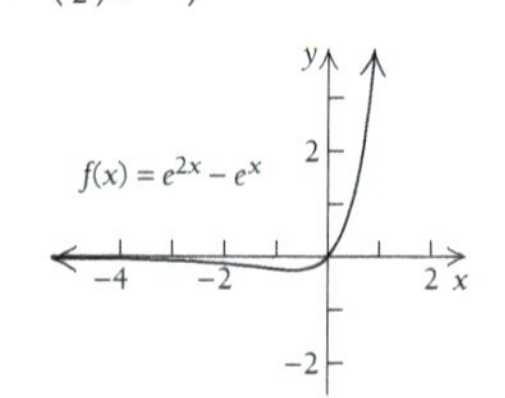

47. Relative minimum $(4, -22)$, relative maximum $(0, 10)$

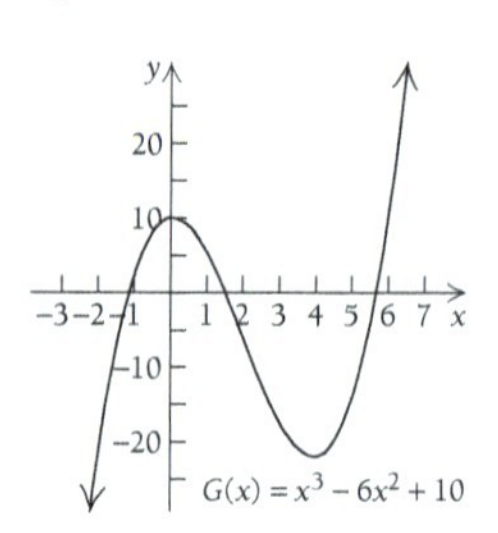

49. Relative maximum $\left(\frac{3}{4}, \frac{27}{256}\right)$

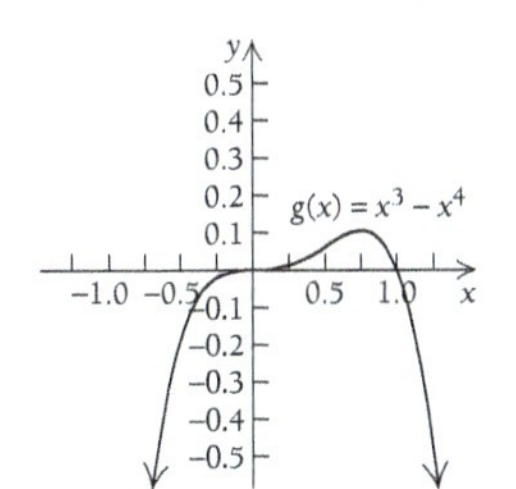

51. No relative extrema

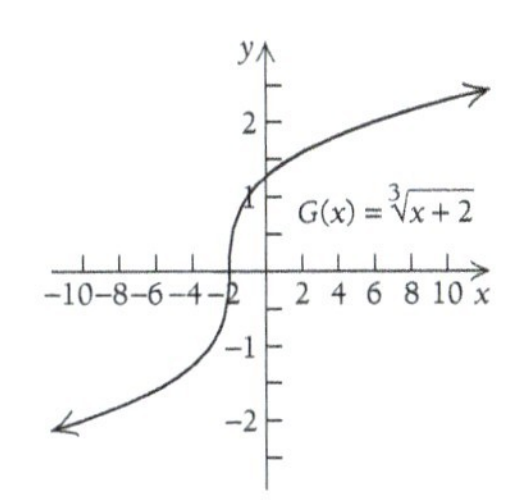

53. Relative maximum $(0, 1)$

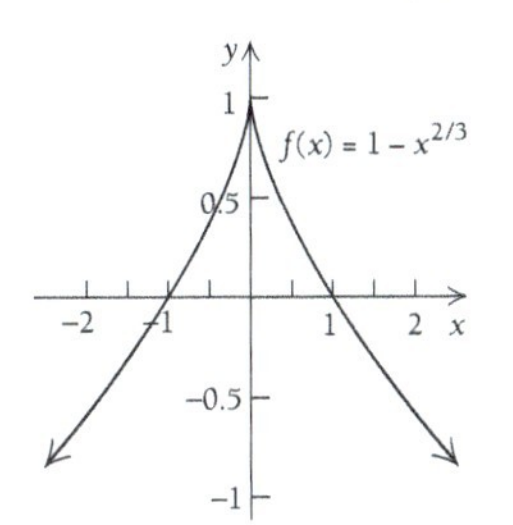

55. Relative minimum $(0, -8)$

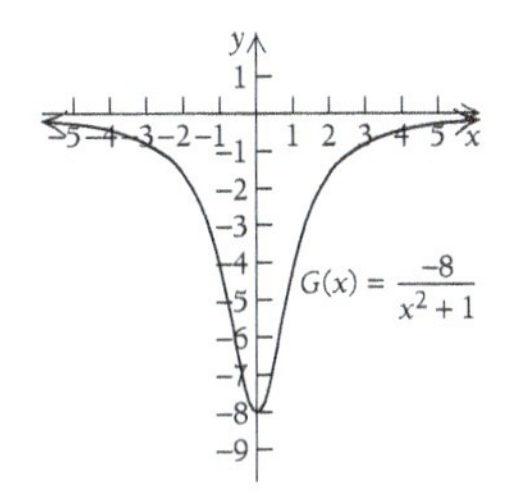

57. Relative minimum $(\ln 2, 2 - 2\ln 2)$

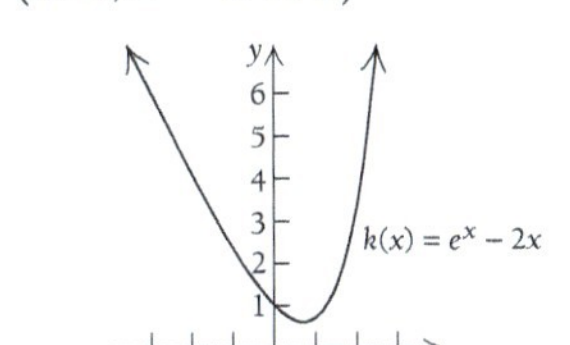

59. Relative minimum $(2, e^{-4})$

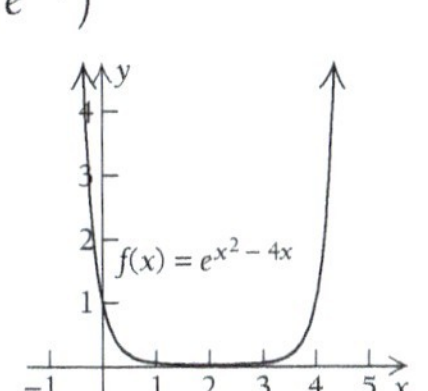

61. Relative minimum $(-1, -e^{-3})$

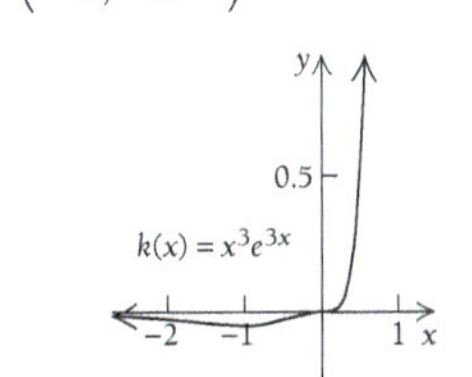

63. Relative minimum $\left(-\frac{1}{2}, \ln\left(\frac{11}{4}\right)\right)$

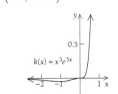

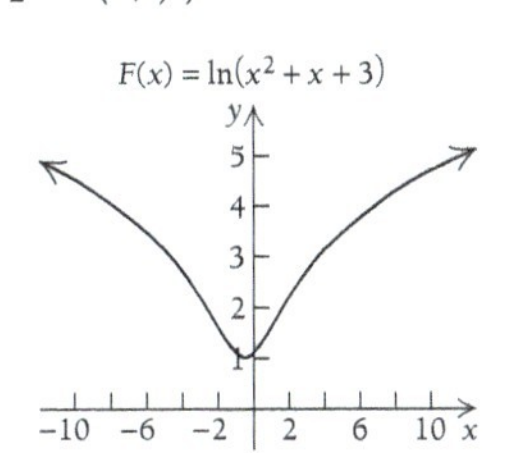

65. Answers may vary. **67. (a)** $R(x) = 200x - 2x^2$; **(b)** relative maximum $(50, 5000)$, which means that when she charges \$50, she maximizes revenue at \$5000
69. (a) $R(x) = 500x - 5x^2$; **(b)** relative maximum $(50, 12{,}500)$, which means that when the price of each sculpture is \$50, a maximum total revenue of \$12,500 is generated
71. 16.08° S **73–77.** Left to the student
79. $f(x) = x^2 - 6x + 16$ **81.** $h(x) = xe^{-5x}$
83. (a) $a = -10$; **(b)** -21; **(c)** relative minimum
85. (a) $a = 4$; **(b)** e^{-4}; **(c)** relative minimum
87. (a) $a = -2$; **(b)** $\frac{1}{2}e^{-1}$; **(c)** relative maximum

89.

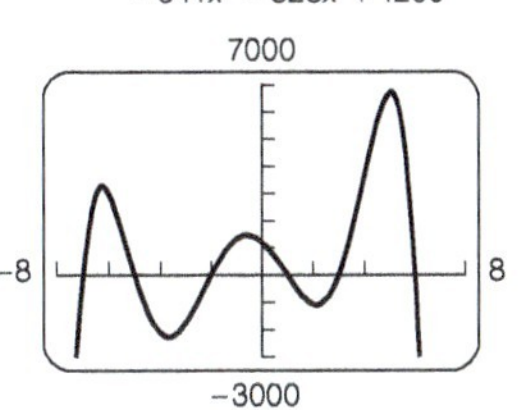

Relative minima $(-3.683, -2288.03)$ and $(2.116, -1083.08)$, relative maxima $(-6.262, 3213.8)$, $(-0.559, 1440.06)$, $(5.054, 6674.12)$

91.

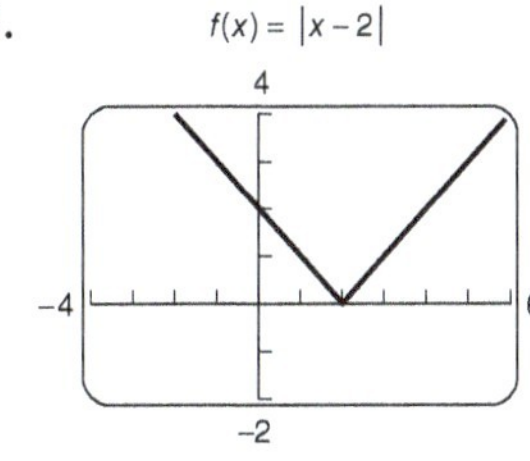

Relative minimum $(2, 0)$, increasing on $(2, \infty)$, decreasing on $(-\infty, 2)$; f' does not exist at $x = 2$.

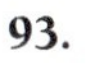

93.

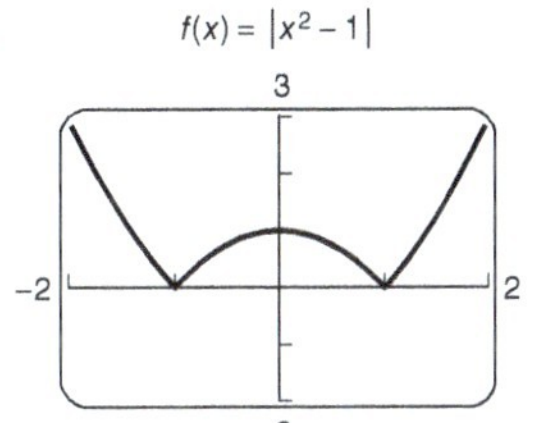

Relative maximum $(0, 1)$, relative minima $(1, 0)$ and $(-1, 0)$, increasing on $(-1, 0)$ and $(1, \infty)$, decreasing on $(-\infty, -1)$ and $(0, 1)$. f' does not exist at $x = -1$ and $x = 1$.

95.

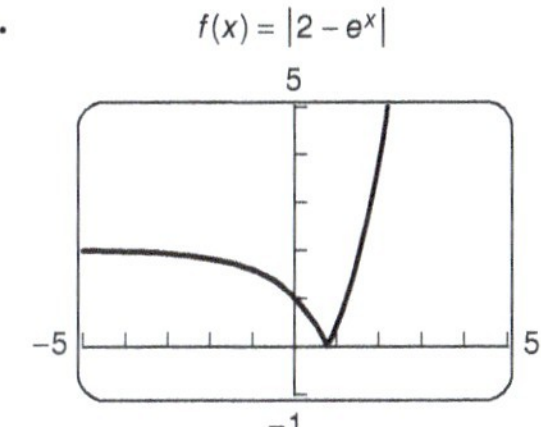

Relative minimum at $(\ln 2, 0)$,decreasing on $(-\infty, \ln 2)$, increasing on $(\ln 2, \infty)$; derivative does not exist at $x = \ln 2$.

97. Answers may vary.

Technology Connection, p. 288

1.

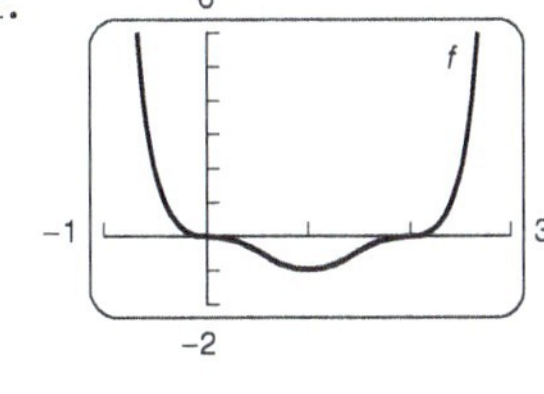

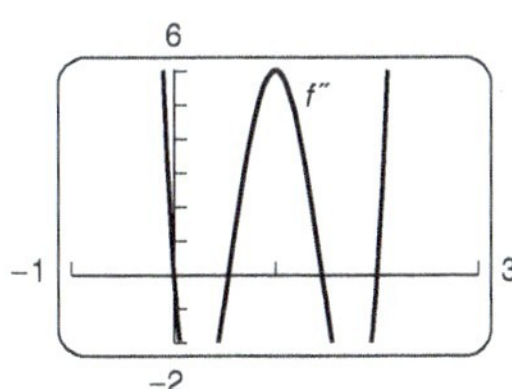

Relative minimum $(1, -1)$, inflection points at $(0, 0)$, $(0.553, -0.512)$, $(1.447, -0.512)$, and $(2, 0)$

Exercise Set 3.2, p. 290

1. (a) $(1, 2)$; **(b)** concave up on $(-\infty, 1)$, concave down on $(1, \infty)$
3. (a) $(-1, 3)$; **(b)** concave down on $(-\infty, -1)$, concave up on $(-1, \infty)$ **5. (a)** $(-1, -1)$ and $(2, -1)$; **(b)** concave up on $(-1, 2)$, concave down on $(-\infty, -1)$ and $(2, \infty)$
7. (a) $(5, -23)$, relative minimum; **(b)** decreasing on $(-\infty, 5)$, increasing on $(5, \infty)$; **(c)** no points of inflection;

(d) concave up on $(-\infty, \infty)$; **(e)**

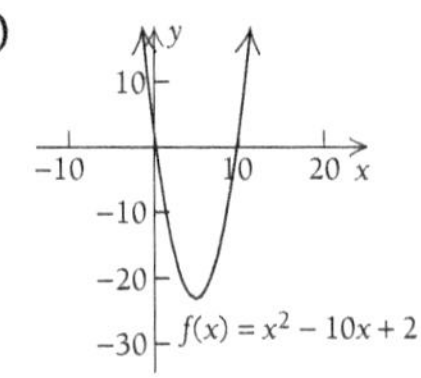

9. **(a)** $(3, 16)$, relative maximum; **(b)** increasing on $(-\infty, 3)$, decreasing on $(3, \infty)$; **(c)** no points of inflection; **(d)** concave down on $(-\infty, \infty)$; **(e)**

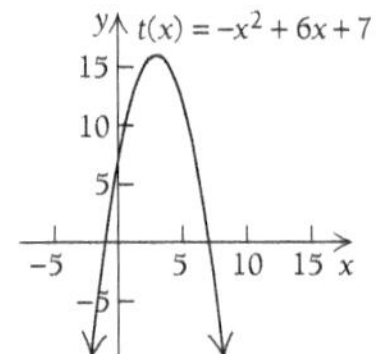

11. **(a)** $\left(-\frac{2}{3}, \frac{2}{3}\right)$, relative minimum; **(b)** decreasing on $\left(-\infty, -\frac{2}{3}\right)$, increasing on $\left(-\frac{2}{3}, \infty\right)$; **(c)** no points of inflection; **(d)** concave up on $(-\infty, \infty)$; **(e)**

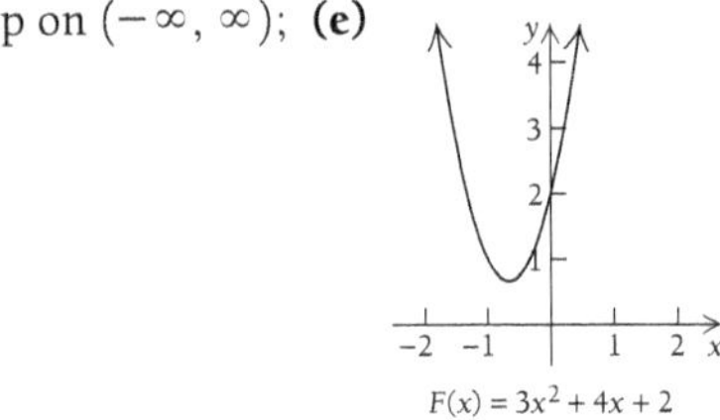

13. **(a)** $(3, -54)$, relative minimum, and $(-3, 54)$ relative maximum; **(b)** increasing on $(-\infty, -3)$ and $(3, \infty)$, decreasing on $(-3, 3)$; **(c)** $(0, 0)$; **(d)** concave down on $(-\infty, 0)$, concave up on $(0, \infty)$; **(e)**

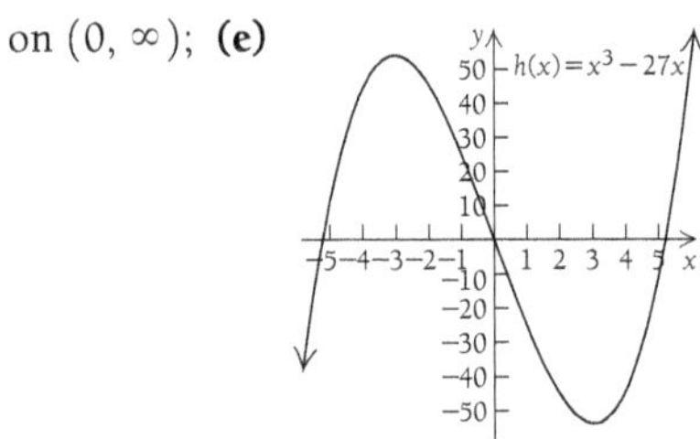

15. **(a)** $\left(-\frac{1}{3}, -\frac{1}{3}e^{-1}\right)$, relative minimum; **(b)** decreasing on $\left(-\infty, -\frac{1}{3}\right)$, increasing on $\left(-\frac{1}{3}, \infty\right)$; **(c)** $\left(-\frac{2}{3}, -\frac{2}{3}e^{-2}\right)$; **(d)** concave down on $\left(-\infty, -\frac{2}{3}\right)$, concave up on $\left(-\frac{2}{3}, \infty\right)$; **(e)**

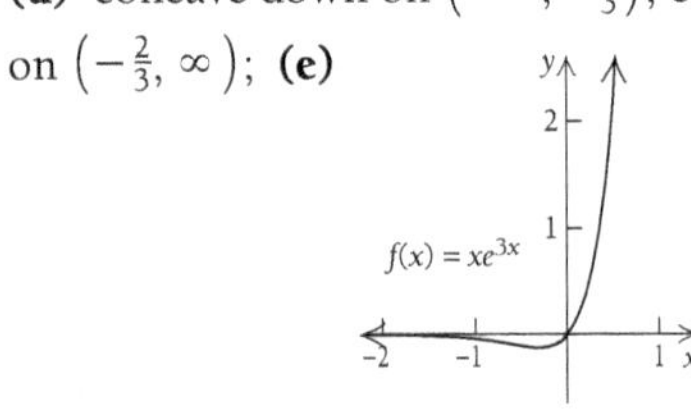

17. **(a)** $(0, \ln 9)$, relative minimum; **(b)** decreasing on $(-\infty, 0)$, increasing on $(0, \infty)$; **(c)** $(-3, \ln 18)$ and $(3, \ln 18)$; **(d)** concave down on $(-\infty, -3)$ and on $(3, \infty)$; concave up on $(-3, 3)$;

(e)

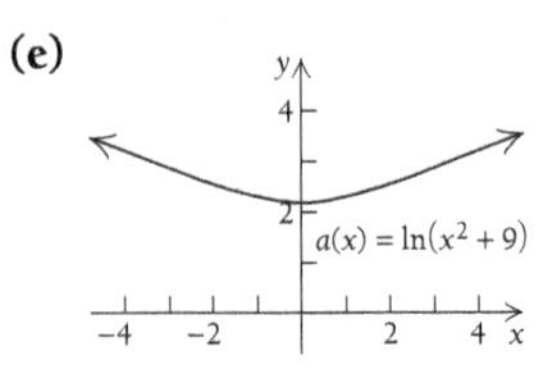

19. **(a)** Relative minimum at $(3, 1)$, relative maximum at $(1, 5)$; **(b)** increasing on $(-\infty, 1)$ and on $(3, \infty)$, decreasing on $(1, 3)$; **(c)** $(2, 3)$; **(d)** concave down on $(-\infty, 2)$, concave up on $(2, \infty)$;

(e)

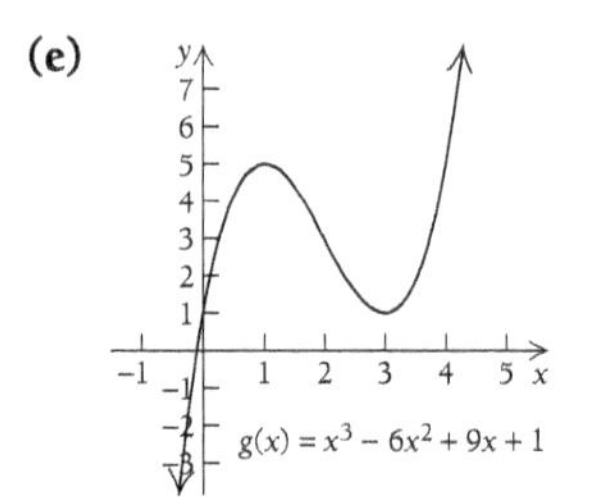

21. **(a)** Relative minimum at $\left(\frac{3}{2}, -\frac{27}{16}\right)$; **(b)** increasing on $\left(\frac{3}{2}, \infty\right)$, decreasing on $\left(-\infty, \frac{3}{2}\right)$; **(c)** $(0, 0)$ and $(1, -1)$; **(d)** concave down on $(0, 1)$, concave up on $(-\infty, 0)$ and on $(1, \infty)$; **(e)**

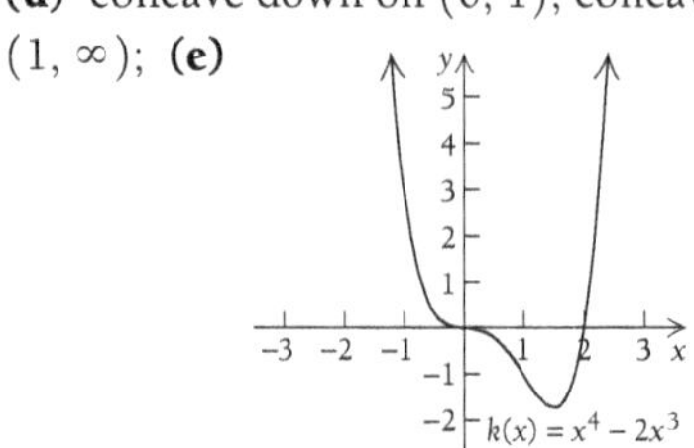

23. **(a)** $\left(\frac{1}{2}\ln\left(\frac{1}{3}\right), -0.385\right)$, relative minimum; **(b)** decreasing on $\left(-\infty, \frac{1}{2}\ln\left(\frac{1}{3}\right)\right)$, increasing on $\left(\frac{1}{2}\ln\left(\frac{1}{3}\right), \infty\right)$; **(c)** $\left(\frac{1}{2}\ln\left(\frac{1}{9}\right), -0.296\right)$; **(d)** concave down on $\left(-\infty, \frac{1}{2}\ln\left(\frac{1}{9}\right)\right)$, concave up on $\left(\frac{1}{2}\ln\left(\frac{1}{9}\right), \infty\right)$; **(e)**

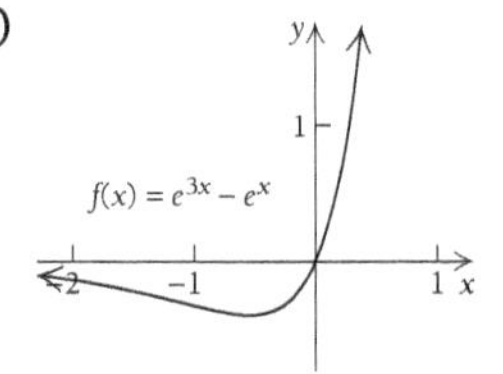

25. **(a)** Relative minimum at $(-1, -4)$, relative maximum at $(1, 4)$; **(b)** increasing on $(-1, 1)$, decreasing on $(-\infty, -1)$ and on $(1, \infty)$; **(c)** $(-\sqrt{3}, -2\sqrt{3})$, $(0, 0)$, and $(\sqrt{3}, 2\sqrt{3})$; **(d)** concave up on $(-\sqrt{3}, 0)$ and on $(\sqrt{3}, \infty)$, concave down on $(-\infty, -\sqrt{3})$ and on $(0, \sqrt{3})$; **(e)**

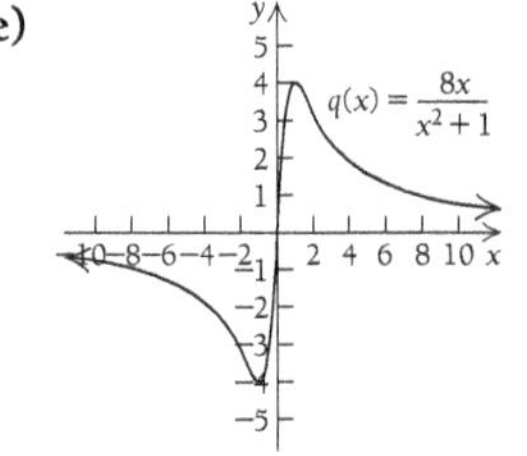

27. **(a)** $\left(e^{-0.5}, -\dfrac{1}{2e}\right)$, relative minimum; **(b)** decreasing on $(0, e^{-0.5})$, increasing on $(e^{-0.5}, \infty)$; **(c)** $\left(e^{-3/2}, -\dfrac{3}{2e^3}\right)$; **(d)** concave down on $(0, e^{-3/2})$, concave up on $(e^{-3/2}, \infty)$; **(e)**

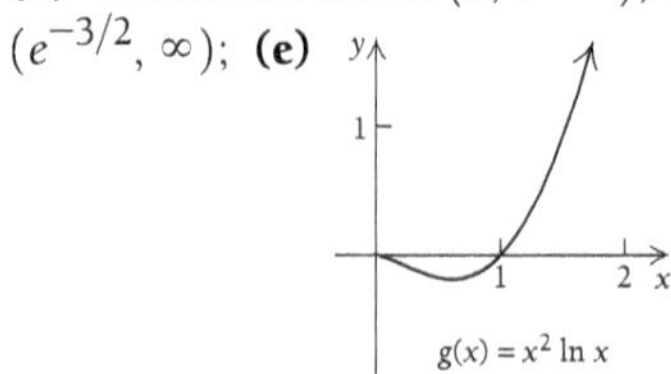

29–37. Left to the student

39. $f(x) = -0.0115x^2 + 0.125x + 81.7$

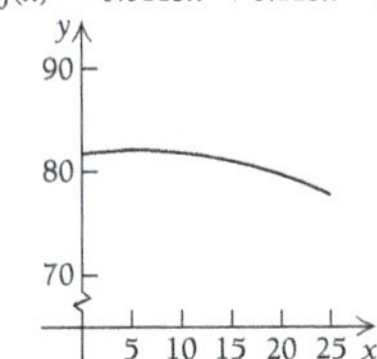

Approximately 1999

41. (a) $(16.82, 97.54)$, at which the rate of change in sales is maximized; **(b)** $s(x) = -0.0131x^3 + 0.661x^2 - 2.021x + 6.865$

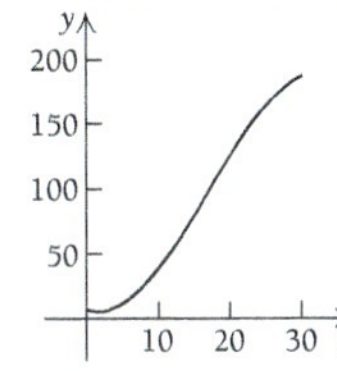

43. $(3.26, 18.36)$; the rate of change of the amount of rainfall is decreasing the fastest at this point.

45. (a) $P(t) = 35{,}000e^{0.05t} + 50{,}000e^{-0.07t}$; **(b)** $(0, 5.78)$; **(c)** $(5.78, \infty)$; **(d)** $(5.78, 80{,}090)$, which means that after 5.78 yr, the combined population is minimized, at about 80,090 people **47–51.** Left to the student **53.** False (explanation may vary) **55.** True **57.** True **59.** True **61.** At about $t = 6$; the rate of change is slowest here.

63.

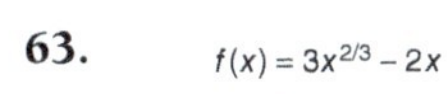

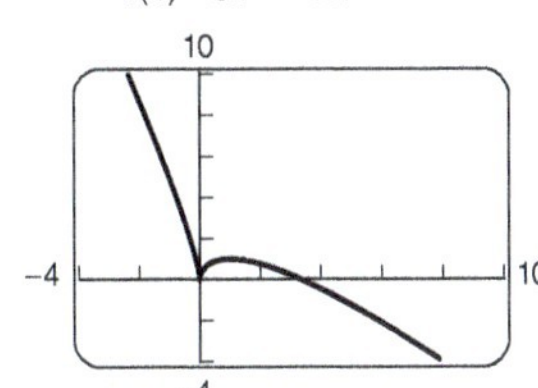

Relative minimum at $(0, 0)$, relative maximum at $(1, 1)$

65.

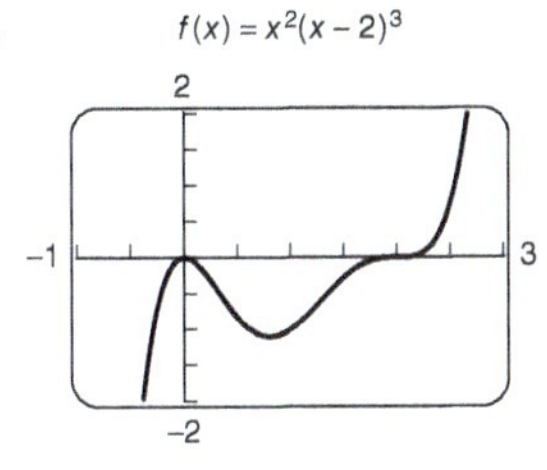

Relative minimum at $(0.8, -1.106)$, relative maximum at $(0, 0)$

67.

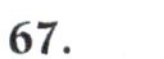

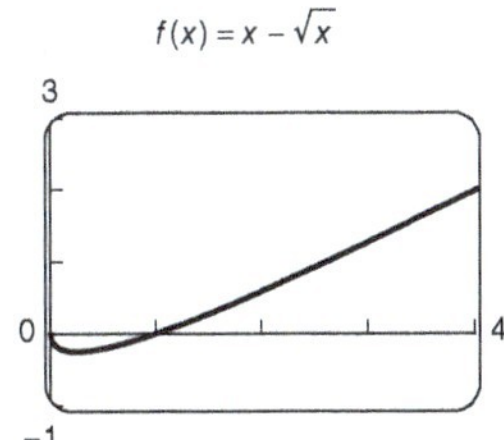

Relative minimum at $(0.25, -0.25)$

69.

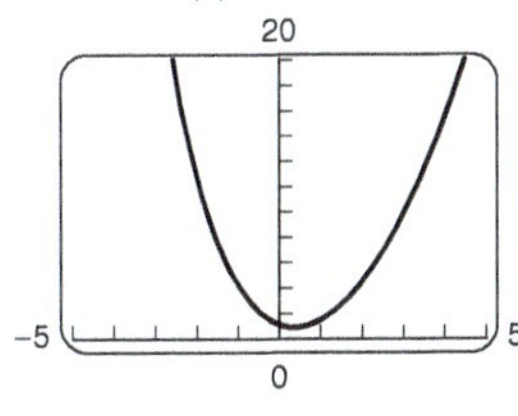

Relative minimum at $(0.352, 0.827)$

71. Left to the student **73.** Left to the student

Technology Connection, p. 294

Graphs are left to the student.

1. Vertical asymptotes at $x = -7$ and $x = 4$ **2.** Vertical asymptote at $x = 0$

Technology Connection, p. 297

Graphs are left to the student.

1. Horizontal asymptote at $y = 3$ **2.** Horizontal asymptote at $y = 0$

Exercise Set 3.3, p. 305

1. $x = 2$ **3.** $x = -5$ and $x = 5$ **5.** $x = -1$, $x = 0$, and $x = 1$ **7.** $x = -4$ **9.** No vertical asymptotes **11.** $x = -7$ **13.** No vertical asymptotes **15.** No vertical asymptotes **17.** $y = \frac{3}{4}$ **19.** $y = 0$ **21.** $y = 4$ **23.** No horizontal asymptote **25.** $y = 4$ **27.** $y = \frac{1}{2}$ **29.** $y = 0$ **31.** $y = 0$ and $y = 25$ **33.** $y = 0$ and $y = 6000$

35.

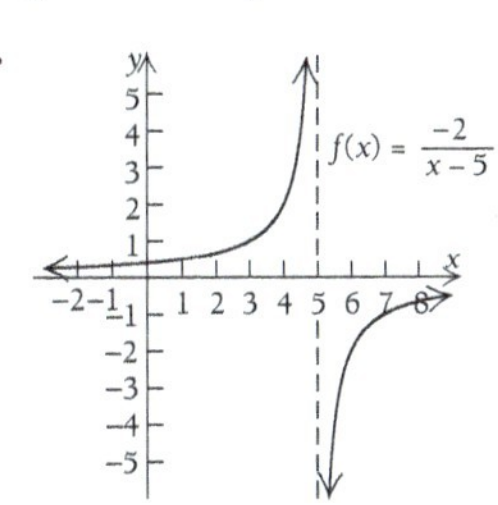

Increasing on $(-\infty, 5)$ and on $(5, \infty)$, no relative extrema, vertical asymptote $x = 5$, horizontal asymptote $y = 0$, concave up on $(-\infty, 5)$, concave down on $(5, \infty)$; no points of inflection; no x-intercept; y-intercept $\left(0, \frac{2}{5}\right)$

37.

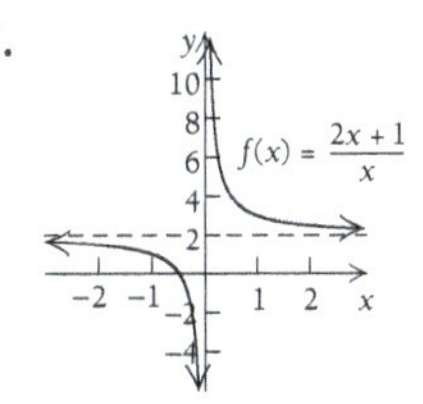

Decreasing on $(-\infty, 0)$ and on $(0, \infty)$, no relative extrema, vertical asymptote $x = 0$, horizontal asymptote $y = 2$, concave up on $(0, \infty)$, concave down on $(-\infty, 0)$; no points of inflection; x-intercept $\left(-\frac{1}{2}, 0\right)$, no y-intercept

39.

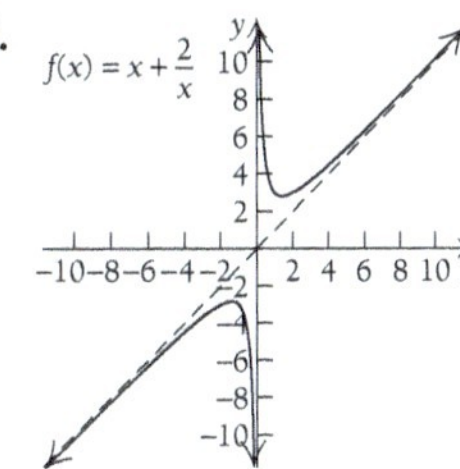

Increasing on $(-\infty, -\sqrt{2})$ and on $(\sqrt{2}, \infty)$, decreasing on $(-\sqrt{2}, 0)$ and on $(0, \sqrt{2})$, relative maximum $(-\sqrt{2}, -2\sqrt{2})$, relative minimum $(\sqrt{2}, 2\sqrt{2})$, vertical asymptote $x = 0$, slant asymptote $y = x$, concave up on $(0, \infty)$, concave down on $(-\infty, 0)$, no points of inflection, no x-intercept or y-intercept

41.

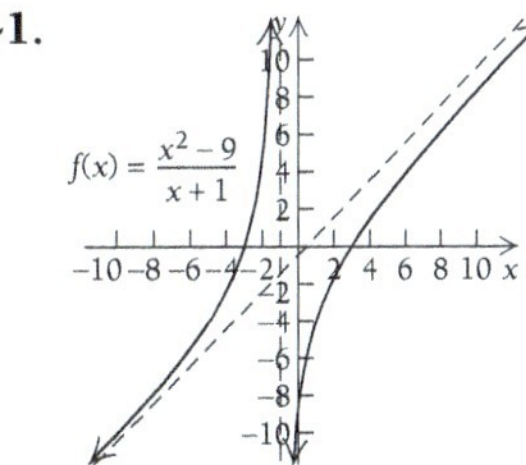

Increasing on $(-\infty, -1)$ and on $(-1, \infty)$, no relative extrema, vertical asymptote $x = -1$, no horizontal asymptote, slant asymptote $y = x - 1$, concave up on $(-\infty, -1)$, concave down on $(-1, \infty)$, no points of inflection, x-intercepts $(-3, 0)$ and $(3, 0)$, y-intercept $(0, -9)$

43.

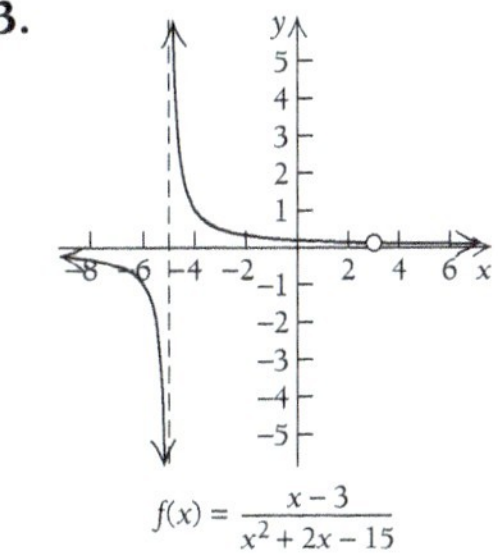

Decreasing on $(-\infty, -5)$ and on $(-5, 3)$ and on $(3, \infty)$, no relative extrema, vertical asymptote $x = -5$, horizontal asymptote $y = 0$, concave up on $(-5, 3)$ and on $(3, \infty)$, concave down on $(-\infty, -5)$, no points of inflection, no x-intercept, y-intercept $\left(0, \frac{1}{5}\right)$

45.

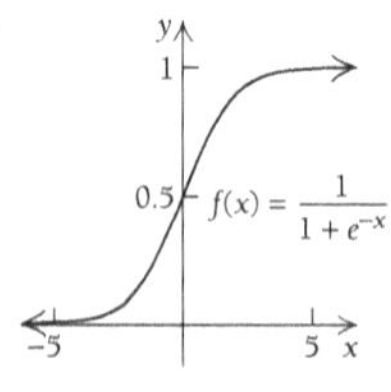

Increasing on $(-\infty, \infty)$, no relative extrema, no vertical asymptote, horizontal asymptotes at $y = 0$ and $y = 1$, concave down on $(0, \infty)$, concave up on $(-\infty, 0)$, point of inflection at $\left(0, \frac{1}{2}\right)$, no x-intercept, y-intercept at $\left(0, \frac{1}{2}\right)$

47.

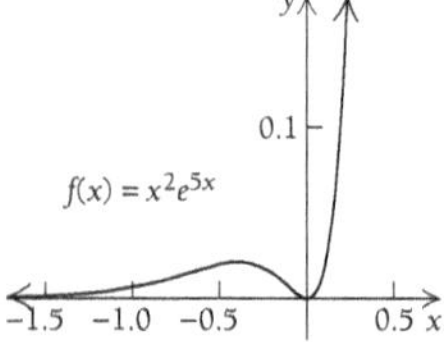

Increasing on $\left(-\infty, -\frac{2}{5}\right)$ and on $(0, \infty)$, decreasing on $\left(-\frac{2}{5}, 0\right)$, relative maximum at $\left(-\frac{2}{5}, \frac{4}{25}e^{-2}\right)$, relative minimum at $(0, 0)$, horizontal asymptote $y = 0$, no vertical asymptote, concave up on $\left(-\infty, -\frac{2}{5} - \frac{\sqrt{2}}{5}\right)$ and on $\left(-\frac{2}{5} + \frac{\sqrt{2}}{5}, \infty\right)$, concave down on $\left(-\frac{2}{5} - \frac{\sqrt{2}}{5}, -\frac{2}{5} + \frac{\sqrt{2}}{5}\right)$, points of inflection at $\left(-\frac{2}{5} - \frac{\sqrt{2}}{5}, 0.01534\right)$ and $\left(-\frac{2}{5} + \frac{\sqrt{2}}{5}, 0.00764\right)$, x-intercept and y-intercept $(0, 0)$

49.

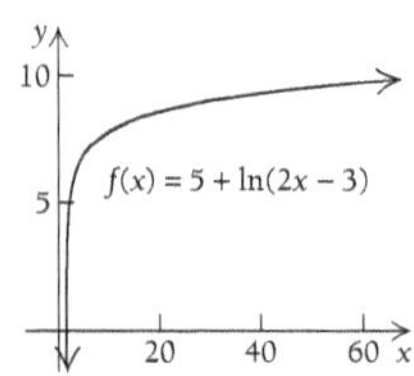

Increasing on $\left(\frac{3}{2}, \infty\right)$, no relative extrema, no horizontal asymptote, vertical asymptote $x = \frac{3}{2}$, concave down on $\left(\frac{3}{2}, \infty\right)$, no point of inflection, no y-intercept, x-intercept $\left(\frac{1}{2}e^{-5} + \frac{3}{2}, 0\right)$

51.

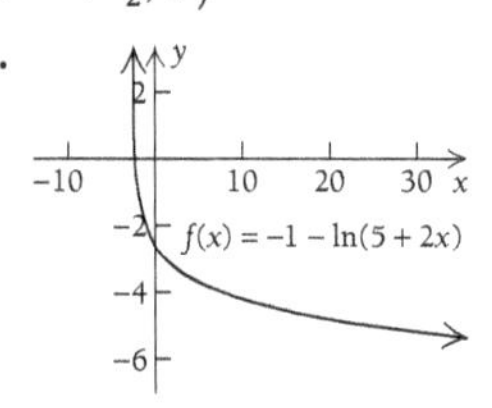

Decreasing on $\left(-\frac{5}{2}, \infty\right)$, no relative extrema, no horizontal asymptote, vertical asymptote $x = -\frac{5}{2}$, concave up on $\left(-\frac{5}{2}, \infty\right)$, no point of inflection, y-intercept $(0, -1 - \ln 5)$, or about $(0, -2.609)$, x-intercept $\left(\frac{e^{-1}}{2} - \frac{5}{2}, 0\right)$, or about $(-2.316, 0)$

53. **(a)** $\overline{C}(x) = 3x + \frac{80}{x}$;

(b)

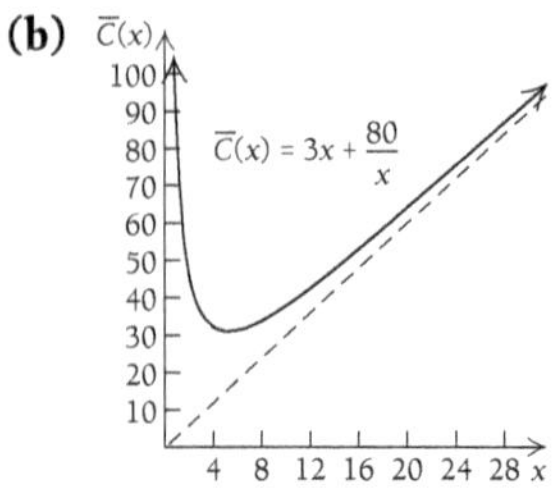

(c) $y = 3x$, which means that as x, the number of units produced, increases, the average cost approaches $3x$

55. **(a)** $P(x) = -\frac{1}{2}x^2 + 400x - 5000$; **(b)** $\overline{P}(x) = -\frac{1}{2}x + 400 - \frac{5000}{x}$; **(c)** $y = -\frac{1}{2}x + 400$;

(d)

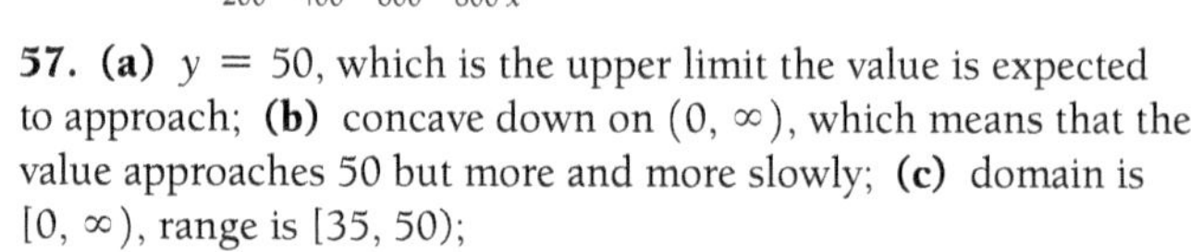

57. **(a)** $y = 50$, which is the upper limit the value is expected to approach; **(b)** concave down on $(0, \infty)$, which means that the value approaches 50 but more and more slowly; **(c)** domain is $[0, \infty)$, range is $[35, 50)$;

(d)

59. **(a)** 100 cc, 50 cc, 20 cc, 2 cc, 0.9901 cc; **(b)** 100 cc at $t = 0$ hr;

(c)

(d) answers may vary. **61.** **(a)** 4.00, 6.00, 12.00, 36.00, 54.00, 108.00; **(b)** 6.00, 9.00, 18.00, 54.00, 81.00, 162.00; **(c)** answers may vary. **63.** Answers may vary. **65.** Answers may vary. **67.** $\frac{2}{3}$ **69.** $\frac{4}{3}$ **71.** Does not exist **73.** -3 **75.** $\frac{3}{2}$

77.

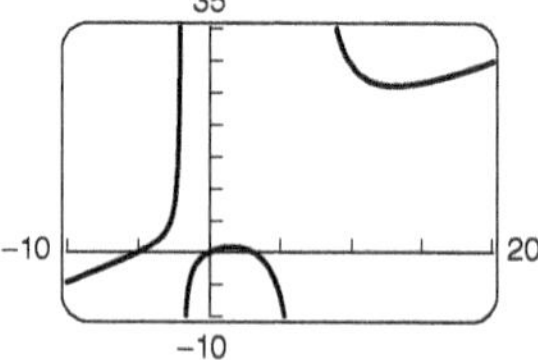

79.

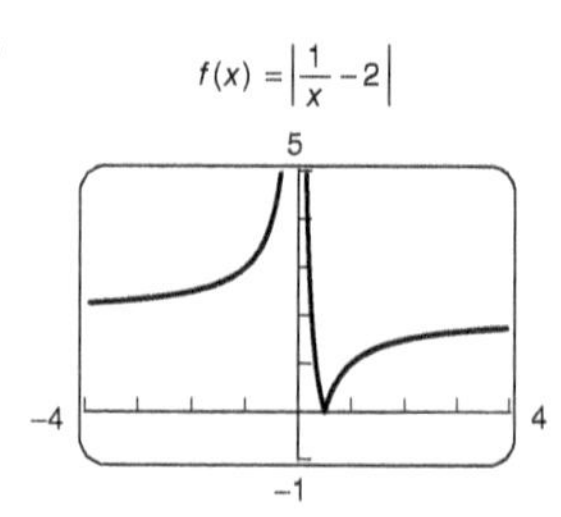

81. $f(x) = \frac{3x - 1}{x}$ **83.** $g(x) = \frac{-3x^2 + 15}{x^2 + 2x}$

85. $h(x) = \frac{x + 3}{4x^2 - 1}$

Exercise Set 3.4, p. 313

1. **(a)** 55 mph; **(b)** 5 mph; **(c)** 25 mpg **3.** Absolute maximum, $\frac{21}{4}$ at $x = \frac{1}{2}$; absolute minimum, 3 at $x = 2$ **5.** Absolute maximum, $\frac{13}{2}$ at $x = -1$; absolute minimum, 3 at $x = -2$ **7.** Absolute maximum, 6 at $x = 1$; absolute minimum, 2 at $x = -1$ **9.** Absolute maximum, 4 at $x = -1$; absolute minimum, -12 at $x = 3$ **11.** Absolute maximum, $\frac{11}{2}$ at $x = -1$; absolute minimum, 2 at $x = -2$ **13.** Absolute maximum, 4 at $x = 1$; absolute minimum, -23 at $x = 4$ **15.** Absolute maximum, $\frac{27}{256}$ at $x = \frac{3}{4}$; absolute minimum, -2 at $x = -1$ **17.** Absolute maximum, 1 at $x = 0$; absolute minimum, -3 at $x = -8$ and $x = 8$ **19.** Absolute maximum, -4 at $x = -2$; absolute minimum, $-\frac{17}{2}$ at $x = -8$ **21.** Absolute maximum, $\frac{4}{5}$ at $x = -2$ and $x = 2$; absolute minimum, 0 at $x = 0$ **23.** Absolute minimum, $-\frac{4}{27}$ at $x = \ln\left(\frac{2}{3}\right)$; absolute maximum, $e^3 - e^2 \approx 12.696$ at $x = 1$ **25.** Absolute maximum, $\ln 6 \approx 1.792$ at $x = -1$; absolute minimum, $\ln 2 \approx 0.693$ at $x = 1$ **27.** Absolute maximum, $4e^{-1} \approx 1.472$ at $x = 4$; absolute minimum, $-e^{1/4} \approx -1.284$ at $x = -1$ **29.** Absolute maximum, $\frac{64}{3}$ at $x = 2$ **31.** Absolute maximum, 5700 at $x = 2400$ **33.** Absolute minimum, 108 at $x = 6$ **35.** Absolute maximum, 2 at $x = 8$; absolute minimum, 0 at $x = 0$ **37.** Absolute maximum, $\dfrac{1}{3e} \approx 0.123$ at $x = \frac{1}{6}$ **39.** Absolute minimum, 60 at $x = 0$ **41.** Absolute minimum, -0.105 at $x = \ln\left(\frac{3}{4}\right)$ **43.** Absolute minimum, 1134.558 at $x = \frac{25}{3}\ln\left(\frac{49}{25}\right) \approx 5.608$ **45.** Absolute minimum, 0 at $x = 1$ **47.** Absolute minimum, $30e^{-0.1} \approx 27.145$ at $x = -10$; absolute maximum, $30e^{0.2} \approx 36.642$ at $x = 20$ **49.** 1430 units after 25 yr **51.** Absolute minimum, \$42,534.55 at $t = \dfrac{1}{0.085}\ln\left(\dfrac{65}{33}\right) \approx 7.975$ yr; absolute maximum, \$47,532.21 at $t = 20$ yr **53.** **(a)** $\overline{C}(x) = 0.2x + 125 + \dfrac{3500}{x}$; **(b)** $x = \sqrt{17{,}500} \approx 132.29$ tons, for an average cost of about \$177.92 per ton **55.** **(a)** $x = \sqrt[4]{2000}$, or about 6.687 in.; **(b)** 178.885 in^2 of material

57. **(a)** $x = 10\sqrt{15}$, or about 38.73 m; **(b)** \$619.68

59. Answers may vary.

61. Absolute maximum point $(1, 3)$; absolute minimum point $(-3, -5)$

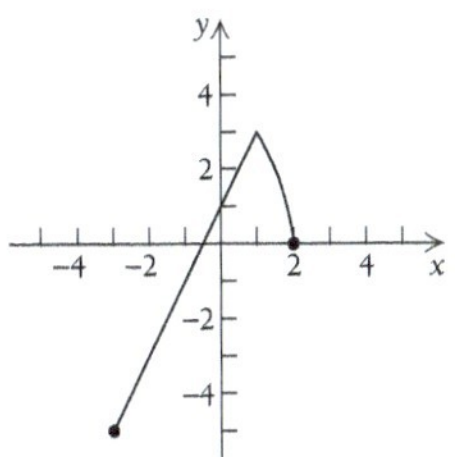

63. Absolute maximum points $(0, 1)$, $(2, 1)$; absolute minimum point $(-4, -15)$

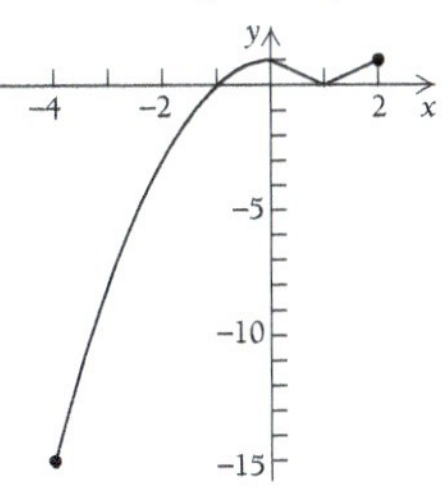

65. Minimum value 2 over $[0, 2]$

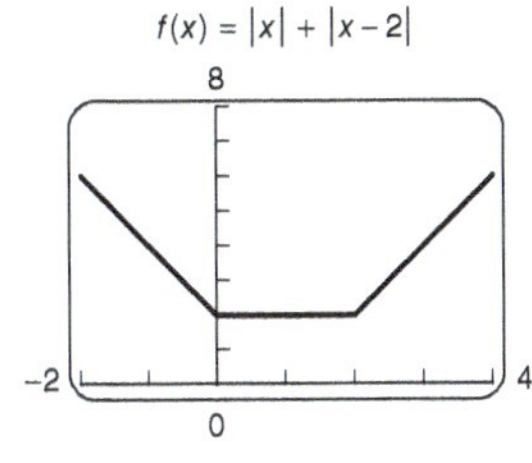

67. Minimum value 9 over $\left(-5, -\frac{1}{2}\right)$

$f(x) = |2x + 1| + |2x + 10|$

69. Absolute minimum point $(-0.141, -1.148)$, no absolute maximum **71.** Absolute minimum point $(-1.706, -7.661)$, absolute maximum point $(1, 5)$ **73.** No absolute minimum, absolute maximum point $(0.216, 2.113)$ **75.** Answers may vary.

Technology Connection, p. 327

1–4. Left to the student

Exercise Set 3.5, p. 328

1. Maximum $Q = 1225$; $x = 35$, $y = 35$ **3.** Minimum $M = -9$; $x = 3$, $y = -3$ **5.** Maximum $B = 4$; $x = 2$, $y = \sqrt{2}$ **7.** Minimum $E = 6$, $x = 2$, $y = 1$ **9.** Maximum $A = \frac{1}{3}$, $x = \frac{2}{3}$, $y = \frac{1}{2}$ **11.** Minimum $V = 2e^{1/2} \approx 3.297$ at $x = \frac{1}{2}$ and $y = \frac{1}{2}$ and $y = 1$ **13.** Maximum $T = e$ at $x = 1$ and $y = 1$ **15.** Maximum area $= 4050$ sq yd (45 yd by 90 yd) **17.** **(a)** 15,000 m^2; **(b)** 22,500 m^2 **19.** Dimensions: $3\frac{1}{3}$ in. by $13\frac{1}{3}$ in. by $13\frac{1}{3}$ in.; volume $= 592.593$ in^3 **21.** 4 ft by 4 ft by 2 ft; 48 ft^2 **23.** 2.08 yd by 4.16 yd by 1.39 yd **25.** \$1048; 46 units **27.** \$19; 70 units **29.** \$5481; 1667 units **31.** **(a)** $R(x) = x(280 - 0.4x)$; **(b)** $P(x) = -x^2 + 280x - 5000$; **(c)** 140 ovens; **(d)** \$14,600; **(e)** \$224 per oven **33.** \$201 per day **35.** 1 fewer patroller **37.** **(a)** $q(x) = 2.13 - 0.04x$; **(b)** \$39.13 **39.** \$11.50 **41.** Chain-link fencing (two long sides and one short side): 76.95 ft; wood fence (short side): 64.98 ft; cost: \$2924 **43.** 6.98 in. by 10.47 in. **45.** Order 20 times/yr, lot size of 10 **47.** Order 12 times/yr, lot size of 30 **49.** Order 12 times/yr, lot size of 30 **51.** $r \approx 5.03$ cm, $h \approx 5.03$ cm **53.** $r \approx 2.88$ cm, $h \approx 15.35$ cm **55.** 6 yd by 8 yd (8 yd side is opposite the side shared with the neighbor) **57.** $x \approx 2.75$ ft; $y \approx 4.92$ ft **59.** **(a)** Radius $= 16.8389$ yd, height $= 0$ yd; **(b)** cost $= \$160{,}343$; **(c)** a hemisphere **61.** 589 µg/dL, at 40 min after administration **63.** **(a)** At the point 3.84 miles west and 2.88 miles north of the farm; **(b)** \$72,000 **65.** S is 3.25 mi downshore from A. **67.** Left to the student **69.** **(a)** $\overline{C}(x) = 8 + \dfrac{20}{x} + \dfrac{x^2}{100}$; **(b)** $C'(x) = \dfrac{3x^2}{100} + 8$, and $\overline{C}'(x) = \dfrac{x}{50} - \dfrac{20}{x^2}$; **(c)** minimum $= \$11$/unit at $x_0 = 10$ units, $C'(10) = \$11$/unit; **(d)** they are equal.

71. Order $\sqrt{\dfrac{aQ}{2b}}$ times, lot size of $\sqrt{\dfrac{2bQ}{a}}$

73. Let $x =$ one number, so the other number is $n - x$ and the product is $P(x) = x(n - x) = nx - x^2$. The derivative is $P'(x) = n - 2x$, which, when set equal to 0, gives $x = n/2$, a critical value. This can be shown to be a maximum, so the two numbers are $n/2$ and $n/2$ and their product is $n^2/4$.

75. $x = 25$, $y = 16.67$, $Q = 416.67$

77. $x = 2.24$, $y = 2.74$, $Q = 45.93$

79. Answers may vary.

Technology Connection, p. 335

1. $P'(50) = \$140$ per unit; $P(51) - P(50) = \$217$ per unit

Exercise Set 3.6, p. 341

1. **(a)** $\Delta y = 0.120601$; **(b)** $dy = 3x^2\,dx$; **(c)** $dy = 0.12$

3. **(a)** $\Delta y = 0.2816$; **(b)** $dy = (1 + 2x)\,dx$; **(c)** $dy = 0.28$

5. **(a)** $\Delta y = -0.16666666\ldots$; **(b)** $dy = -\dfrac{1}{x^2}\,dx$; **(c)** $dy = -0.2$

7. **(a)** $\Delta y = -6$; **(b)** $dy = 3\,dx$; **(c)** $dy = -6$
9. **(a)** $\Delta y = 2.112414358\ldots$; **(b)** $dy = e^x\,dx$;
(c) $dy = 2.008553692\ldots$ **11.** **(a)** $\Delta y = -0.0151136378\ldots$;
(b) $dy = \frac{1}{x}\,dx$; **(c)** $dy = -0.015$ **13.** 5.100 **15.** 10.100
17. 10.017 **19.** **(a)** $L(x) = 6x - 9$; **(b)** 9.6; **(c)** 9.61;
(d) the approximation is 0.01 less than the actual value.
21. **(a)** $L(x) = \frac{1}{8}x + 2$; **(b)** 4.125; **(c)** $4.12310562\ldots$;
(d) the approximation is about 0.00189 greater than the actual value. **23.** **(a)** $L(x) = e^2(x - 1)$; **(b)** $1.1e^2 \approx 8.128$;
(c) $8.16616991\ldots$; **(d)** the approximation is 0.0382 less than the actual value. **25.** **(a)** $P(x) = -0.5x^2 + 46x - 10$;
(b) \$800, \$90, \$710;
(c) $R'(x) = 50 - x$, $C'(x) = 4$, $P'(x) = 46 - x$;
(d) \$30, \$4, \$26; **(e)** left to the student
27. **(a)** \$226,800; **(b)** \$5960; **(c)** \$238,720; **(d)** \$12,057.60
29. **(a)** \$1799; **(b)** \$75.40; **(c)** \$235.88; **(d)** \$1874.40, \$1949.80, \$2025.20 **31.** **(a)** \$3685.03; **(b)** \$276.63;
(c) \$138.20; **(d)** \$3823.23 **33.** If the price increases from \$1000 to \$1001, sales will decrease by 100 units.
35. \$3.21, \$3.20 **37.** \$2.84, \$2.86
39. **(a)** $P(x) = 3000 \ln x - 0.01x^2 - 1.6x - 100$;
(b) \$34.06, \$34.30 **41.** **(a)** $dS/dp = 0.021p^2 - p + 150$;
(b) 3547 units; **(c)** answers may vary; **(d)** answers may vary.
43. **(a)** \$656,000; **(b)** \$80,650/hundred tons; **(c)** \$736,650
45. **(a)** 630, 980, 1430, 630 units; **(b)** $M'(t) = -4t + 100$;
(c) answers may vary. **47.** About 0.0518 billion dollars (about \$51.8 million) **49.** Answers may vary. **51.** About \$0.25 paid in taxes per dollar earned **53.** $dA = 25\text{ ft}^2$
55. **(a)** $dA = 628\text{ ft}^2$; **(b)** 3 extra cans; **(c)** \$90
57. -0.01345 m^2 **59.** **(a)** $L(x) = \frac{1}{12}x + 3$; **(b)** $b = 45.8$
61. **(a)** Left to the student; **(b)** $2\frac{1}{4}, 4\frac{1}{4}, 4\frac{9}{10}, 10\frac{1}{5}$;
(c) answers may vary. **63.** Answers may vary.

Exercise Set 3.7, p. 351

1. **(a)** $E(x) = \frac{x}{400 - x}$; **(b)** $\frac{5}{11}$, inelastic; **(c)** \$200
3. **(a)** $E(x) = \frac{x}{50 - x}$; **(b)** 11.5, elastic; **(c)** \$25
5. **(a)** $E(x) = 1$; **(b)** 1, unit elasticity; **(c)** total revenue is independent of x. **7.** **(a)** $E(x) = \frac{x}{1200 - 2x}$;
(b) $\frac{1}{10}$, inelastic; **(c)** \$400 **9.** **(a)** $E(x) = \frac{2x}{x + 3}$;
(b) $\frac{1}{2}$, inelastic; **(c)** \$3 **11.** **(a)** $E(x) = 0.25x$;
(b) 2.5, elastic; **(c)** \$4 **13.** **(a)** $E(x) = \frac{25x}{967 - 25x}$;
(b) approximately 19¢; **(c)** prices greater than 19¢;
(d) prices less than 19¢; **(e)** about 19¢; **(f)** decrease
15. **(a)** $E(x) = \frac{3}{25}x$; **(b)** $\frac{9}{25}$; **(c)** increase
17. **(a)** $D(x) = 1875 - 15x$; **(b)** $E(x) = \frac{x}{125 - x}$;
(c) $E(45) = \frac{9}{16} < 1$, inelastic; $E(55) = \frac{11}{14} < 1$, inelastic;
(d) $x = \$62.50$ is the price that will result in the maximum monthly revenue of \$58,593.75. **19.** **(a)** $D(x) = 2188.492e^{-0.0134x}$;
(b) $E(x) = 0.0134x$; **(c)** at a price of \$74.63, total revenue will be about \$60,080. **21.** **(a)** $E(x) = \frac{x}{18 - x}$; **(b)** 0.8; **(c)** \$9;
(d) answers may vary. **23.** **(a)** $E(x) = kx$; **(b)** yes; **(c)** at $x = 1/k$ **25.** Answers may vary.
27. **(a)**

Price, x	Quantity, q
8	100
10	95
12	83
14	66
16	45
18	27
20	16
22	6

(b) linear: $q = 165.643 - 7.393x$; cubic:
$q = 0.0606x^3 - 2.775x^2 + 32.702x - 14.981$; logistic:
$q = \frac{106.525}{1 + 0.00265e^{0.389x}}$; **(c)** linear: $E(x) = \frac{7.393x}{165.643 - 7.393x}$;
cubic: $E(x) = -\frac{0.182x^3 - 5.55x^2 + 32.702x}{0.0606x^3 - 2.775x^2 + 32.702x - 14.981}$;
logistic: $E(x) = \frac{0.00103xe^{0.389x}}{1 + 0.00265e^{0.389x}}$; **(d)** \$11.20, \$927.82;
(e) \$11.67, \$992.42; **(f)** \$11.93, \$995.18; **(g)** answers may vary.

Exercise Set 3.8, p. 359

1. $\frac{y + x}{3y - x}$ **3.** $\frac{x}{y}$ **5.** $\frac{5x^4}{3y^2}$ **7.** $\frac{-3xy^2 - 2y}{4x^2y + 3x}$ **9.** $\frac{3}{e^y + 2y}$
11. $2x^2 - 2x + 2y$ **13.** $\frac{y}{1 - 2ye^{2y}}$ **15.** $\frac{9x^2}{2y}$, 4.5
17. $-\frac{3x^2}{4y}$, 3 **19.** $-\frac{x}{y}, -\frac{1}{\sqrt{3}}$ **21.** $-\frac{3y}{2x}$, 4.5
23. $\frac{4x^2 - 2y^3}{3xy^2}, -\frac{7}{3}$ **25.** $\frac{2 - y}{x + 2y}, -\frac{4}{3}$ **27.** $\frac{12x^2 + 5}{4y^3 + 3}, -\frac{17}{29}$
29. $-\frac{2}{2p + 1}$ **31.** $-\frac{p}{3x}$ **33.** $\frac{2 - 2xp - p}{x^2 + x - 1}$ **35.** $-\frac{p + 4}{x + 3}$
37. $y' = (x^2 + 4)^{10}(2x - 5)^8\left(\frac{20x}{x^2 + 4} + \frac{16}{2x - 5}\right)$
39. $y' = (x + 7)^3(2x - 5)^6(x^3 - 2x + 1)^7 \cdot\left(\frac{3}{x + 7} + \frac{12}{2x - 5} + \frac{21x^2 - 14}{x^3 - 2x + 1}\right)$
41. $y' = \frac{(2x - 3)^5}{(3x + 5)^4}\left(\frac{10}{2x - 3} - \frac{12}{3x + 5}\right)$
43. $y' = \frac{\sqrt{5 - 3x}(x^2 + 1)^2}{x^2 + 2x + 5} \cdot\left(-\frac{3}{10 - 6x} + \frac{4x}{x^2 + 1} - \frac{2x + 2}{x^2 + 2x + 5}\right)$
45. $y' = x^5e^{x^2+6x+7}\left(\frac{5}{x} + 2x + 6\right)$

47. $y' = \dfrac{\sqrt{x^2+5x+9}}{e^{x^4+2x^2+2}}\left(\dfrac{2x+5}{2x^2+10x+18} - 4x^3 - 4x\right)$

49. $y' = \dfrac{xe^{\sqrt{x^2+1}}}{2x^3+5x}\left(\dfrac{1}{x} + \dfrac{x}{\sqrt{x^2+1}} - \dfrac{6x^2+5}{2x^3+5x}\right)$

51. $\left(e^{-2}, (e^{-2})^{\sqrt{e^{-2}}}\right) \approx (0.135, 0.479)$

53. **(a)** 9.56 weeks; **(b)** about 568,750 downloads/week; **(c)** 1,750,000 times **55.** **(a)** 81 employees; **(b)** with 81 employees, the rate of change of production is maximized at about 9375 units/yr, but with 101 employees, that rate of change is about 5594 units/yr. **57.** **(a)** 3 days; **(b)** 255 students/day; **(c)** 600 students **59.** **(a)** $R(t) = \dfrac{28{,}000{,}000}{1 + 1119e^{-0.468t}}$; **(b)** by \$3,276,000/week

61. $y'' = e^{3x-2}(3x+1)\left(3 + \dfrac{3}{3x+1}\right)$

63. $y'' = x^{x-1} + x^x(1 + \ln x)^2$ **65.** Answers may vary.

67. $\dfrac{2(y+1)}{(x-2)^2}$ **69.** $\dfrac{y^2 - x^2}{y^3}$ or $-\dfrac{5}{y^3}$ **71.** Answers may vary.

73.

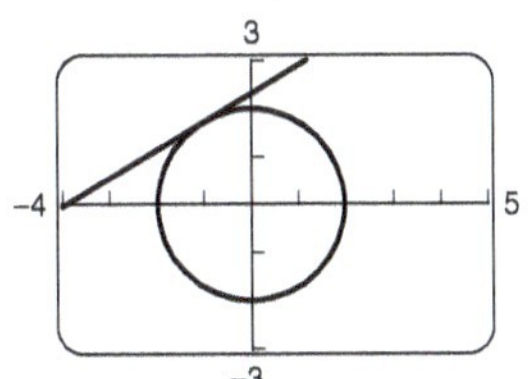

Exercise Set 3.9, p. 364

1. -48 **3.** -22 **5.** $\frac{5}{3}$ **7.** $\frac{5}{31}$ **9.** e^9 **11.** $-\frac{1}{36}$ **13.** 14 **15.** 3 **17.** -50 **19.** 1 **21.** -0.341 cm/min **23.** -0.00764 cm/min **25.** 502.65 cm²/min **27.** -960 cm³/min **29.** -1440 cm²/min **31.** $0, -\dfrac{\sqrt{6}}{4}, -\dfrac{9}{4}$ **33.** \$200/day, \$50/day, \$150/day **35.** \$36,000/day, \$72,000/day, $-$\$36,000/day **37.** -1.18 sales/day **39.** 25 oz/hr **41.** $-31{,}573$ mi²/yr **43.** -0.0256 m²/month **45.** **(a)** $\dfrac{dV}{dt} = 952.38R\dfrac{dR}{dt}$; **(b)** 0.0143 mm/sec² **47.** 65 mph **49.** 70,838.63 m²/yr **51.** 17,000 m³/week **53.** 5 mm²/min **55.** 0.313 in./min **57.** **(a)** π cm/min; **(b)** π cm/min; **(c)** π cm/min; **(d)** answers may vary. **59.** $\dfrac{dy}{dt} = 1.3$

Chapter 3 Review Exercises, p. 376

1. (g) **2.** (e) **3.** (f) **4.** (a) **5.** (b) **6.** (d) **7.** (c) **8.** False **9.** False **10.** True **11.** False **12.** True **13.** False **14.** False **15.** True **16.** False **17.** True

18. Relative maximum $\frac{25}{4}$ at $x = -\frac{3}{2}$

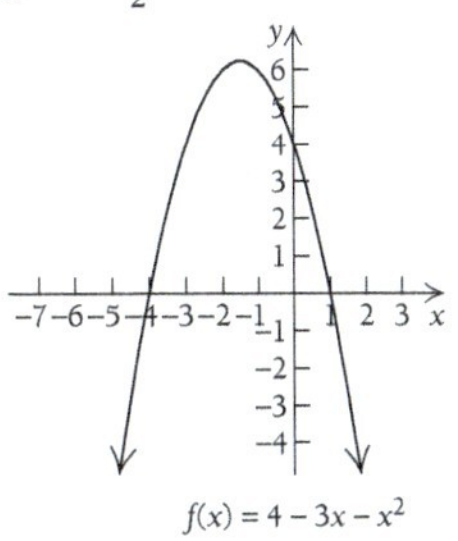

19. Relative minimum -4 at $x = 1$, relative maximum 4 at $x = -1$

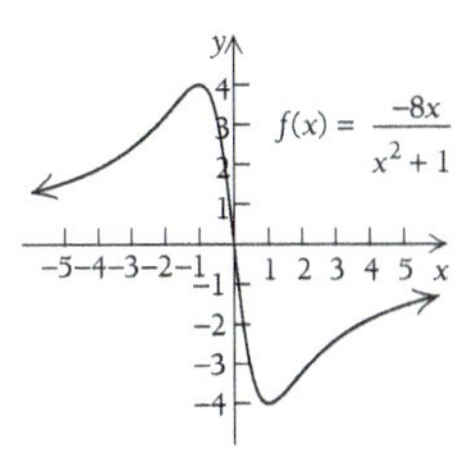

20. Relative maximum $\frac{1}{6}e^{-1}$ at $x = \frac{1}{6}$

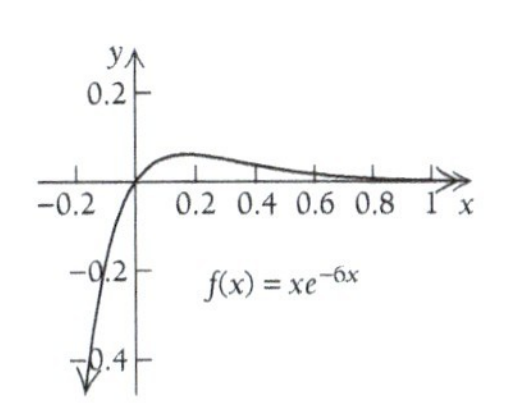

21. Relative minimum $\frac{76}{27}$ at $x = \frac{1}{3}$, relative maximum 4 at $x = -1$

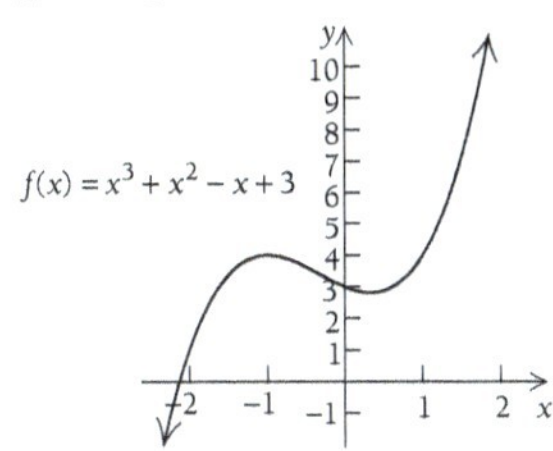

22. Relative minimum 0 at $x = 0$

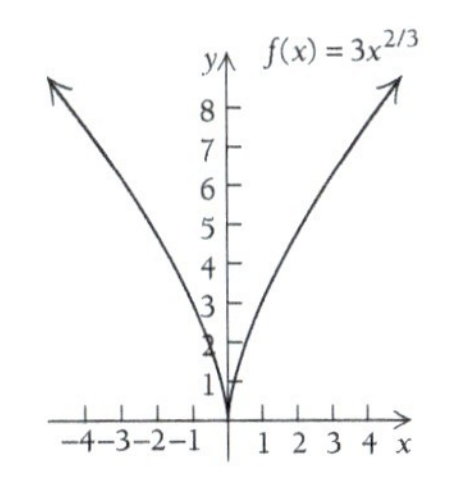

23. Relative minimum -0.326 at

$$x = \frac{\ln\left(\frac{2}{5}\right)}{3} \approx -0.305$$

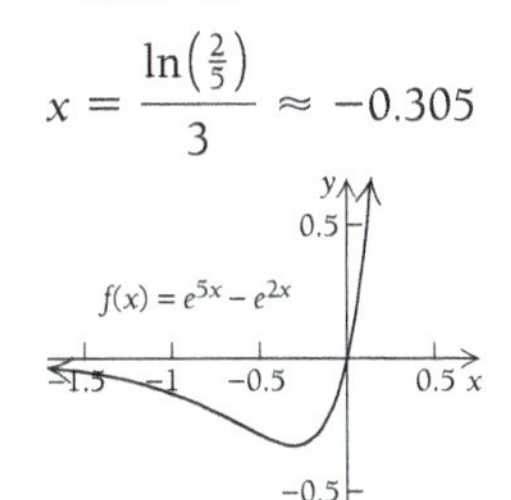

24. Relative maximum 4 at $x = -1$, relative minimum 0 at $x = 1$

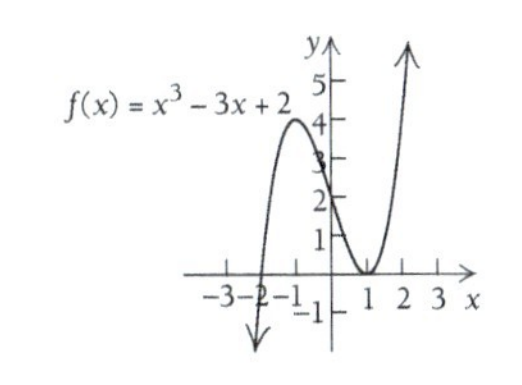

25.

$f(x) = \frac{1}{3}x^3 + 3x^2 + 9x + 2$

No relative extrema, inflection point at $(-3, -7)$, increasing on $(-\infty, \infty)$, concave down on $(-\infty, -3)$ and concave up on $(-3, \infty)$

26.

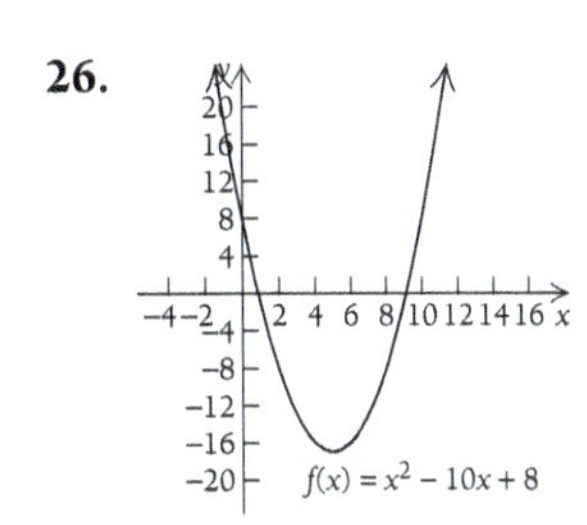

Relative minimum -17 at $x = 5$, decreasing on $(-\infty, 5)$ and increasing on $(5, \infty)$, concave up on $(-\infty, \infty)$

27.

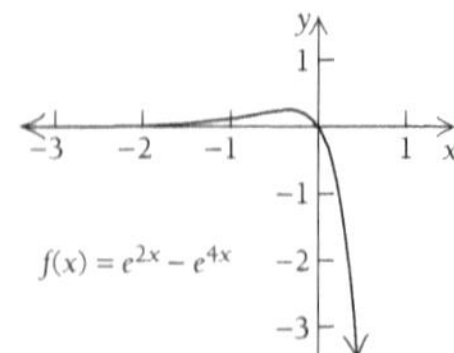

Relative maximum at $\left(-\frac{1}{2}\ln 2, \frac{1}{4}\right)$, increasing on $\left(-\infty, -\frac{1}{2}\ln 2\right)$ and decreasing on $\left(-\frac{1}{2}\ln 2, \infty\right)$, point of inflection at $\left(-\ln 2, \frac{3}{16}\right)$, concave up on $(-\infty, -\ln 2)$ and concave down on $(-\ln 2, \infty)$

28.

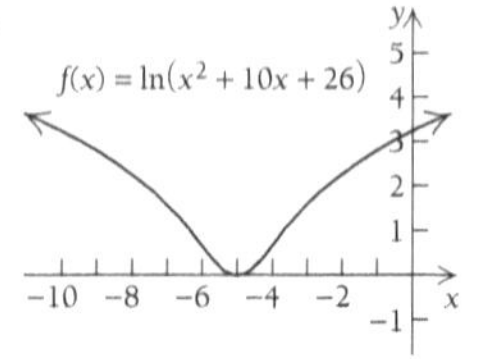

Relative minimum at $(-5, 0)$, decreasing on $(-\infty, -5)$ and increasing on $(-5, \infty)$, points of inflection at $(-6, \ln 2)$ and $(-4, \ln 2)$, concave up on $(-6, -4)$ and concave down on $(-\infty, -6)$ and $(-4, \infty)$

29.

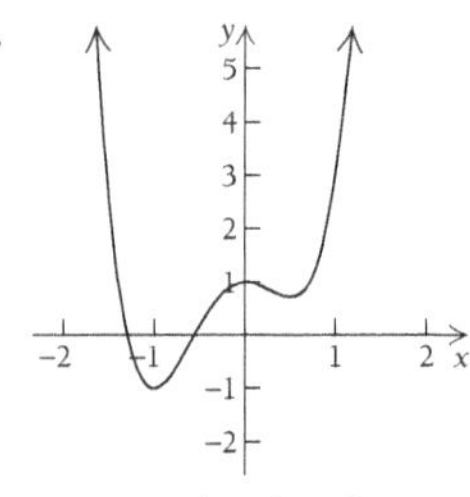

Relative minima -1 at $x = -1$ and $\frac{11}{16}$ at $x = \frac{1}{2}$, relative maximum 1 at $x = 0$, points of inflection at $(-0.608, -0.147)$ and $(0.274, 0.833)$, increasing on $(-1, 0)$ and $\left(\frac{1}{2}, \infty\right)$ and decreasing on $(-\infty, -1)$ and $\left(0, \frac{1}{2}\right)$, concave down on $(-0.608, 0.274)$ and concave up on $(-\infty, -0.608)$ and $(0.274, \infty)$

30.

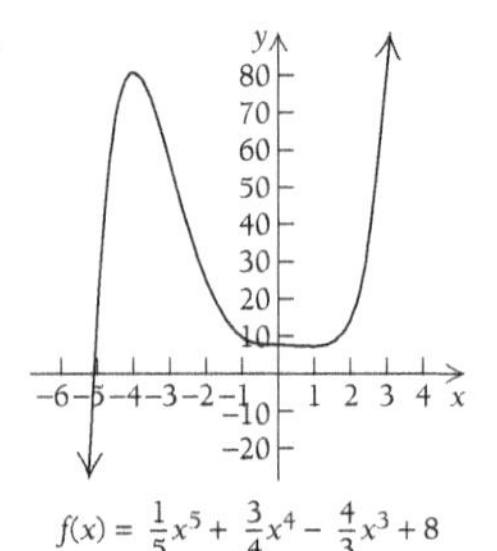

Relative minimum $\frac{457}{60}$ at $x = 1$, relative maximum $\frac{1208}{15}$ at $x = -4$, points of inflection at $(-2.932, 53.701)$, $(0, 8)$, and $(0.682, 7.769)$, increasing on $(-\infty, -4)$ and $(1, \infty)$ and decreasing on $(-4, 1)$, concave down on $(-\infty, -2.932)$ and $(0, 0.682)$ and concave up on $(-2.932, 0)$ and $(0.682, \infty)$

31.

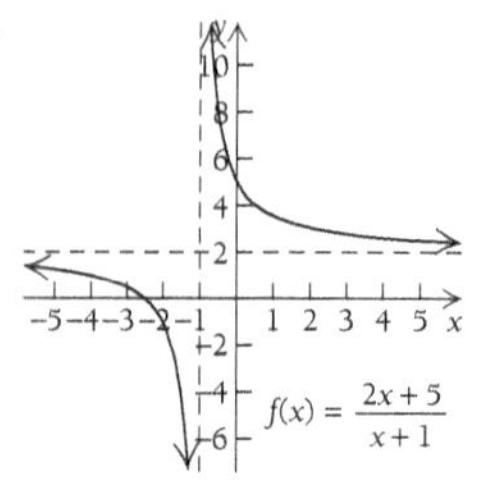

No relative extrema, decreasing on $(-\infty, -1)$ and on $(-1, \infty)$, concave down on $(-\infty, -1)$ and concave up on $(-1, \infty)$, asymptotes at $x = -1$ and $y = 2$, x-intercept at $\left(-\frac{5}{2}, 0\right)$ and y-intercept at $(0, 5)$

32.

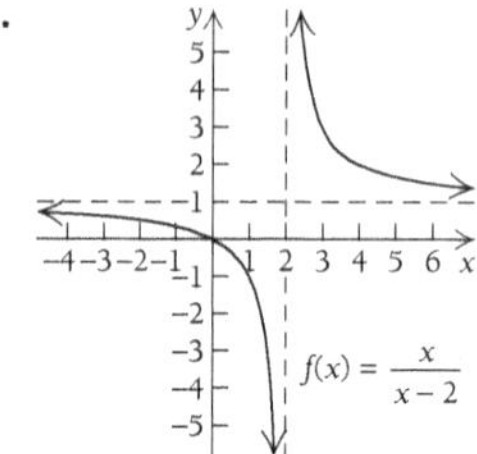

No relative extrema, decreasing on $(-\infty, 2)$ and on $(2, \infty)$, concave down on $(-\infty, 2)$ and concave up on $(2, \infty)$, asymptotes at $x = 2$ and $y = 1$, x-intercept and y-intercept at $(0, 0)$

33.

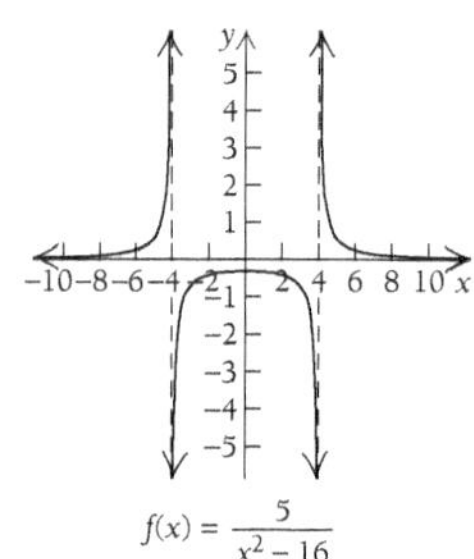

Relative maximum at $\left(0, -\frac{5}{16}\right)$, decreasing on $(0, 4)$ and on $(4, \infty)$ and increasing on $(-\infty, -4)$ and on $(-4, 0)$, concave down on $(-4, 4)$ and concave up on $(-\infty, -4)$ and on $(4, \infty)$, asymptotes at $x = -4$, $x = 4$, and $y = 0$, y-intercept at $\left(0, -\frac{5}{16}\right)$

34.

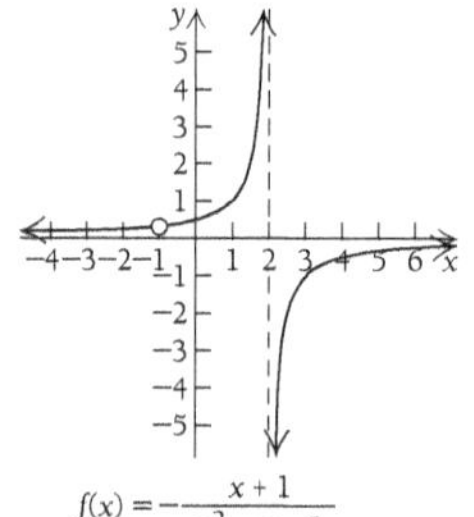

No relative extrema, increasing on $(-\infty, -1)$, $(-1, 2)$, and $(2, \infty)$, concave up on $(-\infty, -1)$ and on $(-1, 2)$ and concave down on $(2, \infty)$, asymptotes at $x = 2$ and $y = 0$, y-intercept at $\left(0, \frac{1}{2}\right)$

35.

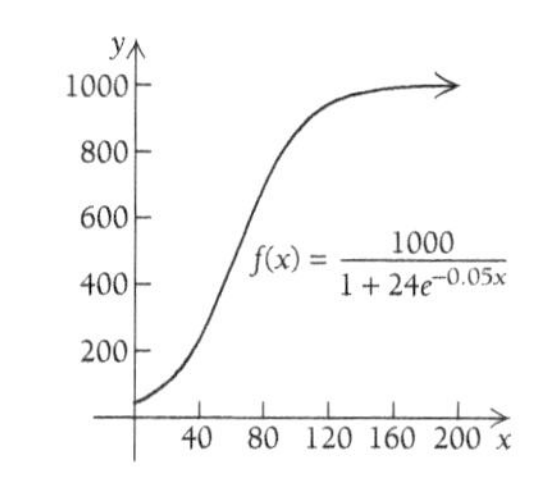

Increasing on $(-\infty, \infty)$, no relative extrema, concave up on $(-\infty, 20\ln 24)$ and concave down on $(20\ln 24, \infty)$, no x-intercept, y-intercept at $(0, 40)$

36.

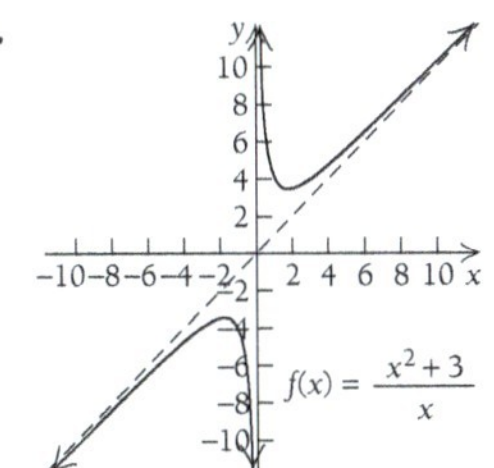

Relative minimum at $(\sqrt{3}, 2\sqrt{3})$, relative maximum at $(-\sqrt{3}, -2\sqrt{3})$, decreasing on $(-\sqrt{3}, 0)$ and on $(0, \sqrt{3})$ and increasing on $(-\infty, -\sqrt{3})$ and on $(\sqrt{3}, \infty)$, concave down on $(-\infty, 0)$ and concave up on $(0, \infty)$, asymptotes at $x = 0$ and $y = x$, no intercepts **37.** Absolute maximum 66 at $x = 3$, absolute minimum 2 at $x = 1$ **38.** Absolute minimum $\frac{8}{3} - \frac{8}{3}\ln\left(\frac{8}{3}\right) \approx 0.0511$ at $x = -\frac{1}{3}\ln\left(\frac{8}{3}\right) \approx -0.327$, absolute maximum $e^{-6} + 16 \approx 16.002$ at $x = 2$
39. Absolute minimum $10\sqrt{2}$ at $x = 5\sqrt{2}$, no absolute maximum
40. Absolute minima 0 at $x = -1$ and $x = 1$, no absolute maximum
41. $Q = 12$ when $x = 4$ and $y = 3$ **42.** $Q = -1$ when $x = -1$ and $y = -1$ **43.** Maximum profit is \$451 when 30 units are produced and sold. **44.** 10 ft by 10 ft by 25 ft; cost = \$1500 **45.** Order 12 times per year with a lot size of 30
46. **(a)** \$108; **(b)** \$1/dinner; **(c)** \$109
47. $\Delta y = -0.335$, $dy = -0.35$ **48.** **(a)** $(6x^2 + 1)\,dx$; **(b)** 0.25 **49.** **(a)** $y = 55x - 108$; **(b)** $L(2.9) = 51.5$, $f(2.9) = 51.678$ **50.** 9.111. . .
51. $\pm 240{,}000$ ft^3 **52.** **(a)** $D(x) = 400 - 5x$; **(b)** $E(x) = \dfrac{x}{80 - x}$; **(c)** $E(20) = \frac{1}{3} < 1$, inelastic; $E(50) = \frac{5}{3} > 1$, elastic; **(d)** \$40 is the price that will maximize weekly revenue at \$8000; **(e)** $y = 476.22e^{-0.0231x}$; **(f)** \$43.29 is the price that will maximize weekly revenue at about \$7584.
53. $\dfrac{dy}{dx} = \dfrac{-3y - 2x^2}{2y^2 + 3x}$; slope $= \dfrac{4}{5}$
54. $\dfrac{dy}{dx} = (x^2 + 1)^8\sqrt{x^4 + 2x - 7}\left(\dfrac{16x}{x^2 + 1} + \dfrac{2x^3 + 1}{x^4 + 2x - 7}\right)$
55. **(a)** 99.87 months; **(b)** 4.5375 deer/month; **(c)** answers may vary. **56.** -5.5 **57.** By about 282.7 mi^2/yr
58. -1.75 ft/sec **59.** \$600/day, \$450/day, \$150/day
60. Absolute maximum 4 at $x = 2$ and $x = 6$, absolute minimum -2 at $x = -2$ **61.** $\dfrac{3x^5 - 2(x - y)^3 - 2(x + y)^3}{2(x + y)^3 - 2(x - y)^3 - 3y^5}$
62. Relative maximum $(0, 0)$, relative minima $(-9, -9477)$ and $(15, -37{,}125)$ **63.** Left to the student. **64.** 630 cm^3/min
65. Relative maximum $(-1.714, 37.445)$, relative minimum $(1.714, -37.445)$ **66.** Relative maximum $(-1, -0.368)$, relative minimum $(-0.5, -0.389)$ **67.** Relative maximum $(-0.941, 0.787)$, relative minimum $(0.396, -0.662)$
68. **(a)** Linear: $y = 6.99818760x - 124.6183581$; quadratic: $y = 0.0439274846x^2 + 2.881202838x - 53.51475166$; cubic: $y = -0.0033441547x^3 + 0.4795643605x^2 - 11.35931622x + 5.276985809$; quartic: $y = -0.00005539834x^4 + 0.0067192294x^3 - 0.0996735857x^2 - 0.8409991942x - 0.246072967$. **(b)** The quartic function fits the best. **(c)** The domain is $[26, 102]$. **(d)** The maximum value is 466 per 100,000 women at $x = 79.0$ yr.

Chapter 3 Test, p. 379

1. Relative minimum -9 at $x = 2$, decreasing on $(-\infty, 2)$ and increasing on $(2, \infty)$

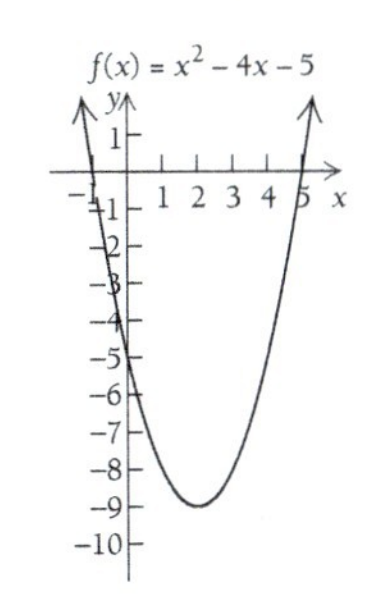

2. Relative maximum $\frac{1}{2}e^{-1} \approx 0.184$ at $x = \frac{1}{4}$, increasing on $\left(-\infty, \frac{1}{4}\right)$ and decreasing on $\left(\frac{1}{4}, \infty\right)$

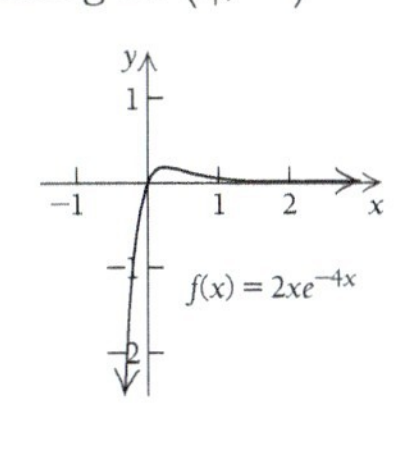

3. Relative minimum -4 at $x = 2$, decreasing on $(-\infty, 2)$ and increasing on $(2, \infty)$

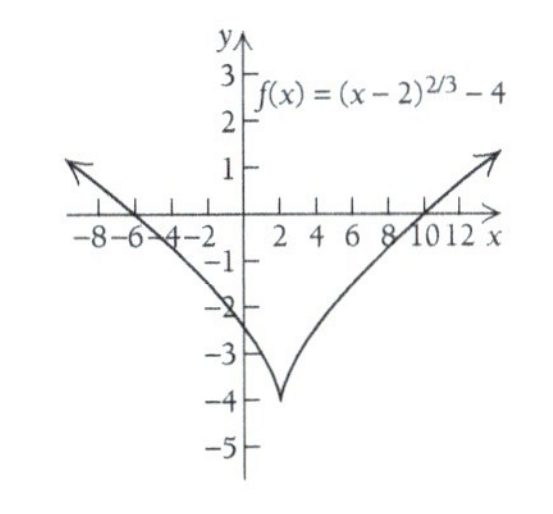

4. Relative maximum 4 at $x = 0$, increasing on $(-\infty, 0)$ and decreasing on $(0, \infty)$

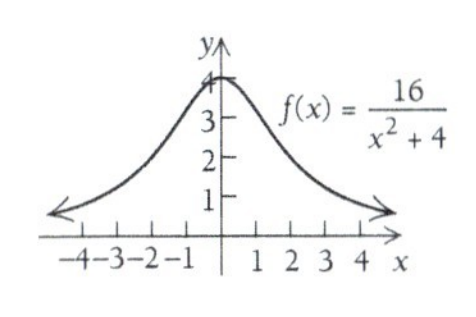

5.

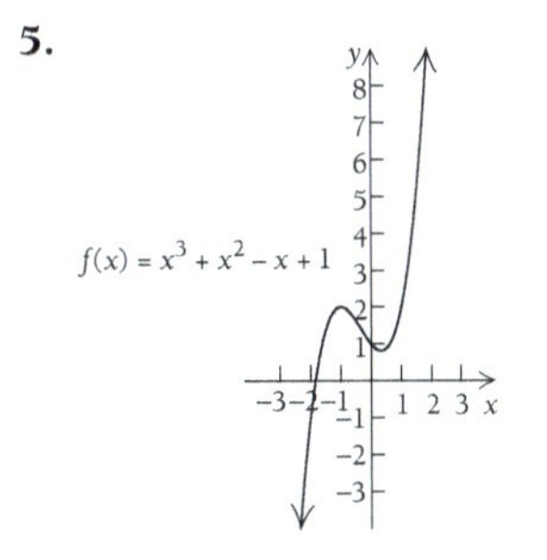

Relative maximum 2 at $x = -1$, relative minimum $\frac{22}{27}$ at $x = \frac{1}{3}$, inflection point at $\left(-\frac{1}{3}, \frac{38}{27}\right)$

6. $f(x) = 2x^4 - 4x^2 + 1$

Relative maximum 1 at $x = 0$, relative minima -1 at $x = -1$ and $x = 1$, inflection points at $\left(-\dfrac{1}{\sqrt{3}}, -\dfrac{1}{9}\right)$ and $\left(\dfrac{1}{\sqrt{3}}, -\dfrac{1}{9}\right)$

7.

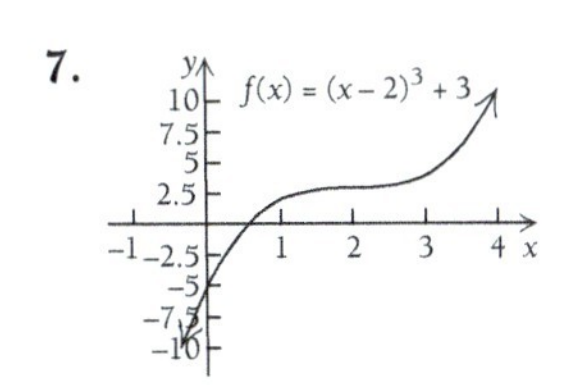

No relative extrema, inflection point at $(2, 3)$

8.

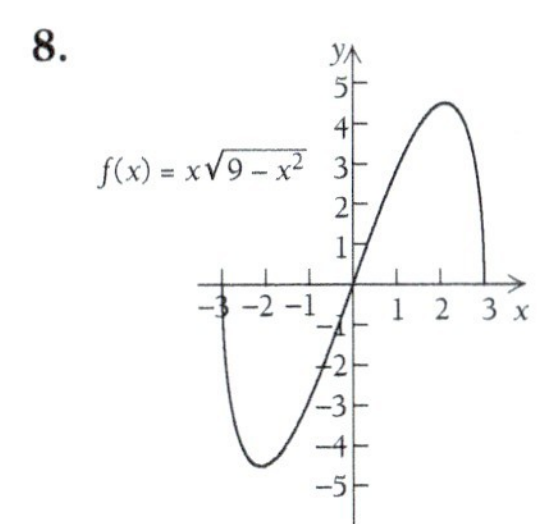

Relative maximum $\dfrac{9}{2}$ at $x = \dfrac{3}{\sqrt{2}}$, relative minimum $-\dfrac{9}{2}$ at $x = -\dfrac{3}{\sqrt{2}}$, inflection point at $(0, 0)$

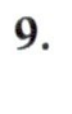

9.

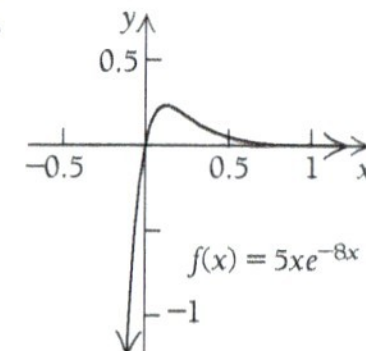

Relative maximum $\frac{5}{8}e^{-1} \approx 0.23$ at $x = \frac{1}{8}$, inflection point at $\left(\frac{1}{4}, \frac{5}{4}e^{-2}\right)$

10.

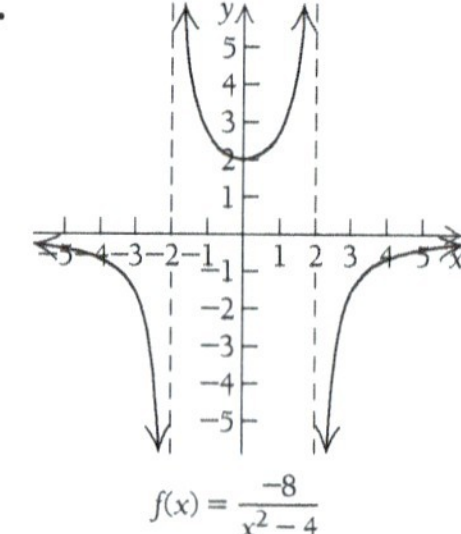

Relative minimum 2 at $x = 0$, asymptotes at $x = -2$, $x = 2$, and $y = 0$

11.

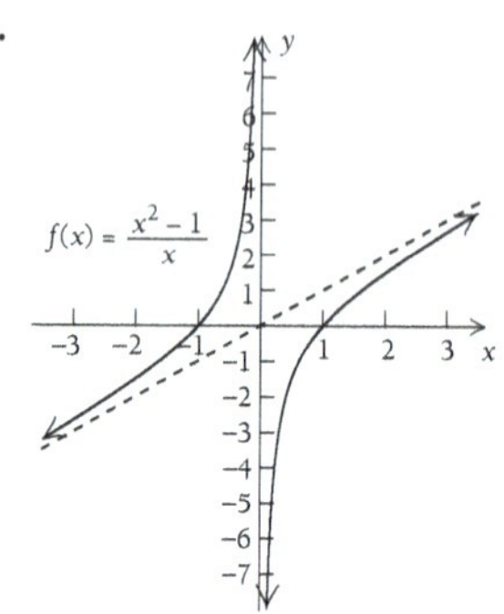

No relative extrema, asymptotes at $x = 0$ and $y = x$

12.

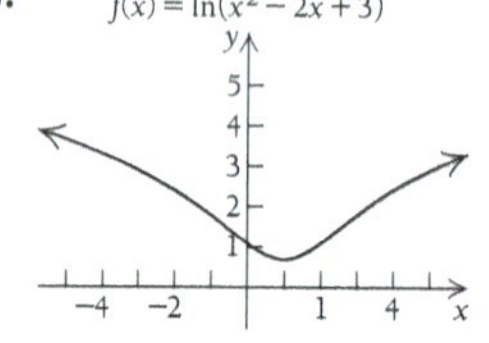

Relative minimum at $(1, \ln 2)$, inflection points at $(1 + \sqrt{2}, 1.386)$ and $(1 - \sqrt{2}, 1.386)$

13. Absolute maximum $(3, 9)$ **14.** Absolute maximum $(-1, 2)$, absolute minimum $(-2, -1)$ **15.** Absolute maximum $(4.3, 28.49)$ **16.** Absolute minimum $\left(-\frac{1}{2}\ln\left(\frac{3}{2}\right), 0.892\right)$, absolute maximum $(-2, 48.598)$ **17.** No absolute extrema **18.** Absolute minimum $\left(\frac{1}{6}, -\frac{13}{12}\right)$ **19.** Absolute minimum $(4, 48)$ **20.** $Q = \frac{125{,}000}{27}$ when $x = \frac{50}{3}$ and $y = \frac{50}{3}$ **21.** $Q = 50$ when $x = 5$ and $y = -5$ **22.** \$24,980; 500 units **23.** **(a)** Chain-link fences 50 ft long, brick wall 40 ft long; **(b)** \$6000 **24.** Order 35 times per year with a lot size of 35 **25.** $\Delta y = 1.01, f'(x)\,\Delta x = 1$

26. 7.0714 **27.** **(a)** $\frac{x}{\sqrt{x^2 + 3}}\,dx$; **(b)** 0.00756

28. **(a)** $L(x) = \frac{1}{8}x + 2$;
(b) $L(15) = \frac{15}{8} + 2 = 3.875, f(15) = 3.87298\ldots$

29. **(a)** $E(x) = \frac{2x}{x + 4}$; **(b)** 0.4, inelastic; **(c)** 1.5, elastic;

(d) decrease; **(e)** \$4 **30.** $-\frac{x^2}{y^2}; -\frac{1}{4}$

31. $y' = \frac{\sqrt{x^3 + 5x}}{e^{x^2+7x+1}}\left(\frac{3x^2 + 5}{2x^3 + 10x} - 2x - 7\right)$

32. **(a)** $(21.29, 22{,}500{,}000)$; **(b)** about \$4,500,000/wk;

(c) \$45,000,000 **33.** 120 shares/day **34.** Absolute maximum $\left(\sqrt[3]{2}, \frac{2^{2/3}}{3}\right)$, absolute minimum $(0, 0)$ **35.** 10,000 units

36. Absolute minimum $(0, 0)$, relative maximum $(1.084, 25.103)$, relative minimum $(2.95, 8.625)$ **37.** Absolute minimum $(-0.448, 0.799)$, absolute maximum $(-2, 3.221)$

38. $Q = 1185.19$ when $x = 2.58$ and $y = 13.33$

39. **(a)** Linear: $y = -0.7707142857x + 12{,}691.60714$; quadratic: $y = -0.9998904762x^2 + 299.1964286x + 192.9761905$; cubic: $y = 0.000084x^3 - 1.037690476x^2 + 303.3964286x + 129.9761905$; quartic: $y = 0.000001966061x^4 + 0.0012636364x^3 - 1.256063636x^2 + 315.8247403x + 66.78138528$. **(b)** Answers may vary. **(c)** The maximum value is about 22,575 bowling balls, and the company should spend \$150,000 on advertising.

Extended Technology Application, p. 382

1. (a)

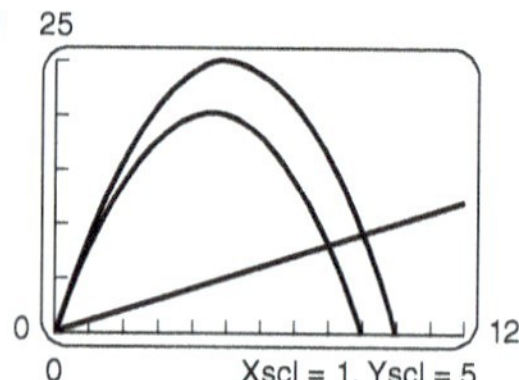

(b) 4500; **(c)** 20,250

2. (a)

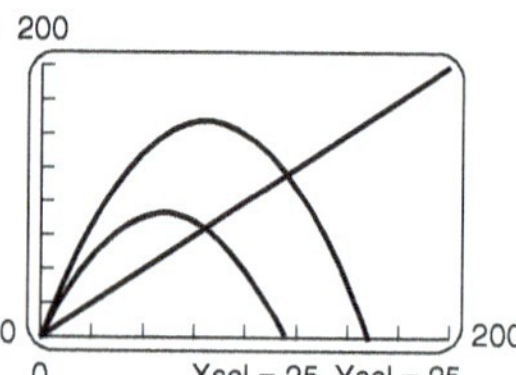

(b) 60,000; **(c)** 90,000

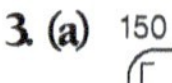

3. (a)

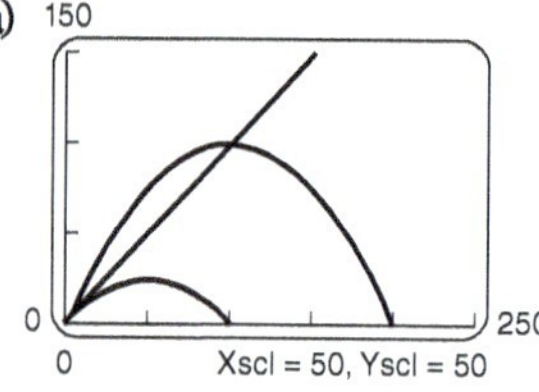

(b) 50,000; **(c)** 25,000

4. (a) 2000 ... 0, 2000, Xscl = 200, Yscl = 200

(b) 400,000; **(c)** 400,000

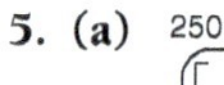

5. (a)

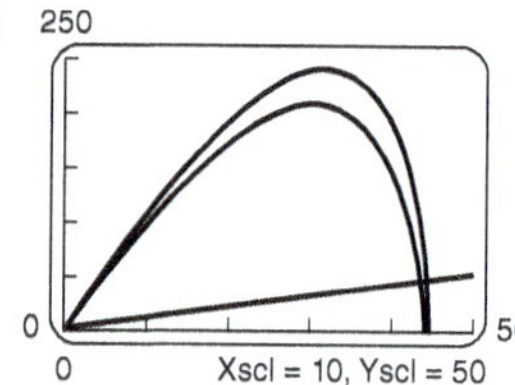

(b) 30,513; **(c)** 205,923

6. **(a)** $y = -0.0011P^3 + 0.0715P^2 - 0.0338P + 4$;
(b)

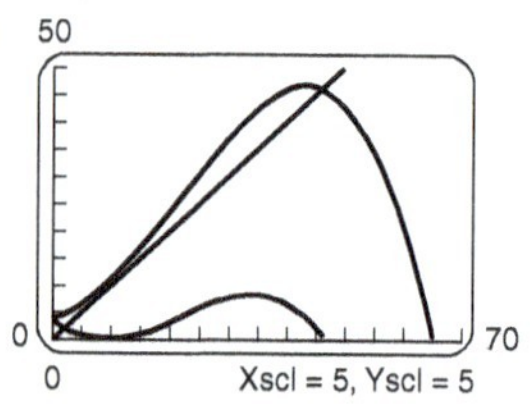

(c) 33,841 **7.** $P'(t) = \frac{d}{dt}\left[\frac{L}{1 + Ce^{-rt}}\right] = \frac{LCre^{-rt}}{(1 + Ce^{-rt})^2}$, which, evaluated at $t = \frac{\ln C}{r}$, gives

$$P\left(\frac{\ln C}{r}\right) = \frac{LCre^{-r(\ln C/r)}}{(1 + Ce^{-r(\ln C/r)})^2} = \frac{LCrC^{-1}}{(1 + CC^{-1})^2} = \frac{Lr}{(1 + 1)^2} = \frac{Lr}{4}$$

8. **(a)** At 47 months; **(b)** 25.3125 pigs/month; **(c)** 25.3125 pigs/month **9.** Answers may vary.

CHAPTER 4

Exercise Set 4.1, p. 391

1. $2x + C$ **3.** $\frac{1}{7}x^7 + C$ **5.** $\frac{4}{5}x^{5/4} + C$
7. $\frac{1}{3}x^3 + \frac{1}{2}x^2 - x + C$ **9.** $\frac{2}{3}t^3 + \frac{5}{2}t^2 - 3t + C$

11. $-\frac{1}{2x^2} + C$ **13.** $\frac{6}{7}\sqrt[6]{x^7} + C$ **15.** $\frac{2}{7}\sqrt{x^7} + C$
17. $-\frac{1}{3x^3} + C$ **19.** $10 \ln|x| + C$ **21.** $3 \ln|x| - \frac{5}{x} + C$
23. $-21\sqrt[3]{x} + C$ **25.** $\frac{1}{3}e^{3x} + C$ **27.** $e^{2x} + C$
29. $12e^{x/2} + C$ **31.** $5000e^{0.02x} + C$ **33.** $\frac{1}{4}e^{4x} - \frac{1}{7}e^{7x} + C$
35. $\frac{1}{4}x^4 + \frac{8}{3}\sqrt{x^3} - \frac{1}{6}e^{-6x} + C$ **37.** $2x^2 - 8x + 3\ln|x| + C$
39. $3x + 2\ln|x| - \frac{5}{x} + C$ **41.** $3x^3 + 6x^2 + 4x + C$
43. $2\sqrt{x} + x + C$ **45.** $9x + 8\sqrt{x^3} + 2x^2 + C$
47. $f(x) = \frac{1}{2}x^2 - 3x + 13$ **49.** $f(x) = \frac{1}{3}x^3 - 4x + 7$
51. $f(x) = \frac{8}{3}x^3 + 2x^2 - 2x + 6$ **53.** $f(x) = \frac{5}{2}e^{2x} - 2$
55. $f(x) = 8\sqrt{x} - 13$ **57.** $D(t) = 6.461t^2 + 11.474t + 848.8$
59. **(a)** $S(t) = 225.5e^{0.427t} - 37.854$; **(b)** about 4441.9 thousand, or about 4.4 million, units
61. **(a)** $P(x) = 0.01x^2 - 1.45x$; **(b)** 145
63. $S(x) = 0.08x^3 + 2x^2 + 10x + 11$
65. **(a)** $E(t) = -5t^2 + 40t - 19$; **(b)** $E(4) = 61\%$, $E(7) = 16\%$
67. **(a)** $M(t) = \frac{1}{10}\sqrt{t^3} + \frac{1}{100}\sqrt{t}$; **(b)** about 47 words
69. **(a)** $h(t) = -16t^2 + 70t + 3$; **(b)** height = 72 ft, velocity = 22 ft/sec; **(c)** 2.19 sec, 79.56 ft; **(d)** −69.1 ft/sec
71. **(a)** $P(t) = 45t + 5000$, $Q(t) = 3500e^{0.03t}$; **(b)** Alphaville: about 5500, Betaburgh: about 4700;
(c)

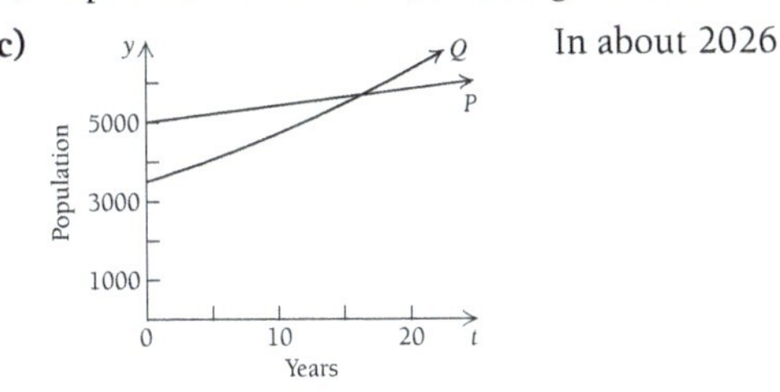

In about 2026

73. $\frac{1}{\ln 3}3^x + C$ **75.** $\frac{1}{\ln 1.25}1.25^x + C$
77. $\frac{1.48}{\ln 1.00325}1.00325^x + C$ **79.** $2\log_3 x + C$
81. $\frac{25}{7}t^7 + \frac{20}{3}t^6 + \frac{16}{5}t^5 + C$
83. $\frac{2}{5}\sqrt{t^5} + 4\sqrt{t^3} + 18\sqrt{t} + C, t > 0$
85. $\frac{1}{4}t^4 + t^3 + \frac{3}{2}t^2 + t + C$ **87.** $3x^4 - \frac{8}{3}x^3 - \frac{17}{2}x^2 - 5x + C$
89. $\frac{1}{2}x^2 - x + C, x \neq -1$
91. $\frac{1}{\ln(1/2)}\left(\frac{1}{2}\right)^x + \frac{1}{\ln(3/4)}\left(\frac{3}{4}\right)^x + C$
93. Answers may vary.

Exercise Set 4.2, p. 401

1. 4 **3.** 12 **5.** $\frac{9}{2}$ **7.** 25 **9.** 36 **11.** 54 **13.** $\frac{9}{4}\pi$
15. **(a)** 3 mi; **(b)** 3 mi; **(c)** 6 mi **17.** **(a)** 4.9 m; **(b)** 14.7 m; **(c)** 19.6 m **19.** **(a)** 1.4914; **(b)** 1.1418 **21.** About 247.68
23. About 124 **25.** About 1240.54 **27.** \$50,625
29. \$1460 **31.** \$2260 **33.** \$8400 **35.** \$2800
37. \$31,662.50 **39.** \$233.02 **41.** \$471.96 **43.** \$306.25
45. 26 **47.** 26 **49.** **(a)** 4; **(b)** 1; **(c)** 2; **(d)** $\frac{9}{2}$; **(e)** $\frac{23}{2}$
51. Answers may vary. **53.** About 20.125; 18

Technology Connection, p. 411

1. 0 **2.** 13.75 **3.** 0.535 **4.** 27.972 **5.** −260

Exercise Set 4.3, p. 412

1. 10 **3.** 7.5 **5.** 9 **7.** 4 **9.** $\frac{4}{3}$ **11.** $e^4 - e^2 \approx 47.21$
13. $2\ln 4 \approx 2.773$ **15.** Total number of miles traveled in *t* hours **17.** Total number of marriages in *t* years
19. Total revenue, in dollars, when *x* units are produced
21. Total sales for *t* days **23.** Total number of words memorized after *t* minutes **25.** 20 **27.** $\frac{59}{6}$ **29.** 12
31. $\frac{1}{3}(e^{15} - e^{-3}) \approx 1{,}089{,}672.44$ **33.** **(a)** 0; **(b)** negative, $-A$
35. 0; the area above the *x*-axis is the same as the area below the *x*-axis. **37.** 0; the area above the *x*-axis is the same as the area below the *x*-axis. **39.** 40 **41.** $\frac{5}{3}$ **43.** $\frac{637}{6}$
45. $e^2 - e^{-5} \approx 7.382$ **47.** $\frac{1}{6}(b^3 - a^3)$ **49.** $\frac{1}{2}(e^{2b} - e^{2a})$
51. 21 **53.** $\frac{16}{21}$ **55.** $\frac{1}{2}(e^2 + 1) \approx 4.195$ **57.** $\frac{8}{3}$
59. \$628.56 **61.** **(a)** \$552.60; **(b)** \$215.40
63. **(a)** \$2948.26; **(b)** \$2913.90 **65.** \$149.272 billion
67. 18.69 hr, 20.12 hr **69.** 7 words **71.** About 5 words
73. $s(t) = t^3 + 4$ **75.** $v(t) = 2t^2 + 20$
77. $s(t) = -\frac{1}{3}t^3 + 3t^2 + 6t + 10$ **79.** **(a)** 104.17 m; **(b)** 229.17 m **81.** $\frac{1}{8}$ mile **83.** **(a)** 16.67 km/hr; **(b)** 0.1875 km **85.** **(a)** $v(t) = -1.76t^2 + 44$; **(b)** 146.67 ft
87. **(a)** $v(t) = 183.4t$; **(b)** 146.72 ft/sec; **(c)** 58.688 ft/sec; **(d)** 100 mi/hr **89.** **(a)** 114,688 lb; **(b)** after 11.5 months
91. 3.5 **93.** $\frac{5392}{15}$ **95.** 30 **97.** 8 **99.** **(a)** 0, 1, 4, 9; **(b)** $f'(t) = 2t$; **(c)** $f'(t) = 2t$; **(d)** answers may vary
101. **(a)** $f'(t) = e^{2t}$; **(b)** $f'(t) = -e^{2t}$ **103.** $f'(t) = 2(2t + 1)^3$
105. Answers may vary. **107.** Answers may vary.
109. 6.283 **111.** 1.507

Exercise Set 4.4, p. 425

1. $\frac{125}{4}$ **3.** $\frac{161}{6}$ **5.** $\frac{275}{6}$ **7.** $\frac{337}{4}$ **9.** 5 **11.** $\frac{3}{2}$ **13.** 9
15. $\frac{3}{10}$ **17.** $\frac{9}{2}$ **19.** $\frac{125}{6}$ **21.** $\frac{1}{3}$ **23.** $\frac{3}{10}$ **25.** $\frac{125}{3}$
27. 2 **29.** 3 **31.** $\frac{125}{6}$ **33.** $\frac{32}{3}$ **35.** 0
37. $-e^{-1} + 1 \approx 0.632$ **39.** $\frac{16}{3}$ **41.** $\frac{1}{2}\ln 3 \approx 0.549$
43. $\frac{3}{5}$ **45.** **(a)** \$1,651,209.94; **(b)** \$165,120.99
47. \$6699.77 **49.** \$23,504.02 **51.** **(a)** Bonnie, 10 more words; **(b)** 7 words/min; **(c)** 8 words/min **53.** **(a)** 90 words/min; **(b)** 96 words/min at $t = 1$ min; **(c)** 70 words/min
55. **(a)** 42.03 μg/mL; **(b)** 22.44 μg/mL **57.** **(a)** 31.7°C; **(b)** −10°C; **(c)** 46.25°C **59.** **(a)** $x = 2$ yr; **(b)** the older engine, by 0.667 billion particulates **61.** **(a)** Beth's car, by 3.472 ft; **(b)** $t = 7.5$ sec; **(c)** Beth's car, by 4.6875 ft
63. 2.67, 3.67, 14.67, 41.67, 90.67, 167.67 **65.** **(a)** \$27,540/month, \$35,890/month, \$37,500/month, \$36,210/month, \$34,900/month, \$35,490/month; **(b)** $P(x) = -0.04x^4 + 1.04x^3 - 8.53x^2 + 26.46x + 10.5$

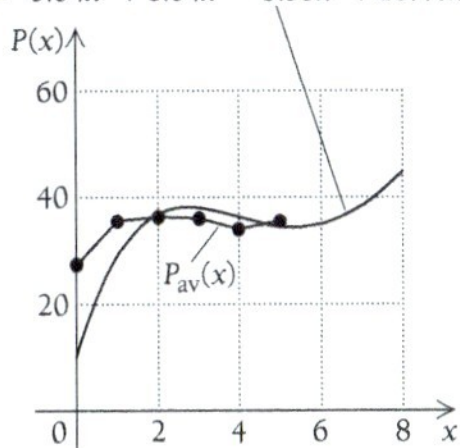

(c) answers may vary **67.** $e^2 + e^{-2} - 2 \approx 5.524$

69. 96 **71.** $Q = \frac{\pi p R^4}{8Lv}$ **73.** After 3 yr
75. (a) After 11.25 sec; **(b)** 31.64 ft **77.** 5.886 **79.** 0.237
81. Answers may vary. With a cubic model, the moving average for months 6 through 8 will be $41,820/month.

Exercise Set 4.5, p. 434

1. $\frac{1}{7}(x^2 - 7)^7 + C$ **3.** $\frac{1}{16}(x^2 - 6)^8 + C$ **5.** $\frac{1}{20}(2t^5 - 3)^2 + C$
7. $\ln|1 + 2x| + C$ **9.** $\frac{1}{8}(\ln x)^8 + C$ **11.** $\frac{1}{3}e^{3x} + C$
13. $2e^{x/2} + C$ **15.** $\frac{1}{5}e^{x^5} + C$ **17.** $-\frac{1}{3}e^{-t^3} + C$
19. $\frac{1}{2}\ln|5 + 2x| + C$ **21.** $\frac{1}{7}\ln|1 + 7x| + C$
23. $-\ln|1 - x| + C$ **25.** $\frac{1}{24}(t^3 - 1)^8 + C$
27. $\frac{1}{8}(x^4 + x^3 + x^2)^8 + C$ **29.** $\ln(3 + e^t) + C$
31. $(\ln x)^2 + C$ **33.** $\frac{1}{2}\ln(\ln x) + C$ **35.** $\frac{1}{3a}(ax^2 + b)^{3/2} + C$
37. $\frac{b}{a}e^{ax} + C$ **39.** $\frac{1}{24(2 - x^4)^6} + C$
41. $-2(1 - x^2)^{5/4} + C$ **43.** $\frac{3}{2}\ln(e^{2x} + 5) + C$ **45.** $e - 1$
47. $\frac{6561}{16}$ **49.** $\frac{1}{4}(e^8 - 1)$ **51.** $\ln\frac{9}{2}$ **53.** $1 - e^{-2b}$
55. $1 - e^{-kb}$ **57.** 39 **59.** $-\frac{21}{512}$ **61.** 5
63. $\ln\frac{3}{2} \approx 0.405$ **65.** $\frac{1}{2}(e^{15} - e^3) \approx 1{,}634{,}498.643$
67. $x + 5\ln|x - 5| + C$ **69.** $-\frac{1}{4}x - \frac{1}{16}\ln|1 - 4x| + C$
71. $\frac{2}{3}x + \frac{13}{9}\ln|3x - 2| + C$
73. $\frac{1}{11}(x + 2)^{11} - \frac{3}{5}(x + 2)^{10} + \frac{4}{3}(x + 2)^9 - (x + 2)^8 + C$
75. $D(x) = 2000\sqrt{25 - x^2} + 5000$ **77.** $1542.47
79. (a) About 170; **(b)** about 136 **81.** $-\frac{64}{3}$ **83.** 0
85. $-\frac{5}{12}(1 - 4x^2)^{3/2} + C$ **87.** $-\frac{1}{3}e^{-x^3} + C$
89. $\frac{3}{4}(x^2 - 6x)^{2/3} + C$ **91.** $\frac{1}{8}[\ln(t^4 + 8)]^2 + C$
93. $x + \frac{9}{x + 3} + C$ **95.** $t - \ln|t - 4| + C$
97. $\ln(e^x + e^{-x}) + C$ **99.** Answers may vary.
101. (a) About 4193; **(b)** about 8386

Exercise Set 4.6, p. 442

1. $\frac{3}{4}xe^{4x} - \frac{3}{16}e^{4x} + C$ **3.** $\frac{1}{5}xe^{5x} - \frac{1}{25}e^{5x} + C$
5. $-\frac{1}{2}xe^{-2x} - \frac{1}{4}e^{-2x} + C$ **7.** $\frac{1}{3}x^3\ln x - \frac{1}{9}x^3 + C$
9. $\frac{1}{4}x^2\ln x - \frac{1}{8}x^2 + C$ **11.** $(x + 5)\ln(x + 5) - x + C$
13. $\left(\frac{1}{2}x^2 + 2x\right)\ln x - \frac{1}{4}x^2 - 2x + C$
15. $\left(\frac{1}{2}x^2 - x\right)\ln x - \frac{1}{4}x^2 + x + C$
17. $\frac{2}{3}x(x + 2)^{3/2} - \frac{4}{15}(x + 2)^{5/2} + C$
19. $\frac{1}{4}x^4\ln(2x) - \frac{1}{16}x^4 + C$ **21.** $e^x(x^2 - 2x + 2) + C$
23. $e^{2x}\left(\frac{1}{2}x^2 - \frac{1}{2}x + \frac{1}{4}\right) + C$
25. $-e^{-2x}\left(\frac{1}{2}x^3 + \frac{3}{4}x^2 + \frac{3}{4}x + \frac{3}{8}\right) + C$
27. $e^{3x}\left(\frac{1}{3}x^4 - \frac{4}{9}x^3 + \frac{4}{9}x^2 - \frac{8}{27}x + \frac{116}{81}\right) + C$
29. $\frac{8}{3}\ln 2 - \frac{7}{9}$ **31.** $\ln 108 - 2 \approx 2.682$ **33.** 1
35. $\frac{1192}{15}$ **37.** $C(x) = \frac{8}{3}x(x + 3)^{3/2} - \frac{16}{15}(x + 3)^{5/2}$
39. (a) $-e^{-kT}\left(\frac{T}{k} + \frac{1}{k^2}\right) + \frac{1}{k^2}$; **(b)** about 14.85 mg
41. $\frac{2}{125}(5x + 1)^{5/2} + \frac{2}{75}(5x + 1)^{3/2} + C$; they are the same.
43. $2\sqrt{x}e^{\sqrt{x}} - 2e^{\sqrt{x}} + C$
45. $\frac{d}{dx}\left[e^{bx}\left(\frac{abx - a}{b^2}\right) + C\right] = e^{bx}\cdot\frac{a}{b} + \left(\frac{abx - a}{b^2}\right)\cdot be^{bx}$
$= \frac{ae^{bx}}{b} + axe^{bx} - \frac{ae^{bx}}{b} = axe^{bx}$
47. $\frac{d}{dx}[x^ne^x - n\int x^{n-1}e^x\,dx] = x^ne^x + nx^{n-1}e^x - nx^{n-1}e^x$
$= x^ne^x$
49. $\frac{d}{dx}\left[\frac{ax + b}{a}\ln(ax + b) - x + C\right]$
$= \frac{ax + b}{a}\cdot\frac{a}{ax + b} + 1\cdot\ln(ax + b) - 1 = \ln(ax + b)$
51. $\left(\frac{3x - 8}{3}\right)\ln(3x - 8) - x + C$
53. $\frac{1}{6}(37\ln 37 - 7\ln 7) - 5$ **55.** $\frac{e^t}{t + 1} + C$
57. $\frac{1}{3}x^3(\ln x)^2 - \frac{2}{9}x^3\ln x + \frac{2}{27}x^3 + C$
59. $\frac{2\cdot 5^x}{\ln 5}\left(x - \frac{1}{\ln 5}\right) + C$ **61.** $\frac{4\cdot 6^{2+3x}}{3\ln 6}\left(x - \frac{1}{3\ln 6}\right) + C$
63. Answers may vary. **65.** $\frac{3^xe^x}{1 + \ln 3} + C$
67. $\frac{10^xe^{3x}}{3 + \ln 10} + C$ **69.** About 355,986

Exercise Set 4.7, p. 453

1. $L_4 = 18$, $R_4 = 34$, average $= 26$
3. $L_6 = 24.375$, $R_6 = 49.875$, average $= 37.125$
5. $L_8 = 0.725$, $R_8 = 0.663$, average $= 0.694$
7. $L_6 = 117.102$, $R_6 = 318.316$, average $= 217.709$
9. $L_8 = 2151.875$, $R_8 = 3839.875$, average $= 2995.875$
11. $M_4 = 25$ **13.** $M_6 = 35.438$ **15.** $M_8 = 0.693$
17. $M_6 = 193.069$ **19.** $M_8 = 2894.109$
21. $T_4 = 2.977$ **23.** $T_8 = 1.325$ **25.** $T_5 = 25.051$
27. $T_4 = 1.155$ **29.** $S_4 = 5.641$ **31.** $S_6 = 2.160$
33. $S_6 = 3.142$ **35.** $S_4 = 1.432$
37. $L_{12} = 0.767$ mi, $R_{12} = 0.867$ mi, average $= 0.817$ mi
39. 336.000 ft^2 **41. (a)** $T_{10} = 7.762$; **(b)** 31.048
43. (a) $M_6 = 1.397$; **(b)** $\pi/2$ **45.** $S_8 = 9.300$
47. About $3192 **49. (a)** About 4700 ft^2; **(b)** about $28,300
51. (a) $<$; **(b)** $>$; **(c)** $>$ **53. (a)** $<$; **(b)** $>$; **(c)** $<$
55.–59. Answers may vary. **61. (a)** 9.255; **(b)** 0.10%
63. (a) 0.091; **(b)** 1.10% **65. (a)** 0.505; **(b)** 0.20%
67. (a) 1.459; **(b)** 0% **69. (a)** 18.534; **(b)** 0%
71. (a) 1.463; **(b)** 0.07% **73. (a)** 3.660; **(b)** 0%
75. (a) 1.152; **(b)** −6.16%

Chapter 4 Review Exercises, p. 463

1. True **2.** False **3.** True **4.** False **5.** False
6. (e) **7.** (d) **8.** (a) **9.** (f) **10.** (b) **11.** (c)
12. $102,500 **13.** $4x^5 + C$ **14.** $\frac{3}{4}e^{4x} + 2x + C$
15. $6t^3 + 3t^2 + \frac{1}{2}\ln t + C$ **16.** 15 **17.** 39
18. Total number of words keyboarded in t minutes
19. Total sales in t days **20.** $\frac{9}{2}$ **21.** $\frac{1}{6}(b^6 - a^6)$ **22.** $-\frac{57}{20}$
23. $\frac{1}{2}e^2$ **24.** $2\ln 4$ **25.** $\frac{22}{3}$ **26.** 0 **27.** Negative
28. Positive **29.** $\frac{1}{6}$ **30.** $\frac{1}{4}e^{x^4} + C$ **31.** $\ln(4t^6 + 3) + C$
32. $\frac{1}{4}(\ln 4x)^2 + C$ **33.** $\frac{1}{2}\ln(e^{2x} + 2) + C$

34. $\frac{3}{4}e^{4x}\left(x - \frac{1}{4}\right) + C$ **35.** $\frac{4x + 9}{4}\ln(4x + 9) - x + C$
36. $\frac{5}{3}x^3 \ln x - \frac{5}{9}x^3 + C$
37. $e^{3x}\left(\frac{1}{3}x^4 - \frac{4}{9}x^3 + \frac{4}{9}x^2 - \frac{8}{27}x + \frac{8}{81}\right) + C$
38. $L_4 = 10.831$, $R_4 = 16.873$, average $= 13.852$
39. $M_4 = 0.323$ **40.** $T_6 = 1.735$ **41.** $S_4 = 3.392$
42. About 435 ft^2 **43.** About \$96,000
44. $\frac{1}{2}(1 - 3e^{-2}) \approx 0.297$ **45.** 80 mi **46.** About \$162,754
47. $\ln|4t^3 + 7| + C$ **48.** $\frac{2}{75}(5x - 8)\sqrt{4 + 5x} + C$
49. $e^{x^5} + C$ **50.** $x - 9\ln|x + 9| + C$ **51.** $\frac{1}{96}(t^8 + 3)^{12} + C$
52. $x\ln|7x| - x + C$ **53.** $\frac{1}{2}x^2 \ln|8x| - \frac{1}{4}x^2 + C$
54. $\frac{1}{10}(\ln(t^5 + 3))^2 + C$ **55.** $-\frac{1}{2}\ln(1 + 2e^{-x}) + C$
56. $\frac{1}{4}(\ln x)^2 + C$ **57.** $\frac{1}{92}x^{92}\ln|x| - \frac{1}{8464}x^{92} + C$
58. $(x - 3)\ln|x - 3| - (x - 4)\ln|x - 4| + C$
59. $-\frac{1}{3(\ln|x|)^3} + C$ **60.** $\frac{3}{7}(x + 3)^{7/3} - \frac{9}{4}(x + 3)^{4/3} + C$
61. $\frac{1}{16}(2x + 1)^2 - \frac{1}{4}(2x + 1) + \frac{1}{8}\ln|2x + 1| + C$ **62.** 1.343

Chapter 4 Test, p. 465

1. 95 **2.** $\frac{2}{3}\sqrt{3}x^{3/2} + C$, or $\frac{2}{9}(3x)^{3/2} + C$ **3.** $50x^6 + C$
4. $\frac{1}{5}e^{5x} + \ln x + \frac{8}{11}x^{11/8} + C$ **5.** $\frac{1}{6}$ **6.** 4 ln 3
7. Total number of miles run in t hours **8.** 21 **9.** $\frac{1 - e^{-2}}{2}$
10. 2 **11.** $\frac{61}{6}$ **12.** $\frac{7}{2}$ **13.** Positive **14.** $\frac{1}{3}\ln|x + 4| + C$
15. $-2e^{-0.5x} + C$ **16.** $\frac{1}{32}(t^4 + 3)^8 + C$ **17.** $\frac{1}{5}e^{5x}\left(x - \frac{1}{5}\right) + C$
18. $\frac{1}{4}x^4(\ln x^4 - 1) + C$ **19.** $T_6 = 6.981$
20. $L_5 = 2.640$, $R_5 = 3.232$; average $= 2.937$
21. $L_9 = 1.15$, $R_9 = 1.05$, average $= 1.10$ mi
22. About \$2305.63 **23.** 6 **24.** $\frac{5}{14}$ **25.** \$118,750
26. 94 words **27.** 7.47 km **28.** $\frac{1}{6}e^{x^6} + C$
29. $-\frac{2}{9}(38 + 8\ln 64 - 27\ln 729) \approx 23.712$
30. $\frac{2}{9}(1 + e^{3x})^{3/2} + C$ **31.** 5.4197
32. $\frac{1}{2}x^2\ln(13x) - \frac{1}{4}x^2 + C$ **33.** $\frac{1}{x + 1} + \ln|x + 1| + C$
34. $\frac{9375}{8}$ **35.** $\frac{48}{\ln 5}\cdot 5^{x/4} + C$ **36.** **(a)** Danah, by $\frac{25}{24} \approx 1.042$ mi; **(b)** 7.5 hr, when both have walked $\frac{225}{32}$, or 7.03125 mi
37. **(a)** $a \approx -0.767$, $b = 2$, $c = 4$; **(b)** 2.106; **(c)** 1.354; **(d)** answers may vary **38.** **(a)** $0, \frac{3}{2}, 6, \frac{27}{2}$; **(b)** $f'(t) = 3t$

Extended Technology Application, p. 468

1. **(a)** 36%; **(b)** 33.3 **2.** **(a)** 16.7%; **(b)** 55.6
3. **(a)** $f(x) = x^{1.75}$, where $0 \le x \le 1$; **(b)** 0.272, 27.2; **(c)** about 59% **4.** **(a)** $f(x) = x^{2.34}$, where $0 \le x \le 1$; **(b)** 0.4, 40; **(c)** about 15.4%; **(d)** about 21.9% **5.** Left to the student **6.** **(a)** $f(x) = x^{2.77}$; **(b)** about 19.1%
7. **(a)** $f(x) = x^{1.86}$; **(b)** about 32.9% **8.** **(a)** 41.5%; **(b)** $f(x) = 0.00033245289 \cdot (1625.403784)^x$, where $0 \le x \le 1$; **(c)** 0.427; **(d)** 0.854, 85.4; **(e)** left to the student

CHAPTER 5

Exercise Set 5.1, p. 479

1. **(a)** (6, \$4); **(b)** \$15; **(c)** \$9 **3.** **(a)** (1, \$4); **(b)** \$2.33; **(c)** \$1.67 **5.** **(a)** (3, \$9); **(b)** \$36; **(c)** \$18
7. **(a)** (40, \$7600); **(b)** \$24,000; **(c)** \$12,000 **9.** **(a)** (2, \$3); **(b)** \$2; **(c)** \$0.35 **11.** **(a)** (899, \$60); **(b)** \$50,460; **(c)** \$17,941.33 **13.** **(a)** (0.8, \$10.24); **(b)** \$2.22; **(c)** \$0.98
15. **(a)** \$81; **(b)** \$30; **(c)** equilibrium point: (3, \$140), consumer surplus: \$137.25, producer surplus: \$67.50; **(d)** answers may vary **17.** **(a)** (22, \$28); **(b)** (14, \$24); **(c)** \$266; **(d)** \$49; **(e)** \$48 **19.** **(a)** (35, \$56.25); **(b)** (16, \$80); **(c)** \$160; **(d)** \$704; **(e)** \$361
21. **(a)** (6.5, \$42.25); **(b)** (5.48, \$30); **(c)** \$302.55; **(d)** \$109.54; **(e)** \$10.40 **23.** **(a)** (60, \$1200); **(b)** consumer surplus: \$9000, producer surplus: \$18,000; **(c)** (40, \$1000); **(d)** new consumer surplus: \$16,000, new producer surplus: \$8000; **(e)** \$3000 **25.** **(a)** (80, \$175); **(b)** consumer surplus: \$4000, producer surplus: \$1600; **(c)** (60, \$200); **(d)** new consumer surplus: \$2250, new producer surplus: \$3000; **(e)** \$350; **(f)** answers may vary **27.** **(a)** (5, \$0.61); **(b)** \$86.36; **(c)** \$2.45 **29.** Answers may vary. **31.** Answers may vary.
33. **(a)** (27, \$6);
(b)

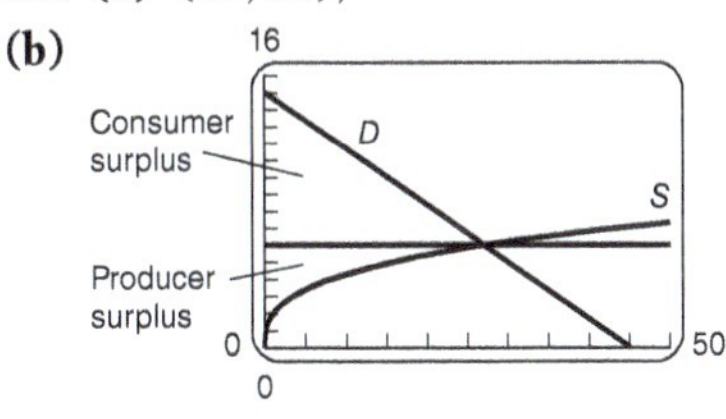

(c) \$121.50; **(d)** \$40.50

Exercise Set 5.2, p. 490

1. \$75,742 **3.** \$125,003 **5.** \$72,615 **7.** \$993,171
9. \$3,463,420 **11.** \$1,511,368 **13.** \$4,959,685
15. \$10,171,803 **17.** \$831,544 **19.** \$6325
21. \$91,923.51 **23.** **(a)** \$2,494,073.38; **(b)** \$12,353,226.33
25. \$174,517.78 **27.** A: \$8,309,596.93. B: \$9,205,617.57; franchise B is the better buy. **29.** **(a)** Program 1: \$48,842.06, program 2: \$46,636.26; **(b)** \$2205.80 **31.** **(a)** \$494,602.93; **(b)** \$31,316.55 **33.** \$22,472,512 **35.** **(a)** \$1,489,330; **(b)** \$803,510 **37.** **(a)** \$1,603,300; **(b)** \$665,019.42; **(c)** 3%: \$751,980.61, 4%: \$688,338.79, 5%: \$632,120.56; **(d)** answers may vary. **39.** \$42,136.19
41. 144.19 trillion cubic feet **43.** 66.52 yr
45. **(a)** 57.27 billion barrels; **(b)** 21.9 yr after 2016
47. 16.031 lb **49.** \$535,847 **51.** \$732,121
53. Answers may vary.

Exercise Set 5.3, p. 497

1. Convergent, $\frac{1}{3}$ **3.** Divergent **5.** Convergent, 1
7. Convergent, $\frac{1}{2}$ **9.** Divergent **11.** Convergent, 2
13. Divergent **15.** Divergent **17.** Divergent
19. Convergent, Q/k **21.** Convergent, 1000
23. Convergent, $\frac{1}{2}$ **25.** Convergent, $\frac{1}{4}$ **27.** Divergent
29. 2 **31.** 1 **33.** \$6,250,000 **35.** 4,761,905 tires
37. \$112,903.23 **39.** \$69,444.44 **41.** \$1,677,198.70
43. 33,333.33 lb **45.** **(a)** 4.20963; **(b)** 0.702858 rem; **(c)** 2.37551 rem **47.** Divergent **49.** Convergent, 2
51. Convergent, 1 **53.** $1/k^2$ is the total dosage of the drug.
55. 4 **57.** 2.5

59.
$$\int_a^\infty \frac{1}{x^n}\,dx = \lim_{b\to\infty}\left[\frac{x^{-n+1}}{-n+1}\right]_a^b = \lim_{b\to\infty}\left[\frac{1}{1-n}\left(b^{-n+1} - a^{-n+1}\right)\right].$$

The term b^{-n+1} will approach 0 only if $-n+1<0$, or $n>1$. The remaining terms are finite, so when $n>1$, the integral is convergent. Otherwise, it diverges. **61–63.** Answers may vary. **65.** 3.142 **67.** 3.142

Exercise Set 5.4, p. 507

1. $\int_3^8 \frac{1}{5}\,dx = \left[\frac{1}{5}x\right]_3^8 = \frac{8}{5}-\frac{3}{5}=1$

3. $\int_1^3 \frac{1}{4}x\,dx = \left[\frac{1}{8}x^2\right]_1^3 = \frac{1}{8}(3)^2-\frac{1}{8}(1)^2=\frac{9}{8}-\frac{1}{8}=1$

5. $\int_0^4 \frac{3}{64}x^2\,dx = \left[\frac{1}{64}x^3\right]_0^4 = \frac{1}{64}(4)^3-\frac{1}{64}(0)^3=\frac{64}{64}-0=1$

7. $\int_{-1}^1 \frac{3}{2}x^2\,dx = \left[\frac{1}{2}x^3\right]_{-1}^1 = \frac{1}{2}(1)^3-\frac{1}{2}(-1)^3=\frac{1}{2}-\left(-\frac{1}{2}\right)=1$

9. $\int_0^\infty 4e^{-4x}\,dx = \lim_{b\to\infty}\left[-e^{-4x}\right]_0^b$

$= \lim_{b\to\infty}\left(-e^{-4b}-(-1)\right)=0-(-1)=1$

11. $\frac{2}{21}$; $f(x)=\frac{2}{21}x$ on $[2,5]$ **13.** $\frac{3}{16}$; $f(x)=\frac{3}{16}x^2$ on $[-2,2]$

15. $\frac{1}{3}$; $f(x)=\frac{1}{3}$ on $[1,4]$ **17.** $\frac{1}{2}$; $f(x)=\frac{2-x}{2}$ on $[0,2]$

19. $\frac{1}{\ln 3}$; $f(x)=\frac{1}{x\ln 3}$ on $[1,3]$

21. $\frac{1}{e^2-1}$; $f(x)=\frac{e^x}{e^2-1}$ on $[0,2]$ **23.** $\frac{8}{25}$ **25.** $\frac{11}{16}$

27. 0.0488 **29.** 0.8647 **31.** 0.3935

33. (a) $\int_0^{10} 0.23\,e^{-0.23t}\,dt = \left[-e^{-0.23t}\right]_0^{10}$

$= -e^{-0.23(10)}-\left(-e^{-0.23(0)}\right)=0.9$;

(b) 0.0286 **35.** 0.950213 **37.** 0.049787

39. We have $\int_k^k 0.02e^{-0.02t}\,dt$, which is 0. **41.** $a=\frac{1}{2}$

43. (a) $k=0.357$, $f(t)=0.357e^{-0.357t}$ on $[0,\infty)$; **(b)** 0.2427

45. (a) $c=\frac{1}{2}$; **(b)** $f(x)=\frac{1}{8}x-\frac{1}{8}$ on $[1,5]$; **(c)** 0.1875

47. $c=\frac{4}{3e^4-e^2}\approx 0.02557$ **49–57.** Left to the student

Exercise Set 5.5, p. 519

1. $\mu=E(x)=5$, $E(x^2)=\frac{79}{3}$, $\sigma^2=\frac{4}{3}$, $\sigma=\frac{2}{\sqrt{3}}$

3. $\mu=E(x)=2$, $E(x^2)=\frac{9}{2}$, $\sigma^2=\frac{1}{2}$, $\sigma=\frac{\sqrt{2}}{2}$

5. $\mu=E(x)=\frac{13}{6}$, $E(x^2)=5$, $\sigma^2=\frac{11}{36}$, $\sigma=\frac{\sqrt{11}}{6}$

7. $\mu=E(x)=-\frac{5}{4}$, $E(x^2)=\frac{11}{5}$, $\sigma^2=\frac{51}{80}$, $\sigma=\frac{1}{4}\sqrt{\frac{51}{5}}$

9. $\mu=E(x)=\frac{6}{\ln 5}$, $E(x^2)=\frac{27}{\ln 5}$, $\sigma^2=\frac{27\ln 5-36}{(\ln 5)^2}$,

$\sigma=\frac{\sqrt{27\ln 5-36}}{\ln 5}$

11. 0.4834 **13.** 0.4778 **15.** 0.6442 **17.** 0.1501

19. 0.1790 **21.** 0.1562 **23. (a)** 0.6826; **(b)** 68.26% **25.** 0.2898 **27.** 0.4514 **29.** 0.3076 **31.** 0.5398 **33.** 0.2119 **35.** 0.3821 **37.** 0.6915 **39. (a)** -0.52; **(b)** 0; **(c)** 1.645 **41. (a)** -15.04; **(b)** -14.44 **43.** 0.62% **45.** 0.7910 **47. (a)** 1007; **(b)** 1128; **(c)** 1347 **49. (a)** 84; **(b)** 71 **51.** 90.8th

53. $\mu=E(x)=\frac{b+a}{2}$, $E(x^2)=\frac{b^2+ab+a^2}{3}$,

$\sigma^2=\frac{(b-a)^2}{12}$, $\sigma=\frac{b-a}{2\sqrt{3}}$

55. $\sqrt{2}$ **57.** $\frac{\ln 2}{k}$ **59.** 7.801 oz

61. $E(x^2+x)=\int_a^b (x^2+x)f(x)\,dx$

$=\int_a^b x^2f(x)\,dx+\int_a^b xf(x)\,dx=E(x^2)+E(x)$

63. $E(\mu^2)=\int_a^b \mu^2 f(x)\,dx$

$=\mu^2\int_a^b f(x)\,dx=\mu^2\cdot 1=\mu^2=E(x)^2$

65. Answers may vary. **67. (a)** 1.056; **(b)** 2.929; **(c)** 6.838

Exercise Set 5.6, p. 525

1. $\frac{\pi}{3}$ **3.** $\frac{15\pi}{2}$ **5.** $\frac{\pi}{2}\left(e^{10}-e^{-4}\right)$ **7.** $\frac{2\pi}{3}$ **9.** $4\pi\ln\frac{9}{4}$

11. 32π **13.** $\frac{32\pi}{5}$ **15.** 56π **17.** $\frac{32\pi}{3}$ **19.** 250π

21. $\frac{81\pi}{2}$ **23.** $2\pi\ln 2$ **25.** $\frac{33\pi}{2}$ **27.** $\frac{762\pi}{7}$

29. $\frac{2\pi}{3}(10^{1.5}-1)$ **31. (a)** 243π; **(b)** 243π; **(c)** answers may vary **33.** $1{,}703{,}704\pi$ cubic feet

35. $\frac{8775}{4}\pi$ cubic feet

37.

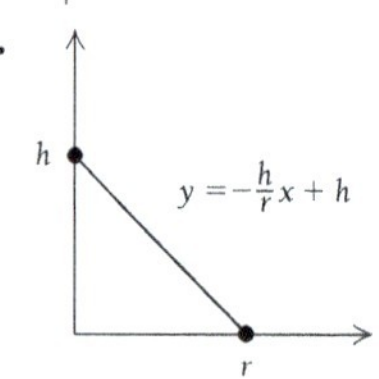

$V=2\pi\int_0^r x\left(-\frac{h}{r}x+h\right)dx=2\pi\left[-\frac{h}{3r}x^3+\frac{h}{2}x^2\right]_0^r$

$=2\pi\left[-\frac{h}{3}r^2+\frac{h}{2}r^2\right]=2\pi\left(\frac{hr^2}{6}\right)=\frac{1}{3}\pi r^2h$

39. $2\pi e^3$ **41.** $\frac{108\pi}{5}$ **43. (a)** $\frac{7\pi}{3}, \frac{5\pi}{3}$, the volume around the x-axis is larger; **(b)** $\frac{26\pi}{3}, \frac{28\pi}{3}$, the volume around the y-axis is larger; **(c)** $a=\sqrt{3}$ **45.** π cubic units

47. $\frac{25}{64}$ **49.** About 0.653 ft

Exercise Set 5.7, p. 535

1. (a) $y=\frac{5}{7}x^7+C$; **(b)** $y=\frac{5}{7}x^7-3$

3. (a) $y=\frac{1}{4}e^{4x}-\frac{1}{2}x^2+2x+C$;

(b) $y = \frac{1}{4}e^{4x} - \frac{1}{2}x^2 + 2x + \frac{15}{4}$
5. (a) $y = 3\ln x + \frac{1}{3}x^3 - \frac{1}{5}x^5 + C$;
(b) $y = 3\ln x + \frac{1}{3}x^3 - \frac{1}{5}x^5 - \frac{62}{15}$
7. (a) $y' = -4e^{-4x}$ so that $(-4e^{-4x}) + 4(e^{-4x}) = 0$;
(b) $y' = Ce^{-4x}$ so that $(-4Ce^{-4x}) + 4(Ce^{-4x}) = 0$
9. $y' = -4 + \ln x$ and $y'' = \frac{1}{x}$, so $\frac{1}{x} - \frac{1}{x} = 0$.
11. $y' = xe^x - e^x$ and $y'' = xe^x$, so $(xe^x) - 2(xe^x - e^x) + (-2e^x + xe^x)$ $= xe^x(1 - 2 + 1) + e^x(2 - 2) = 0$.
13. (a) $y' = 11e^{11x}$, $y'' = 121e^{11x}$ so that $(121e^{11x}) - 7(11e^{11x}) - 44(e^{11x}) = e^{11x}(121 - 77 - 44) = 0$;
(b) $y' = -4e^{-4x}$, $y'' = 16e^{-4x}$ so that $(16e^{-4x}) - 7(-4e^{-4x}) - 44(e^{-4x}) = e^{-4x}(16 + 28 - 44) = 0$;
(c) $y' = 11C_1e^{11x} - 4C_2e^{-4x}$, $y'' = 121C_1e^{11x} + 16C_2e^{-4x}$, so that $(121C_1e^{11x} + 16C_2e^{-4x}) - 7(11C_1e^{11x} - 4C_2e^{-4x}) - 44(C_1e^{11x} + C_2e^{-4x})$ $= C_1e^{11x}(121 - 77 - 44) + C_2e^{-4x}(16 + 28 - 44) = 0$
15. (a) $C(t) = Ce^{0.66t}$; **(b)** $C'(t) = 0.66Ce^{0.66t}$, so that $0.66Ce^{0.66t} = 0.66(Ce^{0.66t})$
17. (a) $V(t) = Ce^{-1.33t}$; **(b)** $V'(t) = -1.33Ce^{-1.33t}$, so that $-1.33Ce^{-1.33t} = -1.33(Ce^{-1.33t})$
19. (a) $h(t) = Ce^{0.023t}$; **(b)** $h'(t) = 0.023Ce^{0.023t}$, so that $0.023Ce^{0.023t} = 0.023(Ce^{0.023t})$ **21.** $y = \frac{1}{3}x^3 + x^2 - 3x + 4$
23. $f(x) = \frac{3}{5}x^{5/3} - \frac{1}{2}x^2 - \frac{61}{10}$ **25.** $B(t) = 500e^{0.03t}$
27. $S(t) = 750e^{-0.125t}$ **29.** $T(t) = 49.26e^{0.015t}$
31. $y = Ce^{x^5}$ **33.** $y = \sqrt[3]{\frac{5}{2}x^2 + C}$ **35.** $y = \pm\sqrt{\frac{1}{2}x^2 + C}$
37. $y = \sqrt[3]{21x + C}$ **39.** $y = 8e^{0.5x^2} - 3$ **41.** $y = \sqrt[3]{15x - 3}$
43. (a) $dA/dt = 0.0375A$, $A(0) = 500$; **(b)** $A(t) = 500e^{0.0375t}$;
(c) $A(5) = \$603.12$, $A'(5) = \$22.62$/yr;
(d) $22.62/603.12 = 0.0375$, which is the continuous growth rate
45. $V(t) = -4.81e^{-kt} + 24.81$ **47. (a)** $I(t) = Ce^{hkt}$;
(b) $I(t) = 500{,}000e^{0.532t}$ **49.** $q(x) = 2e^{4/x-1}$ **51.** $q(x) = \frac{C}{x^2}$
53. (a) $dP/dt = 0.0175P$, $P(0) = 17{,}000$;
(b) $P(t) = 17{,}000e^{0.0175t}$; **(c)** $P(10) = 20{,}251$ people, $P'(10) = 354.4$ people/yr; $354.4/20{,}251 = 0.0175$, which is the continuous growth rate
55. (a) $k = 0.296$, $P(t) = 24e^{0.296t}$;
(b) $P(41) = 4{,}475{,}165$ rabbits, $P'(41) = 1{,}324{,}649$ rabbits/yr;
(c) 0.296 **57.** $R = C \cdot S^k$ **59. (a)** 4.18%/yr;
(b) $A(t) = 3200e^{0.0418t}$; **(c)** \$3200 **61.** $y = -\frac{4}{4x^5 + x^4 + C}$
63. Answers may vary. **65. (a)** $A(t) = 4250e^{0.05t}$;
(b) $dA/dt = 0.05A$, $A(0) = 4250$
67. $y = \sqrt[3]{6x + C}$

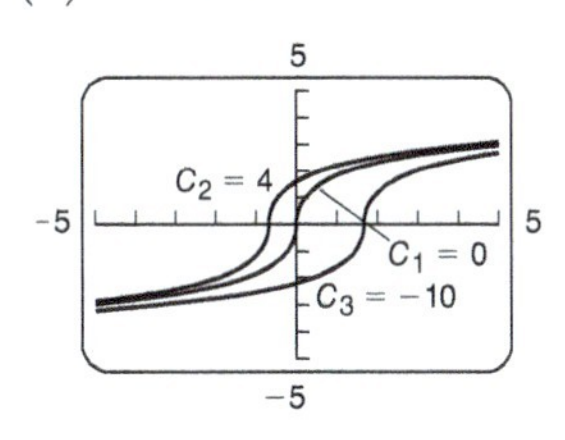

Chapter 5 Review Exercises, p. 545

1. (d) **2.** (e) **3.** (g) **4.** (b) **5.** (c) **6.** (a) **7.** (f) **8.** False **9.** False **10.** False **11.** True **12.** True **13.** False **14.** True **15.** (2, \$16) **16.** \$18.67 **17.** \$5.33 **18. (a)** \$20.06; **(b)** \$1.89; **(c)** \$2.06 **19.** \$6255.36 **20.** \$8065.41 **21.** \$23,820.45 **22.** \$8787.35/yr **23.** \$626,142.24 **24.** 11.52 billion metric tons **25.** In about 33.75 yr **26.** Convergent, 1 **27.** Divergent **28.** Convergent, $\frac{1}{2}$
29. $k = \frac{8}{3}$, $f(x) = \frac{8}{3x^3}$, $1 \le x \le 2$ **30.** 0.6 **31.** $\frac{3}{10}$
32. $\frac{1}{2}$ **33.** $\frac{1}{2}$ **34.** $\frac{1}{20}$ **35.** $\frac{1}{2\sqrt{5}}$ **36.** 0.4678
37. 0.8827 **38.** 0.1002 **39.** 0.5000 **40.** 0.3085
41. \$6199 **42.** $\frac{127\pi}{7}$ **43.** $\frac{\pi}{6}$ **44.** 40π
45. $\pi(e^9 - e)$ **46.** $2\pi\left(\frac{125}{3}\ln 5 - \frac{124}{9}\right)$ **47.** $y = Ce^{x^{11}}$
48. $y = \pm\sqrt{4x + C}$ **49.** $y = 5e^{4x}$ **50.** $y = \sqrt[3]{15t + 19}$
51. $y = \pm\sqrt{3x^2 + C}$ **52.** $y = Ce^{-x^2/2} + 8$
53. $q = 100 - x$ **54.** $V(t) = -6.37e^{-kt} + 36.37$ **55.** $\sqrt[3]{9}$
56. Divergent **57.** Convergent, 3 **58.** 1 **59.** 3.142
60. 30.867π cubic units

Chapter 5 Test, p. 547

1. (3, \$16) **2.** \$45 **3.** \$22.50 **4. (a)** \$33.96; **(b)** \$31.87; **(c)** \$1.67 **5.** \$17,459.90 **6.** \$53,879.14 **7.** 224.29 million metric tons **8.** In 29.13 yr **9.** \$10,540.66/yr
10. \$3,202,050.53 **11.** \$1,350,948.19 **12.** Convergent, $\frac{1}{4}$
13. Divergent **14.** $k = \frac{1}{4}$, $f(x) = \frac{1}{4}x^3$ on $[0, 2]$ **15.** 0.117
16. $\frac{13}{6}$ **17.** 5 **18.** $\frac{13}{6}$ **19.** $\frac{11}{36}$ **20.** $\frac{\sqrt{11}}{6}$ **21.** 0.4032
22. 0.1365 **23.** 0.9071 **24.** 0.3085 **25.** \$14.59/lb
26. $\pi\ln 5$ **27.** $\frac{5\pi}{2}$ **28.** $\frac{512}{15}\pi$ **29.** $\frac{339\pi}{2}$ **30.** $\frac{8000\pi}{3}$
31. $y = Ce^{x^8}$ **32.** $y = \sqrt{18x - 27}$ **33.** $y = 11e^{6t}$
34. $y = Ce^{-x^3/3} + 5$ **35.** $v = \sqrt[4]{8t + 10{,}000}$
36. $y = Ce^{4x + x^2/2}$ **37.** $q = \frac{C}{x^4}$
38. (a) $V(t) = 36(1 - e^{-kt})$; **(b)** $k = 0.12$; **(c)** 14.9 months
39. $\sqrt{2}$ **40.** Convergent, $-\frac{1}{4}$ **41.** 3.628 **42.** 5.4095

Extended Technology Application, p. 549

1. $y = 0.0052548858x^3 - 0.2722052955x^2 + 3.486640971x + 4.056787769$
2. 12,348.28 cm^3
3. $y_1 = 0.00023310023x^4 - 0.0027292152x^3 - 0.0133741259x^2 + 1.074786325x + 1.13986014$
4. 34.703 in^3 **5.** 19.23 fl oz; yes
6. $y_2 = 0.00023310023x^4 - 0.0027292152x^3 - 0.0133741259x^2 + 0.1074786325x + 1.15486014$
7. 0.06983 in^3

CHAPTER 6

Exercise Set 6.1, p. 557

1. 0, 4096, 0 **3.** 28, 5, 12 **5.** $-8, 5, -23$ **7.** $-14, 1$ **9.** $\{(x, y) \mid y \geq 0\}$ **11.** $\{(x, y) \mid y \geq 3x\}$ **13.** 0.62% **15.** \$193,318.20 **17.** **(a)** \$282.60; **(b)** \$23,738.40; **(c)** 6.5%; **(d)** \$254.40 **19.** 0.025 **21.** 1.915 m^2 **23.** **(a)** 314; **(b)** Goldschmidt had 314 total bases during the 2017 season. **25.** **(a)** 65; **(b)** 62; **(c)** about 30%; **(d)** answers may vary. **27.** 4.13 m **29.** Answers may vary. **31.** 0°F **33.** -22°F **35–41.** Left to the student

Exercise Set 6.2, p. 566

1. $2, -3, 2, -3$ **3.** $6x^2 + 3y - 1, 3x, 14, 0$ **5.** 5, 7, 5, 7 **7.** $\frac{x}{\sqrt{x^2 - y^2}}, \frac{-y}{\sqrt{x^2 - y^2}}, -\frac{2}{\sqrt{3}}, \frac{2}{\sqrt{5}}$ **9.** $2e^{2x-y}, -e^{2x-y}$ **11.** $2ye^{2xy}, 2xe^{2xy}$ **13.** $\frac{y}{x + 2y}, \frac{2y}{x + 2y} + \ln(x + 2y)$ **15.** $\frac{y}{x}, 1 + \ln(xy)$ **17.** $\frac{1}{y} + \frac{y}{3x^2}, -\frac{x}{y^2} - \frac{1}{3x}$ **19.** $12(2x + y - 5), 6(2x + y - 5)$ **21.** $-2mb + 10m + 4b - 37, -b^2 + 36m + 10b - 86$ **23.** $5y - 2\lambda, 5x - \lambda, -(2x + y - 8)$ **25.** $9y - 3\lambda, 9x + \lambda, -(3x - y + 7)$ **27.** $f_{xx} = 6y, f_{yy} = 0, f_{xy} = f_{yx} = 6x - 2$ **29.** $f_{xx} = 12x^2y^3 - 2y^3, f_{yy} = 6x^4y - 6x^2y,$ $f_{xy} = f_{yx} = 12x^3y^2 - 6xy^2$ **31.** $f_{xx} = 0, f_{yy} = 0, f_{xy} = f_{yx} = 0$ **33.** $f_{xx} = y^2e^{xy}, f_{yy} = x^2e^{xy}, f_{xy} = f_{yx} = xye^{xy} + e^{xy}$ **35.** $f_{xx} = 0, f_{yy} = -\frac{x}{y^2}, f_{xy} = f_{yx} = \frac{1}{y}$ **37.** **(a)** 1.56; **(b)** 1.571227 **39.** **(a)** 0.24; **(b)** 0.238 **41.** **(a)** 614,400 units; **(b)** $p_x = 960\left(\frac{y}{x}\right)^{3/5}, p_y = 1440\left(\frac{x}{y}\right)^{2/5}$; **(c)** 7680, 360; **(d)** answers may vary. **43.** **(a)** 7200 ft^2; **(b)** 270 ft^2; **(c)** 271 ft^2; **(d)** 1 can **45.** **(a)** \$940,498; **(b)** $P_w = -0.005075w^{-1.638}r^{1.038}s^{0.873}t^{2.468}$; $P_r = 0.008257w^{-0.638}r^{0.038}s^{0.873}t^{2.468}$; $P_s = 0.006945w^{-0.638}r^{1.038}s^{-0.127}t^{2.468}$; $P_t = 0.019633w^{-0.638}r^{1.038}s^{0.873}t^{1.468}$; **(c)** answers may vary. **47.** 117.8°F **49.** Answers may vary. **51.** **(a)** $S_h = \frac{1}{120}\sqrt{\frac{w}{h}}$; **(b)** $S_w = \frac{1}{120}\sqrt{\frac{h}{w}}$; **(c)** -0.0243 m^2 **53.** 78.244 **55.** -0.846 **57.** $f_x = -\frac{4xt^2}{(x^2 - t^2)^2}, f_t = \frac{4x^2t}{(x^2 - t^2)^2}$ **59.** $f_x = 4x^{-1/3} - 2x^{-3/4}t^{1/2} + 6x^{-3/2}t^{3/2}$, $f_t = -4x^{1/4}t^{-1/2} - 18x^{-1/2}t^{1/2}$ **61.** $f_{xx} = -\frac{6y}{x^4}, f_{xy} = f_{yx} = -\frac{2}{y^3} + \frac{2}{x^3}, f_{yy} = \frac{6x}{y^4}$ **63.** **(a)** 8.1; **(b)** 7.76 **65.** $f_{xx} = 4y^3z^4, f_{yy} = 12x^2yz^4, f_{zz} = 24x^2y^3z^2$; $f_{xz} = f_{zx} = 16xy^3z^3$, $f_{xy} = f_{yx} = 12xy^22z^4$, $f_{yz} = f_{zy} = 24x^2y^2z^3$ **67.** **(a)** $-y$; **(b)** x; **(c)** $f_{yx}(0, 0) = 1, f_{xy}(0, 0) = -1$; the mixed second partial derivatives are not equal at this point. **69.** Answers may vary.

Exercise Set 6.3, p. 576

1. Relative minimum $-\frac{25}{3}$ at $\left(-\frac{5}{3}, \frac{10}{3}\right)$ **3.** Relative maximum $\frac{32}{27}$ at $\left(\frac{4}{3}, \frac{4}{3}\right)$ **5.** Relative minimum -1 at $(1, 1)$ **7.** Relative minimum -7 at $(-3, 3)$ **9.** Relative maximum 13 at $(3, 2)$ **11.** No relative extrema **13.** Relative minimum e^{-3} at $(1, 2)$ **15.** Maximum: $\frac{100}{27}$ at $\left(\frac{5}{3}, \frac{10}{3}, \frac{2}{3}\right)$ **17.** Minimum: $\frac{32}{3}$ at $\left(\frac{4}{3}, \frac{8}{3}, \frac{4}{3}\right)$ **19.** 2000 of the \$18 shirt and 3000 of the \$25 shirt **21.** Maximum value of P = \$408 million when a = \$5 million and $n = 1$ thousand items sold **23.** **(a)** $R = 78p_1 - 6p_1^2 - 6p_1p_2 + 66p_2 - 6p_2^2$; **(b)** $p_1 = 5$, or \$50, $p_2 = 3$, or \$30; **(c)** $q_1 = 39$, or 3900 units, $q_2 = 33$, or 3300 units; **(d)** \$294,000 **25.** 729,000 in^3, when length = width = height = 90 in. **27.** Bottom measures 8 ft by 8 ft, height is 5 ft. **29.** Minimum temperature is -18°F at $(4, -1)$; no maximum. **31.** No relative extrema, saddle point at $(0, 0)$ **33.** Relative minimum 0 at $(0, 0)$, saddle points at $(2, 1)$ and $(-2, 1)$ **35.** Answers may vary. **37.** Relative minimum -5 at $(0, 0)$ **39.** No relative extrema

Exercise Set 6.4, p. 582

1. $y = \frac{5}{4}x + \frac{7}{12}$ **3.** $y = \frac{23}{14}x + \frac{3}{2}$ **5.** $y = 9.93(0.76)^x$, or $y = 9.93e^{-0.27x}$ **7.** $y = 34.39(0.66)^x$, or $y = 34.39e^{-0.416x}$ **9.** **(a)** $y = 0.574x + 8.892$; **(b)** \$13.48; **(c)** estimate from regression line for 2024: \$14.63, which is fairly accurate **11.** **(a)** $y = 0.121x + 80.025$; **(b)** 82.57 yr **13.** **(a)** $y = 0.233x + 1.43$; **(b)** 3.76 billion; **(c)** $x = 11.03$ yr, or in 2023 **15.** **(a)** $y = 0.235x + 76.738$; **(b)** 102.12 in., 109.17 in.; **(c)** answers may vary. **17.** **(a)** $y = 26.246e^{0.1735x}$; **(b)** in 7 yr, or in 2019 **19.** **(a)** $y = -0.0079251208x + 10.02244767$; **(b)** 9.53 sec; **(c)** in about 78.5 yr, or in 2046

Exercise Set 6.5, p. 592

1. Maximum: 32 at $(2, 8)$ **3.** Minimum: 17 at $(1, 4)$ **5.** Maximum: -34 at $(1, 6)$ **7.** Minimum: 28 at $(3, 5)$ **9.** Maximum: $\frac{8}{9}$ at $\left(\frac{4}{3}, 1, \frac{2}{3}\right)$ **11.** Minimum: $\frac{4}{3}$ at $\left(\frac{2}{3}, \frac{2}{3}, \frac{2}{3}\right)$ **13.** 35 and 35 **15.** 2 and -2 **17.** $(4, 8, 4)$ **19.** $x = -\frac{20}{29}, y = \frac{50}{29}$ **21.** $\left(\frac{4}{3}, \frac{8}{3}, \frac{4}{3}\right)$ **23.** $9\frac{3}{4}$ in. by $9\frac{3}{4}$ in., $95\frac{1}{16}$ in^2; no **25.** $r = \left(\frac{27}{2\pi}\right)^{1/3} \approx 1.626$ ft, $h \approx 3.251$ ft, about 49.8 ft^2 **27.** Maximum value of $S = 1012.5$ at $L = 22.5$ and $M = 67.5$ **29.** **(a)** $C(x, y, z) = 7xy + 6yz + 6xz$; **(b)** minimum cost: \$75,600, when $x = 60$ ft, $y = 60$ ft, and $z = 70$ ft **31.** 10,000 units on A, 100 units on B **33.** About 0.707 mi, \$5657 **35.** Absolute maximum at $(-1, 2, 9)$ and $(1, 2, 9)$, absolute minimum at $(0, 0, 0)$ **37.** Absolute maximum at $(2, 2, 8)$, absolute minimum at $(0, 6, -12)$ **39.** 125 acres celery, 175 acres lettuce, \$61,562.50 **41.** $\frac{512}{9}\sqrt{3}$ **43.** Minimum: $-\frac{9}{2}$ at $\left(\frac{3}{2}\sqrt{2}, -\frac{3}{2}\sqrt{2}\right)$ and $\left(-\frac{3}{2}\sqrt{2}, \frac{3}{2}\sqrt{2}\right)$ **45.** Maximum: $\sqrt{3}$ at $\left(\frac{1}{3}\sqrt{3}, \frac{1}{3}\sqrt{3}, \frac{1}{3}\sqrt{3}\right)$ **47.** Maximum: 6 at $\left(\frac{2}{3}, \frac{4}{3}, -\frac{4}{3}\right)$ **49.** Absolute minimum at $(1, -2, -5)$, absolute maximum at $(-\sqrt{5}, 2\sqrt{5}, 25 + 10\sqrt{5})$ **51.** Absolute minimum at $(0, 0, 5)$, absolute maximum at $(1.808, 1.2785, 14.789)$ **53.** Absolute minima at $(1, -\sqrt{2}, -\sqrt{2})$ and $(-1, \sqrt{2}, -\sqrt{2})$, absolute maxima at $(1, \sqrt{2}, \sqrt{2})$ and $(-1, -\sqrt{2}, \sqrt{2})$ **55.** $\lambda = \frac{p_x}{c_1} = \frac{p_y}{c_2}$ **57.** Answers may vary. **59.** $x \approx 1.389, y \approx -0.293$

Exercise Set 6.6, p. 599

1. 18 **3.** $-\frac{765}{8}$ **5.** -10 **7.** 5 **9.** $\frac{1}{2}$ **11.** 1 **13.** $\frac{175}{3}$ **15.** $\frac{325}{6}$ **17.** 3 **19.** $-\frac{85}{8}$ **21.** -2 **23.** $\frac{5}{4}$ **25.** $\frac{1}{2(e-2)}$, or about 0.696 **27.** $\frac{2}{3}$ **29.** $\frac{175}{15 \ln 2}$, or about 16.83 **31.** About 9.41938 **33.** $\frac{4}{15}$ **35.** $-\frac{1}{2}$ **37.** $\frac{108}{5}$ **39. (a)** 18,000 fireflies; **(b)** 30 fireflies/yd^2 **41.** 39 **43.** $\frac{13}{240}$ **45. (a)** Left to the student; **(b)** $\frac{5}{12}$; **(c)** $\frac{7}{12}$; **(d)** $\frac{7}{24}$ **47.** $\int_0^{12} \int_{y/4}^{3} f(x, y)\, dx\, dy$ **49.** $\int_0^{16} \int_0^{\sqrt{y}} g(x, y)\, dx\, dy$ **51.** $(2.879, 1.773)$ **53.** $(5.958, 6.459)$ **55.** About 22.5 yards east and 13.333 yards north of the southwest corner of the field **57.** $\left(\frac{8}{3}, 0\right)$ **59.** $\left(0, \frac{8}{3\pi}\right)$, or about $(0, 0.849)$ **61.** At about $(3.522, 2.340)$

Chapter 6 Review Exercises, p. 606

1. (h) **2.** (e) **3.** (f) **4.** (g) **5.** (c) **6.** (b) **7.** (d) **8.** (a) **9.** 1 **10.** $3y^3$ **11.** $e^y + 9xy^2 + 2$ **12.** $9y^2$ **13.** $9y^2$ **14.** 0 **15.** $e^y + 18xy$ **16.** $D = \{(x, y) \mid x \neq 1, y \geq 2\}$ **17.** $6x^2 \ln y + y^2$ **18.** $\frac{2x^3}{y} + 2xy$ **19.** $\frac{6x^2}{y} + 2y$ **20.** $\frac{6x^2}{y} + 2y$ **21.** $12x \ln y$ **22.** $-\frac{2x^3}{y^2} + 2x$ **23. (a)** 2.08; **(b)** 2.09042402 **24.** Relative minimum: $-\frac{549}{20}$ at $\left(5, \frac{27}{2}\right)$ **25.** Relative maximum: $\frac{45}{4}$ at $\left(\frac{3}{2}, -3\right)$ **26.** Relative minimum: 29 at $(-1, 2)$ **27. (a)** $y = -0.4x + 23.1666\ldots$; **(b)** 21.56 million; **(c)** $x = 5.4$, or in 2019 **28. (a)** $y = 19.584x + 121.975$; **(b)** \$416; **(c)** $y = 131.834e^{0.083x}$; **(d)** about \$458 **29.** Minimum: $\frac{125}{4}$ at $\left(-\frac{3}{2}, -3\right)$ **30.** Maximum: 300 at $(5, 10)$ **31.** $\left(\frac{16}{7}, \frac{4}{7}, \frac{8}{7}\right)$ **32.** Absolute maximum: 9 at $x = 3, y = 0$; absolute minimum: -4 at $x = 0, y = 2$ **33.** $\frac{5}{4}$ **34.** $\frac{1}{60}$ **35. (a)** About 1533 students; **(b)** about 767 students/mi^2 **36.** 0 **37.** The cylindrical container, with 4.074 in^2 less surface area **38.** Answers may vary. **39.** $\frac{4}{5} + \frac{3}{8}\sqrt{2}$, or about 1.33

Chapter 6 Test, p. 608

1. -2 **2.** $6x^2y$ **3.** $2x^3 + 1$ **4.** $12xy$ **5.** $6x^2$ **6.** $6x^2$ **7.** 0 **8. (a)** 0.04; **(b)** 0.0391 **9.** Maximum: 18 at $(-1, -2)$; minimum: -18 at $(1, 2)$ **10. (a)** $y = \frac{9}{2}x + \frac{17}{3}$; **(b)** \$23.7 million; **(c)** $y = 7.462e^{0.321x}$; **(d)** \$26.9 million **11.** Maximum: -19 at $(4, 5)$ **12.** 720, 120 **13.** $\frac{45}{8}$ **14.** \$400,000 for labor, \$200,000 for capital **15.** Maximum volume is $\frac{64{,}000}{3}$ in^3, when $x = 40$ in., $y = 40$ in., and $z = \frac{40}{3}$ in. **16.** About 2.467

Extended Technology Application, p. 610

1.

Case	Bldg.	n	k	A	h	$t(h, k)$
1	B1	2	40	3200	15	21.5
	B2	3	32.66	3200	30	19.4
2	B1	2	60	7200	15	31.5
	B2	3	48.99	7200	30	27.5
3	B1	4	40	6400	45	24.5
	B2	5	35.777	6400	60	23.9
4	B1	5	60	18000	60	36
	B2	10	42.426	18000	135	34.7
5	B1	5	150	112500	60	81
	B2	10	106.066	112500	135	66.5
6	B1	10	40	16000	135	33.5
	B2	17	30.679	16000	240	39.3
7	B1	10	80	64000	135	53.5
	B2	17	61.357	64000	240	54.7
8	B1	17	40	27200	240	44
	B2	26	32.344	27200	375	53.7
9	B1	17	50	42500	240	49
	B2	26	40.43	42500	375	57.7
10	B1	26	77	154154	375	76
	B2	50	55.525	154152	735	101.3

2. Yes **3.** $t(h, k) = \frac{h}{10} + \frac{k}{2}$ **4.** $A = \left(1 + \frac{h}{12}\right)k^2 - 40{,}000$ **5.** About 57.7 ft by 57.7 ft by 132.2 ft (11 floors) **6.** Left to the student

CUMULATIVE REVIEW, p. 611

1. $x^2 + 2xh + h^2 - 5$; $2x + h$

2. (a)

(b) 3; **(c)** -3; **(d)** no

3. (a)

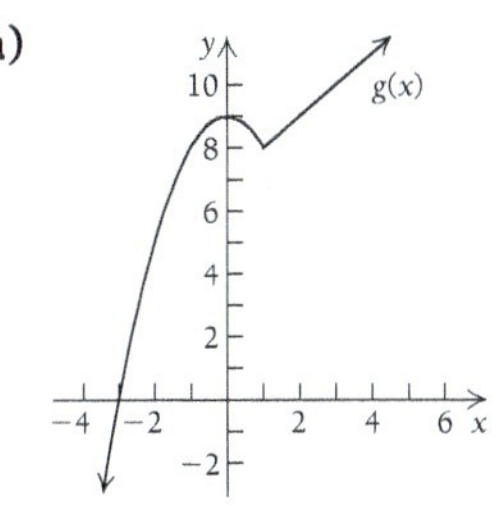

(b) 8; **(c)** 8; **(d)** yes

4. 3 **5.** −8 **6.** Does not exist **7.** 4
8. 0 **9.** $f'(x) = 2x$ **10.** a_6 **11.** a_2, a_6
12. a_2, a_4, a_6 **13.** $2x - 7$ **14.** $\frac{1}{4}x^{-3/4}$ **15.** $-6x^{-7}$
16. $\frac{10}{3}x^4(2x^5 - 8)^{-2/3}$ **17.** $\dfrac{20x^3 - 15x^2 - 8}{(2x-1)^2}$
18. $\dfrac{2x}{x^2+5}$ **19.** $e^{3x}(2x+4) + 3e^{3x}(x^2+4x)$
20. $3e^{3x} + 2x$ **21.** $\dfrac{e^{\sqrt{x-3}}}{2\sqrt{x-3}}$ **22.** $\dfrac{e^x}{e^x - 4}$
23. $2 - 4x^{-3}$ **24.** −\$0.04/pair **25.** $y = x - 2$
26. $x = 1, x = \frac{1}{3}$ **27.** Relative maximum at $(-1, 3)$, relative minimum at $(1, -1)$; point of inflection at $(0, 1)$; increasing on $(-\infty, -1)$ and on $(1, \infty)$, decreasing on $(-1, 1)$; concave down on $(-\infty, 0)$ and concave up on $(0, \infty)$

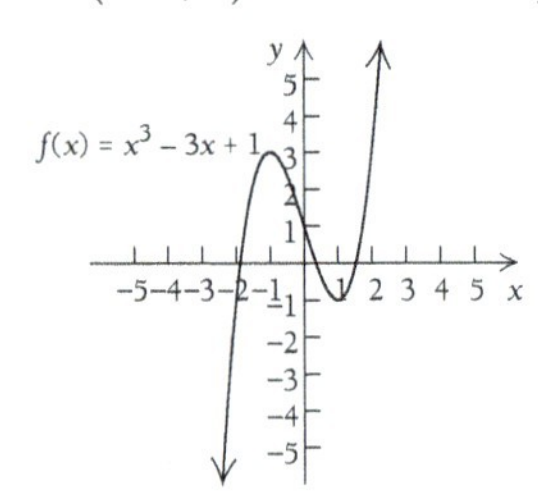

28. Relative minimum at $(-1, \ln 4)$; decreasing on $(-\infty, -1)$ and increasing on $(-1, \infty)$; points of inflection at $(-3, \ln 8)$ and $(1, \ln 8)$; concave down on $(-\infty, -3)$ and on $(1, \infty)$, concave up on $(-3, 1)$

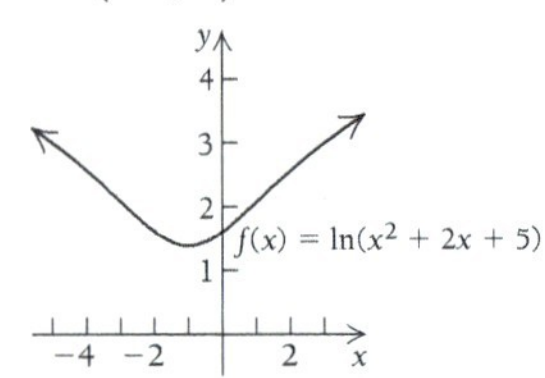

29. Relative maximum at $(1, 4)$, relative minimum at $(-1, -4)$; points of inflection at $(-\sqrt{3}, -2\sqrt{3})$, $(0, 0)$, and $(\sqrt{3}, 2\sqrt{3})$; decreasing on $(-\infty, -1)$ and on $(1, \infty)$, increasing on $(-1, 1)$; concave down on $(-\infty, -\sqrt{3})$ and on $(0, \sqrt{3})$, concave up on $(-\sqrt{3}, 0)$ and $(\sqrt{3}, \infty)$; horizontal asymptote at $y = 0$

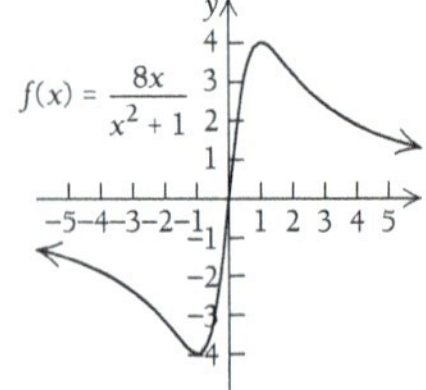

30. Relative maximum at $\left(\frac{1}{3}, \frac{4}{3e}\right)$; increasing on $\left(-\infty, \frac{1}{3}\right)$, decreasing on $\left(\frac{1}{3}, \infty\right)$; point of inflection at $\left(\frac{2}{3}, \frac{8}{3}e^{-2}\right)$; concave down on $\left(-\infty, \frac{2}{3}\right)$, concave up on $\left(\frac{2}{3}, \infty\right)$

31. Absolute minimum: −7 at $x = 1$ **32.** Absolute maximum: 1 at $x = 1$ **33.** Absolute maximum: $6\frac{2}{3}$ at $x = -1$; absolute minimum: $4\frac{1}{3}$ at $x = -2$ **34.** 15 sweatshirts
35. 30 times; lot size of 15 **36.** $\Delta y \approx 0.5$
37. **(a)** $y = 48x - 128$; **(b)** 73.6
38. **(a)** $E(x) = \dfrac{x}{12 - x}$; **(b)** $E(2) = \frac{1}{5}$, inelastic; **(c)** $E(9) = 3$, elastic; **(d)** increase; **(e)** $x = \$6$ **39.** **(a)** $\Delta A \approx \pm 50$ ft²; **(b)** 6 squares, \$48 **40.** $f'(x) = \dfrac{x^5 e^{2x}}{\sqrt{x+4}}\left(\dfrac{5}{x} + 2 + \dfrac{1}{2x+8}\right)$
41. $f'(x) = \dfrac{(x^3 + 2x + 5)\sqrt{3x - e^{3x}}}{e^{4x^2 - 3x}} \cdot \left(\dfrac{3x^2 + 2}{x^3 + 2x + 5} + \dfrac{3 - 3e^{3x}}{6x - 2e^{3x}} - 8x + 3\right)$
42. $3xy^2 + \dfrac{y}{x}$ **43.** $-\dfrac{1}{2\pi}$, or about −0.159 ft/min
44. $3 - \dfrac{2}{e}$ **45.** $\frac{1}{2}x^4 - x^3 + x^2 - 3x + C$ **46.** $\frac{1}{4}e^{x^4} + C$
47. $-\frac{2}{5}xe^{-5x} - \frac{2}{25}e^{-5x} + C$ **48.** $\frac{9279}{10}$ **49.** **(a)** 192; **(b)** 48 **50.** $\frac{125}{6}$ **51.** $L_{10} = \frac{73}{60} \approx 1.217$ mi; $R_{10} = \frac{81}{60} = 1.35$ mi; average $= \frac{77}{60} \approx 1.283$ mi
52. $T_6 = 7.714$ **53.** **(a)** (43.75, 1625); **(b)** consumer surplus: \$3828.13, producer surplus: \$19,140.63; **(c)** (35, 1450); **(d)** new consumer surplus: \$9800, new producer surplus: \$12,250; **(e)** \$918.75 **54.** **(a)** \$28,992.09; **(b)** \$21,007.91
55. \$711,632.48 **56.** Convergent, $\frac{3}{2}$ **57.** **(a)** $\frac{12}{47}$; **(b)** $\frac{27}{47}$; **(c)** $\frac{35}{47}$; **(d)** 0 **58.** 0.12 **59.** **(a)** 0.593; **(b)** 0.105 **60.** **(a)** 0.644; **(b)** 99.4th; **(c)** about \$87,320
61. $-\dfrac{\pi}{2}\left(\dfrac{1}{e^{10}} - 1\right)$, or approximately 1.571
62. $\dfrac{124\pi}{3}$, or approximately 129.85 **63.** $y = \frac{9}{4}e^{2-2x^2} + \frac{3}{4}$
64. **(a)** $\dfrac{dy}{dx} = \sqrt{y}$; **(b)** $y = \left(\dfrac{x}{2} + C\right)^2$ **65.** $8xy^3 + 3$
66. $e^y + 24x^2y$ **67.** Minimum: −10 at (3, −2)
68. Maximum: 4 at (3, 3) **69.** **(a)** $y = 2x + \frac{5}{3}$; **(b)** \$216,666.67; **(c)** $y = 3.05e^{0.275x}$; **(d)** about \$477,100
70. $3(e^3 - 1)$ **71.** **(a)** 100; **(b)** 5 **72.** 1467 shoppers

APPENDIX A

Exercise Set A, p. 625

1. 5·5·5, or 125 **2.** 7·7, or 49 **3.** (−7)(−7), or 49
4. (−5)(−5)(−5), or −125 **5.** 1.0201 **6.** 1.030301
7. $\frac{1}{16}$ **8.** $\frac{1}{64}$ **9.** 1 **10.** $6x$ **11.** $-t$ **12.** −1
13. 1 **14.** $\frac{1}{3}$ **15.** $\frac{1}{9}$ **16.** $\frac{1}{16}$ **17.** 8
18. $\frac{4}{49}$ **19.** 9 **20.** 4 **21.** 0.1 **22.** 0.0001 **23.** $\dfrac{1}{e^b}$
24. $\dfrac{1}{t^k}$ **25.** $\dfrac{1}{b}$ **26.** $\dfrac{1}{h}$ **27.** x^5 **28.** t^7 **29.** x^{-6}, or $\dfrac{1}{x^6}$
30. x^6 **31.** $35x^5$ **32.** $8t^7$ **33.** x^4 **34.** x **35.** 1
36. 1 **37.** x^6 **38.** x^4 **39.** x^{-3}, or $\dfrac{1}{x^3}$ **40.** x^{-4}, or $\dfrac{1}{x^4}$

41. 1 **42.** 1 **43.** e^{t-4} **44.** e^{k-3} **45.** t^{14} **46.** t^{12}

47. t^2 **48.** t^{-4}, or $\frac{1}{t^4}$ **49.** a^6b^5 **50.** x^7y^7 **51.** t^{-6}, or $\frac{1}{t^6}$

52. t^{-12}, or $\frac{1}{t^{12}}$ **53.** e^{4x} **54.** e^{5x} **55.** $8x^6y^{12}$

56. $32x^{10}y^{20}$ **57.** $\frac{1}{81}x^8y^{20}z^{-16}$, or $\frac{x^8y^{20}}{81z^{16}}$

58. $\frac{1}{125}x^{-9}y^{21}z^{15}$, or $\frac{y^{21}z^{15}}{125x^9}$ **59.** $9x^{-16}y^{14}z^4$, or $\frac{9y^{14}z^4}{x^{16}}$

60. $625x^{16}y^{-20}z^{-12}$, or $\frac{625x^{16}}{y^{20}z^{12}}$ **61.** $\frac{c^4d^{12}}{16q^8}$ **62.** $\frac{64x^6y^3}{a^9b^9}$

63. $5x - 35$ **64.** $x + xt$ **65.** $x^2 - 7x + 10$
66. $x^2 - 7x + 12$ **67.** $a^3 - b^3$ **68.** $x^3 + y^3$
69. $2x^2 + 3x - 5$ **70.** $3x^2 + x - 4$ **71.** $a^2 - 4$
72. $9x^2 - 1$ **73.** $25x^2 - 4$ **74.** $t^2 - 1$
75. $a^2 - 2ah + h^2$ **76.** $a^2 + 2ah + h^2$
77. $25x^2 + 10xt + t^2$ **78.** $49a^2 - 14ac + c^2$
79. $5x^5 + 30x^3 + 45x$ **80.** $-3x^6 + 48x^2$
81. $a^3 + 3a^2b + 3ab^2 + b^3$ **82.** $a^3 - 3a^2b + 3ab^2 - b^3$
83. $x^3 - 15x^2 + 75x - 125$ **84.** $8x^3 + 36x^2 + 54x + 27$
85. $x(1 - t)$ **86.** $x(1 + h)$ **87.** $(x + 3y)^2$
88. $(x - 5y)^2$ **89.** $(x - 5)(x + 3)$ **90.** $(x + 5)(x + 3)$
91. $(x - 5)(x + 4)$ **92.** $(x - 10)(x + 1)$
93. $(7x - t)(7x + t)$ **94.** $(3x - b)(3x + b)$
95. $4(3t - 2m)(3t + 2m)$ **96.** $(5y - 3z)(5y + 3z)$
97. $ab(a + 4b)(a - 4b)$ **98.** $2(x^2 + 4)(x + 2)(x - 2)$
99. $(a^4 + b^4)(a^2 + b^2)(a + b)(a - b)$
100. $(6y - 5)(6y + 7)$ **101.** $10x(a + 2b)(a - 2b)$
102. $xy(x + 5y)(x - 5y)$ **103.** $2(1 + 4x^2)(1 + 2x)(1 - 2x)$
104. $2x(y + 5)(y - 5)$ **105.** $(9x - 1)(x + 2)$
106. $(3x - 4)(2x - 5)$ **107.** $(x + 2)(x^2 - 2x + 4)$
108. $(a - 3)(a^2 + 3a + 9)$ **109.** $(y - 4t)(y^2 + 4yt + 16t^2)$
110. $(m + 10p)(m^2 - 10mp + 100p^2)$
111. $(3x^2 - 1)(x - 2)$ **112.** $(y^2 - 2)(5y + 2)$
113. $(x - 3)(x + 3)(x - 5)$ **114.** $(t - 5)(t + 5)(t + 3)$
115. $\frac{7}{4}$ **116.** $\frac{79}{12}$ **117.** -8 **118.** $\frac{4}{5}$ **119.** 120
120. 140 **121.** 200 **122.** 200 **123.** $0, -3, \frac{4}{5}$
124. $0, 2, -\frac{3}{2}$ **125.** 0, 2 **126.** 3, −3 **127.** 0, 3
128. 0, 5 **129.** 0, 7 **130.** 0, 3 **131.** $0, \frac{1}{3}, -\frac{1}{3}$
132. $0, \frac{1}{4}, -\frac{1}{4}$ **133.** 1 **134.** 2 **135.** No solution
136. No solution **137.** −23 **138.** −145 **139.** 5
140. $-\sqrt{7}, \sqrt{7}$ **141.** ± 8 **142.** ± 12 **143.** $\pm\sqrt{30}$

144. $\pm\sqrt{97}$ **145.** $\pm\frac{7}{2}$ **146.** $\pm\frac{13}{10}$ **147.** $\pm\frac{\sqrt{20}}{3}$, or $\pm\frac{2\sqrt{5}}{3}$

148. $\pm\frac{\sqrt{3}}{5}$ **149.** $\pm\frac{2}{\sqrt{5}}$, or $\pm\frac{2\sqrt{5}}{5}$

150. $\pm\frac{12}{\sqrt{3}}$, or $\pm 4\sqrt{3}$ **151.** $1, \frac{1}{3}$ **152.** $\frac{5}{2}, -\frac{25}{6}$

153. $\frac{2 + \sqrt{10}}{5}, \frac{2 - \sqrt{10}}{5}$ **154.** $\frac{1 + \sqrt{2}}{4}, \frac{1 - \sqrt{2}}{4}$

155. $x \geq -\frac{4}{5}$ **156.** $x \geq 3$ **157.** $x > -\frac{1}{12}$
158. $x > -\frac{5}{13}$ **159.** $x > -\frac{4}{7}$ **160.** $x \leq -\frac{6}{5}$
161. $x \leq -3$ **162.** $x \geq -2$ **163.** $x > \frac{2}{3}$ **164.** $x \leq \frac{5}{3}$

165. $x < -\frac{2}{5}$ **166.** $x \leq \frac{5}{4}$ **167.** $2 < x < 4$
168. $2 < x \leq 4$ **169.** $\frac{3}{2} \leq x \leq \frac{11}{2}$ **170.** $\frac{6}{5} \leq x < \frac{16}{5}$
171. $-1 \leq x \leq \frac{14}{5}$ **172.** $-5 \leq x < -2$ **173.** \$650
174. \$800 **175.** More than 7000 units **176.** More than 4200 units **177.** 480 lb **178.** 340 lb
179. 810,000 **180.** 5200 **181.** $60\% \leq x < 100\%$
182. $50\% \leq x < 90\%$ **183.** 18 people **184.** 75 tiles
185. Gina is 16 and Dave is 6. **186.** \$75,000
187. 58, 59, 60 **188.** $\frac{8}{13}$ **189.** 5 **190.** 7 and 24

APPENDIX B

Exercise Set B, p. 632

1. 5 **2.** −4 **3.** $\frac{5}{2}$ **4.** $\frac{13}{3}$ **5.** 0 **6.** 0 **7.** $\frac{19}{2}$
8. $-\frac{1}{2}$ **9.** 2 **10.** $\frac{1}{2}$ **11.** $\frac{2}{3}$ **12.** 1 **13.** $-\frac{5}{4}$
14. $-\frac{9}{2}$ **15.** $\frac{1}{3}$ **16.** 2 **17.** 1 **18.** 1 **19.** e^2
20. e^{-3} **21.** e^{-4} **22.** e^5 **23.** 1 **24.** 1 **25.** $-\frac{1}{2}$
26. $\frac{5}{2}$ **27.** $\frac{1}{3}$ **28.** $\frac{1}{12}$ **29.** Left to the student
30. Left to the student **31.** $\frac{1}{2}$ **32.** $-\frac{1}{3}$ **33.** $-\frac{2}{5}$
34. $-\frac{7}{3}$ **35.** **(a)** 0, 0, 0, 0; **(b)** answers may vary **(c)** answers may vary **36.** **(a)** $e^{2x}/e^{3x} = 1/e^x$, 0; **(b)** answers may vary
37. **(a)** Subtract 0 from numerator and denominator; **(b)** since $x \neq a$, multiply numerator and denominator by $1/(x - a)$; **(c)** property of limits, limit of quotient is quotient of limits; **(d)** definition of derivative at $x = a$; **(e)** differentiability of f and g at $x = a$ **38.** l'Hôpital's Rule does not apply since the first expression is not indeterminate at $x = 3$. The correct limit is 0.

APPENDIX C

Exercise Set C, p. 637

1. $y = 3.45x + 0.6$ **2.** $y = 2.5283x + 13.34$
3. $y = 0.0732x^2 + 2.3x + 11.813$

APPENDIX E

Exercise Set E, p. 645

1. $-\frac{1}{9}e^{-3x}(3x + 1) + C$ **2.** $\frac{2}{9}e^{3x}(3x - 1) + C$ **3.** $\frac{6^x}{\ln 6} + C$

4. $\ln|x + \sqrt{x^2 + 9}| + C$ **5.** $\frac{1}{10}\ln\left|\frac{5 + x}{5 - x}\right| + C$

6. $-\frac{1}{2}\ln\left|\frac{2 + \sqrt{4 + x^2}}{x}\right| + C$ **7.** $-x - 3\ln|3 - x| + C$

8. $\frac{1}{1 - x} + \ln|1 - x| + C$ **9.** $\frac{1}{8(8 - x)} + \frac{1}{64}\ln\left|\frac{x}{8 - x}\right| + C$

10. $\frac{1}{2}[x\sqrt{x^2 + 9} + 9\ln|x + \sqrt{x^2 + 9}|] + C$
11. $x\ln(3x) - x + C$ **12.** $x\ln(\frac{4}{5}x) - x + C$

13. $\frac{x^5}{5}(\ln x) - \frac{x^5}{25} + C$

14. $-\frac{1}{2}x^3e^{-2x} - \frac{3}{4}x^2e^{-2x} - \frac{3}{4}xe^{-2x} - \frac{3}{8}e^{-2x} + C$

15. $\frac{x^4}{4}(\ln x) - \frac{x^4}{16} + C$ **16.** $x^5(\ln x) - \frac{x^5}{5} + C$

17. $\ln|x + \sqrt{x^2 + 7}| + C$ **18.** $-3\ln\left|\frac{1 + \sqrt{1 - x^2}}{x}\right| + C$

19. $\frac{2}{5 - 7x} + \frac{2}{5}\ln\left|\frac{x}{5 - 7x}\right| + C$ **20.** $\frac{1}{5}\ln\left|\frac{x}{7x + 2}\right| + C$

21. $-\frac{5}{4}\ln\left|\frac{x - 1/2}{x + 1/2}\right| + C$

22. $\frac{3}{2}\left[t\sqrt{t^2 - \frac{1}{9}} - \frac{1}{9}\ln\left|t + \sqrt{t^2 + \frac{1}{9}}\right|\right] + C$

23. $m\sqrt{m^2 + 4} + 4\ln\left|m + \sqrt{m^2 + 4}\right| + C$

24. $\frac{3}{x}(-\ln x - 1) + C$ **25.** $\frac{5}{2x^2}(\ln x) + \frac{5}{4x^2} + C$

26. $x(\ln x)^4 - 4x(\ln x)^3 + 12x(\ln x)^2 - 24x(\ln x) + 24 + C$

27. $x^3e^x - 3x^2e^x + 6xe^x - 6e^x + C$

28. $\frac{3}{2}\ln\left|x + \sqrt{x^2 + 25}\right| + C$ **29.** $\frac{1}{15}(3x - 1)(1 + 2x)^{3/2} + C$

30. $\frac{2}{135}(9x - 4)(2 + 3x)^{3/2} + C$

31. $S(x) = 100\left[\frac{20}{20 - x} + \ln(20 - x)\right]$

32. $p(t) = \frac{1}{2(2 + t)} + \frac{1}{4}\ln\left(\frac{t}{2 + t}\right) + 0.8750$

33. $-4\ln\left|\frac{x}{3x - 2}\right| + C$ **34.** $\frac{-3}{4(2x - 3)} + \frac{1}{4}\ln|2x - 3| + C$

35. $\frac{-1}{2(x - 2)} + \frac{1}{4}\ln\left|\frac{x}{x - 2}\right| + C$

36. $\frac{1}{2}\left[e^x\sqrt{e^{2x} + 1} + \ln\left|e^x + \sqrt{e^{2x} + 1}\right|\right] + C$

37. $\frac{-3}{e^{-x} - 3} + \ln\left|e^{-x} - 3\right| + C$

38. $\frac{1}{4}\left[\ln x\sqrt{(\ln x)^2 + 49} + 49\ln\left(\ln x + \sqrt{(\ln x)^2 + 49}\right)\right] + C$

39. When $a = -5$, the antiderivative is $-\frac{1}{10}\ln\left|\frac{x + 5}{x - 5}\right| + C$. Using a property of logarithms, we have

$$\begin{aligned}-\frac{1}{10}\ln\left|\frac{x + 5}{x - 5}\right| &= -\frac{1}{10}(\ln|x + 5| - \ln|x - 5|)\\ &= -\frac{1}{10}\ln|x + 5| + \frac{1}{10}\ln|x - 5|\\ &= \frac{1}{10}(\ln|x - 5| - \ln|x + 5|)\\ &= \frac{1}{10}\ln\left|\frac{x - 5}{x + 5}\right|.\end{aligned}$$

40. Answers may vary. **41.** Answers may vary.

Index of Applications

Business and Economics

Environmental Science

General Interest

Health Care

Life and Physical Sciences

Social Sciences

Sports

Index

Formulas for Differentiation

Derivative of a Constant:

$$\frac{d}{dx}[c] = 0$$

Derivative of a Constant Multiple of a Function:

$$\frac{d}{dx}[cf(x)] = cf'(x)$$

Derivative of a Sum:

$$\frac{d}{dx}[f(x) \pm g(x)] = f'(x) \pm g'(x)$$

Derivative of a Power:

$$\frac{d}{dx}[x^n] = nx^{n-1}$$

Derivative of a Product:

$$\frac{d}{dx}[f(x) \cdot g(x)] = f(x) \cdot g'(x) + g(x) \cdot f'(x), \text{ where } g(x) \neq 0$$

Derivative of a Quotient:

$$\frac{d}{dx}\left[\frac{f(x)}{g(x)}\right] = \frac{g(x) \cdot f'(x) - f(x) \cdot g'(x)}{[g(x)]^2}$$

Derivative of the Composition of Two Functions (the Chain Rule):

$$\frac{d}{dx}[f(g(x))] = f'(g(x)) \cdot g'(x)$$

Derivative of an Exponential Function (Base *e*):

$$\frac{d}{dx}e^x = e^x \qquad \frac{d}{dx}[e^{f(x)}] = e^{f(x)} \cdot f'(x)$$

Derivative of an Exponential Function (Base *a*):

$$\frac{d}{dx}[a^{f(x)}] = a^{f(x)} \cdot \ln a \cdot f'(x), \text{ where } a > 0, a \neq 1$$

Derivative of a Logarithmic Function (Base *e*):

$$\frac{d}{dx}\ln x = \frac{1}{x}, x > 0 \qquad \frac{d}{dx}\ln|x| = \frac{1}{x}, x \neq 0$$

$$\frac{d}{dx}[\ln f(x)] = \frac{f'(x)}{f(x)}, \text{ where } f(x) > 0$$

Derivative of a Logarithmic Function (Base *a*):

$$\frac{d}{dx}[\log_a f(x)] = \frac{f'(x)}{f(x) \cdot \ln a}, \text{ where } f(x) > 0 \text{ and } a > 0, a \neq 1$$

Formulas for Integration

Constant Rule:

$$\int k\,dx = kx + C$$

Power Rule:

$$\int x^n\,dx = \frac{1}{n+1}x^{n+1} + C, n \neq 1$$

Natural Logarithm Rule:

$$\int \frac{1}{x}dx = \ln|x| + C, \text{for } x \neq 0$$

$$\int \frac{1}{x}dx = \ln x + C, \text{for } x > 0$$

Exponential Rule (Base *e*):

$$\int e^x\,dx = e^x + C$$

$$\int e^{ax}\,dx = \frac{1}{a}e^{ax} + C$$

Antiderivative of a Constant Times a Function:

$$\int [c \cdot f(x)]\,dx = c \cdot \int f(x)\,dx.$$

Antiderivative of the Sum or Difference of Two Functions:

$$\int [f(x) \pm g(x)]\,dx = \int f(x)\,dx \pm \int g(x)\,dx.$$

The Fundamental Theorem of Integral Calculus

If a continuous function f has an antiderivative F over $[a, b]$, then

$$\lim_{n \to \infty} \sum_{i=1}^{n} f(x_i)\,\Delta x = \int_a^b f(x)\,dx = F(b) - F(a),$$

where n is the number of subdivisions of $[a, b]$.

For additional integration formulas, see Table 1 in Appendix E.